The APRN and PA's Complete Guide to Prescribing Drug Therapy

2020

Mari J. Wirfs, PhD, MN, RN, APRN, ANP-BC, FNP-BC, CNE, began her career with an ASN (1968, Dekalb College), and subsequently completed a BSN (1970, Georgia State University), MS (1975, Emory University), Post-Masters Certificates in Primary Care of the Adult (1997) and Family (1997, LSU Health Sciences Center), and PhD in Higher Education Administration and Leadership (1991, University of New Orleans). She is a nationally certified Adult Nurse Practitioner (1997, American Nurses Credentialing Center), Family Nurse Practitioner (1998, American Academy of Nurse Practitioners), and Certified Nurse Educator (2008, National League for Nursing). Her career spans 50+ years inclusive of collegiate undergraduate and graduate nursing education and clinical practice in critical care, pediatrics, psychiatric–mental health nursing, and advanced practice primary care nursing. During her academic career, she has achieved the rank of professor with tenure in two university systems. She is a frequent guest lecturer on a variety of advanced practice topics to professional groups and general healthcare topics to community groups.

Dr. Wirfs was a founding member of the medical staff in the establishment of Baptist Community Health Services, a community-based nonprofit primary care clinic founded post-hurricane Katrina in the New Orleans Lower Ninth Ward. Since 2002, Dr. Wirfs has served as clinical director and primary care provider at the Family Health Care Clinic, serving faculty, staff, students, and their families at New Orleans Baptist Theological Seminary (NOBTS). She is also adjunct graduate faculty, teaching neuropsychology and psychopharmacology, in the NOBTS Guidance and Counseling program. She is a long-time member of the National Organization of Nurse Practitioner Faculties (NONPF), Sigma Theta Tau International Honor Society of Nursing, and several other academic honor societies.

Dr. Wirfs has completed, published, and presented six quantitative research studies focusing on academic leadership, nursing education, and clinical practice issues, including one for the Army Medical Department conducted during her 8 years reserve service in the Army Nurse Corps. Her publications include co-authored family primary care certification review books and study materials. Her first prescribing guide, *Clinical Guide to Pharmacotherapeutics for the Primary Care Provider*, was published by Advanced Practice Education Associates (APEA) from 1999 to 2014. *The APRN's Complete Guide to Prescribing Drug Therapy* (launched in 2016), *The APRN's Complete Guide to Prescribing Pediatric Drug Therapy* (launched in 2017), and *The PA's Complete Guide to Prescribing Drug Therapy* (launched in 2017) are published by Springer Publishing Company.

The APRN's Complete Guide to Prescribing Pediatric Drug Therapy 2018 was awarded second place, **Book of the Year 2017** in the Child Health Category, by the *American Journal of Nursing (AJN)*, official publication of the **American Nurses Association (ANA)**. The panel of judges included the co-founder of the nurse practitioner role and first nurse practitioner program, Dr. Loretta C. Ford, Professor Emerita. Dr. Wirfs was the recipient of the **2018 AANP Nurse Practitioner State Award for Excellence from Louisiana** by the **American Association of Nurse Practitioners (AANP)**.

The APRN and PA's Complete Guide to Prescribing Drug Therapy

2020

Mari J. Wirfs, PhD, MN, RN,
APRN, ANP-BC, FNP-BC, CNE

SPRINGER PUBLISHING COMPANY

Copyright © 2019 Springer Publishing Company, LLC

Springer Publishing Company, LLC
11 West 42nd Street
New York, NY 10036
www.springerpub.com

Acquisitions Editor: Margaret Zuccarini
Composition: Exeter Premedia Services Private Ltd.

ISBN: 978-0-8261-7933-3
e-book ISBN: 978-0-8261-7934-0
DOI: 10.1891/9780826179340

19 20 / 5 4 3 2 1

This book is a quick reference for healthcare providers practicing in primary care settings. The information has been extrapolated from a variety of professional sources and is presented in condensed and summary form. It is not intended to replace or substitute for complete and current manufacturer prescribing information, current research, or knowledge and experience of the user. For complete prescribing information, including toxicities, drug interactions, contraindications, and precautions, the reader is directed to the manufacturer's package insert and the published literature. The inclusion of a particular brand name neither implies nor suggests that the author or publisher advises or recommends the use of that particular product or considers it superior to similar products available by other brand names. Neither the author nor the publisher makes any warranty, expressed or implied, with respect to the information, including any errors or omissions, herein.

Library of Congress Cataloging-in-Publication Data
Names: Wirfs, Mari J., author.
Title: The APRN and PA's complete guide to prescribing drug therapy 2020 / Mari J.
   Wirfs.
Description: New York, NY: Springer Publishing Company, LLC, [2020] |
   Includes bibliographical references and index.
Identifiers: LCCN 2017008900| ISBN 9780826179333 | ISBN 9780826179340 (ebook)
Subjects: | MESH: Drug Therapy—nursing | Advanced Practice Nursing—methods
   | Handbooks
Classification: LCC RM301 | NLM WY 49 | DDC 615.1—dc23
LC record available at https://lccn.loc.gov/2017008900

Printed in the United States of America.

CONTENTS

SECTION I: DRUG THERAPY BY CLINICAL DIAGNOSIS

SECTION II: APPENDICES

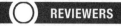
Kelley M. Anderson, PhD, FNP
Assistant Professor of Nursing, Georgetown University School of Nursing and Health Studies, Washington, DC

Kathleen Bradbury-Golas, DNP, RN, FNP-C, ACNS-BC
Associate Clinical Professor, Drexel University, Philadelphia, Pennsylvania; Family Nurse Practitioner, Virtua Medical Group, Hammonton and Linwood, New Jersey

Lori Brien, MS, ACNP-BC
Instructor, Advanced Practice Nursing Department, Georgetown University School of Nursing and Health Studies, Washington, DC

Jill Cash, MSN, APN, CNP
Nurse Practitioner, Logan Primary Care, West Frankfort, Illinois

Catherine M. Concert, DNP, RN, FNP-BC, AOCNP, NE-BC, CNL, CGRN
Nurse Practitioner-Radiation Oncology, Laura and Isaac Perlmutter Cancer Center, New York University Langone Medical Center; Clinical Assistant Professor, Pace University Lienhard School of Nursing, New York, New York

Kate DeMutis, MSN, CRNP
Senior Lecturer, Adult-Gerontology Primary Care Nurse Practitioner Program, Centralized Clinical Site Coordinator-Primary Care, University of Pennsylvania School of Nursing, Philadelphia, Pennsylvania

Gaye M. Douglas, DNP, MEd, APRN-BC
Assistant Professor of Nursing, Francis Marion University, Florence, South Carolina

Brenda Douglass, DNP, APRN, FNP-C, CDE, CTTS
Coordinator of Clinical Faculty, Assistant Clinical Professor, Drexel University College of Nursing and Health Professions, Philadelphia, Pennsylvania

Aileen Fitzpatrick, DNP, RN, FNP-BC
Clinical Assistant Professor, Pace University Lienhard School of Nursing, New York, New York

Nancy M. George, PhD, RN, FNP-BC, FAANP
Director of DNP Program, Associate Clinical Professor, Wayne State University College of Nursing, Detroit, Michigan

Tracy P. George, DNP, APRN-BC, CNE
Assistant Professor of Nursing, Amy V. Cockcroft Fellow 2016-2017, Francis Marion University, Florence, South Carolina

Cheryl Glass, MSN, WHNP, RN-BC
Clinical Research Specialist, KePRO, TennCare's Medical Solutions Unit, Nashville, Tennessee

Kathleen Gray, DNP, FNP-C
Assistant Professor, Georgetown School of Nursing and Health Studies, Washington, DC

Norma Stephens Hannigan, DNP, MPH, FNP-BC, DCC, FAANP
Clinical Professor of Nursing, Coordinator, Accelerated Second Degree (A2D) Program/ Sophomore Honors Program, Hunter College, CUNY Hunter-Bellevue School of Nursing, New York, New York

Ella T. Heitzler, PhD, WHNP, FNP, RNC-OB
Assistant Professor, Georgetown University School of Nursing and Health Studies,
Washington, DC

Mary T. Hickey, EdD, RN
Clinical Professor of Nursing, Hunter College, CUNY Hunter-Bellevue School of Nursing,
New York, New York

Deborah L. Hopla, DNP, APRN-BC
Assistant Professor of Nursing, Director MSN/FNP Track, Amy V. Cockcroft Fellow, Francis
Marion University, Florence, South Carolina

Julia M. Hucks, MN, APRN-BC
Assistant Professor of Nursing, Family Nurse Practitioner, Francis Marion University,
Florence, South Carolina

Honey M. Jones, DNP, ACNP-BC
Acute Care Nurse Practitioner, Duke University Medical Center; Clinical Associate Faculty,
MSN Program, Duke University School of Nursing, Durham, North Carolina

Melissa H. King, DNP, FNP-BC, ENP-BC
Director of Advanced Practice Providers, Director of TelEmergency, Department of
Emergency Medicine, University of Mississippi Medical Center, Jackson, Mississippi

Brittany M. Newberry, PhD, MSN, MPH, APRN, ENP, FNP
Board Certified Emergency and Family Nurse Practitioner; Vice President Education and
Professional Development of Hospital MD; Chair, Practice Committee of American Academy
of Emergency Nurse Practitioners; Adjunct Faculty, Emory University School of Nursing,
Atlanta, Georgia

Andrea Rutherfurd, MS, MPH, FNP-BC
Clinical Faculty Advisor, Adjunct Instructor, FNP Program, Georgetown University School of
Nursing and Health Studies, Washington, DC

Samantha Venable, MSN, RN, FNP
Family Nurse Practitioner, Correctional Nursing, Trabuco Canyon, California

Michael Watson, DNP, APRN, FNP-BC
Lead Family Nurse Practitioner, Wadley Regional Medical Center, Emergency Department,
Texarkana, Texas

The APRN and PA's Complete Guide to Prescribing Drug Therapy 2020 is a prescribing reference intended for use by healthcare providers in all clinical practice settings who are involved in the primary care management of patients of all ages with acute, episodic, and chronic health problems and needs for health promotion and disease prevention. It is organized in a concise and easy-to-read format. Comments are interspersed throughout, including such clinically useful information as laboratory values to be monitored, patient teaching points, safety information, and research notes. If pediatric indications for a drug have not been established or a drug is not recommended for a pediatric subgroup, this information is noted accordingly.

This reference is divided into two major sections. **Section I** presents drug treatment regimens for over 600 clinical diagnoses. Each drug is listed alphabetically by generic name, followed by the FDA pregnancy category (A, B, C, D, X), over-the-counter availability (OTC); DEA schedule (I, II, III, IV, V); generic availability (G); dosing regimens; brand/trade name(s); dose forms; whether tablets, caplets, or chew tabs are single scored (*), cross-scored (**), or tri-scored (***); flavors of chewable, sublingual, buccal, and liquid forms; and information regarding additives (i.e., dye-free, sugar-free, preservative-free or preservative type, alcohol-free or alcohol content). For drugs initially FDA-approved *prior to June 30, 2015*, the former traditional FDA pregnancy categories (A, B, C, D, or X) still apply. Non-pharmaceutical products and drugs that received initial FDA approval on or after June 30, 2015, do not have an FDA pregnancy letter designation. For information regarding special populations, including pregnant and breastfeeding females, refer to the manufacturer's package insert or visit https://www.accessdata.fda.gov/scripts/cder/daf/ to view the product label online. Visit https://www.drugs.com/pregnancy-categories.html to view the FDA Pregnancy and Lactation Labeling Final Rule (PLLR) and new label format.

Section II presents clinically useful information organized in table format, including: the JNC-8 and ASH recommendations for hypertension management, childhood immunization recommendations, brand/trade name drugs (with contents) for the management of common respiratory symptoms, anti-infectives by classification, pediatric dosing by weight for liquid forms, glucocorticosteroids by potency and route of administration, and contraceptives by route of administration and estrogen and/or progesterone content. An alphabetical cross-reference index of drugs by generic and brand/trade name, with FDA pregnancy category and controlled drug schedule, facilitates quick identification of drugs by alternate names and page location(s).

Selected diseases and diagnoses (e.g., angina, ADD/ADHD, growth failure, glaucoma, Parkinson's disease, multiple sclerosis, cystic fibrosis) and selected drugs (e.g., antineoplastics, antipsychotics, antiarrhythmics, anti-HIV drugs, anticoagulants) are included because pediatric patients are frequently referred to primary care providers by specialists for follow-up monitoring and on-going management. Further, the shifting healthcare paradigm is such that with expanding roles and patient empowerment through education, initial diagnosis and initiation of treatment is increasing in primary care with measurable increases in access to quality healthcare and improved patient self-care. Several diseases are included that may not be prevalent in North America but have been identified in other parts of the world. Endemic diseases for which there is no FDA-approved drug treatment are also included with known transmission and treatment interventions. Accordingly, this guide serves primary care providers internationally. Today's healthcare providers are in an era of rapidly expanding knowledge in the field of genomics, and thus, each new edition of this prescribing guide (and quarterly update) contains new drug classes and new FDA-approved drugs as well as brief synopses of recent published research with source reference(s).

For quick reference to weight-based dosing of a drug, the user is directed to the dose by weight table for that drug in the appendices. Potential safe, efficacious, prescribing and monitoring of drug therapy regimens for children and adolescents requires adequate knowledge about (a) the pharmacodynamics and pharmacokinetics of drugs, (b) concomitant therapies, and (c) individual characteristics of the patient (e.g., age, weight, current and past medical history, physical examination findings, hepatic and renal function, and co-morbidities, and risk factors). Users of this clinical guide are encouraged to utilize the manufacturer's package insert, recommendations and guidance of specialists, standard-of-practice protocols, and the current research literature for more comprehensive information about specific drugs (e.g., special precautions, drug-drug and drug-food interactions, risk versus benefit, age-related considerations, potential adverse reactions, and appropriate patient-focused care.

ACKNOWLEDGMENTS

This publication, which we consider to be a "must have" for students, academicians, and practicing clinicians with prescriptive authority, represents the culmination of Springer Publishing Company's collaborative team effort. Margaret Zuccarini, Publisher, Nursing, and the Editorial Committee, shared my vision for a handy pocket prescribing reference for new and experienced prescribers in primary care. Joanne Jay, Vice President, Production and Manufacturing, designed the contents for ease and efficiency of user navigation. The production team at Exeter Premedia Services, on behalf of Springer Publishing Company, understood the critical nature of exactness in this prescribing resource, and faithfully managed the complex files as content was updated and cross-paginated for the final product. The work of the reviewers from academia and clinical practice was essential to the process, and their contributions are greatly appreciated. I am proud of my association with these dedicated professionals, and I thank them on behalf of the medical and advanced practice nursing community worldwide for supporting the end goal of quality healthcare for all.

Most sincerely, Dr. Mari J. Wirfs

ACE-Is and **ARBs** are contraindicated in the 2nd and 3rd trimesters of pregnancy. Addition of a daily ACE-I or ARB is strongly recommended for renal protection in patients with hypertension and/or diabetes. The "ACE inhibitor cough," a dry cough, is an adverse side effect produced by an accumulation of bradykinins that occurs in 5% to 10% of the population and resolves within days of discontinuing the drug.

Alcohol is contraindicated with concomitant **narcotic analgesics, benzodiazepines, SSRIs, antihistamines, TCAs,** and other sedating agents due to risk of over-sedation.

Alpha-1 blockers have a potential adverse side effect of sudden hypotension, especially with first dose. Alert the patient regarding this "first-dose effect" and recommend the patient sit or lie down to take the first dose. Usually start at lowest dose and titrate upward.

Antidepressant monotherapy should be avoided until any presence of (hypo) mania or positive family history for bipolar spectrum disorder has been ruled out as antidepressant monotherapy can induce mania in the bipolar patient.

For patients 65 years-of-age and older, consult the **May 2017 Beers Criteria** for Potentially Inappropriate Medication (PIM) Use in Older Adults, to help improve the safety of prescribing medications for older adults, presented in table format at: https://www.priorityhealth.com/provider/clinical-resources/medication-resources/~/media/documents/pharmacy/cms-high-risk-medications.pdf

Aspirin is contraindicated in children and adolescents with *Varicella* or other viral illness, and 3rd trimester of pregnancy.

Beta-blockers, by all routes of administration, are generally contraindicated in severe COPD, history of <u>or</u> current bronchial asthma, sinus bradycardia, and 2nd <u>or</u> 3rd degree AV block. Use a cardio-specific beta blocker where appropriate in these cases.

A **biosimilar** product is one that has been FDA-approved based on data demonstrating that it is highly similar to a previously FDA-approved biological product, known as the reference product. Accordingly, the FDA has determined that there are no clinically meaningful differences between the biosimilar product and the reference product (e.g., **Cyltezo** [*adalimumab-adbm*] is biosimilar to **Humira** [*adalimumab*]).

The FDA **Breakthrough Therapy Designation (BTD)** is intended to expedite the development and review of a drug candidate that is planned for use, alone or in combination with one or more other drugs, to treat a serious or life-threatening disease or condition when preliminary clinical evidence indicates that the drug may demonstrate substantial improvement over existing therapies on one or more clinically significant endpoints. The benefits of Breakthrough Therapy Designation include the same benefits as Fast Track Designation (FTD), plus an organizational commitment involving the FDA's senior managers with more intensive guidance from the FDA (e.g., *Zulresso [brexanolone]*) received the FDA Breakthrough Therapy Designation for treatment of post-partum depression.

Calcium channel blockers may cause the adverse side effect of pedal edema (feet, ankles, lower legs) that resolves with discontinuation of the drug.

Codeine is known to be excreted in breast milk: <12 years, not recommended; 12-<18, use extreme caution; not recommended for children and adolescents with asthma or other chronic breathing problem. The FDA and the European Medicines Agency (EMA) are investigating the safety of using *codeine*-containing medications to treat pain, cough, and colds in children 12-<18 years because of the potential for serious side effects, including slowed or difficult breathing.

Check **drug interactions** at https://www.drugs.com/drug_interactions.php

Check FDA **drug recalls, market withdrawals, and safety alerts** (http://www.fda.gov/Safety/Recalls/default.htm).

Contraceptives that are estrogen-progesterone combinations and **progesterone-only** are contraindicated in pregnancy (pregnancy category X).

Corticosteroids increase blood sugar in patients with diabetes and decrease immunity; therefore, consider risk versus benefit in susceptible patients, use lowest effective dose, and taper gradually to discontinue.

Erythromycin may increase INR with concomitant warfarin, as well as increase serum level of digoxin, benzodiazepines, and statins.

Finasteride, a 5-alpha reductase inhibitor, is associated with low but increased risk of high-grade prostate cancer. Pregnant females should not touch broken tablets.

Fluoroquinolones and **quinolones** are contraindicated <18 years-of-age, pregnancy, and breastfeeding. *Exception:* in the case of anthrax, *ciprofloxacin* is indicated for patients <18 years-of-age and dosed based on mg/kg body weight. Risk of tendonitis or tendon rupture (ex: *ciprofloxacin, gemifloxacin, levofloxacin, moxifloxacin, norfloxacin, ofloxacin*).

The U.S. Preventive Services Task Force (USPSTF) recommends against using **hormone replacement therapy (HRT)** for primary prevention of chronic conditions among postmenopausal women. The harms associated with combined use of estrogen and a progestin, such as increased risks of invasive breast cancer, venous thromboembolism, and coronary heart disease, far outweigh the benefits.

Ibuprofen is contraindicated in children <6 months of age and in the 3rd trimester of pregnancy.

Live vaccines are contraindicated in patients who are immunosuppressed or receiving immunosuppressive therapy, including immunosuppressive levels of corticosteroid therapy.

Metronidazole and **tinidazole** are contraindicated in the 1st trimester of pregnancy. Alcohol is contraindicated during treatment with oral forms and for 72 hours after therapy due to a possible *disulfiram*-like reaction (nausea, vomiting, flushing, headache).

When prescribing **opioid analgesics,** presumptive urine **drug testing** (UDT) should be performed when opioid therapy for chronic pain is initiated, along with subsequent use as adherence monitoring, using in-office point of service testing to identify patients who are non-compliant or abusing prescription drugs or illicit drugs. American Society of Interventional Pain Physicians (ASIPP)

Orphan Drug designation means the drug is a first-in-class and/or the drug is for treatment of a rare disease and/or the drug is a first and only treatment for a disease and the application for FDA approval received priority review as incentive to assist and encourage the development of drugs for rare diseases.

Oral **PDE5 inhibitors** are contraindicated in patients taking nitrates due to risk of hypotension or syncope (ex: *avanafil, sildenafil, tadalafil, vardenafil*).

Chronic long-term **proton pump inhibitor (PPI)** use carries a risk to renal function (consider risk-benefit and alternative treatment). PPIs should be discontinued, and should not be initiated, in patients with acute kidney injury (AKI) and chronic kidney disease (CKD).

Statins are strongly recommended as adjunctive therapy for patients with diabetes, with or without abnormal lipids.

Sulfonamides (ex: *sulfamethoxazole, trimethoprim*) are not recommended in pregnancy or lactation. CrCl 15-30 mL/min: reduce dose by 1/2; CrCl <15 mL/min: not recommended. Contraindicated with G6PD deficiency. A high fluid intake is indicated during sulfonamide therapy to avoid crystallization in the kidneys.

Tetracyclines are contraindicated in children <8 years-of-age, pregnancy, and breastfeeding (discolors developing tooth enamel). A side effect may be photo-sensitivity (photophobia). Do not take with antacids, calcium supplements, milk or other dairy, or within 2 hours of taking another drug (ex: *doxycycline, minocycline*).

Tramadol is known to be excreted in breast milk. The FDA and the European Medicines Agency (EMA) are investigating the safety of using *tramadol*-containing medications to treat pain in children 12-18 years because of the potential for serious side effects, including slowed or difficult breathing.

The **Transmucosal Immediate Release Fentanyl (TIRF) Risk Evaluation and Mitigation Strategy (REMS)** program is an FDA-required program designed to ensure informed risk-benefit decisions before initiating treatment, and while patients are treated to ensure appropriate use of TIRF medicines. The purpose of the TIRF REMS Access program is to mitigate the risk of misuse, abuse, addiction, overdose, and serious complications due to medication errors with the use of TIRF medicines. You must enroll in the TIRF REMS Access program to prescribe, dispense, or distribute TIRF medicines. To register, call the TIRF REMS Access program at 1-866-822-1483 or register online at https://www.tirfremsaccess.com/TirfUI/rems/home.action

The APRN and PA's Complete Guide to Prescribing Drug Therapy

2020

DRUG THERAPY BY CLINICAL DIAGNOSIS

ACETAMINOPHEN OVERDOSE

ANTIDOTE/CHELATING AGENT

➤ *acetylcysteine* (B)(G) *Loading Dose:* 150 mg/kg administered over 15 minutes; *Maintenance:* 50 mg/kg administered over 4 hours; then 100 mg/kg administered over 16 hours
Pediatric: same as adult

  Acetadote *Vial: soln for IV infusion after dilution:* 200 mg/ml (30 ml; dilute in D₅W) (preservative-free)

Comment: *acetaminophen* overdose is a medical emergency due to the risk of irreversible hepatic injury. An IV infusion of *acetylcysteine* should be started as soon as possible and within 24 hours if the exact time of ingestion is unknown. Use a serum *acetaminophen* nomogram to determine need for treatment. Extreme caution is needed if used with concomitant hepatotoxic drugs.

 ACNE ROSACEA

Comment: All acne rosacea products should be applied sparingly to clean, dry skin as directed. Avoid use of topical corticosteroids.
➤ *ivermectin* (C) apply bid

  Soolantra *Crm:* 1% (30 gm)

  Comment: **Soolantra** is a macrocyclic lactone. Exactly how it works to treat rosacea is unknown.

TOPICAL ALPHA-1A ADRENOCEPTOR AGONIST

➤ *oxymetazoline hcl* (B) apply a pea-sized amount once daily in a thin layer covering the entire face (forehead, nose, cheeks, and chin) avoiding the eyes and lips; wash hands immediately
Pediatric: <18 years: not recommended; ≥18 years: same as adult

  Rhofade *Crm* 1% (30 gm tube)

  Comment: **Rhofade** acts as a vasoconstrictor. Use with caution in patients with cerebral or coronary insufficiency, Raynaud's phenomenon, thromboangiitis obliterans, scleroderma, or Sjögren's syndrome. **Rhofade** may increase the risk of angle closure glaucoma in patients with narrow-angle glaucoma. Advise patients to seek immediate medical care if signs and symptoms of potentiation of vascular insufficiency or acute angle closure glaucoma develop.

TOPICAL ALPHA-2 AGONIST

➤ *brimonidine* (B) apply to affected area once daily
Pediatric: <18 years: not recommended; >18 years: same as adult

  Mirvaso
  Gel: 0.33% (30, 45 gm tube; 30 gm pump)

  Comment: **Mirvaso** is indicated for persistent erythema; *brimonidine* constricts dilated facial blood vessels to reduce redness.

TOPICAL ANTIMICROBIALS

➤ *azelaic acid* (B)(G) apply to affected area bid
  Azelex *Crm:* 20% (30, 50 gm)
  Finacea *Gel:* 15% (30 gm); *Foam:* 15% (50 gm)
➤ *metronidazole* (B) apply to clean dry skin
  MetroCream apply bid
    Emol crm: 0.75% (45 gm)
  MetroGel apply once daily
    Gel: 1% (60 gm tube; 55 gm pump)
  MetroLotion apply bid
    Lotn: 0.75% (2 oz)
➤ *sodium sulfacetamide* (C)(G) apply 1-3 x daily
  Klaron *Lotn:* 10% (2 oz)
➤ *sodium sulfacetamide+sulfur* (C)
  Clenia Emollient Cream apply 1-3 x daily
    Wash: sod sulfa 10%+sulfur 5% (10 oz)

Clenia Foaming Wash wash affected area once or twice daily
Wash: sod sulfa 10%+sulfur 5% (6, 12 oz)
Rosula Gel apply 1-3 x daily
Gel: sod sulfa 10%+sulfur 5% (45 ml)
Rosula Lotion apply tid
Lotn: sod sulfa 10%+sulfur 5% (45 ml) (alcohol-free)
Rosula Wash wash bid
Clnsr: sod sulfa 10%+sulfur 5% (335 ml)

ORAL ANTIMICROBIALS

▷ *doxycycline* (D)(G) 40-100 mg bid
Pediatric: <8 years: not recommended; ≥8 years, <100 lb: 2 mg/lb on first day in 2 divided doses, followed by 1 mg/lb/day in 1-2 divided doses; ≥8 years, ≥100 lb: same as adult; *see page 625 for dose by weight*
Acticlate *Tab:* 75, 150**mg
Adoxa *Tab:* 50, 75, 100, 150 mg ent-coat
Doryx *Tab:* 50, 75, 100, 150, 200 mg del-rel
Doxteric *Tab:* 50 mg del-rel
Monodox *Cap:* 50, 75, 100 mg
Oracea *Cap:* 40 mg del-rel
Vibramycin *Tab:* 100 mg; *Cap:* 50, 100 mg; *Syr:* 50 mg/5 ml (raspberry-apple) (sulfites); *Oral susp:* 25 mg/5 ml (raspberry)
Vibra-Tab *Tab:* 100 mg film-coat
▷ *minocycline* (D)(G) 200 mg on first day; then 100 mg q 12 hours x 9 more days
Pediatric: <8 years: not recommended; ≥8 years, <100 lb: 2 mg/lb on first day in 2 divided doses, followed by 1 mg/lb q 12 hours x 9 more days; ≥8 years, ≥100 lb: same as adult
Dynacin *Cap:* 50, 100 mg
Minocin *Cap:* 50, 75, 100 mg; *Oral susp:* 50 mg/5 ml (60 ml) (custard) (sulfites, alcohol 5%)

ACNE VULGARIS

ORAL CONTRACEPTIVES

see Contraceptives *pages 559–569*
see Progesterone-only Contraceptives (Mini-Pill) *page 567*

Comment: In their 2016 published report, researchers concluded different hormonal contraceptives have significantly varied effects on acne. Women (n = 2,147) who were using a hormonal contraceptive at the time of their first consultation for acne comprised the study sample. Participants completed an assessment at baseline to report how the contraceptive affected their acne. Then the researchers used the Kruskal-Wallis test and logistic regression analysis to compare the outcomes by contraceptive type. On average, the vaginal ring and combined oral contraceptives (COCs) improved acne, whereas depot injections, subdermal implants, and hormonal intrauterine devices worsened acne. In the COC categories, *drospirenone* was the most helpful in improving acne, followed by *norgestimate* and *desogestrel*, and then *levonorgestrel* and *norethindrone*. Although triphasic progestin dosage had a positive effect on acne, estrogen dosage did not.

REFERENCE
Lortscher, D., Admani, S., Satur, N., & Eichenfield, L. F. (2016). Hormonal contraceptives and acne: A retrospective analysis of 2147 patients. *Journal of Drugs in Dermatology, 15*(6), 670–674. http://jddonline.com/articles/dermatology/S1545961616P0670X

TOPICAL ANTIMICROBIALS

Comment: All topical antimicrobials should be applied sparingly to clean, dry skin.
▷ *azelaic acid* (B)(G) apply to affected area bid
Azelex *Crm:* 20% (30, 50 gm)
Finacea *Gel:* 15% (30 gm); *Foam:* 15% (50 gm)
▷ *benzoyl peroxide* (C)(G)
Comment: *benzoyl peroxide* may discolor clothing and linens.

Benzac-W initially apply to affected area once daily; increase to bid-tid as tolerated
    Gel: 2.5, 5, 10% (60 gm)

Benzac-W Wash wash affected area bid
    Wash: 5% (4, 8 oz); 10% (8 oz)

Benzagel apply to affected area one or more x/day
    Gel: 5, 10% (1.5, 3 oz) (alcohol 14%)

Benzagel Wash wash affected area bid
    Gel: 10% (6 oz)

Desquam X⁵ wash affected area bid
    Wash: 5% (5 oz)

Desquam X¹⁰ wash affected area bid
    Wash: 10% (5 oz)

Triaz apply to affected area daily bid
    Lotn: 3, 6, 9% (bottle), 3% (tube); *Pads:* 3, 6, 9% (jar)

ZoDerm apply once or twice daily
    Gel: 4.5, 6.5, 8.5% (125 ml); *Crm:* 4.5, 6.5, 8.5% (125 ml); *Clnsr:* 4.5, 6.5, 8.5% (400 ml)

➤ *clindamycin* topical (**B**) apply to affected area bid
  Pediatric: <12 years: not recommended; ≥12 years: same as adult
    Cleocin T *Pad:* 1% (60/pck; alcohol 50%); *Lotn:* 1% (60 ml); *Gel:* 1% (30, 60 gm); *Soln w. applicator:* 1% (30, 60 ml) (alcohol 50%)
    Clindagel *Gel:* 1% (42, 77 gm)
    Evoclin Foam: 1% (50, 100 gm) (alcohol)

➤ *clindamycin+benzoyl peroxide* topical (**C**) apply to affected area once daily
  Pediatric: <12 years: not recommended; ≥12 years: same as adult
    Acanya (G) apply to affected area once daily-bid
      Gel: clin 1.2%+benz 2.5% (50 gm)
    BenzaClin (G) apply to affected area bid
      Gel: clin 1%+benz 5% (25, 50 gm)
    Duac apply daily in the evening
      Gel: clin 1%+benz 5% (45 gm)
    Onexton Gel (G) apply to affected area once daily
      Gel: clin 1.2%+benz 3.75% (50 gm pump) (alcohol-free) (preservative-free)

➤ *dapsone* topical (**C**)(**G**) apply to affected area bid
  Pediatric: <12 years: not recommended; ≥12 years: same as adult
    Aczone *Gel:* 5, 7.5% (30, 60, 90 gm pump)

➤ *erythromycin+benzoyl peroxide* (**C**) initially apply to affected area once daily; increase to bid as tolerated
    Benzamycin Topical Gel *Gel:* eryth 3%+benz 5% (46.6 gm/jar)

➤ *sodium sulfacetamide* (**C**)(**G**) apply tid
    Klaron *Lotn:* 10% (2 oz)

ORAL ANTIMICROBIALS

➤ *doxycycline* (**D**)(**G**) 100 mg bid
  Pediatric: <8 years: not recommended; ≥8 years, <100 lb: 2 mg/lb on first day in 2 divided doses, followed by 1 mg/lb/day in 1-2 divided doses; ≥8 years, ≥100 lb: same as adult; *see page 625 for dose by weight*
    Acticlate *Tab:* 75, 150**mg
    Adoxa *Tab:* 50, 75, 100, 150 mg ent-coat
    Doryx *Tab:* 50, 75, 100, 150, 200 mg del-rel
    Doxteric *Tab:* 50 mg del-rel
    Monodox *Cap:* 50, 75, 100 mg
    Oracea *Cap:* 40 mg del-rel
    Vibramycin *Tab:* 100 mg; *Cap:* 50, 100 mg; *Syr:* 50 mg/5 ml (raspberry-apple) (sulfites); *Oral susp:* 25 mg/5 ml (raspberry)
    Vibra-Tab *Tab:* 100 mg film coat

➤ *erythromycin base* (**B**)(**G**) 250 mg qid, 333 mg tid or 500 mg bid x 7-10 days; then taper to lowest effective dose
  Pediatric: <45 kg: 30-50 mg in 2-4 divided doses x 7-10 days; ≥45 kg: same as adult
    Ery-Tab *Tab:* 250, 333, 500 mg ent-coat
    PCE *Tab:* 333, 500 mg

Comment: *erythromycin* may increase INR with concomitant *warfarin*, as well as increase serum level of *digoxin*, benzodiazepines, and statins.

➤ *erythromycin ethylsuccinate* (B)(G) 400 mg qid x 7-10 days
   Pediatric: 30-50 mg/kg/day in 4 divided doses x 7-10 days; may double dose with severe
   infection; max 100 mg/kg/day; *see page 626 for dose by weight*
   EryPed *Oral susp:* 200 mg/5 ml (100, 200 ml) (fruit); 400 mg/5 ml (60, 100, 200 ml)
   (banana); *Oral drops:* 200, 400 mg/5 ml (50 ml) (fruit); *Chew tab:* 200 mg wafer (fruit)
   E.E.S. *Oral susp:* 200, 400 mg/5 ml (100 ml) (fruit)
   E.E.S. Granules *Oral susp:* 200 mg/5 ml (100, 200 ml) (cherry)
   E.E.S. 400 Tablets *Tab:* 400 mg
   Comment: *erythromycin* may increase INR with concomitant *warfarin*, as well as increase
   serum level of *digoxin*, benzodiazepines, and statins.

➤ *minocycline* (D)(G) initially 50-200 mg/day in 2 divided doses; reduce dose to once daily
   after improvement
   Pediatric: <8 years: not recommended; ≥8 years: same as adult
   Dynacin *Cap:* 50, 100 mg
   Minocin *Cap:* 50, 75, 100 mg; *Oral susp:* 50 mg/5 ml (60 ml) (custard) (sulfites, alcohol
   5%)
   Minolira *Tab:* 105, 135 mg ext-rel
   Solodyn *Tab:* 55, 65, 80, 105, 115 mg ext-rel
   Comment: Once-daily dosing of **Minolira** or **Solodyn,** extended-release *minocyclines*, is
   approved for inflammatory lesions of non-nodular moderate-to-severe acne vulgaris for
   patients ≥12 years-of-age. The recommended dose of **Solodyn** is 1 mg/kg once daily x 12
   weeks.

➤ *sarecycline* one tab daily based with or without food; <9 years: not recommended; ≥9 years:
   33-54 kg: 60 mg; *55-84 kg:* 100 mg; *85-136 kg:* 150 mg
   Seysara *Tab:* 60, 100, 150 mg
   Comment: **Seysara** is a first-in-class, *tetracycline*-derived, once daily treatment for
   inflammatory lesions of non-nodular moderate-to-severe acne. Efficacy of **Seysara**
   beyond 12 weeks and safety beyond 12 months have not been established. **Seysara**
   has not been evaluated in the treatment of infections. To reduce the development of
   drug-resistant bacteria as well as to maintain the effectiveness of other antibacterial
   drugs, **Seysara** should be used only as indicated. If *Clostridium difficile*-associated
   diarrhea (antibiotic-associated colitis) occurs, discontinue **Seysara**. Central nervous
   system side effects, including light-headedness, dizziness or vertigo, have been reported
   with *tetracycline* use. Patients who experience these symptoms should be cautioned
   about driving vehicles or using hazardous machinery. These symptoms may disappear
   during therapy and may disappear when the drug is discontinued. **Seysara** may cause
   intracranial hypertension; discontinue **Seysara** if symptoms occur. Photosensitivity
   can occur with **Seysara**; minimize or avoid exposure to natural or artificial sunlight.
   tetracycline is contraindicated <8 years-of-age, in pregnancy, and lactation (discolors
   developing tooth enamel). A side effect may be photo-sensitivity (photophobia). Avoid
   co-administration with retinoids and penicillin. Decrease anticoagulant dosage as
   appropriate. Monitor for toxicities of drugs that may require dosage reduction (e.g.,
   P-glycoprotein substrates) and monitor for toxicities. Do not take with antacids,
   calcium supplements, iron preparations, milk or other dairy, or within two hours of
   taking another drug.

➤ *tetracycline* (D)(G) initially 1 gm/day in 2-4 divided doses; after improvement, 125-500 mg
   daily
   Pediatric: <8 years: not recommended; ≥8 years, <100 lb: 25-50 mg/kg/day in 2-4 divided
   doses; ≥8 years, ≥100 lb: same as adult; *see page 630 for dose by weight*
   Achromycin V *Cap:* 250, 500 mg
   Sumycin *Tab:* 250, 500 mg; *Cap:* 250, 500 mg; *Oral susp:* 125 mg/5 ml (100, 200 ml)
   (fruit) (sulfites)
   Comment: *tetracycline* is contraindicated <8 years-of-age, in pregnancy, and lactation
   (discolors developing tooth enamel). A side effect may be photo-sensitivity (photophobia).
   Do not take with antacids, calcium supplements, milk or other dairy, or within two hours of
   taking another drug.

TOPICAL RETINOIDS

Comment: Wash affected area with a soap-free cleanser; pat dry and wait 20 to 30 minutes;
then apply sparingly to affected area; use only once daily in the evening. Avoid applying to
eyes, ears, nostrils, and mouth.

▷ *adapalene* (C) apply once daily at HS
    Pediatric: <12 years: not recommended; ≥12 years: same as adult
        Differin *Crm:* 0.1% (45 gm); *Gel:* 0.1, 0.3% (45 gm) (alcohol-free); *Pad:* 0.1% (30/pck)
        (alcohol 30%); *Lotn:* 0.1% (2, 4 oz)
▷ *tazarotene* (X)(G) apply to affected area once daily at HS
    Pediatric: <12 years: not recommended; ≥12 years: same as adult
        Avage Cream *Crm:* 0.1% (30 gm)
        Tazorac Cream *Crm:* 0.05, 0.1% (15, 30, 60 gm)
        Tazorac Gel *Gel:* 0.05, 0.1% (30, 100 gm)
▷ *tretinoin* (C)(G) apply sparingly to affected area once or twice daily
    Comment: Dryness, pain, erythema, irritation and exfoliation may occur during treatment.
    Avoid paranasal creases and mucous membranes. Minimize exposure to sunlight and
    sunlamps. Use sunscreen and protective clothing when sun exposure cannot be avoided.
    Use with caution if allergic to fish due to potential for allergenicity to fish protein.
    Pediatric: <12 years: not recommended; ≥12 years: same as adult
        Altreno *Lotn:* 0.05% (45 gm tube)
        Comment: **Altreno** is indicated for children >9 years-of-age. Apply a thin film to
        affected area bid.
        Atralin Gel *Gel:* 0.05% (45 gm)
        Avita *Crm:* 0.025% (20, 45 gm); *Gel:* 0.025% (20, 45 gm)
        Retin-A Cream *Crm:* 0.025, 0.05, 0.1% (20, 45 gm)
        Retin-A Gel *Gel:* 0.01, 0.025% (15, 45 gm) (alcohol 90%)
        Retin-A Liquid *Soln:* 0.05% (alcohol 55%)
        Retin-A Micro Gel *Gel:* 0.04, 0.08, 0.1% (20, 45 gm)
        Tretin-X Cream *Crm:* 0.075% (35 gm) (parabens-free, alcohol-free, propylene
        glycol-free)

TOPICAL RETINOID+ANTIMICROBIAL COMBINATIONS

Comment: Wash affected area with a soap-free cleanser; pat dry and wait 20-30 minutes; then
apply sparingly to affected area; use only once daily in the evening. Avoid eyes, ears, nostrils,
and mouth.
▷ *adapalene+benzoyl peroxide* (C)(G) apply a thin film once daily
    Pediatric: <18 years: not recommended
        Epiduo Gel *Gel:* adap 0.1%+benz 2.5% (45 gm)
        Epiduo Forte Gel *Pump gel:* adap 0.3%+benz 2.5% (15, 30, 45, 60 gm)
▷ *tretinoin+clindamycin* (C)(G) apply a thin film once daily
    Pediatric: <18 years: not recommended
        Ziana *Gel:* tret 0.025%+clin 1.2% (30, 60 gm)

ORAL RETINOID

Comment: Oral retinoids are indicated only for severe recalcitrant nodular acne unresponsive
to conventional therapy including systemic antibiotics.
▷ *isotretinoin* (X) initially 0.5-1 mg/kg/day in 2 divided doses; maintenance 0.5-2 mg/kg/
day in 2 divided doses x 4-5 months; repeat only if necessary 2 months following cessation
of first treatment course
    Pediatric: <12 years: not recommended; ≥12 years: same as adult
        Accutane *Cap:* 10, 20, 40 mg (parabens)
        Amnesteem *Cap:* 10, 20, 40 mg (soy)
    Comment: *isotretinoin* is highly teratogenic and, therefore, female patients should
be counseled prior to initiation of treatment as follows: Two negative pregnancy tests
are required prior to initiation of treatment and monthly thereafter. Not for use in
females who are or who may become pregnant or who are breastfeeding. Two effective
methods of contraception should be used for 1 month prior to, during, and continuing
for 1 month following completion of treatment. Low-dose *progestin* (mini-pill) may be
an *inadequate* form of contraception. No refills; a new prescription is required every 30
days and prescriptions must be filled within 7 days. Serum lipids should be monitored
until response is established (usually initially and again after 4 weeks). Bone growth,
serum glucose, ESR, RBCs, WBCs, and liver enzymes should be monitored. Blood
should not be donated during, or for 1 month after, completion of treatment. Avoid

the sun and artificial UV light. *isotretinoin* should be discontinued if any of the following occurs: visual disturbances, tinnitus, hearing impairment, rectal bleeding, pancreatitis, hepatitis, significant decrease in CBC, hyperlipidemia (particularly hypertriglyceridemia).

ACROMEGALY

GROWTH HORMONE RECEPTOR ANTAGONIST

▷ *pegvisomant* (B) *Loading dose:* 40 mg SC; *Maintenance:* 10 mg SC daily; titrate by 5 mg (increments or decrements, based on IGF-1 levels) every 4 to 6 weeks; max 30 mg/day
Pediatric: <12 years: not recommended; ≥12 years: same as adult
   Somavert *Inj:* 10, 15, 20 mg
Comment: Prior to initiation of *pegvisomant*, patients should have baseline fasting serum glucose, HgbA1c, serum K$^+$ and Mg^{++}, liver function tests (LFTs), EKG, and gall bladder ultrasound.

Cyclohexapeptide Somatostatin

▷ *pasireotide* (C) administer SC in the thigh or abdomen; initial dose is 0.6 mg or 0.9 mg bid. Titrate dose based on response and tolerability; for patients with moderate hepatic impairment (Child-Pugh Class B), the recommended initial dosage is 0.3 mg twice daily and max dose 0.6 mg twice daily; avoid use in patients with severe hepatic impairment (Child-Pugh Class C)
Pediatric: <12 years: not recommended; ≥12 years: same as adult
   Signifor LAR *Amp:* 0.3, 0.6, 0.9 mg/ml, single-dose, long-act rel (LAR) susp for inj

ACTINIC KERATOSIS (AK)

▷ *aminolevulinic acid 10%* clean and prepare all lesions prior to applying gel 1 mm thick and include 5 mm of the surrounding skin; max application area 20 cm^2 and max 2 gm per treatment; apply an occlusive dressing x 3 hours; photodynamic therapy involves preparation of lesions, application of the **Ameluz**, occlusion, and illumination with BF-RhodoLED only by a qualified health care provider; remove remaining gel at the end of the treatment; may re-treat in 3 months after the initial treatment; BF-RhodoLED user manual for detailed lamp safety and operating instructions.
Pediatric: <18 years: not recommended; ≥18 years: same as adult
   Ameluz *Gel:* 10% (2 gram tube) 100 mg/gm of *aminolevulinic acid hcl* (equivalent to 78 mg/gm *aminolevulinic acid*) (xanthan gum, soybean phosphatidylcholine, polysorbate 80, medium-chain triglycerides, dibasic sodium phosphate, monobasic sodium phosphate, propylene glycol, sodium benzoate, isopropal alcohol)
   Comment: Ameluz (*aminolevulinic acid*) 10% gel, a porphyrin precursor, in combination with photodynamic therapy using BF-RhodoLED lamp, is indicated for the lesion-directed and field-directed treatment of actinic keratoses of mild-to-moderate severity on the face and scalp. The most common adverse reactions (incidence ≥10%) have been application site erythema, pain/burning, irritation, edema, pruritus, exfoliation, scab formation, induration, and vesicles. Concomitant use of other photosensitizing agents may increase the risk of phototoxic reaction to photodynamic therapy (e.g., St. John's wort, *griseofulvin*, thiazide diuretics, sulfonylureas, phenothiazines, sulfonamides, quinolones, and tetracyclines). Patient and healthcare provider must wear protective eyewear before and during operation of the BF-RhodoLED lamp. Treated lesions should be protected from sunlight exposure for 48 hours post-treatment. Special care should be taken to avoid bleeding during lesion preparation in patients with inherited or acquired a coagulation disorder. Avoid direct contact of **Ameluz** with the eyes and mucous membranes. There are no human or animal reproductive studies of **Ameluz** use in pregnancy to inform a drug-associated risk. Systemic absorption of *aminolevulinic acid* is negligible. No data are available regarding the presence of *aminolevulinic acid* in human milk or effects on the breastfed infant; however, breastfeeding is not expected to result in infant exposure to the drug due to negligible systemic absorption. To report suspected adverse reactions, contact Biofrontera at 1-844-829-7434 or FDA at 1-800-332-1088 or visit www.fda.gov/medwatch.

➤ *diclofenac sodium* 3% (C; D ≥30 wks)(G) apply to lesions bid x 60-90 days
Pediatric: <12 years: not established; ≥12 years: same as adult
    Solaraze Gel *Gel:* 3% (50 gm) (benzyl alcohol)
Comment: *diclofenac* is contraindicated with *aspirin* allergy. As with other NSAIDs,
Solaraze Gel should be avoided in late pregnancy (≥30 weeks) because it may
cause premature closure of the ductus arteriosus; may cause premature closure of the
ductus arteriosus.
    Voltaren Gel apply qid; avoid non-intact skin
      Gel: 1% (100 gm)
➤ *fluorouracil* (X)(G) apply to lesion(s) daily-bid until erosion occurs, usually 2-4 weeks
Pediatric: <12 years: not recommended; ≥12 years: same as adult
    Carac *Crm:* 0.5% (30 gm)
    Efudex (G) *Crm:* 5% (25 gm); *Soln:* 2, 5% (10 ml w. dropper)
    Fluoroplex *Crm:* 1% (30 gm); *Soln:* 1% (30 ml w. dropper)
➤ *imiquimod* (B)
Pediatric: <18 years: not recommended; ≥18 years: same as adult
    Aldara (G) rub into lesions before bedtime and remove with soap and water 8 hours
    later; treat 2 times per week; max 16 weeks
      Crm: 5% (single-use pkts/carton)
    Zyclara rub into lesions before bedtime and remove with soap and water 8 hours later;
    treat for 2-week cycles separated by a 2-week no-treatment cycle; max 2 packs per
    application; max one treatment course per area
      Crm: 3.75% (single-use pkts; 28/carton) (parabens)
➤ *ingenol mebutate* (C) limit application to one contiguous skin area of about 25 cm^2 using
one unit dose tube; allow treated area to dry for 15 minutes; wash hands immediately after
application; may remove with soapy water after 6 hours; *Face and Scalp:* apply 0.015% gel to
lesions daily x 3 days; *Trunk and Extremities:* apply 0.05% gel to lesions daily x 2 days
Pediatric: <18 years: not recommended; ≥18 years: same as adult
    Picato *Gel:* 0.015% (3 single-use tubes), 0.05% (2 single-use tubes)

ALCOHOL DEPENDENCE, DETOXIFICATION/ALCOHOL WITHDRAWAL SYNDROME

ALCOHOL WITHDRAWAL SYNDROME

Comment: Total length of time of a given detoxification regimen and/or length of
treatment at any dose reduction level may be extended based on patient-specific factors,
including potential or actual seizure, hallucinosis, increased sympathetic nervous system
activity (severe anxiety, unwanted elevation in vital signs). If any of these symptoms are
anticipated or occur, revert to an earlier step in the dosing regimen to stabilize the patient,
extend the detoxification timeline and consider appropriate adjunctive drug treatments (e.g.,
anticonvulsants, antipsychotic agents, antihypertensive agents, sedative hypnotics agents).
➤ *clorazepate* (D)(IV)(G) in the following dosage schedule: *Day 1:* 30 mg initially, followed by
30-60 mg in divided doses; *Day 2:* 45-90 mg in divided doses; *Day 3:* 22.5-45 mg in divided
doses; *Day 4:* 15-30 mg in divided doses; *Thereafter*, gradually reduce the daily dose to 7.5-
15 mg; then discontinue when patient's condition is stable; max dose 90 mg/day
Pediatric: <18 years: not recommended; ≥18 years: same as adult
    Tranxene *Tab:* 3.75, 7.5, 15 mg
    Tranxene T-Tab *Tab:* 3.75*, 7.5*, 15*mg
➤ *chlordiazepoxide* (D)(IV)(G)
Pediatric: <18 years: not recommended; ≥18 years: same as adult
    Librium 50-100 mg q 6 hours x 24-72 hours; then q 8 hours x 24-72 hours; then q 12
    hours x 24-72 hours; then daily x 24-72 hours
      Cap: 5, 10, 25 mg
    Librium Injectable 50-100 mg IM or IV; then 25-50 mg IM tid-qid prn; max 300 mg/day
      Inj: 100 mg
➤ *diazepam* (D)(IV)(G) 2-10 mg q 6 hours x 24-72 hours; then q 8 hours x 24-72 hours; then
q 12 hours x 24-72 hours; then daily x 24-72 hours
Pediatric: <18 years: not recommended; ≥18 years: same as adult
    Diastat *Rectal gel delivery system:* 2.5 mg
    Diastat Acu Dial *Rectal gel delivery system:* 10, 20 mg

Valium *Tab:* 2*, 5*, 10*mg
Valium Injectable *Vial:* 5 mg/ml (10 ml); *Amp:* 5 mg/ml (2 ml); *Prefilled syringe:* 5 mg/ml (5 ml)
Valium Intensol Oral Solution *Conc oral soln:* 5 mg/ml (30 ml w. dropper) (alcohol 19%)
Valium Oral Solution *Oral soln:* 5 mg/5 ml (500 ml) (wintergreen-spice)

▷ *oxazepam* (C) 10-15 mg tid-qid x 24-72 hours; decrease dose <u>and/or</u> frequency every 24-72 hours; total length of therapy 5-14 days; max 120 mg/day
   Pediatric: <18 years: not recommended; ≥18 years: same as adult
      Cap: 10, 15, 30 mg

ABSTINENCE THERAPY
GABA Taurine Analog
▷ *acamprosate* (C)(G) 666 mg tid; begin therapy during abstinence; continue during relapse; *CrCl 30-50-mL/min:* max 333 mg tid; *CrCl <30 mL/min:* contraindicated
   Pediatric: <18 years: not recommended; ≥18 years: same as adult
      Campral *Tab:* 333 mg ext-rel
      Comment: **Campral** does <u>not</u> eliminate <u>or</u> diminish alcohol withdrawal symptoms.

AVERSION THERAPY
▷ *disulfiram* (X)(G)
   Pediatric: <18 years: not recommended; ≥18 years: same as adult
      Antabuse 500 mg once daily x 1-2 weeks; then 250 mg once daily
         Tab: 250, 500 mg; *Chew tab:* 200, 500 mg
   Comment: *disulfiram* use requires informed consent. Contraindications: severe cardiac disease, psychosis, concomitant use of *isoniazid*, *phenytoin*, *paraldehyde*, and topical and systemic alcohol-containing products. Approximately 20% remains in the system for 1 week after discontinuation.

⬤ ALLERGIC REACTION: GENERAL

Oral Second Generation Antihistamines *see* **Drugs for the Management of Allergy, Cough, and Cold Symptoms** *pages* 603
Topical Corticosteroids *see page* 574
Parenteral Corticosteroids *see page* 577
Oral Corticosteroids *see page* 577

FIRST GENERATION PARENTERAL ANTIHISTAMINE
▷ *diphenhydramine* (C)(G) 25-50 mg IM immediately; then q 6 hours prn
   Pediatric: <12 years: *See mfr pkg insert:* 1.25 mg/kg up to 25 mg IM x 1 dose; then q 6 hours prn
      Benadryl Injectable *Vial:* 50 mg/ml (1 ml single-use); 50 mg/ml (10 ml multi-dose); *Amp:* 10 mg/ml (1 ml); *Prefilled syringe:* 50 mg/ml (1 ml)

FIRST GENERATION ORAL ANTIHISTAMINES
▷ *diphenhydramine* (B)(G) 25-50 mg q 6-8 hours; max 100 mg/day
   Pediatric: <2 years: not recommended; 2-6 years: 6.25 mg q 4-6 hours; max 37.5 mg/day; >6-12 years: 12.5-25 mg q 4-6 hours; max 150 mg/day; >12 years: same as adult
      Benadryl (OTC) *Chew tab:* 12.5 mg (grape) (phenylalanine); *Liq:* 12.5 mg/5 ml (4, 8 oz); *Cap:* 25 mg; *Tab:* 25 mg; *Dye-free soft gel:* 25 mg; *Dye-free liq:* 12.5 mg/5 ml (4, 8 oz)
▷ *hydroxyzine* (C)(G) 50-100 mg qid; max 600 mg/day
   Pediatric: <6 years: 50 mg/day divided qid; ≥6 years: 50-100 mg/day divided qid
      Atarax *Tab:* 10, 25, 50, 100 mg; *Syr:* 10 mg/5 ml (alcohol 0.5%)
      Vistaril *Cap:* 25, 50, 100 mg; *Oral susp:* 25 mg/5 ml (4 oz) (lemon)

⬤ ALLERGIES: MULTI-FOOD

Comment: Eight food-types cause about 90% of food allergy reactions: *Milk* (mostly in children), *Eggs, Peanuts, Tree nuts,* (e.g., walnuts, almonds, pine nuts, brazil nuts, and pecans),

Soy, Wheat (and other grains with gluten, including barley, rye, and oats), *Fish* (mostly in adults), *Shellfish* (mostly in adults). Combining ***omalizumab*** with oral immunotherapy (OIT) significantly improves the effectiveness of OIT in children with multiple food allergies, according to the results of a recent study. Researchers conducted a blinded, phase 2 clinical trial including children aged 4 to 15 years who had multi-food allergies validated by double-blind, placebo-controlled food challenges. Participants were randomly assigned (3:1) to either receive ***omalizumab*** with multi-food oral immunotherapy or placebo. ***omalizumab*** and placebo were administered for 16 weeks, with oral immunotherapy beginning at 8 weeks. Overall, at week 36, a significantly greater proportion of the ***omalizumab***-treated participants passed double-blind, placebo-controlled food challenges, compared with placebo (83% vs 33%). No serious or severe adverse events were reported. In multi-food allergic patients, ***omalizumab*** improves the efficacy of multi-food oral immunotherapy and enables safe and rapid desensitization.

REFERENCE

Andorf, S., Purington, N., Block, W. M., Long, A. J., Tupa, D., Brittain, E., … Chinthrajah, R. S. (2017). Anti-IgE treatment with oral immunotherapy in multifood allergic participants: A double-blind, randomised, controlled trial. *The Lancet: Gastroenterology & Hepatology, 3*(2), 85–94. doi:10.1016/s2468-1253(17)30392-8

IGE BLOCKER (IGG1K MONOCLONAL ANTIBODY)

▷ *omalizumab* (B) 150-375 mg SC every 2-4 weeks based on body weight and pre-treatment serum total IgE level; max 150 mg/injection site; should be administered <u>only</u> by a qualified health care provider
Pediatric: <12 years: not recommended; 30-90 kg + IgE >30-100 IU/ml 150 mg q 4 weeks; 90-150 kg + IgE >30-100 IU/ml <u>or</u> 30-90 kg + IgE >100-200 IU/ml <u>or</u> 30-60 kg + IgE >200-300 IU/ml 300 mg q 4 hours; >90-150 kg + IgE >100-200 IU/ml <u>or</u> >60-90 kg + IgE >200-300 IU/ml <u>or</u> 30-70 kg + IgE >300-400 IU/ml 225 mg q 2 weeks; >90-150 kg + IgE >200-300 IU/ml <u>or</u> >70-90 kg + IgE >300-400 IU/ml <u>or</u> 30-70 kg + IgE >400-500 IU/ml <u>or</u> 30-60 kg + IgE >500-600 IU/ml <u>or</u> 30-60 kg + IgE >600-700 IU/ml 375 mg q 2 weeks; ≥12 years: same as adult
Xolair *Vial:* 150 mg, single-dose, pwdr for SC injection after reconstitution *Prefilled syringe:* 75 mg/0.5 ml, 150 mg/1 ml single-dose (preservative-free)

⬤ ALZHEIMER'S DISEASE

NUTRITIONAL SUPPLEMENT

▷ *l-methylfolate calcium (as metafolin)+methylcobalamin+n-acetyl cysteine* take 1 cap once daily
Cerefolin *Cap:* metafo 5.6 mg+methyl 2 mg+n-ace cys 600 mg (gluten-free, yeast-free, lactose-free)
Comment: Cerefolin is indicated in the dietary management of patients treated for early memory loss, with emphasis on those at risk for neurovascular oxidative stress, hyper-homocysteinemia, mild to moderate cognitive impairment with <u>or</u> without vitamin B12 deficiency, vascular dementia, <u>or</u> Alzheimer's disease.

REVERSIBLE ANTICHOLINESTERASE INHIBITORS (RAIs)

Comment: The RAI drugs do <u>not</u> halt disease progression. They are indicated for early-stage disease; <u>not</u> effective for severe dementia. If treatment is stopped for more than several days, re-titrate from lowest dose. Side effects include nausea, anorexia, dyspepsia, diarrhea, headache, and dizziness. Side effects tend to resolve with continued treatment. Peak cognitive improvements are seen 12 weeks into therapy (increased spontaneity, reduced apathy, lessened confusion, and improved attention, conversational language, and performance of daily routines).

▷ *donepezil* (C)(G) initially 5 mg q HS, increase to 10 mg after 4-6 weeks as needed; max 23 mg/day
Aricept *Tab:* 5, 10, 23 mg
Aricept ODT *ODT tab:* 5, 10 mg orally-disint

▷ *galantamine* (B) initially 4 mg bid x at least 4 weeks; usual maintenance 8 mg bid; max 16 mg bid
Razadyne *Tab:* 4, 8, 12 mg

Razadyne ER *Tab*: 8, 16, 24 mg ext-rel
Razadyne Oral Solution *Oral soln*: 4 mg/ml (100 ml w. calib pipette)

▷ *rivastigmine* (B)(G)
Exelon initially 1.5 mg bid, increase every 2 weeks as needed; max 12 mg/day; take with food
Cap: 1.5, 3, 4.5, 6 mg
Excelon Oral Solution initially 1.5 mg bid; may increase by 1.5 mg bid at intervals of at least 2 weeks; usual range 6-12 mg/day; max 12 mg/day; if stopped, restart at lowest dose and re-titrate; may take directly from syringe or mix with water, fruit juice, or cola
Oral soln: 2 mg/ml (120 ml w. dose syringe)
Excelon Patch initially apply 4.6 mg/24 hr patch; if tolerated, may increase to 9.5 mg/24 hr patch after 4 weeks; max 13.3 mg/24 hr; change patch daily; apply to clean, dry, hairless, intact skin; rotate application site; allow 14 days before applying new patch to same site
Patch: 4.6, 9.5, 13.3 mg/24 hr trans-sys (30/carton)

▷ *tacrine* (C) initially 10 mg qid, increase 40 mg/day q 4 weeks as needed; max 160 mg/day
Cognex *Cap*: 10, 20, 30, 40 mg
Comment: Transaminase levels should be checked every 3 months while taking Cognex.

N-METHYL-D-ASPARTATE (NMDA) RECEPTOR ANTAGONIST

▷ *memantine* (B)(G)
Namenda initially 5 mg once daily; titrate weekly in 5 mg/day increments; *Week 2*: 5 mg bid; *Week 3*: 5 mg AM and 10 mg PM; *Week 4*: 10 mg bid; *CrCl 5-29 mL/min*: max 5 mg bid
Tab: 5, 10 mg
Namenda Oral Solution initially 5 mg once daily; titrate weekly in 5 mg increments administered bid
Oral soln: 2 mg/ml (360 ml) (peppermint) (sugar-free, alcohol-free)
Namenda Titration Pak
Cap: 7 x 7 mg, 7 x 14 mg, 7 x 21 mg, 7 x 28 mg/pck
Namenda XR initially 7 mg once daily; titrate in 7 mg increments weekly; max 28 mg once daily; do not divide doses
Cap: 7, 14, 21, 28 mg ext-rel
Comment: *memantine* does not halt disease progression. It is indicated for moderate to severe dementia.

N-METHYL-D-ASPARTATE (NMDA) RECEPTOR ANTAGONIST+
ACETYLCHOLIN-ESTERASE INHIBITOR COMBINATION

▷ *memantine+donepezil* (C)(G) initiate one 28/10 dose daily in the evening after stabilized on *memantine* and *donepezil* separately; start the day after the last dose of *memantine* and *donepezil* taken separately; swallow whole or open cap and sprinkle on applesauce; *CrCl 5-29 mL/min*: take one 14/10 dose once daily in the evening
Namzaric
Cap: Namzaric 7/10 mem 7 mg+done 10 mg
Namzaric 14/10 mem 14 mg+done 10 mg
Namzaric 21/10 mem 21 mg+done 10 mg
Namzaric 28/10 mem 28 mg+done 10 mg

ERGOT ALKALOID (DOPAMINE AGONIST)

▷ *ergoloid mesylate* (C) 1 mg tid
Hydergine *Tab*: 1 mg
Hydergine LC *Cap*: 1 mg
Hydergine Liquid *Liq*: 1 mg/ml (100 ml w. calib dropper) (alcohol 28.5%)

◯ AMEBIASIS

AMEBIASIS (INTESTINAL)

▷ *diiodohydroxyquin (iodoquinol)* (C)(G) 650 mg tid pc x 20 days
Pediatric: <6 years: 40 mg/kg/day in 3 divided doses pc x 20 days; max 1.95 gm; 6-12 years: 420 mg tid pc x 20 days
Tab: 210, 650 mg

➤ *metronidazole* (not for use in 1st; B in 2nd, 3rd)(G) 750 mg tid x 5-10 days
    Pediatric: 35-50 mg/kg/day in 3 divided doses x 10 days
        Flagyl *Tab:* 250*, 500*mg
        Flagyl 375 *Cap:* 375 mg
        Flagyl ER *Tab:* 750 mg ext-rel
➤ *tinidazole* (C) 2 gm daily x 3 days; take with food
    Pediatric: <3 years: not recommended; ≥3 years: 50 mg/kg daily x 3 days; take with food;
    max 2 gm/day
        Tindamax *Tab:* 250*, 500*mg
Comment: Other than for use in the treatment of *giardiasis* and *amebiasis* in pediatric
patients older than three years-of-age, safety and effectiveness of *tinidazole* in pediatric
patients have not been established. *tinidazole* is excreted in breast milk in concentrations
similar to those seen in serum and can be detected in breast milk for up to 72 hours
following administration. Interruption of breast-feeding is recommended during *tinidazole*
therapy and for 3 days following the last dose.
➤ *paromomycin* 25-35 mg/kg/day in 3 divided doses x 5-10 days
    Pediatric: same as adult
        Humatin *Cap:* 250 mg

AMEBIASIS (EXTRA-INTESTINAL)

➤ *chloroquine phosphate* (C)(G) 1 gm PO daily x 2 days; then 500 mg daily x 2 to 3 weeks <u>or</u>
200-250 mg IM daily x 10-12 days (when oral therapy is impossible); use with intestinal
amebicide
Pediatric: see mfr pkg insert
        Aralen *Tab:* 500 mg; *Amp:* 50 mg/ml (5 ml)

 AMEBIC LIVER ABSCESS

ANTI-INFECTIVES

➤ *metronidazole* (C)(G) 250 mg tid <u>or</u> 500 mg bid <u>or</u> 750 mg daily x 7 days
    Pediatric: <12 years: not recommended; ≥12 years: same as adult
        Flagyl *Tab:* 250*, 500*mg
        Flagyl 375 *Cap:* 375 mg
        Flagyl ER *Tab:* 750 mg ext-rel
Comment: Alcohol is contraindicated during treatment with oral *metronidazole* and for 72
hours after therapy due to a possible *disulfiram*-like reaction (nausea, vomiting, flushing,
headache).
➤ *tinidazole* (C) 2 gm once daily x 3-5 days; take with food
    Pediatric: <3 years: not recommended; ≥3 years: 50 mg/kg once daily x 3-5 days; take with
    food; max 2 gm/day
        Tindamax *Tab:* 250*, 500*mg
Comment: Other than for use in the treatment of *giardiasis* and *amebiasis* in pediatric
patients older than three years-of-age, safety and effectiveness of *tinidazole* in pediatric
patients have not been established. tinidazole is excreted in breast milk in concentrations
similar to those seen in serum and can be detected in breast milk for up to 72 hours
following administration. Interruption of breast-feeding is recommended during *tinidazole*
therapy and for 3 days following the last dose.

AMENORRHEA: SECONDARY

➤ *estrogen+progesterone* (X)
        Premarin (*estrogen*) 0.625 mg daily x 25 days; then 5 days off; repeat monthly
        Provera (*progesterone*) 5-10 mg last 10 days of cycle; repeat monthly
➤ *estrogen replacement* (X)
    see *Menopause* page 301
➤ *human chorionic gonadotropin* 5,000-10,000 units IM x 1 dose following last dose of
menotropins
        Pregnyl *Vial:* 10,000 units (10 ml) w. diluent (10 ml)

▷ *medroxyprogesterone* (X) *Monthly*: 5-10 mg last 5-10 days of cycle; begin on the 16th or
21st day of cycle; repeat monthly; *One-time only*: 10 mg once daily x 10 days
> Amen *Tab*: 10 mg
> Provera *Tab*: 2.5, 5, 10 mg
▷ *norethindrone* (X) 2.5-10 mg daily x 5-10 days
> Aygestin *Tab*: 5 mg
▷ *progesterone, micronized* (X)(G) 400 mg q HS x 10 days
> Prometrium *Cap*: 100, 200 mg
> Comment: Administration of *progesterone* induces optimum secretory transformation
> of the *estrogen*-primed endometrium. Administration of *progesterone* is contraindicated
> with breast cancer, undiagnosed vaginal bleeding, genital cancer, severe liver dysfunction
> or disease, missed abortion, thrombophlebitis, thromboembolic disorders, cerebral
> apoplexy, and pregnancy.

 AMYOTROPHIC LATERAL SCLEROSIS (ALS, LOU GEHRIG'S DISEASE)

PYRAZOLONE FREE RADICAL SCAVENGER

▷ *edaravone* recommended dosage is 60 mg as an IV infusion administered over 60 minutes;
Initial treatment cycle: daily dosing for 14 days followed by a 14-day drug-free period;
Subsequent treatment cycles: daily dosing for 10 days out of 14-day periods, followed by
14-day drug-free periods
> Radicava *IV soln*: 30 mg/100 ml single-dose polypropylene bag for IV infusion (sodium
> bisulfite)
> Comment: Most common adverse reactions (at least 10%) are confusion, gait
> disturbance, and headache. There are no adequate data on the developmental risk
> associated with the use of Radicava in pregnancy. There are no data on the presence
> of *edaravone* in human milk or the effects on the breastfed infant. However, based
> on animal data, may cause fetal harm. To report suspected adverse reactions, contact
> MT Pharma America at 1-888-292-0058 or FDA at 800-FDA-1088 or www.fda.gov/
> medwatch

 ANAPHYLAXIS

Parenteral Corticosteroids *see page* 577
Oral Corticosteroids *see page* 577

▷ *epinephrine* (C)(G) 0.3-0.5 mg (0.3-0.5 ml of a 1:1000 soln) SC q 20-30 minutes as needed
up to 3 doses
Pediatric: <2 years: 0.05-0.1 ml; 2-6 years: 0.1 ml; ≥6-12 years: 0.2 ml; All: q 20-30 minutes
as needed up to 3 doses; ≥12 years: same as adult

ANAPHYLAXIS EMERGENCY TREATMENT KITS

▷ *epinephrine* (C) 0.3 ml IM or SC in thigh; may repeat if needed
Pediatric: 0.01 mg/kg SC or IM in thigh; may repeat if needed; <15 kg: not established; 15-
30 kg: 0.15 mg; >30 kg: same as adult
> Adrenaclick *Auto-injector*: 0.15, 0.3 mg (1 mg/ml; 1, 2/carton) (sulfites)
> Auvi-Q *Auto-injector*: 0.15, 0.3 mg (1 mg/ml; 1/pck w. 1 non-active training device)
> (sulfites)
> EpiPen *Auto-injector*: 0.3 mg (*epi* 1:1000, 0.3 ml (1, 2/carton) (sulfites)
> EpiPen Jr *Auto-injector*: 0.15 mg (*epi* 1:2000, 0.3 ml) (1, 2/carton) (sulfites)
> Symjepi *Prefilled syringe*: 0.3 mg (0.3 ml) single-dose for manual injection
> Comment: Each Symjepi syringe is over-filled for stability purposes. More than half the
> solution remains in the syringe after use (and the syringe cannot be re-used).
> Twinject *Auto-injector*: 0.15, 0.3 mg (epi 1:1000) (1, 2/carton) (sulfites)
▷ *epinephrine* plus *chlorpheniramine* (C) *epinephrine* 0.3 ml SC or IM *plus* 4 tabs *chlorpheni-*
ramine by mouth
Pediatric: infants to 2 years: 0.05-0.1 ml SC or IM; ≥2-6 years: 0.15 ml SC or IM *plus* 1 tab
chlor; ≥6-12 years: 0.2 ml SC or IM *plus* 2 tabs chlor; ≥12 years: same as adult
> Ana-Kit: *Prefilled injector*: 0.3 ml epi 1:1000 for self-injection *plus* 4 x chlor 2 mg
> chew tabs

ANEMIA OF CHRONIC KIDNEY DISEASE (CKD)/ ANEMIA OF CHRONIC RENAL FAILURE (CRF)

PHOSPHATE BINDER

▶ **ferric citrate** *Iron Deficiency Anemia in Chronic Kidney Disease Not on Dialysis:* starting dose is 1 tablet 3 x/day with meals; adjust dose as needed to achieve and maintain hemoglobin goal, up to max 12 tabs/day; *Hyperphosphatemia in Chronic Kidney Disease on Dialysis:* starting dose is 2 tabs orally 3 x/day with meals; adjust dose by 1 to 2 tabs as needed to maintain serum phosphorus at target levels, up to max 12 tabs/day; dose can be titrated at 1 week or longer intervals

Pediatric: <18 years: not recommended; ≥18 years: same as adult

> **Aurexia** *Tab:* 210 mg *ferric iron* (equivalent to 1 gm *ferric citrate*)

> **Comment:** **Auryxia** is a phosphate binder indicated for the control of serum phosphorus levels in patients ≥18 years-of-age with chronic kidney disease (CKD) on dialysis. Ferric iron binds dietary phosphate in the GI tract and precipitates as ferric phosphate. This compound is insoluble and is excreted in the stool. **Auryxia** is also an iron replacement product indicated for the treatment of iron deficiency anemia in patients >18 years-of-age with chronic kidney (CKD) not on dialysis. Ferric iron is reduced from the ferric to the ferrous form by ferric reductase in the GI tract. After transport through the enterocytes into the blood, oxidized ferric iron circulates bound to the plasma protein transferrin, for incorporation into hemoglobin. **Auryxia** is contraindicated in iron overload syndromes (e.g., hemochromatosis). Monitor ferritin and TSAT. When clinically significant drug interactions are expected, consider separation of the timing of administration. Consider monitoring clinical responses or blood levels of the concomitant medication. The most common adverse reactions (incidence ≥5%) are discolored feces, diarrhea, constipation, nausea, vomiting, cough, abdominal pain, and hyperkalemia. There are no available data on **Auryxia** use in pregnancy to inform a drug-associated risk of major birth defects and miscarriage; however, an overdose of iron may carry a risk for spontaneous abortion, gestational diabetes and fetal malformation. There are no human data regarding effects of **Auryxia** on the breastfed infant. Accidental overdose of iron-containing products is a leading cause of fatal poisoning in children under 6 years-of-age. Keep this product out of reach of children. In case of accidental overdose, contact poison control center immediately and transfer to emergency care.

ERYTHROPOIESIS STIMULATING AGENTS (ESAS)

▶ *darbepoetin alpha* (erythropoiesis stimulating protein) (C) administer IV or SC q 1-2 weeks; do not increase more frequently than once per month; *Not currently receiving epoetin alpha:* initially 0.75 mcg/kg once weekly; adjust based on Hgb levels (target not to exceed 12 gm/dL); reduce dose if Hgb increases more than 1 gm/dL in any 2-week period; suspend therapy if polycythemia occurs; *Converting from epoetin alpha and for dose titration:* see mfr pkg insert

Pediatric: <12 years: not recommended; ≥12 years: same as adult

> **Aranesp** *Vial:* 25, 40, 60, 100, 150, 200, 300, 500 mcg/ml (single-dose) for IV or SC administration (preservative-free, albumin [human] or polysorbate 80)

> **Aranesp Singleject, Aranesp Sureclick Singleject** *Prefilled syringe:* 25, 40, 60, 100, 150, 200, 300, 500 mcg (single-dose) for IV or SC administration (preservative-free, albumin [human] or polysorbate 80)

▶ *peginesatide* (C) use lowest effective dose; initiate when Hgb <10 gm/dL; do not increase dose more often than every 4 weeks; if Hgb rises rapidly (i.e., >1 gm/dL in 2 weeks or >2 gm/dL in 4 weeks), reduce dose by 25% or more; if Hgb approaches or exceeds 11 gm/dL, reduce or interrupt dose and then when Hgb decreases, resume dose at approximately 25% below previous dose; if Hgb does not increase by >1 gm/dL after 4 weeks, increase dose by 25%; if response inadequate after a 12-week escalation period, use lowest dose that will maintain Hgb sufficient to reduce need for RBC transfusion; discontinue if response does not improve; *Not currently on ESA:* initially 0.04 mg/kg as a single IV or SC dose once monthly; *Converting from epoetin alfa:* administer first dose 1 week after last *epoetin alfa; Converting from darbepoetin alfa:* administer first dose at next scheduled dose of *darbepoetin alfa*

Pediatric: <12 years: not established; ≥12 years: use lowest effective dose

> **Omontys** *Vial, single-use:* 2, 3, 4, 5, 6 mg (0.5 ml) (preservative-free); *Vial, multi-use:* 10, 20 mg (2 ml) (preservatives); *Prefilled syringe:* 2, 3, 4, 5, 6 mg (0.5 ml) (preservative-free)

ERYTHROPOIETIN HUMAN, RECOMBINANT

▶ *epoetin alpha* (C) individualize; initially 50-100 units/kg 3 x/week; IV (dialysis or nondialysis) or SC (nondialysis); usual max 200 units/kg 3 x/week (dialysis) or 150 units/kg 3 x/week (non-dialysis); target Hct 30-36%
  Pediatric: <1 month: not recommended; ≥1 month: individualize; *Dialysis:* initially 50 units/kg 3 x/week IV or SC; target Hct 30-36%
    Epogen *Vial:* 2,000, 3,000, 4,000, 10,000, 40,000 units/ml (1 ml) single-use for IV or SC administration (albumin [human]; preservative-free)
    Epogen Multidose *Vial:* 10,000 units/ml (2 ml); 20,000 units/ml, (1 ml) for IV or SC administration (albumin [human]; benzoyl alcohol)
    Procrit *Vial:* 2,000, 3,000, 4,000, 10,000, 40,000 units/ml (1 ml) single-use for IV or SC administration (albumin [human]) (preservative-free)
    Procrit Multidose *Vial:* 10,000 units/ml (2 ml); 20,000 units/ml, (1 ml) for IV or SC administration (albumin [human]; benzoyl alcohol)

▶ *epoetin alfa-epbx* evaluate iron status before and during treatment and maintain iron repletion; correct or exclude other causes of anemia before initiating treatment *Patients with CKD: Initial dose (infants ≥1 month and children):* 50 units/kg 3 times/week; *Initial dose (≥18 years-of-age):* 50 to 100 units/kg 3 x/week; individualize maintenance dose; intravenous route recommended for patients on hemodialysis; *Patients on Zidovudine due to HIV-infection:* 100 units/kg 3 x weekly; *Patients with Cancer on Chemotherapy:* 40,000 units once weekly or 150 units/kg 3 x weekly (adults); 600 Units/kg IV once weekly (pediatric patients >5 years); *Surgery Patients:* 300 units/kg once daily for 15 days or 600 units/kg once weekly
    Retacrit *Vial:* 2,000, 3,000, 4,000, 10,000, 40,000 units/ml (1 ml), single-dose, for SC or IV infusion
    Comment: **Retacrit** *(epoetin alfa-epbx)* is the first FDA-approved biosimilar to **Epogen/Procrit** *(epoetin alfa)* for the SC or IV infusion treatment of anemia caused by chronic kidney disease (CKD), chemotherapy, or *zidovudine* treatment for human immunodeficiency virus infection. **Retacrit** is also approved for use before and after surgery to reduce the potential need for blood transfusions due to blood loss during surgery. Common reported adverse side effects with **Retacrit** include high blood pressure, joint pain, muscle spasm, fever, and dizziness. Contraindications to **Retacrit** include uncontrolled hypertension, pure red cell aplasia (PRCA) that begins after treatment with **Retacrit** or other erythropoietin protein drugs, and serious allergic reactions to **Retacrit** or other *epoetin alfa* products. BBW: ESAs increase the risk of myocardial infarction, stroke, venous thromboembolism, thrombosis of vascular access, and tumor progression or recurrence, and death (see mfr pkg insert for the full BBW). Therefore, use the lowest **Retacrit** dose sufficient to reduce the need for red blood cell (RBC) transfusions and DVT prophylaxis is recommended. The limited available data on *epoetin alfa* use in pregnancy are insufficient to determine a drug-associated risk of adverse developmental outcomes. There is no information regarding the presence of *epoetin alfa* products in human milk or effects on the breastfed infant. Safety and effectiveness in pediatric patients <1 month-of age have not been established.

◯ ANEMIA: FOLIC ACID DEFICIENCY

▶ *folic acid* (A)(OTC) 0.4-1 mg once daily
  Comment: *folic acid (vitamin B9)* 400 mcg daily is recommended during pregnancy to prevent neural tube defects. Women who have had a baby with a neural tube defect should take 400 mcg every day, even when not planning to become pregnant, and if planning to become pregnant should take 4 mg daily during the month before becoming pregnant until at least the 12th week of pregnancy.

◯ ANEMIA: IRON DEFICIENCY

Comment: Hemochromatosis and hemosiderosis are contraindications to iron therapy. **Iron** supplements are best absorbed when taken between meals and with **vitamin C**-rich foods. Excessive *iron* may be extremely hazardous to infants and young children. All vitamin and mineral supplements should be kept out of the reach of children.

IRON PREPARATIONS

▶ *ferrous gluconate* (A)(G) 1 tab once daily
>   *Pediatric:* <12 years: not recommended; ≥12 years: same as adult
>   Fergon (OTC)
>>   *Tab:* iron 27 mg (240 mg as gluconate)

▶ *ferrous sulfate* (A)(G)
>   Feosol Tablets (OTC) 1 tab tid-qid pc and HS
>   *Pediatric:* <6 years: use elixir; ≥6-12 years: 1 tab tid pc
>>   *Tab:* iron 65 mg (200 mg as sulfate)
>   Feosol Capsules (OTC) 1-2 caps daily
>   *Pediatric:* not recommended
>>   *Cap:* iron 50 mg (169 mg as sulfate) sust-rel
>   Feosol Elixir (OTC) 5-10 ml tid between meals
>   *Pediatric:* <1 year: not recommended; >1-11 year: 2.5-5 ml tid between meals; ≥12 years: same as adult
>>   *Elix:* iron 44 mg (220 mg as sulfate) per 5 ml
>   Fer-In-Sol (OTC) 5 ml daily
>   *Pediatric:* <4 years, use drops; ≥4 years: 5 ml once daily
>>   *Syr:* iron 18 mg (90 mg as sulfate) per 5 ml (480 ml)
>   Fer-In-Sol Drops (OTC)
>   *Pediatric:* <4 years: 0.6 ml daily; ≥4 years: use syrup
>>   *Oral drops:* iron 15 mg (75 mg as sulfate) per 5 ml (50 ml)

ANEMIA: PERNICIOUS/MEGALOBLASTIC

Comment: Signs of **vitamin B12** deficiency include megaloblastic anemia, glossitis, paresthesias, ataxia, spastic motor weakness, and reduced mentation.

▶ *vitamin B12 (cyanocobalamin)* (A)(G) 500 mcg intranasally once a week; may increase dose if serum B-12 levels decline; adjust dose in 500 mcg increments
>   Nascobal Nasal Spray *Intranasal gel:* 500 mcg/0.1 ml (1.3 ml, 4 doses) (citric acid, benzalkonium chloride)
>   Comment: **Nascobal Nasal Spray** is indicated for maintenance of hematologic remission following IM B-12 therapy without nervous system involvement. Must be primed before each use.

ANGINA PECTORIS: STABLE

▶ *aspirin* (D) 325 mg (range 75-325 mg) once daily
>   Comment: Daily *aspirin* dose is contingent upon whether the patient is also taking an anticoagulant <u>or</u> antiplatelet agent.

CALCIUM ANTAGONISTS

Comment: Calcium antagonists are contraindicated with history of ventricular arrhythmias, sick sinus syndrome, 2nd <u>or</u> 3rd degree heart block, cardiogenic shock, acute myocardial infarction, and pulmonary congestion.

▶ *amlodipine* (C)(G) 5-10 mg daily
>   *Pediatric:* <12 years: not recommended; ≥12 years: same as adult
>   Norvasc *Tab:* 2.5, 5, 10 mg

▶ *diltiazem* (C)(G)
>   *Pediatric:* <12 years: not recommended; ≥12 years: same as adult
>   Cardizem initially 30 mg qid; may increase gradually every 1-2 days; max 360 mg/day in divided doses
>>   *Tab:* 30, 60, 90, 120 mg
>   Cardizem CD initially 120-180 mg daily; adjust at 1- to 2-week intervals; max 480 mg/day
>>   *Cap:* 120, 180, 240, 300, 360 mg ext-rel
>   Cardizem LA initially 180-240 mg daily; titrate at 2 week intervals; max 540 mg/day
>>   *Tab:* 120, 180, 240, 300, 360, 420 mg ext-rel
>   Cartia XT initially 180 mg <u>or</u> 240 mg once daily; max 540 mg once daily
>>   *Cap:* 120, 180, 240, 300 mg ext-rel

>> **Dilacor XR** initially 180 mg <u>or</u> 240 mg once daily; max 540 mg once daily
>> *Cap:* 180, 240 mg ext-rel
>> **Tiazac** initially 120-180 mg daily; max 540 mg/day
>> *Cap:* 120, 180, 240, 300, 360, 420 mg ext-rel
▷ *nicardipine* (C)(G) initially 20 mg tid; adjust q 3 days; max 120 mg/day
  Pediatric: not recommended
  Cardene *Cap:* 20, 30 mg
▷ *nifedipine* (C)(G)
  Pediatric: <12 years: not recommended; ≥12 years: same as adult
  Adalat CC initially 30 mg once daily; usual range 30-60 mg tid; max 90 mg/day
      Tab: 30, 60, 90 mg ext-rel
  Procardia initially 10 mg tid; titrate over 7-14 days: max 30 mg/dose and 180 mg/day in divided doses
      Cap: 10, 20 mg
  Procardia XL initially 30-60 mg daily; titrate over 7-14 days; max dose 90 mg/day
      Tab: 30, 60, 90 mg ext-rel
▷ *verapamil* (C)(G)
  Pediatric: <12 years: not recommended; ≥12 years: same as adult
  Calan 80-120 mg tid; increase daily <u>or</u> weekly if needed
      Tab: 40, 80*, 120*mg
  Calan SR initially 120 mg once daily; increase weekly if needed
      Tab: 120, 180, 240 mg
  Covera HS initially 180 mg q HS; titrate in steps to 240 mg; then to 360 mg; then to 480 mg if needed
      Tab: 180, 240 mg ext-rel
  Isoptin SR initially 120-180 mg in the AM; may increase to 240 mg in the AM; then 180 mg q 12 hours <u>or</u> 240 mg in the AM and 120 mg in the PM; then 240 mg q 12 hours
      Tab: 120, 180*, 240*mg sust-rel

BETA-BLOCKERS

Comment: Beta-blockers are contraindicated with history of sick sinus syndrome (SSS), 2nd <u>or</u> 3rd degree heart block, cardiogenic shock, pulmonary congestion, asthma, moderate to severe COPD with FEV1 <50% predicted, patients with chronic bronchodilator treatment.
▷ *atenolol* (D)(G) initially 25-50 mg daily; increase weekly if needed; max 200 mg daily
  Pediatric: <12 years: not recommended; ≥12 years: same as adult
  Tenormin *Tab:* 25, 50, 100 mg
▷ *metoprolol succinate* (C)
  Pediatric: <12 years: not recommended; ≥12 years: same as adult
      Toprol-XL initially 100 mg in a single dose once daily; increase weekly if needed; max 400 mg/day
      Tab: 25*, 50*, 100*, 200*mg ext-rel
▷ *metoprolol tartrate* (C)
  Pediatric: <12 years: not recommended; ≥12 years: same as adult
      Lopressor (G) initially 25-50 mg bid; increase weekly if needed; max 400 mg/day
      Tab: 25, 37.5, 50, 75, 100 mg
▷ *nadolol* (C)(G) initially 40 mg daily; increase q 3-7 days; max 240 mg/day
  Pediatric: not recommended
      Corgard *Tab:* 20*, 40*, 80*, 120*, 160*mg
▷ *propranolol* (C)(G)
  Pediatric: <12 years: not recommended; ≥12 years: same as adult
      Inderal LA initially 80 mg daily in a single dose; increase q 3-7 days; usual range 120-160 mg/day; max 320 mg/day in a single dose
      Cap: 60, 80, 120, 160 mg sust-rel
      InnoPran XL initially 80 mg q HS; max 120 mg/day
      Cap: 80, 120 mg ext-rel

NITRATES

Comment: Use a daily nitrate dosing schedule that provides a dose-free period of 14 hours <u>or</u> more to prevent tolerance. *aspirin* and *acetaminophen* may relieve nitrate-induced headache. *Isosorbide* is <u>not</u> recommended for use in MI <u>and/or</u> CHF. Nitrate use is a contraindication for using phosphodiesterase type 5 inhibitors: *sildenafil* (**Viagra**), *tadalafil* (**Cialis**), *vardenafil* (**Levitra**).

▷ *isosorbide dinitrate* (C)
  Pediatric: <12 years: not recommended; ≥12 years: same as adult
    Dilatrate-SR 40 mg once daily; max 160 mg/day
      Cap: 40 mg sust-rel
    Isordil Titradose initially 5-20 mg q 6 hours; maintenance 10-40 mg q 6 hours
      Tab: 5, 10, 20, 30, 40 mg
▷ *isosorbide mononitrate* (C)
  Pediatric: <12 years: not recommended; ≥12 years: same as adult
    Imdur initially 30-60 mg q AM; may increase to 120 mg daily; max 240 mg/day
      Tab: 30*, 60*, 120 mg ext-rel
    Ismo 20 mg upon awakening; then 20 mg 7 hours later
      Tab: 20*mg
▷ *nitroglycerin* (C)(G)
  Pediatric: <12 years: not recommended; ≥12 years: same as adult
    Nitro-Bid Ointment initially 1/2 inch q 8 hours; titrate in 1/2 inch increments
      Oint: 2% (20, 60 gm)
    Nitrodisc initially one 0.2-0.4 mg/Hr patch for 12-14 hours/day
      Transdermal disc: 0.2, 0.3, 0.4 mg/hour (30, 100/carton)
    Nitrolingual Pump Spray 1-2 sprays on o̲r under tongue; max 3 sprays/15 minutes
      Spray: 0.4 mg/dose (14.5 gm, 200 doses)
    Nitromist 1-2 sprays at onset of attack, on o̲r under the tongue while sitting; may repeat q 5 minutes as needed; max 3 sprays/15 minutes; may use prophylactically 5-10 minutes prior to exertion; do not inhale spray; do not rinse mouth for 5-10 minutes after use
      Lingual aerosol spray: 0.4 mg/actuation (230 metered sprays)
    Nitrostat 1 tab SL; may repeat q 5 minutes x 3
      SL tab: 0.3 (1/100 gr), 0.4 (1/150 gr), 0.6 (1/4 gr) mg
    Transderm-Nitro initially one 0.2 mg/hour o̲r 0.4 mg/hour patch for 12-14 hours/day
      Transdermal patch: 0.1, 0.2, 0.4, 0.6, 0.8 mg/hour

NON-NITRATE PERIPHERAL VASODILATOR

▷ *hydralazine* (C)(G) initially 10 mg qid x 2-4 days; then increase to 25 mg qid for remainder of first week; then increase to 50 mg qid; max 300 mg/day
  Pediatric: <12 years: not recommended; ≥12 years: same as adult
    Tab: 10, 25, 50, 100 mg

NITRATE+PERIPHERAL VASODILATOR COMBINATION

▷ *isosorbide+hydralazine HCl* (C) initially 1 tab tid; max 2 tabs tid
  Pediatric: <12 years: not established; ≥12 years: same as adult
    Bidil *Tab:* isosorb 20 mg+hydral 37.5 mg

NON-NITRATE ANTI-ANGINAL

▷ *ranolazine* (C) initially 500 mg bid; may increase to max 1 gm bid
  Pediatric: <12 years: not recommended; ≥12 years: same as adult
    Ranexa *Tab:* 500, 1000 mg ext-rel
    Comment: **Ranexa** is indicated for the treatment chronic angina that is inadequately controlled with other antianginals. Use with amlodipine, beta-blocker, o̲r nitrate.

 ANOREXIA/CACHEXIA

APPETITE STIMULANTS

▷ *cyproheptadine* (B)(G) initially 4 mg tid prn; then adjust as needed; usual range 12-16 mg/day; max 32 mg/day
  Pediatric: <2 years: not recommended; ≥2-6 years: 2 mg bid-tid prn; max 12 mg/day; 7-14 years: 4 mg bid-tid prn; max 16 mg/day; >14 years: same as adult
    Periactin *Tab:* cypro 4*mg; *Syr:* cypro 2 mg/5 ml

▷ *dronabinol* (cannabinoid) (B)(III)
  Pediatric: not established; younger patients may be more sensitive to neurological and psychoactive effects of *dronabinol;* Syndros contains dehydrated alcohol and 5.5% (w/w) propylene glycol; ethanol competitively inhibits the metabolism of propylene glycol, which may lead to elevated concentrations of propylene glycol; preterm neonates may be at increased risk of propylene glycol associated adverse events due to diminished ability to metabolize it, thereby, leading to accumulation; avoid use with preterm infants in the immediate postnatal period

  Marinol initially 2.5 mg bid before lunch and dinner; may reduce to 2.5 mg q HS or increase to 2.5 mg before lunch and 5 mg before dinner; max 20 mg/day in divided doses

   Cap: 2.5, 5, 10 mg (sesame oil)
  Syndros take each dose with 6-8 oz water
  Anorexia/cachexia associated with weight loss in patients with AIDS: inially 2.1 mg twice daily 1 hour before lunch and dinner; if elderly, or severe or persistent CNS effects occur, reduce dose to 2.1 mg once daily 1 hour before dinner or at bedtime; if tolerated, may gradually increase to 2.1 mg 1 hour before lunch and dinner or at bedtime as tolerated; max 8.4 mg twice daily
  Nausea/vomiting associated with chemotherapy: recommended starting dosage is 4.2 mg/m^2, administered 1 to 3 hours prior to chemotherapy; then, every 2 to 4 hours after chemotherapy for a total 4-6 doses/day; administer the first dose on an empty stomach at least 30 minutes prior to eating; subsequent doses can be taken without regard to meals
  Oral soln: 5 mg/ml (50% w/w dehydrated alcohol, 5.5% w/w propylene glycol)
  Comment: *dronabinol* is contraindicated within 14 days before and 7 days after taking *disulfiram* or *metronidazole. dronabinol* is highly protein-bound. Therefore, there is potential for displacement of other drugs from plasma proteins. Monitor for adverse reactions to concomitant narrow therapeutic index drugs (e.g., *warfarin*, *cyclosporine*, *amphotericin B*) when initiating or increasing the dosage of *dronabinol*. Delta-9-THC has been measured in the cord blood of some infants whose mothers reported prenatal use of cannabis, suggesting *dronabinol* may cross the placenta to the fetus during pregnancy. Effects of delta-9-THC on the fetus are not known. There are limited data on the presence of *dronabinol* in human milk and effects on the breastfed infant. The reported effects of inhaled cannabis transferred to the breastfeeding infant have been inconsistent and insufficient to establish causality. Because of the possible adverse effects from *dronabanol* on the breastfed infant, advise females with nausea/vomiting associated with cancer chemotherapy not to breastfeed during treatment with *dronabinol* and for 9 days after the last chemotherapy dose.

▷ *megestrol* (progestin) (X)(G) 40 mg qid
  Pediatric: <12 years: not recommended; ≥12 years: same as adult
    Megace *Tab:* 20*, 40*mg
    Megace ES *Oral susp (concentrate):* 125 mg/ml; 625 mg/5 ml (5 oz) (lemon-lime)
    Megace Oral Suspension *Oral susp:* 40 mg/ml (8 oz); 820 mg/20 ml) (lemon-lime)
    Megestrol Acetate Oral Suspension (G) 125 mg/ml
  Comment: *megestrol* is indicated for the treatment of anorexia, cachexia, or an unexplained, significant weight loss in patients with a diagnosis of AIDS.

ANTHRAX (*BACILLUS ANTHRACIS*)

POST-EXPOSURE PROPHYLAXIS OF INHALATIONAL ANTHRAX AND TREATMENT OF INHALED AND CUTANEOUS ANTHRAX INFECTION

Comment: *B anthracis* spores are resistant to destruction, are easily spread by release into the air, and cause irreversible tissue damage and death. The most lethal form is inhalational anthrax. Even with the most aggressive treatment, the mortality rate is about 45%. People at risk are those who work in slaughterhouses, tanneries, and wood mills who are exposed to infected animals.

Comment: All fourteen members of the Advisory Committee on Immunization Practices (ACIP) voted to approve the anthrax vaccine recommendations for 2018-2019 at their meeting. The recommendations to the committee sought to optimize the use of Anthrax Vaccine Adsorbed (AVA) in post-exposure prophylaxis (PEP) in the event of a wide-area release of *B anthracis* spores. In this event, a mass vaccination effort would be undertaken, requiring expedited administration of AVA. ACIP now recommends that the intramuscular administration may be used over the traditional subcutaneous approach if there are any operational or logistical challenges that delay effective vaccination. Another recommendation from ACIP would allow two full-doses or three half-doses of AVA to be used to expand vaccine coverage for PEP in the event there is an inadequate vaccine supply. The committee also recommended that AbxPEP, an antimicrobial, be stopped 42 days after the first dose of AVA or 2 weeks after the last dose. The committee's recommendations will be used by the CDC to inform state and local health departments to better prepare for an emergency response to a wide-area release of *B anthracis* spores. The committee's recommendations must be approved by the CDC's director before they are considered official recommendations.

REFERENCE

Lacy, I. (published online June 28, 2018). Anthrax vaccine recommendations updated in the event of a wide-area release. *Family Practice News*. https://www.mdedge.com/familypracticenews/article/169178/vaccines/anthrax-vaccine-recommendations-updated-event-wide-area

Immune Globulin

▷ **bacillus anthracis immune globulin intravenous (human)** administer via IV infusion at a maximum rate of 2 ml/min; dose is weight-based as follows, but may be doubled in severe cases if weight >5 kg:

Pediatric: <16 years: not established; 5-<10 kg: 1 vial; 10-<18 kg: 2 vials; 18-<25 kg: 3 vials; 25-<35 kg: 4 vials; 35-<50 kg: 5 vials; 50-<60 kg: 6 vials; ≥60 kg: 7 vials

> **Anthrasil** *Vial:* (60 units) sterile solution of purified human immune globulin gm (IgG) containing polyclonal antibodies that target the anthrax toxins of *Bacillus anthracis* for IV infusion

> **Comment: Anthrasil** is indicated for the emergent treatment of inhaled anthrax in combination with appropriate antibacterial agents

MONOCLONAL ANTIBODIES

Comment: *obiltoxaximab* and *raxibacumab* have no antibacterial activity; rather, they are monoclonal antibodies that neutralize toxins produced by *B. anthracis* by binding to the bacterium's protective antigen, preventing intracellular entry of key enzymatic toxin components. *obiltoxaximab* (**Anthim**) and *raxibacumab* are indicated for treatment of inhalational anthrax in combination with appropriate antibacterial drugs and for prophylaxis of inhalational anthrax when alternative therapies are unavailable or inappropriate. Vials must be refrigerated and protected from light. Do not shake the vials. Pre-medicate the patient with *diphenhydramine*.

▷ **obiltoxaximab** 16 mg/kg diluted in 0.9%NS via IV infusion over 90 minutes

Pediatric: see mfr pkg insert for dosing based on kilograms body weight

> **Anthim** *Vial:* 600 mg in 6 ml (100 mg/ml) single-use, for dilution in 0.9% NS and IV infusion

▷ **raxibacumab** (B)(G) 40 mg/kg diluted in 0.45%NS or 0.9% NS via IV infusion over 2 hours and 15 minutes; see mfr pkg insert for recommended volume of dilution according to weight-based dose

Pediatric: ≤15 kg: 80 mg/kg; >15-50 kg: 60 mg/kg; >50 kg: same as adult

> *Vial:* 1700 mg/34 ml (50 mg/ml), single-use, for dilution and IV infusion

ANTIBACTERIAL AGENTS

▷ **ciprofloxacin** (C) 500 mg (or 10-15 mg/kg/day) q 12 hours for 60 days (start as soon as possible after exposure)

Pediatric: <18 years: 20-40 mg/kg/day divided q 12 hours; ≥18 years: same as adult

> **Cipro** (G) *Tab:* 250, 500, 750 mg; *Oral susp:* 250, 500 mg/5 ml (100 ml) (strawberry)

> **Cipro XR** *Tab:* 500, 1000 mg ext-rel

> **ProQuin XR** *Tab:* 500 mg ext-rel

Comment: *ciprofloxacin* is usually contraindicated <18 years-of-age, and during pregnancy and lactation. Risk of tendonitis or tendon rupture. Risk/benefit must be assessed in the case of anthrax.

▷ **doxycycline** (D)(G) 100 mg daily bid

Pediatric: <8 years: usually contraindicated ≥8 years, <100 lb: 2 mg/lb on first day in 2 divided doses, followed by 1 mg/lb/day in a single or divided doses; ≥8 years, ≥100 lb: same as adult; *see page 625 for dose by weight*

> **Acticlate** *Tab:* 75, 150**mg
> **Adoxa** *Tab:* 50, 75, 100, 150 mg ent-coat
> **Doryx** *Tab:* 50, 75, 100, 150, 200 mg del-rel
> **Doxteric** *Tab:* 50 mg del-rel
> **Monodox** *Cap:* 50, 75, 100 mg
> **Oracea** *Cap:* 40 mg del-rel
> **Vibramycin** *Tab:* 100 mg; *Cap:* 50, 100 mg; *Syr:* 50 mg/5 ml (raspberry-apple) (sulfites); *Oral susp:* 25 mg/5 ml (raspberry)
> **Vibra-Tab** *Tab:* 100 mg film-coat

Comment: *doxycycline,* a tetracycline, is usually contraindicated <8 years-of-age, in pregnancy, and lactation (discolors developing tooth enamel). Risk/benefit must be assessed in the case of anthrax. A side effect may be photosensitivity (photophobia). Do not take with antacids, calcium supplements, milk or other dairy, or within 2 hours of taking another drug.

▷ *minocycline* (D)(G) 2 mg/lb on first day in 2 divided doses, followed by 1 mg/lb q 12 hours x 9 more days; ≥8 years, >100 mg: 100 mg q 12 hours
Pediatric: <8 years: usually not recommended; ≥8 years, <100 lb:

> **Dynacin** *Cap:* 50, 100 mg
> **Minocin** *Cap:* 50, 75, 100 mg; *Oral susp:* 50 mg/5 ml (60 ml) (custard) (sulfites, alcohol 5%)

Comment: *minocycline,* a tetracycline, is usually contraindicated <8 years-of-age, in pregnancy, and lactation (discolors developing tooth enamel). Risk/benefit must be assessed in the case of anthrax. A side effect may be photosensitivity (photophobia). Avoid co-administration with retinoids and penicillin. Decrease anticoagulant dosage as appropriate. Monitor for toxicities of drugs that may require dosage reduction (e.g., P-glycoprotein substrates) and monitor for toxicities. Do not take with antacids, calcium supplements, milk or other dairy, or within two hours of taking another drug.

TREATMENT OF GI & OROPHARYNGEAL ANTHRAX

▷ *ciprofloxacin* (C) 400 mg IV q 12 hours (start as soon as possible); then, switch to 500 mg PO q 12 hours for total 60 days; infuse dose over 60 minutes
Pediatric: <18 years: usually not recommended; 10-15 mg/kg IV q 12 hours (start as soon as possible); then switch to 10-15 mg/kg PO q 12 hours for 60 days

> **Cipro** (G) *Tab:* 250, 500, 750 mg; *Oral susp:* 250, 500 mg/5 ml (100 ml) (strawberry); *IV conc:* 10 mg/ml after dilution (20, 40 ml); *IV premix:* 2 mg/ml (100, 200 ml)
> **Cipro XR** *Tab:* 500, 1000 mg ext-rel
> **ProQuin XR** *Tab:* 500 mg ext-rel

Comment: *ciprofloxacin* is usually contraindicated <18 years-of-age, and during pregnancy and lactation. Risk of tendonitis or tendon rupture. Risk/ benefit must be assessed in the case of anthrax. Infuse IV *ciprofloxacin* over 60 minutes.

▷ *doxycycline* (D)(G) 100 mg daily bid
Pediatric: <8 years: not recommended ≥8 years, <100 lb: 2 mg/lb on first day in 2 divided doses, followed by 1 mg/lb/day in a single or divided doses; ≥8 years, ≥100 lb: same as adult; *see page 625 for dose by weight*

> **Acticlate** *Tab:* 75, 150**mg
> **Adoxa** *Tab:* 50, 75, 100, 150 mg ent-coat
> **Doryx** *Tab:* 50, 75, 100, 150, 200 mg del-rel
> **Doxteric** *Tab:* 50 mg del-rel
> **Monodox** *Cap:* 50, 75, 100 mg
> **Oracea** *Cap:* 40 mg del-rel
> **Vibramycin** *Tab:* 100 mg; *Cap:* 50, 100 mg; *Syr:* 50 mg/5 ml (raspberry-apple) (sulfites); *Oral susp:* 25 mg/5 ml (raspberry)
> **Vibra-Tab** *Tab:* 100 mg film-coat

Comment: *doxycycline* is usually contraindicated <8 years-of-age, in pregnancy, and lactation (discolors developing tooth enamel). Risk/benefit must be assessed in the case of anthrax. A side effect may be photosensitivity (photophobia). Do not take with antacids, calcium supplements, milk or other dairy, or within 2 hours of taking another drug.

▷ *minocycline* (D)(G) 100 mg q 12 hours
Pediatric: <8 years: usually not recommended; ≥8 years, <100 lb: 2 mg/lb on first day in 2 divided doses, followed by 1 mg/lb q 12 hours x 9 more days; ≥8 years, ≥100 lb: same as adult

Dynacin *Cap:* 50, 100 mg
Minocin *Cap:* 50, 75, 100 mg; *Oral susp:* 50 mg/5 ml (60 ml) (custard) (sulfites, alcohol 5%)

Comment: *minocycline* is usually contraindicated <8 years-of-age, in pregnancy, and lactation (discolors developing tooth enamel). Risk/ benefit must be assessed in the case of anthrax. A side effect may be photosensitivity (photophobia). Do not take with antacids, calcium supplements, milk or other dairy, or within two hours of taking another drug.

 ANXIETY DISORDER: GENERALIZED (GAD), ANXIETY DISORDER: SOCIAL (SAD)

FIRST GENERATION ORAL ANTIHISTAMINES

▷ *diphenhydramine* (B)(G) 25-50 mg q 6-8 hours; max 100 mg/day
   Pediatric: <2 years: not recommended; 2-6 years: 6.25 mg q 4-6 hours; max 37.5 mg/day; >6-12 years: 12.5-25 mg q 4-6 hours; max 150 mg/day; ≥12 years: same as adult
      Benadryl (OTC) *Chew tab:* 12.5 mg (grape) (phenylalanine); *Liq:* 12.5 mg/5 ml (4, 8 oz); *Cap:* 25 mg; *Tab:* 25 mg; *Dye-free soft gel:* 25 mg; *Dye-free liq:* 12.5 mg/5 ml (4, 8 oz)

▷ *hydroxyzine* (C)(G) 50-100 mg qid; max 600 mg/day
   Pediatric: <6 years: 50 mg/day divided qid; ≥6 years: 50-100 mg/day divided qid
      Atarax *Tab:* 10, 25, 50, 100 mg; *Syr:* 10 mg/5 ml (alcohol 0.5%)
      Vistaril *Cap:* 25, 50, 100 mg; *Oral susp:* 25 mg/5 ml (4 oz) (lemon)

Comment: *hydroxyzine* is contraindicated in early pregnancy and in patients with a prolonged QT interval. It is not known whether this drug is excreted in human milk; therefore, *hydroxyzine* should not be given to nursing mothers.

AZAPIRONE

▷ *buspirone* (B) initially 7.5 mg bid; may increase by 5 mg/day q 2-3 days; max 60 mg/day
   Pediatric: <6 years: not recommended; ≥6 years: same as adult
      BuSpar *Tab:* 5, 10, 15*, 30*mg

BENZODIAZEPINES

Comment: If possible when considering a benzodiazepine to treat anxiety, a short-acting benzodiazepines should be used only prn to avert intense anxiety and panic for the least time necessary while a different non-addictive antianxiety regimen (e.g., SSRI, SNRI, TCA, *buspirone*, beta-blocker) is established and effective treatment goals achieved. Benzodiazepines have a high addiction potential when they are chronically used and are common drugs of abuse. *Benzodiazepine withdrawal syndrome* may include restlessness, agitation, anxiety, insomnia, tachycardia, tachypnea, diaphoresis, and may be potentially life threatening depending on the benzodiazepine and the length of use. Symptoms of withdrawal from short-acting benzodiazepines, such as *alprazolam* (Xanax), *oxazepam*, *lorazepam* (Ativan), *triazolam* (Halcion), usually appear within 6-8 hours after the last dose and may continue 10-14 days. Symptoms of withdrawal from long-acting benzodiazepines, such as *diazepam* (Valium), *clonazepam* (Klonopin), *chlordiazepoxide* (Librium), usually appear within 24-96 hours after the last dose and may continue from 3-4 weeks to 3 months. People who are heavily dependent on benzodiazepines may experience *protracted withdrawal syndrome* (PAWS), random periods of sharp withdrawal symptoms months after quitting. A closely monitored medical detoxification regimen may be required for a safe withdrawal and to prevent PAWS. Detoxification includes gradual tapering of the benzodiazepine along with other medications to manage the withdrawal symptoms.

Short-Acting Benzodiazepines

▷ *alprazolam* (D)(IV)(G)
   Pediatric: <18 years: not recommended; ≥18 years:
      Niravam initially 0.25-0.5 mg tid; may titrate every 3-4 days; max 4 mg/day
         Tab: 0.25*, 0.5*, 1*, 2*mg orally-disint
      Xanax initially 0.25-0.5 mg tid; may titrate every 3-4 days; max 4 mg/day
         Tab: 0.25*, 0.5*, 1*, 2*mg

Xanax XR initially 0.5-1 mg once daily, preferably in the AM; increase at intervals of at least 3-4 days by up to 1 mg/day. Taper no faster than 0.5 mg every 3 days; max 10 mg/day. When switching from immediate-release *alprazolam*, give total daily dose of immediate-release once daily.
> *Tab:* 0.5, 1, 2, 3 mg ext-rel

▷ *oxazepam* (C)(IV)(G) 10-15 mg tid-qid for moderate symptoms; 15-30 mg tid-qid for severe symptoms
> *Pediatric:* <12 years: not recommended; ≥12 years: same as adult
> *Cap:* 10, 15, 30 mg

Intermediate-Acting Benzodiazepines

▷ *lorazepam* (D)(IV)(G) 1-10 mg/day in 2-3 divided doses
> *Pediatric:* <12 years: not recommended; ≥12 years: same as adult
>> Ativan *Tab:* 0.5, 1*, 2*mg
>> Lorazepam Intensol *Oral conc:* 2 mg/ml (30 ml w. graduated dropper)

Long-Acting Benzodiazepines

▷ *chlordiazepoxide* (D)(IV)(G)
> *Pediatric:* <6 years: not recommended; ≥6 years: 5 mg bid-qid; increase to 10 mg bid-tid
>> Librium 5-10 mg tid-qid for moderate symptoms; 20-25 mg tid-qid for severe symptoms
>>> *Cap:* 5, 10, 25 mg
>> Librium Injectable 50-100 mg IM or IV; then 25-50 mg IM tid-qid prn; max 300 mg/day
>>> *Inj:* 100 mg

▷ *chlordiazepoxide+clidinium* (D)(IV) 1-2 caps tid-qid: max 8 caps/day
> *Pediatric:* not recommended
>> Librax *Cap:* chlor 5 mg+clid 2.5 mg

▷ *clonazepam* (D)(IV)(G) initially 0.25 mg bid; increase to 1 mg/day after 3 days
> *Pediatric:* <18 years: not recommended; ≥18 years: same as adult
>> Klonopin *Tab:* 0.5*, 1, 2 mg
>> Klonopin Wafers dissolve in mouth with or without water
>>> *Wafer:* 0.125, 0.25, 0.5, 1, 2 mg orally-disint

▷ *clorazepate* (D)(IV)(G) 30 mg/day in divided doses; max 60 mg/day
> *Pediatric:* <9 years: not recommended; ≥9 years: same as adult
>> Tranxene *Tab:* 3.75, 7.5, 15 mg
>> Tranxene SD do not use for initial therapy
>>> *Tab:* 22.5 mg ext-rel
>> Tranxene SD Half Strength do not use for initial therapy
>>> *Tab:* 11.25 mg ext-rel
>> Tranxene T-Tab *Tab:* 3.75*, 7.5*, 15*mg

▷ *diazepam* (D)(IV)(G) 2-10 mg bid to qid
> *Pediatric:* <12 years: not recommended; ≥12 years: same as adult
>> Diastat *Rectal gel delivery system:* 2.5 mg
>> Diastat AcuDial *Rectal gel delivery system:* 10, 20 mg
>> Valium *Tab:* 2*, 5*, 10*mg
>> Valium Injectable *Vial:* 5 mg/ml (10 ml); *Amp:* 5 mg/ml (2 ml); *Prefilled syringe:* 5 mg/ml (5 ml)
>> Valium Intensol Oral Solution *Conc oral soln:* 5 mg/ml (30 ml w. dropper) (alcohol 19%)
>> Valium Oral Solution *Oral soln:* 5 mg/5 ml (500 ml) (wintergreen spice)

TRICYCLIC ANTIDEPRESSANTS (TCAs)

Comment: Co-administration of TCAs with SSRIs requires extreme caution.

▷ *amitriptyline* (C)(G) 10-20 mg q HS
> *Pediatric:* <12 years: not recommended; ≥12 years: same as adult
>> *Tab:* 10, 25, 50, 75, 100, 150 mg

▷ *amoxapine* (C) initially 50 mg bid-tid; after 1 week may increase to 100 mg bid-tid; usual effective dose 200-300 mg/day; if total dose exceeds 300 mg/day, give in divided doses (max 400 mg/day); may give as a single bedtime dose (max 300 mg q HS)
> *Pediatric:* <12 years: not recommended; ≥12 years: same as adult
>> *Tab:* 25, 50, 100, 150 mg

▷ *clomipramine* (C)(G) initially 25 mg daily in divided doses; gradually increase to 100 mg during first 2 weeks; max 250 mg/day; total maintenance dose may be given at HS
Pediatric: <10 years: not recommended; 10-<16 years: initially 25 mg daily in divided doses; gradually increase; max 3 mg/kg or 100 mg, whichever is smaller; ≥16 years: same as adult
    Anafranil *Cap:* 25, 50, 75 mg

▷ *desipramine* (C)(G) 100-200 mg/day in single or divided doses; max 300 mg/day
Pediatric: <12 years: not recommended; ≥12 years: same as adult
    Norpramin *Tab:* 10, 25, 50, 75, 100, 150 mg

▷ *doxepin* (C)(G) usual optimum dose 75-150 mg/day; elderly lower initial dose and therapeutic dose; max single dose 150 mg; max 300 mg/day in divided doses
Pediatric: <12 years: not recommended; ≥12 years: same as adult
    Sinequan
    Cap: 10, 25, 50, 75, 100, 150 mg; *Oral conc:* 10 mg/ml (4 oz w. dropper)
Comment: Glaucoma, urinary retention, and bipolar disorder are contraindications to *doxepin*. Separate from MAOIs by at least 14 days. Separate from *fluoxetine* by at least 5 weeks. Avoid abrupt cessation. *doxepin* is potentiated by CYP2D6 inhibitors (e.g., *cimetidine*, SSRIs, phenothiazines, type 1C antiarrhythmics).

▷ *imipramine* (C)(G)
Pediatric: <12 years: not recommended; ≥12 years: same as adult
Tofranil initially 75 mg daily (max 200 mg); adolescents initially 30-40 mg daily (max 100 mg/day); if maintenance dose exceeds 75 mg daily, may switch to **Tofranil PM** for divided or bedtime dose
    Tab: 10, 25, 50 mg
Tofranil PM initially 75 mg daily 1 hour before HS; max 200 mg
    Cap: 75, 100, 125, 150 mg

▷ *nortriptyline* (D)(G) initially 25 mg tid-qid; max 150 mg/day
Pediatric: <12 years: not recommended; ≥12 years: same as adult
    Pamelor *Cap:* 10, 25, 50, 75 mg; *Oral soln:* 10 mg/5 ml (16 oz)

▷ *protriptyline* (C) initially 5 mg tid; usual dose 15-40 mg/day in 3-4 divided doses; max 60 mg/day
Pediatric: <12 years: not recommended; ≥12 years: same as adult
    Vivactil *Tab:* 5, 10 mg

▷ *trimipramine* (C) initially 75 mg/day in divided doses; max 200 mg/day
Pediatric: <12 years: not recommended; ≥12 years: same as adult
    Surmontil *Cap:* 25, 50, 100 mg

PHENOTHIAZINES

▷ *prochlorperazine* (C)(G)
Pediatric: <12 years: not recommended; ≥12 years: same as adult
    Compazine 5 mg tid-qid
        Tab: 5 mg; *Syr:* 5 mg/5 ml (4 oz) (fruit); *Rectal supp:* 2.5, 5, 25 mg
    Compazine Spansule 15 mg q AM or 10 mg q 12 hours
        Spansule: 10, 15 mg sust-rel

▷ *trifluoperazine* (C)(G) 1-2 mg bid; max 6 mg/day; max 12 weeks
Pediatric: <12 years: not recommended; ≥12 years: same as adult
    Stelazine *Tab:* 1, 2, 5, 10 mg

SELECTIVE SEROTONIN REUPTAKE INHIBITORS (SSRIs)

Comment: Co-administration of SSRIs with TCAs requires extreme caution. Concomitant use of MAOIs and SSRIs is absolutely contraindicated. Avoid St. John's wort and other serotonergic agents. A potentially fatal adverse event is *serotonin syndrome*, caused by serotonin excess. Milder symptoms require HCP intervention to avert severe symptoms that can be rapidly fatal without urgent/emergent medical care. Symptoms include restlessness, agitation, confusion, tachycardia, hypertension, dilated pupils, muscle twitching, muscle rigidity, loss of muscle coordination, diaphoresis, diarrhea, headache, shivering, piloerection, hyperpyrexia, cardiac arrhythmias, seizures, loss of consciousness, coma, death. Common symptoms of the *serotonin discontinuation syndrome* include flu-like symptoms (nausea, vomiting, diarrhea, headaches, diaphoresis); sleep disturbances (insomnia, nightmares, constant sleepiness); mood disturbances (dysphoria, anxiety, agitation); cognitive disturbances (mental confusion, hyperarousal); and sensory and movement disturbances (imbalance, tremors, vertigo, dizziness, electric-shock-like sensations in the brain often described by sufferers as "brain zaps").

▷ *citalopram* (C)(G) initially 20 mg once daily; may increase after one week to 40 mg once daily; max 40 mg
  Pediatric: 12 years: not recommended; ≥12 years: same as adult
      Celexa *Tab:* 10, 20, 40 mg; *Oral soln:* 10 mg/5 ml (120 ml) (peppermint) (sugar-free, alcohol-free, parabens)
▷ *escitalopram* (C)(G) initially 10 mg daily; may increase to 20 mg daily after 1 week; *Elderly* o̲r hepatic impairment, 10 mg once daily
  Pediatric: <12 years: not recommended; 12-17 years: initially 10 mg once daily; may increase to 20 mg once daily after 3 weeks
      Lexapro *Tab:* 5, 10*, 20*mg
      Lexapro Oral Solution *Oral soln:* 1 mg/ml (240 ml) (peppermint) (parabens)
▷ *fluoxetine* (C)(G)
      Prozac initially 20 mg daily; may increase after 1 week; doses >20 mg/day may be divided into AM and noon doses; max 80 mg/day
      Pediatric: <8 years: not recommended; 8-17 years: initially 10-20 mg once daily; start lower weight children at 10 mg once daily; if starting at 10 mg once daily, may increase after 1 week to 20 mg once daily
          Cap: 10, 20, 40 mg; *Tab:* 30*, 60*mg; *Oral soln:* 20 mg/5 ml (4 oz) (mint)
      Prozac Weekly following daily *fluoxetine* therapy at 20 mg/day x 13 weeks, may initiate
      Prozac Weekly 7 days after the last 20 mg *fluoxetine* dose
      Pediatric: <12 years: not recommended; ≥12 years: same as adult
          Cap: 90 mg ent-coat del-rel pellets
▷ *paroxetine maleate* (D)(G)
  Pediatric: <12 years: not recommended; ≥12 years: same as adult
      Paxil initially 10-20 mg daily in AM; may increase by 10 mg/day at weekly intervals as needed; max 60 mg/day
          Tab: 10*, 20*, 30, 40 mg
      Paxil CR initially 12.5-25 mg daily in AM; may increase by 12.5 mg at weekly intervals as needed; max 62.5 mg/day
          Tab: 12.5, 25, 37.5 mg ent-coat cont-rel
      Paxil Suspension initially 10-20 mg daily in AM; may increase by 10 mg/day at weekly intervals as needed; max 60 mg/day
          Oral susp: 10 mg/5 ml (250 ml) (orange)
▷ *paroxetine mesylate* (D)(G) initially 7.5 mg daily in AM; may increase by 10 mg/day at weekly intervals as needed; max 60 mg/day
  Pediatric: <12 years: not recommended; ≥12 years: same as adult
      Brisdelle *Cap:* 7.5 mg
▷ *sertraline* (C) initially 50 mg daily; increase at 1 week intervals if needed; max 200 mg daily
  Pediatric: <6 years: not recommended; 6-12 years: initially 25 mg daily; max 200 mg/day; 13-17 years: initially 50 mg daily; max 200 mg/day
      Zoloft *Tab:* 15*, 50*, 100*mg; *Oral conc:* 20 mg per ml (60 ml [dilute just before administering in 4 oz water, ginger ale, lemon-lime soda, lemonade, o̲r orange juice]) (alcohol 12%)

SEROTONIN-NOREPINEPHRINE REUPTAKE INHIBITORS (SNRIs)

▷ *desvenlafaxine* (C)(G) swallow whole; initially 50 mg once daily; max 120 mg/day
  Pediatric: <18 years: not recommended; ≥18 years: same as adult
      Pristiq *Tab:* 50, 100 mg ext-rel
▷ *duloxetine* (C)(G) swallow whole; initially 30 mg once daily x 1 week; then, increase to 60 mg once daily; max 120 mg/day
  Pediatric: <12 years: not recommended; ≥12 years: same as adult
      Cymbalta *Cap:* 20, 30, 40, 60 mg del-rel
▷ *venlafaxine* (C)(G)
      Effexor initially 75 mg/day in 2-3 divided doses; may increase at 4 day intervals in 75 mg increments to 150 mg/day; max 225 mg
      Pediatric: <18 years: not recommended; ≥18 years: same as adult
          Tab: 37.5, 75, 150, 225 mg
      Effexor XR initially 75 mg q AM; may start at 37.5 mg daily x 4-7 days; then increase by increments of up to 75 mg/day at intervals of at least 4 days; usual max 375 mg/day
      Pediatric: <18 years: not recommended; ≥18 years: same as adult
          Tab: Cap: 37.5, 75, 150 mg ext-rel

COMBINATION AGENTS

➤ *chlordiazepoxide+amitriptyline* (D)(G)
  Pediatric: <12 years: not recommended; ≥12 years: same as adult
    Limbitrol 3-4 tabs/day in divided doses
      Tab: chlor 5 mg+amit 12.5 mg
    Limbitrol DS 3-4 tabs/day in divided doses; max 6 tabs/day
      Tab: chlor 10 mg+amit 25 mg
➤ *perphenazine+amitriptyline* (C)(G) 1 tab bid-qid
  Pediatric: <12 years: not recommended; ≥12 years: same as adult
    Tab: **Etrafon 2-10** perph 2 mg+amit 10 mg
      Etrafon 2-25 perph 2 mg+amit 25 mg
      Etrafon 4-25 perph 4 mg+amit 25 mg

 APHASIA, EXPRESSIVE: STROKE-INDUCED

Comment: In a case report published in NEJM, a 52-year-old right-handed woman who sustained an ischemic stroke 3 years prior, the areas of infarction included the left insula, putamen, and superior temporal gyrus. Her stroke resulted in expressive aphasia, leaving her with no intelligible words, but with intact full language comprehension. *zolpidem* 10 mg was prescribed for insomnia. In repeated measures, it was found that the patient consistently demonstrated dramatic speech improvement, durable until HS, and return of the expressive aphasia in the AM. Subsequent single-photon-emission computed tomography (SPECT) scanning of this patient indicated that *zolpidem* increases flow in the Broca area of the brain, an area intimately involved with speech. From these observations, the authors concluded that a select subgroup of patients with aphasia, perhaps with subcortical lesions and spared but hypometabolic cortical structures, might benefit from this treatment. It may be worth trying *zolpidem* in patients who have been labeled with otherwise refractory chronic expressive aphasia. This finding raises the questions, could this intervention help patients earlier in the course, patients with milder disease, <u>and/or</u> patients with other ischemic central nervous system syndromes?

REFERENCE
Cohen, L., Chaaban, B., & Habert, M.-O. (2004). Transient improvement of aphasia with zolpidem. *New England Journal of Medicine, 350*(9), 949–950. doi:10.1056/NEJM200402263500922

➤ *zolpidem* oral solution spray (imidazopyridine hypnotic) (C)(IV)(G) 2 actuations (10 mg) immediately before bedtime; *Elderly, debilitated*, <u>or</u> *hepatic impairment:* 2 actuations (5 mg); max 2 actuations (10 mg)
  Pediatric: <18 years: not recommended; ≥18 years: same adult
    ZolpiMist *Oral soln spray:* 5 mg/actuation (60 metered actuations) (cherry)
    Comment: The lowest dose of *zolpidem* in all forms is recommended for persons >50 years-of-age and women as drug elimination is slower than in men.
➤ *zolpidem* tabs (pyrazolopyrimidine hypnotic) (B)(IV)(G) 5-10 mg <u>or</u> 6.25-12.5 extrel q HS prn; max 12.5 mg/day x 1 month; do not take if unable to sleep for at least 8 hours before required to be active again; delayed effect if taken with a meal
  Pediatric: <18 years: not recommended; ≥18 years: same adult
    Ambien *Tab:* 5, 10 mg
    Ambien CR *Tab:* 6.25, 12.5 mg ext-rel
    Comment: The lowest dose of *zolpidem* in all forms is recommended for persons >50 years-of-age and women as drug elimination is slower than in men.
➤ *zolpidem* sublingual tabs (C)(IV) (imidazopyridine hypnotic) dissolve 1 tab under the tongue; allow to disintegrate completely before swallowing; take only once per night and only if at least 4 hours of bedtime remain before planned time for awakening
  Pediatric: <18 years: not recommended; ≥18 years: same adult
    Edluar *SL Tab:* 5, 10 mg
    Intermezzo *SL Tab:* 1.75, 3.5 mg
    Comment: **Edluar** is indicated for the treatment of insomnia when a middle-of-the-night awakening is followed by difficulty returning to sleep. The lowest dose of *zolpidem* in all forms is recommended for persons >50 years-of-age and women as drug elimination is slower than in men.

APHTHOUS STOMATITIS (MOUTH ULCER, CANKER SORE)

Comment: Aphthous ulcers are very painful sores with an inflamed base and non-viable tissue in the center that appears bacterial or viral. Although the sores are usually neither bacterial nor viral, herpetiform ulcers are most prevalent among the elderly). The sores may be single round/ovoid or several may be coalesced to form larger lesions, and located under the lip, on the buccal membrane, and/or on the tongue. Poor oral hygiene or an underlying immunity impairment can predispose the patient to ulcer formation (e.g., chronic illness, chemotherapy, poor nutrition, vitamin and mineral deficiencies, allergies, local trauma, stress, tobacco use, inflammatory bowel disease). They are frequently the result of local trauma (e.g., orthodontic-ware, chipped tooth) or allergy/irritation to a toothpaste or mouthwash ingredient (e.g. sodium lauryl sulfate). Changing toothpaste and applying dental wax to sharp edges are recommended until dental care is accessed. Debridement of the nonviable tissue by the direct application of salt (osmotic pulling pressure) for a few minutes, thus leaving a healthy tissue crater, speeds healing. Relief of the offending source of tissue trauma and application of a 5 mg prednisone tablet directly to the debrided ulcer are other remedies with reported success. These sores usually first appear in childhood or adolescence. Family history may have a role in the formation of recurrent aphthous stomatitis (RAS). When cases tend to occur in the same family (est 25-40% of the time), the ulcers earlier and with greater severity.

ANTI-INFLAMMATORY AGENTS

▷ **dexamethasone** elixir **(B)** 5 ml swish and spit q 12 hours
  Pediatric: <12 years: not recommended; ≥12 years: same as adult
    Elix: 0.5 mg/ml
▷ **triamcinolone acetonide** 0.1% dental paste **(G)** press (do <u>not</u> rub) a thin film onto lesion at bedtime and, if needed, 2-3 x daily after meals; re-evaluate if no improvement in 7 days
  Pediatric: <12 years: not recommended; ≥12 years: same as adult
    Oralone *Dental paste:* 0.1% (5 gm)
▷ **triamcinolone** 1% in **Orabase (B)** apply 1/4 inch to each ulcer bid-qid until ulcer heals
  Pediatric: <12 years: not recommended; ≥12 years: same as adult
    Kenalog in Orabase *Crm:* 1% (15, 60, 80 gm)

TOPICAL ANESTHETICS

▷ **benzocaine** topical gel **(C)(G)** apply tid-qid
▷ **benzocaine** topical spray **(C)(G)** 1 spray to painful area every 2 hours as needed; retain for 15 seconds, then spit
    Cepacol Spray (OTC), Chloraseptic Spray (OTC)
▷ **lidocaine** viscous soln **(B)(G)** 15 ml gargle <u>or</u> swish, then spit; repeat after 3 hours; max 8 doses/day
  Pediatric: <3 years: not recommended; 3-11 years: 1.25 ml; apply with cotton-tipped applicator; may repeat after 3 hours; max 8 doses/day; ≥12 years: same as adult
    Xylocaine Viscous Solution *Viscous soln:* 2% (20, 100, 450 ml)
▷ **triamcinolone (Kenalog)** in **Orabase (C)** apply with swab

DEBRIDING AGENT/CLEANSER

▷ **carbamide peroxide 10%** **(OTC)** apply 10 drops to affected area; swish x 2-3 minutes, then spit; do not rinse; repeat treatment qid
  Pediatric: <3 years: not recommended; ≥3 years: same as adult
    Gly-Oxide *Liq:* 10% (50, 60 ml squeeze bottle w. applicator)

ANTI-INFECTIVES

▷ **minocycline** **(D)(G)** swish and spit 10 ml susp (50 mg/5 ml) <u>or</u> 1 x 100 mg cap <u>or</u> 2 x 50 mg caps dissolved in 180 ml water, bid x 4-5 days
  Pediatric: <8 years: not recommended; ≥8 years: same as adult
    Dynacin *Cap:* 50, 100 mg
    Minocin *Cap:* 50, 75, 100 mg; *Oral susp:* 50 mg/5 ml (60 ml) (custard) (sulfites, alcohol 5%)
▷ **tetracycline** **(D)** swish and spit 10 ml susp (125 mg/5 ml) <u>or</u> one 250 mg tab/cap dissolved in 180 ml water qid x 4-5 days
  Pediatric: <8 years: not recommended; ≥8 years: same as adult; *see page 630 for dose by weight*
    Achromycin V *Cap:* 250, 500 mg

Sumycin *Tab:* 250, 500 mg; *Cap:* 250, 500 mg; *Oral susp:* 125 mg/5 ml (100, 200 ml) (fruit) (sulfites)

Comment: **tetracycline** is contraindicated <8 years-of-age, in pregnancy, and lactation (discolors developing tooth enamel). A side eff ect may be photo-sensitivity (photophobia). Do not take with antacids, calcium supplements, milk or other dairy, or within two hours of taking another drug.

ASPERGILLOSIS, BLASTOMYCOSIS, HISTOPLASMOSIS

INVASIVE INFECTION

▷ *isavuconazonium* (C) swallow cap whole; *Loading dose:* 372 mg q 8 hours x 6 doses (48 hours); *Maintenance:* 372 mg once daily starting 12-24 hours after last loading dose
Pediatric: <18 years: not established; ≥18 years: same as adult
  Cresemba *Cap:* 186 mg; *Vial:* 372 mg pwdr for reconstitution (7/blister pck) (preservative-free)
  Comment: **Cresemba** is indicated for the treatment of invasive aspergillus and mucormycosis in patients >18-years-old who are at high risk due to being severely compromised.

▷ *itraconazole* take with food; do not break, crush, or chew; 130 mg (2 x 65 mg caps) once daily; if no obvious improvement or there is evidence of progressive fungal disease, the dose should be increased in 65 mg increments to a maximum of 260 mg/day (130 mg [2 x 65 mg capsules] twice daily); doses >130 mg/day should be administered in two divided doses; *Treatment of Life-saving Situations:* although clinical studies did not provide for a loading dose, it is recommended, based on pharmacokinetic data, that a loading dose should be used; a loading dose of 130 mg (2 x 65 mg capsules) 3 x/day (390 mg/day) is recommended to be administered for the first 3 days, followed by the appropriate recommended dosing based on indication; treatment should be continued for a minimum of three months and until clinical parameters and laboratory tests indicate that the active fungal infection has subsided; an inadequate period of treatment may lead to recurrence of active infection
  Tolsura *Gelcap:* 65 mg
  Comment: **Tolsura** is not interchangeable or substitutable with other *itraconazole* products. **Tolsura** is not indicated for the treatment of onychomycosis. **Tolsura** is an azole antifungal indicated for the treatment of blastomycosis (pulmonary and extrapulmonary), histoplasmosis (including chronic cavitary pulmonary disease and disseminated, non-meningeal histoplasmosis) and aspergillosis (pulmonary and extrapulmonary, in patients who are intolerant of or who are refractory to *amphotericin B* therapy). These serious infections most commonly occur in vulnerable or immunocompromised patients, for example, hose with a history of cancer, transplants (solid organ or bone marrow), HIV/AIDS, or chronic rheumatic disorders, and are often associated with high mortality rates or long-term health issues. Most common adverse reactions (incidence ≥1%) are nausea, rash, vomiting, edema, headache, diarrhea, fatigue, fever, pruritus, hypertension, abnormal hepatic function, abdominal pain, dizziness, hypokalemia, anorexia, malaise, decreased libido, somnolence, albuminuria, impotence. *itraconazole* is mainly metabolized through CYP3A4.

▷ *posaconazole* (D)(G) *Oral Therapy:* take with food; swallow tab whole; *Day 1:* 300 mg bid; then 300 mg once daily x 13 days; *IV Infusion Therapy:* must be administered through an in-line filter over approximately 90 minutes via a central venous line. Never administer **Noxafil** as an IV bolus injection; *Loading Dose:* a single 300 mg IV infusion; *Maintenance Dose: a single* 300 mg IV infusion once daily for duration of treatment (e.g., resolution of neutropenia or immunosuppression)
Pediatric: <13 years: not recommended; ≥13 years: same as adult
  Noxafil *Tab:* 100 mg ext-rel; *Oral susp:* 40 mg/ml (105 oz w. dosing spoon) (cherry); *Vial:* 300 mg/16.7 ml (18 mg/ml) soln for IV infusion
  Comment: **Noxafil** is indicated as prophylaxis for invasive aspergillus and candida infections in patients >13-years-old who are at high risk due to being severely compromised.

▷ *voriconazole* (D)(G) *PO:* <40 kg: 100 mg q 12 hours; may increase to 150 mg q 12 hours if inadequate response; >40 kg: 200 mg q 12 hours; may increase to 300 mg q 12 hours if inadequate response; *IV:* 6 mg/kg q 12 hours x 2 doses; then 4 mg/kg q 12 hours; max rate 3 mg/kg/hour over 1-2 hours
Pediatric: <12 years: not recommended; ≥12 years: same as adult
  Vfend *Tab:* 50, 200 mg
  Vfend I.V. for Injection *Vial:* 200 mg pwdr for reconstitution (preservative-free)
  Vfend *Oral susp:* 40 mg/ml pwdr for reconstitution (75 ml) (orange)

ASTHMA

Parenteral Corticosteroids *see page* 577
Oral Corticosteroids *see page* 577

EPINEPHRINE INHALATION AEROSOL (BRONCHODILATOR)

▷ *epinephrine inhalation aerosol* (C)(OTC) shake and spray one time into the air prior to each inhalation; after one inhalation, wait one minute; if inadequate relief, may repeat; 1-2 inhalations constitutes one dose; wait at least 4 hours between doses; max 8 inhalations/24 hours
  Pediatric: <12 years: safety and efficacy not established; ≥12 years: same as adult
    Primatene MIST Pump inhal: *0.125 mg per inhalation spray* (160 sprays) (no sulfites; dehydrated alcohol 1%, hydrofluoroalkane [HFA-134a], polysorbate 80, thymol)
    Comment: **Primatene Mist** *(epinephrine inhalation aerosol)* is indicated for the temporary relief of mild symptoms of intermittent asthma (wheezing, chest tightness, shortness of breath, delivered by a metered-dose inhaler (MDI) with a non-chorofluorocarbon (CFC) propellant. After every 20 sprays, the spray indicator resets (160, 140, 120…20, 0). The spray indicator cannot be manually reset.

INHALED RACEPINEPHRINE (BRONCHODILATOR)

Comment: Inhalation racemic epinephrine is indicated for urgent/emergent acute bronchospasm rescue (e.g., acute asthma attack, laryngospasm, croup, epiglottitis, acute inflammation causing airway obstruction). Inhalational racemic epinephrine is <u>only</u> recommended for use during pregnancy when there are <u>no</u> alternatives and benefit outweighs risk.
▷ *racepinephrine* (C)(OTC)(G) for atomized (nebulizer) treatment.
  Pediatric: <4 years: not recommended; ≥4 years: same as adult
    Asthmanefrin *Starter kit:* 10 x 0.5 ml vials 2.25% solution for atomized inhalation w. EZ Breathe Atomizer; *Refills:* 30 x 0.5 ml vials 2.25% solution for atomized inhalation

INHALED BETA-2 AGONISTS (BRONCHODILATORS)

▷ *albuterol sulfate* (C)(G)
  AccuNeb Inhalation Solution 1 unit-dose vial tid-qid prn by nebulizer; ages 2-12 years only; not for adult
  Pediatric: <2 years: not recommended; 2-12 years: initially 0.63 mg <u>or</u> 1.25 mg tid-qid; 6-12 years: with severe asthma, <u>or</u> >40 kg, <u>or</u> 11-12 years: initially 1.25 mg tid-qid
    Inhal soln: 0.63, 1.25 mg/3 ml (3 ml, 25/carton) (preservative-free)
  Albuterol Inhalation Solution (G) not recommended for adults
  Pediatric: <2 years: not recommended; ≥2 years: 1 vial via nebulizer over 5-15 minutes
    Inhal soln: 0.63 mg/3 ml (0.021%); 1.25 mg/3 ml (0.042%) (25/carton)
  Albuterol Inhalation Solution 0.5% (G) not recommended
  Pediatric: <4 years: not recommended; ≥4 years: same as adult
    Inhal soln: 0.083% (25/carton)
  Albuterol Nebules (G) 2.5 mg (0.5 ml of 5% diluted to 3 ml with sterile NS <u>or</u> 3 ml of 0.083%) tid-qid
  Pediatric: use <12 years: other forms; ≥12 years: same as adult
    Inhal soln: 0.083% (25/carton)
  Proair HFA Inhaler 1-2 inhalations q 4-6 hours prn; 2 inhalations 15 minutes before exercise as prophylaxis for exercise-induced asthma (EIA)
  Pediatric: <4 years: not established; ≥4 years: same as adult
    Inhaler: 90 mcg/actuation (0.65 gm, 200 inh) (CFC-free)
  Proair RespiClick 1-2 inhalations q 4-6 hours prn; 2 inhalations 15-30 minutes before exercise as prophylaxis for exercise-induced asthma (EIA)
  Pediatric: <12 years: not established; ≥12 years: same as adult
    Inhaler: 90 mcg/actuation (8.5 gm, 200 inh)
  Proventil HFA Inhaler 1-2 inhalations q 4-6 hours prn; 2 inhalations 15 minutes before exercise as prophylaxis for exercise-induced asthma (EIA)
  Pediatric: <4 years: use syrup; ≥4 years: same as adult
    Inhaler: 90 mcg/actuation with a dose counter (6.7 gm, 200 inh)
  Proventil Inhalation Solution 2.5 mg diluted to 3 ml with normal saline tid-qid prn by nebulizer

Pediatric: use syrup
  Inhal soln: 0.5% (20 ml w. dropper); 0.083% (3 ml; 25/carton)
Ventolin Inhaler 2 inhalations q 4-6 hours prn; 2 inhalations 15 minutes before exercise as prophylaxis for exercise-induced asthma
Pediatric: <2 years: not recommended; 2-4 years: use syrup; ≥4 years: same as adult
  Inhaler: 90 mcg/actuation (17 gm, 220 inh)
Ventolin Rotacaps 1-2 cap inhalations q 4-6 hours prn; 2 inhalations 15 minutes before exercise as prophylaxis for exercise-induced asthma (EIA)
Pediatric: <4 years: not recommended; ≥4 years 1-2 caps q 4-6 hours prn
  Rotacaps: 200 mcg/rotacap dose (100 doses)
Ventolin 0.5% Inhalation Solution
Pediatric: <2 years: not recommended; ≥2 years: initially 0.1-0.15 mg/kg/dose tid-qid prn; 10-15 kg: 0.25 ml diluted to 3 ml with normal saline by nebulizer tid-qid prn; >15 kg: 0.5 ml diluted to 3 ml with normal saline by nebulizer tid-qid prn
  Inhal soln: 20 ml w. dropper
Ventolin Nebules
Pediatric: <2 years: not recommended; ≥2 years: initially 0.1-0.15 mg/kg/ dose tid-qid prn; 10-15 kg: 1.25 mg <u>or</u> 1/2 nebule tid-qid prn; >15 kg: 2.5 mg <u>or</u> 1 nebule tid-qid prn
  Inhal soln: 0.083% (3 ml; 25/carton)
▷ *isoproterenol* (B) *Rescue:* 1 inhalation prn; repeat if no relief in 2-5 minutes; *Maintenance:* 1-2 inhalations q 4-6 hours
Pediatric: <12 years: not recommended; ≥12 years: same as adult
  Medihaler-ISO *Inhaler:* 80 mcg/actuation (15 ml, 30 inh)
▷ *levalbuterol tartrate* (C)(G) initially 0.63 mg tid q 6-8 hours prn by nebulizer; may increase to 1.25 mg tid at 6-8 hour intervals as needed
Pediatric: <12 years: not recommended; ≥12 years: same as adult
  Xopenex *Inhal soln:* 0.31, 0.63, 1.25 mg/3 ml (24/carton) (preservative-free)
  Xopenex HFA *Inh:* 45 mg (15 gm, 200 inh) (preservative-free)
  Xopenex Concentrate *Vial:* 1.25 mg/0.5 ml (30/carton) (preservative-free)
▷ *metaproterenol* (C)(G)
  Alupent 2-3 inhalations tid-qid prn; max 12 inhalations/day
  Pediatric: <6 years: use syrup; ≥6 years: via nebulizer 0.1-0.2 ml diluted with normal saline to 3 ml, up to q 4 hours prn
    Inhaler: 0.65 mg/actuation (14 gm, 200 doses)
  Alupent Inhalation Solution 5-15 inhalations tid-qid prn; q 4 hours prn for acute attack
  Pediatric: <6 years: use syrup ≥6 years: via nebulizer 0.1-0.2 ml diluted with normal saline to 3 ml, up to q 4 hours prn
    Inhal soln: 5% (10, 30 ml w. dropper)
▷ *pirbuterol* (C) 1-2 inhalations q 4-6 hours prn; max 12 inhalations/day
Pediatric: <12 years: not recommended; ≥12 years: same as adult
  Maxair *Autohaler:* 200 mcg/actuation (14 gm, 400 inh); *Inhaler:* 200 mcg/actuation (25.6 gm, 300 inh)
▷ *terbutaline* (B) 2 inhalations q 4-6 hours prn
Pediatric: <12 years: not recommended; ≥12 years: same as adult
  Inhaler: 0.2 mg/actuation (10.5 gm, 300 inh)

INHALED ANTICHOLINERGICS

▷ *ipratropium bromide* (C)(G)
Pediatric: <12 years: not established; ≥12 years: same as adult
  Atrovent 2 inhalations qid; additional inhalations as required; max 12 inhalations/day
    Inhaler: 18 mcg/actuation (14 gm, 200 inh)
  Atrovent Inhalation Solution 500 mcg tid-qid prn by nebulizer
    Inhal soln: 0.02% (500 mcg in 2.5 ml; 25/carton)

INHALED CORTICOSTEROIDS

Comment: Inhaled corticosteroids are <u>not</u> for primary (rescue) treatment of acute asthma attack. After every inhalation of a steroid <u>or</u> steroid-containing medication treatment, rinse mouth to reduce risk of oral candidiasis. Inhaled corticosteroids are <u>not</u> for primary (rescue) treatment of acute asthma attack. For twice daily dosing, allow 12 hours between doses.

▷ *beclomethasone dipropionate* (C)(G) *Previously using only bronchodilators:* initiate 40-80 mcg bid; max 320 mcg bid; *Previously using inhaled corticosteroid:* initiate 40-160 mcg bid; max 320 mcg/day; *Previously taking a systemic corticosteroid:* attempt to wean off the systemic drug after approximately 1 week after initiating; rinse mouth after use
Pediatric: <12 years: not recommended; ≥12 years: same as adult
  Qvar *Inhal aerosol:* 40, 80 mcg/metered dose actuation (8.7 gm, 120 inh) metered dose inhaler (chlorofluorocarbon [CFC]-free)

▷ *budesonide* (B)
  Pulmicort Flexhaler initially 180-360 mcg bid; max 360 mcg bid; rinse mouth after use
  Pediatric: <6 years: not recommended; ≥6 years: 1-2 inhalations bid
    Flexhaler: 90 mcg/actuation (60 inh); 180 mcg/actuation (120 inh)
  Pulmicort Respules (G) adults and ≥8 years: use flexhaler
  Pediatric: <12 months: not recommended; 12 months-8 years: *Previously using only bronchodilators:* initiate 0.5 mg/day once daily or in 2 divided doses; may start at 0.25 mg daily; *Previously using inhaled corticosteroids:* initiate 0.5 mg once daily or in 2 divided doses; max 1 mg/day; *Previously taking oral corticosteroids:* initiate 1 mg/day daily or in 2 divided doses; ≥8 years: use flexhaler; rinse mouth after use
    Inhal susp: 0.25, 0.5, 1 mg/2 ml (30/carton)

▷ *ciclesonide* (C) initially 80 mcg bid; max 320 mcg/day; rinse mouth after use; *Previously on inhaled corticosteroid:* initially 80 mcg bid; *Previously on oral steroid:* 320 mg bid
Pediatric: <12 years: not recommended; ≥12 years: same as adult
  Alvesco *Inhal aerosol:* 80, 160 mcg/actuation (6.1 gm, 60 inh)

▷ *flunisolide* (C) rinse mouth after use
  AeroBid, AeroBid-M initially 2 inhalations bid; max 8 inhalations/day; rinse mouth after use
  Pediatric: <6 years: not recommended; 6-15 years: 2 inhalations bid; ≥15 years: same as adult
    Inhaler: 250 mcg/actuation (7 gm, 100 inh)
  Aerospan HFA initially 160 mcg bid; max 320 mcg bid
  Pediatric: <6 years: not recommended; 6-11 years: 80 mcg bid; max 160 mcg bid; ≥12 years: same as adult
    Inhaler: 80 mcg (5.1 gm, 60 doses; 80 mcg, 120 doses)

▷ *fluticasone furoate* (C) *currently not on inhaled corticosteroid:* usually initiate at 100 mcg once daily at the same time each day; may increase to 200 mcg once daily if inadequate response after 2 weeks; max 200 mcg/day; rinse mouth after use
Pediatric: <12 years: not established; ≥12 years: same as adult
  Arnuity Ellipta *Inhal:* 100, 200 mcg/dry pwdr per inhalation (30 doses)
  Comment: Arnuity Ellipta is not for primary treatment of status asthmaticus or acute asthma episodes. **Arnuity Ellipta** is contraindicated with severe hypersensitivity to milk proteins.

▷ *fluticasone propionate* (C)
  ArmorAir 1 inhalation bid (12 hours apart); initially 55 mcg bid; *Previously using an inhaled corticosteroid:* see mfr pkg insert; if insufficient response after 2 weeks, may increase the bid dose; max 232 mcg bid; after stability achieved, titrate to lowest effective dose; do not use with spacer or volume-holding chamber
  Pediatric: <12 years: not established; ≥12 years: same as adult
    Inhaler: 55, 113, 232 mcg/actuation (60 inh)
  Flovent, Flovent HFA initially 88 mcg bid; *Previously using an inhaled corticosteroid:* initially 88-220 mcg bid; *Previously taking an oral corticosteroid:* 880 mcg bid; rinse mouth after use
  Pediatric: <11 years: use **Flovent Diskus** ≥12 years: same as adult
    Inhaler: 44 mcg/actuation (7.9 gm, 60 inh; 13 gm, 120 inh); 110 mcg/actuation (13 gm, 120 inh); 220 mcg/actuation (13 gm, 120 inh)
  Flovent Diskus initially 100 mcg bid; max 500 mcg bid; *Previously using an inhaled corticosteroid:* initially 100-250 mcg bid; max 500 mcg bid; *Previously taking an oral corticosteroid:* 1000 mcg bid
  Pediatric: <4 years: not recommended; 4-11 years: initially 50 mcg bid; max 100 mcg bid; rinse mouth after use; ≥12 years: same as adult
    Diskus: 50, 100, 250 mcg/inh dry pwdr (60 blisters w. diskus)

▷ *mometasone furoate* (C) 220-440 mcg once daily or bid; max 880 mcg/day; rinse mouth after use
  Asmanex HFA *Inhaler:* 100, 200 mcg/actuation (13 gm, 120 inh)

Pediatric: <12 years: not established; ≥12 years: same as adult

Asmanex Twisthaler *Inhaler:* 110 mcg/actuation (30 inh), 220 mcg/actuation (30, 60, 120 inh)

Pediatric: <4 years: not recommended; 4-11 years: 110 mcg once daily in the PM; >12 years: may use **Asmanex HFA**; rinse mouth after use

▷ *triamcinolone* (C)

Azmacort 2 inhalations tid-qid or 4 inhalations bid; rinse mouth after use

Pediatric: <6 years: not recommended; 6-12 years: 1-2 inhalations tid or 2-4 inhalations bid; >12 years: same as adult

Inhaler: 100 mcg/actuation (20 gm, 240 inh)

LEUKOTRIENE RECEPTOR ANTAGONISTS (LRAS)

Comment: The LRAs are indicated for prophylaxis and chronic treatment, only. Not for primary (rescue) treatment of acute asthma attack.

▷ *montelukast* (B)(G) 10 mg once daily in the PM; for EIB, take at least 2 hours before exercise; max 1 dose/day

Pediatric: <12 months: not recommended; 12-23 months: one 4 mg granule pkt daily; 2-5 years: one 4 mg chew tab or granule pkt daily; 6-14 years: one 5 mg chew tab daily; ≥15 years: same as adult

Singulair *Tab:* 10 mg

Singulair Chewable *Chew tab:* 4, 5 mg (cherry) (phenylalanine)

Singulair Oral Granules *Granules:* 4 mg/pkt; take within 15 minutes of opening pkt; may mix with applesauce, carrots, rice, or ice cream

▷ *zafirlukast* (B) 20 mg bid, 1 hour ac or 2 hours pc

Pediatric: <7 years: not recommended; 7-11 years: 10 mg bid 1 hour ac or 2 hours pc; ≥12 years: same as adult

Accolate *Tab:* 10, 20 mg

▷ *zileuton* (C)(G)

Pediatric: <12 years: not recommended; ≥12 years: same as adult

Zyflo 1 tab qid (total 2400 mg/day)

Tab: 600 mg

Zyflo CR 2 tabs bid (total 2400 mg/day)

Tab: 600 mg ext-rel

IGE BLOCKER (IGG1K MONOCLONAL ANTIBODY)

▷ *omalizumab* (B) 150-375 mg SC every 2-4 weeks based on body weight and pre-treatment serum total IgE level; max 150 mg/injection site; should be administered only by a qualified health care provider

Pediatric: <12 years: not recommended; 30-90 kg + IgE >30-100 IU/ml 150 mg q 4 weeks; 90-150 kg + IgE >30-100 IU/ml or 30-90 kg + IgE >100-200 IU/ml or 30-60 kg + IgE >200-300 IU/ml 300 mg q 4 hours; >90-150 kg + IgE >100-200 IU/ml or >60-90 kg + IgE >200-300 IU/ml or 30-70 kg + IgE >300-400 IU/ml 225 mg q 2 weeks; >90-150 kg + IgE >200-300 IU/ml or >70-90 kg + IgE >300-400 IU/ml or 30-70 kg + IgE >400-500 IU/ml or 30-60 kg + IgE >500-600 IU/ml or 30-60 kg + IgE >600-700 IU/ml 375 mg q 2 weeks

Xolair *Vial:* 150 mg, single-dose, pwdr for SC injection after reconstitution; *Prefilled syringe:* 75 mg/0.5 ml, 150 mg/1 ml single-dose (preservative-free)

INHALED MAST CELL STABILIZERS (PROPHYLAXIS)

Comment: IMCSs are for prophylaxis and chronic treatment, only. Not for primary (rescue) treatment of acute asthma attack.

▷ *cromolyn sodium* (B)(G)

Intal 2 inhalations qid; 2 inhalations up to 10-60 minutes before precipitant as prophylaxis; rinse mouth after use

Pediatric: <2 years: not recommended; 2-5 years: use inhal soln via nebulizer; >5 years: 2 inhalations qid via inhaler

Inhaler: 0.8 mg/actuation (8.1, 14.2 gm; 112, 200 inh)

Intal Inhalation Solution 20 mg by nebulizer qid; 20 mg up to 10-60 minutes before precipitant as prophylaxis

Pediatric: <2 years: not recommended; ≥2 years: same as adult

Inhal soln: 20 mg/2 ml (60, 120/carton)

▷ *nedocromil sodium* (B)

   Tilade 2 sprays qid; rinse mouth after use
   Pediatric: <6 years: not recommended; ≥6 years: 2 sprays qid
   Inhaler: 1.75 mg/spray (16.2 gm; 104 sprays)
   Tilade Nebulizer Solution 0.5% 1 amp qid by nebulizer
   Pediatric: <2 years: not recommended; ≥2 years: initially 1 amp qid by nebulizer; 2-5
   years: initially 1 amp tid by nebulizer; ≥5 years: same as adult
   Inhal soln: 11 mg/2.2 ml (2 ml; 60, 120/carton)

INHALED LONG-ACTING ANTICHOLINERGIC

▷ *tiotropium (as bromide monohydrate)* (C) 2 inhalations once daily using inhalation device;
do not swallow caps
   Pediatric: <12 years: not recommended; ≥12 years: same as adult
   Spiriva HandiHaler *Inhal device:* 18 mcg/cap pwdr for inhalation (5, 30, 90 caps w.
   inhalation device)
   Spiriva Respimat *Inhal device:* 1.25, 2.5 mcg/actuation cartridge w. inhalation device
   (4 gm, 60 metered actuations) (benzylkonian chloride)
   Comment: *tiotropium* is for prophylaxis and chronic treatment, only. Not for primary
   (rescue) treatment of acute attack. Avoid getting powder in eyes. Caution with narrow-
   angle glaucoma, BPH, bladder neck obstruction, and pregnancy. Contraindicated with
   allergy to *atropine* or its derivatives (e.g., *ipratropium*).

INHALED ANTICHOLINERGIC+BETA-2 AGONIST

▷ *ipratropium bromide+albuterol sulfate* (C) 2 inhalations qid
   Pediatric: <12 years: not recommended; ≥12 years: same as adult
   Combivent 2 inhalations qid; additional inhalations as required; max 12 inhalations/day
   Inhaler: ipra 18 mcg+albu 90 mcg/actuation (14.7 gm, 200 inh)
   Duoneb 1 vial via nebulizer 4-6 times daily prn
   Inhal soln: ipra 0.5 mg (0.017%)+albu 2.5 mg (0.083%) per 3 ml (23/carton)

INHALED LONG-ACTING BETA-2 AGONIST (LABA)

Comment: LABA agents are not for primary (rescue) treatment of acute asthma attack. For
twice daily dosing, allow 12 hours between doses.

▷ *arformoterol* (C) 15 mcg bid via nebulizer
   Pediatric: <12 years: not recommended; ≥12 years: same as adult
   Brovana *Inhal soln:* 15 mcg/2 ml (2 ml; 30/carton)
   Comment: *arformoterol* is indicated for the treatment of COPD but is used off-label for the
   treatment of asthma. It is used for prophylaxis and chronic treatment, only. Not for primary
   (rescue) treatment of acute attack.
▷ *formoterol fumarate* (C)
   Foradil Aerolizer 12 mcg q 12 hours
   Pediatric: <5 years: not recommended; ≥5 years: same as adult
   Inhaler: 12 mcg/cap (12, 60 caps w. device)
   Perforomist 20 mcg q 12 hours
   Pediatric: <12 years: not recommended; ≥12 years: same as adult
   Inhal soln: 20 mcg/2 ml (60/carton)
   Comment: *formoterol* is for prophylaxis and chronic treatment, only. Not for primary
   (rescue) treatment of acute attack. Do not mix *formoterol* with other drugs. Use of
   formoterol is off-label for asthma.
▷ *olodaterol* (C) 12 mcg q 12 hours
   Pediatric: <12 years: not established; ≥12 years: same as adult
   Striverdi Respimat
   Inhal soln: 2.5 mcg/cartridge (metered actuation) (40 gm, 60 metered actuations)
   (benzalkonium chloride)
   Comment: Striverdi Respimat is contraindicated in persons with asthma without
   concomitant use of long-term control medication.
▷ *salmeterol* (C)(G) 2 inhalations q 12 hours prn; 2 inhalations at least 30-60 minutes before
exercise as prophylaxis for exercise-induced asthma; do not use extra doses for exercise-
induced bronchospasm if already using regular dose

Pediatric: <4 years: not recommended; 4-<12 years: 1 inhalation q 12 hours prn; 1 inhalation at least 30-60 minutes before exercise as prophylaxis for exercise-induced asthma; do not use extra doses for exercise-induced bronchospasm if already using regular dose; ≥12 years: same as adult

Serevent Diskus *Diskus (pwdr):* 50 mcg/actuation (60 doses/diskus)

INHALED CORTICOSTEROID+LONG-ACTING BETA-2 AGONIST (LABA)

Comment: Inhaled corticosteroids and LABA agents are not for primary (rescue) treatment of acute asthma attack. For twice daily dosing, allow 12 hours between doses. After every inhalation of a steroid or steroid-containing medication treatment, rinse mouth to reduce risk of oral candidiasis.

▷ *budesonide+formoterol* (C) 1 inhalation bid; rinse mouth after use
   Pediatric: <12 years: not established; ≥12 years: same as adult
      Symbicort 80/4.5 *Inhaler:* bud 80 mcg+for 4.5 mcg
      Symbicort 160/4.5 *Inhaler:* bud 160 mcg+for 4.5 mcg
▷ *fluticasone propionate+salmeterol* (C)
   Advair HFA *Not previously using inhaled steroid:* start with 2 inh 45/21 or 115/21 bid; if insufficient response after 2 weeks, use next higher strength; max 2 inh 230/50 bid; allow 12 hours between doses; *Already using inhaled steroid;* see mfr pkg insert
      Advair HFA 45/21 1 inhalation bid; rinse mouth after use
      Pediatric: <12 years: not recommended; ≥12 years: same as adult
         Inhaler: flu pro 45 mcg+sal 21 mcg/actuation (CFC-free)
      Advair HFA 115/21 1 inhalation bid; rinse mouth after use
      Pediatric: <12 years: not established; ≥12 years: same as adult
         Inhaler: flu pro 115 mcg+sal 21 mcg/actuation (CFC-free)
      Advair HFA 230/21 1 inhalation bid; rinse mouth after use
      Pediatric: <12 years: not established; ≥12 years: same as adult
         Inhaler: flu pro 230 mcg+sal 21 mcg/actuation (CFC-free)
      Advair Diskus (G) *Not previously using inhaled steroid:* start with 1 inh 100/50 bid; *Already using inhaled steroid:* see mfr pkg insert; rinse mouth after use
      Advair Diskus (G) 100/50 1 inhalation bid; rinse mouth after use
      Pediatric: <4 years: not recommended; 4-11 years: 1 bid; >11 years: 1 inhalation bid
         Diskus: flu pro 100 mcg+sal 50 mcg/actuation (60 blisters)
      Advair Diskus (G) 250/50 1 inhalation bid; rinse mouth after use
      Pediatric: <4 years: not recommended; 4-12 years: use 100/50 strength; >12 years: same as adult
         Diskus: flu pro 250 mcg+sal 50 mcg/actuation (60 blisters)
      Advair Diskus (G) 500/50 1 inhalation bid; rinse mouth after use
      Pediatric: <4 years: not recommended; 4-12 years: use 100/50 strength; >12 years: same as adult
         Diskus: flu pro 500 mcg+sal 50 mcg/actuation (60 blisters)
      AirDuo RespiClick pwdr for oral inhalation; *Not previously using an inhaled steroid:* 1 inh 55/14 bid; *Already using an inhaled steroid:* see mfr pkg insert; if insufficient response after 2 weeks, titrate with a higher strength; max inh 232/14 bid
      Pediatric: <12 years: not established; ≥12 years: same as adult
         AirDuo RespiClick 55/14 flu pro 55 mcg+sal (as xinafoate) 14 mcg dry pwdr/actuation (60 actuations)
         AirDuo RespiClick 113/14 flu pro 113 mcg+sal (as xinafoate) 14 mcg dry pwdr/actuation (60 actuations)
         AirDuo RespiClick 232/14 flu pro 232 mcg+sal (as xinafoate) 14 mcg dry pwdr/actuation (60 actuations)
▷ *fluticasone furoate+vilanterol* (C) 1 inhalation 100/25 once daily at the same time each day
   Pediatric: <17 years: not established; ≥17 years: same as adult
      Breo Ellipta
         Breo Ellipta 100/25 flu 100 mcg+vil 25 mcg dry pwdr per inhalation (30 doses)
         Breo Ellipta 200/25 flu 200 mcg+vil 25 mcg dry pwdr per inhalation (30 doses)
         Comment: **Breo Ellipta** is contraindicated with severe hypersensitivity to milk proteins.
▷ *mometasone furoate+formoterol fumarate* (C) 2 inhalations bid; rinse mouth after use
   Pediatric: <12 years: not established; ≥12 years: same as adult

Dulera
> **Dulera 100/5** *Inhaler:* mom 100 mcg/for 5 mcg (HFA)
> **Dulera 200/5** *Inhaler:* mom 200 mcg/for 5 mcg (HFA)
> Comment: **Dulera** is not a rescue inhaler.

INHALED ANTICHOLINERGIC+LONG-ACTING BETA-2 AGONIST (LABA)

▷ *glycopyrrolate+formoterol fumarate* (C) 2 inhalations bid (AM & PM)
> *Pediatric:* <18 years: not established; ≥18 years: same as adult
> **Bevespi Aerosphere 9/4.8** *Metered dose inhaler:* gly 9 mcg+for 4.8 mcg/inhalation (10.7 gm, 120 inh)

ORAL BETA-2 AGONISTS (BRONCHODILATORS)

▷ *albuterol* (C)
> **Albuterol Syrup (G)** *Adult:* 2-4 mg tid-qid; may increase gradually; max 8 mg qid;
> *Elderly:* initially 2-3 mg tid-qid; may increase gradually; max 8 mg qid
> *Pediatric:* <2 years: not recommended; ≥2-6 years: 0.1 mg/kg tid; initially max 2 mg tid; may increase gradually to 0.2 mg/kg tid; max 4 mg tid; >6-12 years: 2 mg tid-qid; may increase gradually; max 6 mg qid; ≥12 years: same as adult
> > *Syr:* 2 mg/5 ml
> **Proventil** 2-4 mg tid-qid prn
> *Pediatric:* <6 years: not recommended; ≥6 years: same as adult
> > *Tab:* 2, 4 mg
> **Proventil Repetabs** 4-8 mg q 12 hours prn
> *Pediatric:* use syrup
> > *Repetab:* 4 mg sust-rel
> **Proventil Syrup** 5-10 ml tid-qid prn; may increase gradually; max 20 ml qid prn
> *Pediatric:* <2 years: not recommended; ≥2-6 years: 0.1 mg/kg tid prn; max initially 5 ml tid prn; may increase gradually to 0.2 mg/kg tid prn; max 10 ml tid; >6-14 years: 5 ml tid-qid prn; may increase gradually; max 60 ml/day in divided doses; >14 years: same as adult
> > *Syr:* 2 mg/5 ml
> **Ventolin** 2-4 mg tid-qid prn; may increase gradually; max 8 mg qid
> *Pediatric:* <2 years: not recommended; ≥2-6 years: 0.1 mg/kg tid prn; max initially 2 mg tid prn; may increase gradually to 0.2 mg/kg tid; max 4 mg tid; >6-14 years: 2 mg tid-qid prn; may increase gradually; max 6 mg tid
> > *Tab:* 2, 4 mg; *Syr:* 2 mg/5 ml (strawberry)
> **VoSpire ER** 4-8 mg q 12 hours prn; max 32 mg/day divided q 12 hours; swallow whole; do not crush or chew
> *Pediatric:* <6 years: not recommended; ≥6-12 years: 4 mg q 12 hours; max 24 mg/day q 12 hours; >12 years: same as adult
> > *Tab:* 4, 8 mg ext-rel
▷ *metaproterenol* (C) 20 mg tid-qid prn
> *Pediatric:* <6 years: not recommended (doses of 1.3-2.6 mg/kg/day have been used); ≥6-9 years (<60 lb): 10 mg tid-qid prn; >9-12 years (>60 lb): 20 mg tid-qid prn; >12 years: same as adult
> **Alupent** *Tab:* 10, 20 mg; *Syr:* 10 mg/5 ml

METHYLXANTHINES

Comment: Check serum theophylline level just before 5th dose is administered. Therapeutic theophylline level: 10-20 mcg/ml.
▷ *theophylline* (C)(G)
> **Theo-24** initially 300-400 mg once daily at HS; after 3 days, increase to 400-600 mg once daily at HS; max 600 mg/day
> *Pediatric:* <45 kg: initially 12-14 mg/kg/day; max 300 mg/day; increase after 3 days to 16 mg/kg/day to max 400 mg; after 3 more days increase to 30 mg/kg/day to max 600 mg/day; ≥45 kg: same as adult
> > *Cap:* 100, 200, 300, 400 mg ext-rel
> **Theo-Dur** initially 150 mg bid; increase to 200 mg bid after 3 days; then to 300 mg bid after 3 more days
> *Pediatric:* <6 years: not recommended; 6-15 years: initially 12-14 mg/kg/day in 2 divided doses; max 300 mg/day; then increase to 16 mg/kg in 2 divided doses; max 400 mg/day; then to 20 mg/kg/day in 2 divided doses; max 600 mg/day; ≥15 years: same as adult
> > *Tab:* 100, 200, 300 mg ext-rel

Theolair-SR
Pediatric: not recommended
    Tab: 200, 250, 300, 500 mg sust-rel
Uniphyl 400-600 mg daily with meals
Pediatric: not recommended
    Tab: 400*, 600*mg cont-rel

METHYLXANTHINE+EXPECTORANT COMBINATION

➤ *dyphylline+guaifenesin* (C) 1 tab qid
    Lufyllin GG *Tab:* dyphy 200 mg+guaif 200 mg; Elix: dyphy 100 mg+guaif 100 mg per 15 ml

INTERLEUKIN-4 RECEPTOR ALPHA ANTAGONIST

➤ *dupilumab* administer SC into the upper arm, abdomen, or thigh; rotate sites; initially 600 mg (2 x 300 mg injections at different sites) followed by 300 mg SC once every other week; may use with or without topical corticosteroids; may use with calcineurin inhibitors, but reserve only for problem areas (e.g., face, neck, intertriginous, and genital areas); avoid live vaccines.
Pediatric: <12 years: not recommended; ≥12 years: same as adult
    Dupixent *Prefilled syringe:* 300 mg/2 ml (2/pck without needle) (preservative-free)
    Comment: *dupilumab* is a human monoclonal IgG4 antibody that inhibits interleukin-4 (IL-4) and interleukin-13 (IL-13) signaling by specifically binding to the IL4Ra sub-unit shared by the IL-4 and IL-13 receptor complexes, thereby inhibiting the release of pro-inflammatory cytokines, chemokines, and IgE. *dupilumab* is indicated as an add-on maintenance therapy for patients ≥12 years-of-age with moderate-to-severe asthma with an eosinophilic subtype or with oral corticosteroid-dependent asthma.

HUMANIZED INTERLEUKIN-5 ANTAGONIST MONOCLONAL ANTIBODY

➤ *mepolizumab* 100 mg SC once every 4 weeks in upper arm, abdomen, or thigh
Pediatric: <12 years: not recommended; ≥12 years: same as adult
    Nucala *Vial:* 100 mg pwdr for reconstitution, single-use (preservative-free)
    Comment: **Nucala** is an add-on maintenance treatment for severe asthma. There is a pregnancy exposure registry that monitors pregnancy outcomes in women exposed to **Nucala** during pregnancy. Healthcare providers can enroll patients or encourage patients to enroll themselves by calling 1-877-311-8972 or visiting www.mothertobaby. org/asthma.

⬭ ASTHMA-COPD OVERLAP SYNDROME (ACOS)

Comment: An estimated 16% of patients with asthma or COPD have asthma- COPD overlap syndrome (ACOS), a poorly understood disease with an increasing morbidity and mortality. PROSPRO (Prospective Study to Evaluate Predictors of Clinical Effectiveness in Response to Omalizumab), a 48-week, prospective, multicenter, observational study, included patients (n = 806) who were 12 years-of-age and older who were initiating *omalizumab* treatment for moderate to severe allergic asthma, including patient with co-morbid COPD (n = 78). Researchers reported that *omalizumab* (**Xolair**) decreased asthma exacerbations and improved symptom control to a similar extent in patients with ACOS as seen in patients with asthma but no COPD. While patients with COPD typically experience annual declines in lung function, at least some of the ACOS patients in this study, which included one of the largest observational cohorts to date of patients with ACOS, showed preserved lung function after 48 weeks of *omalizumab* treatment (as demonstrated by improved post-bronchodilator FEV_1 at end of stud and asthma exacerbations numbers reduced from baseline though month 12, from 3 or more exacerbations in both ACOS and non-ACOS groups to 1.1 or less

REFERENCE
Hanania, N. (2017, November). *Omalizumab helps asthma COPD overlap patients.* Presented at the 2017 CHEST Annual Meeting in Toronto, Canada, as reported by Beck, DL. Family Practice News. http:// www.mdedge.com/familypracticenews/article/151778/copd/omalizumab-helps-asthma-copd-overlap-patients?channel=41038&utm_source=News_FPN_eNL_111617_F&utm_medium=email&utm_content=Omalizumab for asthma COPD overlap patients

IGE BLOCKER (IGG1K MONOCLONAL ANTIBODY)

▷ *omalizumab* (B) 150-375 mg SC every 2-4 weeks based on body weight and pre-treatment serum total IgE level; max 150 mg/injection site; should be administered only by a qualified health care provider
Pediatric: <12 years: not recommended; 30-90 kg + IgE >30-100 IU/ml 150 mg q 4 weeks; 90-150 kg + IgE >30-100 IU/ml or 30-90 kg + IgE >100-200 IU/ml or 30-60 kg + IgE >200-300 IU/ml 300 mg q 4 hours; >90-150 kg + IgE >100-200 IU/ml or >60-90 kg + IgE >200-300 IU/ml or 30-70 kg + IgE >300-400 IU/ml 225 mg q 2 weeks; >90-150 kg + IgE >200-300 IU/ml or >70-90 kg + IgE >300-400 IU/ml or 30-70 kg + IgE >400-500 IU/ml or 30-60 kg + IgE >500-600 IU/ml or 30-60 kg + IgE >600-700 IU/ml 375 mg q 2 weeks
  Xolair *Vial:* 150 mg, single-dose, pwdr for SC injection after reconstitution; *Prefilled syringe:* 75 mg/0.5 ml, 150 mg/1 ml, single-dose (preservative-free)

ASTHMA: SEVERE, EOSINOPHILIA

Comment: *tezepelumab* is a human IgG2 monoclonal antibody that binds to thymic stromal lymphopoietin (TSLP), which is a cytokine produced in response to environmental and pro-inflammatory stimuli. It is an important potential mechanism because it works high up in the inflammatory cascade appears to have a beneficial effect in patients across different asthma phenotypes. Currently available therapies for patients with severe asthma include anti-IgE therapy (*omalizumab*), and anti-interleukin-5 monoclonal antibodies (*mepolizumab* [**Nucala**], *reslizumab* [**Xolair**], and *benralizumab* [**Cinqair**]). The data on pregnancy exposure from the clinical trials are insufficient to inform on drug-associated risk. Monoclonal antibodies are transported across the placenta in a linear fashion as pregnancy progresses; therefore, potential effects on a fetus are likely to be greater during the second and third trimester of pregnancy. IgG is known to be present in human milk; however, effects on the breast fed infant are unknown.

INTERLEUKIN-4 RECEPTOR ALPHA ANTAGONIST

▷ *dupilumab* administer SC into the upper arm, abdomen, or thigh; rotate sites; initially 600 mg (2 x 300 mg injections at different sites) followed by 300 mg SC once every other week; may use with or without topical corticosteroids; may use with calcineurin inhibitors, but reserve only for problem areas (e.g., face, neck, intertriginous, and genital areas); avoid live vaccines.
Pediatric: <12 years: not recommended; ≥12 years: same as adult
  Dupixent *Prefilled syringe:* 300 mg/2 ml (2/pck without needle)(preservative-free)
  Comment: *dupilumab* is a human monoclonal IgG4 antibody that inhibits interleukin-4 (IL-4) and interleukin-13 (IL-13) signaling by specifically binding to the IL4Ra sub-unit shared by the IL-4 and IL-13 receptor complexes, thereby inhibiting the release of pro-inflammatory cytokines, chemokines, and IgE. *dupilumab* is indicated as an add-on maintenance therapy for patients ≥12 years-of-age with moderate-to-severe asthma with an eosinophilic subtype or with oral corticosteroid-dependent asthma.

HUMANIZED INTERLEUKIN-5 ANTAGONIST MONOCLONAL ANTIBODY

Interleukin-5 Antagonist Monoclonal Antibody (IgG1 Kappa)

▷ *mepolizumab* 100 mg SC once every 4 weeks in upper arm, abdomen, or thigh
Pediatric: <12 years: not recommended; ≥12 years: same as adult
  Nucala *Vial:* 100 mg pwdr for reconstitution, single-use (preservative-free)
  Comment: Nucala is an interleukin-5 antagonist monoclonal antibody (IgG1 kappa). It is an add-on maintenance treatment for patients ≥12 years-of-age with severe asthma and with an eosinophilic phenotype. **Nucala** is also indicated for the treatment of patients >18 years-of-age with eosinophilic granulomatosis with polyangiitis (EGPA). **Nucala** is not for relief of acute bronchospasm or status asthmaticus. Hypersensitivity reactions (e.g., anaphylaxis, angioedema, bronchospasm, hypotension, urticaria, rash) have occurred after administration of **Nucala**; discontinue **Nucala** in the event of a hypersensitivity reaction. Herpes zoster infections have occurred in patients receiving **Nucala**. Consider vaccination if medically appropriate. Do not discontinue systemic or inhaled corticosteroids abruptly upon initiation of therapy with **Nucala**. Decrease corticosteroids gradually, if appropriate. Treat patients with pre-existing parasitic helminth infections before therapy with **Nucala**. If patients become infected while receiving treatment with **Nucala** and do not respond to anti-helminth treatment,

discontinue **Nucala** until parasitic infection resolves. The most common adverse reactions (incidence ≥5%) include headache, injection site reaction, back pain, and fatigue. Formal drug interaction trials have not been performed with **Nucala**. The data on pregnancy exposure are insufficient to inform on drug-associated risk. Monoclonal antibodies, such as *mepolizumab*, are transported across the placenta in a linear fashion as pregnancy progresses; therefore, potential effects on a fetus are likely to be greater during the second and third trimester of pregnancy. There is a pregnancy exposure registry that monitors pregnancy outcomes in patients exposed to **Nucala** during pregnancy. Healthcare providers can enroll patients or encourage patients to enroll themselves by calling 1-877-311-8972 or visiting www.mothertobaby.org/asthma. There is no information regarding the presence of *mepolizumab* in human milk or effects on the breastfed infant. To report suspected adverse reactions, contact GlaxoSmithKline at 1-888-825-5249 or FDA at 1-800-FDA-1088 or www.fda.gov/medwatch.

Interleukin-5 Antagonist Monoclonal Antibody (IgG4 Kappa)

▶ **resilumab** should be administered by a qualified healthcare professional and, in line with clinical practice, monitoring of patients after administration of biologic agents is recommended; recommended dose is 3 mg/kg once every 4 weeks via IV infusion over 20-50 minutes; do not administer as an IV push (IVP) or bolus
Pediatric: <18 years: not established; ≥18 years: same as adult
  Cinqair *Vial:* 100 mg/10 ml (10 mg/ml) soln single-use (preservative-free)
  Comment: **Nucala** is an interleukin-5 antagonist monoclonal antibody (IgG1 kappa). It is an add-on maintenance treatment for patients ≥12 years-of-age with severe asthma and with an eosinophilic phenotype. **Nucala** is also indicated for the treatment of patients >18 years-of-age with eosinophilic granulomatosis with polyangiitis (EGPA). **Nucala** is not for relief of acute bronchospasm or status asthmaticus. Hypersensitivity reactions (e.g., anaphylaxis, angioedema, bronchospasm, hypotension, urticaria, rash) have occurred after administration of **Nucala**; discontinue **Nucala** in the event of a hypersensitivity reaction. Herpes zoster infections have occurred in patients receiving **Nucala**. Consider vaccination if medically appropriate. Do not discontinue systemic or inhaled corticosteroids abruptly upon initiation of therapy with **Nucala**. Decrease corticosteroids gradually, if appropriate. Treat patients with pre-existing parasitic helminth infections before therapy with **Nucala**. If patients become infected while receiving treatment with **Nucala** and do not respond to anthelminth treatment, discontinue **Nucala** until parasitic infection resolves. The most common adverse reactions (incidence ≥5%) include headache, injection site reaction, back pain, and fatigue. Formal drug interaction trials have not been performed with **Nucala**. The data on pregnancy exposure are insufficient to inform on drug-associated risk. Monoclonal antibodies, such as *mepolizumab*, are transported across the placenta in a linear fashion as pregnancy progresses; therefore, potential effects on a fetus are likely to be greater during the second and third trimester of pregnancy. There is a pregnancy exposure registry that monitors pregnancy outcomes in patients exposed to **Nucala** during pregnancy. Healthcare providers can enroll patients or encourage patients to enroll themselves by calling 1-877-311-8972 or visiting www.mothertobaby.org/asthma. There is no information regarding the presence of *mepolizumab* in human milk or effects on the breastfed infant. To report suspected adverse reactions, contact GlaxoSmithKline at 1-888-825-5249 or FDA at 1-800-FDA-1088 or www.fda.gov/medwatch.

INTERLEUKIN-5 RECEPTOR ALPHA-DIRECTED CYTOLYTIC MONOCLONAL ANTIBODY (IGG1, KAPPA)

▶ **benralizumab** should be administered by a qualified healthcare professional and, in line with clinical practice, monitoring of patients after administration of biologic agents is recommended; recommended dose is 30 mg SC every 4 weeks for the first 3 doses; then, once every 8 weeks thereafter; inject SC into the upper arm, abdomen, or thigh. Store in refrigerator; do not freeze; prior to administration, warm **Fasenra** by leaving carton at room temperature for about 30 minutes. Administer within 24 hours or discard into sharps container.
Pediatric: <12 years: not established; ≥12 years: same as adult
  Fasenra *Prefilled syringe:* 30 mg/ml single-dose
  Comment: Fasenra (*benralizumab*) is FDA approved for the add-on maintenance treatment of patients with severe asthma and an eosinophilic phenotype aged ≥12 years-of-age. The approval was based on the results of the WINDWARD program,

which included Phase 3 exacerbation trials and a Phase 3 oral corticosteroid-sparing trial. The trials showed that patients assigned to an 8-week *benralizumab* dosing regimen experienced up to a 51% reduction in annual asthma exacerbation rate, compared with placebo, significant improvement in lung function as measured by forced expiratory volume in one second compared with placebo, and a 75% median reduction in daily oral corticosteroid use and a discontinuation of oral corticosteroid use in 52% of eligible patients.

INTERLEUKIN-5 ANTAGONIST MONOCLONAL ANTIBODY (IGG4 KAPPA)

▷ *reslizumab* <18 years: not recommended; ≥18 years: 3 mg/kg once every 4 weeks by IV infusion over 20-50 minutes; do not administer as an IV push or bolus; should be administered in a healthcare setting by a qualified healthcare professional prepared to manage anaphylaxis

Cinqair *Vial:* 100 mg/10 ml (10 mg/ml) single-dose

Comment: Anaphylaxis occurred with **Cinqair** infusion in 0.3% of patients in placebo-controlled studies. Patients should be observed for an appropriate period of time after **Cinqair** infusion; healthcare professionals should be prepared to manage anaphylaxis. Discontinue **Cinqair** immediately if the patient experiences anaphylaxis. The most common adverse reaction (incidence greater than or equal to 2%) includes oropharyngeal pain.

IGE BLOCKER (IGG1K MONOCLONAL ANTIBODY)

▷ *omalizumab* (B) 150-375 mg SC every 2-4 weeks based on body weight and pre-treatment serum total IgE level; max 150 mg/injection site; should be administered only by a qualified health care provider
Pediatric: <12 years: not recommended; 30-90 kg + IgE >30-100 IU/ml 150 mg q 4 weeks; 90-150 kg + IgE >30-100 IU/ml or 30-90 kg + IgE >100-200 IU/ml or 30-60 kg + IgE >200-300 IU/ml 300 mg q 4 hours; >90-150 kg + IgE >100-200 IU/ml or >60-90 kg + IgE >200-300 IU/ml or 30-70 kg + IgE >300-400 IU/ml 225 mg q 2 weeks; >90-150 kg + IgE >200-300 IU/ml or >70-90 kg + IgE >300-400 IU/ml or 30-70 kg + IgE >400-500 IU/ml or 30-60 kg + IgE >500-600 IU/ml or 30-60 kg + IgE >600-700 IU/ml 375 mg q 2 weeks

Xolair *Vial:* 150 mg, single-dose, pwdr for SC injection after reconstitution; *Prefilled syringe:* 75 mg/0.5 ml, 150 mg/1 ml, single-dose (preservative-free)

INTERLEUKIN-5 RECEPTOR ALPHA-DIRECTED CYTOLYTIC MONOCLONAL ANTIBODY (IGG1,KAPPA)

▷ *benralizumab* should be administered by a qualified healthcare professional and, in line with clinical practice, monitoring of patients after administration of biologic agents is recommended; recommended dose is 30 mg SC every 4 weeks for the first 3 doses; then, once every 8 weeks thereafter; inject SC into the upper arm, abdomen, or thigh. Store in refrigerator; do not freeze; prior to administration, warm **Fasenra** by leaving carton at room temperature for about 30 minutes. Administer within 24 hours or discard into sharps container.
Pediatric: <12 years: not established; ≥12 years: same as adult

Fasenra *Prefilled syringe:* 30 mg/ml soln, single-dose (preservative-free)

Comment: *benralizumab* is an interleukin-5 receptor alpha-directed cytolytic monoclonal antibody (IgG1, kappa) produced in Chinese hamster ovary cells by recombinant DNA technology. **Fasenra** is indicated for the add-on maintenance treatment of patients with severe asthma ≥12 years-of-age, and with an neosinophilic phenotype. It is not for treatment of other eosinophilic conditions: Discontinue systemic or inhaled corticosteroids abruptly upon initiation of therapy with **Fasenra**; decrease corticosteroids gradually, if appropriate. Treat patients with pre-existing parasitic helminth infection before therapy with **Fasenra**. If patients become infected while receiving **Fasenra** and do not respond to anti-helminth treatment, discontinue **Fasenra** until the parasitic infection resolves. The most common adverse reactions (incidence ≥5%) include headache and pharyngitis. No formal drug interaction studies have been conducted. The data on pregnancy exposure from the clinical trials are insufficient to inform on drug-associated risk. Monoclonal antibodies such as *benralizumab* are transported across the placenta during the third trimester of pregnancy; therefore, potential effects on a fetus are likely to be greater during the third trimester of pregnancy.

In women with poorly or moderately controlled asthma, evidence demonstrates that there is an increased risk of preeclampsia in the mother and neonate prematurity, low birth weight, and small for gestational age. The level of asthma control should be closely monitored in pregnant females and treatment adjusted as necessary to maintain optimal control. There is no information regarding the presence of *benralizumab* in human or animal milk, and the effects of *benralizumab* on the breastfed infant and on milk production are not known. To report suspected adverse reactions, contact AstraZeneca at 1-800-236-9933 or FDA at 1-800-FDA-1088 or visit www.fda.gov/medwatch.

IgE BLOCKER (igG1K MONOCLONAL ANTIBODY)

➤ *omalizumab* (B) 150-375 mg SC every 2-4 weeks based on body weight and pre-treatment serum total IgE level; max 150 mg/injection site; should be administered only by a qualified health care provider
Pediatric: <12 years: not recommended; 30-90 kg + IgE >30-100 IU/ml 150 mg q 4 weeks; 90-150 kg + IgE >30-100 IU/ml or 30-90 kg + IgE >100-200 IU/ml or 30-60 kg + IgE >200-300 IU/ml 300 mg q 4 hours; >90-150 kg + IgE >100-200 IU/ml or >60-90 kg + IgE >200-300 IU/ml or 30-70 kg + IgE >300-400 IU/ml 225 mg q 2 weeks; >90-150 kg + IgE >200-300 IU/ml or >70-90 kg + IgE >300-400 IU/ml or 30-70 kg + IgE >400-500 IU/ml or 30-60 kg + IgE >500-600 IU/ml or 30-60 kg + IgE >600-700 IU/ml 375 mg q 2 weeks
    Xolair *Vial:* 150 mg pwdr single-dose for SC injection after reconstitution; *Prefilled syringe:* 75 mg/0.5 ml, 150 mg/1 ml single-dose (preservative-free)

INTERLEUKIN-4 RECEPTOR ALPHA ANTAGONIST

➤ *dupilumab* administer SC into the upper arm, abdomen, or thigh; rotate sites; initially 600 mg (2 x 300 mg injections at different sites) followed by 300 mg SC once every other week; may use with or without topical corticosteroids; may use with calcineurin inhibitors, but reserve only for problem areas (e.g., face, neck, intertriginous, and genital areas); avoid live vaccines
Pediatric: <12 years: not recommended; ≥12 years: same as adult
    Dupixent *Prefilled syringe:* 300 mg/2 ml (2/pck without needle) (preservative-free)
    Comment: *dupilumab* is a human monoclonal IgG4 antibody that inhibits interleukin-4 (IL-4) and interleukin-13 (IL-13) signaling by specifically binding to the IL4Ra subunit shared by the IL-4 and IL-13 receptor complexes, thereby inhibiting the release of pro-inflammatory cytokines, chemokines, and IgE. *dupilumab* is indicated as an add-on maintenance therapy for patients ≥12 years-of-age with moderate-to-severe asthma with an eosinophilic subtype or with oral corticosteroid-dependent asthma.

 ATROPHIC VAGINITIS

Oral Estrogens *see Menopause page* 301

VAGINAL ESTROGEN PREPARATIONS

➤ *estradiol* (X)(G)
    Vagifem Vaginal Tablet 1 tab intravaginally daily x 2 weeks; then 1 tab intravaginally twice weekly
      Vag tab: 10 mcg (15 tabs w. applicators)
    Yuvafem Vaginal Tablet 1 tab intravaginally daily x 2 weeks; then 1 tab intravaginally twice weekly
      Vag tab: 10 mcg (15 tabs w. applicators)
➤ *estradiol* (X)(G)
    Estrace Vaginal Cream 2-4 gm daily x 1-2 weeks; then gradually reduce to 1/2 initial dose x 1-2 weeks; then maintenance dose of 1 gm 1-3 x/week
      Vag crm: 0.01% (1 oz tube w. calib applicator)
➤ *estrogens, conjugated* (X)
    Premarin Cream 2 gm/day intravaginally
      Vag crm: 1.5 oz w. applicator marked in 1/2 gm increments to max 2 gm
➤ *estropipate* (X)
    Ogen Cream 2-4 gm intravaginally daily x 3 weeks; discontinue 4th week; continue in this cyclical pattern
      Vag crm: 1.5 mg/gm (42.5 gm w. calib applicator)

SELECTIVE NOREPINEPHRINE REUPTAKE INHIBITORS (SNRIs)

▷ *atomoxetine* (C)(G) take one dose daily in the morning or in two divided doses in the morning and late afternoon or early evening; initially 40 mg/kg; increase after at least 3 days to 80 mg/kg; then after 2-4 weeks may increase to max 100 mg/day
Pediatric: <6 years: not recommended; ≥6 years, <70 kg: initially 0.5 mg/kg/day: increase after at least 3 days to 1.2 mg/kg/day; max 1.4 mg/kg/day or 100 mg/day (whichever is less); ≥6 years, >70 kg: same as adult

Strattera *Cap:* 10, 18, 25, 40, 60, 80, 100 mg

Comment: **Strattera** is not associated with stimulant or euphoric effects. May discontinue without tapering. Common adverse effects associated with *atomoxetine* in children and adolescents included upset stomach, decreased appetite, nausea or vomiting, dizziness, tiredness, and mood swings. For adult patients, the most common adverse side effects included constipation, dry mouth, nausea, decreased appetite, sexual side effects, problems passing urine, and dizziness. Other adverse effects associated with *atomoxetine* included severe liver damage and potential for serious cardiovascular events. In addition, *atomoxetine* increases the risk of suicidal ideation in children and adolescents. Health Care providers should monitor patients taking this medication for clinical worsening, suicidality, and unusual changes in behavior, particularly within the first few months of initiation or during dose changes.

STIMULANTS

▷ *amphetamine, mixed salts of single entity amphetamine* (C)(II)

Adzenys ER initially 12.5 mg (10 ml) once daily in the morning; take with or without food; individualize the dosage according to the therapeutic needs and response
Pediatric: <6 years: not recommended; 6-17 years: take with or without food; individualize the dosage according to the therapeutic needs and response; 6-12 years: initially 6.3 mg (5 ml) once daily in the morning; max dose 18.8 mg (15 ml); 13-17 years:12.5 mg (10 ml) once daily in the morning; ≥17 years: same as adult

Oral susp: 125 mg/ml ext-rel (450 ml) (orange)

Comment: Patients taking **Adderall XR** may be switched to **Adzenys ER** at the equivalent dose taken once daily; switching from any other amphetamine products (e.g., **Adderall** immediate-release), discontinue that treatment, and titrate with **Adzenys ER** using the titration schedule (see mfr pkg insert). To avoid substitution errors and overdosage, do not substitute for other amphetamine products on a mg-per-mg basis because of different amphetamine salt compositions and differing pharmacokinetic profiles. No dosage adjustments for renal or hepatic insufficiency are provided in the manufacturer's labeling.

Adzenys XR-ODT take with or without food; individualize the dosage according to the therapeutic needs and response; initially 12.5 mg once daily; max recommended dose 18.8 mg once daily
Pediatric: <6 years: not recommended; ≥6 years: take with or without food; individualize the dosage according to the therapeutic needs and response; 6-12 years: initially 6.3 mg once daily in the morning; increase in increments of 3.1 mg or 6.3 mg at weekly intervals; max recommended dose 18.8 mg once daily; ≥13 years: 12.5 mg (10 ml) once daily in the morning

Comment: Patients taking **Adderall XR** may be switched to **Adzenys XR-ODT** at the equivalent dose taken once daily; switching from any other amphetamine products (e.g., **Adderall** immediate-release), discontinue that treatment, and titrate with **Adzenys XR-ODT** using the titration schedule (see mfr pkg insert). To avoid substitution errors and overdosage, do not substitute for other amphetamine products on a mg-per-mg basis because of different amphetamine salt compositions and differing pharmacokinetic profiles. No dosage adjustments for renal or hepatic insufficiency are provided in the manufacturer's labeling.

Dyanavel XR Oral Suspension <6 years: not recommended; ≥6 years: initially 2.5 mg or 5 mg once daily in the morning; may increase in increments of 2.5 mg to 5 mg per day every 4-7 days; max 20 mg per day; shake bottle prior to administration

Oral susp: 2.5 mg/ml (464 ml) ext-rel

Evekeo <3 years: not recommended; ≥3-5 years: initially 2.5 mg once or twice daily at the same time(s) each day; may increase by 2.5 mg/day at weekly intervals; max 40 mg/day; >5 years: initially 5 mg once or twice daily at the same time(s) each day; may increase by 5 mg/day at weekly intervals; max 40 mg/day

Tab: 5, 10 mg

Mydayis initially 12.5 mg once daily in the morning; may titrate at weekly intervals; max 50 mg/day

Pediatric: <13 years: not recommended; 13-17 years: initially 12.5 mg once daily in the morning; may titrate at weekly intervals; max 25 mg/day; >17 years: same as adult

Cap: 12.5, 25, 37.5, 50 mg ext-rel

▷ *dexmethylphenidate* (C)(II)(G) not indicated for adults

Focalin <6 years: not established; ≥6 years: initially 2.5 mg bid; allow at least 4 hours between doses; may increase at 1 week intervals; max 20 mg/day

Tab: 2.5, 5, 10*mg (dye-free)

Focalin ER <6 years: not established; ≥6 years: initially 5 mg weekly; usual dose 10-30 mg/day

Cap: 15, 30 mg ext-rel

Focalin XR <6 years: not established; ≥6 years: initially 5 mg weekly; usual dose 10-30 mg/day

Cap: 5, 10, 15, 20, 25, 30, 35, 40 mg ext-rel

▷ *dextroamphetamine sulfate* (C)(II)(G) initially start with 10 mg daily; increase by 10 mg at weekly intervals if needed; may switch to daily dose with sust-rel spansules when titrated

Pediatric: <3 years: not recommended; ≥3-5 years: 2.5 mg daily; may increase by 2.5 mg daily at weekly intervals if needed; 6-12 years: initially 5 mg daily or bid; may increase by 5 mg/day at weekly intervals; usual max 40 mg/day; >12 years: initially 10 mg daily; may increase by 10 mg/day at weekly intervals; max 40 mg/day

Dexedrine *Tab:* 5*mg (tartrazine)

Dexedrine Spansule *Cap:* 5, 10, 15 mg ext-rel

Dextrostat *Tab:* 5, 10 mg (tartrazine)

▷ *dextroamphetamine saccharate+dextroamphetamine sulfate+amphetamine aspartate+amphetamine sulfate* (C)(II)(G) not indicated for adults

Adderall initially 10 mg daily; may increase weekly by 10 mg/day; usual max 60 mg/day in 2-3 divided doses; first dose on awakening; then q 4-6 hours prn

Pediatric: <6 years: not indicated; ≥6-12 years: initially 5 mg daily; may increase by 5 mg/day at weekly intervals; >12 years: same as adult

Tab: 5**, 7.5**, 10**, 12.5**, 15**, 20**, 30**mg

Adderall XR 20 mg by mouth once daily in AM; may increase by 10 mg/day at weekly intervals; max: 60 mg/day

Pediatric: <6 years: not recommended; ≥6 years: initially 10 mg daily in the AM; may increase by 10 mg/day at weekly intervals; max 30 mg/day; 13-17 years: 10-20 mg by mouth daily in the AM; may increase by 10 mg/day at weekly intervals; max 40 mg/day; Do not chew; may sprinkle on apple sauce

Cap: 5, 10, 15, 20, 25, 30 mg ext-rel

▷ *lisdexamfetamine dimesylate* (C)(II) 30 mg once daily in the AM; may increase by 10-20 mg/day at weekly intervals; max 70 mg/day

Pediatric: <6 years: not recommended; ≥6 years: same as adult

Vyvanse *Cap:* 20, 30, 40, 50, 60, 70 mg

Comment: May dissolve **Vyvanse** capsule contents in water; take immediately.

▷ *methylphenidate (regular-acting)* (C)(II)(G)

Methylin, Methylin Chewable, Methylin Oral Solution usual dose 20-30 mg/day in 2-3 divided doses 30-45 minutes before a meal; max 60 mg/day

Pediatric: <6 years: not recommended; ≥6 years: initially 5 mg bid ac (breakfast and lunch); may increase 5-10 mg/day at weekly intervals; max 60 mg/day

Tab: 5, 10*, 20*mg; *Chew tab:* 2.5, 5, 10 mg; (grape) (phenylalanine); *Oral soln:* 5, 10 mg/5 ml (grape)

Ritalin 10-60 mg/day in 2-3 divided doses 30-45 minutes ac; max 60 mg/day

Pediatric: <6 years: not recommended; ≥6 years: initially 5 mg bid ac (breakfast and lunch); may increase by 5-10 mg/day at weekly intervals as needed; max 60 mg/day

Tab: 5, 10*, 20*mg

▷ *methylphenidate (long-acting)* (C)(II)
    Concerta initially 18 mg q AM; may increase in 18 mg increments as needed; max 54 mg/day; do not crush or chew
    Pediatric: <6 years: not recommended; ≥6-12 years: initially 18 mg daily; max 54 mg/day; ≥13-17 years: initially 18 mg daily; max 72 mg/day or 2 mg/kg, whichever is less
      Tab: 18, 27, 36, 54 mg sust-rel
    Cotempla XR-ODT take consistently with or without food in the morning
    Pediatric: <6 years: not recommended; 6-17 years: initially 8.6 mg; may increase as needed and tolerated by 8.6 mg/day; daily dosage >51.8 mg is not recommended.
      ODT: 8.6, 17.3, 25.9 mg ext-rel orally-disint
    Metadate CD (G) 1 cap daily in the AM; may sprinkle on food; do not crush or chew
    Pediatric: <6 years: not recommended; ≥6 years: initially 20 mg daily; may gradually increase by 20 mg/day at weekly intervals as needed; max 60 mg/day
      Cap: 10, 20, 30, 40, 50, 60 mg immed- and ext-rel beads
    Metadate ER 1 tab daily in the AM; do not crush or chew
    Pediatric: <6 years: not recommended; ≥6 years: use in place of regular-acting *methylphenidate* when the 8-hour dose of **Metadate-ER** corresponds to the titrated 8-hour dose of regular-acting *methylphenidate*
      Tab: 10, 20 mg ext-rel (dye-free)
    QuilliChew ER (G) initially 1 x 10 mg chew tab once daily in the AM
    Pediatric: <6 years: not recommended; initially 10 mg daily; may gradually increase by 20 mg/day at weekly intervals as needed; max 60 mg/day
      Chew tab: 20*, 30*40 mg ext-rel
    Quillivant XR (G) initially 20 mg once daily in the AM, with or without food; may be titrated in increments of 10-20 mg/day at weekly intervals; daily doses above 60 mg have not been studied and are not recommended; shake the bottle vigorously for at least 10 seconds to ensure that the correct dose is administered
    Pediatric: <6 years: not recommended; ≥6 years: same as adult
      Bottle: 5 mg/ml, 25 mg/5 ml pwdr for reconstitution; 300 mg (60 ml), 600 mg (120 ml), 750 mg (150 ml), 900 mg (180 ml)
    Comment: Quillivant XR must be reconstituted by a pharmacist, not by the patient or caregiver.
    Ritalin LA (G) 1 cap daily in the AM
    Pediatric: <6 years: not recommended; ≥6 years: use in place of regular-acting *methylphenidate* when the 8-hour dose of **Ritalin LA** corresponds to the titrated 8-hour dose of regular-acting *methylphenidate*; max 60 mg/day
      Cap: 10, 20, 30, 40 mg ext-rel (immed- and ext-rel beads)
    Ritalin SR 1 cap daily in the AM
    Pediatric: <6 years: not recommended; ≥6 years: use in place of regular-acting *methylphenidate* when the 8-hour dose of **Ritalin SR** corresponds to the titrated 8-hour dose of regular-acting *methylphenidate*; max 60 mg/day
      Tab: 20 mg sust-rel (dye-free)
▷ *methylphenidate* (transdermal patch) (C)(II)(G)
    Pediatric: <6 years: not recommended; ≥6-17 years: initially 10 mg patch applied to hip 2 hours before desired effect daily in the AM; may increase by 5-10 mg at weekly intervals; max 60 mg/day; >17 years: not applicable
      Daytrana *Transdermal patch:* 10, 15, 20, 30 mg
▷ *pemoline* (B)(IV) 18.75-112.5 mg/day; usually start with 37.5 mg in AM; may increase 18.75 mg/day at weekly intervals; max 112.5 gm/day
    Pediatric: <6 years: not recommended; ≥6 years: same as adult
      Cylert *Tab:* 18.75*, 37.5*, 75*mg
      Cylert Chewable *Chew tab:* 37.5*mg
    Comment: Check baseline serum ALT and monitor every 2 weeks thereafter.

CENTRAL ALPHA-2 AGONIST

▷ *guanfacine* (B)(G)
    Pediatric: <6 years: not recommended; ≥6-17 years: initially 1 mg once daily; may increase by 1 mg/day at weekly intervals; usual max 4 mg/day; >17 years: not applicable
    Intuniv *Tab:* 1, 2, 3, 4 mg ext-rel
    Comment: Take **Intuniv** with water, milk, or other liquid. Do not take with a high-fat meal. Withdraw gradually by 1 mg every 3-7 days.

TRICYCLIC ANTIDEPRESSANTS (TCAs)
see Depression page 117

OTHER AGENTS
▶ *clonidine* (C)(G)
>
> **Catapres** 4-5 mcg/kg/day
> *Pediatric:* <12 years: not recommended; ≥12 years: same as adult
>> *Tab:* 0.1*, 0.2*, 0.3*mg
>
> **Catapres-TTS** <12 years: not recommended; ≥12 years: initially 0.1 mg patch weekly;
> increase after 1-2 weeks if needed; max 0.6 mg/day
>> *Patch:* 0.1, 0.2 mg/day (12/carton); 0.3 mg/day (4/carton)
>
> **Kapvay** not indicated for adults
> *Pediatric:* <6 years: not recommended; ≥6-12 years: initially 0.1 mg at bedtime x 1
> week; then 0.1 mg bid x 1 week; then 0.1 mg AM and 0.2 mg PM x 1 week; then 0.2 mg
> bid; withdraw gradually by 0.1 mg/day at 3-7 day intervals
>> *Tab:* 0.1, 0.2 mg ext-rel
>
> **Nexiclon XR** initially 0.18 mg (2 ml) suspension or 0.17 mg tab once daily; usual max
> 0.52 mg (6 ml suspension) once daily
> *Pediatric:* <12 years: not recommended; ≥12 years: same as adult
>> *Tab:* 0.17, 0.26 mg ext-rel; *Oral susp:* 0.09 mg/ml ext-rel (4 oz)

AMINOKETONES (FOR THE TREATMENT OF ADHD)
▶ *bupropion HBr* (C)(G) initially 100 mg bid for at least 3 days; may increase to 375 or 400
mg/day after several weeks; then after at least 3 more days, 450 mg in 4 divided doses; max
450 mg/day, 174 mg/single dose
Pediatric: <18 years: not recommended; ≥18 years: Safety and effectiveness in the pediatric
population have not been established. When considering the use of **Aplenzin** in a child or
adolescent, balance the potential risks with the clinical need
> **Aplenzin** *Tab:* 174, 348, 522 mg

▶ *bupropion HCl* (C)(G)
Forfivo XL do not use for initial treatment; use immediate-release *bupropion* forms for
initial titration; switch to **Forfivo XL** 450 mg once daily when total dose/day reaches 450
mg; may switch to **Forfivo XL** when total dose/day reaches 300 mg for 2 weeks and patient
needs 450 mg/day to reach therapeutic target; swallow whole, do not crush or chew
> *Pediatric:* <18 years: not recommended; >18 years: same as adult; Safety and effective-
> ness of long-acting and extended-release *bupropion* in the pediatric population have
> not been established. When considering the use of **Forfivo XL** in a child or adolescent,
> balance the potential risks with the clinical need
>> *Tab:* 450 mg ext-rel
>
> **Wellbutrin** initially 100 mg bid for at least 3 days; may increase to 375 or 400 mg/day
> after several weeks; then after at least 3 more days, 450 mg in 4 divided doses; max 450
> mg/day, 150 mg/single dose
> *Pediatric:* <12 years: not recommended; ≥12 years: same as adult
>> *Tab:* 75, 100 mg
>
> **Wellbutrin SR** initially 150 mg in AM for at least 3 days; may increase to 150 mg bid if
> well tolerated; usual dose 300 mg/day; max 400 mg/day
> *Pediatric:* <12 years: not recommended; ≥12 years: same as adult
>> *Tab:* 100, 150 mg sust-rel
>
> **Wellbutrin XL** initially 150 mg in AM for at least 3 days; increase to 150 mg bid if well
> tolerated; usual dose 300 mg/day; max 400 mg/day
> *Pediatric:* <12 years: not recommended; ≥12 years: same as adult
>> *Tab:* 150, 300 mg sust-rel

BACTERIAL ENDOCARDITIS: PROPHYLAXIS

Comment: Bacterial endocarditis prophylaxis is appropriate for persons with a history of
previous infective endocarditis, persons with a prosthetic cardiac valve or prosthetic material
used for valve repair, cardiac transplant patients who develop cardiac valvulopathy, congenital
heart disease (CHD), unrepaired cyanotic CHD including palliative shunts and conduits,

completely repaired congenital heart defect(s) with prosthetic material or device, whether placed by surgery or by catheter intervention, during the first 6 months after the procedure, repaired CHD with residual defects at the site or adjacent to the site of a prosthetic patch or prosthetic device (which may inhibit endothelialization), or any other condition deemed to place a patient at high risk.

DENTAL, ORAL, RESPIRATORY TRACT, ESOPHAGEAL PROCEDURES

▷ *amoxicillin* (B)(G) 2 gm PO 30-60 minutes before procedure as a single dose or 3 gm 1 hour before procedure and 1.5 gm 6 hours later
Pediatric: 50 mg/kg as a single dose or 50 mg/kg (max 3 gm) 1 hour before procedure and (max 1.5 gm) 25 mg/kg 6 hours later; ≥40 kg: same as adult; *see pages 617–618 for dose by weight*
    Amoxil *Cap:* 250, 500 mg; *Tab:* 875*mg; *Chew tab:* 125, 200, 250, 400 mg (cherry-banana-peppermint) (phenylalanine); *Oral susp:* 125, 250 mg/5 ml (80, 100, 150 ml) (strawberry); 200, 400 mg/5 ml (50, 75, 100 ml) (bubble gum); *Oral drops:* 50 mg/ml (30 ml) (bubble gum)
    Trimox *Tab:* 125, 250 mg; *Cap:* 250, 500 mg; *Oral susp:* 125, 250 mg/5 ml (80, 100, 150 ml) (raspberry-strawberry)

▷ *ampicillin* (B)(G) 2 gm PO/IM/IV 30-60 minutes before procedure
Pediatric: <12 years: 50 mg/kg PO/IM/IV 30-60 minutes before procedure; ≥12 years: same as adult
    Omnipen, Principen *Cap:* 250, 500 mg; *Oral susp:* 125, 250 mg/5 ml (100, 150, 200 ml) (fruit)
    Unasyn *Vial:* 1.5, 3 gm

▷ *azithromycin* (B)(G) 500 mg 30-60 minutes before procedure
Pediatric: <12 years: 15 mg/kg 30-60 minutes before procedure; max 500 mg; *see page 619 for dose by weight*; ≥12 years: same as adult
    Zithromax *Tab:* 250, 500, 600 mg; *Oral susp:* 100 mg/5 ml (15 ml); 200 mg/5 ml (15, 22.5, 30 ml) (cherry)

▷ *cefazolin* (B) 1 gm IM/IV 30-60 minutes before procedure
Pediatric: <12 years: 25 mg/kg IM/IV 30-60 minutes before procedure; ≥12 years: same as adult
    Ancef *Vial:* 250, 500 mg; 1, 5 gm
    Kefzol *Vial:* 500 mg; 1 gm

▷ *ceftriaxone* (B)(G) 1 gm IM/IV as a single dose
Pediatric: <12 years: 50 mg/kg IM/IV as a single dose; ≥12 years: same as adult
    Rocephin *Vial:* 250, 500 mg; 1, 2 gm

▷ *cephalexin* (B)(G) 2 gm as a single dose 30-60 minutes before procedure
Pediatric: 50 mg/kg as a single dose 30-60 minutes before procedure; *see page 623 for dose by weight*
    Keflex *Cap:* 250, 333, 500, 750 mg; *Oral susp:* 125, 250 mg/5 ml (100, 200 ml) (strawberry) w

▷ *clarithromycin* (C)(G) 500 mg or 500 mg ext-rel as a single dose 30-60 minutes before procedure
Pediatric: 15 mg/kg as a single dose 30-60 minutes before procedure; *see page 624 for dose by weight*
    Biaxin *Tab:* 250, 500 mg
    Biaxin Oral Suspension *Oral susp:* 125, 250 mg/5 ml (50, 100 ml) (fruit-punch)
    Biaxin XL *Tab:* 500 mg ext-rel

Comment: The FDA is advising caution before prescribing *clarithromycin* to patients with heart disease because of a potential increased risk of heart problems or death that can occur years later. This recommendation is based on a review of the results of a 10-year follow-up study of patients with coronary heart disease from a large clinical trial that first observed this safety issue. Consider risk benefit and the use of other antibiotics in such patients.

▷ *clindamycin* (B)(G) 600 mg PO as a one-time single-dose or 300 mg 30-60 minutes before procedure and 150 mg 6 hours later; take with a full glass of water
Pediatric: <12 years: 20 mg/kg (max 300 mg) 1 hour before procedure and 10 mg/kg (max 150 mg) 6 hours later; take with a full glass of water; *see page 624 for dose by weight*; ≥12 years: same as adult
    Cleocin (G) *Cap:* 75 (tartrazine), 150 (tartrazine), 300 mg; *Vial:* 150 mg/ml (2, 4 ml) (benzyl alcohol)
    Cleocin Pediatric Granules (G) *Oral susp:* 75 mg/ml (100 ml) (cherry)

➤ **erythromycin estolate** (B)(G) 1 gm 1 hour before procedure; then 500 mg 6 hours later
  Pediatric: <12 years: 20 mg/kg 1 hour before procedure; then 10 mg/kg 6 hours later; *see page 625 for dose by weight*; ≥12 years: same as adult
  Ilosone *Pulvule:* 250 mg; *Tab:* 500 mg; *Liq:* 125, 250 mg/5 ml (100 ml)
  Comment: *erythromycin* may increase INR with concomitant *warfarin*, as well as increase serum level of *digoxin*, benzodiazepines, and statins.
➤ **penicillin v potassium** (B)(G) 2 gm 1 hour before procedure; then 1 gm 6 hours later or 2 gm 1 hour before procedure; then 1 gm q 6 hours x 8 doses
  Pediatric: <12 years, <60 lb: 1 gm 1 hour before procedure; then 500 mg 6 hours later or 1 gm 1 hour before procedure; then 500 mg q 6 hours x 8 doses; *see page 629 for dose by weight*; ≥12 years: same as adult
  Pen-Vee K *Tab:* 250, 500 mg; *Oral soln:* 125 mg/5 ml (100, 200 ml); 250 mg/5 ml (100, 150, 200 ml)

BACTERIAL VAGINOSIS (BV, *GARDNERELLA VAGINALIS*)

PROPHYLAXIS AND RESTORATION OF VAGINAL ACIDITY

➤ **acetic acid+oxyquinolone** (C) one full applicator intravaginally bid for up to 30 days
  Pediatric: <12 years: not recommended; ≥12 years: same as adult
  Relagard *Gel:* acet acid 0.9%+oxyq 0.025% (50 gm tube w. applicator)
  Comment: The following treatment regimens for *bacterial vaginosis* are published in the 2015 CDC **Sexually Transmitted Diseases Treatment Guidelines**. Treatment regimens are presented by generic drug name first, followed by information about brands and dose forms. BV is associated with adverse pregnancy outcomes, including premature rupture of the membranes, preterm labor, preterm birth, intra-amniotic infection, and postpartum endometritis. Therefore, treatment is recommended for all pregnant women with symptoms or positive screen.

RECOMMENDED REGIMENS
Regimen 1
➤ **metronidazole** 500 mg bid x 7 days or **metronidazole** ext-rel 750 mg once daily x 7 days

Regimen 2
➤ **metronidazole** gel 0.75% one applicatorful (5 gm) once daily x 5 days

Regimen 3
➤ **clindamycin** cream 2% one full applicatorful (5 gm) intravaginally once daily at bedtime x 5 days

ALTERNATE REGIMENS
Regimen 1
➤ **tinidazole** 2 gm once daily x 2 days

Regimen 2
➤ **tinidazole** 1 gm once daily x 5 days

Regimen 3
➤ **clindamycin** 300 mg bid x 7 days

Regimen 4
➤ **clindamycin** ovules 100 mg intravaginally once daily at bedtime x 3 days

Regimen 5
➤ **secnidazole** one 2 gm packet as a single dose

Drug Brands and Dose Forms
➤ **clindamycin** (B)
  Cleocin (G) *Cap:* 75 (tartrazine), 150 (tartrazine), 300 mg
  Cleocin Pediatric Granules (G) *Oral susp:* 75 mg/5 ml (100 ml) (cherry)

Cleocin Vaginal Cream *Vag crm:* 2% (21, 40 gm tubes w. applicator)
Cleocin Vaginal Ovules *Vag supp:* 100 mg

▷ *metronidazole* (not for use in 1st; B in 2nd, 3rd)
Flagyl *Tab:* 250*, 500*mg
Flagyl 375 *Cap:* 375 mg
Flagyl ER *Tab:* 750 mg ext-rel
MetroGel-Vaginal, Vandazole *Vag gel:* 0.75% (70 gm w. applicator) (parabens)

▷ *secnidazole*
Solosec *Oral granules:* 2 gm/pkt
Comment: Solosec is a nitromidazole antimicrobial. Do not dissolve **Solosec** in liquid. Sprinkle contents onto applesauce, yogurt or pudding. Consume within 30 mins without chewing or crunching. May follow with a glass of water. Potential adverse side effects are vulvovaginal pruritus, vulvovaginal candidiasis, headache, nausea, dysgeusia, vomiting, diarrhea, and abdominal pain. Not recommended in pregnancy. Breast-feeding is not recommended during and for 96 hours after dose; may pump and discard milk during this time period.

▷ *tinidazole* (C)
Tindamax *Tab:* 250*, 500*mg
Comment: Other than for use in the treatment of *giardiasis* and *amebiasis* in pediatric patients >3 years-of-age, safety and effectiveness of *tinidazole* in pediatric patients have not been established. *tinidazole* is excreted in breast milk in concentrations similar to those seen in serum and can be detected in breast milk for up to 72 hours following administration. Interruption of breast-feeding is recommended during *tinidazole* therapy and for 3 days following the last dose.

BALDNESS: MALE PATTERN

TYPE II 5-ALPHA-REDUCTASE SPECIFIC INHIBITOR

▷ *finasteride* (X)(G) 1 mg daily
Propecia *Tab:* 1 mg
Comment: Pregnant women should not touch broken *finasteride* tabs. Use of **Propecia**, a 5-alpha reductase inhibitor, is associated with low but increased risk of high-grade prostate cancer.

PERIPHERAL VASODILATOR

▷ *minoxidil* topical soln (C)(G) 1 ml from dropper or 6 sprays bid
Pediatric: <18 years: not recommended; ≥18 years: same as adult
Rogaine for Men (OTC) *Regular soln:* 2% (60 ml w. applicator) (alcohol 60%); *Extra strength soln:* 5% (60 ml w. applicator) (alcohol 30%)
Rogaine for Women (OTC) *Regular soln:* 2% (60 ml w. applicator) (alcohol 60%); *Topical aerosol:* 5%
Comment: Do not use *minoxidil* on abraded or inflamed scalp.

BELL'S PALSY

▷ *prednisone* (C)(G) 80 mg once daily x 3 days; then 60 mg daily x 3 days; then 40 mg daily x 3 days; then 20 mg x 1 dose; then discontinue
Pediatric: <18 years: oral suspension options by weight
Deltasone *Tab:* 2.5*, 5*, 10*, 20*, 50*mg

BENIGN ESSENTIAL TREMOR

ANTI-PARKINSON'S AGENT

▷ *amantadine* (C)(G) 200 mg daily or 100 mg bid; 4 tsp of syrup once daily or 2 tsp bid
Symmetrel *Tab:* 100 mg; *Syr:* 50 mg/5 ml (raspberry)

BETA-BLOCKER

▷ *propranolol* (C)(G)
Inderal initially 40 mg bid; usual range 160-240 mg/day
Tab: 10*, 20*, 40*, 60*, 80*mg

Inderal LA initially 80 mg once daily in a single dose; increase q 3-7 days; usual range 120-160 mg/day; max 320 mg/day in a single dose
Cap: 60, 80, 120, 160 mg sust-rel
InnoPran XL initially 80 mg q HS; max 120 mg/day
Cap: 80, 120 mg ext-rel

BENIGN PROSTATIC HYPERPLASIA (BPH)

ALPHA-1 BLOCKERS

Comment: Educate patient regarding potential side effect of hypotension especially with first dose. Usually start at lowest dose and titrate upward.

▷ *doxazosin* (C)
   Cardura initially 1 mg daily; may double dose every 1-2 weeks; max 8 mg/day
   Tab: 1*, 2*, 4*, 8*mg
   Cardura XL initially 4 mg once daily with breakfast; may titrate after 3-4 weeks; max 8 mg/day
   Tab: 4, 8 mg ext-rel
▷ *silodosin* (B)(G) 8 mg once daily; *CrCl 30-50 mL/min:* 4 mg once daily
   Rapaflo *Cap:* 4, 8 mg
▷ *terazosin* (C)(G) initially 1 mg q HS; titrate up to 10 mg once daily; max 20 mg/day
   Hytrin *Cap:* 1, 2, 5, 10 mg

ALPHA-1A BLOCKERS

▷ *alfuzosin* (B)(G) 10 mg once daily taken immediately after the same meal each day
   UroXatral *Tab:* 10 mg ext-rel
▷ *tamsulosin* (B)(G) initially 0.4 mg once daily; may increase to 0.8 mg daily after 2-4 weeks if needed
   Flomax *Cap:* 0.4 mg
   Comment: May take **Flomax** 0.4 mg plus **Imitrex** 0.5 mg once daily as combination therapy.

TYPE II 5-ALPHA-REDUCTASE INHIBITOR

Comment: Pregnant women and women of childbearing age should not handle *finasteride*. Monitor for potential side effects of decreased libido and/or impotence. Low, but increased risk of being diagnosed with high-grade prostate cancer.
▷ *finasteride* (X) 5 mg once daily
   Proscar *Tab:* 5 mg

TYPES I AND II 5-ALPHA-REDUCTASE INHIBITOR

Comment: Pregnant women and women of childbearing age should not handle *dutasteride*. Monitor for potential side effects of decreased libido and/or impotence. Low, but increased risk of being diagnosed with high-grade prostate cancer.
▷ *dutasteride* (X)(G) 0.5 mg once daily
   Avodart *Cap:* 0.5 mg
   Comment: May take **Avodart** 0.5 mg with **Flomax** 0.4 mg once daily as combination therapy.

TYPE I AND II 5-ALPHA-REDUCTASE INHIBITOR+ALPHA-1A BLOCKER

▷ *dutasteride+tamsulosin* (X)(G) take 1 cap once daily after the same meal each day
   Jalyn *Cap:* duta 0.5 mg+tam 0.4 mg

PHOSPHODIESTERASE TYPE 5 (PDE5) INHIBITORS, CGMP-SPECIFIC

Comment: Oral PDE5 inhibitors are contraindicated in patients taking nitrates. Caution with history of recent MI, stroke, life-threatening arrhythmia, hypotension, hypertension, cardiac failure, unstable angina, retinitis pigmentosa, CYP3A4 inhibitors (e.g., *cimetidine*, the azoles, *erythromycin*, grapefruit juice), protease inhibitors (e.g., *ritonavir*), CYP3A4 inducers (e.g., *rifampin, carbamazepine, phenytoin, phenobarbital*), alcohol, antihypertensive agents. Side effects include headache, flushing, nasal congestion, rhinitis, dyspepsia, and diarrhea.

▷ **tadalafil** (B)(G) 5 mg once daily at the same time each day; *CrCl 30-50 mL/min:* initially 2.5 mg; *CrCl <30 mL/min:* not recommended; *Concomitant alpha blockers:* not recommended

    Cialis *Tab:* 2.5, 5, 10, 20 mg

 BILE ACID DEFICIENCY

BILE ACID

▷ **ursodiol** (B)
    Dissolution of radiolucent non-calcified gallstones <20 mm diameter: 8-10 mg/kg/day in 2-3 divided doses; *Prevention:* 13-15 mg/kg/day in 4 divided doses
    Pediatric: <12 years: not recommended; ≥12 years: same as adult
      Actigall *Cap:* 300 mg
    Comment: *ursodiol* decreases the amount of cholesterol produced by the liver and absorbed by the intestines. It helps break down cholesterol that has formed into stones in the gallbladder. *ursodiol* increases bile flow in patients with primary biliary cirrhosis. It is used to treat small gallstones in people who cannot have cholecystectomy surgery and to prevent gallstones in overweight patients undergoing rapid weight loss. *ursodiol* is not for treating gallstones that are calcified.

BINGE EATING DISORDER

CENTRAL NERVOUS SYSTEM (CNS) STIMULANT

▷ **lisdexamfetamine dimesylate** (C)(II) swallow whole or may open and mix/dissolve contents of cap in yogurt, water, orange juice and take immediately; 30 mg once daily in the AM; may adjust in increments of 20 mg at weekly intervals; target dose 50-70 mg/day; max 70 mg/day; *GFR 15-<30 mL/min:* max 50 mg/day; *GFR <15 mL/min, ESRD:* max 30 mg/day
    Pediatric: <18 years: not established; ≥18 years: same as adult
      Vyvanse *Cap:* 10, 20, 30, 40, 50, 60 70 mg
      Comment: Vyvanse is not approved or recommended for weight loss treatment of obesity.

BIPOLAR DISORDER

Comment: Bipolar I Disorder is characterized by one or more manic episodes that last at least a week or require hospitalization. Severe mania may manifest symptoms of psychosis. Bipolar II Disorder is characterized by one or more depressive episodes accompanied by at least one hypomanic episode. When one parent has Bipolar Disorder, the risk to each child of developing the disorder is estimated to be 15-30%. When both parents have the disorder, the risk to each child increases to 50-75%. Symptoms of mood disorders may be difficult to diagnose in children and adolescents because they can be mistaken for age-appropriate emotions and behaviors or overlap with symptoms of other conditions such as ADHD. However, since anxiety and depression in children may be precursers to Bipolar Disorder, these behaviors should be carefully monitored and evaluated. The cornerstone of treatment for Bipolar Disorder is mood-stabilizers (*lithium* and *valproate*). Common adjunctive agents include antiepileptics, antipsychotics, and combination agents. Mounting evidence suggests that antidepressants aren't effective in the treatment of bipolar depression. A major study funded by the National Institute of Mental Health (NIMH) showed that adding an antidepressant to a mood stabilizer was no more effective in treating bipolar depression than using a mood stabilizer alone. Another NIMH study found that antidepressants work no better than placebo. If antidepressants are used at all, they should be combined with a mood stabilizer such as *lithium* or *valproic acid*. Antidepressants, without a concomitant mood stabilizer, can increase the frequency of mood cycling and trigger a manic episode. Many experts believe that over time, antidepressant use as monotherapy (i.e., without a mood stabilizer) in people with Bipolar Disorder has a mood destabilizing effect, increasing the frequency of manic and depressive episodes. Drugs and conditions that can mimic Bipolar Disorder include thyroid disorders, corticosteroids, antidepressants, adrenal disorders (e.g., Addison's disease, Cushing's syndrome), antianxiety drugs, drugs for Parkinson's disease, vitamin B12 deficiency, neurological disorders (e.g., epilepsy, multiple sclerosis).

MOOD STABILIZERS

Lithium Salts Mood Stabilizer

▷ *lithium carbonate* (D)(G) swallow whole; *Usual maintenance:* 900-1200 mg/day in 2-3 divided doses
Pediatric: <12 years: not recommended; ≥12 years: same as adult
Lithobid *Tab:* 300 mg slow-rel

Comment: Signs and symptoms of *lithium* toxicity can occur below 2 mEq/L and include blurred vision, tinnitus, weakness, dizziness, nausea, abdominal pains, vomiting, diarrhea to (severe) hand tremors, ataxia, muscle twitches, nystagmus, seizures, slurred speech, decreased level of consciousness, coma, death.

Valproate Mood Stabilizer

▷ *divalproex sodium* (D)(G) take once daily; swallow ext-rel form whole; initially 25 mg/kg/day in divided doses; max 60 mg/kg/day; *Elderly:* reduce initial dose and titrate slowly
Pediatric: <12 years: not recommended; ≥12 years: same as adult
Depakene *Cap:* 250 mg; *Syr:* 250 mg/5 ml (16 oz)
Depakote *Tab:* 125, 250 mg
Depakote ER *Tab:* 250, 500 mg ext-rel
Depakote Sprinkle *Cap:* 125 mg

ANTIEPILEPTICS

▷ *carbamazepine* (D) ext-rel oral forms should be swallowed whole; may open caps and sprinkle on applesauce (do not crush or chew beads); initially 400 mg/day in 2 divided doses; adjust in increments of 200 mg/day; max 1.6 gm/day. *Elderly:* reduce initial dose and titrate slowly; oral doses are preferred; IV administration is recommended when the patient is unable to swallow an oral form (see **Carnexiv**)
Pediatric: <12 years: not recommended; ≥12 years: same as adult
Carbatrol (G) *Cap:* 200, 300 mg ext-rel
Carnexiv *Vial:* 10 mg/ml (20 ml)
Comment: The total daily dose of **Carnexiv** is 70% of the total daily oral *carbamazepine* dose (see mfr pkg insert for dosage conversion table). The total daily dose should be equally divided into four 30-minute infusions, separated by 6 hours. Must be diluted prior to administration. Patients should be switched back to oral *carbamazepine* at their previous total daily oral dose and frequency of administration as soon as clinically appropriate. The use of **Carnexiv** for more than 7 consecutive days has not been studied.
Equetro (G) *Cap:* 100, 200, 300 mg ext-rel
Tegretol (G) *Tab:* 200*mg; *Chew tab:* 100*mg; *Oral susp:* 100 mg/5 ml (450 ml; citrus-vanilla)
Tegretol XR (G) *Tab:* 100, 200, 400 mg ext-rel
Comment: *carbamazepine* is indicated in mixed episodes in bipolar I disorder.

▷ *lamotrigine* (C)(G) Not taking an enzyme-inducing antiepileptic drug (EIAED) (e.g., *phenytoin, carbamazepine, phenobarbital, primidone, valproic acid*): 25 mg once daily x 2 weeks; then 50 mg once daily x 2 weeks; then 100 mg once daily x 2 weeks; then target dose 200 mg once daily; *Concomitant valproic acid:* 25 mg every other day x 2 weeks; then 25 mg once daily x 2 weeks; then 50 mg once daily x 1 week; then target dose 100 mg once daily; *Concomitant EIAED, not valproic acid:* 50 mg once daily x 2 weeks; then 100 mg daily in divided doses; then increase weekly by 100 mg in divided doses to target dose 400 mg/day in divided doses daily
Pediatric: <12 years: not recommended; ≥12 years: same as adult
Lamictal *Tab:* 25*, 100*, 150*, 200*mg
Lamictal Chewable Dispersible Tab *Chew tab:* 2, 5, 25, 50 mg (black current)
Lamictal ODT *ODT:* 25, 50, 100, 200 mg
Lamictal XR *Tab:* 25, 50, 100, 200 mg ext-rel
Comment: *lamotrigine* is indicated for maintenance treatment of bipolar I disorder. See mfr pkg insert for drug interactions, interactions with contraceptives and hormone replacement therapy, and discontinuation protocol

ANTIPSYCHOTICS

Comment: Common side effects of antipsychotic drugs include drowsiness, weight gain, sexual dysfunction, dry mouth, constipation, blurred vision. *Neuroleptic Malignant*

Syndrome (NMS) and *Tardive Dyskinesia* (TD) are adverse side effects (ASEs) most often associated with the older antipsychotic drugs. Risk is decreased with the newer "atypical" antipsychotic drugs. However, these syndromes can develop, although much less commonly, after relatively brief treatment periods at low doses. Given these considerations, antipsychotic drugs should be prescribed in a manner that is most likely to minimize the occurrence. NMS, a potentially fatal symptom complex, is characterized by hyperpyrexia, muscle rigidity, altered mental status and evidence of autonomic instability (irregular pulse or blood pressure, tachycardia, diaphoresis, and cardiac dysrhythmia). Additional signs may include elevated creatine phosphokinase (CPK), myoglobinuria (rhabdomyolysis), and acute renal failure (ARF). TD is a syndrome consisting of potentially irreversible, involuntary, dyskinetic movements that can develop in patients with antipsychotic drugs. Characteristics include repetitive involuntary movements, usually of the jaw, lips and tongue, such as grimacing, sticking out the tongue and smacking the lips. Some affected people also experience involuntary movement of the extremities or difficulty breathing. The syndrome may remit, partially or completely, if antipsychotic treatment is withdrawn. If signs and symptoms of NMS and/or TD appear in a patient, management should include immediate discontinuation of antipsychotic drugs and other drugs not essential to concurrent therapy, intensive symptomatic treatment, medical monitoring, and treatment of any concomitant serious medical problems. The risk of developing NMS and/or TD, and the likelihood that either syndrome will become irreversible, is believed to increase as the duration of treatment and the total cumulative dose of antipsychotic drugs administered to the patient increase. The first and only FDA-approved treatment for TD is *valbenazine* (Ingrezza) (*see page* 473)

▶ *aripiprazole* (C)(G) initially 15 mg once daily; may increase to max 30 mg/day
  Pediatric: <10 years: not recommended; ≥10-17 years: initially 2 mg/day in a single dose for 2 days; then increase to 5 mg/day in a single dose for 2 days; then increase to target dose of 10 mg/day in a single dose; may increase by 5 mg/day at weekly intervals as needed to max 30 mg/day
    Abilify *Tab:* 2, 5, 10, 15, 20, 30 mg
    Abilify Discmelt *Tab:* 15 mg orally-disint (vanilla) (phenylalanine)
    Abilify Maintena *Vial:* 300, 400 mg ext-rel pwdr for IM injection after reconstitution; 300, 400 mg single dose prefilled dual-chamber syringes w. supplies
    Comment: **Abilify** is indicated for acute and maintenance treatment of mixed episodes in bipolar I disorder, as monotherapy or as adjunct to *lithium* or *valproic acid.*

▶ *asenapine* (C)(G) allow SL tab to dissolve on tongue; do not split, crush, chew, or swallow; do not eat or drink for 10 minutes after administration; *Monotherapy:* 10 mg bid; *Adjunctive therapy:* 5 mg bid; may increase to max 10 mg bid
  Pediatric: <10 years: not established; 10-17 years: *Monotherapy:* initially 2.5 mg bid; may increase to 5 mg bid after 3 days; then to 10 mg bid after 3 more days; max 10 mg bid
    Saphris *SL tab:* 2, 5, 5, 10 mg (black cherry)
    Comment: **Saphris** is indicated for acute treatment of manic or mixed episodes in bipolar I disorder, as monotherapy or as adjunct to *lithium* or *valproic acid.*

▶ *cariprazine* initially 1.5 mg once daily; recommended therapeutic dose 3-6 mg/day
  Pediatric: <12 years: not established; ≥12 years: same as adult
    Vraylar *Cap:* 1.5, 3, 4.5, 6 mg; 7-count (1 x 1.5 mg, 6 x 3 mg) mixed blister pck
    Comment: **Vraylar** is an atypical antipsychotic with partial agonist activity at D2 and 5-HT1A receptors and antagonist activity at 5-HT2A receptors. It is indicated for acute treatment of mixed episodes in bipolar I disorder. There is a **Vraylar** pregnancy exposure registry that monitors pregnancy outcomes in women exposed to **Vraylar** during pregnancy. For more information, contact the National Pregnancy Registry for Atypical Antipsychotics at 1-866-961-2388 or visit https://womensmentalhealth. org/clinical-and-research-programs/pregnancyregistry. Safety and effectiveness in pediatric patients have not been established.

▶ *lurasidone* (B)(G) initially 20 mg once daily; usual range 20 to max 120 mg/day; take with food; *CrCl <50 mL/min, moderate hepatic impairment (Child-Pugh 7-9):* max 80 mg/day; *Child-Pugh 10-15):* max 40 mg/day
  Pediatric: <10 years: not established; 10-17 years: initially 20 mg once daily; may titrate up to max 80 mg/day; >17 years: same as adult
    Latuda *Tab:* 20, 40, 60, 80, 120 mg
    Comment: **Latuda** is indicated for major depressive episodes associated with bipolar I disorder as monotherapy and as adjunctive therapy with *lithium* or *valproic* acid.

Contraindicated with concomitant strong CYP3A4 inhibitors (e.g., *ketoconazole, voriconazole, clarithromycin, ritonavir*) and inducers (e.g., *phenytoin, carbamazepine, rifampin, St. John's wort*); see mfr pkg insert if patient taking moderate CYP3A4 inhibitors (e.g., *diltiazem, atazanavir, erythromycin, fluconazole, verapamil*). The efficacy of **Latuda** in the treatment of mania associated with bipolar disorder has not been established.

▷ *quetiapine fumarate* (C)(G)

SeroQUEL initially 25 mg bid, titrate q 2nd or 3rd day in increments of 25-50 mg bid-tid; usual maintenance 400-600 mg/day in 2-3 divided doses

Pediatric: <10 years: not recommended; ≥10-17 years: initially 25 mg bid, titrate q 2nd or 3rd day in increments of 25-50 mg bid-tid; max 600 mg/day in 2-3 divided doses

Tab: 25, 50, 100, 200, 300, 400 mg

SeroQUEL XR swallow whole; administer once daily in the PM; *Day 1:* 50 mg; *Day 2:* 100 mg; *Day 3:* 200 mg; *Day 4:* 300 mg; usual range 400-600 mg/day

Pediatric: <18 years: not recommended; ≥18 years: same as adult

Tab: 50, 150, 200, 300, 400 mg ext-rel

▷ *risperidone* (C) *Tab:* initially 2-3 mg once daily; may adjust at 24 hour intervals by 1 mg/day; usual range 1-6 mg/day; max 6 mg/day; *Oral soln:* do not take with cola or tea; *M-tab:* dissolve on tongue with or without fluid; *Consta:* administer deep IM in the deltoid or gluteal; give with oral *risperidone* or other antipsychotic x 3 weeks; then stop oral form; 25 mg IM every 2 weeks; max 50 mg every 2 weeks

Risperdal

Pediatric: <5 years: not established; 5-10 years: initially 0.5 mg once daily at the same time each day adjust at 24 hour intervals by 0.5-1 mg to target dose 1-2.5 mg/day; usual range 1-6 mg/day; max 6 mg/day; >10 years: same as adult

Tab: 0.25, 0.5, 1, 2, 3, 4 mg; *Oral soln:* 1 mg/ml (100 ml)

Risperdal Consta

Pediatric: <18 years: not established; ≥18 years: same as adult

Vial: 12.5, 25, 37.5, 50 mg pwdr for long-acting IM inj after reconstitution, single-use, w. diluent and supplies

Risperdal M-Tab

Pediatric: <10 years: not established; ≥10 years: same as adult

Tab: 0.5, 1, 2, 3, 4 mg orally-disint (phenylalanine)

Comment: **Risperdol** tabs, oral solution, and M-tabs are indicated for the short-term monotherapy of acute mania or mixed episodes associated with bipolar I disorder, or in combination with *lithium* or *valproic acid* in adults

Risperdol Consta is indicated as monotherapy or adjunctive therapy to *lithium* or *valproic acid* for the maintenance treatment of mania and mixed episodes in bipolar I disorder.

▷ *ziprasidone* (C)(G) *Adult:* take with food; initially 40 mg bid; on day 2, may increase to 60-80 mg bid; *Elderly:* lower initial dose and titrate slowly

Pediatric: <12 years: not recommended; ≥12 years: same as adult

Geodon *Cap:* 20, 40, 60, 80 mg

Comment: **Geodon** is indicated for acute and maintenance treatment of mixed episodes in bipolar I disorder, as monotherapy or as adjunct to *lithium* or *valproic acid*.

COMBINATION AGENTS

Thienobenzodiazepine+Selective Serotonin Reuptake Inhibitor (SSRI) Combinations

▷ *olanzapine+fluoxetine* (C) initially 1 x 6/25 cap once daily in the PM; titrate; max 1 x 12/50 cap once daily in the PM

Pediatric: <10 years: not recommended; 10-17 years: initially 1 x 3/25 cap once daily in the PM; max 1 x 12/50 cap once daily in the PM

Symbyax

Cap: **Symbyax 3/25** olan 3 mg+fluo 25 mg

Symbyax 6/25 olan 6 mg+fluo 25 mg

Symbyax 6/50 olan 6 mg+fluo 50 mg

Symbyax 12/25 olan 12 mg+fluo 25 mg

Symbyax 12/50 olan 12 mg+fluo 50 mg

Comment: **Symbyax** is indicated for the treatment of depressive episode associated with bipolar I disorder and treatment-resistant depression (TRD).

BITE: CAT

TETANUS PROPHYLAXIS

▷ *tetanus toxoid* vaccine (C) 0.5 ml IM x 1 dose if previously immunized; *see* **Tetanus** *page* 478 for patients not previously immunized
> *Vial:* 5 Lf units/0.5 ml (0.5, 5 ml); *Prefilled syringe:* 5 Lf units/0.5 ml (0.5 ml)

ANTI-INFECTIVES

▷ *amoxicillin+clavulanate* (B)(G)
> **Augmentin** 500 mg tid or 875 mg bid x 10 days
> *Pediatric:* 40-45 mg/kg/day divided tid x 10 days or 90 mg/kg/day divided bid x 10 days
> *see pages 618 for dose by weight*
>> *Tab:* 250, 500, 875 mg; *Chew tab:* 125, 250 mg (lemon-lime); 200, 400 mg (cherry-banana) (phenylalanine); *Oral susp:* 125 mg/5 ml (banana), 250 mg/5 ml (75, 100, 150 ml) (orange); 200, 400 mg/5 ml (50, 75, 100 ml) (orange) (phenylalanine)
> **Augmentin ES-600** not recommended for adults
> *Pediatric:* <3 months: not recommended; ≥3 months, <40 kg: 90 mg/kg/day in 2 divided doses x 10 days; ≥40 kg: not recommended
>> *Oral susp:* 42.9 mg/5 ml (50, 75, 100, 125, 150, 200 ml) (strawberry cream) (phenylalanine)
> **Augmentin XR** 2 tabs q 12 hours x 10 days
> *Pediatric:* <16 years: use other forms; ≥16 years: same as adult
>> *Tab:* 1000*mg ext-rel
▷ *doxycycline* (D)(G) 100 mg bid day 1; then 100 mg daily x 10 days
> *Pediatric:* <8 years: not recommended ≥8 years, <100 lb: 2 mg/lb on first day in 2 divided doses, followed by 1 mg/lb/day in 1-2 divided doses; *see page 625 for dose by weight;* ≥8 years, ≥100 lb: same as adult
>> **Acticlate** *Tab:* 75, 150**mg
>> **Adoxa** *Tab:* 50, 75, 100, 150 mg ent-coat
>> **Doryx** *Tab:* 50, 75, 100, 150, 200 mg del-rel
>> **Doxteric** *Tab:* 50 mg del-rel
>> **Monodox** *Cap:* 50, 75, 100 mg
>> **Oracea** *Cap:* 40 mg del-rel
>> **Vibramycin** *Tab:* 100 mg; *Cap:* 50, 100 mg; *Syr:* 50 mg/5 ml (raspberry-apple) (sulfites); *Oral susp:* 25 mg/5 ml (raspberry)
>> **Vibra-Tab** *Tab:* 100 mg film-coat
> Comment: *doxycycline* is contraindicated <8 years-of-age, in pregnancy, and lactation (discolors developing tooth enamel). A side effect may be photosensitivity (photophobia). Do not take with antacids, calcium supplements, milk or other dairy, or within 2 hours of taking another drug.
▷ *penicillin v potassium* (B)(G) 500 mg PO qid x 3 days
> *Pediatric:* <12 years: 15-50 mg/kg/day in 3-6 divided doses x 3 days; *see page 629 for dose by weight;* ≥12 years: same as adult
>> **Pen-Vee K** *Tab:* 250, 500 mg; *Oral soln:* 125 mg/5 ml (100, 200 ml); 250 mg/5 ml (100, 150, 200 ml)

 BITE: DOG

TETANUS PROPHYLAXIS

▷ *tetanus toxoid* vaccine (C) 0.5 ml IM x 1 dose if previously immunized; *see* **Tetanus** *page* 478 for patients not previously immunized
> *Vial:* 5 Lf units/0.5 ml (0.5, 5 ml); *Prefilled syringe:* 5 Lf units/0.5 ml (0.5 ml)

ANTI-INFECTIVES

▷ *amoxicillin+clavulanate* (B)(G)
> **Augmentin** 500 mg tid or 875 mg bid x 10 days
> *Pediatric:* 40-45 mg/kg/day divided tid x 10 days or 90 mg/kg/day divided bid x 10 days
> *see pages 618 for dose by weight*

Tab: 250, 500, 875 mg; *Chew tab:* 125, 250 mg (lemon-lime); 200, 400 mg (cherry-banana) (phenylalanine); *Oral susp:* 125 mg/5 ml (banana), 250 mg/5 ml (75, 100, 150 ml) (orange); 200, 400 mg/5 ml (50, 75, 100 ml) (orange) (phenylalanine)

Augmentin ES-600 not recommended for adults

Pediatric: <3 months: not recommended; ≥3 months, <40 kg: 90 mg/kg/day in 2 divided doses x 10 days; ≥40 kg: not recommended

Oral susp: 42.9 mg/5 ml (50, 75, 100, 125, 150, 200 ml) (strawberry cream) (phenylalanine)

Augmentin XR 2 tabs q 12 hours x 10 days

Pediatric: <16 years: use other forms; ≥16 years: same as adult

Tab: 1000*mg ext-rel

➤ *clindamycin* (B) (administer with fluoroquinolone in adult and TMP-SMX in children) 300 mg qid x 10 days

Pediatric: 8-16 mg/kg/day in 3-4 divided doses x 10 days; *see page 624 for dose by weight*

Cleocin (G) *Cap:* 75 (tartrazine), 150 (tartrazine), 300 mg

Cleocin Pediatric Granules (G) *Oral susp:* 75 mg/5 ml (100 ml) (cherry)

➤ *doxycycline* (D)(G) 100 mg bid

Pediatric: <8 years: not recommended ≥8 years, <100 lb: 2 mg/lb on first day in 2 divided doses, followed by 1 mg/lb/day in 1-2 divided doses; ≥8 years, ≥100 lb: same as adult; *see page 625 for dose by weight*

Acticlate *Tab:* 75, 150**mg

Adoxa *Tab:* 50, 75, 100, 150 mg ent-coat

Doryx *Tab:* 50, 75, 100, 150, 200 mg del-rel

Doxteric *Tab:* 50 mg del-rel

Monodox *Cap:* 50, 75, 100 mg

Oracea *Cap:* 40 mg del-rel

Vibramycin *Tab:* 100 mg; *Cap:* 50, 100 mg; *Syr:* 50 mg/5 ml (raspberry-apple) (sulfites); *Oral susp:* 25 mg/5 ml (raspberry)

Vibra-Tab *Tab:* 100 mg film-coat

Comment: *doxycycline* is contraindicated <8 years-of-age, in pregnancy, and lactation (discolors developing tooth enamel). A side effect may be photosensitivity (photophobia). Do not take with antacids, calcium supplements, milk or other dairy, or within 2 hours of taking another drug.

➤ *penicillin v potassium* (B)(G) 500 mg PO qid x 3 days

Pediatric: 50 mg/kg/day in 4 divided doses x 3 days; ≥12 years: same as adult; *see page 629 for dose by weight*

Pen-Vee K *Tab:* 250, 500 mg; *Oral soln:* 125 mg/5 ml (100, 200 ml); 250 mg/5 ml (100, 150, 200 ml)

BITE: HUMAN

TETANUS PROPHYLAXIS

➤ *tetanus toxoid* vaccine (C) 0.5 ml IM x 1 dose if previously immunized; *see Tetanus page 478* for patients not previously immunized

Vial: 5 Lf units/0.5 ml (0.5, 5 ml); *Prefilled syringe:* 5 Lf units/0.5 ml (0.5 ml)

ANTI-INFECTIVES

➤ *amoxicillin+clavulanate* (B)(G)

Augmentin 500 mg tid or 875 mg bid x 10 days

Pediatric: 40-45 mg/kg/day divided tid x 10 days or 90 mg/kg/day divided bid x 10 days *see pages 618 for dose by weight*

Tab: 250, 500, 875 mg; *Chew tab:* 125, 250 mg (lemon-lime); 200, 400 mg (cherry-banana) (phenylalanine); *Oral susp:* 125 mg/5 ml (banana), 250 mg/5 ml (75, 100, 150 ml) (orange); 200, 400 mg/5 ml (50, 75, 100 ml) (orange) (phenylalanine)

Augmentin ES-600 not recommended for adults

Pediatric: <3 months: not recommended; ≥3 months, <40 kg: 90 mg/kg/day in 2 divided doses x 10 days; ≥40 kg: not recommended

Oral susp: 42.9 mg/5 ml (50, 75, 100, 125, 150, 200 ml) (strawberry cream) (phenylalanine)

Augmentin XR 2 tabs q 12 hours x 10 days

Pediatric: <16 years: use other forms; ≥16 years: same as adult
    Tab: 1000*mg ext-rel

➤ *cefoxitin* (B) 80-160 mg/kg/day IM in 3-4 divided doses x 10 days; max 12 gm/day
Pediatric: <3 months: not recommended; ≥3 months: same as adult
    Mefoxin *Injectable Vial:* 1, 2 g

➤ *ciprofloxacin* (C) 500 mg bid x 10 days
Pediatric: <18 years: not recommended; ≥18 years: same as adult
    Cipro (G) *Tab:* 250, 500, 750 mg; *Oral susp:* 250, 500 mg/5 ml (100 ml) (strawberry)
    Cipro XR *Tab:* 500, 1000 mg ext-rel
    ProQuin XR *Tab:* 500 mg ext-rel

➤ *erythromycin base* (B)(G) 250 mg qid x 10 days
Pediatric: <45 kg: 30-40 mg/kg/day in 4 divided doses x 10 days; ≥45 kg: same as adult
    Ery-Tab *Tab:* 250, 333, 500 mg ent-coat
    PCE *Tab:* 333, 500 mg

Comment: *erythromycin* may increase INR with concomitant *warfarin*, as well as increase serum level of *digoxin,* benzodiazepines, and statins.

➤ *erythromycin ethylsuccinate* (B)(G) 400 mg qid x 10 days
Pediatric: 30-50 mg/kg/day in 4 divided doses x 10 days; may double dose with severe infection; max 100 mg/kg/day; *see page 626 for dose by weight*
    EryPed *Oral susp:* 200 mg/5 ml (100, 200 ml) (fruit); 400 mg/5 ml (60, 100, 200 ml) (banana); *Oral drops:* 200, 400 mg/5 ml (50 ml) (fruit); *Chew tab:* 200 mg wafer (fruit)
    E.E.S. *Oral susp:* 200, 400 mg/5 ml (100 ml) (fruit)
    E.E.S. Granules *Oral susp:* 200 mg/5 ml (100, 200 ml) (cherry)
    E.E.S. 400 Tablets *Tab:* 400 mg

Comment: *erythromycin* may increase INR with concomitant *warfarin,* as well as increase serum level of *digoxin,* benzodiazepines, and statins.

➤ *trimethoprim+sulfamethoxazole (TMP-SMX)*(D)(G) bid x 10 days
Pediatric: <2 months: not recommended; ≥2 months: 40 mg/kg/day of *sulfamethoxazole* in 2 divided doses bid x 10 days; *see page 630 for dose by weight*
    Bactrim, Septra 2 tabs bid x 10 days
        Tab: trim 80 mg+sulfa 400 mg*
    Bactrim DS, Septra DS 1 tab bid x 10 days
        Tab: trim 160 mg+sulfa 800 mg*
    Bactrim Pediatric Suspension, Septra Pediatric Suspension
        Oral susp: trim 40 mg+sulfa 200 mg per 5 ml (100 ml) (cherry) (alcohol 0.3%)

Comment: Sulfonamides are contraindicated in the first trimester of pregnancy, the final month of pregnancy, and infants <8 weeks-of-age. *CrCl 15-30 mL/min:* reduce dose by 1/2; *CrCl <15 mL/min:* not recommended. Contraindicated with G6PD deficiency. A high fluid intake is indicated during sulfonamide therapy to avoid crystallization in the kidneys.

BLEPHARITIS

OPHTHALMIC AGENTS

➤ *erythromycin* ophthalmic ointment (B) apply 1/2 inch bid-qid x 14 days; then q HS x 10 days
Pediatric: same as adult
    Ilotycin *Oint:* 5 mg/gm (1/2 oz)

➤ *polymyxin b+bacitracin* ophthalmic ointment (C) apply 1/2 inch bid-qid x 14 days; then q HS
Pediatric: same as adult
    Polysporin *Oint:* poly b 10,000 U+baci 500 U (3.75 gm)

➤ *polymyxin b+bacitracin+neomycin* ophthalmic ointment (C) apply 1/2 inch bid-qid x 14 days; then q HS
Pediatric: same as adult
    Neosporin *Oint:* poly b 10,000 U+baci 400 U+neo 3.5 mg/gm (3.75 gm)

➤ *sodium sulfacetamide* (C)
    Bleph-10 Ophthalmic Solution 2 drops q 4 hours x 7-14 days
        Pediatric: <2 years: not recommended; ≥2 years: 1-2 drops q 2-3 hours during the day x 7-14 days
        Ophth soln: 10% (2.5, 5, 15 ml) (benzalkonium chloride)

Bleph-10 Ophthalmic Ointment apply 1/2 inch qid and HS x 7-14 days
Pediatric: <2 years: not recommended; ≥2 years: same as adult
Ophth oint: 10% (3.5 gm) (phenylmercuric acetate)

SYSTEMIC AGENTS

➤ *tetracycline* (D)(G) 250 mg qid x 7 days
Pediatric: <8 years: not recommended; ≥8 years, <100 lb: 25-50 mg/kg/day in 2-4 divided doses x 7-10 days; ≥100 lb: same as adult; *see page 630 for dose by weight*
Achromycin V *Cap:* 250, 500 mg
Sumycin *Tab:* 250, 500 mg; *Cap:* 250, 500 mg; *Oral susp:* 125 mg/5 ml (100, 200 ml) (fruit) (sulfites)
Comment: *tetracycline* is contraindicated <8 years-of-age, in pregnancy, and lactation (discolors developing tooth enamel). A side effect may be photo-sensitivity (photophobia). Do not take with antacids, calcium supplements, milk or other dairy, or within two hours of taking another drug.

BOWEL RESECTION WITH PRIMARY ANASTOMOSIS

➤ *alvimopan* (B) administer 12 mg 30 minutes to 5 hours prior to surgery; then, 12 mg bid for up to 7 days; max 15 doses
Pediatric: <18 years: not established; ≥18 years: same as adult
Entereg *Cap:* 12 mg
Comment: **Entereg** is a peripherally acting μ-opioid receptor antagonist indicated to accelerate the time to upper and lower gastrointestinal recovery following partial large or small bowel resection surgery with primary anastomosis. Therapeutic doses of opioids for more than 7 consecutive days prior to **Entereg** is contraindicated. A higher number of myocardial infarctions was reported in patients treated with *alvimopan* 0.5 mg twice daily compared with placebo in a 12-month study in patients treated with opioids for chronic pain, although a causal relationship has not been established. **Entereg** is not recommended for patients with severe hepatic impairment and end stage renal disease (ESRD). Dosage adjustment is not required in patients with mild to severe renal impairment but they should be monitored for adverse effects. The most common adverse reactions (incidence ≥3%) in patients undergoing bowel resection were anemia, dyspepsia, hypokalemia, back pain, and urinary retention. **Entereg** is available only for short-term (15 doses) use in hospitalized patients and only hospitals that have registered in and met all of the requirements for the ENTEREG Access Support and Education (E.A.S.E.) program may use **Entereg**. To report suspected adverse reactions, contact Adolor at 1-866-4ADOLOR (1-866-423-6567) or FDA at 1-800FDA-1088 or www.fda.gov/medwatch.

BREAST CANCER

NONSTEROIDAL ANTI-ESTROGEN AGENTS

➤ *fulvestrant* (D) 250 mg IM once monthly; administer 2.5 ml IM in each buttock concurrently
Faslodex *Prefilled syringe:* 50 mg/ml (2 x 2.5 ml, 1 x 5 ml)
➤ *letrozole* (D)(G) 2.5 mg daily
Femara *Tab:* 2.5 mg film-coat

KINASE INHIBITOR

➤ *abemaciclib Starting dose in combination with fulvestrant or an aromatase inhibitor:* 150 mg twice daily; *Starting dose as monotherapy:* 200 mg twice daily; dosing interruption and/or dose reductions may be required based on individual safety and tolerability
Pediatric: <18 years: not recommended; >18 years: same as adult
Verzenio *Tab:* 50, 100, 150, 200 mg
Comment: **Verzenio** *(abemaciclib)* is indicated (1) in combination with an aromatase inhibitor as initial endocrine-based therapy for the treatment of postmenopausal women with hormone receptor (HR)-positive, human epidermal growth factor receptor 2 (HER2)-negative advanced or metastatic breast cancer, (2) in combination

with *fulvestrant* for the treatment of women with hormone receptor (HR)-positive, human epidermal growth factor receptor 2 (HER2)-negative advanced or metastatic breast cancer with disease progression following endocrine therapy, and (3) as monotherapy for the treatment of adult patients with HR-positive, HER2-negative advanced or metastatic breast cancer with disease progression following endocrine therapy and prior chemotherapy in the metastatic setting. **Verzenio** can cause embryo-fetal harm. Advise patients of potential risk to a fetus and to use effective contraception. There are no data on the presence of *abemaciclib* in human milk or its effects on the breastfed infant. However, breastfeeding is not recommended. Reduce the dosing frequency when administering **Verzenio** to patients with severe hepatic impairment (Child-Pugh C). The most common adverse reactions (incidence ≥20%) have been diarrhea, neutropenia, nausea, abdominal pain, infections, fatigue, anemia, leukopenia, decreased appetite, vomiting, headache, alopecia, and thrombocytopenia.

POLY ADP-RIBOCE POLYMERASE (PARP) INHIBITOR

▷ *talazoparib* recommended dose 1 mg once daily with unacceptable toxicity occurs; for adverse reactions, consider dose interruption or dose reduction CrCl30-59 mL/min: 0.75 mg once daily without food; treat until disease progression
Pediatric: <18 years: not recommended; >18 years: same as adult
  Talzenna *Cap:* 0.25, 1 mg
  Comment: Talzenna *(talazoparib)* is a poly (ADP-ribose) polymerase (PARP) inhibitor indicated for the treatment of adult patients with deleterious or suspected deleterious germline BRCA-mutated (*gBRCAm*) HER2-negative locally advanced or metastatic breast cancer. Select patients for therapy based on an FDA-approved companion diagnostic for **Talzenna**. Most common (incidence ≥20%) adverse reactions of any grade were fatigue, anemia, nausea, neutropenia, headache, thrombocytopenia, vomiting, alopecia, diarrhea, decreased appetite. Most common laboratory abnormalities (incidence ≥25%) were *decreases* in hemoglobin, platelets, neutrophils, lymphocytes, leukocytes, and calcium and *increases* Increases in glucose, alanine aminotransferase, aspartate aminotransferase, and alkaline phosphatase. Reduce **Talzenna** dose with certain P-gp inhibitors. Monitor for potential increased adverse reactions with concomitant BCRP Inhibitors. There are no available data on **Talzenna** use in pregnant women to inform drug-associated embryo-fetal risk. However, animal studies have demonstrated embryo-fetal harm. Breastfeeding is not advisable.

HER2/NEU RECEPTOR ANTAGONISTS
Trastuzumab Products

Comment: Exposure to *trastuzumab* products during pregnancy can result in embryo-fetal toxicity including oligohydramnios, in some cases complicated by pulmonary hypoplasia and neonatal death. Verify the pregnancy status of females prior to initiation. Advise patients of these risks and the need for effective contraception. There is no information regarding the presence of *trastuzumab* products in human milk or effects on the breastfed infant. Treatment with a *trastuzumab* product can result in subclinical and clinical cardiac failure manifesting as CHF, and decreased LVEF, with greatest risk when administered concurrently with anthracyclines. Evaluate cardiac function prior to and during treatment. Discontinue for cardiomyopathy, anaphylaxis, angioedema, interstitial pneumonitis, or acute respiratory distress syndrome (ARDS). Monitor patient for exacerbation of chemotherapy-induced neutropenia (CIN). Do not substitute a *trastuzumab* product for or with **Kadcyla** (*ado-trastuzumab emtansine*). *Adjuvant Breast Cancer Treatment ASEs:* most common incidence (incidence ≥5%) are headache, diarrhea, nausea, and chills. *Metastatic Breast Cancer Treatment ASEs:* most common (incidence ≥10%) are fever, chills, headache, infection, congestive heart failure, insomnia, cough, and rash.

Dosing of *trastuzumab* Products:
  Adjuvant Treatment of HER2-Overexpressing Breast Cancer: Administer initial dose of 4 mg/kg over 90 minutes via IV infusion; then, 2 mg/kg over 30 minute IV infusion once weekly x 12 weeks (with *paclitaxel* or *docetaxel*) or x 18 weeks (with *docetaxel* and *carboplatin*); then, one week after the last weekly dose of the *trastuzument* product, administer 6 mg/kg via IV infusion over 30 to 90 minutes once every 3 weeks to complete a total of 52 weeks of therapy

or
Administer initial dose of 8 mg/kg over 90 minutes via IV infusion, then, 6 mg/kg over 30 to 90 minutes via IV infusion once every 3 weeks x 52 weeks *Treatment of Metastatic HER2-Overexpressing Breast Cancer:* Administer initial dose of 4 mg/kg over 90 minutes via IV infusion; then, once weekly doses of 2 mg/kg via 30 minute IV infusions

▷ **trastuzumab**
Herceptin for Injection *Vial:* 150 mg, single-dose; 420 mg multi-dose, pwdr for reconstitution, dilution, and IV infusion
▷ **trastuzumab-dkst**
Ogivri for Injection *Vial:* 420 mg, multi-dose, pwdr for reconstitution, dilution, and IV infusion
Comment: Ogivri *(trastuzumab-dkst)* is a HER2/neu receptor antagonist biosimilar to Herceptin *(trastuzumab).*
▷ **trastuzumab-dttb**
Ontruzant for Injection *Vial:* 150 mg, powder, single-dose, pwdr for reconstitution, dilution, and IV infusion
Comment: Ontruzant *(trastuzumab-dttb)* is a HER2/neu receptor antagonist biosimilar to Herceptin *(trastuzumab).*
▷ **trastuzumab-pkrb**
Herzuma *Vial:* 420 mg, multi-dose, pwdr for reconstitution, dilution, and IV infusion
Comment: Herzuma *(trastuzumab-pkrb)* is an HER2/neu receptor antagonist biosimilar to Herceptin *(trastuzumab).*

NONSTEROIDAL ANTI-ESTROGEN

▷ **tamoxifen citrate** (D)
Ductal Carcinoma in Situ (DCIS): 20 mg once daily x 5 years
Reduction in Breast Cancer Incidence in High Risk Women: 20 mg once daily x 5 years
Tab: 10, 20 mg
Comment: *tamoxifen citrate* is an orally administered nonsteroidal antiestrogen. *tamoxifen* is effective in the treatment of metastatic breast cancer in women and men. In females with ductal carcinoma in situ (DCIS), following breast surgery and radiation, *tamoxifen* is indicated to reduce the risk of developing invasive breast cancer. *tamoxifen* is indicated to reduce the incidence of breast cancer in females at high risk for breast cancer (high risk is defined as women at least 35 years-of-age with a 5-year predicted risk of breast cancer ≥1.67%, as calculated by the Gail Model). For premenopausal women with metastatic breast cancer, *tamoxifen* is an alternative to oophorectomy or ovarian irradiation. Available evidence indicates that patients whose tumors are estrogen receptor-positive are more likely to benefit from *tamoxifen* therapy. *tamoxifen* is indicated for the treatment of node-positive breast cancer in women following total mastectomy or segmental mastectomy, axillary dissection, and breast irradiation. In some *tamoxifen* adjuvant studies, most of the benefit to date has been in the subgroup with four or more positive axillary nodes. *tamoxifen* is indicated for the treatment of axillary node-negative breast cancer in women following total mastectomy or segmental mastectomy, axillary dissection, and breast irradiation. *tamoxifen* has demonstrated effectiveness in the palliative treatment of male breast cancer. *tamoxifen* reduces the occurrence of contralateral breast cancer in patients receiving adjuvant *tamoxifen* therapy for breast cancer. Reduction in recurrence and mortality has been greater in studies using *tamoxifen* for about 5 years than in those that used *tamoxifen* for a shorter period of therapy. Serious and life-threatening events associated with *tamoxifen* in the risk reduction setting (women at high risk for cancer and women with DCIS) include uterine malignancies, stroke and pulmonary embolism. The benefits of *tamoxifen* outweigh its risks in women already diagnosed with breast cancer. The effects of age, gender and race on the pharmacokinetics of *tamoxifen* have not been determined. Safety and efficacy of *tamoxifen* in girls aged 2 to 10 years with McCune-Albright Syndrome and precocious puberty have not been studied beyond one year of treatment. Effects of reduced liver function on the metabolism and pharmacokinetics of tamoxifen have not been determined. *In vitro* studies have shown that **erythromycin, cyclosporin, nifedipine** and **diltiazem** competitively inhibited formation of N-desmethyl tamoxifen. The clinical significance of these *in vitro* studies is unknown. *tamoxifen* is contraindicated in females who require concomitant coumarin-type anticoagulant therapy or in females with a history of deep vein thrombosis (DVT) or pulmonary embolus (PE). *tamoxifen* may cause

fetal harm in pregnancy. Patients should be advised not to become pregnant while taking *tamoxifen* or within 2 months of discontinuation and should use barrier or non-hormonal contraceptive measures. *tamoxifen* does not cause infertility. Patients should be apprised of the potential risks to the fetus including the potential long-term risk of a DES-like syndrome. For sexually active patients of child-bearing potential, *tamoxifen* should be initiated during menstruation. In patients with menstrual irregularity, a negative B-HCG immediately prior to the initiation of therapy is sufficient. *tamoxifen* has been reported to inhibit lactation. There are no data that address whether *tamoxifen* is excreted into human milk or effects on the breastfed infant. Because of the potential for serious adverse reactions in breastfed, patients taking tamoxifen should not breast feed. Although adverse reactions to *tamoxifen* are relatively mild and rarely severe enough to require discontinuation, loss of libido and impotence resulting in male discontinuation has been reported. In oligospermic males treated with *tamoxifen*, LH, FSH, testosterone and estrogen levels were elevated. However, no significant clinical changes have been reported.

SELECTIVE ESTROGEN RECEPTOR MODULATOR (SERM)

▷ *toremifene* (D)(G) 60 mg once daily
> Fareston *Tab*: 60 mg
> Comment: Fareston *(toremifene)* is an estrogen agonist/antagonist indicated for the treatment of metastatic breast cancer (MBC) in postmenopausal women with estrogen-receptor positive or unknown tumors. Most common adverse reactions are hot flashes, sweating, nausea, and vaginal discharge. Fetal harm may occur when administered to a pregnant woman. Women should be advised not to become pregnant when taking **Fareston**. Females of childbearing potential should use effective non-hormonal contraception during **Fareston** therapy. Discontinue drug or nursing taking into account the importance of the drug to the mother.

BRONCHIOLITIS

Inhaled Beta-2 Agonists (Bronchodilators) *see Asthma page* 30
Oral Beta-2 Agonists (Bronchodilators) *see Asthma page* 36
Inhaled Corticosteroids *see Asthma page* 31
Parenteral Corticosteroids *see page* 577
Oral Corticosteroids *see page* 577

BRONCHITIS: ACUTE & ACUTE EXACERBATION OF CHRONIC BRONCHITIS (AECB)

Comment: Antibiotics are seldom needed for treatment of acute bronchitis because the etiology is usually viral.
Inhaled Beta-2 Agonists (Bronchodilators) *see Asthma page* 30
Oral Beta-2 Agonists (Bronchodilators) *see Asthma page* 36
Decongestants *see page* 603
Expectorants *see page* 603
Antitussives *see page* 603

ANTI-INFECTIVES FOR SECONDARY BACTERIAL INFECTION

 amoxicillin (B)(G) 500-875 mg bid or 250-500 mg tid x 10 days
> *Pediatric:* <40 kg (88 lb): 20-40 mg/kg/day in 3 divided doses x 10 days or 25-45 mg/kg/day in 2 divided doses x 10 days; ≥40 kg: same as adult; *see page* 617 *for dose by weight*
>> Amoxil *Cap*: 250, 500 mg; *Tab*: 875*mg; *Chew tab*: 125, 200, 250, 400 mg (cherry-banana-peppermint) (phenylalanine); *Oral susp*: 125, 250 mg/5 ml (80, 100, 150 ml) (strawberry); 200, 400 mg/5 ml (50, 75, 100 ml) (bubble gum); *Oral drops:* 50 mg/ml (30 ml) (bubble gum)
>> Moxatag *Tab*: 775 mg ext-rel
>> Trimox *Tab*: 125, 250 mg; *Cap*: 250, 500 mg; *Oral susp*: 125, 250 mg/5 ml (80, 100, 150 ml) (raspberry-strawberry)
▷ *amoxicillin+clavulanate* (B)(G)
>> Augmentin 500 mg tid or 875 mg bid x 7-10 days

Pediatric: 40-45 mg/kg/day divided tid x 10 days or 90 mg/kg/day divided bid x 10 days *see pages 618 for dose by weight*

    Tab: 250, 500, 875 mg; *Chew tab:* 125, 250 mg (lemon-lime); 200, 400 mg (cherry-banana) (phenylalanine); *Oral susp:* 125 mg/5 ml (banana), 250 mg/5 ml (75, 100, 150 ml) (orange); 200, 400 mg/5 ml (50, 75, 100 ml) (orange) (phenylalanine)

Augmentin ES-600 not recommended for adults

Pediatric: <3 months: not recommended; ≥3 months, <40 kg: 90 mg/kg/day in 2 divided doses x 7-10 days; ≥40 kg: not recommended

    Oral susp: 42.9 mg/5 ml (50, 75, 100, 125, 150, 200 ml) (strawberry cream) (phenylalanine)

Augmentin XR 2 tabs q 12 hours x 7-10 days

Pediatric: <16 years: use other forms; ≥16 years: same as adult

    Tab: 1000*mg ext-rel

▷ *ampicillin* (B) 250-500 mg qid x 10 days

Pediatric: not recommended for bronchitis in children

    Omnipen, Principen *Cap:* 250, 500 mg; *Oral susp:* 125, 250 mg/5 ml (100, 150, 200 ml) (fruit)

▷ *azithromycin* (B)(G) 500 mg x 1 dose on day 1, then 250 mg daily on days 2-5 or 500 mg once daily x 3 days or 2 gm in a single dose

Pediatric: not recommended for bronchitis in children

    Zithromax *Tab:* 250, 500, 600 mg; *Oral susp:* 100 mg/5 ml (15 ml); 200 mg/5 ml (15, 22.5, 30 ml) (cherry); *Pkt:* 1 gm for reconstitution (cherry-banana)

    Zithromax Tri-pak *Tab:* 3 x 500 mg tabs/pck

    Zithromax Z-pak *Tab:* 6 x 250 mg tabs/pck

    Zmax *Oral susp:* 2 gm ext-rel for reconstitution (cherry-banana) (148 mg Na^+)

▷ *cefaclor* (B)(G) 250-500 mg q 8 hours x 10 days; max 2 gm/day

    Tab: 500 mg; *Cap:* 250, 500 mg; *Susp:* 125 mg/5 ml (75, 150 ml) (strawberry); 187 mg/5 ml (50, 100 ml) (strawberry); 250 mg/5 ml (75, 150 ml) (strawberry); 375 mg/5 ml (50, 100 ml) (strawberry)

Pediatric: <16 years: ext-rel not recommended; ≥16 years: same as adult

    Cefaclor Extended Release *Tab:* 375, 500 mg ext-rel

▷ *cefadroxil* (B) 1-2 gm in 1-2 divided doses x 10 days

Pediatric: 30 mg/kg/day in 2 divided doses x 10 days; *see page 620 for dose by weight*

    Duricef *Tab:* 1 gm; *Cap:* 500 mg; *Oral susp:* 250 mg/5 ml (100 ml); 500 mg/5 ml (75, 100 ml) (orange-pineapple)

▷ *cefdinir* (B) 300 mg bid x 5-10 days or 600 mg daily x 10 days

Pediatric: <6 months: not recommended; 6 months-12 years: 14 mg/kg/day in 1-2 divided doses x 10 days; ≥12 years: same as adult; *see page 621 for dose by weight*

    Omnicef *Cap:* 300 mg; *Oral susp:* 125 mg/5 ml (60, 100 ml) (strawberry)

▷ *cefditoren pivoxil* (B) 400 mg bid x 10 days

Pediatric: <12 years: not recommended; ≥12 years: same as adult

    Spectracef *Tab:* 200 mg

    Comment: Spectracef is contraindicated with milk protein allergy or carnitine deficiency.

▷ *cefixime* (B)(G)

Pediatric: <6 months: not recommended; ≥6 months-12 years, <50 kg: 8 mg/kg/day in 1-2 divided doses x 10 days; ≥12 years, >50 kg: same as adult; *see page 621 for dose by weight*

    Suprax *Tab:* 400 mg; *Cap:* 400 mg; *Oral susp:* 100, 200, 500 mg/5 ml (50, 75, 100 ml) (strawberry)

▷ *cefpodoxime proxetil* (B) 200 mg bid x 10 days

Pediatric: <2 months: not recommended; ≥2 months-12 years: 10 mg/kg/day (max 400 mg/dose) or 5 mg/kg/day bid (max 200 mg/dose) x 10 days; >12 years: same as adult; *see page 622 for dose by weight*

    Vantin *Tab:* 100, 200 mg; *Oral susp:* 50, 100 mg/5 ml (50, 75, 100 mg) (lemon creme)

▷ *cefprozil* (B) 500 mg q 12 hours x 10 days

Pediatric: <2 years: not recommended; 2-12 years: 15 mg/kg q 12 hours x 10 days; *see page 622 for dose by weight;* >12 years: same as adult

    Cefzil *Tab:* 250, 500 mg; *Oral susp:* 125, 250 mg/5 ml (50, 75, 100 ml) (bubble gum) (phenylalanine)

▷ *ceftibuten* (B) 400 mg daily x 10 days

Pediatric: 9 mg/kg daily x 10 days; max 400 mg/day; *see page 623 for dose by weight*

    Cedax *Cap:* 400 mg; *Oral susp:* 90 mg/5 ml (30, 60, 90, 120 ml); 180 mg/5 ml (30, 60, 120 ml) (cherry)

▷ *ceftriaxone* (B)(G) 1-2 gm IM daily continued 2 days after signs of infection have disappeared; max 4 gm/day
    Pediatric: 50 mg/kg IM daily and continued 2 days after clinical stability
        Rocephin *Vial:* 250, 500 mg; 1, 2 gm

▷ *cephalexin* (B)(G) 250-500 mg qid or 500 mg bid x 10 days
    Pediatric: 25-50 mg/kg/day in 4 divided doses x 10 days; ≥12 years: same as adult; *see page 623 for dose by weight*
        Keflex *Cap:* 250, 333, 500, 750 mg; *Oral susp:* 125, 250 mg/5 ml (100, 200 ml) (strawberry)

▷ *clarithromycin* (C)(G) 500 mg bid or 500 mg ext-rel once daily x 7 days
    Pediatric: <6 months: not recommended; ≥6 months: 7.5 mg/kg bid x 7 days; *see page 624 for dose by weight*; ≥12 years: same as adult
        Biaxin *Tab:* 250, 500 mg
        Biaxin Oral Suspension *Oral susp:* 125, 250 mg/5 ml (50, 100 ml) (fruit-punch)
        Biaxin XL *Tab:* 500 mg ext-rel

Comment: The FDA is advising caution before prescribing *clarithromycin* to patients with heart disease because of a potential increased risk of heart problems or death that can occur years later. This recommendation is based on a review of the results of a 10-year follow-up study of patients with coronary heart disease from a large clinical trial that first observed this safety issue. Consider risk benefit and the use of other antibiotics in such patients.

▷ *dirithromycin* (C)(G) 500 mg daily x 7 days
    Pediatric: <12 years: not recommended; ≥12 years: same as adult
        Dynabac *Tab:* 250 mg

▷ *doxycycline* (D)(G) 100 mg bid x 10 days
    Pediatric: <8 years: not recommended; ≥8 years, <100 lb: 2 mg/lb on first day in 2 divided doses, followed by 1 mg/lb/day in 1-2 divided doses; ≥8 years, ≥100 lb: same as adult; *see page 625 for dose by weight*
        Acticlate *Tab:* 75, 150**mg
        Adoxa *Tab:* 50, 75, 100, 150 mg ent-coat
        Doryx *Tab:* 50, 75, 100, 150, 200 mg del-rel
        Doxteric *Tab:* 50 mg del-rel
        Monodox *Cap:* 50, 75, 100 mg
        Oracea *Cap:* 40 mg del-rel
        Vibramycin *Tab:* 100 mg; *Cap:* 50, 100 mg; *Syr:* 50 mg/5 ml (raspberry-apple) (sulfites); *Oral susp:* 25 mg/5 ml (raspberry)
        Vibra-Tab *Tab:* 100 mg film-coat

Comment: *doxycycline* is contraindicated <8 years-of-age, in pregnancy, and lactation (discolors developing tooth enamel). A side effect may be photosensitivity (photophobia). Do not take with antacids, calcium supplements, milk or other dairy, or within 2 hours of taking another drug.

▷ *erythromycin ethylsuccinate* (B)(G) 400 mg qid x 7 days
    Pediatric: 30-50 mg/kg/day in 4 divided doses x 7 days; may double dose with severe infection; max 100 mg/kg/day; *see page 626 for dose by weight*
        EryPed *Oral susp:* 200 mg/5 ml (100, 200 ml) (fruit); 400 mg/5 ml (60, 100, 200 ml) (banana); *Oral drops:* 200, 400 mg/5 ml (50 ml) (fruit); *Chew tab:* 200 mg wafer (fruit)
        E.E.S. *Oral susp:* 200, 400 mg/5 ml (100 ml) (fruit)
        E.E.S. Granules *Oral susp:* 200 mg/5 ml (100, 200 ml) (cherry)
        E.E.S. 400 Tablets *Tab:* 400 mg

Comment: *erythromycin* may increase INR with concomitant *warfarin*, as well as increase serum level of *digoxin*, benzodiazepines, and statins.

▷ *gemifloxacin* (C) 320 mg daily x 5 days
    Pediatric: <18 years: not recommended; ≥18 years: same as adult
        Factive *Tab:* 320*mg

Comment: *gemifloxacin* is contraindicated <18 years-of-age and during pregnancy and lactation. Risk of tendonitis or tendon rupture.

▷ *levofloxacin* (C) *Uncomplicated:* 500 mg daily x 7 days; *Complicated:* 750 mg daily x 7 days
    Pediatric: <18 years: not recommended; ≥18 years: same as adult

Levaquin *Tab:* 250, 500, 750 mg

Comment: *levofloxacin* is contraindicated <18 years-of-age and during pregnancy and lactation. Risk of tendonitis or tendon rupture.

▷ *loracarbef* (B) 200-400 mg bid x 7 days
Pediatric: 30 mg/kg/day in 2 divided doses x 7 days; ≥12 years: same as adult; *see page 628 for dose by weight*
Lorabid *Pulvule:* 200, 400 mg; *Oral susp:* 100 mg/5 ml (50, 100 ml); 200 mg/5 ml (50, 75, 100 ml) (strawberry bubble gum)

▷ *moxifloxacin* (C)(G) 400 mg daily x 5 days
Pediatric: <18 years: not recommended; ≥18 years: same as adult
Avelox *Tab:* 400 mg; IV soln: 400 mg/250 mg (latex-free, preservative-free)

Comment: *moxifloxacin* is contraindicated <18 years-of-age and during pregnancy and lactation. Risk of tendonitis or tendon rupture.

▷ *ofloxacin* (C)(G) 400 mg bid x 10 days
Pediatric: <18 years: not recommended; ≥18 years: same as adult
Floxin *Tab:* 200, 300, 400 mg

Comment: *ofloxacin* is contraindicated <18 years-of-age and during pregnancy and lactation. Risk of tendonitis or tendon rupture.

▷ *telithromycin* (C) 800 mg once daily x 7-10 days; *Severe renal impairment including dialysis:* 600 mg once daily; *Severe renal impairment with coexisting hepatic impairment:* 400 mg once daily.
Pediatric: <18 years: not recommended; ≥18 years: same as adult
Ketek *Tab:* 400, 500 mg

Comment: *telithromycin* is a ketolide indicated for the treatment of mild-to-moderate CAP). Fatal acute liver injury has been reported; discontinue immediately if signs and symptoms of hepatitis occur. There is increased risk for ventricular arrhythmias, including ventricular tachycardia and *torsades de pointes* with fatal outcomes; avoid use in patients with known QT prolongation, hypokalemia, and with class IA and III antiarrhythmics. Fatalities with *colchicine*, rhabdomyolysis with HMG-CoA reductase inhibitors (statins), and hypotension with calcium channel blockers (CCBs) have been reported; therefore, avoid concomitant use. Monitor for toxicity and consider dose reduction of the concomitant medication, if concomitant use is unavoidable. Evaluate for *C. difficile* if diarrhea occurs. Contraindications include: myasthenia gravis, concomitant *cisapride* or *pimozide*, history of hepatitis or jaundice with any macrolide.

▷ *tetracycline* (D)(G) 250-500 mg qid x 7 days
Pediatric: <8 years: not recommended; ≥8 years, <100 lb: 25-50 mg/kg/day in 2-4 divided doses x 7 days; ≥8 years, ≥100 lb: same as adult; *see page 630 for dose by weight*
Achromycin V *Cap:* 250, 500 mg
Sumycin *Tab:* 250, 500 mg; *Cap:* 250, 500 mg; *Oral susp:* 125 mg/5 ml (100, 200 ml) (fruit) (sulfites)

Comment: *tetracycline* is contraindicated <8 years-of-age, in pregnancy, and lactation (discolors developing tooth enamel). A side effect may be photo-sensitivity (photophobia). Do not take with antacids, calcium supplements, milk or other dairy, or within two hours of taking another drug.

▷ *trimethoprim+sulfamethoxazole (TMP-SMX)*(D)(G) bid x 10 days
Pediatric: <2 months: not recommended; ≥2 months: 40 mg/kg/day of *sulfamethoxazole* in 2 divided doses bid x 10 days; *see page 630 for dose by weight*; ≥12 years: same as adult
Bactrim, Septra 2 tabs bid x 10 days
Tab: trim 80 mg+sulfa 400 mg*
Bactrim DS, Septra DS 1 tab bid x 10 days
Tab: trim 160 mg+sulfa 800 mg*
Bactrim Pediatric Suspension, Septra Pediatric Suspension
Oral susp: trim 40 mg+sulfa 200 mg per 5 ml (100 ml) (cherry) (alcohol 0.3%)

Comment: Sulfonamides are contraindicated in the first trimester of pregnancy, the final month of pregnancy, and infants <8 weeks-of-age. *CrCl 15-30 mL/min:* reduce dose by 1/2; *CrCl <15 mL/min:* not recommended. Contraindicated with G6PD deficiency. A high fluid intake is indicated during sulfonamide therapy to avoid crystallization in the kidneys.

BRONCHITIS: CHRONIC/CHRONIC OBSTRUCTIVE PULMONARY DISEASE (COPD)

Oral Beta-2 Agonists (Bronchodilators) *see Asthma page* 36
Inhaled Corticosteroids *see Asthma page* 31
Parenteral Corticosteroids *see page* 577
Oral Corticosteroids *see page* 577
Inhaled Beta-2 Agonists (Bronchodilators) *see Asthma page* 30

LONG-ACTING INHALED BETA-2 AGONIST (LABA)

▶ *indacaterol* (C) inhale contents of one 75 mcg cap daily
   Pediatric: <12 years: not recommended; ≥12 years: same as adult
      Arcapta Neohaler *Neohaler Device/Cap:* 75 mcg pwdr for inhalation (5 blister cards, 6 caps/card)
   Comment: Remove cap from blister cap immediately before use. For oral inhalation with **Neohaler** device only. *indacaterol* is indicated for the long-term maintenance treatment of bronchoconstriction in patients with COPD. Not indicated for treating asthma, for primary treatment of acute symptoms, or for acute deterioration of COPD.
▶ *indacaterol+glycopyrrolate* (C) inhale the contents of one cap twice daily
   Pediatric: <18 years: not recommended; ≥18 years: same as adult
      Utibron Neohaler *Neohaler Device/Cap:* inda 27.5 mcg+glyco 15.6 mcg pwdr for inhalation (1, 10 blister cards, 6 caps/card)
▶ *olodaterol* (C) 12 mcg q 12 hours
   Pediatric: <12 years: not recommended; ≥12 years: same as adult
      Striverdi Respimat *Inhal soln:* 2.5 mcg/cartridge (metered actuation) (40 gm, 60 metered actuations) (benzalkonium chloride)
▶ *salmeterol* (C)(G) 1 inhalation q 12 hours
   Pediatric: <4 years: not recommended; ≥4 years: same as adult
      Serevent Diskus *Diskus (pwdr):* 50 mcg/actuation (60 doses/diskus)

ANTICHOLINERGIC

▶ *glycopyrrolate inhalation solution* administer the contents of one vial via **Magnair** handset twice daily
   Pediatric: <18 years: not indicated
      Lonhala Magnair *Vial:* 25 mcg/ml (1 ml) unit dose for use with **Magnair** handset; *Starter Kit:* 60 unit-dose vials w. **Magnair** handset; *Refill Kit:* 60 unit-dose vials w. **Magnair** handset
   Comment: For oral inhalation only. Do not swallow **Lonhala** solution. Only use **Lonhala** vials with **Magnair**. Do not initiate in acutely deteriorating COPD or to treat acute symptoms. If paradoxical bronchospasm occurs, discontinue **Lonhala Magnair** immediately and institute alternative therapy. Worsening of narrow-angle glaucoma may occur; use with caution in patients with narrow-angle glaucoma and instruct patients to contact a physician immediately if symptoms occur. Worsening of urinary retention may occur. Use with caution in patients with prostatic hyperplasia (BPH) or bladder neck obstruction (BNO) and instruct patients to consult a physician immediately if symptoms occur. Avoid administration with other anticholinergic drugs. Consider risk versus benefit in patients with severe renal impairment. Most common adverse reactions (incidence ≥ 2.0%) are dyspnea and urinary tract infection. There are no adequate and well-controlled studies in pregnancy. **Lonhala Magnair** should only be used during pregnancy if the expected benefit to the patient outweighs the potential risk to the fetus. There are no data on the presence of *glycopyrrolate* or its metabolites in human milk or effects on the breastfed infant. The developmental and health benefits of breastfeeding should be considered along with the mother's clinical need for **Lonhala Magnair** and any potential adverse effects on the breastfed infant from **Lonhala Magnair** or from the underlying maternal condition. To report suspected adverse reactions, contact Sunovion Pharmaceuticals at 1 877-737-7226 or FDA at 1-800-FDA-1088 or www.fda.gov/medwatch.

INHALED ANTICHOLINERGICS

▷ *glycopyrrolate inhalation solution* (C) inhale the contents of 1 capsule twice daily at the same time of day, AM and PM, using the **Neohaler**; do not swallow caps
Pediatric: not indicated
> **Seebri Neohaler** *Inhal cap:* 15.6 mcg (60/blister pck) dry pwdr for inhalation w. 1 Neo- haler device (lactose)

▷ *ipratropium bromide* (B)(G)
Pediatric: <12 years: not recommended; ≥12 years: same as adult
> **Atrovent** 2 inhalations qid; max 12 inhalations/day
> > *Inhaler:* 14 gm (200 inh)
> **Atrovent Inhalation Solution** 500 mcg by nebulizer tid-qid
> > *Inhal soln:* 0.02% (2.5 ml)

Comment: *ipratropium bromide* is contraindicated with severe hypersensitivity to milk proteins.

▷ *umeclidinium* (C) 1 inhalation once daily at the same time each day
Pediatric: <12 years: not recommended; ≥12 years: same as adult
> **Incruse Ellipta** *Inhal pwdr:* 62.5 mcg/inhalation (30 doses) (lactose)
> Comment: **Incruse Ellipta** is contraindicated with allergy to *atropine* or its derivatives.

INHALED LONG-ACTING ANTI-CHOLINERGICS (LAA) (ANTIMUSCARINICS)

Comment: Inhaled LAAs are for prophylaxis and chronic treatment, only. Not for primary (rescue) treatment of acute attack. Avoid getting powder in eyes. Caution with narrow-angle glaucoma, BPH, bladder neck obstruction, and pregnancy. Contraindicated with allergy to atropine or its derivatives (e.g., *ipratropium*). Avoid other anticholinergic agents.

▷ *aclidinium bromide* (C) 1 inhalation twice daily using inhaler
Pediatric: <12 years: not recommended; ≥12 years: same as adult
> **Tudorza Pressair** *Inhal device:* 400 mcg/actuation (60 doses per inhalation device)

▷ *glycopyrrolate inhalation solution* (C) administer the contents of one vial twice daily at the same times of day, AM and PM, via the **Magnair** neb inhal device; do not swallow solution; do not use **Magnair** with any other medicine; length of treatment is 2-3 minutes; do not use 2 vials/treatment or more than 2 vials/day
Pediatric: not indicated
> **Lonhala Magnair** *Vial:* 25 mcg/ml (1 ml) unit dose for use with **Magnair** hand-set; *Starter Kit:* 60 unit-dose vials w. **Magnair** handset; *Refill Kit:* 60 unit-dose vials (low-density polyethylene [LDPE]) w. **Magnair** handset (preservative-free)
> Comment: **Lonhala Magnair** is the first nebulizing long-acting muscarinic antago-nist (LAMA) approved for the treatment of COPD in the United States. Its approval was based on data from clinical trials in the Glycopyrrolate for Obstructive Lung Disease via Electronic Nebulizer (GOLDEN) program, including GOLDEN-3 and GOLDEN-4, 2 Phase 3, 12-week, randomized, double-blind, placebo-controlled, parallel-group, multicenter study. Do not initiate **Lonhala Magnair** in acutely deteriorating COPD or to treat acute symptoms. If paradoxical bronchospasm occurs, discontinue **Lonhala Magnair** immediately and institute alternative therapy. Worsening of narrow-angle glaucoma may occur; use with caution in patients with narrow-angle glaucoma and instruct patients to contact a physician immediately if symptoms occur. Worsening of urinary retention may occur. Use with caution in patients with prostatic hyperplasia (BPH) or bladder neck obstruction (BNO) and instruct patients to seek medical care immediately if symptoms occur. Avoid admin-istration with other anticholinergic drugs. Consider risk versus benefit in patients with severe renal impairment. Most common adverse reactions (incidence ≥ 2.0%) have been dyspnea and urinary tract infection. There are no adequate and well-con-trolled studies in pregnancy. **Lonhala Magnair** should only be used during pregnancy if the expected benefit to the patient outweighs the potential risk to the fetus. There are no data on the presence of *glycopyrrolate* or its metabolites in human milk or effects on the breastfed infant. The developmental and health benefits of breastfeed-ing should be considered along with the mother's clinical need for **Lonhala Magnair** and any potential adverse effects on the breastfed infant from **Lonhala Magnair** or from the underlying maternal condition. To report suspected adverse reactions, contact Sunovion Pharmaceuticals at 1 877-737-7226 or FDA at 1-800-FDA-1088 or visit www.fda.gov/medwatch.

▷ *revefenacin inhalation solution* administer the contents of one vial via nebulizer once daily
at the same times of day; do not swallow solution; do not use more than 1 vial/day; do not
use **Yupelri** with any other medicine
Pediatric: not indicated
  Yupelri *Vial:* 175 mcg/3 ml (3 ml) unit-dose solution for nebulizer
  Comment: **Yupelri** is the first and only long-acting muscarinic antagonist (LAMA)
  solution for once daily nebulized administration. **Yupelri** is indicated for maintenance treatment of moderate-to-severe. Do not initiate **Yupelri** in acutely deteriorating COPD or to treat acute symptoms. If paradoxical bronchospasm occurs,
  discontinue **Yupelri** immediately and institute alternative therapy. Worsening of
  narrow-angle glaucoma may occur; use with caution in patients with narrow-angle
  glaucoma and instruct patients to contact a healthcare provider immediately if symptoms occur. Use with caution in patients with prostatic hyperplasia or bladder-neck
  obstruction and instruct patients to contact a healthcare provider immediately
  if symptoms occur. May interact additively with other concomitantly used anticholinergic medications; avoid administration of **Yupelri** with other anticholinergic-containing drugs. Co-administration of **Yupelri** with OATP1B1 and OATP1B3
  inhibitors (e.g. rifampicin, cyclosporine) may lead to an increase in exposure of the
  active metabolite; co-administration with **Yupelri** is not recommended. Avoid use
  of **Yupelri** in patients with hepatic impairment. Most common adverse reactions
  (incidence ≥2%) include cough, nasopharyngitis, upper respiratory tract infection,
  headache, and back pain. There are no adequate and well-controlled studies with
  Yupelri in pregnancy and no information regarding the presence of *revefenacin* in
  human milk or effects on the breastfed infant. To report suspected adverse reactions,
  contact Mylan at 1-877-446-3679 (1-877-4-INFO-RX) or FDA at 1-800-FDA-1088 or
  visit www.fda.gov/medwatch.
▷ *tiotropium (as bromide monohydrate)* (C) 1 inhalation daily using inhaler; do not swallow
caps
Pediatric: <12 years: not recommended; ≥12 years: same as adult
  Spiriva HandiHaler *Inhal device:* 18 mcg/cap (5, 30, 90 caps w. inhalation device)

INHALED ANTI-CHOLINERGIC+LONG-ACTING BETA-2 AGONIST (LABA) COMBINATIONS

▷ *ipratropium/albuterol* (C) 1 inhalation qid; max 6 inhalations/day
Pediatric: <12 years: not established; ≥12 years: same as adult
  Combivent Respimat *Inhal soln:* ipra 20 mcg+alb 100 mcg per inhalation (4 gm,
  120 inhal)
  Comment: **Combivent Respimat** is contraindicated with *atropine* allergy.
▷ *tiotropium+olodaterol* (C) 2 inhalations once daily at the same time each day; max 2
inhalations/day
Pediatric: <12 years: not recommended; ≥12 years: same as adult
  Stiolto Respimat *Inhal soln:* tio 2.5 mcg+olo 2.5 mcg per actuation (4 gm, 60 inh)
  (benzalkonium chloride)
  Comment: **Stiolto Respimat** is not for treating asthma, for relief of acute bronchospasm, or acutely deteriorating COPD.
▷ *umeclidinium+vilanterol* (C) 1 inhalation once daily at the same time each day
Pediatric: <12 years: not recommended; ≥12 years: same as adult
  Anoro Ellipta *Inhal soln:* ume 62.5 mcg+vila 25 mcg per inhalation (30 doses)
  Comment: **Anoro Ellipta** is contraindicated with severe hypersensitivity to milk proteins.

INHALED CORTICOSTEROID+LONG-ACTING BETA-2 AGONIST (LABA) COMBINATION

▷ *fluticasone furoate+vilanterol* (C) 1 inhalation 100/25 once daily at the same time each
day
Pediatric: <17 years: not recommended; ≥17 years: same as adult
  Breo Ellipta 100/25 *Inhal pwdr:* flu 100 mcg+vil 25 mcg dry pwdr per inhalation
  (30 doses)
  Breo Ellipta 200/25 *Inhal pwdr:* flu 200 mcg+vil 25 mcg dry pwdr per inhalation
  (30 doses)
  Comment: **Breo Ellipta** is contraindicated with severe hypersensitivity to milk proteins.

INHALED CORTICOSTEROID+ANTICHOLINERGIC+LONG-ACTING BETA-2 AGONIST (LABA) COMBINATION

▷ *fluticasone furoate+umeclidinium+vilanterol* one inhalation once daily

Trelegy Ellipta flutic furo 100 mcg/umec 62.5 mcg/vilan 25 mcg dry pwdr

Comment: **Trelegy Ellipta** is maintenance therapy for patients with COPD, including chronic bronchitis and emphysema, who are receiving fixed-dose *furoate* and *vilanterol* for airflow obstruction and to reduce exacerbations, or receiving *umeclidinium* and a fixed-dose combination of *fluticasone furoate* and *vilanterol*. **Trelegy Ellipta** is the first FDA-approved once-daily single-dose inhaler that combines *fluticasone furoate*, a corticosteroid, *umeclidinium*, a long-acting muscarinic antagonist, and *vilantero*, a long-acting beta-2 adrenergic agonist. Common adverse reactions reported with **Trelegy Ellipta** included headache, back pain, dysgeusia, diarrhea, cough, oropharyngeal pain, and gastroenteritis. **Trelegy Ellipta** has been found to increase the risk of pneumonia in patients with COPD, and increase the risk of asthma-related death in patients with asthma. **Trelegy Ellipta** is not indicated for the treatment of asthma or acute bronchospasm.

METHYLXANTHINES

Comment: Check serum theophylline level just before 5th dose is administered. Therapeutic theophylline level: 10-20 mcg/ml.

▷ *theophylline* (C)(G)

Theo-24 initially 300-400 mg once daily at HS; after 3 days, increase to 400-600 mg once daily at HS; max 600 mg/day

Pediatric: <45 kg: initially 12-14 mg/kg/day; max 300 mg/day; increase after 3 days to 16 mg/kg/day to max 400 mg; after 3 more days increase to 30 mg/kg/day to max 600 mg/day; ≥45 kg: same as adult

Cap: 100, 200, 300, 400 mg ext-rel

Theo-Dur initially 150 mg bid; increase to 200 mg bid after 3 days; then increase to 300 mg bid after 3 more days

Pediatric: <6 years: not recommended; ≥6-15 years: initially 12-14 mg/kg/day in 2 divided doses; max 300 mg/day; then increase to 16 mg/kg in 2 divided doses; max 400 mg/day; then to 20 mg/kg/day in 2 divided doses; max 600 mg/day

Tab: 100, 200, 300 mg ext-rel

Theolair-SR

Pediatric: <12 years: not recommended; ≥12 years: same as adult

Tab: 200, 250, 300, 500 mg sust-rel

Uniphyl 400-600 mg daily with meals

Pediatric: <12 years: not recommended; ≥12 years: same as adult

Tab: 400*, 600*mg cont-rel

METHYLXANTHINE+EXPECTORANT COMBINATION

▷ *dyphylline+guaifenesin* (C)

Lufyllin GG 1 tab qid or 15-30 ml qid

Tab: dyphy 200 mg+guaif 200 mg; *Elix:* dyphy 100 mg+guaif 100 mg per 15 ml

SELECTIVE PHOSPHODIESTERASE 4 (PDE4) INHIBITOR

▷ *roflumilast* (C)(G) 500 mcg once daily

Pediatric: <12 years: not recommended; ≥12 years: same as adult

Daliresp *Tab:* 500 mcg

Comment: *roflumilast* is indicated to reduce the risk of COPD exacerbations in severe COPD patients with chronic bronchitis and a history of exacerbations.

LONG-ACTING MUSCARINIC ANTAGONISTS (LAMA)

▷ *glycopyrrolate* (C)

Comment: There are no data on the safety of *glycopyrrolate* use in pregnancy or presence of *glycopyrrolate* or its metabolites in human milk or effects on the breastfed infant.

Lonhala Magnair inhale the contents of 1 vial twice daily at the same times of day, AM and PM, via Magnair neb inhal device; do not swallow solution; do not use **Magnair**

with any other medicine; length of treatment is 2-3 minutes; do not use 2 vials/treatment or more than 2 vials/day
Pediatric: not indicated for use in children
   Neb soln: Vial: 25 mcg/1 ml single-dose for administration with Magnair neb inhal device; *Starter Kit:* 30 day supply (2 vials/pouch, 30 foil pouches/carton) and 1 complete MAGNAIR Nebulizer System; *Refill Kit:* (2 vials/pouch, 30 foil pouches/carton) and 1 complete MAGNAIR refill handset
Comment: **Lonhala Magnair** is the first nebulizing long-acting muscarinic antagonist (LAMA) approved for the treatment of COPD in the United States. Its approval was based on data from clinical trials in the Glycopyrrolate for Obstructive Lung Disease via Electronic Nebulizer (GOLDEN) program, including GOLDEN-3 and GOLDEN-4, 2 Phase 3, 12-week, randomized, double-blind, placebo-controlled, parallel-group, multicenter study.
Seebri Neohaler inhale the contents of 1 capsule twice daily at the same time of day, AM and PM, using the neohaler; do not swallow caps
Pediatric: not indicated for use in children
   Inhal cap: 15.6 mcg (60/blister pck) dry pwdr for inhalation w. 1 Neohaler device (lactose)

BULIMIA NERVOSA

SELECTIVE SEROTONIN REUPTAKE INHIBITOR (SSRI)
▷ *fluoxetine* (C)(G)
   Prozac initially 20 mg daily; may increase after 1 week; doses >20 mg/day may be divided into AM and noon doses; usual daily dose 60 mg; max 80 mg/day
   Pediatric: <8 years: not recommended; 8-17 years: initially 10-20 mg/day; start lower weight children at 10 mg/day; if starting at 10 mg daily, may increase after 1 week to 20 mg/day; >17 years: same as adult
      Cap: 10, 20, 40 mg; *Tab:* 30*, 60*mg; *Oral soln:* 20 mg/5 ml (4 oz) (mint)
   Prozac Weekly following daily *fluoxetine* therapy at 20 mg/day for 13 weeks, may initiate **Prozac Weekly** 7 days after the last 20 mg *fluoxetine* dose
   Pediatric: <12 years: not recommended; ≥12 years: same as adult
      Cap: 90 mg ent-coat del-rel pellets

BURN: MINOR

▷ *silver sulfadiazine* (C)(G) apply topically to burn 1-2 x daily
   Pediatric: <12 years: not recommended; ≥12 years: same as adult
      Silvadene *Crm:* 1% (20, 50, 85, 400, 1000 gm jar; 20 gm tube)
   Comment: *silver sulfadiazine* is contradicted in sulfa allergy.

TOPICAL AND TRANSDERMAL ANESTHETICS
Comment: *lidocaine* should not be applied to non-intact skin.
▷ *lidocaine* cream (B) apply to affected area bid prn
   Pediatric: <12 years: not recommended; ≥12 years: same as adult
      LidaMantle *Crm:* 3% (1, 2 oz)
      Lidoderm *Crm:* 3% (85 gm)
      ZTlido *lidocaine* topical system 1% (30/carton)
      Comment: Compared to **Lidoderm** (*lidocaine* patch 5%) which contains 700 mg/patch, **ZTlido** only requires 35 mg per topical system to achieve the same therapeutic dose.
▷ *lidocaine* lotion (B) apply to affected area bid prn
   Pediatric: <12 years: not recommended; ≥12 years: same as adult
      LidaMantle *Lotn:* 3% (177 ml)
▷ *lidocaine* 5% patch (B)(G) apply up to 3 patches at one time for up to 12 hours/24-hour period (12 hours on/12 hours off); patches may be cut into smaller sizes before removal of the release liner; do not re-use

Pediatric: <12 years: not recommended; ≥12 years: same as adult
Lidoderm *Patch:* 5% (10x14 cm; 30/carton)
▷ *lidocaine+dexamethasone* **(B)**
Pediatric: <12 years: not recommended; ≥12 years: same as adult
Decadron Phosphate with Xylocaine *Lotn:* dexa 4 mg+lido 10 mg per ml (5 ml)
▷ *lidocaine+hydrocortisone* **(B)(G)** apply to affected area bid prn
Pediatric: <12 years: not recommended; ≥12 years: same as adult
LidaMantle HC *Crm:* lido 3%+hydro 0.5% (1, 3 oz); *Lotn:* (177 ml)
▷ *lidocaine 2.5%+prilocaine 2.5%* apply sparingly to the burn bid-tid prn
Pediatric: <12 years: not recommended; ≥12 years: same as adult
Emla Cream (B) 5, 30 gm/tube

 BURSITIS

Acetaminophen for IV Infusion *see Pain page* 352
NSAIDs *see page* 571
Opioid Analgesics *see Pain page* 354
Topical & Transdermal Analgesics *see Pain page* 352
Parenteral Corticosteroids *see page* 577
Oral Corticosteroids *see page* 577
Topical Analgesic and Anesthetic Agents *see page* 569

CANDIDIASIS: ABDOMEN, BLADDER, ESOPHAGUS, KIDNEY

▷ *voriconazole* **(D)(G)** *PO:* <40 kg: 100 mg q 12 hours; may increase to 150 mg q 12 hours
if inadequate response; ≥40 kg: 200 mg q 12 hours; may increase to 300 mg q 12 hours if
inadequate; *IV:* 6 mg/kg q 12 hours x 2 doses; then 4 mg/kg q 12 hour; max rate 3 mg/kg/
hour over 1-2 hours; response
Pediatric: <12 years: not recommended; ≥12 years: same as adult
Vfend *Tab:* 50, 200 mg
Vfend I.V. for Injection *Vial:* 200 mg pwdr for reconstitution (preservative-free)
Vfend *Oral susp:* 40 mg/ml pwdr for reconstitution (75 ml) (orange)

CANDIDIASIS: ORAL (THRUSH)

ORAL ANTIFUNGALS

▷ *clotrimazole* **(C)** *Prophylaxis:* 1 troche dissolved in mouth tid; *Treatment:* 1 troche dissolved
in mouth 5 x/day x 10-14 days
Pediatric: <3 years: not recommended; ≥3 years: same as adult
Mycelex Troches *Troche:* 10 mg
▷ *fluconazole* **(C)** 200 mg x 1 dose first day; then 100 mg once daily x 13 days
Pediatric: >2 weeks: 6 mg/kg x 1 day; then 3 mg/kg/day for at least 3 weeks; *see page* 627 *for
dose by weight*
Diflucan *Tab:* 50, 100, 150, 200 mg; *Oral susp:* 10, 40 mg/ml (35 ml) (orange) (sucrose)
▷ *gentian violet* **(G)** apply to oral mucosa with a cotton swab tid x 3 days
▷ *itraconazole* **(C)(G)** 200 mg daily x 7-14 days
Pediatric: 5 mg/kg daily x 7-14 days; max 200 mg/day; *see page* 628 *for dose by weight*
Sporanox *Oral soln:* 10 mg/ml (150 ml) (cherry-caramel)
▷ *miconazole* **(C)** One buccal tab once daily x 14 days; apply to upper gum region; hold in
place 30 seconds; do not crush, chew, *or* swallow
Pediatric: <16 years: not recommended; ≥16 years: same as adult
Oravig *Buccal tab:* 50 mg (14/pck)
▷ *nystatin* **(C)(G)**
Mycostatin 1-2 pastilles dissolved slowly in mouth 4-5 x/day x 10-14 days; max 14 days
Pediatric: same as adult
Pastille: 200,000 units (30 pastilles/pck)
Mycostatin Suspension 4-6 ml qid swish and swallow
Pediatric: Infants: 1 ml in each cheek qid after feedings; *Older children:* same as adult
Oral susp: 100,000 units/ml (60 ml w. dropper)

INVASIVE INFECTION

▷ *posaconazole* (D)(G) *Oral Therapy:* take with food; 100 mg bid on day one; then 100 mg once daily x 13 days; refractory, 400 mg bid x 13 days; *IV Infusion Therapy:* must be administered through an in-line filter over approximately 90 minutes via a central venous line. <u>Never</u> administer **Noxafil** as an IV bolus injection; *Loading Dose:* a single 300 mg IV infusion; *Maintenance Dose: a single* 300 mg IV infusion once daily; duration of therapy is based on recovery from neutropenia <u>or</u> immunosuppression.
   Pediatric: <13 years: not recommended; ≥13 years: same as adult
     Noxafil *Tab:* 100 mg ext-rel; *Oral susp:* 40 mg/ml (105 ml) (cherry); *Vial:* 300 mg/16.7 ml (18 mg/ml) soln for IV infusion
     Comment: **Noxafil** is indicated as prophylaxis for invasive aspergillus and candida infections in patients >13-years-old who are at high risk due to being severely compromised.

CANDIDIASIS: SKIN

TOPICAL ANTIFUNGALS

▷ *butenafine* (B)(G) apply bid x 1 week <u>or</u> once daily x 4 weeks
   Pediatric: <12 years: not recommended; ≥12 years: same as adult
     Lotrimin Ultra (C)(OTC) *Crm:* 1% (12, 24 gm)
     Mentax *Crm:* 1% (15, 30 gm)
   Comment: *butenafine* is a benzylamine, not an azole. Fungicidal activity continues for at least 5 weeks after the last application.

▷ *ciclopirox* (B)
     Loprox Cream apply bid; max 4 weeks
       Pediatric: <10 years: not recommended; ≥10 years: same as adult
       Crm: 0.77% (15, 30, 90 gm)
     Loprox Lotion apply bid; max 4 weeks
       Pediatric: <10 years: not recommended; ≥10 years: same as adult
       Lotn: 0.77% (30, 60 ml)
     Loprox Gel apply bid; max 4 weeks
       Pediatric: <16 years: not recommended; ≥16 years: same as adult
       Gel: 0.77% (30, 45 gm)

▷ *clotrimazole* (B) apply bid x 7 days
   Pediatric: <12 years: not recommended; ≥12 years: same as adult
     Lotrimin *Crm:* 1% (15, 30, 45 gm)
     Lotrimin AF (OTC) *Crm:* 1% (12 gm); *Lotn:* 1% (10 ml); *Soln:* 1% (10 ml)

▷ *econazole* (C) apply bid x 14 days
   Pediatric: <12 years: not recommended; ≥12 years: same as adult
     Spectazole *Crm:* 1% (15, 30, 85 gm)

▷ *ketoconazole* (C) apply once daily x 14 days
   Pediatric: <12 years: not recommended; ≥12 years: same as adult
     Nizoral Cream *Crm:* 2% (15, 30, 60 gm)

▷ *miconazole* 2% (C) apply once daily x 2 weeks
   Pediatric: <12 years: not recommended; ≥12 years: same as adult
     Lotrimin AF Spray Liquid (OTC) *Spray liq:* 2% (113 gm) (alcohol 17%)
     Lotrimin AF Spray Powder (OTC) *Spray pwdr:* 2% (90 gm) (alcohol 10%)
     Monistat-Derm *Crm:* 2% (1, 3 oz); *Spray liq:* 2% (3.5 oz); *Spray pwdr:* 2% (3 oz)

▷ *nystatin* (C) dust affected skin freely bid-tid
     Nystop Powder *Pwdr:* 100,000 U/gm (15 gm)

ORAL ANTIFUNGALS

▷ *amphotericin b* (B)
     Fungizone *Oral susp:* 100 mg/ml (24 ml w. dropper)

▷ *ketoconazole* (C) 400 mg once daily x 1-2 weeks
   Pediatric: <2 years: not recommended; ≥2 years: 3.3-6.6 mg/kg once daily
     Nizoral *Tab:* 200 mg

INVASIVE INFECTION

▷ *posaconazole* (D)(G) *Oral Therapy:* take with food; 100 mg bid on day one; then 100 mg once daily x 13 days; refractory, 400 mg bid x 13 days *IV Infusion Therapy:* must be administered through an in-line filter over approximately 90 minutes via a central venous line. <u>Never</u> administer **Noxafil** as an IV bolus injection; *Loading Dose: a single* 300 mg IV infusion; *Maintenance Dose: a single* 300 mg IV infusion once daily; duration of therapy is based on recovery from neutropenia <u>or</u> immunosuppression.

Pediatric: <13 years: not recommended; ≥13 years: same as adult

Noxafil *Tab:* 100 mg ext-rel; *Oral susp:* 40 mg/ml (105 ml) (cherry); *Vial:* 300 mg/16.7 ml (18 mg/ml) soln for IV infusion

Comment: **Noxafil** is indicated as prophylaxis for invasive aspergillus and candida infections in patients >13 years old who are at high risk due to being severely compromised.

 CANDIDIASIS: VULVOVAGINAL (MONILIASIS)

PROPHYLAXIS

▷ *acetic acid+oxyquinolone* (C) one full applicator intravaginally bid for up to 30 days
Pediatric: <12 years: not recommended; ≥12 years: same as adult

Relagard *Gel:* acetic acid 0.9%+oxyquin 0.025% (50 gm tube w. applicator)

Comment: The following treatment regimens for vulvovaginal candidiasis (VVC) are published in the **2015 CDC Sexually Transmitted Diseases Treatment Guidelines**. Treatment regimens are presented by generic drug name first, followed by information about brands and dose forms. Complicated VVC (recurrent, severe, non-albicans, <u>or</u> women with uncontrolled diabetes, debilitation, <u>or</u> immunosuppression) may require more intensive treatment <u>and/or</u> longer duration of treatment. VVC frequently occurs during pregnancy. Only topical azole therapies, applied for 7 days, are recommended during pregnancy.

RX ORAL AGENT

▷ *fluconazole* 150 mg in a single dose; complicated VVC, 150 mg x 3 doses on days 1, 4, 7 <u>or</u> weekly x 6 months

Rx INTRAVAGINAL AGENTS

Regimen 1
▷ *butoconazole* 2% cream (bioadhesive product) 5 gm intravaginally in a single dose

Regimen 2
▷ *nystatin* 100,000-unit vaginal tablet once daily x 14 days

Regimen 3
▷ *terconazole* 0.4% cream 5 gm intravaginally once daily x 7 days

Regimen 4
▷ *terconazole* 0.8% cream 5 gm intravaginally once daily x 3 days

Regimen 5
▷ *terconazole* 80 mg vaginal suppository intravaginally once daily x 3 days

OTC INTRAVAGINAL AGENTS

Regimen 1
▷ *butoconazole* 2% cream 5 gm intravaginally once daily x 3 days

Regimen 2
▷ *clotrimazole* 1% cream intravaginally once daily x 7-14 days

Regimen 3
▷ *clotrimazole* 2% cream intravaginally once daily x 3 days

Regimen 4
▷ *miconazole* 2% cream intravaginally once daily x 7 days

Regimen 5

▷ *miconazole* 4% cream intravaginally once daily x 3 days

Regimen 6

▷ *miconazole* 100 mg vaginal suppository intravaginally once daily x 7 days

Regimen 7

▷ *miconazole* 200 mg vaginal suppository intravaginally once daily x 3 days

Regimen 8

▷ *miconazole* 1,200 mg vaginal suppository intravaginally in a single application

Regimen 9

▷ *tioconazole* 6.5% ointment 5 gm intravaginally in a single application

DRUG BRANDS AND DOSE FORMS

▷ *butoconazole* cream 2% (C)

Gynazole-12% Vaginal Cream *Prefilled vag applicator:* 5 g
Femstat-3 Vaginal Cream (OTC) *Vag crm:* 2% (20 gm w. 3 applicators); *Prefilled vag applicator:* 5 gm (3/pck)

▷ *clotrimazole* (B)(OTC)

Gyne-Lotrimin Vaginal Cream (OTC) *Vag crm:* 1% (45 gm w. applicator)
Gyne-Lotrimin Vaginal Suppository (OTC) *Vag supp:* 100 mg (7/pck)
Gyne-Lotrimin 3 Vaginal Suppository (OTC) *Vag supp:* 200 mg (3/pck)
Gyne-Lotrimin Combination Pack (OTC) *Combination pck:* 7-100 mg supp <u>with</u> 7 gm 1% cream
Gyne-Lotrimin 3 Combination Pack (OTC) *Combination pck:* 200 mg supp (7/pck) <u>plus</u> 1% cream (7 gm)
Mycelex-G Vaginal Cream *Vag crm:* 1% (45, 90 gm w. applicator)
Mycelex-G Vaginal Tab 1 *Tab:* 500 mg (1/pck)
Mycelex Twin Pack *Twin pck:* 500 mg tab (7/pck) <u>with</u> 1% crm (7 gm)
Mycelex-7 Vaginal Cream (OTC) *Vag crm:* 1% (45 gm w. applicator)
Mycelex-7 Vaginal Inserts (OTC) *Vag insert:* 100 mg insert (7/pck)
Mycelex-7 Combination Pack (OTC) *Combination pck:* 100 mg inserts (7/pck) <u>plus</u> 1% crm (7 gm)

▷ *fluconazole* (C)

Diflucan *Tab:* 50, 100, 150, 200 mg; *Oral susp:* 10, 40 mg/ml (35 ml) (orange)

▷ *miconazole* (B)

Monistat-3 Combination Pack (OTC) *Combination pck:* 200 mg supp (3/pck) <u>plus</u> 2% crm (9 gm)
Monistat-7 Combination Pack (OTC) *Combination pck:* 100 mg supp (7/pck) <u>plus</u> 2% crm (9 gm)
Monistat-7 Vaginal Cream (OTC) *Vag crm:* 2% (45 gm w. applicator)
Monistat-7 Vaginal Suppositories (OTC) *Vag supp:* 100 mg (7/pck)
Monistat-3 Vaginal Suppositories (OTC) *Vag supp:* 200 mg (3/pck)

▷ *nystatin* (C)

Mycostatin *Vag tab:* 100,000 U (1/pck)

▷ *terconazole* (C)

Terazol-3 Vaginal Cream *Vag crm:* 0.8% (20 gm w. applicator)
Terazol-3 Vaginal Suppositories *Vag supp:* 80 mg supp (3/pck)
Terazol-7 Vaginal Cream *Vag crm:* 0.4% (45 gm w. applicator)

▷ *tioconazole* (C)

1-Day (OTC) *Vag oint:* 6.5% (prefilled applicator x 1)
Monistat 1 Vaginal Ointment (OTC) *Vag oint:* 6.5% (prefilled applicator x 1)
Vagistat-1 Vaginal Ointment (OTC) *Vag oint:* 6.5% (prefilled applicator x 1)

INVASIVE INFECTION

▷ *posaconazole* (D)(G) *Oral Therapy:* take with food; 100 mg bid on day 1; then 100 mg once daily x 13 days; refractory, 400 mg bid x 13 days; *IV Infusion Therapy:* must be administered through an in-line filter over approximately 90 minutes via a central venous line. <u>Never</u> administer **Noxafil** as an IV bolus injection; *Loading Dose: a single* 300 mg IV infusion;

Maintenance Dose: a single 300 mg IV infusion once daily; duration of therapy is based on recovery from neutropenia <u>or</u> immunosuppression.
Pediatric: <13 years: not recommended; ≥13 years: same as adult
    Noxafil *Tab:* 100 mg ext-rel; *Oral susp:* 40 mg/ml (105 ml) (cherry); *Vial:* 300 mg/ 16.7 ml (18 mg/ml) soln for IV infusion
    Comment: **Noxafil** is indicated as prophylaxis for invasive aspergillus and candida infections in patients >13-years-old who are at high risk due to being severely compromised.

CANNABINOID HYPEREMESIS SYNDROME (CHS)

Comment: cannabinoid hyperemesis syndrome (CHS) is indicated by recurrent episodes of refractory nausea and vomiting with vague diffuse abdominal pain (accompanied by compulsive, frequent, hot baths <u>or</u> showers for relief of abdominal pain; these behaviors are thought to be learned through their cyclical periods of emesis) in the setting of chronic cannabis use (at least weekly for >2 years. The nausea and vomiting typically do not respond to antiemetic medications. 5HT3 (e.g., *ondansetron*), D2 (e.g., *prochlorperazine*), H1 (e.g., *promethazine*), <u>or</u> neurokinin-1 receptor antagonists (e.g., *aprepitant*) can be tried, but these therapies often are ineffective. The recovery phase can last weeks to months despite continued cannabis use prior to returning to the hyperemetic phase. Symptoms that are worse in the morning, with normal bowel habits, and negative evaluation, including laboratory, radiography, and endoscopy. Resolution requires cannabis cessation from 1 to 3 months. Returning to cannabis use often results in the returning of CHS.

REFERENCE
Fleming, J. E., & Lockwood, S. (2017). Cannabinoid hyperemesis syndrome. *Federal Practitioner, 34*(10),
    33–36. Retrieved from https://www.mdedge.com/fedprac/article/148661/hospital-medicine/cannabinoid-hyperemesis-syndrome

PHENOTHIAZINES

▷ *chlorpromazine* (C)(G) 10-25 mg PO q 4 hours prn <u>or</u> 50-100 mg rectally q 6-8 hours prn
Pediatric: <6 months: not recommended; ≥6 months: 0.25 mg/lb orally q 4-6 hours prn <u>or</u> 0.5 mg/lb rectally q 6-8 hours prn
    Thorazine *Tab:* 10, 25, 50, 100, 200 mg; *Spansule:* 30, 75, 150 mg sust-rel; *Syr:* 10 mg/5 ml (4 oz; orange custard); *Conc:* 30 mg/ml (4 oz); 100 mg/ml (2, 8 oz); *Supp:* 25, 100 mg
▷ *perphenazine* (C) 5 mg IM (may repeat in 6 hours) <u>or</u> 8-16 mg/day PO in divided doses; max 15 mg/day IM; max 24 mg/day PO
Pediatric: <12 years: not recommended; ≥12 years: same as adult
    Trilafon *Tab:* 2, 4, 8, 16 mg; *Oral conc:* 16 mg/5 ml (118 ml); *Amp:* 5 mg/ml (1 ml)
▷ *prochlorperazine* (C)(G) 5-10 mg tid-qid prn; usual max 40 mg/day
    Compazine
    Pediatric: <2 years <u>or</u> <20 lb: not recommended; 20-29 lb: 2.5 mg daily bid prn; max 7.5 mg/day; 30-39 lb: 2.5 mg bid-tid prn; max 10 mg/day; 40-85 lb: 2.5 mg tid <u>or</u> 5 mg bid prn; max 15 mg/day
        Tab: 5, 10 mg; *Syr:* 5 mg/5 ml (4 oz) (fruit)
    Compazine Suppository 25 mg rectally bid prn; usual max 50 mg/day
    Pediatric: <2 years <u>or</u> <20 lb: not recommended; 20-29 lb: 2.5 mg daily-bid prn; max 7.5; mg/day; 30-39 lb: 2.5 mg bid-tid prn; max 10 mg/day; 40-85 lb: 2.5 mg tid <u>or</u> 5 mg bid prn; max 15 mg/day
        Rectal supp: 2.5, 5, 25 mg
    Compazine Injectable 5-10 mg tid <u>or</u> qid prn
    Pediatric: <2 years <u>or</u> <20 lb: not recommended; ≥2 years <u>or</u> ≥20 lb: 0.06 mg/kg x 1 dose
        Vial: 5 mg/ml (2, 10 ml)
    Compazine Spansule 15 mg q AM prn <u>or</u> 10 mg q 12 hours prn usual max 40 mg/day
    Pediatric: <12 years: not recommended; ≥12 years: same as adult
        Spansule: 10, 15 mg sust-rel
▷ *promethazine* (C)(G) 25 mg PO <u>or</u> rectally q 4-6 hours prn
Pediatric: <2 years: not recommended; ≥2 years: 0.5 mg/lb <u>or</u> 6.25-25 mg q 4-6 hours prn
    Phenergan *Tab:* 12.5*, 25*, 50 mg; *Plain syr:* 6.25 mg/5 ml; *Fortis syr:* 25 mg/5 ml; *Rectal supp:* 12.5, 25, 50 mg
Comment: *promethazine* is contraindicated in children with uncomplicated nausea, dehydration, Reye's syndrome, history of sleep apnea, asthma, and lower respiratory disorders in children. *promethazine* lowers the seizure threshold in children, may cause cholestatic

jaundice, anticholinergic effects, extrapyramidal effects, and potentially fatal respiratory depression.

SUBSTANCE P/NEUROKININ 1 RECEPTOR ANTAGONIST

▷ *aprepitant* (B)(G) administer with 5HT-3 receptor antagonist; *Day 1:* 125 mg x 1 dose; *Starting Day 2:* 80 mg once daily in the morning
Pediatric: <6 months: years: not recommended; ≥6 months: use oral suspension (see mfr pkg insert for dose by weight
  Emend *Cap:* 40, 80, 125 mg (2 x 80 mg bi-fold pck; 1 x 25 mg/2 x 80 mg tri-fold pck); *Oral susp:* 125 mg pwdr for oral suspension, single-dose pouch w. dispenser; *Vial:* 150 mg pwdr for reconstitution and IV infusion

SEROTONIN (5HT-3) RECEPTOR ANTAGONISTS

▷ *dolasetron* (B) administer 100 mg IV over 30 seconds; max 100 mg/dose
Pediatric: <2 years: not recommended; 2-16 years: 1.8 mg/kg; >16 years: same as adult
  Anzemet *Tab:* 50, 100 mg; *Amp:* 12.5 mg/0.625 ml; *Prefilled carpuject syringe:* 12.5 mg (0.625 ml); *Vial:* 100 mg/5 ml (single-use); *Vial:* 500 mg/25 ml (multi-dose)
▷ *granisetron*
  Kytril (B) administer IV over 30 seconds; max 1 dose/week
  Pediatric: <2 years: not recommended; ≥2 years: 10 mcg/kg
    Tab: 1 mg; *Oral soln:* 2 mg/10 ml (30 ml) (orange); *Vial:* 1 mg/ml (1 ml single-dose) (preservative-free); 1 mg/ml (4 ml multi-dose) (benzyl alcohol)
  Sancuso (B) apply 1 patch; remove 24 hours (minimum) to 7 days (maximum)
    Transdermal patch: 3.1 mg/day
▷ *granisetron extended-release injection* administer SC over 20-30 seconds (due to drug viscosity) on Day 1 of chemotherapy and not more frequently than once every 7 days; *CrCl 30-59 mL/min:* repeat dose no more than every 14th day; *CrCl <30 mL/min:* not recommended; for patients receiving MEC, the recommended *dexamethasone* dosage is 8 mg IV on Day 1; for patients receiving AC combination chemotherapy regimens, the recommended *dexamethasone* dosage is 20 mg IV on Day 1, followed by 8 mg PO bid on Days 2, 3 and 4; if Sustol is administered with an NK₁ receptor antagonist, see that drug's mfr pkg insert for the recommended *dexamethasone* dosing
Pediatric: <12 years: not established; ≥12 years: same as adult
  Sustol *Syringe:* 10 mg/0.4 ml ext-rel; prefilled single-dose/kit
  Comment: At least 60 minutes prior to administration, remove the Sustol kit from refrigeration; activate a warming pouch and wrap the syringe in the warming pouch for 5-6 minutes to warm it to room temperature.
▷ *ondansetron* (C)(G) Oral Forms: 8 mg q 8 hours x 2 doses; then 8 mg q 12 hours
Pediatric: <4 years: not recommended; 4-11 years: 4 mg q 4 hours x 3 doses; then 4 mg q 8 hours
  Zofran *Tab:* 4, 8, 24 mg
  Zofran ODT *ODT:* 4, 8 mg (strawberry) (phenylalanine)
  Zofran Oral Solution *Oral soln:* 4 mg/5 ml (50 ml) (strawberry) (phenylalanine); *Parenteral form:* see mfr pkg insert
  Zofran Injection *Vial:* 2 mg/ml (2 ml single-dose); 2 mg/ml (20 ml muti-dose); 32 mg/50 ml (50 ml multi-dose); *Prefilled syringe:* 4 mg/2 ml, single-use (24/ carton)
  Zuplenz Oral Soluble Film: 4, 8 mg oral-dis (10/carton) (peppermint)
  Comment: The FDA has issued an updated warning against *ondansetron* use in pregnancy *ondansetron* is a 5-HT3 receptor antagonist approved by the FDA for preventing nausea and vomiting related to cancer chemotherapy and surgery. However, it has been used "off label" to treat the nausea and vomiting of pregnancy. The FDA has cautioned against the use of *ondansetron* in pregnancy in light of studies of *ondansetron* in early pregnancy and associated with congenital cardiac malformations and oral clefts (i.e., cleft lip and cleft palate). Further, there are potential maternal risks in pregnancy with electrolyte imbalance caused by severe nausea and vomiting (as with hyperemesis gravidarum). These risks include serotonin syndrome (a triad of cognitive and behavioral changes including confusion, agitation, autonomic instability, and neuromuscular changes). Therefore, *ondansetron* should not be taken during pregnancy.
▷ *palonosetron* (B)(G) administer 0.25 mg IV over 30 seconds; max 1 dose/week
Pediatric: <1 month: not recommended; 1 month to 17 years: 20 mcg/kg; max 1.5 mg/ single dose; infuse over 15 minutes
  Aloxi *Vial (single-use):* 0.075 mg/1.5 ml; 0.25 mg/5 ml (mannitol)

CARCINOID SYNDROME DIARRHEA (CSD)

TRYPTOPHAN HYDROXYLASE

▷ *telotristat* take with food; 250 mg tid
  Pediatric: <12 years: not established; ≥12 years: same as adult
    Xermelo *Tab:* 250 mg (4 x 7 daily dose pcks/carton)
  Comment: Take **Xermelo** in combination with somatostatin analog (SSA) therapy to treat patients inadequately controlled by SSA therapy. Breastfeeding females should monitor the infant for constipation.

 CARPAL TUNNEL SYNDROME (CTS)

Acetaminophen for IV Infusion *see Pain page* 352
NSAIDs *see page* 571
Opioid Analgesics *see Pain page* 354
Topical & Transdermal Analgesics *see Pain page* 352
Parenteral Corticosteroids *see page* 577
Oral Corticosteroids *see page* 577
Topical Analgesic and Anesthetic Agents *see page* 569

CAT SCRATCH FEVER (*BARTONELLA* INFECTION)

Comment: Cat scratch fever is usually self-limited. Treatment should be limited to severe or debilitating cases.

ANTI-INFECTIVES

▷ *azithromycin* (B)(G) 500 mg x 1 dose on day 1, then 250 mg daily on days 2-5 or 500 mg daily x 3 days or **Zmax** 2 gm in a single dose
  Pediatric: 12 mg/kg/day x 5 days; max 500 mg/day; *see page* 619 *for dose by weight*
    Zithromax *Tab:* 250, 500, 600 mg; *Oral susp:* 100 mg/5 ml (15 ml); 200 mg/5 ml (15, 22.5, 30 ml) (cherry); *Pkt:* 1 gm for reconstitution (cherry-banana)
    Zithromax Tri-pak *Tab:* 3 x 500 mg tabs/pck
    Zithromax Z-pak *Tab:* 6 x 250 mg tabs/pck
    Zmax *Oral susp:* 2 gm ext-rel for reconstitution (cherry-banana) (148 mg Na⁺)
▷ *doxycycline* (D)(G) 100 mg daily bid
  Pediatric: <8 years: not recommended ≥8 years, <100 lb: 2 mg/lb on first day in 2 divided doses, followed by 1 mg/lb/day in 1-2 divided doses; ≥8 years, ≥100 lb: same as adult; *see page* 625 *for dose by weight*
    Acticlate *Tab:* 75, 150**mg
    Adoxa *Tab:* 50, 75, 100, 150 mg ent-coat
    Doryx *Tab:* 50, 75, 100, 150, 200 mg del-rel
    Doxteric *Tab:* 50 mg del-rel
    Monodox *Cap:* 50, 75, 100 mg
    Oracea *Cap:* 40 mg del-rel
    Vibramycin *Tab:* 100 mg; *Cap:* 50, 100 mg; *Syr:* 50 mg/5 ml (raspberry-apple) (sulfites); *Oral susp:* 25 mg/5 ml (raspberry)
    Vibra-Tab *Tab:* 100 mg film-coat
  Comment: *doxycycline* is contraindicated <8 years-of-age, in pregnancy, and lactation (discolors developing tooth enamel). A side effect may be photosensitivity (photophobia). Do not give with antacids, calcium supplements, milk or other dairy, or within 2 hours of taking another drug.
▷ *erythromycin base* (B)(G) 500-1000 mg qid x 4 weeks
  Pediatric: <45 kg: 30-50 mg in 2-4 divided doses x 4 weeks; ≥45 kg: same as adult
    Ery-Tab *Tab:* 250, 333, 500 mg ent-coat
    PCE *Tab:* 333, 500 mg
  Comment: *erythromycin* may increase INR with concomitant *warfarin*, as well as increase serum level of *digoxin*, benzodiazepines, and statins.

➤ *erythromycin ethylsuccinate* (B)(G) 400 mg qid x 4 weeks
Pediatric: 30-50 mg/kg/day in 4 divided doses x 4 weeks; may double dose with severe infection; max 100 mg/kg/day; *see page 626 for dose by weight*

> **EryPed** *Oral susp:* 200 mg/5 ml (100, 200 ml) (fruit); 400 mg/5 ml (60, 100, 200 ml) (banana); *Oral drops:* 200, 400 mg/5 ml (50 ml) (fruit); *Chew tab:* 200 mg wafer (fruit)
> **E.E.S.** *Oral susp:* 200, 400 mg/5 ml (100 ml) (fruit)
> **E.E.S. Granules** *Oral susp:* 200 mg/5 ml (100, 200 ml) (cherry)
> **E.E.S. 400 Tablets** *Tab:* 400 mg

Comment: *erythromycin* may increase INR with concomitant *warfarin*, as well as increase serum level of *digoxin*, benzodiazepines, and statins.

➤ *trimethoprim+sulfamethoxazole (TMP-SMX)*(D)(G) bid x 10 days
Pediatric: <2 months: not recommended; ≥2 months: 40 mg/kg/day of *sulfamethoxazole* in 2 divided doses bid x 10 days; *see page 630 for dose by weight*

> **Bactrim, Septra** 2 tabs bid x 10 days
> *Tab:* trim 80 mg+sulfa 400 mg*
> **Bactrim DS, Septra DS** 1 tab bid x 10 days
> *Tab:* trim 160 mg+sulfa 800 mg*
> **Bactrim Pediatric Suspension, Septra Pediatric Suspension**
> *Oral susp:* trim 40 mg+sulfa 200 mg per 5 ml (100 ml) (cherry) (alcohol 0.3%)

Comment: Sulfonamides are contraindicated in the first trimester of pregnancy, the final month of pregnancy, and infants <8 weeks-of-age. *CrCl 15-30 mL/min:* reduce dose by 1/2; *CrCl <15 mL/min:* not recommended. Contraindicated with G6PD deficiency. A high fluid intake is indicated during sulfonamide therapy to avoid crystallization in the kidneys.

CELLULITIS, ACUTE BACTERIAL SKIN AND SKIN STRUCTURE INFECTION (ABSSSI)

Comment: Duration of treatment should be 10-30 days. Obtain culture from site. Consider blood cultures.

ANTI-INFECTIVES

➤ *amoxicillin* (B)(G) 500-875 mg bid or 250-500 mg tid x 10 days
Pediatric: <40 kg (88 lb): 20-40 mg/kg/day in 3 divided doses x 10 days or 25-45 mg/kg/day in 2 divided doses x 10 days; ≥40 kg: same as adult; *see page 617 for dose by weight*

> **Amoxil** *Cap:* 250, 500 mg; *Tab:* 875*mg; *Chew tab:* 125, 200, 250, 400 mg (cherry-banana-peppermint) (phenylalanine); *Oral susp:* 125, 250 mg/5 ml (80, 100, 150 ml) (strawberry); 200, 400 mg/5 ml (50, 75, 100 ml) (bubble gum); *Oral drops:* 50 mg/ml (30 ml) (bubble gum)
> **Moxatag** *Tab:* 775 mg ext-rel
> **Trimox** *Tab:* 125, 250 mg; *Cap:* 250, 500 mg; *Oral susp:* 125, 250 mg/5 ml (80, 100, 150 ml) (raspberry-strawberry)

➤ *amoxicillin+clavulanate* (B)(G)

> **Augmentin** 500 mg tid or 875 mg bid x 7-10 days
> *Pediatric:* 40-45 mg/kg/day divided tid x 10 days or 90 mg/kg/day divided bid x 10 days *see pages 618 for dose by weight*
>> *Tab:* 250, 500, 875 mg; *Chew tab:* 125, 250 mg (lemon-lime); 200, 400 mg (cherry-banana) (phenylalanine); *Oral susp:* 125 mg/5 ml (banana), 250 mg/5 ml (75, 100, 150 ml) (orange); 200, 400 mg/5 ml (50, 75, 100 ml) (orange) (phenylalanine)
> **Augmentin ES-600** not recommended for adults
> *Pediatric:* <3 months: not recommended; ≥3 months, <40 kg: 90 mg/kg/day in 2 divided doses x 7-10 days; ≥40 kg: not recommended
>> *Oral susp:* 42.9 mg/5 ml (50, 75, 100, 125, 150, 200 ml) (strawberry cream) (phenylalanine)
> **Augmentin XR** 2 tabs q 12 hours x 7-10 days
> *Pediatric:* <16 years: use other forms; ≥16 years: same as adult
>> *Tab:* 1000*mg ext-rel

➤ *azithromycin* (B)(G) 500 mg x 1 dose on day 1, then 250 mg daily on days 2-5 or 500 mg daily x 3 days or **Zmax** 2 gm in a single dose

Pediatric: 12 mg/kg/day x 5 days; max 500 mg/day; *see page 619 for dose by weight*
    Zithromax *Tab:* 250, 500, 600 mg; *Oral susp:* 100 mg/5 ml (15 ml); 200 mg/5 ml (15, 22.5, 30 ml) (cherry); *Pkt:* 1 gm for reconstitution (cherry-banana)
    Zithromax Tri-pak *Tab:* 3 x 500 mg tabs/pck
    Zithromax Z-pak *Tab:* 6 x 250 mg tabs/pck
    Zmax *Oral susp:* 2 gm ext-rel for reconstitution (cherry-banana) (148 mg Na⁺)

► *cefaclor* (B)(G) 250-500 mg q 8 hours x 10 days; max 2 gm/day
Pediatric: <1 month: not recommended; 20-40 mg/kg bid <u>or</u> q 12 hours x 10 days; max 1 gm/day; *see page 620 for dose by weight*
Tab: 500 mg; *Cap:* 250, 500 mg; *Susp:* 125 mg/5 ml (75, 150 ml) (strawberry); 187 mg/5 ml (50, 100 ml) (strawberry); 250 mg/5 ml (75, 150 ml) (strawberry); 375 mg/5 ml (50, 100 ml) (strawberry)
    Cefaclor Extended Release
    Pediatric: <16 years: ext-rel not recommended; ≥16 years: same as adult
    Tab: 375, 500 mg ext-rel

► *cefpodoxime proxetil* (B) 400 mg bid x 7-14 days
Pediatric: ≥2 months-12 years: 10 mg/kg/day (max 400 mg/dose) <u>or</u> 5 mg/kg/day bid (max 200 mg/dose) x 7-14 days; *see page 622 for dose by weight;* >12 years: same as adult
    Vantin *Tab:* 100, 200 mg; *Oral susp:* 50, 100 mg/5 ml (50, 75, 100 mg) (lemon creme)

► *cefprozil* (B) 500 mg q 12 hours x 10 days
Pediatric: <2 years: not recommended; 2-12 years: 15 mg/kg q 12 hours x 10 days; *see page 622 for dose by weight;* >12 years: same as adult
    Cefzil *Tab:* 250, 500 mg; *Oral susp:* 125, 250 mg/5 ml (50, 75, 100 ml) (bubble gum) (phenylalanine)

► *ceftaroline fosamil* (B) administer 600 mg once every 12 hours, by IV infusion over 5-60 minutes, x 5-14 days
Pediatric: <18 years: not established; ≥18 years: same as adult
    Teflaro *Vial:* 400, 600 mg pwdr for reconstitution, single-use (10/carton)
    Comment: Teflaro is indicated for the treatment of adults with acute bacterial skin and skin structures infection (ABSSSI).

► *ceftriaxone* (B)(G) 1-2 gm daily x 5-14 days IM; max 4 gm daily
Pediatric: 50-75 mg/kg IM in 1-2 divided doses x 5-14 days; max 2 gm/day
    Rocephin *Vial:* 250, 500 mg; 1, 2 gm

► *cephalexin* (B)(G) 500 mg bid x 10 days
Pediatric: 25-50 mg/kg/day in 4 divided doses x 10 days; *see page 623 for dose by weight*
    Keflex *Cap:* 250, 333, 500, 750 mg; *Oral susp:* 125, 250 mg/5 ml (100, 200 ml) (strawberry)

► *clarithromycin* (C)(G) 500 mg q 12 hours <u>or</u> 500 mg ext-rel once daily x 10 days
Pediatric: <6 months: not recommended; ≥6 months: 7.5 mg/kg bid x 10 days; *see page 624 for dose by weight*
    Biaxin *Tab:* 250, 500 mg
    Biaxin Oral Suspension *Oral susp:* 125, 250 mg/5 ml (50, 100 ml) (fruit-punch)
    Biaxin XL *Tab:* 500 mg ext-rel
Comment: The FDA is advising caution before prescribing *clarithromycin* to patients with heart disease because of a potential increased risk of heart problems <u>or</u> death that can occur years later. This recommendation is based on a review of the results of a 10-year follow-up study of patients with coronary heart disease from a large clinical trial that first observed this safety issue. Consider risk benefit and the use of other antibiotics in such patients.

► *dalbavancin* (C) 1000 mg administered once as a single dose via IV infusion over 30 minutes <u>or</u> initially 1,000 mg once, followed by 500 mg 1 week later; infuse over 30 minutes; *CrCl <30 mL/min:* not receiving dialysis: initially 750 mg, followed by 375 mg 1 week later
Pediatric: <18 years: not established; ≥18 years: same as adult
    Dalvance *Vial:* 500 mg pwdr for reconstitution, single-use (preservative-free)
    Comment: Dalvance is a lipoglycopeptide indicated for the treatment of acute bacterial skin and skin structures infection (ABSSSI) caused by gram-positive bacteria.

► *delafloxacin IV infusion:* administer 300 mg every 12 hours over 60 minutes x 5-14 days; *Tablet:* 450 mg every 12 hours x 5-14 days; dosage for patients with renal impairment is based on eGFR (see mfr pkg insert)
Pediatric: <18 years: not recommended; ≥18 years: same as adult
    Baxdela *Tab:* 450 mg; *Vial:* 300 mg pwdr for reconstitution and IV infusion

Comment: **Baxdela**, a fluoroquinolone, is indicated for the treatment of acute bacterial skin and skin structure infections (ABSSSI) caused by designated susceptible bacteria. Fluoroquinolones have been associated with disabling and potentially irreversible serious adverse reactions that have occurred together, including tendinitis and tendon rupture, peripheral neuropathy, and central nervous system effects. Discontinue **Baxdela** immediately and avoid the use of fluoroquinolones, including **Baxdela**, in patients who experience any of these serious adverse reactions. Fluoroquinolones may exacerbate muscle weakness in patients with myasthenia gravis. Therefore, avoid **Baxdela** in patients with known history of myasthenia gravis. Most common adverse reactions are nausea, diarrhea, headache, transaminase elevations and vomiting. Closely monitor SCr in patients with severe renal impairment (eGFR 15-29 mL/min/1.73 m^2) receiving intravenous *delafloxacin*. If SCr level increases occur, consider changing to oral *delafloxacin*. Discontinue **Baxdela** if eGFR decreases to <15 mL/min/1.73 m^2. The limited available data with **Baxdela** use in pregnant females are insufficient to inform a drug-associated risk of major birth defects and miscarriages. There are no data available on the presence of *delafloxacin* in human milk or effects on the breast-fed infant. To report suspected adverse reactions, contact Melinta Therapeutics at (844) 635-4682 or FDA at 1-800FDA-1088 or www.fda.gov/medwatch.

▷ *dicloxacillin* (B)(G) 500 mg q 6 hours x 10 days
  Pediatric: 12.5-25 mg/kg/day in 4 divided doses x 10 days; *see page 624 for dose by weight*
    Dynapen *Cap:* 125, 250, 500 mg; *Oral susp:* 62.5 mg/5 ml (80, 100, 200 ml)
▷ *dirithromycin* (C)(G) 500 mg once daily x 5-7 days
  Pediatric: <12 years: not recommended; ≥12 years: same as adult
    Dynabac *Tab:* 250 mg
▷ *erythromycin base* (B)(G) 250 mg qid or 333 mg tid or 500 mg bid x 7-10 days; then taper to lowest effective dose
  Pediatric: <45 kg: 30-50 mg in 2-4 divided doses x 7-10 days; ≥45 kg: same as adult
    Ery-Tab *Tab:* 250, 333, 500 mg ent-coat
    PCE *Tab:* 333, 500 mg

Comment: *erythromycin* may increase INR with concomitant *warfarin*, as well as increase serum level of *digoxin*, benzodiazepines, and statins.

▷ *erythromycin ethylsuccinate* (B)(G) 400 mg qid x 7-10 days
  Pediatric: 30-50 mg/kg/day in 4 divided doses x 7-10 days; may double dose with severe infection; max 100 mg/kg/day; *see page 626 for dose by weight*
    EryPed *Oral susp:* 200 mg/5 ml (100, 200 ml) (fruit); 400 mg/5 ml (60, 100, 200 ml) (banana); *Oral drops:* 200, 400 mg/5 ml (50 ml) (fruit); *Chew tab:* 200 mg wafer (fruit)
    E.E.S. *Oral susp:* 200, 400 mg/5 ml (100 ml) (fruit)
    E.E.S. Granules *Oral susp:* 200 mg/5 ml (100, 200 ml) (cherry)
    E.E.S. 400 Tablets *Tab:* 400 mg

Comment: *erythromycin* may increase INR with concomitant *warfarin*, as well as increase serum level of *digoxin*, benzodiazepines, and statins.

▷ *linezolid* (C)(G) 600 mg q 12 hours x 10-14 days
  Pediatric: <5 years: 10 mg/kg q 8 hours x 10-14 days; 5-11 years: 10 mg/kg q 12 hours x 10-14 days; >11 years: same as adult
    Zyvox *Tab:* 400, 600 mg; *Oral susp:* 100 mg/5 ml (150 ml) (orange) (phenylalanine)

Comment: *linezolid* is indicated to treat susceptible vancomycin-resistant *E. faecium* infections of skin and skin structures, including diabetic foot without osteomyelitis.

▷ *loracarbef* (B) 200 mg bid x 10 days
  Pediatric: 15 mg/kg/day in 2 divided doses x 10 days; *see page 628 for dose by weight*
    Lorabid *Pulvule:* 200, 400 mg; *Oral susp:* 100 mg/5 ml (50, 100 ml); 200 mg/5 ml (50, 75, 100 ml) (strawberry bubble gum)
▷ *moxifloxacin* (C)(G) 400 mg once daily x 5 days
  Pediatric: <18 years: recommended; ≥18 years: same as adult
    Avelox *Tab:* 400 mg; *IV soln:* 400 mg/250 mg (latex-free, preservative-free)

Comment: *moxifloxacin* is contraindicated <18 years-of-age and during pregnancy and lactation. Risk of tendonitis or tendon rupture.

▷ *omadacycline* <u>before</u> oral dosing, fast x at least 4 hours and then take tablets with water; <u>after</u> oral dosing, <u>no</u> food <u>or</u> drink (except water) x 2 hours and <u>no</u> dairy products, antacids, <u>or</u> multivitamins x 4 hours; total treatment duration 7-14 days
  OPTION 1, *Loading Dose, Day 1:* 200 mg via IV infusion over 60 minutes or 100 mg via IV

infusion over 30 minutes twice; *Maintenance:* 100 mg via IV infusion over 30 minutes once daily or 300 mg orally once daily

OPTION 2 (tablets only): Day 1 and Day 2: 450 mg orally once daily; then, reduce dose to 300 mg orally once daily

Pediatric: <18 years: not recommended; ≥18 years: same as adult

> Nuzyra *Tab:* 150 mg; *Vial:* 100 mg single dose for reconstitution, dilution, and IV infusion
> Comment: **Nuzyra** *(omadacycline)* is an aminomethylcycline tetracycline antibiotic for the treatment of community-acquired bacterial pneumonia (CABP) and acute bacterial skin and skin structure infection (ABSSSI). The most common adverse reactions (incidence ≥2%) are nausea, vomiting, infusion site reactions, alanine aminotransferase (ALT) increased, aspartate aminotransferase (AST) increased, gamma-glutamyl transferase (GGT) increased, hypertension, headache, diarrhea, insomnia, and constipation. Like other tetracycline-class antibacterial drugs, **Nuzyra** may cause discoloration of deciduous teeth and reversible inhibition of bone growth when administered during the second and third trimester of pregnancy. The limited available data of **Nuzyra** use in pregnancy is insufficient to inform drug-associated risk of major birth defects and miscarriages. There is no information on the presence of *omadacycline* in human milk or effects on the breastfed infant.

▷ *oritavancin* (C) administer 1,200 mg as a single dose by IV infusion over 3 hours
  Pediatric: <18 years: not established; ≥18 years: same as adult
    Orbactiv *Vial:* 400 mg pwdr for reconstitution, single-use (10/carton) (mannitol; preservative-free)
    Comment: **Orbactiv** is indicated for the treatment of acute bacterial skin and skin structures infection (ABSSSI).

▷ *penicillin v potassium* (B) 250-500 mg q 6 hours x 5-7 days
  Pediatric: <12 years: *see page 629 for dose by weight;* >12 years: same as adult
    Pen-Vee K *Tab:* 250, 500 mg; *Oral soln:* 125 mg/5 ml (100, 200 ml); 250 mg/5 ml (100, 150, 200 ml)

▷ *tedizolid phosphate* (C) administer 200 mg once daily x 6 days, via PO or IV infusion over 1 hour
  Pediatric: <18 years: not established; ≥18 years: same as adult
    Sivextro *Tab:* 200 mg (6/blister pck)
    Comment: **Sivextro** is indicated for the treatment of adults with acute bacterial skin and skin structures infection (ABSSSI).

▷ *tigecycline* (D)(G) 100 mg as a single dose; then 50 mg q 12 hours x 5-14 days; with severe hepatic impairment (Child-Pugh Class C), 100 mg as a single dose; then 25 mg q 12 hours
  Pediatric: <18 years: not recommended; ≥18 years: same as adult
    Tygacil *Vial:* 50 mg pwdr for reconstitution and IV infusion (preservative-free)
    Comment: **Tygacil** is contraindicated in pregnancy, and lactation (discolors developing tooth enamel). A side effect may be photo-sensitivity (photophobia). Do not give with antacids, calcium supplements, milk or other dairy, or within two hours of taking another drug.

CERUMEN IMPACTION

OTIC ANALGESIC

▷ *antipyrine+benzocaine+zinc acetate dihydrate* otic (C) fill ear canal with solution; then moisten cotton plug with solution and insert into meatus; may repeat every 1-2 hours prn
  Pediatric: same as adult
    Otozin *Otic soln:* antipyr 5.4%+benz 1%+zinc 1% per ml (10 ml w. dropper)

CERUMINOLYTICS

▷ *triethanolamine* (OTC)(G) fill ear canal and insert cotton plug for 15-30 minutes before irrigating with warm water
    Cerumenex *Soln:* 10% (6, 12 ml)

▷ *carbamide peroxide* (OTC)(G) instill 5-10 drops in ear canal; keep drops in ear several minutes; then irrigate with warm water; repeat bid for up to 4 days
    Debrox *Soln:* 15, 30 ml squeeze bottle w. applicator

CHAGAS DISEASE (AMERICAN TRYPANOSOMIASIS)

Comment: Chagas Disease is a protozoal parasite (*Trypanosoma cruzi*) infection with increasing prevalence in the US attributed to immigration from *T. cruzi*-endemic areas of South and Central Latin America. Approximately 300,000 persons in the US have chronic Chagas Disease and up to 30% of them will develop clinically evident cardiovascular and/or gastrointestinal disease. Chagas Disease is one of the five neglected parasitic infections (NPIs) targeted by CDC for public health action. Transmitted by the bite of the triatomine bug ("kissing bug") which feeds on human blood, maternal-fetus vertical transmission, blood transfusion, consumption of contaminated food, and organ donation. A clinical marker is Romaña sign (periorbital swelling), chagoma (skin nodule), Schizotrypanides (nonpruritic morbilliform rash). Only two antiparasitic drugs, *benznidazole* and *nifurtimox*, have demonstrated effectiveness altering the progression of this chronic disease. These drugs are not FDA approved and are available only from CDC under investigational protocols. Treatment is indicated for all cases of acute or reactivated Chagas Disease and for chronic *Trypanosoma cruzi* infection in children ≤18. Congenital infections are considered acute disease. Treatment is strongly recommended up to 50 years old with chronic infection who do not already have advanced Chagas cardiomyopathy. For adults older than 50 years with chronic *T. cruzi* infection, the decision to treat with antiparasitic drugs should be individualized, weighing the potential benefits and risks for the patient. Patients taking either of these drugs should have a CBC and CMP at the start of treatment and then bi-monthly for the duration of treatment to monitor for rare bone marrow suppression. Contraindications for treatment include severe hepatic and/or renal disease. As safety for infants exposed through breastfeeding has not been documented, withholding treatment while breastfeeding is also recommended. For emergencies (for example, acute Chagas Disease with severe manifestations, Chagas Disease in a newborn, or Chagas Disease in an immunocompromised person) outside of regular business hours, call the CDC Emergency Operations Center (770-488-7100) and ask for the person on call for Parasitic Diseases. For more detailed information about screening, assessment, and treatment of this public health threat, see McDonald, J, & Mattingly, J. (November, 2016). Chagas disease: Creeping into family practice in the United States, *Clinician Reviews*, pp. 38-45, or call 404-718-4745 or e-mail questions to chagas@cdc.gov.

ANTI-PARASITIC AGENTS

➤ *benznidazole* (NR)(G) take with a meal to avoid GI upset; <12 years: 5-7.5 mg/kg/day divided bid x 60 days; ≥12 years: 5-7 mg/kg/day divided bid x 60 days

Comment: Common side effects of *benznidazole* are allergic dermatitis, peripheral neuropathy, insomnia, anorexia with weight loss.

➤ *nifurtimox* (NR)(G) take with a meal to avoid GI upset; ≤10 years: 15-20 mg/kg/day divided tid-qid x 90 days; 11-16 years: 12.5-15 mg/kg/day divided tid-qid x 90 days; ≥17 years: 8-10 mg/kg/day divided tid-qid x 90 days

Comment: Common side effects of *nifurtimox* are anorexia and weight loss, nausea, vomiting, polyneuropathy, headache, dizziness or vertigo.

 CHANCROID

ANTI-INFECTIVES

➤ *azithromycin* (B)(G) 500 mg x 1 dose on day 1, then 250 mg daily on days 2-5 or 500 mg daily x 3 days or **Zmax** 2 gm in a single dose

Pediatric: 12 mg/kg/day x 5 days; max 500 mg/day; *see page* 619 *for dose by weight*

Zithromax *Tab:* 250, 500, 600 mg; *Oral susp:* 100 mg/5 ml (15 ml); 200 mg/5 ml (15, 22.5, 30 ml) (cherry); *Pkt:* 1 gm for reconstitution (cherry-banana)

Zithromax Tri-pak *Tab:* 3 x 500 mg tabs/pck

Zithromax Z-pak *Tab:* 6 x 250 mg tabs/pck

Zmax *Oral susp:* 2 gm ext-rel for reconstitution (cherry-banana) (148 mg Na⁺)

➤ *ceftriaxone* (B)(G) 250 mg IM in a single dose

Pediatric: <45 kg: 125 mg IM in a single dose; ≥45 kg: same as adult

Rocephin *Vial:* 250, 500 mg; 1, 2 gm

▷ *ciprofloxacin* (C) 500 mg bid x 3 days
  Pediatric: <18 years: not recommended; ≥18 years: same as adult
    Cipro *Tab:* 250, 500, 750 mg; *Oral susp:* 250, 500 mg/5 ml (100 ml) (strawberry)
    Cipro XR *Tab:* 500, 1000 mg ext-rel
    ProQuin XR *Tab:* 500 mg ext-rel
▷ *erythromycin base* (B)(G) 500 mg qid x 7 days
  Pediatric: 30-50 mg/kg/day divided bid-qid; max 100 mg/kg/day
    Ery-Tab *Tab:* 250, 333, 500 mg ent-coat
    PCE *Tab:* 333, 500 mg

Comment: *erythromycin* may increase INR with concomitant *warfarin*, as well as increase serum level of *digoxin*, benzodiazepines, and statins.

▷ *erythromycin ethylsuccinate* (B)(G) 400 mg qid x 7 days
  Pediatric: 30-50 mg/kg/day in 4 divided doses x 7 days; may double dose with severe infection; max 100 mg/kg/day; *see page* 626 *for dose by weight*
    EryPed *Oral susp:* 200 mg/5 ml (100, 200 ml) (fruit); 400 mg/5 ml (60, 100, 200 ml) (banana); *Oral drops:* 200, 400 mg/5 ml (50 ml) (fruit); *Chew tab:* 200 mg wafer (fruit)
    E.E.S. *Oral susp:* 200, 400 mg/5 ml (100 ml) (fruit)
    E.E.S. Granules *Oral susp:* 200 mg/5 ml (100, 200 ml) (cherry)
    E.E.S. 400 Tablets *Tab:* 400 mg

Comment: *erythromycin* may increase INR with concomitant *warfarin*, as well as increase serum level of *digoxin*, benzodiazepines, and statins.

CHEMOTHERAPY-INDUCED NAUSEA/VOMITING (CINV)

PHENOTHIAZINES

▷ *chlorpromazine* (C)(G) 10-25 mg PO q 4 hours prn or 50-100 mg rectally q 6-8 hours prn
  Pediatric: <6 months: not recommended; ≥6 months: 0.25 mg/lb orally q 4-6 hours prn or 0.5 mg/lb rectally q 6-8 hours prn; >12 years: same as adult
    Thorazine *Tab:* 10, 25, 50, 100, 200 mg; *Spansule:* 30, 75, 150 mg sust-rel; *Syr:* 10 mg/5 ml (4 oz; orange custard); *Conc:* 30 mg/ml (4 oz); 100 mg/ml (2, 8 oz); *Supp:* 25, 100 mg
▷ *perphenazine* (C) 5 mg IM (may repeat in 6 hours) or 8-16 mg/day PO in divided doses; max 15 mg/day IM; max 24 mg/day PO
  Pediatric: <12 years: not recommended; ≥12 years: same as adult
    Trilafon *Tab:* 2, 4, 8, 16 mg; *Oral conc:* 16 mg/5 ml (118 ml); *Amp:* 5 mg/ml (1 ml)
▷ *prochlorperazine* (C)(G) 5-10 mg tid-qid prn; usual max 40 mg/day
    Compazine
    Pediatric: <2 years or <20 lb: not recommended; 20-29 lb: 2.5 mg daily bid prn; max 7.5 mg/day; 30-39 lb: 2.5 mg bid-tid prn; max 10 mg/day; 40-85 lb: 2.5 mg tid or 5 mg bid prn; max 15 mg/day; >85 lb: same as adult
      Tab: 5, 10 mg; *Syr:* 5 mg/5 ml (4 oz) (fruit)
    Compazine Suppository 25 mg rectally bid prn; usual max 50 mg/day
    Pediatric: <2 years or <20 lb: not recommended; 20-29 lb: 2.5 mg daily-bid prn; max 7.5; mg/day; 30-39 lb: 2.5 mg bid-tid prn; max 10 mg/day; 40-85 lb: 2.5 mg tid or 5 mg bid prn; max 15 mg/day; >85 lb: same as adult
      Rectal supp: 2.5, 5, 25 mg
    Compazine Injectable 5-10 mg tid or qid prn
    Pediatric: <2 years or <20 lb: not recommended; ≥2 years or ≥20 lb: 0.06 mg/kg x 1 dose; >12 years: same as adult
      Vial: 5 mg/ml (2, 10 ml)
    Compazine Spansule 15 mg q AM prn or 10 mg q 12 hours prn usual max 40 mg/day
    Pediatric: <12 years: not recommended; ≥12 years: same as adult
      Spansule: 10, 15 mg sust-rel
▷ *promethazine* (C)(G) 25 mg PO or rectally q 4-6 hours prn
  Pediatric: <2 years: not recommended; ≥2 years: 0.5 mg/lb or 6.25-25 mg q 4-6 hours prn; >12 years: same as adult
    Phenergan *Tab:* 12.5*, 25*, 50 mg; *Plain syr:* 6.25 mg/5 ml; *Fortis syr:* 25 mg/5 ml; *Rectal supp:* 12.5, 25, 50 mg

Comment: *promethazine* is contraindicated in children with uncomplicated nausea, dehydration, Reye's syndrome, history of sleep apnea, asthma, and lower respiratory disorders in children. *promethazine* lowers the seizure threshold in children, may cause cholestatic jaundice, anticholinergic effects, extrapyramidal effects, and potentially fatal respiratory depression.

SUBSTANCE P/NEUROKININ 1 RECEPTOR ANTAGONIST

▷ *aprepitant* (B)(G) administer with corticosteroid and 5HT-3 receptor antagonist; *Day 1 of chemotherapy cycle:* 125 mg 1 hour prior to chemotherapy *Day 2 and 3:* 80 mg in the morning
Pediatric: <6 months: years: not recommended; ≥6 months-12 years: use oral suspension (see mfr pkg insert for dose by weight); >12 years: same as adult
   Emend *Cap:* 40, 80, 125 mg (2 x 80 mg bi-fold pck; 1 x 25 mg/2 x 80 mg tri-fold pck); *Oral susp:* 125 mg pwdr for oral suspension, single-dose pouch w. dispenser; *Vial:* 150 mg pwdr for reconstitution and IV infusion

SUBSTANCE P/NEUROKININ-1 (NK-1) RECEPTOR ANTAGONIST AND SEROTONIN-3 (5-HT3) RECEPTOR ANTAGONIST COMBINATION

▷ *fosnetupitant+palonosetron*
Comment: **Akynzeo** capsules and **Akynzeo for Injection** are indicated in combination with *dexamethasone* for the prevention of acute and delayed nausea and vomiting associated with initial and repeat courses of cancer chemotherapy. The most common adverse reactions (incidence ≥3%) are headache, asthenia, dyspepsia, fatigue, constipation and erythema. Avoid concomitant CYP3A4 substrates for one week; if not avoidable, consider dose reduction of the CYP3A4 substrate because inhibition of CYP3A4 by *netupitant* can result in increased plasma concentrations of the concomitant drug for 6 days after single dosage administration of **Akynzeo**. CYP3A4 inducers (e.g., *rifampin*) decrease plasma concentrations of *netupitant*.
Pediatric: <18 years: not recommended; ≥18 years: same as adult
   Akynzeo administer a single dose approximately 1 hour prior to the start of chemotherapy, with or without food, with concurrent administration of *dexamethasone* 12 mg; on days 2-4, omit *dexamethasone*
      Cap: netu 300 mg+palo 0.5 mg
   Akynzeo for Injection reconstitute in 50 ml of D$_5$0.9% NaCl and administer via IV infusion over 30 minutes starting approximately 30 minutes prior to the start of chemotherapy with concurrent administration of *dexamethasone* 12 mg; on days 2-4, decrease *dexamethasone* to 8 mg each day
      Vial: fosn 235 mg+palo 0.25 mg single-dose pwdr for reconstitution and IV infusion

5HT-3 RECEPTOR ANTAGONISTS

Comment: The selective 5HT-3 receptor antagonists indicated for prevention of nausea and vomiting associated with moderately to highly emetogenic chemotherapy.
▷ *dolasetron* (B) administer 100 mg IV over 30 seconds, 30 min prior to administration of chemotherapy or 2 hours before surgery; max 100 mg/dose
Pediatric: <2 years: not recommended; 2-16 years: 1.8 mg/kg; >16 years: same as adult
   Anzemet *Tab:* 50, 100 mg; *Amp:* 12.5 mg/0.625 ml; *Prefilled carpuject syringe:* 12.5 mg (0.625 ml); *Vial:* 100 mg/5 ml (single-use); *Vial:* 500 mg/25 ml (multi-dose)
▷ *granisetron*
   Kytril (B) 10 mcg/kg as a single dose; administer IV over 30 seconds, 30 min prior to administration of chemotherapy; max 1 dose/week
   Pediatric: <2 years: not recommended; ≥2 years: same as adult
      Tab: 1 mg; *Oral soln:* 2 mg/10 ml (30 ml; orange); *Vial:* 1 mg/ml (1 ml single-dose) (preservative-free); 1 mg/ml (4 ml multi-dose) (benzyl alcohol)
   Sancuso (B) apply 1 patch 24-48 hours before chemo; remove 24 hours (minimum) to 7 days (maximum) after completion of treatment
   Pediatric: <2 years: not recommended; ≥2 years: same as adult
      Transdermal patch: 3.1 mg/day
▷ *granisetron extended release injection* administer SC over 20-30 seconds (due to drug viscosity) on Day 1 of chemotherapy and not more frequently than once every 7 days;

CrCl 30-59 mL/min: repeat dose no more than every 14th day; *CrCl <30 mL/min:* not recommended; for patients receiving MEC, the recommended *dexamethasone* dosage is 8 mg IV on Day 1; for patients receiving AC combination chemotherapy regimens, the recommended *dexamethasone* dosage is 20 mg IV on Day 1, followed by 8 mg PO bid on Days 2, 3 and 4; if **Sustol** is administered with an NK₁ receptor antagonist, see that drug's mfr pkg insert for the recommended *dexamethasone* dosing

Pediatric: <18 years: not recommended; ≥18 years: same as adult

    Sustol *Syringe:* 10 mg/0.4 ml ext-rel; prefilled single-dose/kit

    Comment: At least 60 minutes prior to administration, remove the **Sustol** kit from refrigeration; activate a warming pouch and wrap the syringe in the warming pouch for 5-6 minutes to warm it to room temperature.

▷ *ondansetron* (C)(G) Oral Forms: *Highly emetogenic chemotherapy:* 24 mg x 1 dose 30 min prior to start of single-day chemotherapy; *Moderately emetogenic chemotherapy:* 8 mg q 8 hours x 2 doses beginning 30 minutes prior to start of chemotherapy; then 8 mg q 12 hours x 1-2 days following

Pediatric: <4 years: not recommended; 4-11 years: *Moderately emetogenic chemotherapy:* 4 mg q 4 hours x 3 doses beginning 30 min prior to start; then 4 mg q 8 hours x 1-2 days following

    Zofran *Tab:* 4, 8, 24 mg

    Zofran ODT *ODT:* 4, 8 mg (strawberry) (phenylalanine)

    Zofran Oral Solution *Oral soln:* 4 mg/5 ml (50 ml) (strawberry) (phenylalanine); *Parenteral form:* see mfr pkg insert

    Zofran Injection *Vial:* 2 mg/ml (2 ml single-dose); 2 mg/ml (20 ml multi-dose); 32 mg/50 ml (50 ml multi-dose); *Prefilled syringe:* 4 mg/2 ml, single-use (24/carton)

    Zuplenz Oral Soluble Film: 4, 8 mg oral-dis (10/carton) (peppermint)

    Comment: The FDA has issued an updated warning against *ondansetron* use in pregnancy *ondansetron* is a 5-HT3 receptor antagonist approved by the FDA for preventing nausea and vomiting related to cancer chemotherapy and surgery. However, it has been used "off label" to treat the nausea and vomiting of pregnancy. The FDA has cautioned against the use of *ondansetron* in pregnancy in light of studies of *ondansetron* in early pregnancy and associated with congenital cardiac malformations and oral clefts (i.e., cleft lip and cleft palate). Further, there are potential maternal risks in pregnancy with electrolyte imbalance caused by severe nausea and vomiting (as with hyperemesis gravidarum). These risks include serotonin syndrome (a triad of of cognitive and behavioral changes including confusion, agitation, autonomic instability, and neuromuscular changes). Therefore, *ondansetron* should <u>not</u> be taken during pregnancy.

▷ *palonosetron* (B)(G) *Chemotherapy:* administer 0.25 mg IV over 30 seconds, 30 min prior to administration of chemo; max 1 dose/week <u>or</u> 1 cap 1 hour before chemo; *Post-op:* administer 0.075 mg IV over 10 seconds immediately before induction of anesthesia

Pediatric: <1 month: not recommended; 1 month-17 years: 20 mcg/kg; max 1.5 mg single dose; infuse over 15 minutes beginning 30 minutes prior to administration of chemo

    Aloxi *Vial (single-use):* 0.075 mg/1.5 ml; 0.25 mg/5 ml (mannitol)

CANNABINOIDS

▷ *dronabinol* (C)(III) initially 5 mg/m² 1-3 hours before chemotherapy; then q 2-4 hours prn; max 4-6 doses/day, 15 mg/m²

Pediatric: <18 years: not recommended; ≥18 years: same as adult

    Marinol *Cap:* 2.5, 5, 10 mg (sesame seed oil)

▷ *nabilone* (C)(II) 1-2 mg bid; max 6 mg/day in 3 divided doses; initially 1-3 hours before chemotherapy; may give 1-2 mg the night before chemo; may continue 48 hours after each chemo cycle

Pediatric: <18 years: not recommended; ≥18 years: same as adult

    Cesamet *Cap:* 1 mg (sesame seed oil)

 CHICKENPOX (VARICELLA)

PROPHYLAXIS

▷ *Varicella virus* vaccine, live, attenuated (C)

    Varivax 0.5 ml SC; repeat 4-8 weeks later

Pediatric: <12 months: not recommended; 12 months-12 years: 1 dose of 0.5 ml SC; repeat 4-6 weeks later

> *Vial:* 1350 PFU/0.5 ml single-dose w. diluent (preservative-free)

Comment: Administer **Varivax** SC in the deltoid for adults and children.

IMMUNE GLOBULIN

▷ *immune globulin (human)* administer via intramuscular injection <u>only</u> (<u>never</u> intravenously); ensure adequate hydration prior to administration

Household and Institutional Varicella Case Contacts: promptly administer 0.6-1.2 ml/kg IM as a single dose (if Varicella-Zoster Immune Globulin (Human) is unavailable

Planned Travel to Varicella Endemic Area: administer 0.6-1.2 ml/kg as a single dose at least 6 days prior to travel (if Varicella-Zoster Immune Globulin (Human) is unavailable

Pediatric: 0.25 ml/kg IM (0.5 mg/kg in immunocompromised children)

> **GamaSTAN S/D** *Vial:* 2, 10 ml single-dose
>
> Comment: **GamaSTAN S/D** is the only *gammaglobulin* product FDA-approved for measles and HAV post-exposure prophylaxis (PEP). **GamaSTAN S/D** is also FDA-approved for varicella post-exposure prophylaxis (PEP). Other **GamaSTAN S/D** indications: to prevent <u>or</u> modify measles in a susceptible person exposed fewer than 6 days previously; to modify varicella; to modify rubella in exposed women who will <u>not</u> consider a therapeutic abortion. **GamaSTAN S/D** is <u>not</u> indicated for routine prophylaxis <u>or</u> treatment of viral hepatitis B, rubella, poliomyelitis, mumps <u>or</u> varicella. Contraindications to **GamaSTAN S/D** include persons with cancer, chronic liver disease, and persons allergic to *gammaglobulin*, the HAV vaccine, <u>or</u> a component of the HAV vaccine. Dosage is higher for HAV PEP than for measles and varicella PEP based on recently observed decreasing concentrations of HAV antibodies in **GamaSTAN S/D**, attributed to the decreasing prevalence of previous HAV infection among plasma donors.

TREATMENT

Antipyretics *see Fever page* 163
Infants and young children: No aspirin

ORAL ANTIPRURITICS

▷ *diphenhydramine* (B)(OTC)(G) 25-50 mg q 6-8 hours; max 100 mg/day

Pediatric: <2 years: not recommended; 2-6 years: 6.25 mg q 4-6 hours; max 37.5 mg/day; >6-12 years: 12.5-25 mg q 4-6 hours; max 150 mg/day; >12 years: same as adult

> **Benadryl (OTC)** *Chew tab:* 12.5 mg (grape; phenylalanine); *Liq:* 12.5 mg/5 ml (4, 8 oz); *Cap:* 25 mg; *Tab:* 25 mg; *dye-free soft gel:* 25 mg; *Dye-free liq:* 12.5 mg/5 ml (4, 8 oz)

▷ *hydroxyzine* (C)(G) 50-100 mg qid; max 600 mg/day

Pediatric: <6 years: 50 mg/day divided qid; ≥6 years: 50-100 mg/day divided qid

> **AtaraxR** *Tab:* 10, 25, 50, 100 mg; *Syr:* 10 mg/5 ml (alcohol 0.5%)
>
> **Vistaril** *Cap:* 25, 50, 100 mg; *Oral susp:* 25 mg/5 ml (4 oz) (lemon)

ANTIVIRALS

▷ *acyclovir* (B)(G) 800 mg qid x 5 days

Pediatric: <2 years: not recommended; ≥2 years, <40 kg: 20 mg/kg qid x 5 days; ≥2 years, >40 kg: 800 mg qid x 5 days; *see page 616 for dose by weight*

> **Zovirax** *Cap:* 200 mg; *Tab:* 400, 800 mg
>
> **Zovirax Oral Suspension** *Oral susp:* 200 mg/5 ml (banana)

◯ CHIKUNGUNYA VIRUS/CHIKUNGUNYA-RELATED ARTHRITIS

Comment: Chikungunya is a mosquito-borne viral disease first described during an outbreak in southern Tanzania in 1952. It is an RNA virus that belongs to the alphavirus genus of the family *Togaviridae.* The name "chikungunya" derives from a word in the Kimakonde language, meaning "to become contorted," and describes the stooped appearance of sufferers with joint pain (arthralgia). Acute infection with *chikungunya virus* is associated with fever, rash, headache, and muscle and joint pain, with outbreaks having been reported in

Africa, Asia, the Indian and Pacific Ocean islands, and Europe. In 2013 for the first time the virus was first detected in the Caribbean region, and more than 1.2 million peoples in the Americas have now been infected. After transmission by an *Aedes aegypti* or *Aedes albopictus* mosquito bite, *chikungunya virus* undergoes local replication and then dissemination to lymphoid tissue," the researchers explained. Viremia is detectable for only 5 to 12 days, but animal studies have indicated that the virus can be found in lymphoid organs, joints, and muscles for several months and that viral RNA can be detected in muscle, liver, and spleen for long periods. But it is not known whether the remnants of the virus actually persist in humans and, if so, whether this can be causatively linked with chronic arthritis, which has implications for treatment. With no evidence of viral persistence, potential mechanisms for arthritis included epigenetic changes to host DNA, as has been observed with *Epstein Barr virus* infection, modification of macrophages, and molecular mimicry. There is currently cure and no standard treatment for acute *chikungunya virus* infection or chikungunya-related arthritis, but various immunosuppressants such as **methotrexate** and **hydroxychloroquine** and biologics such as **adalimumab** (**Humira**) and **etanercept** (**Enbrel**) have been tried, despite concerns of renewed viral replication in the synovium and relapse of systemic viral infection. However, no relapses have been reported, and the lack of evidence of viral persistence in the joint seen in this analysis may provide some reassurance that treatment with immunosuppressant anti-rheumatic medications 2 years after infection is a viable option.

REFERENCES

Chang, A. Y., Encinales, L., Porras, A., Pachecho, N., Reid, S. P., Martins, K. A. O., . . . Simon, G. L. (2018). Frequency of chronic joint pain following chikungunya infection: A Colombian cohort study. *Arthritis & Rheumatology, 70*(4), 578–584. doi:10.1002/art.40384

Chang, A. Y., Martins, K. A. O., Encinales, L., Reid, S. P., Acuña, M., Encinales, C., . . . Firestein, G. S. (2017). A cross-sectional analysis of chikungunya arthritis patients 22-months post-infection demonstrating no detectable viral persistence in synovial fluid. *Arthritis & Rheumatology, 70*(4), 585–593. doi:10.1002/art.40383

CHLAMYDIA TRACHOMATIS

Comment: The following treatment regimens for *C. trachomatis* are published in the **2015 CDC Sexually Transmitted Diseases Treatment Guidelines**. Treatment regimens are presented by generic drug name first, followed by information about brands and dose forms. Treat all sexual contacts. Patients who are HIV-positive should receive the same treatment as those who are HIV-negative. Sexual abuse must be considered a cause of chlamydial infection in preadolescent children, although perinatally transmitted *C. trachomatis* infections of the nasopharynx, urogenital tract, and rectum may persist for >1 year.

RECOMMENDED REGIMENS: ADOLESCENT & >18 YEARS, NON-PREGNANT
Regimen 1
➢ *azithromycin* 1 gm in a single dose

Regimen 2
➢ *doxycycline* 100 mg bid x 7 days

ALTERNATIVE REGIMENS: ADOLESCENT AND ADULT, NON-PREGNANT
Regimen 1
➢ *erythromycin base* 500 mg qid x 7 days

Regimen 2
➢ *erythromycin ethylsuccinate* 800 mg qid x 7 days

Regimen 3
➢ *levofloxacin* 500 mg once daily x 7 days

Regimen 4
➢ *ofloxacin* 300 mg bid x 7 days

RECOMMENDED REGIMENS: PREGNANCY

Regimen 1

▷ *azithromycin* 1 gm in a single dose

Regimen 2

▷ *amoxicillin* 500 mg tid x 7 days

ALTERNATE REGIMENS: PREGNANCY

Regimen 1

▷ *erythromycin base* 500 mg qid x 7 days

Regimen 2

▷ *erythromycin base* 250 mg qid x 14 days

Regimen 3

▷ *erythromycin ethylsuccinate* 800 mg qid x 7 days

Regimen 4

▷ *erythromycin ethylsuccinate* 400 mg qid x 14 days

ALTERNATE REGIMENS: CHILDREN (>8 YEARS)

Regimen 1

▷ *azithromycin* 1 gm in a single dose

Regimen 2

▷ *doxycycline* 100 mg bid x 7 days

ALTERNATE REGIMEN: CHILDREN (>45 KG; <8 YEARS)

Regimen 1

▷ *azithromycin* 1 gm in a single dose

ALTERNATE REGIMENS: INFANTS

Regimen 1

▷ *erythromycin base* 50 mg/kg/day in divided doses qid x 14 days

Regimen 2

▷ *erythromycin ethylsuccinate* 50 mg/kg/day divided qid x 14 days

DRUG BRANDS AND DOSE FORMS

▷ *azithromycin* (B)(G) 500 mg x 1 dose on day 1, then 250 mg daily on days 2-5 or 500 mg daily x 3 days or **Zmax** 2 gm in a single dose
   Pediatric: 12 mg/kg/day x 5 days; max 500 mg/day; *see page* 619 *for dose by weight*
   Zithromax *Tab:* 250, 500, 600 mg; *Oral susp:* 100 mg/5 ml (15 ml); 200 mg/5 ml (15, 22.5, 30 ml) (cherry); *Pkt:* 1 gm for reconstitution (cherry-banana)
   Zithromax Tri-pak *Tab:* 3 x 500 mg tabs/pck
   Zithromax Z-pak *Tab:* 6 x 250 mg tabs/pck
   Zmax *Oral susp:* 2 gm ext-rel for reconstitution (cherry-banana) (148 mg Na$^+$)
▷ *doxycycline* (D)(G)
   Acticlate *Tab:* 75, 150**mg
   Adoxa *Tab:* 50, 75, 100, 150 mg ent-coat
   Doryx *Tab:* 50, 75, 100, 150, 200 mg del-rel
   Doxteric *Tab:* 50 mg del-rel
   Monodox *Cap:* 50, 75, 100 mg
   Oracea *Cap:* 40 mg del-rel
   Vibramycin *Tab:* 100 mg; *Cap:* 50, 100 mg; *Syr:* 50 mg/5 ml (raspberry-apple) (sulfites); *Oral susp:* 25 mg/5 ml (raspberry)
   Vibra-Tab *Tab:* 100 mg film-coat

Comment: *doxycycline* is contraindicated <8 years-of-age, in pregnancy, and lactation (discolors developing tooth enamel). A side effect may be photosensitivity (photophobia). Do not take with antacids, calcium supplements, milk or other dairy, or within 2 hours of taking another drug.

▷ *erythromycin base* (B)(G)
  Ery-Tab *Tab:* 250, 333, 500 mg ent-coat
  PCE *Tab:* 333, 500 mg
  Comment: *erythromycin* may increase INR with concomitant *warfarin*, as well as increase serum level of *digoxin,* benzodiazepines, and statins.

▷ *erythromycin ethylsuccinate* (B)(G)
  EryPed *Oral susp:* 200 mg/5 ml (100, 200 ml) (fruit); 400 mg/5 ml (60, 100, 200 ml) (banana); *Oral drops:* 200, 400 mg/5 ml (50 ml) (fruit); *Chew tab:* 200 mg wafer (fruit)
  E.E.S. *Oral susp:* 200, 400 mg/5 ml (100 ml) (fruit)
  E.E.S. Granules *Oral susp:* 200 mg/5 ml (100, 200 ml) (cherry)
  E.E.S. 400 Tablets *Tab:* 400 mg
  Comment: *erythromycin* may increase INR with concomitant *warfarin*, as well as increase serum level of *digoxin,* benzodiazepines, and statins.

▷ *levofloxacin* (C)
  Levaquin *Tab:* 250, 500, 750 mg
  Comment: *levofloxacin* is contraindicated; <18 years-of-age, and during pregnancy and lactation. Risk of tendonitis or tendon rupture.

▷ *ofloxacin* (C)(G)
  Floxin *Tab:* 200, 300, 400 mg
  Comment: *ofloxacin* is contraindicated <18 years-of-age, and during pregnancy and lactation. Risk of tendonitis or tendon rupture.

CHOLANGITIS, PRIMARY BILIARY (PBC)

Comment: Monitor intensity of pruritis and administer antihistamines as appropriate for dermal pruritis. **Ocaliva** (*obeticholic acid*), a farnesoid X receptor (FXR) agonist, is indicated for the treatment of primary biliary cholangitis (PBC) in combination with *ursodeoxycholic acid* (UDCA), in adults with an inadequate response to UDCA, or as monotherapy in adults unable to tolerate UDCA. This indication is approved under accelerated approval based on a reduction in alkaline phosphatase (ALP). An improvement in survival or disease-related symptoms has not been established. Continued approval for this indication may be contingent upon verification and description of clinical benefit in confirmatory trials.

FARNESOID X RECEPTOR (FXR) AGONIST

▷ *obeticholic acid* initially 5 mg once daily (this lower starting dose is recommended to reduce pruritis); then after 3 months of treatment, if an adequate reduction in ALP and/or total bilirubin is not achieved, and if the patient is tolerating the drug, increase the dose to 10 mg once daily; take with or without food
  Pediatric: <18 years: not recommended; ≥18 years: same as adult
  Ocaliva *Tab:* 5, 10 mg
  Comment: **Ocalvia** is contraindicated in patients with complete biliary obstruction. If this complication develops, discontinue **Ocaliva**. Because PBC management strategies include bile acid binding resin (e.g., *cholestyramine, colestipol,* or *colesevelam*), concurrent use with *obeticholic acid* should be separated by at least 4 hours. Concurrent use of *obeticholic acid* and *warfarin* may reduce the international normalized ratio (INR), monitor INR and adjust the *warfarin* dose as necessary. Monitor concentrations of CYP1A2 substrates with a narrow therapeutic index (e.g., *theophylline* and *tizanidine*) as *obeticholic acid* a CYP1A2 inhibitor). Reduce the dose of **Ocaliva** in patients with moderate or severe hepatic impairment, and monitor LFTs and lipid levels (especially reduction in HDL).

URSODEOXYCHOLIC ACID (UDCA)

▷ *ursodeoxycholic acid* (UDCA) (G) in the first 3 months of treatment, the total daily dose should be divided tid (morning, midday, evening); as liver function values improve, the total daily dose may be taken once a day at bedtime; (see mfr pkg insert for dose table based on kilograms weight); monitor hepatic function every 4 weeks for the first 3 months; then, monitor hepatic function once every 3 months

Pediatric: same as adult

    Ursofalk *Tab:* 500 mg film-coat; *Cap:* 250 mg, *Oral susp:* 250 mg/5 ml

    Comment: *ursodeoxycholic acid* (UDCA) is indicated for the dissolution of cholesterol gall stones that are radioluscent (not visible on plain x-ray), ≤15 mm, and the gall bladder must still be functioning despite the gall stones.

BILE ACID BINDING RESINS

Comment: This drug class may produce or severely worsen pre-existing constipation. The dosage should be increased gradually in patients to minimize the risk of developing fecal impaction. Increased fluid and fiber intake should be encouraged to alleviate constipation and a stool softener may occasionally be indicated. If the initial dose is well tolerated, the dose may be increased as needed in one dose/day (at monthly intervals) with periodic monitoring of serum lipoproteins. If constipation worsens or the desired therapeutic response is not achieved at one to six doses/day, combination therapy or alternate therapy should be considered. Bile acid sequestrants may decrease absorption of fat-soluble vitamins. Use caution in patients susceptible to fat-soluble vitamin deficiencies.

▷ *cholestyramine* (C)(G) starting dose: 1 packet or 1 scoopful of powder once daily for 5 to 7 days; then, increase to twice daily with monitoring of constipation and of serum lipoproteins, at least twice, 4 to 6 weeks apart; empty one packet into a glass or cup; add 1/2 to 1 cup (4 to 8 ounces) of water, fruit juice, or diet soft drink; stir well and drink immediately; do not swallow dry form; take with meals

Pediatric: 240 mg/kg/day of anhydrous cholestyramine resin in two to three divided doses, normally not to exceed 8 gm/day with dose titration based on response and tolerance.

    Prevalite *Pwdr:* 4 gm/pkt, 4 gm/scoopful (1 level tsp) for oral suspension

▷ *colestipol* (C)(G)

Starting dose tabs: 2 gm once or twice daily; then, increases should occur at one or two month intervals; usual dose is 2 to 16 gm/day given once daily or in divided doses *Starting dose granules:* 1 packet or 1 scoopful (1 level tsp) of granules once daily for 5 to 7 days, increasing to twice daily with monitoring of constipation and of serum lipoproteins, at least twice, 4 to 6 weeks apart; empty one packet or one scoopful (1 level tsp) of granules into a glass or cup; add 1/2 to 1 cup (4 to 8 ounces) of water, fruit juice, or diet soft drink; stir well and drink immediately; do not swallow dry form; take with meals

Pediatric: <12 years: not established; ≥12 years: same as adult

    Colestid *Tab:* 1 gm; *Granules:* 5 gm/pkt, 5 gm/scoopful (1 level tsp) for oral suspension

    Flavored Colestid *Granules:* 5 gm/pkt, 5 gm/scoopful (1 level tsp) for oral suspension (orange)

▷ *colesevelam* (B)(G)

WelChol recommended dose is 6 tablets once daily or 3 tablets twice daily; take with a meal and liquid

Pediatric: <10 years: not recommended; ≥10 years: same as adult

    Tab: 625 mg

WelChol for Oral Suspension recommended dose is one 3.75 gm packet once daily or one 1.875 gm packet twice daily; empty one packet into a glass or cup; add 1/2 to 1 cup (4 to 8 ounces) of water, fruit juice, or diet soft drink; stir well and drink immediately; do not swallow dry form; take with meals

Pediatric: <12 years: not established; ≥12 years: same as adult

    Pwdr: 3.75 gm/pkt (30 pkt/carton), 1.875 gm/pkt (60 pkt/carton) for oral suspension

    Comment: **WelChol** is indicated as adjunctive therapy to improve glycemic control in adults with type 2 diabetes. It can be added to *metformin*, sulfonylureas, or insulin alone or in combination with other antidiabetic agents.

CHOLELITHIASIS

▷ *ursodeoxycholic acid* (UDCA) (G) in the first 3 months of treatment, the total daily dose should be divided tid (morning, midday, evening); as liver function values improve, the total daily dose may be taken once a day at bedtime; (see mfr pkg insert for dose table based on kilograms weight); monitor hepatic function every 4 weeks for the first 3 months; then, monitor hepatic function once every 3 months

Pediatric: same as adult

Ursofalk *Tab:* 500 mg film-coat; *Cap:* 250 mg, *Oral susp:* 250 mg/5 ml

Comment: *ursodeoxycholic* (UDCA) is indicated for the dissolution of cholesterol gall stones that are radioluscent (not visible on plain x-ray), ≤15 mm, and the gall bladder must still be functioning despite the gall stones

▷ *ursodiol* (B) 8-10 mg/kg/day in 2-3 divided doses

Pediatric: <12 years: not recommended; ≥12 years: same as adult

Actigall *Cap:* 300 mg

Comment: **Actigall** is indicated for the dissolution of radiolucent, noncalciferous, gallstones <20 mm in diameter and for prevention of gallstones during rapid weight loss.

BILE ACID BINDING RESINS

Comment: This drug class may produce or severely worsen pre-existing constipation. The dosage should be increased gradually in patients to minimize the risk of developing fecal impaction. Increased fluid and fiber intake should be encouraged to alleviate constipation and a stool softener may occasionally be indicated. If the initial dose is well tolerated, the dose may be increased as needed by one dose/day (at monthly intervals) with periodic monitoring of serum lipoproteins. If constipation worsens or the desired therapeutic response is not achieved at one to six doses/day, combination therapy or alternate therapy should be considered. Bile acid sequestrants may decrease absorption of fat-soluble vitamins. Use caution in patients susceptible to fat-soluble vitamin deficiencies.

▷ *cholestyramine* (C)(G) starting dose: 1 packet or 1 scoopful of powder once daily for 5 to 7 days; then, increase to twice daily with monitoring of constipation and of serum lipoproteins, at least twice, 4 to 6 weeks apart; empty one packet into a glass or cup; add 1/2 to 1 cup (4 to 8 ounces) of water, fruit juice, or diet soft drink; stir well and drink immediately; do not swallow dry form; take with meals

Pediatric: <12 years: 240 mg/kg/day of anhydrous cholestyramine resin in 2 to 3 divided doses, normally not to exceed 8 gm/day with dose titration based on response and tolerance.

Prevalite *Pwdr:* 4 gm/pkt, 4 gm/scoopful (1 level tsp) for oral suspension

▷ *colestipol* (C)(G)

Starting dose tabs: 2 gm once or twice daily; then, increases should occur at one or two month intervals; usual dose is 2 to 16 gm/day given once daily or in divided doses

Starting dose granules: 1 packet or 1 scoopful (1 level tsp) of granules once daily for 5 to 7 days, increasing to twice daily with monitoring of constipation and of serum lipoproteins, at least twice, 4 to 6 weeks apart; empty one packet or one scoopful (1 level tsp) of granules into a glass or cup; add 1/2 to 1 cup (4 to 8 ounces) of water, fruit juice, or diet soft drink; stir well and drink immediately; do not swallow dry form; take with meals

Pediatric: <12 years: not established; ≥12 years: same as adult

Colestid *Tab:* 1 gm; *Granules:* 5 gm/pkt, 5 gm/scoopful (1 level tsp) for oral suspension

Flavored Colestid *Granules:* 5 gm/pkt, 5 gm/scoopful (1 level tsp) for oral suspension (orange)

▷ *colesevelam* (B)(G)

WelChol recommended dose is 6 tablets once daily or 3 tablets twice daily; take with a meal and liquid

Pediatric: <10 years: not recommended; ≥10 years: same as adult

Tab: 625 mg

WelChol for Oral Suspension recommended dose is one 3.75 gm packet once daily or one 1.875 gm packet twice daily; empty one packet into a glass or cup; add 1/2 to 1 cup (4 to 8 ounces) of water, fruit juice, or diet soft drink; stir well and drink immediately; do not swallow dry form; take with meals

Pediatric: <12 years: not established; ≥12 years: same as adult

Pwdr: 3.75 gm/pkt (30 pkt/carton), 1.875 gm/pkt (60 pkt/carton) for oral suspension

Comment: **WelChol** is indicated as adjunctive therapy to improve glycemic control in adults with type 2 diabetes. It can be added to *metformin*, sulfonylureas, or insulin alone or in combination with other antidiabetic agents

CHOLERA (*VIBRIO CHOLERAE*)

Comment: On June 10, 2016, the FDA approved the first vaccine for the prevention of cholera caused by serogroup O1 (the most predominant cause of cholera globally [WHO]) in adults age 18-64 years traveling to cholera-affected areas. https://www.drugs.com/newdrugs/fda-approves-vaxchora-cholera-vaccine-live-oral-prevent-cholera-travelers-4396.html. **Vaxchora** (R) is the only FDA approved vaccine for the prevention of cholera. The bacterium *Vibrio cholerae* is acquired by ingesting contaminated water or food and causes nausea, vomiting, and watery diarrhea that may be mild to severe. Profuse fluid loss may cause life-threatening dehydration if antibiotics and fluid replacement are not initiated promptly.

VACCINE PROPHYLAXIS

▷ *Vibrio cholerae* vaccine

> **Vaxchora** reconstitute the buffer component in 100 ml purified bottled water; then add the active component (lyophilized V. cholerae CVD 103-HgR); total dose after reconstitution is 100 ml; instruct the patient to avoid eating or drinking fluids for 60 minutes before and after ingestion of the dose

> **Comment:** **Vaxchora** is a live, attenuated vaccine that is taken as a single oral dose at least 10 days before travel to a cholera-affected area and at least 10 days before starting antimalarial prophylaxis. Diminished immune response when taken concomitantly with *chloroquine*. Avoid concomitant administration with systemic antibiotics since these agents may be active against the vaccine strain. Do not administer to patients who have received an oral or parental antibiotic within 14 days prior to vaccination. **Vaxchora** may be shed in the stool of recipients for at least 7 days. There is potential for transmission of the vaccine strain to non-vaccinated and immunocompromised close contacts. The CDC and several health professional organizations state that vaccines given to a nursing mother do not affect the safety of breastfeeding for mothers or infants and that breastfeeding is not a contraindication to cholera vaccine. **Vaxchora** is not absorbed systemically, and maternal use is not expected to result in fetal exposure to the drug. The **Vaxchora** pregnancy exposure registry for reporting adverse events is 800-533-5899. There are 0 disease interactions, but at least 165 drug-drug interactions with **Vaxchora** (see mfr pkg insert).

TREATMENT

Comment: The first line treatment for *V. cholerae* is oral rehydration therapy (ORT) and intravenous fluid replacement as indicated. Antibiotic therapy may shorten the duration and severity of symptoms, but is optional in other than severe cases. Although *doxycycline* is contraindicated in pregnancy and in children under 7 years-of-age, the benefits may outweigh the risks (WHO, CDC, UNICEF). Although *ciprofloxacin* is contraindicated in children under 18 years-of-age, the benefits may outweigh the risks (WHO, CDC, UNICEF). Cholera is not transmitted from person to person, but rather the fecal-oral route. Therefore, chemoprophylaxis is not usually required with strict hand hygiene and sanitation measures, and avoidance of contaminated food and water. Drugs and dosages for chemoprophylaxis are the same as for treatment.

NON-PREGNANT FEMALES ≥15 YEARS
Regimen 1

▷ *doxycycline* (D)(G) 300 mg in a single dose

> **Acticlate** *Tab:* 75, 150**mg
> **Adoxa** *Tab:* 50, 75, 100, 150 mg ent-coat
> **Doryx** *Tab:* 50, 75, 100, 150, 200 mg del-rel
> **Doxteric** *Tab:* 50 mg del-rel
> **Monodox** *Cap:* 50, 75, 100 mg
> **Oracea** *Cap:* 40 mg del-rel
> **Vibramycin** *Tab:* 100 mg; *Cap:* 50, 100 mg; *Syr:* 50 mg/ml (raspberry-apple) (sulfites); *Oral susp:* 25 mg/5 ml (raspberry)
> **Vibra-Tab** *Tab:* 100 mg film-coat

Regimen 2

▷ *azithromycin* (B)(G) 1000 mg in a single dose
    Zithromax *Tab:* 250, 500, 600 mg
    Zmax *Oral susp:* 2 gm ext-rel for reconstitution (cherry-banana) (148 mg Na⁺)
      or
▷ *ciprofloxacin* (C)(G) 1000 mg in a single dose
    Cipro *Tab:* 250, 500, 750 mg;
    Cipro XR *Tab:* 500, 1000 mg ext-rel
    ProQuin XR *Tab:* 500 mg ext-rel

PREGNANT FEMALES ≥15 YEARS

▷ *azithromycin* (B)(G) 1000 mg in a single dose
    Zithromax *Tab:* 250, 500, 600 mg
    Zmax *Oral susp:* 2 gm ext-rel for reconstitution (cherry-banana) (148 mg Na⁺)
      or
▷ *erythromycin* (B)(G) 500 mg q 6 hours x 3 days
    E.E.S. 400 Tablets *Tab:* 400 mg
    Ery-Tab *Tab:* 250, 333, 500 mg ent-coat
    PCE *Tab:* 333, 500 mg

CHILDREN 3-15 YEARS WHO CAN SWALLOW TABLETS
Regimen 1

▷ *erythromycin* (B)(G) 12.5 mg/kg q 6 hours x 3 days
    E.E.S. 400 Tablets *Tab:* 400 mg
    Ery-Tab *Tab:* 250, 333, 500 mg ent-coat
    PCE *Tab:* 333, 500 mg
      or
▷ *azithromycin* (B)(G) 20 mg/kg in a single dose; max 1 gm
    Zithromax *Tab:* 250, 500, 600 mg
    Zmax *Oral susp:* 2 gm ext-rel for reconstitution (cherry-banana) (148 mg Na⁺)

Regimen 2

▷ *ciprofloxacin* (D)(G) <18 years usually not recommended; *erythromycin* or *azithromycin* preferred; consider risk/benefit; 20 mg/kg in a single dose
    Cipro *Tab:* 250, 500, 750 mg;
    Cipro XR *Tab:* 500, 1000 mg ext-rel
    ProQuin XR *Tab:* 500 mg ext-rel
      or
▷ *doxycycline* (D)(G) <8 years usually not recommended; *erythromycin* or *azithromycin* preferred; consider risk benefit; >8 years: 2-4 mg/kg in a single dose
    Acticlate *Tab:* 75, 150**mg
    Adoxa *Tab:* 50, 75, 100, 150 mg ent-coat
    Doryx *Tab:* 50, 75, 100, 150, 200 mg del-rel
    Doxteric *Tab:* 50 mg del-rel
    Monodox *Cap:* 50, 75, 100 mg
    Oracea *Cap:* 40 mg del-rel
    Vibramycin *Tab:* 100 mg; *Cap:* 50, 100 mg; *Syr:* 50 mg/ml (raspberry-apple) (sulfites); *Oral susp:* 25 mg/5 ml (raspberry)
    Vibra-Tab *Tab:* 100 mg film-coat

CHILDREN <3 YEARS
Regimen 1

▷ *erythromycin ethylsuccinate* (B)(G) 12.5 mg/kg q 6 hours x 3 days; use suspension
    E.E.S. *Oral susp:* 200, 400 mg/5 ml (100 ml) (fruit)
    E.E.S. Granules *Oral susp:* 200 mg/5 ml (100, 200 ml) (cherry, fruit); *Chew tab:* 200 mg wafer (fruit)
    EryPed *Oral susp:* 200 mg/5 ml (100, 200 ml) (fruit); 400 mg/5 ml (60, 100, 200 ml) (banana); *Oral drops:* 200, 400 mg/5 ml (50 ml) (fruit); *Chew tab:* 200 mg wafer (fruit)
      or

▷ *azithromycin* (B)(G) 20 mg/kg in a single dose; max 1 gm; use suspension
   Zithromax *Tab:* 250, 500, 600 mg; *Oral susp:* 100 mg/5 ml (15 ml); 200 mg/5 ml (15, 22.5, 30 ml) (cherry)
   Zmax *Oral susp:* 2 gm ext-rel for reconstitution (cherry-banana) (148 mg Na⁺)

Regimen 2

▷ *ciprofloxacin* (C)(G) <18 years usually not recommended; *erythromycin* or *azithromycin* preferred; consider risk benefit; 20 mg/kg in a single dose; use suspension
   Cipro *Oral susp:* 250, 500 mg/5 ml (100 ml) (strawberry)
         or
▷ *doxycycline* (D)(G) <8 years usually not recommended; *erythromycin* or *azithromycin* preferred; consider risk benefit; 2-4 mg/kg in a single dose; use suspension or syrup
   Vibramycin *Syr:* 50 mg/5 ml (raspberry-apple) (sulfites); *Oral susp:* 25 mg/5 ml (raspberry)

⚪ CLOSTRIDIUM DIFFICILE/PSEUDOMEMBRANOUS COLITIS

Comment: Acid-suppressing drugs including proton pump inhibitors (PPIs), third- and fourth-generation cephalosporins, carbapenems, and *piperacillin-tazobactam* significantly increase the risk of hospital-onset *Clostridium difficile* infection (CDI), according to the results of a recent study. Patients who received tetracyclines, macrolides, or clindamycin had lower risk of developing hospital-onset CDI.

REFERENCE
Watson, T., Hickok, J., Fraker, S., Korwek, K., Poland, R. E., & Septimus, E. (2017). Evaluating the risk factors for hospital-onset *Clostridium difficile* infections in a large healthcare system. *Clinical Infectious Diseases, 66*(12), 1957–1957. doi:10.1093/cid/cix1112

MACROLIDE ANTIBACTERIAL AGENT

▷ *fidaxomicin* (B) 200 mg bid x 10 days with or without food.
   Pediatric: <18 years: not established; ≥18 years: same as adult
   Dificid *Tab:* 200 mg film-coat
   Comment: **Dificid** *(fidaxomicin)* is a macrolide antibacterial agent, FDA-approved for treatment of *C. difficile*–associated diarrhea (CDAD). **Dificid** should not be used for treatment of systemic infections. Only use **Dificid** for infection proven or strongly suspected to be caused by *C. difficile*. Prescribing **Dificid** in the absence of a proven or strongly suspected *C. difficile* infection is unlikely to provide benefit to the patient and increases the risk of development of drug-resistant bacteria. Acute hypersensitivity reactions, including dyspnea, rash pruritus, and angioedema of the mouth, throat, and face have been reported with *fidaxomicin*. If a severe hypersensitivity reaction occurs, **Dificid** should be discontinued and appropriate therapy should be instituted. The most common adverse reactions reported in clinical trials are nausea (11%), vomiting (7%), abdominal pain (6%), gastrointestinal hemorrhage (4%), anemia (2%), and neutropenia (2%). Among patients receiving **Dificid**, 5.9% withdrew from trials as a result of adverse reactions. Vomiting was the primary adverse reaction leading to discontinuation of dosing (incidence of 0.5% for both **Dificid** and *vancomycin* patients). No dose adjustment is recommended for patients ≥65 years-of-age. No dose adjustment is recommended for patients with renal impairment. No dosage adjustments are recommended when co-administering *fidaxomicin* with substrates of P-gp or CYP enzymes. The impact of hepatic impairment on the pharmacokinetics of *fidaxomicin* has not been evaluated; however, because *fidaxomicin* and its active metabolite (OP-1118) do not appear to undergo significant hepatic metabolism, elimination of *fidaxomicin* and OP-1118 is not expected to be significantly affected by hepatic impairment. There are no adequate and well-controlled studies in pregnancy; **Dificid** should be used during pregnancy only if clearly needed. It is not known whether fidaxomicin is excreted in human milk.

GLYCOPEPTIDE ANTIBACTERIAL AGENTS

▷ *vancomycin hcl capsule* (B)(G) 500 mg to 2 gm in 3-4 doses x 7-10 days; max 2 gm/day
Pediatric: 40 mg/kg/day in 3-4 doses x 7-10 days; max 2 gm/day;use caps or oral solution as
appropriate
Vancocin *Cap:* 125, 250 mg

▷ *vancomycin hcl oral solution* see mfr pkg insert for preparation and important administration information; <18 years: *CDAD and Staphylococcal enterocolitis:* 40 mg/kg orally in 3 or
4 divided doses x 7-10 days; total daily dosage max 2 gm; ≥18 years: *CDAD* 125 mg orally
4 x/day x 10 days; *Staphylococcal enterocolitis:* 500 mg to 2 gm orally in 3 or 4 divided doses
x 7-10 days
Firvanq *Kit w. pwdr for oral soln:* 25, 50 mg/ml (150, 300 ml) equivalent to 3.75, 7.5,
10.5, or 15 gm *vancomycin hcl*, plus grape-flavored diluent

Comment: *vancomycin hcl,* a glycopeptide antibacterial agent, is FDA approved for treatment
of *C. difficile*-associated diarrhea (CDAD) and enterocolitis caused by *Staphylococcus aureus*,
including methicillin-resistant strains (MRSA). *vancomycin hcl* should be used only to
treat or prevent infections that are proven or strongly suspected to be caused by susceptible
bacteria. Orally administered *vancomycin hcl* is not effective for treatment of other types
of infections. Prescribing *vancomycin hcl* in the absence of a proven or strongly suspected
bacterial infection is unlikely to provide benefit to the patient and increases the risk of
the development of drug-resistant bacteria. Nephrotoxicity has occurred following oral
vancomycin hcl therapy and can occur either during or after completion of therapy. The risk
is increased in geriatric patients. Monitor renal function. Ototoxicity has occurred in patients
receiving *vancomycin hcl.* Assessment of auditory function may be appropriate in some
instances. The most common adverse reactions ≥10%) have been nausea (17%), abdominal
pain (15%) and hypokalemia (13%). There are no available data on **Firvanq** use in the first
trimester of pregnancy to inform a drug associated risk of major birth defects or miscarriage.
Available published data on *vancomycin hcl* use in pregnancy during the second and third
trimesters have not shown an association with adverse pregnancy-related outcomes. There
are insufficient data to inform the levels of *vancomycin hcl* in human milk. However, systemic
absorption of *vancomycin hcl* following oral administration is expected to be minimal. There
are no data on effects of **Firvanq** on the breastfed infant.

HUMAN IGG1 MONOCLONAL ANTIBODY

Comment: *bezlotoxumab* is a human IgG1 monoclonal antibody that inhibits the binding
of *Clostridium difficile* toxin B, preventing its effects on mammalian cells. *bezlotoxumab*
does not bind to *C. difficile* toxin A. *bezlotoxumab* is indicated to reduce the recurrence of
CDI in patients who are receiving antibacterial drug treatment of CDI and are at high risk
for CDI recurrence. CDI recurrence is defined as a new episode of diarrhea associated with
a positive stool test for toxigenic *C. difficile* following a clinical cure of the presenting CDI
episode. It is not indicated for the primary treatment of CDI infection. It is to be used only
in conjunction with appropriate primary drug treatment of CDI. Patients at high risk for
CDI recurrence, studied in clinical trials establishing efficacy, include those ≥65 years-of-
age, with a history of CDI in the previous 6 months, immunocompromised state, severe
CDI at presentation, and *C. difficile* ribotype 027.

▷ *bezlotoxumab* (C) administer a single dose of 10 mg/kg via IV infusion over 60 minutes
Pediatric: <18 years: not established; ≥18 years: same as adult
Zinplava *Vial:* 1,000 mg/40 ml (40 ml, 25 mg/ml) single-use

COLIC: INFANTILE

▷ *hyoscyamine* (C)(G)
Levsin Drops
Pediatric: 3-4 kg: 4 drops q 4 hours prn; max 24 drops/day; 5 kg: 5 drops q 4 hours
prn; max 30 drops/day; 7 kg: 6 drops q 4 hours prn; max 36 drops/day; 10 kg: 8
drops q 4 hours prn; max 40 drops/day; *Oral drops:* 0.125 mg/ml (15 ml) (orange)
(alcohol 5%)
▷ *simethicone* (C) 0.3 ml qid pc and HS
Mylicon Drops (OTC) *Oral drops:* 40 mg/0.6 ml (30 ml)

COLONOSCOPY PREP/COLON CLEANSE

▷ *polyethylene glycol 3350 with electrolytes* two doses of **Plenvu** are required for a complete preparation for colonoscopy, using a One-Day <u>or</u> Two-Day dosing regimen; reconstitute in water prior to ingestion; additional clear liquids must be consumed after each dose for both dosing regimens; do <u>not</u> take oral medications within 1 hour of starting each dose; for complete information on dosing, preparation, and administration see mfr pkg insert

One-Day Regimen: Dose 1 the morning of the colonoscopy (approximately 3 am to 7 am) <u>and</u> *Dose 2* (Pouch A and B) a minimum of 2 hours after the start of Dose 1

Two-Day Regimen: Dose 1 the evening before the colonoscopy (approximately 4 pm to 8 pm) <u>and</u> *Dose 2* (Pouch A and B) the next morning approximately 12 hours after the start of Dose 1)

    Plenvu *Oral soln:* polyethylene glycol 3350 (140 gm), sodium ascorbate (48.11 gm), sodium sulfate (9 gm), ascorbic acid (7.54 gm), sodium chloride (5.2 gm), and potassium chloride (2.2 gm); *Dose 1:* PEG 3350 (100 gm), sodium sulfate (9 gm), sodium chloride (2 gm), potassium chloride (1 gm) ; *Dose 2, Pouch A:* PEG 3350 (40 gm), sodium chloride (3.2 gm), potassium chloride (1.2 gm); *Dose 2, Pouch B:* sodium ascorbate (48.11 gm), ascorbic acid (7.54 gm)

    Comment: **Plenvu for Oral Solution** is a lower-volume, polyethylene glycol-based osmotic laxative indicated for cleansing of the colon (bowel prepara- to any ingredient in **Plenvu**. Patients with glucose-6-phosphate dihydrogenase deficiency (G6PD) should use with caution. **Plenvu** contains phenylalanine; there is risk for patients with phenylketonuria (PKA). Most common adverse reactions (incidence ≥2%) are nausea, vomiting, dehydration and abdominal pain/discomfort.

▷ *sodium picosulfate+magnesium oxide+citric acid* reconstitute pwdr with cold water right before use; two dosing regimen options—each requires two separate dosing times; *Split Dose Method* (preferred): 1st dose during evening before the colonoscopy and 2nd dose the next day during the morning prior to the colonoscopy; *Day Before Method* (alternative, if split dose is not appropriate): 1st dose during afternoon <u>or</u> early evening before the colonoscopy and 2nd dose 6 hours later during evening before colonoscopy; additional clear liquids (no solid food or milk) must be consumed after every dose in both dosing regimens

Pediatric: <18 years: not recommended; ≥18 years: same as adult

    Prepopik *Pwdr:* sod picos 10 mg+mag oxide 3.5 gm+anhy cit acid 12 gm/pkt pwdr for oral solution (2 pkts)

    Comment: **Prepopik** is a combination of sodium picosulfate, a stimulant laxative, and magnesium oxide and anhydrous citric acid which form magnesium citrate, an osmotic laxative, indicated for cleansing of the colon as a preparation for colonoscopy in adults. Rule out diagnosis of suspected GI obstruction <u>or</u> perforation diagnosis before administration. **Prepopik** should be used during pregnancy only if clearly needed. **Prepopik** is contraindicated with severely reduced renal function (CrCl< 30 mL/min), GI obstruction <u>or</u> ileus, bowel perforation, toxic colitis <u>or</u> toxic megacolon, and gastric retention for any reason.

COMMON COLD (VIRAL UPPER RESPIRATORY INFECTION, URI)

Drugs for the Management of Allergy, Cough, and Cold Symptoms *see page* 603
Oral Decongestants *see page* 603
Oral Expectorants *see page* 603
Oral Antitussives *see page* 603
Oral Antipyretic-Analgesics *see Fever page* 163

NASAL SALINE DROPS & SPRAYS

Comment: Homemade saline nose drops: 1/4 tsp salt added to 8 oz boiled water, then cool water.

▷ *saline* nasal spray (G)

    Afrin Saline Mist w. Eucalyptol and Menthol (OTC) 2-6 sprays in each nostril prn

Pediatric: 1 month-2 years: 1-2 sprays in each nostril prn; >2-12 years: 1-4 sprays in each nostril prn; >12 years: same as adult
    Squeeze bottle: 45 ml
Afrin Moisturizing Saline Mist (OTC) 2-6 sprays in each nostril prn
Pediatric: 1 month-2 years: 1-2 sprays in each nostril prn; 2-12 years: 1-4 sprays in each nostril prn; >12 years: same as adult
    Squeeze bottle: 45 ml
Ocean Mist (OTC) 2-6 sprays in each nostril prn
Pediatric: 1 month-2 years: 1-2 sprays in each nostril prn; >2-12 years: 1-4 sprays in each nostril prn; >12 years: same as adult
    Squeeze bottle: saline 0.65% (45 ml) (alcohol-free)
Pediamist (OTC) 2-6 sprays in each nostril prn
Pediatric: 1 month-2 years: 1-2 sprays in each nostril prn; >2-12 years: 1-4 sprays in each nostril prn; >12 years: same as adult
    Squeeze bottle: saline 0.5% (15 ml) (alcohol-free)

NASAL SYMPATHOMIMETICS

▷ *oxymetazoline* (C)(OTC)
    4-Hour Formulation: 2-3 drops or sprays in each nostril q 10-12 hours prn; max 2 doses/day; max duration 5 days
    Pediatric: <6 years: not recommended; ≥6 years: same as adult
    Afrin 4-Hour:
    12-hour Formulation: 2-3 drops or sprays q 4 hours prn; max duration 5 days
    Pediatric: <12 years: not recommended; ≥12 years: same as adult
    Afrin 12-Hour Extra Moisturizing Nasal Spray
    Afrin 12-Hour Nasal spray Pump Mist
    Afrin 12-Hour Original Nasal spray
    Afrin 12-Hour Original Nose Drops
    Afrin 12-Hour Severe Congestion Nasal Spray
    Afrin 12-Hour Sinus Nasal Spray
        Nasal spray: 0.05% (45 ml); *Nasal drops:* 0.05% (45 ml)
    Afrin 4-Hour Nasal Spray
    Neo-Synephrine 12 Hour Nasal Spray
    Neo-Synephrine 12 Hour Extra Moisturizing Nasal Spray
        Nasal spray: 0.05% (15 ml)
▷ *phenylephrine* (C)
    Afrin Allergy Nasal Spray (OTC) 2-3 sprays in each nostril q 4 hours prn; max duration 5 days
    Pediatric: <12 years: not recommended; ≥12 years: same as adult
        Nasal spray: 0.5% (15 ml)
    Afrin Nasal Decongestant Children's Pump **Mist (OTC)**
    Pediatric: <6 years: not recommended; ≥6 years: 2-3 sprays in each nostril q 4 hours prn; max duration 5 days
        Nasal spray: 0.25% (15 ml)
    Neo-Synephrine Extra Strength (OTC) 2-3 sprays or drops in each nostril q 4 hours prn; max duration 5 days
    Pediatric: <12 years: not recommended; ≥12 years: same as adult
        Nasal spray: 0.1% (15 ml); *Nasal drops:* 0.1% (15 ml)
    Neo-Synephrine Mild Formula (OTC) 2-3 sprays or drops in each nostril q 4 hours prn; max duration 5 days
    Pediatric: <6 years: not recommended; ≥6 years: same as adult
        Nasal spray: 0.25% (15 ml)
    Neo-Synephrine Regular Strength (OTC) 2-3 sprays or drops in each nostril q 4 hours prn; max duration 5 days
    Pediatric: <12 years: not recommended; ≥12 years: same as adult
        Nasal spray: 0.5% (15 ml); *Nasal drops:* 0.5% (15 ml)
▷ *tetrahydrozoline* (C)
    Tyzine 2-4 drops or 3-4 sprays in each nostril q 3-8 hours prn; max duration 5 days
    Pediatric: <6 years: not recommended; ≥6 years: same as adult
        Nasal spray: 0.1% (15 ml); *Nasal drops:* 0.1% (30 ml)
    Tyzine Pediatric Nasal Drops 2-3 sprays or drops in each nostril q 3-6 hours prn
        Nasal drops: 0.05% (15 ml)

COMPLICATED URINARY TRACT INFECTION (cUTI), PYELONEPHRITIS

▷ *plazomicin* recommended dose is 15 mg/kg once every 24 hours by IV infusion over 30 minutes x 4-7 days in patients with CrCl ≥90 mL/min; *CrCl ≥60 to <90 mL/min:* 15 mg/kg every 24 hours; *CrCl ≥30 to <60 mL/min:* 10 mg/kg every 24 hours; CrCl ≥15 to <30 mL/min: 10 mg/kg every 48 hours
Pediatric: <18 years: not recommended; ≥18 years: same as adult
   Zemdri Injection *Vial:* 500 mg/10 ml (50 mg/ml) single-dose
   Comment: **Zemdri** (*plazomicin*) is an aminoglycoside antibacterial for the treatment of complicated urinary tract infection (cUTI) including pyelonephritis. As only limited clinical safety and efficacy data are available, reserve **Zemdri** for use in patients who have limited <u>or</u> no alternative treatment options. Assess creatinine clearance in all patients prior to initiating therapy and daily during therapy. Adjustment of initial dose and therapeutic drug monitoring (TDM) is recommended in patients with renal impairment. There is insufficient information to recommend a dosing regimen in patients with CrCl < 15 mL/min <u>or</u> on hemodialysis <u>or</u> continuous renal replacement therapy. For patients with CrCl ≥ 15 mL/min and < 90 mL/min, TDM is recommended in order to avoid *plazomicin*-induced nephrotoxicity. Monitor *plazomicin* trough concentrations and adjust **Zemdri** as described in the mfr pkg insert. BBW: Aminoglycosides are associated with nephrotoxicity, ototoxicity, and neuromuscular blockade; therefore, administer **Zamdri** no faster than 30 minutes, monitor for adverse reactions, and stop the infusion if any of these adverse events occur.
   Aminoglycosides can cause fetal harm in pregnancy. There are no available data on the use of **Zamdri** in pregnancy to inform a drug-related risk of adverse developmental outcomes. *streptomycin*, an aminoglycoside, can cause total and irreversible in children whose mothers received *streptomycin* in pregnancy. There are no data on the presence of **Zemdri** in human milk <u>or</u> effects on the breastfed infant; therefore, potential risk/benefit should be discussed with the mother. The most common adverse reactions (incidence ≥ 1%) are decreased renal function, diarrhea, hypertension, headache, nausea, vomiting and hypotension. To report suspected adverse side effects, contact Achogen at 1-833-252-6402 <u>or</u> FDA at 1-800-FDA-1088 <u>or</u> visit www.fda.gov/medwatch.

CONJUNCTIVITIS/BLEPHAROCONJUNCTIVITIS: BACTERIAL

OPHTHALMIC ANTI-INFECTIVES
▷ *azithromycin* **(B)(G)** ophthalmic solution **(B)(G)** 1 drop to affected eye(s) bid x 2 days; then 1 drop once daily for the next 5 days
Pediatric: <1 year: not recommended; ≥1 year: same as adult
   AzaSite Ophthalmic Solution *Ophth susp:* 1% (2.5 ml) (benzalkonium chloride)
▷ *bacitracin* ophthalmic ointment **(C)(G)** apply 1/2 inch ribbon to the lower conjunctival sac of affected eye(s) 1-3 x daily x 7 days
Pediatric: same as adult
   Bacitracin Ophthalmic Ointment *Ophth oint:* 500 units/gm (3.5 gm)
▷ *besifloxacin* ophthalmic solution **(C)** 1 drop to affected eye(s) tid x 7 days
Pediatric: <1 year: not recommended; ≥1 year: same as adult
   Besivance Ophthalmic Solution *Ophth susp:* 0.6% (5 ml) (benzalkonium chloride)
▷ *ciprofloxacin* ophthalmic ointment **(C)** apply 1/2 inch ribbon to the lower conjunctival sac of affected eye(s) tid x 2 days; then bid x 5 days
Pediatric: <2 years: not recommended; ≥2 years: same as adult
   Ciloxan Ophthalmic Ointment *Ophth oint:* 0.3% (3.5 gm)
▷ *ciprofloxacin* ophthalmic solution **(C)** 1-2 drops to affected eye(s) q 2 hours while awake x 2 days; then, q 4 hours while awake x 5 days
Pediatric: <1 years: not recommended; ≥1 year: same as adult
   Ciloxan Ophthalmic Solution *Ophth soln:* 0.3% (2.5, 5, 10 ml) (benzalkonium chloride)
▷ *erythromycin* ophthalmic ointment **(B)** apply 1/2 inch ribbon to the lower conjunctival sac of affected eye(s) up to 6 x/day
Pediatric: same as adult
   Ilotycin Ophthalmic Ointment *Ophth oint:* 5 mg/gm (1/8 oz)

➤ *gatifloxacin* ophthalmic solution (C)
  Pediatric: <1 years: not recommended; ≥1 year: same as adult
    Zymar Ophthalmic Solution initially 1 drop to affected eye(s) q 2 hours while awake up to 8 x/day for 2 days; then 1 drop qid while awake x 5 more days
      Ophth soln: 0.3% (5 ml) (benzalkonium chloride)
    Zymaxid Ophthalmic Solution (G) initially 1 drop to affected eye(s) q 2 hours while awake up to 8 x/day on day 1; then 1 drop bid-qid while awake on days 2-7
      Ophth soln: 0.5% (2.5 ml) (benzalkonium chloride)
➤ *gentamicin sulfate* ophthalmic ointment (C)(G) apply 1/2 inch ribbon to the lower conjunctival sac of affected eye(s) bid-tid
  Pediatric: same as adult
    Garamycin Ophthalmic Ointment *Ophth oint:* 3 mg/gm (3.5 gm) (preservative-free formulation available)
    Genoptic Ophthalmic Ointment *Ophth oint:* 3 mg/gm (3.5 gm)
    Gentacidin Ophthalmic Ointment *Ophth oint:* 3 mg/gm (3.5 gm)
➤ *gentamicin sulfate* ophthalmic solution (C)(G) 1-2 drops to affected eye(s) q 4 hours x 7-14 days; max 2 drops q 1 h
  Pediatric: same as adult
    Garamycin Ophthalmic Solution *Ophth soln:* 0.3% (5 ml) (benzalkonium chloride)
    Genoptic Ophthalmic Solution *Ophth soln:* 0.3% (3, 5 ml)
➤ *levofloxacin* ophthalmic solution (C) 1-2 drops to affected eye(s) q 2 hours while awake on days 1 and 2 (max 8 x/day); then 1-2 drops q 4 hours while awake on days 3-7; max 4 x/day
  Pediatric: <1 years: not recommended; ≥1 years: same as adult
    Quixin Ophthalmic Solution *Ophth soln:* 0.5% (2.5, 5 ml) (benzalkonium chloride)
➤ *moxifloxacin* ophthalmic solution (C)(G) 1 drop to affected eye(s) tid x 7 days
  Pediatric: <1 years: not recommended; ≥1 year: same as adult
    Moxeza Ophthalmic Solution (G) *Ophth soln:* 0.5% (3 ml)
    Vigamox Ophthalmic Solution *Ophth soln:* 0.5% (3 ml)
➤ *ofloxacin* ophthalmic solution (C) 1-2 drops to affected eye(s) q 2-4 hours x 2 days; then qid x 5 days
  Pediatric: <1 years: not recommended; ≥1 year: same as adult
    Ocuflox Ophthalmic Solution *Ophth soln:* 0.3% (5, 10 ml) (benzalkonium chloride)
➤ *sulfacetamide* ophthalmic solution and ointment (C)
    Bleph-10 Ophthalmic Solution 1-2 drops to affected eye(s) q 2-3 hours x 7-10 days
    Pediatric: <2 months: not recommended; ≥2 months: 1-2 drops q 2-3 hours during the day x 7-10 days
      Ophth soln: 10% (2.5, 5, 15 ml) (benzalkonium chloride)
    Bleph-10 Ophthalmic Ointment apply 1/2 inch ribbon to the lower conjunctival sac of affected eye(s) q 3-4 hours and HS x 7-10 days
    Pediatric: <2 years: not recommended; ≥2 years: same as adult
      Ophth oint: 10% (3.5 gm) (phenylmercuric acetate)
    Cetamide Ophthalmic Solution initially 1-2 drops to affected eye(s) q 2-3 hours; then increase dosing interval as condition improves
    Pediatric: <2 years: not recommended; ≥2 years: same as adult
      Ophth soln: 15% (5, 15 ml)
    Isopto Cetamide Ophthalmic Ointment initially 1/2 inch ribbon in lower conjunctival sac of affected eye(s) q 3-4 hours; then increase dosing interval as condition improves
    Pediatric: <2 years: not recommended; ≥2 years: same as adult
      Ophth oint: 10% (3.5 gm)
    Isopto Cetamide Ophthalmic Solution initially 1-2 drops to affected eye(s) q 2-3 hours; then increase dosing interval as condition improves
    Pediatric: <2 years: not recommended; ≥2 years: same as adult
      Ophth soln: 15% (5, 15 ml)
➤ *tobramycin* (B)
    Tobrex Ophthalmic Solution 1-2 drops to affected eye(s) q 4 hours
    Pediatric: same as adult
      Ophth soln: 0.3% (5 ml) (benzalkonium chloride)
    Tobrex Ophthalmic Ointment apply 1/2 inch ribbon to the lower conjunctival sac of affected eye(s) bid-tid
    Pediatric: same as adult
      Ophth oint: 0.3% (3.5 gm) (chlorobutanol)

OPHTHALMIC ANTI-INFECTIVE COMBINATIONS

▶ *polymyxin b sulfate+bacitracin* ophthalmic ointment (C) apply 1/2 inch ribbon to the lower conjunctival sac of affected eye(s) q 3-4 hours x 7-10 days
Pediatric: same as adult
> **Polysporin Ophthalmic Ointment** *Ophth oint:* poly b 10,000 U+bac 500 U (3.75 gm)

▶ *polymyxin b sulfate+bacitracin zinc+neomycin sulfate* ophthalmic ointment (C) apply 1/2 inch ribbon to the lower conjunctival sac of affected eye(s) q 3-4 hours x 7-10 days
Pediatric: same as adult
> **Neosporin Ophthalmic Ointment** *Ophth oint:* poly b 10,000 U+bac 400 U+neo 3.5 mg/gm (3.75 gm)

▶ *polymyxin b sulfate+gramicidin+neomycin* ophthalmic solution (C) 1-2 drops to affected eye(s) q 1 hour x 2-3 doses; then 1-2 drops bid-qid x 7-10 days
Pediatric: <2 years: not recommended; ≥12 years: same as adult
> **Neosporin Ophthalmic Solution** *Ophth soln:* poly b 10,000 U+grami 0.025 mg+neo 1.7 mg/gm (10 ml)

▶ *trimethoprim+polymyxin b sulfate* ophthalmic solution (C) 1 drop to affected eye(s) q 3 hours x 7-10 days; max 6 doses/day
Pediatric: <2 years: not recommended; ≥2 years: same as adult
> **Polytrim** *Ophth soln:* trim 1 mg+poly b 10,000 U/ml (10 ml) (benzalkonium chloride)

OPHTHALMIC ANTI-INFECTIVE+STEROID COMBINATIONS

Comment: Ophthalmic corticosteroids are contraindicated after removal of a corneal foreign body, epithelial herpes simplex keratitis, *varicella*, other viral infections of the cornea or conjunctiva, fungal ocular infections, and mycobacterial ocular infections. Limit ophthalmic steroid use to 2-3 days if possible; usual max 2 weeks. With prolonged or frequent use, there is risk of corneal and scleral thinning and cataract formation.

▶ *gentamicin sulfate+prednisolone acetate* ophthalmic suspension (C)
Pediatric: <12 years: not recommended; ≥12 years: same as adult
> **Pred-G Ophthalmic Suspension** 1 drop to affected eye(s) bid-qid; max 20 ml/therapeutic course
> *Ophth susp:* gent 0.3%+pred 1%/ml (2, 5, 10 ml) (benzalkonium chloride)
> **Pred-G Ophthalmic Ointment** apply 1/2 inch ribbon to the lower conjunctival sac of affected eye(s) once daily-tid; max 8 gm/therapeutic course
> *Ophth oint:* gent 0.3%+pred 0.6%/gm (3.5 gm)

▶ *neomycin sulfate+polymyxin b sulfate+dexamethasone* ophthalmic suspension (C)
Pediatric: <12 years: not recommended; ≥12 years: same as adult
> **Maxitrol Ophthalmic Suspension** 1-2 drops to affected eye(s) q 1 hour (severe infection) or qid (mild to moderate infection)
> *Ophth susp:* neo 0.35%+poly b 10,000 U+dexa 1%/ml (5 ml) (benzalkonium chloride)
> **Maxitrol Ophthalmic Ointment** apply 1/2 inch ribbon to the lower conjunctival sac of affected eye(s) q 1 hour (severe infection) or qid (mild to moderate infection)
> *Ophth oint:* neo 0.35%+poly b 10,000 U+dexa 0.1%/gm (3.5 gm)

▶ *neomycin sulfate+polymyxin b sulfate+prednisolone acetate ophthalmic suspension* (C)
Pediatric: <12 years: not recommended; ≥12 years: same as adult
> **Poly-Pred Ophthalmic Suspension** 1-2 drops to affected eye(s) q 3-4 hours; more often as necessary; max 20 ml/therapeutic course.
> *Ophth susp:* neo 0.35%+poly b 10,000 U+pred 0.5%/ml (10 ml)

▶ *polymyxin b sulfate+neomycin sulfate+hydrocortisone* ophthalmic suspension (C)
Pediatric: <12 years: not recommended; ≥12 years: same as adult
> **Cortisporin Ophthalmic Suspension** 1-2 drops to affected eye(s) tid-qid; more often if necessary; max 20 ml/therapeutic course
> *Ophth susp:* poly b 10,000 U+neo 0.35%+hydro 1%/ml (7.5 ml) (thimerosal)

▶ *polymyxin b sulfate+neomycin sulfate+bacitracin zinc+hydrocortisone* ophthalmic ointment (C)
Pediatric: <12 years: not recommended; ≥12 years: same as adult
> **Cortisporin Ophthalmic Ointment** apply 1/2 inch ribbon to the lower conjunctival sac of affected eye(s) tid-qid; more often if necessary; max 8 gm/therapeutic course
> *Ophth oint:* poly b 10,000 U+neo 0.35%+bac 400 U+hydro 1%/gm (3.5 gm)

▶ *sulfacetamide sodium+fluorometholone* suspension **(C)** 1 drop to affected eye(s) qid; max 20 ml/therapeutic course
  Pediatric: <12 years: not recommended; ≥12 years: same as adult
    FML-S *Ophth susp:* sulfa 10%+fluoro 0.1%+ml (5, 10, 15 ml) (benzalkonium chloride)
▶ *sulfacetamide sodium+prednisolone acetate* ophthalmic suspension and ointment **(C)**
  Pediatric: <6 years: not recommended; ≥6 years: same as adult
    Blephamide Liquifilm 2 drops to affected eye(s) qid and HS
      Ophth susp: sulfa 10%+pred 0.2%/ml (5, 10 ml) (benzalkonium chloride)
    Blephamide S.O.P. Ophthalmic Ointment apply 1/2 inch ribbon to the lower conjunctival sac of affected eye(s) tid-qid
      Ophth oint: sulfa 10%+pred 0.2%/gm (3.5 gm) (benzalkonium chloride)
▶ *sulfacetamide sodium+prednisolone sodium phosphate* ophthalmic solution **(C)** 2 drops to affected eye(s) q 4 hours
  Pediatric: <6 years: not recommended; ≥6 years: same as adult
    Vasocidin Ophthalmic Solution *Ophth soln:* sulfa 10%+pred 0.25%/ml (5, 10 ml)
▶ *tobramycin+dexamethasone* ophthalmic solution and ointment **(C)**
    TobraDex Ophthalmic Solution 1-2 drops to affected eye(s) q 2-6 hours x 24-48 hours; then 4-6 hours; reduce frequency of dose as condition improves; max 20 ml per therapeutic course
  Pediatric: ≤2 years: not recommended; ≥2 years: 1-2 drops q 4-6 hours; may start with 1-2 drops q 2 hours first 1-2 days
      Ophth susp: tobra 0.3%+dexa 0.1%/ml (2.5, 5 ml) (benzalkonium chloride)
    TobraDex Ophthalmic Ointment apply 1/2 inch ribbon to the lower conjunctival sac of affected eye(s) tid-qid; may use at HS in conjunction with daytime drops; max 8 gm/therapeutic course
  Pediatric: <2 years: not recommended; ≥2 years: apply 1/2 inch ribbon to lower conjunctival sac tid-qid
      Ophth oint: tobra 0.3%/dexa 0.1%/gm (3.5 gm) (chlorobutanol chloride)
    TobraDex ST 1-2 drops to affected eye(s) q 2-6 hours x 24-48 hours; then 4-6 hours; reduce frequency of dose as condition improves; max 20 ml per therapeutic course
  Pediatric: <12 years: not recommended; ≥12 years: same as adult
      Ophth susp: tobra 0.3%/dexa 0.05%/ml (2.5, 5, 10 ml) (benzalkonium chloride)
▶ *tobramycin+loteprednol etabonate* ophthalmic suspension **(C)**
  Pediatric: <12 years: not recommended; ≥12 years: same as adult
    Zylet 1-2 drops to affected eye(s) q 1-2 hours first 24-48 hours; reduce frequency of dose to q 4-6 hours as condition improves; max 20 ml per therapeutic course
      Ophth susp: tobra 0.3%+lote etab 0.5%/ml (2.5, 5, 10 ml) (benzalkonium chloride)

CONJUNCTIVITIS: CHLAMYDIAL

Comment: A chlamydial etiology should be considered for all infants aged ≤30 days that have conjunctivitis, especially if the mother has a history of chlamydia infection. Topical antibiotic therapy alone is inadequate for treatment for *ophthalmia neonatorum* caused by chlamydia and is unnecessary when systemic treatment is administered.

RECOMMENDED FIRST LINE REGIMEN

▶ *erythromycin base* (B)(G) 250 mg qid x 14 days or 500 mg qid x 7 days
  Pediatric: <45 kg: 50 mg/kg/day in 4 divided doses x 14 days; ≥45 kg: same as adult
    Ery-Tab *Tab:* 250, 333, 500 mg ent-coat
    PCE *Tab:* 333, 500 mg
  Comment: *erythromycin* may increase INR with concomitant *warfarin*, as well as increase serum level of *digoxin*, benzodiazepines, and statins.
    OR
▶ *erythromycin ethylsuccinate* (B)(G) 400 mg qid x 14 days or 800 mg qid x 7 days
  Pediatric: 50 mg/kg/day in 4 divided doses x 7 days; max 100 mg/kg/day; *see page 626 for dose by weight*
    EryPed *Oral susp:* 200 mg/5 ml (100, 200 ml) (fruit); 400 mg/5 ml (60, 100, 200 ml) (banana); *Oral drops:* 200, 400 mg/5 ml (50 ml) (fruit); *Chew tab:* 200 mg wafer (fruit)
    E.E.S. *Oral susp:* 200, 400 mg/5 ml (100 ml) (fruit)
    E.E.S. Granules *Oral susp:* 200 mg/5 ml (100, 200 ml) (cherry)
    E.E.S. 400 Tablets *Tab:* 400 mg

Comment: *erythromycin* may increase INR with concomitant *warfarin*, as well as increase serum level of *digoxin*, benzodiazepines, and statins.

ALTERNATE REGIMEN

▷ *azithromycin* (B)(G) 500 mg x 1 dose on day 1; then 250 mg once daily on days; 2-5 or 500 mg daily x 3 days or 2 gm in a single dose
  Pediatric: 20 mg/kg in a single dose once daily x 3 days
    Zithromax *Tab:* 250, 500, 600 mg; *Oral susp:* 100 mg/5 ml (15 ml); 200 mg/5 ml (15, 22.5, 30 ml) (cherry); *Pkt:* 1 gm for reconstitution (cherry-banana)
    Zithromax Tri-pak *Tab:* 3 x 500 mg tabs/pck
    Zithromax Z-pak *Tab:* 6 x 250 mg tabs/pck
    Zmax *Oral susp:* 2 gm ext-rel for reconstitution (cherry-banana) (148 mg Na⁺)

CONJUNCTIVITIS: FUNGAL

▷ *natamycin* ophthalmic suspension (C) 1 drop q 1-2 hours x 3-4 days; then 1 drop every 6 hours; treat for 14-21 days; withdraw dose gradually at 4- to 7-day intervals
  Pediatric: <1 year: not recommended; ≥1 year: same as adult
    Natacyn Ophthalmic Suspension *Ophth susp:* 0.5% (15 ml) (benzalkonium chloride)

CONJUNCTIVITIS: GONOCOCCAL

RECOMMENDED REGIMENS

Regimen 1

▷ *ceftriaxone* (B)(G) 250 mg IM x 1 dose
  Pediatric: <45 kg: 50 mg/kg IM x 1 dose; max 125 mg IM
    Rocephin *Vial:* 250, 500 mg; 1, 2 gm

Regimen 2

▷ *erythromycin base* (B)(G) 250 mg qid x 10-14 days
  Pediatric: <45 kg: 50 mg/kg/day in 4 divided doses x 10-14 days; ≥45 kg: same as adult
    Ery-Tab *Tab:* 250, 333, 500 mg ent-coat
    PCE *Tab:* 333, 500 mg
  Comment: *erythromycin* may increase INR with concomitant *warfarin*, as well as increase serum level of *digoxin*, benzodiazepines, and statins.
▷ *erythromycin ethylsuccinate* (B)(G) 400 mg qid x 14 days or 800 mg qid x 7 days
  Pediatric: 50 mg/kg/day in 4 divided doses x 7 days; max 100 mg/kg/day; *see page 626 for dose by weight*
    EryPed *Oral susp:* 200 mg/5 ml (100, 200 ml) (fruit); 400 mg/5 ml (60, 100, 200 ml) (banana); *Oral drops:* 200, 400 mg/5 ml (50 ml) (fruit); *Chew tab:* 200 mg wafer (fruit)
    E.E.S. *Oral susp:* 200, 400 mg/5 ml (100 ml) (fruit)
    E.E.S. Granules *Oral susp:* 200 mg/5 ml (100, 200 ml) (cherry)
    E.E.S. 400 Tablets *Tab:* 400 mg
  Comment: *erythromycin* may increase INR with concomitant *warfarin*, as well as increase serum level of *digoxin*, benzodiazepines, and statins.

ALTERNATE REGIMEN

▷ *azithromycin* (B)(G) 500 mg x 1 dose on day 1; then 250 mg once daily on days; 2-5 or 500 mg daily x 3 days or 2 gm in a single dose
  Pediatric: not recommended for bronchitis in children
    Zithromax *Tab:* 250, 500, 600 mg; *Oral susp:* 100 mg/5 ml (15 ml); 200 mg/5 ml (15, 22.5, 30 ml) (cherry); Pkt: 1 gm for reconstitution (cherry-banana)
    Zithromax Tri-pak *Tab:* 3 x 500 mg tabs/pck
    Zithromax Z-pak *Tab:* 6 x 250 mg tabs/pck
    Zmax *Oral susp:* 2 gm ext-rel for reconstitution (cherry-banana) (148 mg Na⁺)

CONJUNCTIVITIS/KERATITIS/KERATOCONJUNCTIVITIS: ALLERGIC (VERNAL)

Oral Antihistamines *see* **Drugs for the Management of Allergy, Cough, and Cold Symptoms** *page* 603

OPHTHALMIC CORTICOSTEROIDS

Comment: Concomitant contact lens wear is contraindicated during therapy. Ophthalmic steroids are contraindicated with ocular, fungal, mycobacterial, viral (except herpes zoster), and untreated bacterial infection. Ophthalmic steroids may mask or exacerbate infection, and may increase intraocular pressure, optic nerve damage, cataract formation, or corneal perforation. Limit ophthalmic steroid use to 2-3 days if possible; usual max 2 weeks. With prolonged or frequent use, there is risk of corneal and scleral thinning and cataract formation.

▷ *dexamethasone* (C) initially 1-2 drops hourly during the day and q 2 hours at night; then prolong dosing interval to 4-6 hours as condition improves
  Pediatric: <12 years: not recommended; ≥12 years: same as adult
    Maxidex *Ophth susp:* 0.1% (5, 15 ml) (benzalkonium chloride)

▷ *dexamethasone phosphate* (C) initially 1-2 drops hourly during the day and q 2 hours at night; then 1 drop q 4-8 hours or more as condition improves
  Pediatric: <12 years: not recommended; ≥12 years: same as adult
    Decadron *Ophth soln:* 0.1% (5 ml) (sulfites)

▷ *fluorometholone* (C) 1 drop bid-qid or 1/2 inch of ointment once daily-tid; may increase dose frequency during initial 24-48 hours
  Pediatric: <2 years: not recommended; ≥2 years: same as adult
    FML *Ophth susp:* 0.1% (5, 10, 15 ml) (benzalkonium chloride)
    FML Forte *Ophth susp:* 0.25% (5, 10, 15 ml) (benzalkonium chloride)
    FML S.O.P. Ointment *Ophth oint:* 0.1% (3.5 gm)

▷ *fluorometholone acetate* (C) initially 2 drops q 2 hours during the first 24-48 hours; then 1-2 drops qid as condition improves
  Pediatric: <12 years: not recommended; ≥12 years: same as adult
    Flarex *Ophth susp:* 0.1% (2.5, 5 10 ml) (benzalkonium chloride)

▷ *loteprednol etabonate* (C)
  Pediatric: <12 years: not recommended; ≥12 years: same as adult
    Alrex 1 drop qid
      Ophth susp: 0.2% (5, 10 ml) (benzalkonium chloride)
    Lotemax 1-2 drops qid
      Ophth susp: 0.5% (5, 10, 15 ml) (benzalkonium chloride)

▷ *medrysone* (C) 1 drop up to q 4 hours
  Pediatric: <12 years: not recommended; ≥12 years: same as adult
    HMS *Ophth susp:* 1% (5, 10 ml) (benzalkonium chloride)

▷ *rimexolone* (C) initially 1-2 drops hourly while awake x 1 week; then 1 drop q 2 hours while awake x 1 week; then taper as condition improves
  Pediatric: <12 years: not recommended; ≥12 years: same as adult
    Vexol *Ophth susp:* 0.1% (5, 10 ml) (benzalkonium chloride)

▷ *prednisolone acetate* (C)(G)
  Pediatric: <12 years: not recommended; ≥12 years: same as adult
    Econopred 2 drops qid
      Ophth susp: 0.125% (5, 10 ml)
    Econopred Plus 2 drops qid
      Ophth susp: 1% (5, 10 ml)
    Pred Forte initially 2 drops hourly x 24-48 hours; then 1-2 drops bid-qid
      Ophth susp: 1% (1, 5, 10, 15 ml) (benzalkonium chloride, sulfites)
    Pred Mild initially 2 drops hourly x 24-48 hours; then 1-2 drops bid-qid
      Ophth susp: 0.12% (5, 10 ml) (benzalkonium chloride)

▷ *prednisolone sodium phosphate* (C) initially 1-2 drops hourly during the day and q 2 hours at night; then 1 drop q 4 hours; then 1 drop tid-qid as condition improves
  Pediatric: <12 years: not recommended; ≥12 years: same as adult
    Inflamase Forte *Ophth soln:* 1% (5, 10, 15 ml) (benzalkonium chloride)
    Inflamase Mild *Ophth soln:* 1/8% (5, 10 ml) (benzalkonium chloride)

OPHTHALMIC H1 ANTAGONISTS (ANTIHISTAMINES)

Comment: May insert contact lens 10 minutes after administration of ophthalmic antihistamine.
▷ *cetirizine* (C) 1 drop bid prn
  Pediatric: <2 years: not established; ≥2 years: same as adult
    Zerviate *Ophth soln:* 0.24%/ml (5 ml [7.5 ml bottle]; 7.5 ml [10 ml bottle])

▷ *emedastine* (C) 1 drop qid prn
  Pediatric: <3 years: not recommended; ≥3 years: same as adult
    Emadine *Ophth soln:* 0.05% (5 ml) (benzalkonium chloride)

▷ *levocabastine* (C) 1 drop qid prn
  Pediatric: <12 years: not recommended; ≥12 years: same as adult
    Livostin *Ophth susp:* 0.05% (2.5, 5, 10 ml) (benzalkonium chloride)

OPHTHALMIC MAST CELL STABILIZERS

Comment: Concomitant contact lens wear is contraindicated during treatment.
▷ *cromolyn sodium* (B) 1-2 drops 4-6 x/day at regular intervals
  Pediatric: <4 years: not recommended; ≥4 years: same as adult
    Crolom *Ophth soln:* 4% (10 ml) (benzalkonium chloride)
▷ *lodoxamide tromethamine* (B) 1-2 drops qid up to 3 months
  Pediatric: <2 years: not recommended; ≥2 years: same as adult
    Alomide *Ophth soln:* 1% (10 ml) (benzalkonium chloride)
▷ *nedocromil* (B) 1-2 drops bid
  Pediatric: <3 years: not recommended; ≥3 years: same as adult
    Alocril *Ophth soln:* 2% (5 ml) (benzalkonium chloride)
▷ *pemirolast potassium* (C) 1-2 drops qid
  Pediatric: <3 years: not recommended; ≥3 years: same as adult
    Alamast *Ophth soln:* 0.1% (10 ml) (lauralkonium chloride)

OPHTHALMIC ANTIHISTAMINE+MAST CELL STABILIZER COMBINATIONS

▷ *alcaftadine* (B) 1 drop each eye daily
  Pediatric: <2 years: not recommended; ≥2 years: same as adult
    Lastacaft *Ophth soln:* 0.25% (6 ml) (benzalkonium chloride)
  Comment: May insert contact lens 10 minutes after ophthalmic administration.
▷ *azelastine* (C) 1 drop each eye bid
  Pediatric: <3 years: not recommended; ≥3 years: same as adult
    Optivar *Ophth soln:* 0.05% (6 ml) (benzalkonium chloride)
  Comment: May insert contact lens 10 minutes after ophthalmic administration.
▷ *bepotastine besilate* (C) 1 drop each eye bid
  Pediatric: <2 years: not recommended; ≥2 years: same as adult
    Bepreve *Ophth soln:* 1.5% (10 ml) (benzalkonium chloride)
  Comment: May insert contact lens 10 minutes after ophthalmic administration.
▷ *epinastine* (C)(G) 1 drop each eye bid
  Pediatric: <3 years: not recommended; ≥3 years: same as adult
    Elestat *Ophth soln:* 0.05% (5 ml) (benzalkonium chloride)
  Comment: May insert contact lens 10 minutes after administration.
▷ *ketotifen fumarate* (C) 1 drop each eye q 8-12 hours
  Pediatric: <3 years: not recommended; ≥3 years: same as adult
    Alaway (OTC) *Ophth soln:* 0.025% (10 ml) (benzalkonium chloride)
    Claritin Eye (OTC) *Ophth soln:* 0.025% (5 ml) (benzalkonium chloride)
    Refresh Eye Itch Relief (OTC) *Ophth soln:* 0.025% (5 ml) (benzalkonium chloride)
    Zaditor (OTC) *Ophth soln:* 0.025% (5 ml) (benzalkonium chloride)
    Zyrtec Itchy Eye (OTC) *Ophth soln:* 0.025% (5 ml) (benzalkonium chloride)
  Comment: May insert contact lens 10 minutes after administration.
▷ *olopatadine* (C) 1 drop each eye bid
  Pediatric: <3 years: not recommended; ≥3 years: same as adult
    Pataday (G) *Ophth soln:* 0.2% (2.5 ml) (benzalkonium chloride)
    Patanol (G) *Ophth soln:* 0.1% (5 ml) (benzalkonium chloride)
    Pazeo *Ophth soln:* 0.7% (2.5 ml) (benzalkonium chloride)
  Comment: May insert contact lens 10 minutes after administration.

OPHTHALMIC VASOCONSTRICTORS

Comment: Concomitant contact lens wear is contraindicated during treatment.
▷ *naphazoline* (C) 1-2 drops each eye qid prn
  Pediatric: <12 years: not recommended; ≥12 years: same as adult
    Vasocon-A *Ophth soln:* 0.1% (15 ml) (benzalkonium chloride)
▷ *oxymetazoline* (OTC) 1-2 drops each eye qid prn
  Pediatric: <6 years: not recommended; ≥6 years: same as adult
    Visine L-R *Ophth soln:* 0.025% (15, 30 ml)
▷ *tetrahydrozoline* (OTC)(G) 1-2 drops each eye qid prn
  Pediatric: <6 years: not recommended; ≥6 years: same as adult
    Visine *Ophth soln:* 0.05% (15, 22.5, 30 ml)

OPHTHALMIC VASOCONSTRICTOR+MOISTURIZER COMBINATION

Comment: Concomitant contact lens wear is contraindicated during treatment.
▷ *tetrahydrozoline+polyethylene glycol 400+povidone+dextran 70* (OTC) 1-2 drops each eye qid prn
  Pediatric: <6 years: not recommended; ≥6 years: same as adult
    Advanced Relief Visine *Ophth soln:* tetra 0.025%+poly 1%+pov 1%+dex 0.1% (15, 30 ml)

OPHTHALMIC VASOCONSTRICTOR+ASTRINGENT COMBINATION

Comment: Concomitant contact lens wear is contraindicated during treatment.
▷ *tetrahydrozoline+zinc sulfate* (OTC) 1-2 drops each eye qid prn
  Pediatric: <6 years: not recommended; ≥6 years: same as adult
    Visine AC *Ophth soln:* tetra 0.025%+zinc 0.05% (15, 30 ml)

OPHTHALMIC VASOCONSTRICTOR+ANTI HISTAMINE COMBINATIONS

Comment: Concomitant contact lens wear is contraindicated during treatment.
▷ *naphazoline+pheniramine* (C) 1-2 drops each eye qid
  Pediatric: <6 years: not recommended; ≥6 years: same as adult
    Naphcon-A (OTC) *Ophth soln:* naph 0.025%+phen 0.3% (15 ml) (benzalkonium chloride)

OPHTHALMIC NSAIDs

Comment: Concomitant contact lens wear is contraindicated during treatment.

▷ *bromfenac* (C)(G) 1 drop affected eye(s) bid
    Bromday Ophthalmic Solution *Ophth soln:* 0.09% (2.5 ml in 7.5 ml dropper bottle; 7.5 ml in 10 ml dropper bottle)
    Xibrom Ophthalmic Solution *Ophth soln:* 0.09% (2.5 ml in 7.5 ml dropper bottle; 7.5 ml in 10 ml dropper bottle)
▷ *diclofenac* (B) 1 drop affected eye(s) qid
  Pediatric: <12 years: not recommended; ≥12 years: same as adult
    Voltaren Ophthalmic Solution *Ophth soln:* 0.1% (2.5, 5 ml)
▷ *ketorolac tromethamine* (C) 1 drop affected eye(s) qid; max x 4 days
  Pediatric: <3 years: not recommended; ≥3 years: same as adult
    Acular *Ophth soln:* 0.5% (3, 5, 10 ml) (benzalkonium chloride)
    Acular LS *Ophth soln:* 0.4% (5 ml) (benzalkonium chloride)
    Acular PF *Ophth soln:* 0.5% (0.4 ml; 12 single-use vials/carton) (preservative-free)
▷ *nepafenac* (C) 1 drop affected eye(s) tid
  Pediatric: <10 years: not recommended; ≥10 years: same as adult
    Nevanac Ophthalmic Suspension *Ophth susp:* 0.1% (3 ml) (benzalkonium chloride)

CONJUNCTIVITIS: VIRAL

Comment: For prevention of secondary bacterial infection, see agents listed under bacterial conjunctivitis. Ophthalmic corticosteroids are contraindicated with herpes simplex, keratitis, *Varicella*, and other viral infections of the cornea.
▷ *trifluridine* ophthalmic suspension (C) 1 drop q 2 hours while awake; max 9 drops/day; after re-epithelialization, 1 drop q 4 h x 7 days (at least 5 drops/day); max 21 days of therapy
  Pediatric: <6 years: not recommended; ≥6 years: same as adult
    Viroptic Ophthalmic Solution *Ophth soln:* 1% (7.5 ml) (thimerosal)

CONSTIPATION: CHRONIC IDIOPATHIC (CIC)

GUANYLATE CYCLASE-C AGONISTS

Comment: Guanylate cyclase-c agonists increase intestinal fluid and intestinal transit time may induce diarrhea and bloating and therefore, are contraindicated with known or suspected mechanical GI obstruction.

▷ *linaclotide* (C) 145 mcg orally once daily or 72 mcg orally once daily based on individual presentation or tolerability; take on an empty stomach at least 30 minutes before the first meal of the day; swallow whole, do not crush or chew cap or cap contents; may open cap and administer with applesauce or water (e.g., NGT, PEG tube)
Pediatric: ≤18 years: not established (<6 years: contraindicated; 6-18 years: avoid); >18 years: same as adult
   Linzess *Cap:* 72, 145, 290 mcg
   Comment: *linaclotide* and its active metabolite are negligibly absorbed systemically following oral administration and maternal use is not expected to result in fetal exposure to the drug. There is no information regarding the presence of *plecanatide* in human milk or its effects on the breastfed infant.
▷ *plecanatide* take one tab once daily; if necessary, may crush and administer with applesauce or water (e.g., NGT, PEG tube)
Pediatric: ≤18 years: not established (<6 years: contraindicated; 6-18 years: avoid); >18 years: same as adult
   Trulance *Tab:* 3 mg
   Comment: Suspend *plecanatide* dosing and rehydrate if severe diarrhea occurs. Most common adverse reactions in CIC are sinusitis, URI, diarrhea, abdominal distension and tenderness, flatulence, increased liver enzymes. *plecanatide* and its active metabolite are negligibly absorbed systemically following oral administration and maternal use is not expected to result in fetal exposure to the drug. There is no information regarding the presence of *plecanatide* in human milk or its effects on the breastfed infant.

CHLORIDE CHANNEL ACTIVATOR

▷ *lubiprostone* (C) **one** 24 mcg cap bid with food and water; swallow whole, do not break apart or chew
Pediatric: <18 years: not recommended; ≥18 years: same as adult
   Amitiza *Cap:* 8, 24 mcg
   Comment: **Amitiza** increases intestinal fluid and intestinal transit time. Suspend dosing and rehydrate if severe diarrhea occurs. **Amitiza** is contraindicated with known or suspected mechanical GI obstruction. Most common adverse reactions in CIC are nausea, diarrhea, headache, abdominal pain, abdominal distension, and flatulence.

Selective Serotonin Type 4 (5HT4) Receptor Agonist

▷ *prucalopride* 2 mg once daily; *CrCl <30 mL/min:* 1 mg once daily; *ESRD:* avoid
Pediatric: <18 years: not established; ≥18 years: same as adult
   Motegrity *Tab:* 1, 2 mg film-coat
   Comment: **Motegrity** (*prucalopride*) is a selective serotonin type 4 (5HT4) receptor agonist for the treatment of chronic idiopathic constipation (CIC) in adults. *prucalopride* is a gastrointestinal (GI) prokinetic agent that stimulates colonic peristalsis (high-amplitude propagating contractions [HAPCs]), which increases bowel motility. The most common adverse reactions (incidence ≥2%) have been headache, abdominal pain, nausea, diarrhea, abdominal distension, dizziness, vomiting, flatulence, and fatigue. Contraindications include intestinal perforation or obstruction due to structural or functional disorder of the gut wall, obstructive ileus, severe inflammatory conditions of the intestinal tract such as Crohn's disease, ulcerative colitis, and toxic megacolon/megarectum. Monitor patients for persistent worsening of depression and emergence of suicidal thoughts and behavior. Instruct patients to discontinue **Motegrity** immediately and contact their healthcare provider if their depression is persistently worse, or they experience emerging suicidal thoughts or behaviors. Available data from case reports with *prucalopride* use in pregnancy are insufficient to identify any drug-associated risks of miscarriage, major birth defects, or adverse maternal or fetal outcomes. *prucalopride* is present in breast milk. There are no data on effects of *prucalopride* on the breastfed infant.

 CONSTIPATION: OCCASIONAL, INTERMITTENT

BULK-FORMING AGENTS

▷ *calcium polycarbophil* (C) 2 tabs once daily to qid
Pediatric: <6 years: not recommended; 6-12 years: 1 tab daily to qid

FiberCon (OTC) *Cplt:* 625 mg
Konsyl Fiber Tablets (OTC) *Tab:* 625 mg
▷ *methylcellulose*
Citrucel 1 heaping tbsp in 8 oz cold water tid
Pediatric: <6 years: not recommended; 6-12 years: 1/2 adult dose
Oral pwdr: 16, 24, 30 oz and single-dose pkts (orange)
Citrucel Sugar-Free 1 heaping tbsp in 8 oz cold water tid
Pediatric: <6 years: not recommended; 6-12 years: 1/2 adult dose
Oral pwdr: 16, 24, 30 oz and single-dose pkts (orange) (sugar-free, phenylalanine)
▷ *psyllium husk* (B)
Pediatric: <6 years: not recommended; 6-12 years: 1/2 adult dose in 8 oz liquid tid
Metamucil (OTC) wafer or cap or 1 pkt or 1 rounded tsp (1 rounded tbsp for sug-ar-containing form) in 8 oz liquid tid
Cap: psyllium husk 5.2 gm (100, 150/carton); Wafer: *psyllium husk* 3.4 gm/rounded tsp (24/carton) (apple crisp, cinnamon spice); *Plain and flavored pwdr:* 3.4 gm/rounded tsp (15, 20, 24, 29, 30, 36, 44, 48 oz); *Efferv sugar-free flav pkts:* 3.4 gm/pkt (30/carton) (phenylalanine)
▷ *psyllium* hydrophilic mucilloid (B) 2 rounded tsp in 8 oz water qid
Pediatric: <6 years: not recommended; 6-12 years: 1 rounded tsp in 8 oz liquid tid
Konsyl (OTC) *Pwdr:* 6 gm/rounded tsp (10.6, 15.9 oz); *Pwdr pkt:* 6 gm/rounded tsp (30/carton)
Konsyl-D (OTC) *Pwdr:* 3.4 gm/rounded tsp (11.5, 17.59 oz); *Pwdr pkt:* 3.4 gm/rounded tsp (30/carton)
Konsyl Easy Mix Formula (OTC) *Pwdr:* 3.4 gm/rounded tsp (8 oz) (sugar-free, low sodium)
Konsyl Orange (OTC) *Pwdr:* 3.4 gm/rounded tsp (19 oz); *Pwdr pkt:* 3.4 gm/rounded tsp (30/carton)
Konsyl Orange SF (OTC) *Pwdr:* 3.5 gm/rounded tsp (15 oz) (phenylalanine); *Pwdr pkt:* 3.5 gm/rounded tsp (30/carton) (phenylalanine)

STOOL SOFTENERS

▷ *docusate sodium* (OTC) 50-200 mg/day
Pediatric: <3 years: 10-40 mg/day; 3-6 years: 20-60 mg/day; >6 years: 40-120 mg/day
Cap: 50, 100 mg; *Liq:* 10 mg/ml (30 ml w. dropper); *Syr:* 20 mg/5 ml (8 oz) (alcohol ≤1%)
Dialose 1 tab q HS
Pediatric: <6 years: not recommended; ≥6 years: same as adult
Tab: 100 mg
Surfak (OTC) 240 mg/day
Pediatric: <12 years: not recommended; ≥12 years: same as adult
Cap: 240 mg

OSMOTIC LAXATIVES

▷ *lactulose* (B)(G) take 10-20 gm dissolved in 4 oz water once daily prn; max 40 gm/day
Pediatric: <12 years: not recommended; ≥12 years: same as adult
Kristalose *Crystals for oral soln:* 10, 20 gm single-dose pkts (30/carton)
▷ *magnesium citrate* (B)(G) 1 full bottle (120-300 ml) once daily prn
Pediatric: <2 years: not recommended; 2-6 years: 4-12 ml once daily prn; ≥6-12 years: 50-100 ml once daily prn
Citrate of Magnesia (OTC) *Oral soln:* 300 ml
▷ *magnesium hydroxide* (B) 30-60 ml/day in a single or divided doses prn
Pediatric: 2-5 years: 5-15 ml/day in a single or divided doses; 6-11 years: 15-30 ml/day in a single or divided doses; ≥12 years: same as adult
Milk of Magnesia *Liq:* 390 mg/5 ml (10, 15, 20, 30, 100, 120, 180, 360, 720 ml)
▷ *polyethylene glycol (PEG)* (C)(OTC)(G) 1 tbsp (17 gm) dissolved in 4-8 oz water per day for up to max 7 days; may need 2-4 days for results
Pediatric: ≤17: <12 years: not recommended; ≥12 years: same as adult
GlycoLax Powder for Oral Solution *Oral pwdr:* 7, 14, 30, and 45 dose bottles w. 17 gm dosing cup (gluten-free, sugar-free); 17 gm single-dose pkts (20/ carton)
MiraLAX Powder for Oral Solution *Oral pwdr:* 7, 14, 30, and 45 dose bottles w. 17 gm dosing cup (gluten-free, sugar-free)

Polyethylene Glycol 3350 Powder for Oral Solution (G) *Oral pwdr:* 3350 gm w. dosing cup; 17 gm/scoop

Comment: *PEG* is an osmotic indicated for occasional constipation without affecting glucose and electrolyte levels. Contraindicated with suspected or known bowel obstruction.

STIMULANTS

▷ *bisacodyl* (B) 2-3 tabs or 1 suppository bid prn

Dulcolax, Gentlax *Tab:* 5 mg; *Rectal supp:* 10 mg
Pediatric: <12 years: 1/2 suppository once daily prn; 6-12 years: 1 tablet or 1/2 suppository once daily prn; >12 years: same as adult
Senokot (OTC) initially 2-4 tabs or 1 level tsp at HS prn; max 4 tabs or 2 tsp bid
Pediatric: <2 years: not recommended; 2-6 years: 1/4 tab or 1/2 tsp once daily prn; max 1 tab or 1/2 tsp bid; 6-12 years: 1 tab or 1/2 tsp once daily prn; max 2 tabs or 1 tsp once daily
   Tab: 8.6*mg; *Granules:* 15 mg/tsp (2, 6, 12 oz) (cocoa)
Senokot Syrup (OTC) initially 10-15 ml at HS prn; max 15 ml bid
Pediatric: use Childrens Syrup
   Syr: 8.8 mg/5 ml (2, 8 oz) (chocolate) (alcohol-free)
Senokot Childrens Syrup (OTC)
Pediatric: <2 years: not recommended; 2-6 years: 2.5-3.75 ml once daily prn; max 3.75 ml bid prn; ≥6-12 years: 5-7.5 ml once daily prn; max 7.5 ml bid
   Syr: 8.8 mg/5 ml (2.5 oz) (chocolate) (alcohol-free)
Senokot Xtra (OTC) 1 tab at HS prn; max 2 tabs bid
Pediatric: <2 years: not recommended; 2-6 years: use Childrens Syrup; 6-12 years: 1/2 tab once daily at HS; max 1 tab bid
   Tab: 17*mg

BULK FORMING AGENT+STIMULANT COMBINATIONS

▷ *psyllium+senna* (B)

Perdiem (OTC) 1-2 rounded tsp swallowed with 8 oz cool liquid daily bid
Pediatric: <7 years: not recommended; 7-11 years: 1 rounded tsp swallowed with 8 oz cool liquid once daily-bid; ≥12 years: same as adult
   Canister: 8.8, 14 oz; *Individual pkt:* 6 gm (6/pck)
SennaPrompt (OTC) initially 2-5 caps bid
Pediatric: <12 years: not recommended; ≥12 years: same as adult
   Cap: psyl 500 mg+senna 9 mg

STOOL SOFTENER+STIMULANT COMBINATIONS

▷ *docusate+casanthranol* (C)

Doxidan (OTC) 1-3 caps/day; max 1 week
Pediatric: <2 years: not recommended; ≥2 years: 1 cap/day
   Cap: doc 60 mg+cas 30 mg
Peri-Colace (OTC) 1-2 caps or 15-30 ml q HS; max 2 caps or 30 ml bid or 3 caps q HS
Pediatric: 5-15 ml q HS
   Cap: doc 100 mg+cas 30 mg; *Syr:* doc 60 mg+cas 30 mg per 15 ml (8, 16 oz)
▷ *docusate+senna* concentrate (C)

Senokot S (OTC) 2 tabs q HS; max 4 tabs bid
   Pediatric: <2 years: not recommended; 2-6 years: 1/2 tab daily; max 1 tab bid; >6-12 years: 1 tab daily; max 2 tabs bid
      Tab: doc 50 mg+senna 8.6 mg

ENEMAS AND OTHER AGENTS

▷ *sodium biphosphate+sodium phosphate* enema (C)(OTC)

Fleets Adult 59-118 ml rectally
Pediatric: <2 years: not recommended; ≥2-12 years: 59 ml rectally
   Enema: sod biphos 19 gm+sod phos 7 gm (59, 118 ml w. applicator)
Fleets Pediatric 59 ml
Pediatric: rectally
   Enema: sod biphos 19 gm+sod phos 7 gm (59 ml w. applicator)

▷ *glycerin* suppositories (C)(OTC) 1 adult suppository
Pediatric: <6 years: 1 pediatric suppository; ≥6 years: 1 adult suppository

CORNEAL EDEMA

▷ *sodium chloride* (G)
Pediatric: same as adult 1-2 drops or 1 inch ribbon q 3-4 hours prn; reduce frequency as edema subsides
  Various (OTC)
   Ophth soln: 2, 5% (15, 30 ml); *Ophth oint:* 5% (3.5 gm)

CORNEAL ULCERATION

ANTIBACTERIAL OPHTHALMIC SOLUTION/OINTMENT
see Conjunctivitis/Blepharoconjunctivitis: Bacterial page 96

COSTOCHONDRITIS (CHEST WALL SYNDROME)

Acetaminophen for IV Infusion *see Pain page 352*
NSAIDs *see page 571*
Opioid Analgesics *see Pain page 354*
Topical & Transdermal Analgesics *see Pain page 352*
Parenteral Corticosteroids *see page 577*
Oral Corticosteroids *see page 577*
Topical Analgesic and Anesthetic Agents *see page 569*

CRAMPS: ABDOMINAL, INTESTINAL

ANTISPASMODIC-ANTICHOLINERGIC AGENTS

▷ *dicyclomine* (B)(G) initially 20 mg bid-qid; may increase to 40 mg qid PO; usual IM dose 80 mg/day divided qid; do not use IM route for more than 1-2 days
Pediatric: <12 years: not recommended; ≥12 years: same as adult
  Bentyl *Tab:* 20 mg; *Cap:* 10 mg; *Syr:* 10 mg/5 ml (16 oz); *Vial:* 10 mg/ml (10 ml); *Amp:* 10 mg/ml (2 ml)
▷ *methscopolamine bromide* (B) 1 tab q 6 hours prn
Pediatric: <12 years: not recommended; ≥12 years: same as adult
  Pamine *Tab:* 2.5 mg
  Pamine Forte *Tab:* 5 mg

ANTICHOLINERGICS

▷ *hyoscyamine* (C)(G)
  Anaspaz 1-2 tabs q 4 hours prn; max 12 tabs/day
  Pediatric: <2 years: not recommended; 2-12 years: 0.0625-0.125 mg q 4 hours prn; max 0.75 mg/day; ≥12 years: same as adult
    Tab: 0.125*mg
  Levbid 1-2 tabs q 12 hours prn; max 4 tabs/day
  Pediatric: <12 years: not recommended; ≥12 years: same as adult
    Tab: 0.375*mg ext-rel
  Levsin 1-2 tabs q 4 hours prn; max 12 tabs/day
  Pediatric: <6 years: not recommended; ≥6-12 years: 1 tab q 4 hours prn
    Tab: 0.125*mg
  Levsinex SL 1-2 tabs q 4 hours SL or PO; max 12 tabs/day
  Pediatric: 2-12 years: 1 tab SL or PO q 4 hours; max 6 tabs/day
    Tab: 0.125 mg sublingual
  Levsinex Timecaps 1-2 caps q 12 hours; may adjust to 1 cap q 8 hours
  Pediatric: 2-12 years: 1 cap q 12 hours; max 2 caps/day
    Cap: 0.375 mg time-rel
  NuLev dissolve 1-2 tabs on tongue, with or without water, q 4 hours prn; max 12 tabs/day

Pediatric: <2 years: not recommended; 2-12 years: dissolve 1 tab on tongue, with <u>or</u> without water, q 4 hours prn; max 6 tabs/day; >12 years: same as adult
   ODT: 0.125 mg (mint) (phenylalanine)
▷ *simethicone* (C)(G) 0.3 ml qid pc and HS
   Mylicon Drops (OTC) *Oral drops:* 40 mg/0.6 ml (30 ml)
▷ *phenobarbital+hyoscyamine+atropine+scopolamine* (C)(IV)(G)
   Donnatal 1-2 tabs ac and HS
   Pediatric: <12 years: not recommended; ≥12 years: same as adult
      Tab: pheno 16.2 mg+hyo 0.1037 mg+atro 0.0194 mg+scop 0.0065 mg
   Donnatal Elixir 1-2 tsp ac and HS
   Pediatric: 20 lb: 1 ml q 4 hours <u>or</u> 1.5 ml q 6 hours; 30 lb: 1.5 ml q 4 hours <u>or</u> 2 ml q 6 hours; 50 lb: 1/2 tsp q 4 hours <u>or</u> 3/4 tsp q 6 hours; 75 lb: 3/4 tsp q 4 hours <u>or</u> 1 tsp q 6 hours; 100 lb: 1 tsp q 4 hours <u>or</u> 1 tsp q 6 hours
      Elix: pheno 16.2 mg+hyo 0.1037 mg+atro 0.0194 mg+scop 0.0065 mg per 5 ml (4, 16 oz)
   Donnatal Extentabs 1 tab q 12 hours
   Pediatric: <12 years: not recommended; ≥12 years: same as adult
      Tab: pheno 48.6 mg+hyo 0.3111 mg+atro 0.0582 mg+scop 0.0195 mg ext-rel

ANTICHOLINERGIC+SEDATIVE COMBINATION

▷ *chlordiazepoxide+clidinium* (D)(IV) 1-2 caps ac and HS; max 8 caps/day
   Pediatric: <12 years: not recommended; ≥12 years: same as adult
      Librax *Cap:* chlor 5 mg+clid 2.5 mg

 CROHN'S DISEASE

Parenteral Corticosteroids *see page 577*
Oral Corticosteroids *see page 577*

Comment: Standard treatment regimen for active disease (flare) is: antibiotic, antispasmodic, and bowel rest; progress to clear liquids; then progress to high-fiber diet. Long term management of chronic disease includes salicylates, immune modulators, and tumor necrosis factor (TNF) blockers.

ORAL ANTI-INFECTIVES

▷ *metronidazole* (G) 500 mg tid <u>or</u> 750 mg bid; max 8 weeks
   Pediatric: 35-50 mg/kg/day in 3 divided doses x 10 days
      Flagyl *Tab:* 250*, 500*mg
      Flagyl 375 *Cap:* 375 mg
      Flagyl ER *Tab:* 750 mg ext-rel
   Comment: Alcohol is contraindicated during treatment with oral *metronidazole* and for 72 hours after therapy due to a possible *disulfiram*-like reaction (nausea, vomiting, flushing, headache).

SALICYLATES

▷ *mesalamine* (B)(G)
      Asacol 800 mg tid x 6 weeks; maintenance 1.6 gm/day in divided doses; swallow whole, do not crush <u>or</u> chew
   Pediatric: <12 years: not recommended; ≥12 years: same as adult
      Tab: 400 mg del-rel
   Comment: 2 x **Asacol** 400 mg tabs are <u>not</u> bioequivalent to 1 x **Asacol HD** 800 mg tab.
      Asacol HD 1600 mg tid x 6 weeks; swallow whole, do not crush <u>or</u> chew
   Pediatric: <12 years: not recommended; ≥12 years: same as adult
      Tab: 800 mg del-rel
   Comment: 1 x **Asacol HD** 800 mg tab is <u>not</u> bioequivalent to 2 x **Asacol** 400 mg tabs
      Canasa 1 gm qid for up to 8 weeks
   Pediatric: <12 years: not recommended; ≥12 years: same as adult
      Rectal supp: 1 gm del-rel (30, 42/pck)
      Delzicol *Treatment:* 800 mg tid x 6 weeks; maintenance 1.6 gm/day in 2-4 divided doses daily; swallow whole; do not crush <u>or</u> chew
   Pediatric: <5 years: not established; ≥5 years: same as adult
      Cap: 400 mg del-rel

Comment: 2 x **Delzicol** 400 mg caps are <u>not</u> bioequivalent to 1 x *mesalamine* 800 mg del-rel tab

Lialda 2.4-4.8 gm daily in a single dose for up to 8 weeks; swallow whole, do not crush <u>or</u> chew

Pediatric: <18 years: not recommended; ≥18 years: same as adult

   Tab: 1.2 gm del-rel

Pentasa 1 gm qid for up to 8 weeks; swallow whole, do not crush <u>or</u> chew

Pediatric: <12 years: not recommended; ≥12 years: same as adult

   Cap: 250 mg cont-rel

Rowasa Enema 4 gm rectally by enema q HS; retain for 8 hours x 3-6 weeks

Pediatric: <12 years: not recommended; ≥12 years: same as adult

   Enema: 4 gm/60 ml (7, 14, 28/pck; kit, 7, 14, 28/pck w. wipes)

Rowasa Suppository 1 suppository rectally bid x 3-6 weeks; retain for 1-3 hours <u>or</u> longer

   Rectal supp: 500 mg

Sulfite-Free Rowasa Rectal Suspension 4 gm rectally by enema q HS; retain for 8 hours x 3-6 weeks

   Enema: 4 gm/60 ml (7, 14, 28/pck; kit, 7, 14, 28/pck w. wipes)

▷ *olsalazine* (C)

Dipentum 1 gm/day in 2 divided doses; max 2 gm/day

   Cap: 250 mg

Comment: Indicated in persons who cannot tolerate *sulfasalazine*.

▷ *sulfasalazine* (B)(G)

Azulfidine initially 1-2 gm/day; increase to 3-4 gm/day in divided doses pc until clinical symptoms controlled; maintenance 2 gm/day; max 4 gm/day

   Tab: 500*mg

   Pediatric: <2 years: not recommended; 2-16 years: initially 40-60 mg/kg/day in 3-6 divided doses; max 2 gm/day

Azulfidine EN initially 500 mg in the PM x 7 days; then 500 mg bid x 7 days; then 500 mg in the AM and 1 gm in the PM x 7 days; then 1 gm bid; max 4 gm/day

   Pediatric: <12 years: not recommended; ≥12 years: same as adult

   Tab: 500 mg ent-coat

▷ *budesonide micronized* (C) (G)

Pediatric: <12 years: not recommended; ≥12 years: same as adult

Entocort EC *Treatment* 9 mg once daily in the AM for up to 8 weeks; may repeat an 8-week course; *Maintenance of remission*: 6 mg once daily for up to 3 months

   Cap: 3 mg ent-coat ext-rel granules

Comment: Taper other systemic steroids when transferring to **Entocort EC**. When corticosteroids are used chronically, systemic effects such as hypercorticism and adrenal suppression may occur. Corticosteroids can reduce the response of the hypothalamus-pituitary-adrenal (HPA) axis to stress. In situations where patients are subject to surgery <u>or</u> other stress situations, supplementation with a systemic corticosteroid is recommended. General precautions concerning corticosteroids should be followed.

PURINE ANTIMETABOLITE IMMUNOSUPPRESSANT

▷ *azathioprine* (D)(G)

Imuran *Tab:* 50*mg; *Injectable:* 100 mg

Comment: **Imuran** is usually administered on a daily basis. The initial dose should be approximately 1.0 mg/kg (50 to 100 mg) as a single dose <u>or</u> divided bid. Dose may be increased beginning at 6-8 weeks, and thereafter at 4-week intervals, if there are no serious toxicities and if initial response is unsatisfactory. Dose increments should be 0.5 mg/kg/day, up to max 2.5 mg/kg per day. Therapeutic response usually occurs after 6-8 weeks of treatment. An adequate trial should be a minimum of 12 weeks. Patients not improved after 12 weeks can be considered refractory. **Imuran** may be continued long-term in patients with clinical response, but patients should be monitored carefully, and gradual dosage reduction should be attempted to reduce risk of toxicities. Maintenance therapy should be at the lowest effective dose, and the dose given can be lowered decrementally with changes of 0.5 mg/kg <u>or</u> approximately 25 mg daily every 4 weeks while other therapy is kept constant. The optimum duration of maintenance **Imuran** has not been determined. **Imuran** can be discontinued abruptly, but delayed effects are possible.

TUMOR NECROSIS FACTOR (TNF) BLOCKERS

▷ *adalimumab* (B) 40 mg SC once every other week; may increase to once weekly without MTX; administer in abdomen or thigh; rotate sites
Pediatric: <2 years, <10 kg: not recommended; 10-<15 kg: 10 mg every other week; 15-<30 kg: 20 mg every other week; ≥30 kg: 40 mg every other week; 2-17 years, supervise first dose
   Humira *Prefilled syringe:* 20 mg/0.4 ml; 40 mg/0.8 ml single-dose (2/pck; 2, 6/starter pck) (preservative-free)
   Comment: May use with *methotrexate* (MTX), DMARDS, corticosteroids, salicylates, NSAIDs, or analgesics.

▷ *adalimumab-adaz* (B) *First dose (Day 1):* 160 mg SC (4 x 40 mg injections in one day or 2 x 40 mg injections per day for two consecutive days); *Second dose two weeks later (Day 15):* 80 mg SC; *Two weeks later (Day 29):* begin a maintenance dose of 40 mg SC every other week
Pediatric: <18 years: not recommended; ≥18 years: same as adult
   Hyrimoz *Prefilled syringe:* 40 mg/0.8 ml single-dose (preservative-free)
   Comment: Hyrimoz is biosimilar to Humira (*adalimumab*).

▷ *adalimumab-adbm* (B) *First dose (Day 1):* 160 mg SC (4 x 40 mg injections in one day or 2 x 40 mg injections per day for two consecutive days); *Second dose two weeks later (Day 15):* 80 mg SC; *Two weeks later (Day 29):* begin a maintenance dose of 40 mg SC every other week
Pediatric: <18 years: not recommended; ≥18 years: same as adult
   Cyltezo *Prefilled syringe:* 40 mg/0.8 ml single-dose (preservative-free)
   Comment: Cyltezo is biosimilar to Humira (*adalimumab*).

▷ *certolizumab* (B) 400 mg SC (2 x 200 mg inj at two different sites on day 1); then, 400 mg SC at weeks 2 and 4; maintenance 400 mg SC every 4 weeks; administer in abdomen or thigh; rotate sites
Pediatric: <12 years: not recommended; ≥12 years: same as adult
   Cimzia *Vial:* 200 mg (2/pck); *Prefilled syringe:* 200 mg/ml single-dose (2/pck; 2, 6/ starter pck) (preservative-free)

▷ *infliximab* (*tumor necrosis factor-alpha blocker*) must be refrigerated at 2°C to 8°C (36°F to 46°F); administer dose intravenously over a period of not less than 2 hours; do not use beyond the expiration date as this product contains no preservative; 5 mg/kg at 0, 2 and 6 weeks, then every 8 weeks.
Pediatric: <6 years: not studied; ≥6-17 years: mg/kg at 0, 2 and 6 weeks, then every 8 weeks; ≥18 years: same as adult
   Remicade *Vial:* 100 mg for reconstitution to 10 ml administration volume, single-dose (preservative-free)
   Comment: Remicade is indicated to reduce signs and symptoms, and induce and maintain clinical remission, in adults and children ≥6 years-of-age with moderately to severely active disease who have had an inadequate response to conventional therapy and reduce the number of draining enterocutaneous and rectovaginal fistulas, and maintain fistula closure, in adults with fistulizing disease. Common adverse effects associated with Remicade included abdominal pain, headache, pharyngitis, sinusitis, and upper respiratory infections. In addition, Remicade might increase the risk for serious infections, including tuberculosis, bacterial sepsis, and invasive fungal infections. Available data from published literature on the use of *infliximab* products during pregnancy have not reported a clear association with *infliximab* products and adverse pregnancy outcomes. *infliximab* products cross the placenta and infants exposed *in utero* should not be administered live vaccines for at least 6 months after birth. Otherwise, the infant may be at increased risk of infection, including disseminated infection which can become fatal. Available information is insufficient to inform the amount of *infliximab* products present in human milk or effects on the breast-fed infant. To report suspected adverse reactions, contact Merck Sharp & Dohme Corp., a subsidiary of Merck & Co. at 1-877-888-4231 or FDA at 1-800-FDA1088 or www.fda.gov/medwatch.

▷ *infliximab-abda* (*tumor necrosis factor-alpha blocker*) (B)
   Renflexis: see *infliximab* (Remicade) above for full prescribing information
   Comment: Renflexis is a biosimilar to Remicade for the treatment of immune disorders including Crohn's disease, ulcerative colitis, rheumatoid arthritis, ankylosing spondylitis, psoriatic arthritis and plaque psoriasis. Renflexis was approved under the FDA category for biosimilars and demonstrated no clinically meaningful differences for use, dosing regimens, strengths, dosage forms, and routes of administration from the FDA-approved biological product Remicade.

▷ **infliximab-qbtx** *(tumor necrosis factor-alpha blocker)* **(B)**
    Ifixi: see **infliximab** (**Remicade**) above for full prescribing information
    Comment: Ifixi is a biosimilar to **Remicade** for the treatment of immune disorders
    including Crohn's disease, ulcerative colitis, rheumatoid arthritis, ankylosing
    spondylitis, psoriatic arthritis and plaque psoriasis. **Ifixi** was approved under the FDA
    category for biosimilars and demonstrated no clinically meaningful differences for use,
    dosing regimens, strengths, dosage forms, and routes of administration from the FDA-
    approved biological product **Remicade.**

▷ **infliximab-qbtx** *(tumor necrosis factor-alpha blocker)* **(B)**
    Ifixi: see **infliximab** (**Remicade**) above for full prescribing information
    Comment: Ifixi is a biosimilar to **Remicade** for the treatment of immune disorders
    including Crohn's disease, ulcerative colitis, rheumatoid arthritis, ankylosing
    spondylitis, psoriatic arthritis and plaque psoriasis. **Ifixi** was approved under the FDA
    category for biosimilars and demonstrated no clinically meaningful differences for use,
    dosing regimens, strengths, dosage forms, and routes of administration from the FDA-
    approved biological product **Remicade.**

INTEGRIN RECEPTOR ANTAGONIST (IMMUNOMODULATOR)

▷ **natalizumab** **(C)** administer by IV infusion over 1 hour; monitor during and for 1 hour
    post-infusion; 300 mg every 4 weeks; discontinue after 12 weeks if no therapeutic response,
    or if unable to taper off chronic concomitant steroids within 6 months; may continue
    aminosalicylates
    Pediatric: <18 years: not established; ≥18 years: same as adult
    Tysabri *Vial:* 300 mg single-dose, soln after dilution for IV infusion (preservative-free)

▷ **vedolizumab** **(B)** administer by IV infusion over 30 minutes; 300 mg at weeks 0, 2, 6; then
    once every 8 weeks
    Pediatric: <18 years: not established; ≥18 years: same as adult
    Entyvio *Vial:* 300 mg (20 ml) single-dose, pwdr for IV infusion after reconstitution
    (preservative-free)
    Comment: To report suspected adverse reactions, contact Takeda Pharmaceuticals at
    1-877-TAKEDA-7 (1-877-825-3327) or FDA at 1800-FDA-1088 or www.fda.gov/medwatch.

CRYPTOSPORIDIOSIS (*CRYPTOSPORIDIUM PARVUM*)

▷ **nitazoxanide** **(B)** 500 mg by mouth q 12 hours x 3 days
    Pediatric: 12-47 months: 5 ml q 12 hours x 3 days; 4-11 years: 10 ml q 12 hours x 3 days;
    ≥12 years: same as adult
    Alinia *Oral susp:* 100 mg/5 ml (60 ml)
    Comment: **Alinia** is an antiprotozoal for the treatment of diarrhea due to *G. lamblia* or
    C. parvum.

CYCLOSPORIASIS (*CYCLOSPORA CAVETANENSIS*)

Comment: The CDC, state and local health departments, and the US Food and Drug
Administration have issued a Health Alert Network advisory after an increase in reported
cases of cyclosporiasis, an intestinal illness caused by the parasite *Cyclospora cayetanensis*.
Clinicians should consider a diagnosis of cyclosporiasis in patients who experience
prolonged or remitting-relapsing diarrhea. Since May 1, 2017, 206 cases have been
identified, more than twice the 88 cases reported from May 1 to August 3, 2016. Most
laboratories in the United States do not routinely test for *Cyclospora*, even when a stool
sample has been tested for parasites, so providers must specifically order the test. Several
stool specimens may be required because *Cyclospora* oocysts may be shed intermittently
and at low levels, even in persons with profuse diarrhea. Symptoms include watery diarrhea,
which can be profuse, anorexia, fatigue, weight loss, nausea, flatulence, stomach cramps,
myalgia, vomiting, and low-grade fever. Symptoms begin from 2 days to more than 2
weeks (average 7 days) after ingestion of the parasite. *Cyclospora* is food- and water-borne;
it is not transmitted directly from person to person. The recommended treatment is
trimethoprim-sulfamethoxazole (TMP/SMX). There are no effective alternatives for people
who are allergic to or who cannot tolerate TMP/SMX; observation and symptomatic care is
recommended for those patients. If untreated, illness may last for a few days to a month or
longer.

▷ **trimethoprim+sulfamethoxazole (TMP-SMX)(C)(G)** bid x 10 days
Pediatric: <2 months: not recommended; ≥2 months: 40 mg/kg/day of *sulfamethoxazole* in 2 divided doses x 10 days; *see page 630 for dose by weight*
   Bactrim, Septra 2 tabs bid x 10 days
      Tab: trim 80 mg+sulfa 400 mg*
   Bactrim DS, Septra DS 1 tab bid x 10 days
      Tab: trim 160 mg+sulfa 800 mg*
   Bactrim Pediatric Suspension, Septra Pediatric Suspension
      Oral susp: trim 40 mg+sulfa 200 mg per 5 ml (100 ml) (cherry) (alcohol 0.3%)
Comment: Sulfonamides are contraindicated in the first trimester of pregnancy, the final month of pregnancy, and infants <8 weeks-of-age. *CrCl 15-30 mL/min:* reduce dose by 1/2; *CrCl <15 mL/min:* not recommended. Contra-indicated with G6PD deficiency. A high fluid intake is indicated during sulfonamide therapy to avoid crystallization in the kidneys.

CYSTIC FIBROSIS (CF)

▷ **acetylcysteine (B)(G)** administer via face mask, mouth piece, tracheostomy T-piece, mist tent, or croupette; routine tracheostomy care, 1 to 2 ml of a 10% to 20% solution may be administered by direct instillation into the tracheostomy every 1 to 4 hours
Pediatric: same as adult
   Mucomyst *Vial:* 10, 20% (4, 10, 30 ml) soln for inhalation
      Comment: **Mucomyst** is a mucolytic. For inhalation, the 10% concentration may be used undiluted; the 20% concentration should be diluted with sterile water or normal saline (either for injection or inhalation).

CYSTIC FIBROSIS TRANSMEMBRANE CONDUCTANCE REGULATOR (CFTR) POTENTIATOR

▷ **ivacaftor (B)** 150 mg every 12 hours; administer with fat-containing food (e.g., eggs, butter, peanut butter, cheese pizza); avoid food and juices containing grapefruit or Seville oranges.
Pediatric: <12 months: not established; 12-<24 months (if ≥1 mutation in the CFTR gene that is responsive to **Kalydeco** based on clinical and/or *in-vitro* assay data) and 2-6 years, <14 kg: one 50 mg packet mixed with 1 tsp (5 ml) soft food or liquid every 12 hours with fat-containing food; 2-6 years, ≥14 kg: one 75 mg packet mixed with 1 tsp (5 ml) soft food or liquid every 12 hours with fat-containing food; >6 years: same as adult
   Kalydeco *Tab:* 150 mg film-coat; *Oral granules:* 50, 75 mg unit dose pkts (56 pkt/carton)
Comment: ivacaftor is indicated for the treatment of CF in patients who have a *G551D* co-mutation in the *CFTR* gene. If the patient's genotype is unknown, an FDA-cleared CF mutation test should be used to detect the presence of the *G551D* mutation. **Kalydeco** is not effective in patients with CF who are homozygous for the *F508del* mutation in the *CFTR* gene. Transaminases (ALT and AST) should be assessed prior to initiating **Kalydeco**, every 3 months during the first year of treatment, and annually thereafter. Patients who develop increased transaminase levels should be closely monitored until the abnormalities resolve. Dosing should be interrupted in patients with ALT or AST greater than 5 times the upper limit of normal (ULN). Following resolution of transaminase elevations, consider the benefits and risks of resuming **Kalydeco**. Concomitant use with strong CYP3A inducers (e.g., *rifampin*, St. John's wort) substantially decreases exposure of *Kalydeco* (which may diminish effectiveness); therefore, co-administration is not recommended. Reduce dose to 150 mg twice weekly when co-administered with strong CYP3A inhibitors (e.g., *ketoconazole*). Reduce dose to 150 mg once daily when co-administered with moderate CYP3A inhibitors. Caution is recommended in patients with severe renal impairment (CrCl ≤30 mL/min) or ESRD. No dose adjustment is necessary for patients with mild hepatic impairment (Child-Pugh Class A). A reduced dose of 150 mg once daily is recommended in patients with moderate hepatic impairment (Child-Pugh Class B). No studies have been conducted in patients with severe hepatic impairment (Child-Pugh Class C). The most commonly reported adverse reactions are headache, sore throat, nasopharyngitis, URI, nasal congestion, abdominal pain, nausea, diarrhea, dizziness, and rash. Excretion of **Kalydeco** into human milk is probable. To report suspected adverse reactions, contact Vertex Pharmaceuticals Incorporated at 1-877-752-5933 or FDA at 1-800-FDA-1088 or www.fda.gov/medwatch.

(CFTR) POTENTIATOR COMBINATIONS

▷ *lumacaftor+ivacaftor* (B) <6years: not recommended; 6-11 years: 2 x 100/125 tabs q 12 hours; ≥12 years: 2 x 200/125 tabs q 12 hours

Orkambi *Tab:* luma 100 mg+iva 125 mg; luma 200 mg+iva 125 mg film-coat
Comment: **Orkambi** is indicated for the treatment of CF in patients age ≥6 years-of-age who are homozygous for the F508del mutation in the CFTR gene. The efficacy and safety of **Orkambi** have not been established in patients with CF other than those homozygous for the F508del mutation. If the patient's genotype is unknown, an FDA-cleared CF mutation test should be used to detect the presence of the F508del mutation on both alleles of the CFTR gene. Reduce the dose of **Orkambi** in patients with moderate-to severe-hepatic impairment. In patients with advanced liver disease, with caution and only if the benefits are expected to outweigh the risks. When initiating **Orkambi** in patients taking strong CYP3A inhibitors, reduce the dose of **Orkambi** for the first week of treatment. There are limited and incomplete human data from clinical trials and postmarketing reports on use of **Orkambi** or its individual components in pregnancy to inform a drug-associated risk. There is no information regarding the presence of *lumacaftor* or *ivacaftor* in human milk or effects on the breastfed infant. To report suspected adverse reactions, contact Vertex Pharmaceuticals at 1-877-634-8789 or FDA at 1-800-FDA-1088 or visit www.fda.gov/medwatch.

▷ *tezacaftor+ivacaftor plus ivacaftor* (B) <12 years: not established; ≥12 years: 1 x 100/150 fixed dose tab in the morning and 1 x 150 mg *ivacaflor* tab in the evening, approximately 12 hours later. Take with fat-containing food. Avoid grapefruit and Seville oranges.

Symdeko *Tab:* teza 100 mg+iva 150 mg, fixed-dose combination *plus Tab:* iva 150 mg (4-week supply/carton)
Comment: **Symdeko** is indicated for the treatment of the underlying cause of CF in patients ≥12 years-of-age who have two copies of the F508del mutation in the CFTR gene or who have ≥1 mutation that is responsive to *tevacaftor+ivacaftor*. If the patient's genotype is unknown, an FDA-cleared CF mutation test should be used to detect the presence of a CFTR mutation followed by verification with bi-directional sequencing when recommended by the mutation test instructions for use. Reduce dose with moderate to severe hepatic impairment. Reduce dose when co-administered with drugs that are moderate or strong CYP3A inhibitors. There are limited and incomplete human data from clinical trials and post-marketing reports on the use of **Symdeko** in pregnancy to inform a drug-associated risk. There is no information regarding the presence of *tezacaftor* or *ivacaftor* in human milk or effects on the breastfed infant. To report suspected adverse reactions, contact Vertex Pharmaceuticals at 1-877-634-8789 or FDA at 1-800-FDA-1088 or visit www.fda.gov/medwatch.

URSODEOXYCHOLIC ACID (UDCA)

Comment: *ursodeoxycholic acid (UDCA)* is indicated for liver disease associated with cystic fibrosis in children 6-18 years-of-age.

▷ *ursodeoxycholic acid (UDCA)* (G) in the first 3 months of treatment, the total daily dose should be divided tid (morning, midday, evening); as liver function values improve, the total daily dose may be taken once a day at bedtime; (see mfr pkg insert for dose table based on kilograms weight); monitor hepatic function every 4 weeks for the first 3 months; then, monitor hepatic function once every 3 months
Pediatric: 6-18 years: same as adult

Ursofalk *Tab:* 500 mg film-coat; *Cap:* 250 mg, *Oral susp:* 250 mg/5 ml
Comment: **ursodeoxycholic (UDCA)** is indicated for the dissolution of cholesterol gall stones that are radioluscent (not visible on plain x-ray), <15 mm, and the gall bladder must still be functioning despite the gall stones.

ANTI-INFECTIVE

▷ *ciprofloxacin* (C)(G) <18 years: 20-40 mg/kg/day divided q 12 hours; ≥18 years: 500 mg bid x 7-10 days; max 1.5 gm/day

Cipro *Tab:* 250, 500, 750 mg; *Oral susp:* 250, 500 mg/5 ml (100 ml) (strawberry)
Cipro XR *Tab:* 500, 1000 mg ext-rel
ProQuin XR *Tab:* 500 mg ext-rel

DEEP VEIN THROMBOSIS (DVT) PROPHYLAXIS

Anticoagulation Therapy *see page* 596

 DEHYDRATION

ORAL REHYDRATION AND ELECTROLYTE REPLACEMENT THERAPY
▷ *oral electrolyte replacement* (OTC)(G)
    KaoLectrolyte 1 pkt dissolved in 8 oz water q 3-4 hours
    Pediatric: not indicated <2 years
        Pkt: sodium 12 mEq+potassium 5 mEq+chloride 10 mEq+citrate 7 mEq+dextrose 5 gm+calories 22 per 6.2 gm
    Pedialyte
    Pediatric: <2 years: as desired and as tolerated; ≥2 years: 1-2 liters/day
        Oral soln: dextrose 20 gm+fructose 5 gm+sodium 25 mEq+potassium 20 mEq+chloride 35 mEq+citrate 30 mEq+calories 100 per liter (8 oz, 1 L)
    Pedialyte Freezer Pops
    Pediatric: as desired and as tolerated
        Pops: dextrose 1.6 gm+sodium 2.8 mEq+potassium 1.25 mEq+chloride 2.2 mEq+citrate 1.88 mEq+calories 6.25 per 62.5 ml (2.1 fl oz) pop

 DELIRIUM: END-OF-LIFE

Comment: "Ultimately ... it is essential for clinicians to focus on the humanness of medicine; to keep dying patients comfortable and as awake as they and their families would like them to be so they can make the last few hours or days of life meaningful; and to make reasonable efforts not to cloud their sensorium unless essential to alleviate patient pain or other severe symptoms" (Pandharipande & Ely, 2017). In a preliminary randomized control study, Hui et al (2017) demonstrated that adding the benzodiazepine *lorazepam* to background *haloperidol* therapy significantly reduced agitated delirium at 8 hours compared with *haloperidol* alone in patients admitted to an acute palliative care unit with advanced cancer and a very short life-expectancy. Moreover, most of the effect the combination had on delirium was achieved in the first 30 minutes following administration (Hui, et al., 2017).

REFERENCES
Hui, D., Frisbee-Hume, S., Wilson, A., Dibaj, S. S., Nguyen, T., De La Cruz, M., ... Bruera, E. (2017). Effect of lorazepam with haloperidol vs haloperidol alone on agitated delirium in patients with advanced cancer receiving palliative care. *Journal of the American Medical Association, 318*(11), 1047–1056. doi:10.1001/jama.2017.11468
Pandharipande, P. P., & Ely, E. W. (2017). Humanizing the treatment of hyperactive delirium in the last days of life. *Journal of the American Medical Association, 318*(11), 1014–1015. doi:10.1001/jama.2017.11466

BENZODIAZEPINE: INTERMEDIATE-ACTING
▷ *lorazepam* (D)(IV)(G) 1-10 mg/day in 2-3 divided doses
    Pediatric: <12 years: not recommended; ≥12 years: same as adult
        Ativan *Tab:* 0.5, 1*, 2*mg
        Lorazepam Intensol *Oral conc:* 2 mg/ml (30 ml w. graduated dropper)

ANTIPSYCHOSIS AGENTS
▷ *haloperidol* (C)(G)
    Oral route of administration: Moderate Symptomology: 0.5 to 2 mg orally 2 to 3 times a day; Severe symptomology: 3 to 5 mg orally 2 to 3 times a day; initial doses of up to 100 mg/day have been necessary in some severely resistant cases;
    Maintenance: after achieving a satisfactory response, the dose should be adjusted as practical to achieve optimum control
    Parenteral route of administration: Prompt control of acute agitation: 2 to 5 mg IM every 4 to 8 hours; *Maintenance:* frequency of IM administration should be determined by patient response and may be given as often as every hour; max: 20 mg/day
        Haldol *Tab:* 0.5*, 1*, 2*, 5*, 10*, 20*mg
        Haldol Lactate *Vial:* 5 mg for IM injection, single-dose

➤ *mesoridazine* (C) initially 25 mg tid; max 300 mg/day
　　Serentil *Tab:* 10, 25, 50, 100 mg; *Conc:* 25 mg/ml (118 ml)
➤ *olanzapine* (C) initially 2.5-10 mg daily; increase to 10 mg/day within a few days; then by 5 mg/day at weekly intervals; max 20 mg/day
　　Zyprexa *Tab:* 2.5, 5, 7.5, 10 mg
　　Zyprexa Zydis *ODT:* 5, 10, 15, 20 mg (phenylalanine)
➤ *quetiapine fumarate* (C)(G)
　　SeroQUEL initially 25 mg bid, titrate q 2nd <u>or</u> 3rd day in increments of 25-50 mg bid-tid; usual maintenance 400-600 mg/day in 2-3 divided doses
　　　Tab: 25, 50, 100, 200, 300, 400 mg
　　SeroQUEL XR administer once daily in the PM; *Day 1:* 50 mg; *Day 2:* 100 mg; *Day 3:* 200 mg; *Day 4:* 300 mg; usual range 400-600 mg/day
　　　Tab: 50, 150, 200, 300, 400 mg ext-rel
➤ *risperidone* (C) 0.5 mg bid x 1 day; adjust in increments of 0.5 mg bid; usual range 0.5-5 mg/day
　　Risperdal *Tab:* 1, 2, 3, 4 mg; *Oral soln:* 1 mg/ml (100 ml)
　　Risperdal M-Tab *Tab:* 0.5, 1, 2 mg
➤ *thioridazine* (C)(G) 10-25 mg bid
　　Mellaril *Tab:* 10, 15, 25, 50, 100, 150, 200 mg; *Oral susp:* 25 mg/5 ml, 100 mg/5 ml; *Oral conc:* 30 mg/ml, 100 mg/ml (4 oz)

 DEMENTIA

Alzheimer's Disease *see page* 11
Antidepressants *see Depression page* 117
Hypnotics/Sedatives *see Insomnia page* 273

ANTIPSYCHOTICS

Comment: Underlying cause should be explored, accurately diagnosed, and addressed. All antipsychotic agents are associated with increased risk of mortality in elderly patients with dementia-related psychosis (Black Box Warning.) APA recommends that non-emergency antipsychotic medication should only be used for the treatment of agitation <u>or</u> psychosis in patients with dementia when symptoms are severe, are dangerous <u>and/or</u> cause significant distress to the patient. APA recommends that before non-emergency treatment with an antipsychotic is initiated in patients with dementia, the potential risks and benefits are discussed with the patient and the patient's surrogate decision maker with input from family <u>or</u> others involved with the patient. *haloperidol injection* is <u>not</u> approved for the treatment of patients with dementia-related psychosis.
➤ *haloperidol* (C)(G) 0.5-1 mg q HS
　　Haldol *Tab:* 0.5, 1, 2, 5, 10, 20 mg
➤ *mesoridazine* (C) initially 25 mg tid; max 300 mg/day
　　Serentil *Tab:* 10, 25, 50, 100 mg; *Conc:* 25 mg/ml (118 ml)
➤ *olanzapine* (C) initially 2.5-10 mg daily; increase to 10 mg/day within a few days; then by 5 mg/day at weekly intervals; max 20 mg/day
　　Zyprexa *Tab:* 2.5, 5, 7.5, 10 mg
　　Zyprexa Zydis *ODT:* 5, 10, 15, 20 mg (phenylalanine)
➤ *quetiapine fumarate* (C)(G)
　　SeroQUEL initially 25 mg bid, titrate q 2nd <u>or</u> 3rd day in increments of 25-50 mg bid-tid; usual maintenance 400-600 mg/day in 2-3 divided doses
　　　Tab: 25, 50, 100, 200, 300, 400 mg
　　SeroQUEL XR administer once daily in the PM; *Day 1:* 50 mg; *Day 2:* 100 mg; *Day 3:* 200 mg; *Day 4:* 300 mg; usual range 400-600 mg/day
　　　Tab: 50, 150, 200, 300, 400 mg ext-rel
➤ *risperidone* (C) 0.5 mg bid x 1 day; adjust in increments of 0.5 mg bid; usual range 0.5-5 mg/day
　　Risperdal *Tab:* 1, 2, 3, 4 mg; *Oral soln:* 1 mg/ml (100 ml)
　　Risperdal M-Tab *Tab:* 0.5, 1, 2 mg
➤ *thioridazine* (C)(G) 10-25 mg bid
　　Mellaril *Tab:* 10, 15, 25, 50, 100, 150, 200 mg; *Oral susp:* 25 mg/5 ml, 100 mg/5 ml; *Oral conc:* 30 mg/ml, 100 mg/ml (4 oz)

DENGUE FEVER (*DENGUE VIRUS*)

Dengue is the most common arthropod-borne viral (arboviral) illness in humans. The CDC reports that cases of dengue in returning US travelers have increased steadily during the past 20 years, and dengue has become the leading cause of acute febrile illness in US travelers returning from the Caribbean, South America, and Asia. Dengue is transmitted by mosquitoes of the genus *Aedes*, which are widely distributed in subtropical and tropical areas of the world. A small percentage of persons who have previously been infected by one dengue serotype develop bleeding and endothelial leak upon infection with another dengue serotype. This syndrome is termed "dengue hemorrhagic fever." Dengue fever is typically a self-limited disease, with a mortality rate of less than 1%. When treated, dengue hemorrhagic fever has a mortality rate of 2%-5%, but when left untreated, the mortality rate is as high as 50%. Dengue fever is usually a self-limited illness. Supportive care with analgesics, fluid replacement, and bed rest is usually sufficient. Acetaminophen may be used to treat fever and relieve other symptoms. *aspirin*, nonsteroidal anti-inflammatory drugs (NSAIDs), and corticosteroids should be avoided. Management of severe dengue requires careful attention to fluid management and proactive treatment of hemorrhage. Single dose methylprednisolone showed no mortality benefit in the treatment of dengue shock syndrome in a prospective, randomized, double-blind, placebo-controlled trial. **There is no specific antiviral treatment currently available for dengue fever. No vaccine is currently approved or in drug trials for the prevention of dengue infection.** Because lack of immunity to a single dengue strain is the major risk factor for dengue hemorrhagic fever and dengue shock syndrome, a vaccine must provide high levels of immunity to all 4 dengue strains to be clinically useful.

A live attenuated tetravalent vaccine against dengue was effective against all four serotypes of the virus and well-tolerated among children, according to researchers. Interim results from a phase II study showed that children at four study sites in dengue-endemic areas of Asia and Latin America who received the vaccine all had significantly higher levels of antibody titers 18 months later. The vaccine (TAK-003 or TDV) is comprised of a molecularly cloned attenuated strain of dengue serotype 2 (DENV-2), and engineered strains of dengue serotypes 1, 3 and 4 (DENV-1, DENV-3 and DENV-4). Prior phase I and phase II data found the vaccine was well-tolerated and immunogenic against all four dengue serotypes. The trial will take 48 months to complete. The trial is ongoing at three sites in the Dominican Republic (n = 535), Panama (n = 935), and the Philippines (n = 330). Participants are "healthy" children, ages 2 to 17 years, randomized into three groups plus a placebo group. A phase III efficacy trial for the vaccine, entitled Tetravalent Immunization against Dengue Efficacy Study (TIDES) is currently being conducted in eight dengue-endemic countries, with data available in late 2018.

REFERENCES

Sáez-Llorens, X., Tricou, V., Yu, D., Rivera, L., Jimeno, J., Villarreal, A. C., . . . Wallace, D. (2018). Immunogenicity and safety of one versus two doses of tetravalent dengue vaccine in healthy children aged 2–17 years in Asia and Latin America: 18-month interim data from a phase 2, randomised, placebo-controlled study. *The Lancet: Infectious Diseases, 18*(2), 162–170. doi:10.1016/s1473-3099(17)30632-1

Tricou, V., Sáez-Llorens, X., Yu, D., Rivera, L., Borkowski, A., & Wallace, D. (2017, November 6). *Progress in development of Takeda's tetravalent dengue vaccine candidate.* Paper presented at the 66th annual meeting of the American Society of Tropical Medicine & Hygiene, Baltimore, MD. Retrieved from http://www.abstractsonline.com/pp8/#!/4395/presentation/1438

Yoon, I.-K., & Thomas, S. J. (2018). Encouraging results but questions remain for dengue vaccine. *The Lancet: Infectious Diseases, 18*(2), 125–126. doi:10.1016/s1473-3099(17)30634-5

 DENTAL ABSCESS

ANTI-INFECTIVES

➤ *amoxicillin+clavulanate* (B)(G)
    Augmentin 500 mg tid or 875 mg bid x 7-10 days
        Pediatric: 40-45 mg/kg/day divided tid x 10 days or 90 mg/kg/day divided bid x 10 days
        see pages 618 *for dose by weight*
            Tab: 250, 500, 875 mg; *Chew tab:* 125, 250 mg (lemon-lime); 200, 400 mg (cherry-banana) (phenylalanine); *Oral susp:* 125 mg/5 ml (banana), 250 mg/5 ml (75, 100, 150 ml) (orange); 200, 400 mg/5 ml (50, 75, 100 ml) (orange) (phenylalanine)
    Augmentin ES-600 not recommended for adults

Pediatric: <3 months: not recommended; ≥3 months, <40 kg: 90 mg/kg/day in 2 divided doses x 7-10 days; ≥40 kg: not recommended
> *Oral susp:* 42.9 mg/5 ml (50, 75, 100, 125, 150, 200 ml) (strawberry cream) (phenylalanine)

Augmentin XR 2 tabs q 12 hours x 7-10 days
Pediatric: <16 years: use other forms; ≥16 years: same as adult
> *Tab:* 1000*mg ext-rel

➤ *clindamycin* (B) (administer with fluoroquinolone in adults and TMP-SMX in children) 300 mg qid x 10 days
Pediatric: 8-16 mg/kg/day in 3-4 divided doses x 10 days
Cleocin (G) *Cap:* 75 (tartrazine), 150 (tartrazine), 300 mg
Cleocin Pediatric Granules (G) *Oral susp:* 75 mg/5 ml (100 ml) (cherry)

➤ *erythromycin base* (B)(G) 500 mg q 6 hours x 10 days
Pediatric: 30-40 mg/kg/day in 4 divided doses x 10 days
Ery-Tab *Tab:* 250, 333, 500 mg ent-coat
PCE *Tab:* 333, 500 mg

Comment: *erythromycin* may increase INR with concomitant *warfarin*, as well as increase serum level of *digoxin*, benzodiazepines, and statins.

➤ *erythromycin ethylsuccinate* (B)(G) 400 mg qid x 7 days
Pediatric: 30-50 mg/kg/day in 4 divided doses x 7 days; may double dose with severe infection; max 100 mg/kg/day; *see page 626 for dose by weight*
EryPed *Oral susp:* 200 mg/5 ml (100, 200 ml) (fruit); 400 mg/5 ml (60, 100, 200 ml) (banana); *Oral drops:* 200, 400 mg/5 ml (50 ml) (fruit); *Chew tab:* 200 mg wafer (fruit)
E.E.S. *Oral susp:* 200, 400 mg/5 ml (100 ml) (fruit)
E.E.S. Granules *Oral susp:* 200 mg/5 ml (100 ml) (cherry)
E.E.S. 400 Tablets *Tab:* 400 mg

Comment: *erythromycin* may increase INR with concomitant *warfarin*, as well as increase serum level of *digoxin*, benzodiazepines, and statins.

➤ *penicillin v potassium* (B) 250-500 mg q 6 hours x 5-7 days
Pediatric: <12 years: 25-50 mg/kg/day divided q 6 hours x 5-7 days; *see page 629 for dose by weight*; ≥12 years: same as adult
Pen-Vee K *Tab:* 250, 500 mg; *Oral soln:* 125 mg/5 ml (100, 200 ml); 250 mg/5 ml (100, 150, 200 ml)

 DENTURE IRRITATION

DEBRIDING AGENT/CLEANSER

➤ *carbamide peroxide 10%* (OTC) apply 10 drops to affected area; swish x 2-3 minutes, then spit; do not rinse; repeat treatment qid
Pediatric: with adult supervision only
Gly-Oxide *Liq:* 10% (15, 60 ml, squeeze bottle w. applicator)

DEPRESSION/MAJOR DEPRESSIVE DISORDER (MDD)

Comment: Antidepressant monotherapy should be avoided until any presence of (hypo) mania or positive family history for bipolar spectrum disorder has been ruled out as antidepressant monotherapy can induce mania in the bipolar patient. Abrupt withdrawal or interruption of treatment with an antidepressant medication is sometimes associated with an antidepressant discontinuation syndrome which may be mediated by gradually tapering the drug over a period of two weeks or longer, depending on the dose strength and length of treatment. Common symptoms of antidepressant withdrawal include flu-like symptoms, insomnia, nausea, imbalance, sensory disturbances, and hyperarousal. These medications include SSRIs, TCAs, MAOIs, and atypical agents such as *venlafaxine* **(Effexor)**, *mirtazapine* **(Remeron)**, *trazodone* **(Desyrel)**, and *duloxetine* **(Cymbalta)**. Common symptoms of the serotonin discontinuation syndrome include flu-like symptoms (nausea, vomiting, diarrhea, headaches, sweating), sleep disturbances (insomnia, nightmares, constant sleepiness), mood disturbances (dysphoria, anxiety, agitation), cognitive disturbances (mental confusion, hyperarousal), sensory and movement disturbances (imbalance, tremors, vertigo, dizziness, electric-shock-like sensations in the brain, often described by sufferers as "brain zaps."

SELECTIVE SEROTONIN REUPTAKE INHIBITORS (SSRIs)

Comment: Co-administration of SSRIs with TCAs requires extreme caution. Concomitant use of MAOIs and SSRIs is absolutely contraindicated. Avoid St. John's wort and other serotonergic agents. A potentially fatal adverse event is *serotonin syndrome*, caused by serotonin excess. Milder symptoms require HCP intervention to avert severe symptoms which can be rapidly fatal without urgent/emergent medical care. Symptoms include restlessness, agitation, confusion, tachycardia, hypertension, dilated pupils, muscle twitching, muscle rigidity, loss of muscle coordination, diaphoresis, diarrhea, headache, shivering, piloerection, hyperpyrexia, cardiac arrhythmias, seizures, loss of consciousness, coma, death. Common symptoms of the *serotonin discontinuation syndrome* include flu-like symptoms (nausea, vomiting, diarrhea, headaches, sweating), sleep disturbances (insomnia, nightmares, constant sleepiness), mood disturbances (dysphoria, anxiety, agitation), cognitive disturbances (mental confusion, hyperarousal, hallucinations), sensory and movement disturbances (imbalance, tremors, vertigo, dizziness, electric-shock-like sensations in the brain, often described by sufferers as "brain zaps."

➤ *citalopram* (C)(G) initially 20 mg daily; may increase after one week to 40 mg; max 40 mg
  Pediatric: <12 years: not recommended; ≥12 years: same as adult
    Celexa *Tab:* 10, 20, 40 mg; *Oral soln:* 10 mg/5 ml (120 ml) (peppermint) (sugar-free, alcohol-free, parabens)

➤ *escitalopram* (C)(G) initially 10 mg daily; may increase to 20 mg daily after 1 week; elderly or hepatic impairment, 10 mg once daily
  Pediatric: <12 years: not recommended; 12-17 years: initially 10 mg daily; may increase to 20 mg daily after 3 weeks
    Lexapro *Tab:* 5, 10*, 20*mg
    Lexapro Oral Solution *Oral soln:* 1 mg/ml (240 ml) (peppermint) (parabens)

➤ *fluoxetine* (C)(G)
    Prozac initially 20 mg daily; may increase after 1 week; doses >20 mg/day should be divided into AM and noon doses; max 80 mg/day
    Pediatric: <8 years: not recommended; 8-17 years: initially 10 mg/day; may increase after 1 week to 20 mg/day; range 20-60 mg/day; range for lower weight children, 20-30 mg/day; >17 years: same as adult
      Cap: 10, 20, 40 mg; *Tab:* 30*, 60*mg; *Oral soln:* 20 mg/5 ml (4 oz) (mint)
    Prozac Weekly following daily fluoxetine therapy at 20 mg/day for 13 weeks, may initiate **Prozac Weekly** 7 days after the last 20 mg fluoxetine dose
    Pediatric: <12 years: not recommended; ≥12 years: same as adult
      Cap: 90 mg ent-coat del-rel pellets

➤ *levomilnacipran* (C) swallow whole; initially 20 mg once daily for 2 days; then increase to 40 mg once daily; may increase dose in 40 mg increments at intervals of ≥2 days; max 120 mg once daily; *CrCl 30-59 mL/min:* max 80 mg once daily; *CrCl 15-29 mL/min:* max 40 mg once daily
    Fetzima
    Pediatric: <12 years: not recommended; ≥12 years: same as adult
      Cap: 20, 40, 80, 120 mg ext-rel

➤ *paroxetine maleate* (D)(G)
  Pediatric: <12 years: not recommended; ≥12 years: same as adult
    Paxil initially 20 mg daily in AM; may increase by 10 mg/day at weekly intervals as needed; max 60 mg/day
      Tab: 10*, 20*, 30, 40 mg
    Paxil CR initially 25 mg daily in AM; may increase by 12.5 mg at weekly intervals as needed; max 62.5 mg/day
      Tab: 12.5, 25, 37.5 mg cont-rel ent-coat
    Paxil Suspension initially 20 mg daily in AM; may increase by 10 mg/day at weekly intervals as needed; max 60 mg/day
      Oral susp: 10 mg/5 ml (250 ml) (orange)

➤ *paroxetine mesylate* (D)(G) initially 7.5 mg daily in AM; may increase by 10 mg/day at weekly intervals as needed; max 60 mg/day
  Pediatric: <12 years: not established; ≥12 years: same as adult
    Brisdelle *Cap:* 7.5 mg

➤ *sertraline* (C)(G) initially 50 mg daily; increase at 1 week intervals if needed; max 200 mg daily; dilute oral concentrate immediately prior to administration in 4 oz water, ginger ale, lemon-lime soda, lemonade, or orange juice

Pediatric: <6 years: not recommended; 6-12 years: initially 25 mg daily; max 200 mg/day; 13-17 years: initially 50 mg daily; max 200 mg/day; >17 years: same as adult
    Zoloft *Tab:* 25*, 50*, 100*mg; *Oral conc:* 20 mg per ml (60 ml) (alcohol 12%)

SEROTONIN-NOREPINEPHRINE REUPTAKE INHIBITORS (SNRIs)

➤ *desvenlafaxine* (C)(G) swallow whole; initially 50 mg once daily; max 120 mg/day
    Pediatric: <12 years: not recommended; ≥12 years: same as adult
        Pristiq *Tab:* 50, 100 mg ext-rel
➤ *duloxetine* (C)(G) swallow whole; initially 30 mg once daily x 1 week; then, increase to 60 mg once daily; max 120 mg/day
    Pediatric: <12 years: not recommended; ≥12 years: same as adult
        Cymbalta *Cap:* 20, 30, 40, 60 mg del-rel
➤ *levomilnacipran* (C) swallow whole; initially 20 mg once daily for 2 days; then increase to 40 mg once daily; may increase dose in 40 mg increments at intervals of ≥2 days; max 120 mg once daily; *CrCl 30-59 mL/min:* max 80 mg once daily; *CrCl 15-29 mL/min:* max 40 mg once daily
    Pediatric: <12 years: not recommended; ≥12 years: same as adult
        Fetzima *Cap:* 20, 40, 80, 120 mg ext-rel
➤ *venlafaxine* (C)(G)
        Effexor initially 75 mg/day in 2-3 divided doses; may increase at 4 day intervals in 75 mg increments to 150 mg/day; max 225 mg/day
    Pediatric: <18 years: not recommended; ≥18 years: same as adult
      Tab: 37.5, 75, 150, 225 mg
        Effexor XR initially 75 mg q AM; may start at 37.5 mg daily x 4-7 days, then increase by increments of up to 75 mg/day at intervals of at least 4 days; usual max 375 mg/day
    Pediatric: <18 years: not recommended; ≥18 years: same as adult
      Tab/Cap: 37.5, 75, 150 mg ext-rel
➤ *vortioxetine* (C) initially 10 mg once daily; max 30 mg/day
    Pediatric: <18 years: not established; ≥18 years: same as adult
        Brintellix *Tab:* 5, 10, 15, 20 mg

SELECTIVE SEROTONIN REUPTAKE INHIBITOR (SSRI)+5HT-14 RECEPTOR PARTIAL AGONIST COMBINATION

➤ *vilazodone* (C) take with food; initially 10 mg once daily x 7 days; then, 20 mg once daily x 7 days; then, 40 mg once daily
    Pediatric: <18 years: not established; ≥18 years: same as adult
        Viibryd *Tab:* 10, 20, 40 mg

THIENOBENZODIAZEPINE+SSRI COMBINATION

➤ *olanzapine+fluoxetine* (C) initially one 6/25 cap in the PM; titrate; max one 18/75 cap once daily in the PM
    Pediatric: <10 years: not established; ≥10 years: same as adult
        Symbyax
            Cap: **Symbyax 3/25** olan 3 mg+fluo 25 mg
                Symbyax 6/25 olan 6 mg+fluo 25 mg
                Symbyax 6/50 olan 6 mg+fluo 50 mg
                Symbyax 12/25 olan 12 mg+fluo 25 mg
                Symbyax 12/50 olan 12 mg+fluo 50 mg
    Comment: Symbyax is a thienobenzodiazepine-SSRI indicated for the treatment of depressive episodes associated with bipolar depression disorder and treatment resistant depression (TRD).

TRICYCLIC ANTIDEPRESSANTS (TCAs)

Comment: Co-administration of TCAs with SSRIs requires extreme caution.
➤ *amitriptyline* (C)(G) initially 75 mg/day in divided doses <u>or</u> 50-100 mg in a single dose at HS; max 300 mg/day
    Pediatric: <12 years: not recommended; ≥12 years: same as adult
      Tab: 10, 25, 50, 75, 100, 150 mg
➤ *amoxapine* (C) initially 50 mg bid-tid; after 1 week may increase to 100 mg bid-tid; usual effective dose 200-300 mg/day; if total dose exceeds 300 mg/day, give in divided doses (max 400 mg/day); may give as a single bedtime dose (max 300 mg q HS)

Pediatric: <12 years: not recommended; ≥12 years: same as adult
  Tab: 25, 50, 100, 150 mg
▷ ***desipramine*** **(C)(G)** 100-200 mg/day in single or divided doses; max 300 mg/day
  Pediatric: <12 years: not recommended; ≥12 years: same as adult
    Norpramin *Tab:* 10, 25, 50, 75, 100, 150 mg
▷ ***doxepin*** **(C)(G)** 75 mg/day; max 150 mg/day
  Pediatric: <12 years: not recommended; ≥12 years: same as adult
    Cap: 10, 25, 50, 75, 100, 150 mg; *Oral conc:* 10 mg/ml (4 oz w. dropper)
▷ ***imipramine*** **(C)(G)**
  Pediatric: <12 years: not recommended; ≥12 years: same as adult
    Tofranil initially 75 mg daily (max 200 mg); adolescents initially 30-40 mg daily (max 100 mg/day); if maintenance dose exceeds 75 mg daily, may switch to **Tofranil PM** for divided or bedtime dose
      Tab: 10, 25, 50 mg
    Tofranil PM initially 75 mg daily 1 hour before HS; max 200 mg
      Cap: 75, 100, 125, 150 mg
    Tofranil Injection 50 mg IM; lower dose for adolescents; switch to oral form as soon as possible
      Amp: 25 mg/2 ml (2 ml)
▷ ***nortriptyline*** **(D)(G)** initially 25 mg tid-qid; max 150 mg/day
  Pediatric: <12 years: not recommended; ≥12 years: same as adult
    Pamelor *Cap:* 10, 25, 50, 75 mg; *Oral soln:* 10 mg/5 ml (16 oz)
▷ ***protriptyline*** **(C)** initially 5 mg tid; usual dose 15-40 mg/day in 3-4 divided doses; max 60 mg/day
  Pediatric: <12 years: not recommended; ≥12 years: same as adult
    Vivactil *Tab:* 5, 10 mg
▷ ***trimipramine*** **(C)** initially 75 mg/day in divided doses; max 200 mg/day
  Pediatric: not recommended
    Surmontil *Cap:* 25, 50, 100 mg

AMINOKETONES

▷ ***bupropion HBr*** **(C)(G)**
  Pediatric: Safety and effectiveness of ***bupropion*** in the pediatric population have not been established; when considering the use of **bupropion** in a child or adolescent, balance the potential risks with the clinical need
    Aplenzin initially 100 mg bid for at least 3 days; may increase to 375 or 400 mg/day after several weeks; then after at least 3 more days, 450 mg in 4 divided doses; max 450 mg/day, 174 mg/single dose
      Tab: 174, 348, 522 mg
▷ ***bupropion HCl*** **(C)(G)**
  Pediatric: Safety and effectiveness of ***bupropion*** in the pediatric population have not been established; when considering the use of **bupropion** in a child or adolescent, balance the potential risks with the clinical need
    Forfivo XL do not use for initial treatment; use immediate-release ***bupropion*** forms for initial titration; switch to **Forfivo XL** 450 mg once daily when total dose/day reaches 450 mg; may switch to **Forfivo XL** when total dose/day reaches 300 mg for 2 weeks and patient needs 450 mg/day to reach therapeutic target; swallow whole, do not crush or chew
      Tab: 450 mg ext-rel
    Wellbutrin initially 100 mg bid for at least 3 days; may increase to 375 or 400 mg/day after several weeks; then after at least 3 more days, 450 mg in 4 divided doses; max 450 mg/day, 150 mg/single dose
      Tab: 75, 100 mg
    Wellbutrin SR initially 150 mg in AM for at least 3 days; increase to 150 mg bid if well tolerated; usual dose 300 mg/day; max 400 mg/day
      Tab: 100, 150 mg sust-rel
    Wellbutrin XL initially 150 mg in AM for at least 3 days; increase to 150 mg bid if well tolerated; usual dose 300 mg/day; max 450 mg/day
      Tab: 150, 300 mg sust-rel

MONOAMINE OXIDASE INHIBITORS (MAOIs)

Comment: Many drug and food interactions with this class of drugs, use cautiously. Should be reserved for refractory depression that has not responded to other classes of antidepressants.

Concomitant use of MAOIs and SSRIs is an absolute contraindication. See mfr pkg insert for drug and food interactions.

▷ **isocarboxazid** (C)(G) initially 10 mg bid; increase by 10 mg every 2-4 days up to 40 mg/day; may increase by 20 mg/week to max 60 mg/day divided bid-qid
   Pediatric: <16 years: not recommended; ≥16 years: same as adult
      Marplan *Tab:* 10 mg
▷ **phenelzine** (C)(G) initially 15 mg tid; max 90 mg/day
   Pediatric: <16 years: not recommended; ≥16 years: same as adult
      Nardil *Tab:* 15 mg
▷ **selegiline** (C) initially 10 mg tid; max 60 mg/day
      Emsam *Transdermal patch:* 6 mg/24 Hr, 9 mg/24 Hr, 12 mg/24 Hr
      Comment: With the **Emsam** transdermal patch 6 mg/24 h dose, the dietary restrictions commonly required when using nonselective MAOIs are not necessary.
▷ **tranylcypromine** (C) initially 10 mg tid; may increase in 10 mg/day every 1-3 weeks; max 60 mg/day
      Parnate *Tab:* 10 mg

TETRACYCLICS

▷ **maprotiline** (B)(G) initially 75 mg/day for 2 weeks then change gradually as needed in 25 mg increments; max 225 mg/day
   Pediatric: <18 years: not recommended; ≥18 years: same as adult
      Ludiomil *Tab:* 25, 50, 75 mg
▷ **mirtazapine** (C) initially 15 mg q HS; increase at intervals of 1-2 weeks; usual range 15-45 mg/day; max 45 mg/day
   Pediatric: <12 years: not recommended; ≥12 years: same as adult
      Remeron *Tab:* 15*, 30*, 45*mg
      Remeron SolTab *ODT:* 15, 30, 45 mg (orange) (phenylalanine)
▷ **chlordiazepoxide+amitriptyline** (C)(IV)
   Pediatric: <12 years: not recommended; ≥12 years: same as adult
      Limbitrol 3-4 tabs in divided doses
         Tab: chlor 5 mg+amit 12.5 mg
      Limbitrol DS 3-4 tabs in divided doses; max 6 tabs/day
         Tab: chlor 10 mg+amit 25 mg
▷ **trazodone** (C)(G) initially 150 mg/day in divided doses with food; increase by 50 mg/day q 3-4 days; max 400 mg/day in divided doses
   Pediatric: <18 years: not recommended; ≥18 years: same as adult
      Oleptro *Tab:* 50, 100*, 150*, 200, 250, 300 mg

ATYPICAL ANTIPSYCHOTICS

▷ **aripiprazole** (C)(G) initially 15 mg daily; may increase to max 30 mg/day
   Pediatric: <10 years: not recommended; 10-17 years: initially 2 mg/day for 2 days; then, increase to 5 mg/day for 2 days; then, increase to target dose of 10 mg/day; may increase by 5 mg/day at 1 week intervals as needed to max 30 mg/day
      Abilify *Tab:* 2, 5, 10, 15, 20, 30 mg
      Abilify Discmelt *Tab:* 15 mg orally disintegrating (vanilla) (phenylalanine)
      Abilify Maintena *Vial:* 300, 400 mg ext-rel pwdr for IM injection after reconstitution; 300, 400 mg single-dose prefilled dual-chamber syringes w. supplies
      Comment: Abilify is indicated for acute and maintenance treatment of manic or mixed episodes in bipolar I disorder, as monotherapy or as an adjunct to **lithium** or **valproate**, as adjunct to antidepressants for major depressive disorder (MDD), and for irritability associated with autistic disorder.
▷ **brexpiprazole** (C) initially 0.5 or 1 mg once daily; titrate weekly up to target 2 mg/day; max 3 mg/day; *Moderate-severe hepatic impairment, renal impairment*, or *ESRD*, max 2 mg/day
   Pediatric: <12 years: not established; ≥12 years: same as adult
      Rexulti *Tab:* 0.25, 0.5, 1, 2, 3, 4 mg

 DERMATITIS: ATOPIC (ECZEMA)

Parenteral Corticosteroids *see page* 577
Oral Corticosteroids *see page* 577
Topical Corticosteroids *see page* 574

PHOSPHODIESTERASE 4 INHIBITOR

▷ *crisaborole 2%* (C) apply sparingly bid; max 4 weeks
  Pediatric: <2 years: not recommended; ≥2 years: same as adult
    Eucrisa *Oint:* 2% (60 gm)

MOISTURIZING AGENTS

  Aquaphor Healing Ointment (OTC) *Oint:* 1.75, 3.5, 14 oz (alcohol)
  Eucerin Daily Sun Defense (OTC) *Lotn:* 6 oz (fragrance-free)
  Comment: Eucerin Daily Sun Defense is a moisturizer with SPF-15 sunscreen.
  Eucerin Facial Lotion (OTC) *Lotn:* 4 oz
  Eucerin Light Lotion (OTC) *Lotn:* 8 oz
  Eucerin Lotion (OTC) *Lotn:* 8, 16 oz
  Eucerin Original Creme (OTC) *Crm:* 2, 4, 16 oz (alcohol)
  Eucerin Plus Creme (OTC) *Crm:* 4 oz
  Eucerin Plus Lotion (OTC) *Lotn:* 6, 12 oz
  Eucerin Protective Lotion (OTC) *Lotn:* 4 oz (alcohol)
  Comment: Eucerin Protective Lotion is a moisturizer with SPF-25 sunscreen.
  Lac-Hydrin Cream (OTC) *Crm:* 280, 385 gm
  Lac-Hydrin Lotion (OTC) *Lotn:* 25, 400 gm
  Lubriderm Dry Skin Scented (OTC) *Lotn:* 6, 10, 16, 32 oz
  Lubriderm Dry Skin Unscented (OTC) *Lotn:* 3.3, 6, 10, 16 oz (fragrance-free)
  Lubriderm Sensitive Skin Lotion (OTC) *Lotn:* 3.3, 6, 10, 16 oz (lanolin-free)
  Lubriderm Dry Skin (OTC) *Lotn (scented):* 2.5, 6, 10, 16 oz;
    Lotn (fragrance-free): 1, 2.5, 6, 10, 16 oz
  Lubriderm Bath 1-2 capfuls in bath or rub onto wet skin as needed, then rinse
    Oil: 8 oz
  Moisturel (OTC) apply as needed
    Crm: 4, 16 oz; *Lotn:* 8, 12 oz; *Clnsr:* 8.75 oz

OATMEAL COLLOIDS

  Aveeno (OTC) add to bath as needed
    Regular: 1.5 oz (8/pck); *Moisturizing:* 0.75 oz (8/pck)
  Aveeno Oil (OTC) add to bath as needed
    Oil: 8 oz
  Aveeno Moisturizing (OTC) apply as needed
    Lotn: 2.5, 8, 12 oz; *Crm:* 4 oz
  Aveeno Cleansing Bar (OTC) *Bar:* 3 oz
  Aveeno Gentle Skin Cleanser (OTC) *Liq clnsr:* 6 oz

TOPICAL OIL

▷ *fluocinolone acetonide* 0.01% topical oil (C)
  Pediatric: <6 years: not recommended; ≥6 years: apply sparingly bid for up to 4 weeks
    Derma-Smoothe/FS Topical Oil apply sparingly tid
    Topical oil: 0.01% (4 oz) (peanut oil)

TOPICAL STEROIDS

Comment: Topical steroids should be applied sparingly and for the shortest time necessary.
Do not use in the diaper area. Do not use an occlusive dressing. Systemic absorption of topical
corticosteroids can induce reversible hypothalamic-pituitary-adrenal (HPA) axis suppression
with the potential for clinical corticosteroid insufficiency.
▷ *desonide* 0.05% topical gel (C) apply sparingly bid-tid; max 4 weeks
  Pediatric: <3 months: not recommended; ≥3 months: same as adult
    Desonate *Gel:* 0.05% (60 gm) (89% purified water; fragrance-free, surfactant-free,
    alcohol-free)

SECOND GENERATION ORAL ANTIHISTAMINES

Comment: The following drugs are second generation antihistamines. As such they minimally
sedating, much less so than the first generation antihistamines. All antihistamines are excreted
into breast milk.

➤ *cetirizine* (C)(OTC)(G) initially 5-10 mg once daily; 5 mg once daily; >65 years: use with caution
  Pediatric: <6 years: not recommended; ≥6 years: same as adult
    cetirizine Cap: 10 mg
    Children's Zyrtec Chewable *Chew tab:* 5, 10 mg (grape)
    Children's Zyrtec Allergy Syrup *Syr:* 1 mg/ml (4 oz) (grape, bubble gum) (sugar-free, dye-free)
    Zyrtec *Tab:* 10 mg
    Zyrtec Hives Relief *Tab:* 10 mg
    Zyrtec Liquid Gels *Liq gel:* 10 mg
➤ *desloratadine* (C)
    Clarinex 1/2-1 tab once daily
    Pediatric: <6 years: not recommended; ≥6 years: same as adult
      Tab: 5 mg
    Clarinex RediTabs 5 mg once daily
    Pediatric: <6 years: not recommended; 6-12 years: 2.5 mg once daily; ≥12 years: same as adult
      ODT: 2.5, 5 mg (tutti-frutti) (phenylalanine)
    Clarinex Syrup 5 mg (10 ml) once daily
    Pediatric: <6 months: not recommended; 6-11 months: 1 mg (2 ml) once daily; 1-5 years: 1.25 mg (2.5 ml) once daily; 6-11 years: 2.5 mg (5 ml) once daily; ≥12 years: same as adult
      Syr: 0.5 mg per ml (4 oz) (tutti-frutti) (phenylalanine)
    Desloratadine ODT 1 tab once daily
    Pediatric: <6 years: not recommended; 6-11 years: 1/2 tab once daily; ≥12 years: same as adult
      ODT: 5 mg
➤ *fexofenadine* (C)(OTC)(G) 60 mg once daily-bid <u>or</u> 180 mg once daily; *CrCl <90 mL/min:* 60 mg once daily
  Pediatric: <6 months: not recommended; 6 months-2 years: 15 mg bid; *CrCl ≤90 mL/min:* 15 mg once daily; 2-11 years: 30 mg bid; *CrCl ≤90 mL/min:* 30 mg once daily; ≥12 years: same as adult
    Allegra *Tab:* 30, 60, 180 mg film-coat
    Allegra Allergy *Tab:* 60, 180 mg film-coat
    Allegra ODT *ODT:* 30 mg (phenylalanine)
    Allegra Oral Suspension *Oral susp:* 30 mg/5 ml (6 mg/ml) (4 oz)
➤ *levocetirizine* (B)(OTC)(G) administer dose in the PM; *Seasonal Allergic Rhinitis:* <2 years: not recommended; may start at ≥2 years; *Chronic Idiopathic Urticaria (CIU), Perennial Allergic Rhinitis:* <6 months: not recommended; may start at ≥ 6 months; *Dosing by Age:* 6 months-5 years: max 1.25 mg once daily; 6-11 years: max 2.5 mg once daily; ≥12 years: 2.5-5 mg once daily; *Renal Dysfunction <12 years:* contraindicated; *Renal Dysfunction ≥12 years:* CrCl 50-80 ml/min: 2.5 mg once daily; *CrCl* 30-50 mL/min: 2.5 mg every other day; CrCl: 10-30 mL/min: 2.5 mg twice weekly (every 3-4 days); CrCl <10 mL/min, ESRD <u>or</u> hemodialysis: contraindicated
    Children's Xyzal Allergy 24HR *Oral Soln:* 0.5 mg/ml (150 ml)
    Xyzal Allergy 24HR *Tab:* 5*mg
➤ *loratadine* (C)(OTC)(G) 5 mg bid <u>or</u> 10 mg once daily; *Hepatic <u>or</u> Renal Insufficiency:* see mfr pkg insert
  Pediatric: <2 years: not recommended; 2-5 years: 5 mg once daily; ≥6 years: same as adult
    Children's Claritin Chewables *Chew tab:* 5 mg (grape) (phenylalanine)
    Children's Claritin Syrup 1 mg/ml (4 oz) (fruit) (sugar-free, alcohol-free, dye-free; sodium 6 mg/5 ml)
    Claritin *Tab:* 10 mg
    Claritin Hives Relief *Tab:* 10 mg
    Claritin Liqui-Gels *Liq gel:* 10 mg
    Claritin RediTabs 12 Hours *ODT:* 5 mg (mint)
    Claritin RediTabs 24 Hours *ODT:* 10 mg (mint)

FIRST GENERATION ANTIHISTAMINES

➤ *diphenhydramine* (B)(G) 25-50 mg q 6-8 hours; max 100 mg/day
  Pediatric: <2 years: not recommended; 2-6 years: 6.25 mg q 4-6 hours; max 37.5 mg/day; >6-12 years: 12.5-25 mg q 4-6 hours; max 150 mg/day; >12 years: same as adult
    Benadryl (OTC) *Chew tab:* 12.5 mg (grape) (phenylalanine); *Liq:* 12.5 mg/5 ml (4, 8 oz); *Cap:* 25 mg; *Tab:* 25 mg; *Dye-free soft gel:* 25 mg; *Dye-free liq:* 12.5 mg/5 ml (4, 8 oz)

▶ *diphenhydramine injectable* (B)(G) 25-50 mg IM immediately; then q 6 hours prn
Pediatric: <12 years: *See mfr pkg insert:* 1.25 mg/kg up to 25 mg IM x 1 dose; then q 6 hours prn; ≥12 years: same as adult
Benadryl Injectable *Vial:* 50 mg/ml (1 ml single-use); 50 mg/ml (10 ml multi-dose);
Amp: 10 mg/ml (1 ml); *Prefilled syringe:* 50 mg/ml (1 ml)
▶ *hydroxyzine* (C)(G) 50 mg/day divided qid prn; 50-100 mg/day divided qid prn
Pediatric: <6 years: 50 mg/day divided qid prn; ≥6 years: same as adult
Atarax *Tab:* 10, 25, 50, 100 mg; *Syr:* 10 mg/5 ml (alcohol 0.5%)
Vistaril *Cap:* 25, 50, 100 mg; *Oral susp:* 25 mg/5 ml (4 oz) (lemon)
Comment: *hydroxyzine* is contraindicated in early pregnancy and in patients with a prolonged QT interval. It is not known whether this drug is excreted in human milk; therefore, *hydroxyzine* should not be given to nursing mothers.

TOPICAL ANALGESICS

▶ *capsaicin* cream (B)(G) apply tid-qid prn
Pediatric: <2 years: not recommended; ≥2 years: apply sparingly tid-qid prn
Axsain *Crm:* 0.075% (1, 2 oz)
Capsin (OTC) *Lotn:* 0.025, 0.075% (59 ml)
Capzasin-HP (OTC) *Crm:* 0.075% (1.5 oz); *Lotn:* 0.075% (2 oz)
Capzasin-P (OTC) *Crm:* 0.025% (1.5 oz); *Lotn:* 0.025% (2 oz)
Dolorac *Crm:* 0.025% (28 gm)
Double Cap (OTC) *Crm:* 0.05% (2 oz)
R-Gel *Gel:* 0.025% (15, 30 gm)
Zostrix (OTC) *Crm:* 0.025% (0.7, 1.5, 3 oz)
Zostrix HP (OTC) *Emol crm:* 0.075% (1, 2 oz)

TOPICAL & TRANSDERMAL ANALGESICS

▶ *capsaicin* 8% patch (B) apply up to 4 patches for one 60-minute application to clean dry skin; may prep area with topical anesthetic; wear non-latex gloves; patches may be cut to size/shape; treatment may be repeated every 3 months
Pediatric: <18 years: not recommended; ≥18 years: same as adult
Qutenza *Patch:* 8% 1640 mcg/cm (179 mg) (1 or 2 patches w. 1-50 gm tube cleansing gel/carton)
▶ *diclofenac sodium* (C; D ≥30 wks)(G) apply qid prn to intact skin
Pediatric: <12 years: not established; ≥12 years: same as adult
Pennsaid 1.5% in 10 drop increments, dispense and rub into front, side, and back of knee: usually; 40 drops (40 mg) qid
Topical soln: 1.5% (150 ml)
Pennsaid 2% apply 2 pump actuations (40 mg) and rub into front, side, and back of knee bid
Topical soln: 2% (20 mg/pump actuation, 112 gm)
Solaraze Gel massage in to clean skin bid prn
Gel: 3% (50 gm) (benzyl alcohol)
Voltaren Gel (G) apply qid prn to intact skin
Gel: 1% (100 gm)
Comment: *diclofenac* is contraindicated with *aspirin* allergy. As with other NSAIDs, should be avoided in late pregnancy (≥30 weeks) because it may cause premature closure of the ductus arteriosus.
▶ *doxepin* (B) cream apply to affected area qid at intervals of at least 3-4 hours; max 8 days
Pediatric: <12 years: not recommended; >12 years: same as adult
Prudoxin *Crm:* 5% (45 gm)
Zonalon *Crm:* 5% (30, 45 gm)
▶ *pimecrolimus* 1% cream (C)(G) <2 years: not recommended; ≥2 years: apply to affected area bid; do not apply an occlusive dressing
Elidel *Crm:* 1% (30, 60, 100 gm)
Comment: *pimecrolimus* is indicated for short-term and intermittent long-term use. Discontinue use when resolution occurs. Contraindicated if the patient is immunosuppressed. Change to the 0.1% preparation or if secondary bacterial infection is present.
▶ *trolamine salicylate* apply tid-qid
Pediatric: <2 years: not recommended; ≥2 years: same as adult
Mobisyl Creme *Crm:* 10% (100 gm)

TOPICAL AND TRANSDERMAL ANESTHETICS

Comment: *lidocaine* should not be applied to non-intact skin.

▷ *lidocaine* cream (B) apply to affected area bid prn
Pediatric: <12 years: not recommended; ≥12 years: same as adult
LidaMantle *Crm:* 3% (1, 2 oz)
Lidoderm *Crm:* 3% (85 gm)
ZTlido *lidocaine* topical system 1% (30/carton)
Comment: Compared to **Lidoderm** (*lidocaine* patch 5%) which contains 700 mg/patch, **ZTlido** only requires 35 mg per topical system to achieve the same therapeutic dose.

▷ *lidocaine* lotion (B) apply to affected area bid prn
Pediatric: <12 years: not recommended; ≥12 years: same as adult
LidaMantle *Lotn:* 3% (177 ml)

▷ *lidocaine* 5% patch (B)(G) apply up to 3 patches at one time for up to 12 hours/24-hour period (12 hours on/12 hours off); patches may be cut into smaller sizes before removal of the release liner; do not re-use
Pediatric: <12 years: not recommended; ≥12 years: same as adult
Lidoderm *Patch:* 5% (10x14 cm; 30/carton)

▷ *lidocaine+dexamethasone* (B)
Pediatric: <12 years: not recommended; ≥12 years: same as adult
Decadron Phosphate with Xylocaine *Lotn:* dexa 4 mg+lido 10 mg per ml (5 ml)

▷ *lidocaine+hydrocortisone* (B)(G) apply to affected area bid prn
Pediatric: <12 years: not recommended; ≥12 years: same as adult
LidaMantle HC *Crm:* lido 3%+hydro 0.5% (1, 3 oz); *Lotn:* (177 ml)

▷ *lidocaine 2.5%+prilocaine 2.5%* apply sparingly to the burn bid-tid prn
Pediatric: <12 years: not recommended; ≥12 years: same as adult
Emla Cream (B) 5, 30 gm/tube

INTERLEUKIN-4 RECEPTOR ALPHA ANTAGONIST

▷ *dupilumab* administer SC into the upper arm, abdomen, or thigh; rotate sites; initially 600 mg (2 x 300 mg injections at different sites) followed by 300 mg SC once every other week; may use with or without topical corticosteroids; may use with calcineurin inhibitors, but reserve only for problem areas (e.g., face, neck, intertriginous, and genital areas); avoid live vaccines.
Pediatric: <12 years: not recommended; ≥12 years: same as adult
Dupixent *Prefilled syringe:* 300 mg/2 ml (2/pck without needle) (preservative-free)
Comment: *dupilumab* is a human monoclonal IgG4 antibody that inhibits interleukin-4 (IL-4) and interleukin-13 (IL-13) signaling by specifically binding to the IL4Rα subunit shared by the IL-4 and IL-13 receptor complexes, thereby inhibiting the release of pro-inflammatory cytokines, chemokines, and IgE. *dupilumab* is indicated as an add-on maintenance therapy for patients ≥12 years-of-age with moderate-to-severe atopic dermatitis who are not adequately controlled with topical prescription therapies or when they are not advisable.

 DERMATITIS: CONTACT

Topical Corticosteroids *see page* 574
Parenteral Corticosteroids *see page* 577
Oral Corticosteroids *see page* 577
OTC diphenhydramine cream

PROPHYLAXIS

▷ *bentoquatam* apply as a wet film to exposed skin at least 15 minutes prior to possible contact; reapply at least q 4 hours; remove with soap and water
Pediatric: <6 years: not recommended; ≥6 years: same as adult
IvyBlock (OTC) *Soln:* 120 ml
Comment: Provides protection against genus *Rhus* (poison ivy, oak, and sumac).

TREATMENT

Oatmeal Colloids

Aveeno (OTC) add to bath as needed
Regular: 1.5 oz (8/pck); *Moisturizing:* 0.75 oz (8/pck)

Aveeno Oil (OTC) add to bath as needed
> *Oil:* 8 oz
Aveeno Moisturizing (OTC) apply as needed
> *Lotn:* 2.5, 8, 12 oz; *Crm:* 4 oz
Aveeno Cleansing Bar (OTC) *Bar:* 3 oz
Aveeno Gentle Skin Cleanser (OTC) *Liq clnsr:* 6 oz

SECOND GENERATION ORAL ANTIHISTAMINES

Comment: The following drugs are second generation antihistamines. As such they minimally sedating, much less so than the first generation antihistamines. All antihistamines are excreted into breast milk.

▷ *cetirizine* (C)(OTC)(G) initially 5-10 mg once daily; 5 mg once daily; ≥65 years: use with caution
Pediatric: <6 years: not recommended; ≥6 years: same as adult
> cetirizine *Cap:* 10 mg
> Children's Zyrtec Chewable *Chew tab:* 5, 10 mg (grape)
> Children's Zyrtec Allergy Syrup *Syr:* 1 mg/ml (4 oz) (grape, bubble gum) (sugar-free, dye-free)
> Zyrtec *Tab:* 10 mg
> Zyrtec Hives Relief *Tab:* 10 mg
> Zyrtec Liquid Gels *Liq gel:* 10 mg

▷ *desloratadine* (C)
> Clarinex 1/2-1 tab once daily
> *Pediatric:* <6 years: not recommended; ≥6 years: same as adult
> > *Tab:* 5 mg
> Clarinex RediTabs 5 mg once daily
> *Pediatric:* <6 years: not recommended; 6-12 years: 2.5 mg once daily; ≥12 years: same as adult
> > *ODT:* 2.5, 5 mg (tutti-frutti) (phenylalanine)
> Clarinex Syrup 5 mg (10 ml) once daily
> *Pediatric:* <6 months: not recommended; 6-11 months: 1 mg (2 ml) once daily; 1-5 years: 1.25 mg (2.5 ml) once daily; 6-11 years: 2.5 mg (5 ml) once daily; ≥12 years: same as adult
> > *Syr:* 0.5 mg per ml (4 oz) (tutti-frutti) (phenylalanine)
> Desloratadine ODT 1 tab once daily
> *Pediatric:* <6 years: not recommended; 6-11 years: 1/2 tab once daily; ≥12 years: same as adult
> > *ODT:* 5 mg

▷ *fexofenadine* (C)(OTC)(G) 60 mg once daily-bid <u>or</u> 180 mg once daily; *CrCl <90 mL/min:* 60 mg once daily
Pediatric: <6 months: not recommended; 6 months-2 years: 15 mg bid; *CrCl ≤90 mL/min:* 15 mg once daily; 2-11 years: 30 mg bid; *CrCl ≤90 mL/min:* 30 mg once daily; ≥12 years: same as adult
> Allegra *Tab:* 30, 60, 180 mg film-coat
> Allegra Allergy *Tab:* 60, 180 mg film-coat
> Allegra ODT *ODT:* 30 mg (phenylalanine)
> Allegra Oral Suspension *Oral susp:* 30 mg/5 ml (6 mg/ml) (4 oz)

▷ *levocetirizine* (B)(OTC)(G) administer dose in the PM; *Seasonal Allergic Rhinitis:* <2 years: not recommended; may start at ≥2 years; *Chronic Idiopathic Urticaria (CIU), Perennial Allergic Rhinitis:* <6 months: not recommended; may start at ≥ 6 months; *Dosing by Age:* 6 months-5 years: max 1.25 mg once daily; 6-11 years: max 2.5 mg once daily; ≥12 years: 2.5-5 mg once daily; *Renal Dysfunction <12 years:* contraindicated; *Renal Dysfunction ≥12 years:* CrCl 50-80 ml/min: 2.5 mg once daily; CrCl 30-50 mL/min: 2.5 mg every other day; CrCl: 10-30 mL/min: 2.5 mg twice weekly (every 3-4 days); CrCl <10 mL/min, ESRD <u>or</u> hemodialysis: contraindicated
> Children's Xyzal Allergy 24HR *Oral Soln:* 0.5 mg/ml (150 ml)
> Xyzal Allergy 24HR *Tab:* 5*mg

▷ *loratadine* (C)(OTC)(G) 5 mg bid <u>or</u> 10 mg once daily; *Hepatic or Renal Insufficiency:* see mfr pkg insert
Pediatric: <2 years: not recommended; 2-5 years: 5 mg once daily; ≥6 years: same as adult
> Children's Claritin Chewables *Chew tab:* 5 mg (grape) (phenylalanine)

Children's Claritin Syrup 1 mg/ml (4 oz) (fruit) (sugar-free, alcohol-free, dye-free; sodium 6 mg/5 ml)
Claritin *Tab:* 10 mg
Claritin Hives Relief *Tab:* 10 mg
Claritin Liqui-Gels *Liq gel:* 10 mg
Claritin RediTabs 12 Hours *ODT:* 5 mg (mint)
Claritin RediTabs 24 Hours *ODT:* 10 mg (mint)

FIRST GENERATION ORAL ANTIHISTAMINES

▷ *diphenhydramine* (B)(G) 25-50 mg q 6-8 hours; max 100 mg/day
Pediatric: <2 years: not recommended; 2-6 years: 6.25 mg q 4-6 hours; max 37.5 mg/day; >6-12 years: 12.5-25 mg q 4-6 hours; max 150 mg/day; >12 years: same as adult
    Benadryl (OTC) *Chew tab:* 12.5 mg (grape) (phenylalanine); *Liq:* 12.5 mg/5 ml (4, 8 oz); *Cap:* 25 mg; *Tab:* 25 mg; *Dye-free soft gel:* 25 mg; *Dye-free liq:* 12.5 mg/5 ml (4, 8 oz)
▷ *hydroxyzine* (C)(G) 50 mg/day divided qid prn; 50-100 mg/day divided qid prn
Pediatric: <6 years: 50 mg/day divided qid prn; ≥6 years: same as adult
    Atarax *Tab:* 10, 25, 50, 100 mg; *Syr:* 10 mg/5 ml (alcohol 0.5%)
    Vistaril *Cap:* 25, 50, 100 mg; *Oral susp:* 25 mg/5 ml (4 oz) (lemon)
Comment: *hydroxyzine* is contraindicated in early pregnancy and in patients with a prolonged QT interval. It is not known whether this drug is excreted in human milk; therefore, *hydroxyzine* should not be given to nursing mothers.

FIRST GENERATION PARENTERAL ANTIHISTAMINE

▷ *diphenhydramine* injectable (B)(G) 25-50 mg IM immediately; then q 6 hours prn
Pediatric: <12 years: *See mfr pkg insert:* 1.25 mg/kg up to 25 mg IM x 1 dose; then q 6 hours prn; ≥12 years: same as adult
    Benadryl Injectable *Vial:* 50 mg/ml (1 ml single-use); 50 mg/ml (10 ml multi-dose); *Amp:* 10 mg/ml (1 ml); *Prefilled syringe:* 50 mg/ml (1 ml)

 DERMATITIS: GENUS *RHUS* (POISON OAK, POISON IVY, POISON SUMAC)

Topical Corticosteroids *see page* 574
Parenteral Corticosteroids *see page* 577
Oral Corticosteroids *see page* 577
OTC Calamine Lotion
OTC diphenhydramine cream

PROPHYLAXIS

▷ *bentoquatam* <6 years: not recommended; ≥6 years: apply as a wet film to exposed skin at least 15 minutes prior to possible contact; reapply at least q 4 hours; remove with soap and water
    IvyBlock (OTC) *Soln:* 120 ml
Comment: Provides protection against genus *Rhus* (poison oak, poison ivy, and poison sumac).

TREATMENT

Oatmeal Colloids
Aveeno (OTC) add to bath as needed
Regular: 1.5 oz (8/pck); *Moisturizing:* 0.75 oz (8/pck)
Aveeno Oil (OTC) add to bath as needed
Oil: 8 oz
Aveeno Moisturizing (OTC) apply as needed
Lotn: 2.5, 8, 12 oz; *Crm:* 4 oz
Aveeno Cleansing Bar (OTC) *Bar:* 3 oz
Aveeno Gentle Skin Cleanser (OTC) *Liq clnsr:* 6 oz

SECOND GENERATION ORAL ANTIHISTAMINES

Comment: The following drugs are second generation antihistamines. As such they are minimally sedating, much less so than the first generation antihistamines. All antihistamines are excreted into breast milk.

▷ *cetirizine* (C)(OTC)(G) initially 5-10 mg once daily; 5 mg once daily; ≥65 years: use with caution
Pediatric: <6 years: not recommended; ≥6 years: same as adult
    cetirizine Cap: 10 mg
    Children's Zyrtec Chewable *Chew tab:* 5, 10 mg (grape)
    Children's Zyrtec Allergy Syrup *Syr:* 1 mg/ml (4 oz) (grape, bubble gum) (sugar-free, dye-free)
    Zyrtec *Tab:* 10 mg
    Zyrtec Hives Relief *Tab:* 10 mg
    Zyrtec Liquid Gels *Liq gel:* 10 mg

▷ *desloratadine* (C)
    Clarinex 1/2-1 tab once daily
    Pediatric: <6 years: not recommended; ≥6 years: same as adult
      Tab: 5 mg
    Clarinex RediTabs 5 mg once daily
    Pediatric: <6 years: not recommended; 6-12 years: 2.5 mg once daily; ≥12 years: same as adult
      ODT: 2.5, 5 mg (tutti-frutti) (phenylalanine)
    Clarinex Syrup 5 mg (10 ml) once daily
    Pediatric: <6 months: not recommended; 6-11 months: 1 mg (2 ml) once daily; 1-5 years: 1.25 mg (2.5 ml) once daily; 6-11 years: 2.5 mg (5 ml) once daily; ≥12 years: same as adult
      Syr: 0.5 mg per ml (4 oz) (tutti-frutti) (phenylalanine)
    Desloratadine ODT 1 tab once daily
    Pediatric: <6 years: not recommended; 6-11 years: 1/2 tab once daily; ≥12 years: same as adult
      ODT: 5 mg

▷ *fexofenadine* (C)(OTC)(G) 60 mg once daily-bid <u>or</u> 180 mg once daily; *CrCl <90 mL/min:* 60 mg once daily
Pediatric: <6 months: not recommended; 6 months-2 years: 15 mg bid; *CrCl ≤90 mL/min:* 15 mg once daily; 2-11 years: 30 mg bid; *CrCl ≤90 mL/min:* 30 mg once daily; ≥12 years: same as adult
    Allegra *Tab:* 30, 60, 180 mg film-coat
    Allegra Allergy *Tab:* 60, 180 mg film-coat
    Allegra ODT *ODT:* 30 mg (phenylalanine)
    Allegra Oral Suspension *Oral susp:* 30 mg/5 ml (6 mg/ml) (4 oz)

▷ *levocetirizine* (B)(OTC)(G) administer dose in the PM; *Seasonal Allergic Rhinitis:* <2 years: not recommended; may start at ≥2 years; *Chronic Idiopathic Urticaria (CIU), Perennial Allergic Rhinitis:* <6 months: not recommended; may start at ≥ 6 months; *Dosing by Age:* 6 months-5 years: max 1.25 mg once daily; 6-11 years: max 2.5 mg once daily; ≥12 years: 2.5-5 mg once daily; *Renal Dysfunction <12 years:* contraindicated; *Renal Dysfunction ≥12 years:* CrCl 50-80 ml/min: 2.5 mg once daily; CrCl 30-50 mL/min: 2.5 mg every other day; CrCl: 10-30 mL/min: 2.5 mg twice weekly (every 3-4 days); CrCl <10 mL/min, ESRD <u>or</u> hemodialysis: contraindicated
    Children's Xyzal Allergy 24HR *Oral Soln:* 0.5 mg/ml (150 ml)
    Xyzal Allergy 24HR *Tab:* 5*mg

▷ *loratadine* (C)(OTC)(G) 5 mg bid <u>or</u> 10 mg once daily; *Hepatic <u>or</u> Renal Insufficiency:* see mfr pkg insert
Pediatric: <2 years: not recommended; 2-5 years: 5 mg once daily; ≥6 years: same as adult
    Children's Claritin Chewables *Chew tab:* 5 mg (grape) (phenylalanine)
    Children's Claritin Syrup 1 mg/ml (4 oz) (fruit) (sugar-free, alcohol-free, dye-free, sodium 6 mg/5 ml)
    Claritin *Tab:* 10 mg
    Claritin Hives Relief *Tab:* 10 mg
    Claritin Liqui-Gels *Liq gel:* 10 mg
    Claritin RediTabs 12 Hours *ODT:* 5 mg (mint)
    Claritin RediTabs 24 Hours *ODT:* 10 mg (mint)

FIRST GENERATION ANTIHISTAMINES

▷ *diphenhydramine* (B)(G) 25-50 mg q 6-8 hours; max 100 mg/day
Pediatric: <2 years: not recommended; 2-6 years: 6.25 mg q 4-6 hours; max 37.5 mg/day; >6-12 years: 12.5-25 mg q 4-6 hours; max 150 mg/day; >12 years: same as adult

Benadryl (OTC) *Chew tab:* 12.5 mg (grape) (phenylalanine); *Liq:* 12.5 mg/5 ml (4, 8 oz); *Cap:* 25 mg; *Tab:* 25 mg; *Dye-free soft gel:* 25 mg; *Dye-free liq:* 12.5 mg/5 ml (4, 8 oz)

➤ *diphenhydramine* injectable (B)(G) 25-50 mg IM immediately; then q 6 hours prn
Pediatric: <12 years: *See mfr pkg insert:* 1.25 mg/kg up to 25 mg IM x 1 dose; then q 6 hours prn; ≥12 years: same as adult

Benadryl Injectable *Vial:* 50 mg/ml (1 ml single-use); 50 mg/ml (10 ml multi-dose); *Amp:* 10 mg/ml (1 ml); *Prefilled syringe:* 50 mg/ml (1 ml)

➤ *hydroxyzine* (C)(G) 50 mg/day divided qid prn; 50-100 mg/day divided qid prn
Pediatric: <6 years: 50 mg/day divided qid prn; ≥6 years: same as adult

Atarax *Tab:* 10, 25, 50, 100 mg; *Syr:* 10 mg/5 ml (alcohol 0.5%)

Vistaril *Cap:* 25, 50, 100 mg; *Oral susp:* 25 mg/5 ml (4 oz) (lemon)

Comment: *hydroxyzine* is contraindicated in early pregnancy and in patients with a prolonged QT interval. It is not known whether this drug is excreted in human milk; therefore, *hydroxyzine* should not be given to nursing mothers.

DERMATITIS: SEBORRHEIC

ANTIFUNGAL SHAMPOOS AND TOPICAL AGENTS

➤ *chloroxine* shampoo (C) massage onto wet scalp; wait 3 minutes, rinse, repeat, and rinse thoroughly; use twice weekly
Pediatric: <12 years: not recommended; ≥12 years: same as adult

Capitrol Shampoo *Shampoo:* 2% (4 oz)

➤ *ciclopirox* (B) apply gel once daily or apply cream or lotion twice daily, x 4 weeks or shampoo twice weekly; massage shampoo onto wet scalp; wait 3 minutes, rinse, repeat, and rinse thoroughly; shampoo twice weekly

Loprox Cream
Pediatric: <10 years: not recommended; ≥10 years: same as adult
Crm: 0.77% (15, 30, 90 gm)

Loprox Gel
Pediatric: <16 years: not recommended; ≥16 years: same as adult
Gel: 0.77% (30, 45 gm)

Loprox Lotion
Pediatric: <10 years: not recommended; ≥10 years: same as adult
Lotn: 0.77% (30, 60 ml)

Loprox Shampoo *Shampoo:* 1% (120 ml)

➤ *coal tar* (C)(G)
Pediatric: same as adult

Scytera (OTC) apply once daily-qid; use lowest effective dose
Foam: 2%

T/Gel Shampoo Extra Strength (OTC) use every other day; max 4 x/week; massage into wet scalp for 5 minutes; rinse; repeat *Shampoo:* 1%

T/Gel Shampoo Original Formula (OTC) use every other day; max 7 x/week; massage into wet scalp for 5 minutes; rinse; repeat
Shampoo: 0.5%

T/Gel Shampoo Stubborn Itch Control (OTC) use every other day; max 7 x/week; massage into wet scalp for 5 minutes; rinse; repeat
Shampoo: 0.5%

➤ *fluocinolone acetonide* (C)
Derma-Smoothe/FS Shampoo apply up to 1 oz to scalp daily, lather, and leave on x 5 minutes, then rinse twice
Pediatric: <12 years: not recommended; ≥12 years: same as adult
Shampoo: 0.01% (4 oz)

Derma-Smoothe/FS Topical Oil *fluocinolone acetonide* 0.01% topical oil (C) apply sparingly tid; for scalp psoriasis wet or dampen hair or scalp, then apply a thin film, massage well, cover with a shower cap and leave on for at least 4 hours or overnight, then wash hair with regular shampoo and rinse
Pediatric: <6 years: not recommended; ≥6 years: apply sparingly bid for up to 4 weeks
Topical oil: 0.01% (4 oz) (peanut oil)

➤ *ketoconazole* (C) apply cream or gel once daily x 4 week or apply up to 1 oz shampoo to scalp daily, lather, leave on x 5 minutes, then rinse twice
Pediatric: <12 years: not recommended; ≥12 years: same as adult
Nizoral Cream *Crm:* 2% (15, 30, 60 gm)

Nizoral Shampoo *Shampoo:* 2% (4 oz)
Xolegel *Gel:* 2% (45 gm)
Xolegel Duo *Kit:* **Xolegel** *Gel:* 2% (45 gm) + **Xolex** *Shampoo:* 2% (4 oz)
 selenium sulfide (C) massage cream into scalp twice weekly x 2 weeks <u>or</u> massage into wet scalp, wait 2-3 minutes, rinse; repeat twice weekly x 2 weeks; may continue treatment with lotion of shampoo 1-2 x weekly as needed
Pediatric: <12 years: not recommended; ≥12 years: same as adult
Exsel Shampoo *Shampoo:* 2.5% (4 oz)
Selsun Rx *Lotn:* 2.5% (4 oz)
Selsun Shampoo *Shampoo:* 1% (120, 210, 240, 330 ml); 2.5% (120 ml)
 sodium sulfacetamide+sulfur (C)
Clenia Emollient Cream apply daily tid
Emol crm: sod sulfa 10%+sulfur 5% (10 oz)
Clenia Foaming Wash wash 1-2 x/day
Wash: sod sulfa 10%+sulfur 5% (6, 12 oz)
Rosula Gel apply daily tid
Gel: sod sulfa 10%+sulfur 5% (45 ml)
Rosula Lotion apply daily tid
Lotn: sod sulfa 10%+sulfur 5% (45 ml) (alcohol-free)
Rosula Wash wash bid
Clnsr: sod sulfa 10%+sulfur 5% (335 ml)

TOPICAL STEROID

 betamethasone valerate 0.12% foam (C)(G) apply twice daily in AM and PM; invert can and dispense a small amount of foam onto a clean saucer <u>or</u> other cool surface (do not apply directly to hand) and massage a small amount into affected area until foam disappears
Pediatric: <12 years: not recommended; ≥12 years: same as adult
Luxiq *Foam:* 100 gm

OXIDIZING AGENT

 hydrogen peroxide 40% apply 4 times to targeted lesion(s) approx 1 min apart during a single session; repeat if lesions have not cleared after 3 weeks; treatments must be applied by a qualified health care provider
Pediatric: not applicable
Eskata *Pen applicator:* 1.5, 2.2 ml/pen (1, 3, 12/carton)
Comment: Not for oral, ophthalmic, or intravaginal use. Avoid open <u>or</u> infected seborrheic keratoses, lesions within the orbital rim, eyes and mucous membranes. The most common adverse reactions include erythema (99%), stinging (97%), edema (91%), scaling (90%), crusting (81%), and pruritus (58%).

DIABETIC PERIPHERAL NEUROPATHY (DPN)

Other Oral Analgesics *see Pain page 352*

NUTRITIONAL SUPPLEMENT

 L-methylfolate calcium (as metafolin)+pyridoxyl 5-phosphate+methylcobalamin 1 cap twice daily <u>or</u> 2 caps once daily
Pediatric: <12 years: not recommended; ≥12 years: same as adult
Metanx *Cap:* meta 3 mg+pyr 35 mg+methyl 2 mg
Comment: **Metanx** is indicated as adjunct treatment for patients with endothelial cell dysfunction, who have loss of protective sensation and neuropathic pain associated with diabetic peripheral neuropathy.

ORAL ANALGESICS

 acetaminophen (B)(G) *see Fever page 163*
 aspirin (D)(G) *see Fever page 164*
Comment: *aspirin*-containing medications are contraindicated with history of allergic-type reaction to *aspirin*, children and adolescents with *Varicella* <u>or</u> other viral illness, and 3rd trimester of pregnancy.

▷ *tramadol* (C)(IV)(G)
  Comment: *tramadol* is known to be excreted in breast milk. The FDA and the European Medicines Agency (EMA) are investigating the safety of using *tramadol*-containing medications to treat pain in children 12-18 years because of the potential for serious side effects, including slowed or difficult breathing.
  Rybix ODT initially 100 mg once daily; may increase by 100 mg every 5 days; max 300 mg/day; *CrCl <30 mL/min* or *severe hepatic impairment*: not recommended; *Cirrhosis*: max 50 mg q 12 hours
  Pediatric: <18 years: not recommended; ≥18 years: same as adult
    ODT: 50 mg (mint) (phenylalanine)
  Ryzolt initially 100 mg once daily; may increase by 100 mg every 5 days; max 300 mg/day; *CrCl <30 mL/min* or *severe hepatic impairment*: not recommended
  Pediatric: <18 years: not recommended; ≥18 years: same as adult
    Tab: 100, 200, 300 mg ext-rel
  Ultram 50-100 mg q 4-6 hours prn; max 400 mg/day; *CrCl <30 mL/min*, max 100 mg q 12 hours; cirrhosis, max 50 mg q 12 hours
  Pediatric: <18 years: not recommended; ≥18 years: same as adult
    Tab: 50*mg
  Ultram ER initially 100 mg once daily; may increase by 100 mg every 5 days; max 300 mg/day; *CrCl <30 mL/min* or *severe hepatic impairment*: not recommended
    Pediatric: <18 years: not recommended; ≥18 years: same as adult
    Tab: 100, 200, 300 mg ext-rel
▷ *tramadol+acetaminophen* (C)(IV)(G) 2 tabs q 4-6 hours; max 8 tabs/day x 5 days; *CrCl <30 mL/min:* max 2 tabs q 12 hours; max 4 tabs/day x 5 days
  Pediatric: <18 years: not recommended; ≥18 years: same as adult
  Ultracet *Tab:* tram 37.5+acet 325 mg
  Comment: *Tramadol* is known to be excreted in breast milk. The FDA and the European Medicines Agency (EMA) are investigating the safety of using *tramadol*-containing medications to treat pain in children 12-18 years because of the potential for serious side effects, including slowed or difficult breathing.

TOPICAL ANALGESICS

▷ *capsaicin* cream (B)(G) apply tid-qid after lesions have healed
  Pediatric: <2 years: not recommended; ≥2 years: same as adult
    Axsain *Crm:* 0.075% (1, 2 oz)
    Capsin *Lotn:* 0.025, 0.075% (59 ml)
    Capzasin-HP (OTC) *Crm:* 0.075% (1.5 oz); 0.025% (45, 90 gm); *Lotn:* 0.075% (2 oz); 0.025% (45, 90 gm)
    Capzasin-P (OTC) *Crm:* 0.025% (1.5 oz); *Lotn:* 0.025% (2 oz)
    Capsaicin-HP (OTC) *Crm:* 0.075% (1.5 oz); *Lotn:* 0.075% (2 oz); *Crm:* 0.025%
    Dolorac *Crm:* 0.025% (28 gm)
    Double Cap (OTC) *Crm:* 0.05% (2 oz)
    R-Gel *Gel:* 0.025% (15, 30 gm)
    Zostrix (OTC) *Crm:* 0.025% (0.7, 1.5, 3 oz)
    Zostrix HP *Emol crm:* 0.075% (1, 2 oz)
▷ *capsaicin* 8% patch (B) apply up to 4 patches for one 60-minute application to clean dry skin; may prep area with topical anesthetic; wear non-latex gloves; patches may be cut to size/shape; treatment may be repeated every 3 months
  Pediatric: <18 years: not recommended; ≥18 years: same as adult
    Qutenza *Patch:* 8% 1640 mcg/cm (179 mg) (1 or 2 patches w. 1-50 gm tube cleansing gel/carton)
▷ *diclofenac sodium* (C; D ≥30 wks)(G) apply qid prn to intact skin
  Pediatric: <12 years: not established; ≥12 years: same as adult
    Pennsaid 1.5% in 10 drop increments, dispense and rub into front, side, and back of knee: usually; 40 drops (40 mg) qid
      Topical soln: 1.5% (150 ml)
    Pennsaid 2% apply 2 pump actuations (40 mg) and rub into front, side, and back of knee bid
      Topical soln: 2% (20 mg/pump actuation, 112 gm)
    Solaraze Gel massage in to clean skin bid prn
      Gel: 3% (50 gm) (benzyl alcohol)

Voltaren Gel (G) apply qid prn to intact skin
    Gel: 1% (100 gm)
Comment: *diclofenac* is contraindicated with *aspirin* allergy. As with other NSAIDs, should be avoided in late pregnancy (≥30 weeks) because it may cause premature closure of the ductus arteriosus.

▷ *doxepin* (B) cream apply to affected area qid at intervals of at least 3-4 hours; max 8 days
    Pediatric: <12 years: not recommended; ≥12 years: same as adult
        Prudoxin *Crm:* 5% (45 gm)
        Zonalon *Crm:* 5% (30, 45 gm)

▷ *pimecrolimus* 1% cream (C)(G) <2 years: not recommended; ≥2 years: apply to affected area bid; do not apply an occlusive dressing
        Elidel *Crm:* 1% (30, 60, 100 gm)
Comment: *pimecrolimus* is indicated for short-term and intermittent long-term use. Discontinue use when resolution occurs. Contraindicated if the patient is immunosuppressed. Change to the 0.1% preparation or if secondary bacterial infection is present.

▷ *trolamine salicylate* apply tid-qid
    Pediatric: <2 years: not recommended; ≥2 years: same as adult
        Mobisyl Creme *Crm:* 10% (100 gm)

TOPICAL AND TRANSDERMAL ANESTHETICS

Comment: *lidocaine* should not be applied to non-intact skin.

▷ *lidocaine* cream (B) apply to affected area bid prn
    Pediatric: <12 years: not recommended; ≥12 years: same as adult
        LidaMantle *Crm:* 3% (1, 2 oz)
        Lidoderm *Crm:* 3% (85 gm)
        ZTlido *lidocaine* topical system 1% (30/carton)
        Comment: Compared to **Lidoderm** (*lidocaine* patch 5%) which contains 700 mg/patch, **ZTlido** only requires 35 mg per topical system to achieve the same therapeutic dose.

▷ *lidocaine* lotion (B) apply to affected area bid prn
    Pediatric: <12 years: not recommended; ≥12 years: same as adult
        LidaMantle *Lotn:* 3% (177 ml)

▷ *lidocaine* 5% patch (B)(G) apply up to 3 patches at one time for up to 12 hours/24-hour period (12 hours on/12 hours off); patches may be cut into smaller sizes before removal of the release liner; do <u>not</u> re-use
    Pediatric: <12 years: not recommended; ≥12 years: same as adult
        Lidoderm *Patch:* 5% (10x14 cm; 30/carton)

▷ *lidocaine+dexamethasone* (B)
    Pediatric: <12 years: not recommended; ≥12 years: same as adult
        Decadron Phosphate with Xylocaine *Lotn:* dexa 4 mg+lido 10 mg per ml (5 ml)

▷ *lidocaine+hydrocortisone* (B)(G) apply to affected area bid prn
    Pediatric: <12 years: not recommended; ≥12 years: same as adult
        LidaMantle HC *Crm:* lido 3%+hydro 0.5% (1, 3 oz); *Lotn:* (177 ml)

▷ *lidocaine* 2.5%+*prilocaine* 2.5% apply sparingly to the burn bid-tid prn
    Pediatric: <12 years: not recommended; ≥12 years: same as adult
        Emla Cream (B) 5, 30 gm/tube

ANTICONVULSANTS

Gamma Aminobutyric Acid Analog

▷ *gabapentin* (C)
    Pediatric: <3 years: not recommended; 3-12 years: initially 10-15 mg/kg/day in 3 divided doses; max 12 hours between doses; titrate over 3 days; 3-4 years: titrate to 40 mg/kg/day; 5-12 years: titrate to 25-35 mg/kg/day; max 50 mg/kg/day
        Gralise (C) initially 300 mg on Day 1; then 600 mg on Day 2; then 900 mg on Days 3-6; then 1200 mg on Days 7-10; then 1500 mg on Days 11-14; titrate up to 1800 mg on Day 15; take entire dose once daily with the evening meal; do not crush, split, or chew
        Tab: 300, 600 mg
        Neurontin (G) *Tab:* 600*, 800*mg; *Cap:* 100, 300, 400 mg; *Oral soln:* 250 mg/5 ml (480 ml) (strawberry-anise)

▷ *gabapentin enacarbil* (C) 600 mg once daily at about 5:00 PM; if dose not taken at recommended time, next dose should be taken the following day; swallow whole; take with food; *CrCl 30-59 mL/min:* 600 mg on Day 1, Day 3, and every day thereafter; *CrCl <30 mL/min:* or on hemodialysis: not recommended

Pediatric: <12 years: not recommended; ≥12 years: same as adult
    Horizant *Tab:* 300, 600 mg ext-rel
Comment: Avoid abrupt cessation of *gabapentin* and *gabapentin enacarbil*. To discontinue, withdraw gradually over 1 week or longer.
▷ *pregabalin (GABA analog)* **(C)(V)**
  Pediatric: <12 years: not recommended; ≥12 years: same as adult
    Lyrica initially 50 mg tid; may titrate to 100 mg tid within one week; max 600 mg divided tid; discontinue over 1 week
      Cap: 25, 50, 75, 100, 150, 200, 225, 300 mg; *Oral soln:* 20 mg/ml
    Lyrica CR *Tab:* usual dose: 165 mg once daily; may increase to 330 mg/day within 1 week; max 660 mg/day
      Tab: 82.5, 165, 330 mg ext-rel

TRICYCLIC ANTIDEPRESSANTS (TCAs)

Comment: Co-administration of TCAs with SSRIs requires extreme caution.
▷ *amitriptyline* **(C)(G)** titrate to achieve pain relief; max 300 mg/day
  Pediatric: <12 years: not recommended; ≥12 years: same as adult
    Tab: 10, 25, 50, 75, 100, 150 mg
▷ *amoxapine* **(C)** titrate to achieve pain relief; if total dose exceeds 300 mg/day, give in divided doses; max 400 mg/day
  Pediatric: <12 years: not recommended; ≥12 years: same as adult
    Tab: 25, 50, 100, 150 mg
▷ *desipramine* **(C)(G)** titrate to achieve pain relief; max 300 mg/day
  Pediatric: <12 years: not recommended; ≥12 years: same as adult
    Norpramin *Tab:* 10, 25, 50, 75, 100, 150 mg
▷ *doxepin* **(C)(G)** titrate to achieve pain relief; max 150 mg/day
  Pediatric: <12 years: not recommended; ≥12 years: same as adult
    Cap: 10, 25, 50, 75, 100, 150 mg; *Oral conc:* 10 mg/ml (4 oz w. dropper)
▷ *imipramine* **(C)(G)**
  Pediatric: <12 years: not recommended; ≥12 years: same as adult
    Tofranil titrate to achieve pain relief; max 200 mg/day; adolescents max 100 mg/day; if maintenance dose exceeds 75 mg/day, may switch to **Tofranil PM** at bedtime
      Tab: 10, 25, 50 mg
    Tofranil PM titrate to achieve pain relief; initially 75 mg at HS; max 200 mg at HS
      Cap: 75, 100, 125, 150 mg
    Tofranil Injection 50 mg IM; lower dose for adolescents; switch to oral form as soon as possible
      Amp: 25 mg/2 ml (2 ml)
▷ *nortriptyline* **(D)(G)** titrate to achieve pain relief; initially 10-25 mg tid-qid; max 150 mg/day; lower doses for elderly and adolescents
  Pediatric: <12 years: not recommended; ≥12 years: same as adult
    Pamelor titrate to achieve pain relief; max 150 mg/day
      Cap: 10, 25, 50, 75 mg; *Oral soln:* 10 mg/5 ml (16 oz)
▷ *protriptyline* **(C)** titrate to achieve pain relief; initially 5 mg tid; max 60 mg/day
  Pediatric: <12 years: not recommended; ≥12 years: same as adult
    Vivactil *Tab:* 5, 10 mg
▷ *trimipramine* **(C)** titrate to achieve pain relief; max 200 mg/day
  Pediatric: <12 years: not recommended; ≥12 years: same as adult
    Surmontil *Cap:* 25, 50, 100 mg

 DIABETIC RETINOPATHY, MACULAR EDEMA, MACULAR DEGENERATION

VASCULAR ENDOTHELIAL GROWTH FACTOR (VEGF) INHIBITOR

Comment: Diabetic retinopathy is the leading cause of blindness among working-age adults in the US. **Lucentis** *(ranibizumab)* is only one FDA-approved drug for the treatment of diabetic retinopathy. Additional labeled indications include treatment of diabetic macular edema (DME), treatment of neovascular (wet) age-related macular degeneration (AMD), treatment of macular edema following retinal vein occlusion (RVO), and treatment of myopic choroidal neovascularization (mCNV).
▷ *aflibercept intravitreal injection* **(C)** 2 mg (0.05 ml) administered by intravitreal injection, with a 30-gauge x ½-inch injection needle, every 4 weeks (monthly) for the first 3 months, followed by 2 mg (0.05 mL) via intravitreal injection once every 8 weeks (2 months); although **Eylea** may

be dosed as frequently as 2 mg every 4 weeks (monthly), additional efficacy has not been demonstrated; *Age-related Macular Degeneration (AMD):* although not as effective as the every 8 week dosing regimen, patients with AMD may also be treated with one dose every 12 weeks after one year of effective therapy; must only be administered by a qualified physician
Pediatric: <18 years: not established; ≥18 years: same as adult

    Eylea *(aflibercept)* **Injection** *Vial:* 40 mg/ml solution for intravitreal injection, single-use
    Comment: **Eylea** *(aflibercept)* is indicated for the treatment of patients with neovascular (wet) age-related macular degeneration, macular edema following retinal vein occlusion, diabetic macular edema, and diabetic retinopathy. It is designed to block the growth of new blood vessels and decrease the ability of fluid to pass through blood vessels (vascular permeability) in the eye by blocking VEGF-A and placental growth factor (PLGF), two growth factors involved in angiogenesis.

▶ *ranibizumab* **(D)**
Pediatric: <18 years: not established; ≥18 years: same as adult
    DR: Diabetic retinopathy: Intravitreal: 0.3 mg once a month (approximately every 28 days)
    DME: Diabetic macular edema: Intravitreal: 0.3 mg once a month (approximately every 28 days); in clinical trials, monthly doses of 0.5 mg were also studied
    AMD: Neovascular (wet) Age-related Macular Degeneration: Intravitreal: 0.5 mg once a month (approximately every 28 days). Frequency may be reduced (e.g., 4 to 5 injections over 9 months) after the first 3 injections or may be reduced after the first 4 injections to once every 3 months if monthly injections are not feasible. *Note:* A regimen averaging 4 to 5 doses over 9 months is expected to maintain visual acuity and an every 3-month dosing regimen has reportedly resulted in a ~5 letter (1 line) loss of visual acuity over 9 months, as compared to monthly dosing which may result in an additional ~1 to 2 letter gain
    RVO: macular edema following retinal vein occlusion: Intravitreal: 0.5 mg once a month (approximately every 28 days)
    mCNV: myopic choroidal neovascularization: Intravitreal: 0.5 mg once a month (approximately every 28 days) for up to 3 months; may re-treat if necessary
    Lucentis *Prefilled Syringe:* 0.3 mg/0.05 ml (0.05 ml); 0.5 mg/0.05 ml (0.05 ml); single-use for intravitreal injection (preservative free); *Vial:* 10 mg/ml (**Lucentis** 0.5 mg); 6 mg/ml solution (**Lucentis** 0.3 mg); single-use; a 5-micron sterile filter needle (19 gauge x 1½ inch) is required for preparation, but not included; keep refrigerated; do not freeze; protect vial from light; see mfr pkg insert for other precautions

Comment: *ranibizumab* is a recombinant humanized monoclonal antibody fragment which binds to and inhibits human vascular endothelial growth factor A (VEGF-A). **Lucentis** inhibits VEGF from binding to its receptors and thereby suppressing neovascularization and slowing vision loss. Contraindications include ocular or periocular infection, and active intraocular inflammation. For ophthalmic intravitreal injection only. Each vial or prefilled syringe should only be used for the treatment of a single eye. If the contralateral eye requires treatment, a new vial or prefilled syringe should be used and the sterile field, syringe, gloves, drapes, eyelid speculum, filter, and injection needles should be changed before **Lucentis** is administered to the other eye. Adequate anesthesia and a topical broad-spectrum antimicrobial agent should be administered prior to the procedure. Refer to manufacturer labeling for additional detailed information. Based on its mechanism of action, adverse effects on pregnancy would be expected. Information related to use in pregnancy is limited. The intravitreal injection procedure should be carried out under controlled aseptic conditions, which include the use of sterile gloves, a sterile drape, and a sterile eyelid speculum (or equivalent). Adequate anesthesia and a broad-spectrum microbicide should be given prior to the injection. Prior to and 30 minutes following the intravitreal injection, patients should be monitored for elevation in intraocular pressure using tonometry. Each prefilled syringe or vial should only be used for the treatment of a single eye. If the contralateral eye requires treatment, a new prefilled syringe or vial should be used and the sterile field, syringe, gloves, drapes, eyelid speculum, filter needle (vial only), and injection needles should be changed.

REFERENCE

Solomon, S. D., Chew, E., Duh, E. J., Sobrin, L., Sun, J. K., VanderBeek, B. L., . . . Gardner, T. W. (2017). Diabetic retinopathy: A position statement by the American Diabetes Association. *Diabetes Care, 40*(3), 412–418. doi:10.2337/dc16-2641

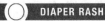 **DIAPER RASH**

Topical Corticosteroids *see page 574*
Comment: Low to intermediate potency topical corticosteroids are indicated if inflammation is present.

BARRIER AGENTS

▷ *aloe+vitamin e+zinc oxide* ointment apply at each diaper change after thoroughly cleansing skin
   Balmex *Oint:* 2, 4 oz tube; 16 oz jar
▷ *vitamin a and e* (G) ointment apply at each diaper change after thoroughly cleansing skin
   A&D Ointment *Oint:* 1.5, 4 oz
▷ *zinc oxide* (G) cream and ointment apply at each diaper change after thoroughly cleansing the skin
   A&D Ointment with Zinc Oxide *Oint:* 10% (1.5, 4 oz)
   Desitin *Oint:* 40% (1, 2, 4, 9 oz)
   Desitin Cream *Crm:* 10% (2, 4 oz)

TOPICAL ANTIFUNGALS

Comment: Use if caused by *Candida albicans*.
▷ *butenafine* (B)(G) apply bid x 1 week <u>or</u> once daily x 4 weeks
   Pediatric: <12 years: not recommended; ≥12 years: same as adult
   Lotrimin Ultra (C)(OTC) *Crm:* 1% (12, 24 gm)
   Mentax *Crm:* 1% (15, 30 gm)
   Comment: *butenafine* is a benzylamine, not an azole. Fungicidal activity continues for at least 5 weeks after last application.
▷ *clotrimazole* (B) apply to affected area bid x 7 days
   Pediatric: same as adult
   Lotrimin (OTC) *Crm:* 1% (15, 30, 45 gm)
   Lotrimin AF (OTC) *Crm:* 1% (12 gm); *Lotn:* 1% (10 ml); *Soln:* 1% (10 ml)
▷ *econazole* (C) apply bid x 7 days
   Spectazole *Crm:* 1% (15, 30, 85 gm)
▷ *ketoconazole* (C)(G)
   Nizoral Cream *Crm:* 2% (15, 30, 60 gm)
▷ *miconazole* 2% (C)(G) apply bid x 7 days
   Pediatric: same as adult
   Lotrimin AF Spray Liquid (OTC) *Spray liq:* 2% (113 gm) (alcohol 17%)
   Lotrimin AF Spray Powder (OTC) *Spray pwdr:* 2% (90 gm) (alcohol 10%)
   Monistat-Derm *Crm:* 2% (1, 3 oz); *Spray liq:* 2% (3.5 oz); *Spray pwdr:* 2% (3 oz)
▷ *nystatin* (C)(G) apply bid x 7 days
   Mycostatin *Crm:* 100,000 U/gm (15, 30 gm)

COMBINATION AGENT

▷ *clotrimazole+betamethasone* (C)(G) cream apply bid x 7 days
   Lotrisone *Crm:* 15, 45 g

 DIARRHEA: ACUTE

▷ *attapulgite* (C)
   Donnagel (OTC) 30 ml after each loose stool; max 7 doses/day x 2 days
   Pediatric: <3 years: not recommended; 3-6 years: 7.5 ml; >6-12 years: 15 ml; >12 years: same as adult
      Liq: 600 mg/15 ml (120, 240 ml)
   Donnagel Chewable Tab (OTC) 2 tabs after each loose stool; max 14 tabs/day
   Pediatric: <3 years: not recommended; 3-6 years: 1/2 tab after each loose stool; max 7 doses/day; >6-12 years: 1 tab after each loose stool; max 7 tabs/day
      Chew tab: 600 mg
   Kaopectate (OTC) 30 ml after each loose stool; max 7 doses/day x 2 days
   Pediatric: <3 years: not recommended; 3-6 years: 7.5 ml after each loose stool; >6-12 years: 15 ml after each loose stool; >12 years: same as adult
      Liq: 600 mg/15 ml (120, 240 ml)

▷ *bismuth subsalicylate* (C; D in 3rd)(G)

    Pepto-Bismol (OTC) 2 tabs or 30 ml q 30-60 minutes as needed; max 8 doses/day

    Pediatric: <3 years (14-18 lb): 2.5 ml q 4 hours; max 6 doses/day; <3 years (18-28 lb): 5 ml q 4 hours; max 6 doses/day; 3-6 years: 1/3 tab or 5 ml q 30-60 minutes; max 8 doses/day; >6-9 years: 2/3 tab or 10 ml q 30-60 minutes; max 8 doses/day; >9-12 years: 1 tab or 15 ml q 30-60 minutes; max 8 doses/day

    Chew tab: 262 mg; *Liq:* 262 mg/15 ml (4, 8, 12, 16 oz)

    Pepto-Bismol Maximum Strength (OTC) 30 ml q 60 minutes; max 4 doses/day

    Pediatric: <3 years: not recommended; 3-6 years: 5 ml q 60 minutes; max 4 doses/day; >6-9 years: 10 ml q 60 minutes; max 4 doses/day; >9-12 years: 15 ml q 60 minutes; max 4 doses/day

    Liq: 525 mg/15 ml (4, 8, 12, 16 oz)

Comment: *aspirin*-containing medications are contraindicated with history of allergic-type reaction to *aspirin*, children and adolescents with *Varicella* or other viral illness, and 3rd trimester of pregnancy.

▷ *calcium polycarbophil* (C)

    Pediatric: <6 years: not recommended; 6-12 years: 1 tab daily qid; >12 years: same as adult

    Fibercon (OTC) 2 tabs daily qid

    Cplt: 625 mg

▷ *crofelemer* (C) 2 tabs once daily; swallow whole with or without food; do not crush or chew

    Pediatric: <12 years: not established; ≥12 years: same as adult

    Mytesi *Tab:* 125 mg del-rel

Comment: *crofelemer* is indicated for the symptomatic relief of non-infectious diarrhea in adult patients with HIV/AIDS on antiretroviral therapy.

▷ *difenoxin+atropine* (C)

    Pediatric: <2 years: not recommended; ≥2 years: same as adult

    Motofen 2 tabs, then 1 tab after each loose stool or 1 tab q 3-4 hours as needed; max 8 tab/day x 2 days

    Tab: dif 1 mg+atro 0.025 mg

▷ *diphenoxylate+atropine* (C)(V)(G)

    Pediatric: <2 years: not recommended; 2-12 years: initially 0.3-0.4 mg/kg/day in 4 divided doses; >12 years: same as adult

    Lomotil 2 tabs or 10 ml qid until diarrhea is controlled

    Tab: diphen 2.5 mg+atrop 0.025 mg; *Liq:* diphen 2.5 mg+atrop 0.025 mg per 5 ml (2 oz)

▷ *loperamide* (B)(OTC)(G)

    Imodium 4 mg initially, then 2 mg after each loose stool; max 16 mg/day x 2 days

    Pediatric: <5 years: not recommended; ≥5 years: same as adult

    Cap: 2 mg

    Imodium A-D 4 mg initially, then 2 mg after each loose stool; usual max 8 mg/day x 2 days

    Pediatric: <2 years: not recommended; 2-5 years (24-47 lb): 1 mg up to tid x 2 days; 6-8 years (48-59 lb): 2 mg initially, then 1 mg after each loose stool; max 4 mg/day x 2 days; 9-11 years (60-95 lb): 2 mg initially, then 1 mg after each loose stool; max 6 mg/day x 2 days

    Cplt: 2 mg; *Liq:* 1 mg/5 ml (2, 4 oz) (cherry-mint) (alcohol 0.5%)

▷ *loperamide+simethicone* (B)(OTC)(G)

    Imodium Advanced 2 tabs chewed after loose stool, then 1 after the next loose stool; max 4 tabs/day

    Pediatric: 6-8 years: chew 1 tab after loose stool, then chew 1/2 tab after next loose stool; 9-11 years: chew 1 tab after loose stool, then chew 1/2 tab after next loose stool; max 3 tabs/day; ≥12 years: same as adult

    Chew tab: loper 2 mg+simeth 125 mg (vanilla-mint)

ORAL REHYDRATION AND ELECTROLYTE REPLACEMENT THERAPY

▷ *oral electrolyte replacement* (OTC)

    CeraLyte 50 dissolve in 8 oz water

    Pediatric: <4 years: not indicated; ≥4 years, same as adult

    Pkt: sodium 50 mEq+potassium 20 mEq+chloride 40 mEq+citrate 30 mEq+rice syrup solids 40 gm+calories 190 per liter (mixed berry) (gluten-free)

    CeraLyte 70 dissolved in 8 oz water

    Pediatric: <4 years: not indicated; ≥4 years: same as adult

Pkt: sodium 70 mEq+potassium 20 mEq+chloride 60 mEq+citrate 30 mEq+rice syrup solids 40 gm+calories 165 per liter (natural, lemon) (gluten-free)

KaoLectrolyte 1 pkt dissolved in 8 oz water q 3-4 hours
Pediatric: <2 years: not indicated; ≥2 years: same as adult
Pkt: sodium 12 mEq+potassium 5 mEq+chloride 10 mEq+citrate 7 mEq+ dextrose 5 gm+calories 22 per 6.2 gm

Pedialyte
Pediatric: <2 years: as desired and as tolerated; ≥2 years: 1-2 L/day
Oral soln: dextrose 20 gm+fructose 5 gm+sodium 25 mEq+potassium 20 mEq+chloride 35 mEq+citrate 30 mEq+calories 100 per liter (8 oz, 1 L)

Pedialyte Freezer Pops
Pediatric: as desired and as tolerated
Pops: dextrose 1.6 gm+sodium 2.8 mEq+potassium 1.25 mEq+chloride 2.2 mEq+citrate 1.88 mEq+calories 6.25 per 6.25 ml pop (8 oz, 1 L)

 DIARRHEA: CARCINOID SYNDROME (CSD)

TRIPTOPHAN HYDROXYLASE

▷ *telotristat* take with food; 250 mg tid
Pediatric: <18 years: not established; ≥18 years: same as adult
Xermelo *Tab:* 250 mg (4 x 7 daily dose pcks/carton)
Comment: Take **Xermelo** in combination with somatostatin analog (SSA) therapy to treat patients inadequately controlled by SSA therapy. Breastfeeding females should monitor the infant for constipation. ESRD requiring dialysis not studied.

 DIARRHEA: CHRONIC

▷ *cholestyramine* (C)
Questran Powder for Oral Suspension initially 1 pkt or scoop daily; usual maintenance 2-4 pkts or scoops daily in 2 doses; max 6 pkts or scoops daily
Oral pwdr: 9 gm pkts; 9 gm equal 4 gm *anhydrous cholestyramine resin* (60/pck); *Bulk can:* 378 gm w. scoop
Questran Light initially 1 pkt or scoop daily; usual maintenance 2-4 pkts or scoops daily in 2 doses
Light: 5 gm pkts; 5 gm equals 4 gm *anhydrous cholestyramine resin* (60/pck); *Bulk can:* 210 gm w. scoop
Comment: Use *cholestyramine* only if diarrhea is due to bile salt malabsorption.

▷ *crofelemer* (C) 2 tabs once daily; swallow whole with or without food; do not crush or chew
Pediatric: <12 years: not established; ≥12 years: same as adult
Mytesi *Tab:* 125 mg del-rel
Comment: *crofelemer* is indicated for the symptomatic relief of non-infectious diarrhea in adult patients with HIV/AIDS on antiretroviral therapy.

▷ *difenoxin+atropine* (C) 2 tabs, then 1 tab after each loose stool or 1 tab q 3-4 hours prn; max 8 tab/day x 2 days
Pediatric: <2 years: not recommended; ≥2 years: same as adult
Motofen *Tab:* dif 1 mg+atrop 0.025 mg

▷ *diphenoxylate+atropine* (B)(V)(G)
Pediatric: <2 years: not recommended; 2-12 years: initially 0.3-0.4 mg/kg/day in 4 divided doses; >12 years: same as adult
Lomotil 5-20 mg/day in divided doses
Tab: diphen 2.5 mg+atrop 0.025 mg; *Liq:* diphen 2.5 mg+atrop 0.025 mg per 5 ml (2 oz w. dropper)

▷ *attapulgite* (C)(G)
Donnagel (OTC) 30 ml after each loose stool; max 7 doses/day
Pediatric: <2 years: not recommended; 2-6 years: 7.5 ml after each loose stool; >6 years: same as adult
Liq: 600 mg/15 ml (120, 240 ml)
Donnagel Chewable Tab 2 tabs after each loose stool; max 14 tabs/day
Pediatric: <3 years: not recommended; 3-6 years: 1/2 tab after each stool; max 7 doses/day; >6-12 years: 1 tab after each loose stool; max 7 tabs/day; >12 years: same as adult

▷ *loperamide* (B)(OTC)(G)
Imodium (OTC) 4-16 mg/day in divided doses
Pediatric: <5 years: not recommended; ≥5 years: same as adult
Cap: 2 mg
Imodium A-D (OTC) 4-16 mg/day in divided doses
Pediatric: <2 years: not recommended; 2-5 years (24-47 lb): 1 mg up to tid x 2 days; 6-8 years (48-59 lb): 2 mg initially, then 1 mg after each loose stool; max 4 mg/day x 2 days; 9-11 years (60-95 lb): 2 mg initially, then 1 mg after each loose stool; max 6 mg/day x 2 days; ≥12 years: same as adult
Cplt: 2 mg; *Liq:* 1 mg/5 ml (2, 4 oz)
▷ *loperamide+simethicone* (B)(OTC)(G)
Imodium Advanced 2 tabs chewed after loose stool, then 1 after the next loose stool; max 4 tabs/day
Pediatric: 6-8 years: chew 1 tab after loose stool, then chew 1/2 tab after next loose stool; 9-11 years: chew 1 tab after loose stool, then chew 1/2 tab after next loose stool; max 3 tabs/day
Chew tab: loper 2 mg+simeth 125 mg

DIARRHEA: TRAVELERS'

Comment: Travelers' diarrhea is the most common travel-related illness, affecting an estimated 10-40% of travelers worldwide each year. Travelers' diarrhea is defined by having ≥3 unformed stools in 24 hours, in a person who is traveling. It is caused by a variety of pathogens, but most commonly bacteria found in food and water. The highest-risk destinations are in most of Asia as well as the Middle East, Africa, Mexico, and Central and South America.

ANTI-INFECTIVES

▷ *ciprofloxacin* (C) 500 mg bid x 3 days
Pediatric: <18 years: not recommended; ≥18 years: same as adult
Cipro (G) *Tab:* 250, 500, 750 mg; *Oral susp:* 250, 500 mg/5 ml (100 ml) (strawberry)
Cipro XR *Tab:* 500, 1000 mg ext-rel
ProQuin XR *Tab:* 500 mg ext-rel
▷ *rifamycin* (C) take 388 mg (2 x 194 mg tabs) bid x 3 days; may be taken with or without food; swallow whole; do not crush, break, or chew; contraindicated with concomitant alcohol; discontinue if diarrhea worsens or persists more than 24 hours; not for use if diarrhea is accompanied by fever or blood in the stool or if causative organism other than *E. coli* is suspected
Pediatric: <18 years: not recommended; ≥18 years: same as adult
Aemcolo *Tab:* 194 mg del-rel
Comment: FDA-approved in November, 2018, **Aemcolo** *(rifamycin)* is an antibacterial drug indicated for the treatment of adult patients with traveler's diarrhea caused by noninvasive strains of *Escherichia coli* (*E. coli*), not complicated by fever or blood in the stool. **Aemcolo** is a broad spectrum, semi-synthetic, orally administered, minimally absorbed antibiotic. Mechanism of action is inhibition of bacterial DAN-dependent RNA synthesis. **Aemcolo** has the potential to be used for the treatment of other bacterial infections of the colon, such as infectious colitis, *Clostridium difficile*-associated disease, diverticulitis and also as supportive treatment of inflammatory bowel diseases and hepatic encephalopathy. **Aemcolo** should not be used in patients with a known hyper-sensitivity to *rifamycin* or any of the other *rifamycin*-class antimicrobial agents (e.g. *rifaximin*). Most common adverse reactions (incidence > 2%) have been headache and constipation. There are no available data on **Aemcolo** use in pregnancy to inform any drug-associated risks for major birth defects, miscarriage, or adverse maternal or fetal outcomes. Systemic absorption of **Aemcolo** in humans is negligible; however, there is no information regarding the presence of **Aemcolo** in human milk, the effects on the breastfed infant.
▷ *rifaximin* (C) 200 mg tid x 3 days; discontinue if diarrhea worsens or persists more than 24 hours; not for use if diarrhea is accompanied by fever or blood in the stool or if causative organism other than *E. coli* is suspected
Pediatric: <12 years: not recommended; ≥12 years: same as adult
Xifaxan *Tab:* 200 mg

▷ *trimethoprim+sulfamethoxazole (TMP-SMX)* **(C)(G)** bid x 10 days
  Pediatric: <2 months: not recommended; ≥2 months: 40 mg/kg/day of *sulfamethoxazole* in 2 divided doses x 10 days; *see page 630 for dose by weight*
  Bactrim, Septra 2 tabs bid x 10 days
    Tab: trim 80 mg+sulfa 400 mg*
  Bactrim DS, Septra DS 1 tab bid x 10 days
    Tab: trim 160 mg+sulfa 800 mg*
  Bactrim Pediatric Suspension, Septra Pediatric Suspension
    Oral susp: trim 40 mg+sulfa 200 mg per 5 ml (100 ml) (cherry) (alcohol 0.3%)
  Comment: Sulfonamides are contraindicated in the first trimester of pregnancy, the final month of pregnancy, and infants <8 weeks-of-age. *CrCl 15-30 mL/min:* reduce dose by 1/2; *CrCl <15 mL/min:* not recommended. Contraindicated with G6PD deficiency. A high fluid intake is indicated during sulfonamide therapy to avoid crystallization in the kidneys.

DIGITALIS TOXICITY

Comment: The digitalis therapeutic index is narrow, 0.8-1.2 ng/mL. Whether acute or chronic toxicity, the patient should be treated in the emergency department and/or admitted to in-patient service for continued monitoring and care. Signs and symptoms of digitalis toxicity include: loss of appetite, nausea, vomiting, abdominal pain, diarrhea, visual disturbances (diplopia, blurred, or yellow vision, yellow-green halos around lights and other visual images, spots, blind spots), decreased urine output, generalized edema, orthopnea, confusion, delirium, decreased consciousness, potentially lethal cardiac arrhythmias (ranging from ventricular tachycardia (VT) and ventricular fibrillation (VF) to sino-atrial heart block AVB). Treatment measures include repeated doses of charcoal via NG tube administered after gastric lavage for acute ingestion (methods to induce vomiting are usually discouraged because vomiting can worsen bradyarrhythmias), digitalis binders. Monitoring includes: serial ECGs, serum digitalis level, chemistries, potassium (hyperkalemia), magnesium (hypomagnesemia), BUN and creatinine.

DIGOXIN BINDER

▷ *digoxin (immune fab [ovine])* **(B)**
  Digibind contents of one vial of **Digibind** neutralizes 0.5 mg digoxin; dose based on amount of *digoxin* or *digitoxin* to be neutralized; see mfr pkg insert
  Pediatric: see mfr pkg insert
    Vial: 38 mg
  Digifab dose is based on amount of digoxin or digitoxin to be neutralized (see mfr pkg insert for dosage; contents of 1 vial neutralizes 0.5 mg digoxin.
  Pediatric: see mfr pkg insert
    Vial: 40 mg for IV injection after reconstitution (preservative-free)

DIPHTHERIA (*CORYNEBACTERIUM DIPHTHERIAE*)

Prophylaxis *see Childhood Immunizations page 557*

POST-EXPOSURE PROPHYLAXIS FOR NON-IMMUNIZED PERSONS

▷ *erythromycin base* **(B)(G)** 500 mg qid x 14 days
  Pediatric: <45 kg: 50 mg/kg/day in 4 divided doses x 14 days; ≥45 kg: same as adult
  Ery-Tab *Tab:* 250, 333, 500 mg ent-coat
  PCE *Tab:* 333, 500 mg
  Comment: *erythromycin* may increase INR with concomitant *warfarin*, as well as increase serum level of *digoxin*, benzodiazepines, and statins.
▷ *erythromycin ethylsuccinate* **(B)(G)** 400 mg qid x 14 days
  Pediatric: 30-50 mg/kg/day in 4 divided doses x 14 days; may double dose with severe infection; max 100 mg/kg/day; *see page 626 for dose by weight*
  EryPed *Oral susp:* 200 mg/5 ml (100, 200 ml) (fruit); 400 mg/5 ml (60, 100, 200 ml) (banana); *Oral drops:* 200, 400 mg/5 ml (50 ml) (fruit); *Chew tab:* 200 mg wafer (fruit)
  E.E.S. *Oral susp:* 200, 400 mg/5 ml (100 ml) (fruit)
  E.E.S. Granules *Oral susp:* 200 mg/5 ml (100, 200 ml) (cherry)
  E.E.S. 400 Tablets *Tab:* 400 mg

Comment: *erythromycin* may increase INR with concomitant *warfarin*, as well as increase serum level of *digoxin*, benzodiazepines, and statins.
▷ *Immunization Series*
    See *Childhood Immunizations* page 557

POST-EXPOSURE PROPHYLAXIS FOR IMMUNIZED PERSONS
▷ *Diphtheria* immunization booster

 DIVERTICULITIS

ANTI-INFECTIVES
▷ *amoxicillin* (B)(G) 500 mg q 8 hours <u>or</u> 875 mg q 12 hours x 7 days
    Amoxil *Cap:* 250, 500 mg; *Tab:* 875*mg; *Chew tab:* 125, 200, 250, 400 mg (cherry-banana-peppermint) (phenylalanine); *Oral susp:* 125, 250 mg/5 ml (80, 100, 150 ml) (strawberry); 200, 400 mg/5 ml (50, 75, 100 ml) (bubble gum); *Oral drops:* 50 mg/ml (30 ml) (bubble gum)
    Moxatag *Tab:* 775 mg ext-rel
    Trimox *Tab:* 125, 250 mg; *Cap:* 250, 500 mg; *Oral susp:* 125, 250 mg/5 ml (80, 100, 150 ml) (raspberry-strawberry)
▷ *amoxicillin+clavulanate* (B)(G)
    Augmentin 500 mg tid or 875 mg bid x 7-10 days
    Pediatric: 40-45 mg/kg/day divided tid x 10 days or 90 mg/kg/day divided bid x 10 days *see pages 618 for dose by weight*
        Tab: 250, 500, 875 mg; *Chew tab:* 125, 250 mg (lemon-lime); 200, 400 mg (cherry-banana) (phenylalanine); *Oral susp:* 125 mg/5 ml (banana), 250 mg/5 ml (75, 100, 150 ml) (orange); 200, 400 mg/5 ml (50, 75, 100 ml) (orange) (phenylalanine)
    Augmentin ES-600 not recommended for adults
    Pediatric: <3 months: not recommended; ≥3 months, <40 kg: 90 mg/kg/day in 2 divided doses x 7-10 days; ≥40 kg: not recommended
        Oral susp: 42.9 mg/5 ml (50, 75, 100, 125, 150, 200 ml) (strawberry cream) (phenylalanine)
    Augmentin XR 2 tabs q 12 hours x 7-10 days
    Pediatric: <16 years: use other forms; ≥16 years: same as adult
        Tab: 1000*mg ext-rel
▷ *ciprofloxacin* (C) 500 mg bid x 7 days
    Cipro (G) *Tab:* 250, 500, 750 mg; *Oral susp:* 250, 500 mg/5 ml (100 ml) (strawberry)
    Cipro XR *Tab:* 500, 1000 mg ext-rel
    ProQuin XR *Tab:* 500 mg ext-rel
▷ *metronidazole* (not for use in 1st; B in 2nd, 3rd)(G) 250-500 mg q 8 hours <u>or</u> 750 mg q 12 hours x 7 days
    Flagyl *Tab:* 250*, 500*mg
    Flagyl 375 *Cap:* 375 mg
    Flagyl ER *Tab:* 750 mg ext-rel
▷ *trimethoprim+sulfamethoxazole (TMP-SMX)* (D)(G) bid x 7 days
    Bactrim, Septra 2 tabs bid x 7 days
        Tab: trim 80 mg+sulfa 400 mg*
    Bactrim DS, Septra DS 1 tab bid x 7 days
        Tab: trim 160 mg+sulfa 800 mg*
    Bactrim Pediatric Suspension, Septra Pediatric Suspension 20 ml bid x 7 days
        Oral susp: trim 40 mg+sulfa 200 mg per 5 ml (100 ml) (cherry) (alcohol 0.3%)
Comment: Sulfonamides are contraindicated in the first trimester of pregnancy, the final month of pregnancy, and infants <8 weeks-of-age. *CrCl 15-30 mL/min:* reduce dose by 1/2; *CrCl <15 mL/min:* not recommended. Contraindicated with G6PD deficiency. A high fluid intake is indicated during sulfonamide therapy to avoid crystallization in the kidneys.

 DIVERTICULOSIS

BULK-PRODUCING AGENTS
See *Constipation* page 103

DRY EYE SYNDROME (KERATOCONJUNCTIVITIS SICCA)

▷ **lifitegrast** instill 1 drop in each eye twice daily q 12 hours; use one single-use container to dose both eyes and discard unused portion; contacts may be reinserted after 15 minutes
Pediatric: <17 years: not recommended; ≥17 years: same as adult

   Xiidra *Ophth soln* 5% (50 mg/ml) (foil pouch containing 5 low density polyethylene 0.2 mL single-use containers, 60 single-use containers/carton) (preservative-free)
   Comment: The exact mechanism of action of **lifitegrast** in dry eye disease is *not* known. However, it is known *that lifitegrast* binds to the integrin lymphocyte function-associated antigen-1 (LFA-1), a cell surface protein found on leukocytes and blocks the interaction of LFA-1 with its cognate ligand intercellular adhesion molecule-1 (ICAM-1). ICAM-1 may be overexpressed in corneal and conjunctival tissues in dry eye disease. LFA-1/ICAM-1 interaction can contribute to the formation of an immunological synapse resulting in T-cell activation and migration to target tissues. *In vitro* studies demonstrated that lifitegrast may inhibit T-cell adhesion to ICAM-1 in a human T-cell line and may inhibit secretion of inflammatory cytokines in human peripheral blood mononuclear cells.

OPHTHALMIC IMMUNOMODULATOR/ANTI-INFLAMMATORY

Comment: Ophthalmic immunomodulators are contraindicated with active ocular infection. Allow at least 15 minutes between doses of artificial tears. May re-insert contact lenses 15 minutes after treatment.

▷ **cyclosporine** (C) using 1 single-use disposable vial, instill 1 drop in each eye twice daily q 12 hours
Pediatric: <16 years: not recommended; ≥16 years: same as adult

   Cequa *Ophth soln:* 0.09% single-use vials (0.25 ml, 6 pouches, 10 vials/pouch per carton) (preservative-free)
   Comment: **Cequa** ophthalmic solution is a calcineurin inhibitor immune-suppressant indicated to increase tear production in patients with kerato-conjunctivitis sicca. It is the first cyclosporine product to utilize nano-micellar technology, facilitating the drug molecule to penetrate the eye's aqueous layer, and preventing the release of active lipophilic molecule prior to penetration.
   Restasis *Ophth emul:* 0.05% (0.4 ml) (preservative-free)

OCULAR LUBRICANTS

Comment: Remove contact lens prior to using an ocular lubricant.
▷ **dextran 70+hypromellose** 1-2 drops prn
Pediatric: same as adult
   Bion Tears (OTC) *Ophth soln:* single-use containers (28/pck) (preservative-free)
▷ **hydroxypropyl cellulose** apply 1/2 inch ribbon or 1 insert in each inferior cul-de-sac 1-2 x/day prn
Pediatric: same as adult
   Lacrisert *Ophth inserts:* 5 mg (60/pck) (preservative-free)
   Hypotears Ophthalmic Ointment (OTC) *Ophth oint:* 1% (3.5 gm) (preservative-free)
   Comment: Place insert in the inferior cul-de-sac of the eye, beneath the base of the tarsus, not in apposition to the cornea nor beneath the eyelid at the level of the tarsal plate.
▷ **hydroxypropyl methylcellulose** 1-2 drops prn
Pediatric: same as adult
   GenTeal Mild, GenTeal Moderate (OTC) *Ophth soln:* (15 ml) (perborate)
   GenTeal Severe (OTC) *Ophth soln:* (15 ml) (carbopol 980, perborate)
▷ **petrolatum+mineral oil** apply 1/2 inch ribbon prn
Pediatric: same as adult
   Hypotears Ophthalmic Ointment (OTC) *Ophth oint:* 1% (3.5 gm) (benzalkonium chloride, alcohol 1%)
   Hypotears PF Ophthalmic Ointment (OTC) *Ophth oint:* 1% (3.5 gm) (preservative-free, alcohol 1%)
   Lacri-Lube (OTC) *Ophth oint:* 1% (3.5, 7 gm)
   Lacri-Lube NP (OTC) *Ophth oint:* 1% (0.7 gm, 24/pck) (preservative-free)
▷ **petrolatum+lanolin+mineral oil** apply 1/4 inch ribbon prn
Pediatric: same as adult
   Duratears Naturale (OTC) *Ophth oint:* 3.5 gm (preservative-free)

▷ *polyethylene glycol+glycerin+hydroxypropyl methylcellulose* 1-2 drops prn
  Pediatric: same as adult
      Visine Tears (OTC) *Ophth soln:* 1% (15, 30 ml)
▷ *polyethylene glycol* 400 0.4%+*propylene glycol* 0.3% 1-2 drops prn
  Pediatric: same as adult
      Systane (OTC) *Ophth soln:* (15, 30, 40 ml) (polyquaternium-1, zinc chloride); *Vial:* 0.01
      oz (28) (preservative-free)
      Systane Ultra (OTC) *Ophth soln:* (10, 20 ml) (aminomethylpropanol, polyquaterni-
      um-1, sorbitol (zinc chloride); *Vial:* 0.01 oz (24) (preservative-free)
▷ *polyvinyl alcohol* 1-2 drops prn
  Pediatric: same as adult
      Hypotears (OTC) *Ophth soln:* 1% (15, 30 ml)
      Hypotears PF (OTC) 1-2 drops q 3-4 hours prn
        Ophth soln: 1% (0.02 oz single-use containers, 30/pck) (preservative-free)
▷ *propylene glycol* 0.6% 1-2 drops prn
  Pediatric: same as adult
      Systane Balance (OTC) *Ophth soln:* (10 ml) (polyquaternium-1)

DUCHENNE MUSCULAR DYSTROPHY (DMD)

▷ *deflazacort* (B) 0.9 mg/kg/day administered once daily; take with <u>or</u> without food; may
  crush and mix with applesauce (then take immediately)
  Pediatric: <5 years: not established; ≥ 5 years: same as adult
      Emflaza *Tab:* 6, 18, 30, 36 mg; *Oral susp:* 22.75 mg/ml (13 ml)
      Comment: **Emflaza** is the first and only FDA-approved indicated for DMD
      to decrease inflammation and reduce the activity of the immune system. The
      side effects caused by **Emflaza** are similar to those experienced with other
      corticosteroids. The most common side effects include facial puffiness (cushingoid
      appearance), weight gain, increased appetite, upper respiratory tract infection,
      cough, extraordinary daytime urinary frequency (pollakiuria), hirsutism, and
      central obesity. Other side effects that are less common include problems with
      endocrine function, increased susceptibility to infection, elevation in blood
      pressure, risk of gastrointestinal perforation, serious skin rashes, behavioral and
      mood changes, decrease in the density of the bones and vision problems such as
      cataracts. Patients receiving immunosuppressive doses of corticosteroids should
      not be given live <u>or</u> live attenuated vaccines (LAVs). Moderate <u>or</u> strong CYP3A4
      inhibitors, give one third of the recommended dosage of **Emflaza**. Avoid use of
      moderate <u>or</u> strong CYP3A4 inducers with **Emflaza**, as they may reduce efficacy.
      Dosage must be decreased gradually if the drug has been administered for more
      than a few days. Use only the oral dispenser provided with the product. After
      withdrawing the appropriate dose into the oral dispenser, slowly add the oral
      suspension into 3 to 4 ounces of juice <u>or</u> milk and mix well and then the dose should
      then be administered immediately. Do not administer with grapefruit. Discard any
      unused **Emflaza** oral suspension remaining after 1 month of first opening the bottle.

REFERENCE

U.S. Food & Drug Administration. (2017). *FDA approves drug to treat Duchenne muscular dystrophy* [Press
    release]. Retrieved from https://www.fda.gov/NewsEvents/Newsroom/PressAnnouncements/ucm540945.htm

▷ *eteplirsen* 30 mg/kg via IV infusion over 35-60 minutes once weekly
  Pediatric: same as adult
      Exondys *Vial:* 100 mg/2 ml (50 mg/ml), 500 mg/10 ml
      Comment: **Exondys** is indicated for patients who have a confirmed mutation of the
      dystrophin gene amenable to exon 51 skipping (which affects about 13% of patients
      with DMD. There are <u>no</u> controlled data to inform safety in human pregnancy,
      lactation, <u>or</u> effects on the breastfed infant.

DUST MITE ALLERGY

ALLERGEN EXTRACT

▷ *dermatophagoides farinae+dermatophagoides pteronyssinus allergen extract* 1 tab SL
  daily; dissolves in 10 seconds; do not swallow for at least minute; the; *First Dose:* should be

administered under the supervision of a physician with experience in the diagnosis and treatment of allergic diseases and the patient should be observed in the office for at least 30 minutes; Prescribe auto-injectable epinephrine, instruct and train patients on its appropriate use, and instruct patients to seek immediate medical care upon its use

Pediatric: <18 years: not recommended; ≥18 years: same as adult

    Odactra *SL tab:* 12 SQ-HDM

    Comment: **Odactra** can cause life-threatening allergic reactions such as anaphylaxis and severe laryngopharyngeal restriction. **Odactra** may not be suitable for patients with certain underlying medical conditions that may reduce their ability to survive a serious allergic reaction. **Odactra** may not be suitable for patients who may be unresponsive to epinephrine or inhaled bronchodilators, such as those taking beta-blockers. Contraindications to **Odactra** include: severe, unstable or uncontrolled asthma; history of any severe systemic allergic reaction or any severe local reaction to sublingual allergen immunotherapy; history of eosinophilic esophagitis. The most common solicited adverse reactions reported in ≥10% of subjects treated with **Odactra** were throat irritation/tickle, itching in the mouth, itching in the ear, swelling of the uvula/back of the mouth, swelling of the lips, swelling of the tongue, nausea, tongue pain, throat swelling, tongue ulcer/sore on the tongue, stomach pain, mouth ulcer/sore in the mouth, and taste alteration/food tastes different. Available data on **Odactra** are insufficient to inform associated risks in pregnancy or effects on the breastfed infant. To report suspected adverse reactions, contact Merck Sharp & Dohme, a subsidiary of Merck at 1-877-888-4231 or FDA at 1-800-FDA-1088 or www.fda.gov/medwatch.

DYSFUNCTIONAL UTERINE BLEEDING (DUB)

NSAIDs *see page* 571
Opioid Analgesics *see Pain page* 354
Oral and Injectable Progesterone-only Contraceptives *page* 567
Combined Oral Contraceptives *page* 559

➢ *medroxyprogesterone acetate* **(X)** 10 mg daily x 10-13 days
    Provera *Tab:* 2.5, 5, 10 mg
➢ *combined oral contraceptive* **(X)** with 35 mcg estrogen equivalent

DYSHIDROSIS (DYSHIDROTIC ECZEMA, POMPHYLOX)

Topical Corticosteroids *see page* 574
Comment: Intermediate to high potency ophthalmic steroid treatment is indicated for dyshidrosis.

DYSLIPIDEMIA (HYPERCHOLESTEROLEMIA, HYPERLIPIDEMIA, MIXED DYSLIPIDEMIA)

Comment: As recommended by the American Heart, Lung, and Blood Institute, children and adolescents should be screened for dyslipidemia once between 9 and 11 years and once between 17 and 21 years.

OMEGA 3-FATTY ACID ETHYL ESTERS

Comment: *Vascepa, Lovaza,* and *Epanova* are indicated for the treatment of TG ≥500 mg/dL.

➢ *icosapent ethyl (omega 3-fatty acid ethyl ester of EPA)* **(C)** 2 caps bid with food; max 4 gm/day; swallow whole, do not crush or chew
    Pediatric: <18 years: not recommended; ≥18 years: same as adult
    Vascepa *sgc:* 0.5, 1 gm (α-tocopherol 4 mg/cap)
➢ *omega 3-acid ethyl esters* **(C)(G)** 2 gm bid or 4 gm once daily; swallow whole, do not crush or chew
    Pediatric: <18 years: not recommended; ≥18 years: same as adult
    Lovaza *Soft gel cap:* 1 gm (α-tocopherol 4 mg/cap)
    Epanova *Gelcap:* 1 gm

MICROSOMAL TRIGLYCERIDE-TRANSFER PROTEIN (MTP) INHIBITOR

▷ *lomitapide mesylate* (X) 10 mg daily
  Pediatric: <12 years: not established; ≥12 years: same as adult
   Juxtapid *Cap:* 5, 10, 20 mg
   Comment: **Juxtapid** is an adjunct to low-fat diet and other lipid-lowering treatments,
   including LDL apheresis where available, to reduce LDL-C, total cholesterol, apoB, and
   non-HDL-C in patients with homozygous familial hypercholesterolemia (HoFH); not
   for patients with hypercholesterolemia who do not have HoFH.

OLIGONUCLEOTIDE INHIBITOR OF APO B-100 SYNTHESIS

▷ *mipomersen* (B) administer 200 mg SC once weekly, on the same day, in the upper arm, abdomen, or thigh; administer 1st injection under appropriate professional supervision
  Pediatric: <12 years: not established; ≥12 years: same as adult
   Kynamro *Vial/Prefilled syringe:* 200 mg mg/ml soln for SC inj single-use vial (preservative-free)
   Comment: **Kynamro** is an adjunct to low-fat diet and other lipid-lowering treatments,
   to reduce LDL-C, apo-B, total cholesterol (TC), non-HDL-C in patients with
   homozygous familial hypercholesterolemia (HoFH).

CHOLESTEROL ABSORPTION INHIBITOR

▷ *ezetimibe* (C)(G) 10 mg daily
  Pediatric: <10 years: not recommended; ≥10 years: same as adult
   Zetia *Tab:* 10 mg
   Comment: *ezetimibe* is contraindicated with concomitant statins in liver disease, persistent
   elevations in serum transaminase, pregnancy, and nursing mothers. Concomitant fibrates
   are not recommended. Potentiated by *fenofibrate*, *gemfibrozil*, and possibly *cyclosporine*.
   Separate dosing of bile acid sequestrants is required; take *ezetimibe* at least 2 hours before
   or 4 hours after.

PROPROTEIN CONVERTASE SUBTILISIN KEXIN TYPE 9 (PCSK9) INHIBITOR

Comment: PCSK9 inhibitors are an adjunct to maximally tolerated statin therapy in persons
who require additional lowering of LDL-C. There is currently no information regarding the
use of PCSK9 inhibitors in pregnancy or the presence of PCSK9 inhibitors in human milk.
▷ *alirocumab* administer SC in the upper outer arm, abdomen, or thigh; initially 75 mg
  SC once every 2 weeks; measure LDL 4-8 weeks after initiation or titration; if inadequate
  response, may increase to 150 mg SC every 2 weeks or 300 mg SC once monthly
  Pediatric: <18 years: not established; ≥18 years: same as adult
   Praluent *Soln for SC inj:* 75, 150 mg/ml single-use prefilled syringe (preservative-free)
   Comment: The FDA has approved a new once-monthly 300 mg dosing option for
   Praluent injection, for the treatment of patients with high low-density lipoprotein
   (LDL) cholesterol. The drug is indicated as an adjunct to diet and statin therapy
   for patients with heterozygous familial hypercholesterolemia (HeFH) or clinical
   atherosclerotic cardiovascular disease (ASCVD) who require additional LDL lowering.
   The most common side effects of **Praluent** include injection site reactions, symptoms
   of the common cold, and flu-like symptoms. Each 150 mg pen delivers the dose over 20
   seconds. A 300 mg once monthly dose = administration of 2 x 150 mg pens. **Praluent** is
   contraindicated in the 2nd and 3rd trimester of pregnancy.
▷ *evolocumab* administer SC in the upper outer arm, elbow, or thigh; measure LDL 4-8 weeks
  after initiation; *HeFH or primary hyperlipidemia:* 140 mg SC once every 2 weeks or 420 mg
  once monthly; *HoFH:* 420 mg once monthly
  Pediatric: HeFH, primary hyperlipidemia: not established; HoFH: <13 years: not established; ≥13 years: same as adult
   Repatha *Soln for SC inj:* single-use prefilled syringe; 140 mg/syringe; single-use prefilled
   SureClick autoinjector (140 mg/syringe preservative-free)
   Comment: To achieve 420 mg of **Repatha**, administer 150 mg SC x 3 within
   30 minutes. Although **Repatha**, does not have an assigned pregnancy category, it is
   contraindicated in pregnancy.

HMG-COA REDUCTASE INHIBITORS (STATINS)

Comment: The statins decrease total cholesterol, LDL-C, TG, and apo-B, and increase
HDL-C. Before initiating and at 4-6 weeks, 3 months, and 6 months of therapy, check fasting

lipid profile and LFTs. Side effects include myopathy and increased liver enzymes. Relative contraindications include concomitant use of cyclosporine, a macrolide antibiotic, various oral antifungal agents, and CYP-450 inhibitors. An absolute contraindication is active or chronic liver disease.

▷ *atorvastatin* (X)(G) initially 10 mg daily; usual range 10-80 mg/day
  Pediatric: <10 years: not recommended; ≥10 years (female post-menarche): same as adult
    Lipitor *Tab*: 10, 20, 40, 80 mg
▷ *fluvastatin* (X)(G) initially 20-40 mg q HS; usual range 20-80 mg/day
  Pediatric: <18 years: not recommended; ≥18 years: same as adult
    Lescol *Cap*: 20, 40 mg
    Lescol XL *Tab*: 80 mg ext-rel
▷ *lovastatin* (X)
    Mevacor initially 20 mg daily at evening meal; may increase at 4-week intervals; max 80 mg/day in single or divided doses; if concomitant fibrates, *niacin,* or *CrCl <30 mL/min*, usual max 20 mg/day
    Pediatric: <10 years: not recommended; 10-17 years: initially 10-20 mg daily at evening meal; may increase at 4-week intervals; max 40 mg daily
      Tab: 10, 20, 40 mg
    Altoprev initially 20 mg daily at evening meal; may increase at 4-week intervals; max 60 mg/day; if concomitant fibrates, or *niacin*; >1 gm/day, usual max 40 mg/day; if concomitant *cyclosporine, amiodarone*, or *verapamil*, or *CrCl <30 mL/min*, usual max 20 mg/day
    Pediatric: <20 years: not recommended
      Tab: 10, 20, 40, 60 mg ext-rel
▷ *pitavastatin* (X)(G) initially 2 mg q HS; may increase to 4 mg after 4 weeks; max 4 mg/day; if concomitant *erythromycin* or *CrCl <60 ml/min;* 1 mg/day with usual max 2 mg/day; if concomitant rifampin, max 2 mg once daily
  Pediatric: <12 years: not established; ≥12 years: same as adult
    Livalo *Tab*: 1, 2, 4 mg
    Nikita *Tab*: 1, 2, 4 mg
    Zypitamag *Tab*: 1, 2, 4 mg
▷ *pravastatin* (X) initially 10-20 mg q HS; usual range 10-40 mg/day; may start at 40 mg/day
  Pediatric: <8 years: not recommended; 8-13 years: 20 mg daily; 14-18 years: 40 mg daily
    Pravachol *Tab*: 10, 20, 40, 80 mg
▷ *rosuvastatin* (X)(G) initially 10-20 mg q HS; usual range 5-40 mg/day; adjust at 4-week intervals
  Pediatric: <10 years: not recommended; 10-17 years: 5-20 mg/day; max 20 mg/day
    Crestor *Tab*: 5, 10, 20, 40 mg
▷ *simvastatin* (X) initially 20 mg q PM; usual range 5-80 mg/day; adjust at 4-week intervals
  Pediatric: <10 years: not recommended; ≥10 years (female post-menarche): same as adult
    Zocor *Tab*: 5, 10, 20, 40, 80 mg

CHOLESTEROL ABSORPTION INHIBITOR+HMG-COA REDUCTASE INHIBITOR COMBINATIONS

▷ *ezetimibe+atorvastatin* (X)(G) Take once daily in the PM; may start at 10/40; swallow whole, do not cut, crush, or chew
  Pediatric: <17 years: not recommended; ≥17 years: same as adult
    Tab: **Liptruzet 10/10** ezet 10 mg+atorva 10 mg
          Liptruzet 10/20 ezet 10 mg+atorva 20 mg
          Liptruzet 10/40 ezet 10 mg+atorva 40 mg
          Liptruzet 10/80 ezet 10 mg+atorva 80 mg
▷ *ezetimibe+simvastatin* (X)(G) Take once daily in the PM; may start at 10/40; swallow whole, do not cut, crush, or chew
  Pediatric: <17 years: not recommended; ≥17 years: same as adult
    Tab: **Vytorin 10/10** ezet 10 mg+simva 10 mg
          Vytorin 10/20 ezet 10 mg+simva 20 mg
          Vytorin 10/40 ezet 10 mg+simva 40 mg
          Vytorin 10/80 ezet 10 mg+simva 80 mg
  Comment: These agents decrease total cholesterol, LDL-C, and TG; increase HDL-C. They are indicated when the primary problem is very high TG level. Side effects include epigastric discomfort, dyspepsia, abdominal pain, cholelithiasis, myopathy, and

neutropenia. Before initiating, and at 4-6 weeks, 3 months, and 6 months of therapy, check fasting CBC, lipid profile, LFT, and serum creatinine. Absolute contraindications include severe renal disease and severe hepatic disease.

ISOBUTYRIC ACID DERIVATIVES

▷ *gemfibrozil* (C)(G) 600 mg bid 30 minutes before AM and PM meal
 Pediatric: <12 years: not recommended; ≥12 years: same as adult
   Lopid *Tab:* 600*mg

FIBRATES (FIBRIC ACID DERIVATIVES)

▷ *fenofibrate* (C)(G) take with meals; adjust at 4- to 8-week intervals; discontinue if inade-quate response after 2 months; lowest dose or contraindicated with renal impairment and the elderly
 Pediatric: <12 years: not recommended; ≥12 years: same as adult
   Antara 43-130 mg daily; max 130 mg/day
     Cap: 43, 87, 130 mg
   Fenoglide 40-120 mg daily; max 120 mg/day
     Tab: 40, 120 mg
   FibriCor 30-105 mg daily; max 105 mg/day
     Tab: 30, 105 mg
   TriCor 48-145 mg daily; max 145 mg/day
     Tab: 48, 145 mg
   TriLipix 45-135 mg daily; max 135 mg/day
     Cap: 45, 135 mg del-rel
   Lipofen 50-150 mg daily; max 150 mg/day
     Cap: 50, 150 mg
   Lofibra 67-200 mg daily; max 200 mg/day
     Tab: 67, 134, 200 mg

NICOTINIC ACID DERIVATIVES

Comment: Nicotinic acid derivatives decrease total cholesterol, LDL-C, and TG; increase HDL-C. Before initiating and at 4-6 weeks, 3 months, and 6 months of therapy, check fasting lipid profile, LFT, glucose, and uric acid. Side effects include hyperglycemia, upper GI distress, hyperuricemia, hepatotoxicity, and significant transient skin flushing. Take with food and take *aspirin* 325 mg 30 minutes before *niacin* dose to decrease flushing. *Relative contraindications:* diabetes, hyperuricemia (gout), and PUD Absolute contraindications severe gout and chronic liver disease.

▷ *niacin* (C)
   Niaspan (G) 375 mg daily for 1st week, then 500 mg daily for 2nd week, then 750 mg daily for 3rd week, then 1 gm daily for weeks 4-7; may increase by 500 mg q 4 weeks; usual range 1-2 gm/day; max 2 gm/day
 Pediatric: <21 years: not recommended; ≥21 years: same as adult
     Tab: 500, 750, 1000 mg ext-rel
   Slo-Niacin one 250 or 500 mg tab q AM or HS or one-half 750 mg tab q AM or HS
 Pediatric: <12 years: not recommended; ≥12 years: same as adult
     Tab: 250, 500, 750 mg cont-rel

BILE ACID SEQUESTRANTS

Comment: Bile acid sequestrants decrease total cholesterol, LDL-C, and increase HDL-C, but have no effect on triglycerides. A relative contraindication is TG ≥200 mg/dL and an absolute contraindication is TG ≥400 mg/dL. Before initiating and at 4-6 weeks, 3 months, and 6 months of therapy, check fasting lipid profile. Side effects include sandy taste in mouth, abdominal gas, abdominal cramping, and constipation. These agents decrease the absorption of many other drugs.

▷ *cholestyramine* (C)
 Pediatric: see mfr pkg insert
   Questran Powder for Oral Suspension initially 1 pkt or scoop daily; usual mainte-nance 2-4 pkts or scoops daily in 2 divided doses; max 6 pkts or scoops daily
     Pwdr: 9 gm pkts; 9 gm equals 4 gm anhydrous *cholestyramine* resin for reconstitu-tion (60/pck); *Bulk can:* 378 gm w. scoop

Questran Light initially 1 pkt or scoop daily; usual maintenance 2-4 pkts or scoops daily in 2 doses
   Light: 5 gm pkts; 5 gm equals 4 gm anhydrous *cholestyramine* resin (60/pck): *Bulk can:* 210 gm w. scoop
▷ *colesevelam* (B)(G)
WelChol recommended dose is 6 tablets once daily or 3 tablets twice daily; take with a meal and liquid
Pediatric: <10 years: not recommended; ≥10 years: same as adult
   Tab: 625 mg
WelChol for Oral Suspension recommended dose is one 3.75 gm packet once daily or one 1.875 gm packet twice daily; empty one packet into a glass or cup; add 1/2 to 1 cup (4 to 8 ounces) of water, fruit juice, or diet soft drink; stir well and drink immediately; do not swallow dry form; take with meals
Pediatric: <12 years: not established; ≥12 years: same as adult
   Pwdr: 3.75 gm/pkt (30 pkt/carton), 1.875 gm/pkt (60 pkt/carton) for oral suspension
Comment: **WelChol** is indicated as adjunctive therapy to improve glycemic control in adults with type 2 diabetes. It can be added to *metformin*, sulfonylureas, or insulin alone or in combination with other antidiabetic agents
▷ *colestipol* (C)
Comment: *colestipol* lowers LDL and total cholesterol.
Pediatric: <12 years: not recommended; ≥12 years: same as adult
   Colestid tabs: 2-16 gm daily in a single or divided doses; granules: 5-30 gm daily in a single or divided dose
      Tabs: 1 gm (120); *Granules:* unflavored: 5 gm pkt (30, 90/carton); unflavored bulk: 300, 500 gm w. scoop; orange-flavored: 7.5 gm pkt (60/carton) (aspartame); orange-flavored bulk: 450 gm w. scoop (aspartame) flavored: 7.5 gm pkt; flavored bulk: 450 gm w. scoop
   Colestid Tab initially 2 gm bid; increase by 2 gm bid at 1-2-month intervals; usual maintenance 2-16 gm/day
      Tab: 1 gm

ANTILIPID COMBINATIONS

Nicotinic Acid Derivative+HMG-CoA Reductase Inhibitors Combinations
Comment: Nicotinic acid derivatives decrease total cholesterol, LDL-C, and TG; increase HDL-C. Before initiating and at 4-6 weeks, 3 months, and 6 months of therapy, check fasting lipid profile, LFT, glucose, and uric acid. Side effects include hyperglycemia, upper GI distress, hyperuricemia, hepatotoxicity, and significant transient skin flushing. Take with food and take *aspirin* 325 mg 30 minutes before *niacin* dose to decrease flushing. Relative contraindications: diabetes, hyperuricemia (gout), and peptic ulcer disease (PUD). *Absolute contraindications:* severe gout and chronic liver disease.
▷ *niacin+lovastatin* (X)
Pediatric: <18 years: not recommended; ≥18 years: same as adult
   Advicor swallow whole at bedtime with a low-fat snack; may pretreat with aspirin; start at lowest niacin dose; may titrate niacin by no more than 500 mg/day every 4 weeks; max 2000/40 daily
      Tab: **Advicor 500/20** nia 500 mg ext-rel+lova 20 mg
         Advicor 750/20 nia 750 mg ext-rel+lova 20 mg
         Advicor 1000/20 nia 1000 mg ext-rel+lova 20 mg
         Advicor 1000/40 nia 1000 mg ext-rel+lova 40 mg
▷ *niacin+simvastatin* (X)
Pediatric: <18 years: not recommended; ≥18 years: same as adult
   Simcor swallow whole at bedtime with a low-fat snack; may pretreat with *aspirin*; to reduce niacin reaction. Start at lowest *niacin* dose; may titrate *niacin* by no more than 500 mg/day every 4 weeks; max 2000/40 daily; take *aspirin* 325 mg 30 minutes before dose to decrease niacin flushing
      Tab: **Simcor 500/20** nia 500 mg ext-rel+simva 20 mg
         Simcor 750/20 nia 750 mg ext-rel+simva 20 mg
         Simcor 1000/20 nia 1000 mg ext-rel+simva 20 mg
         Simcor 500/40 nia 500 mg ext-rel+simva 40 mg
         Simcor 1000/40 nia 1000 mg ext-rel+simva 40 mg

ANTIHYPERTENSIVE+ANTILIPID COMBINATIONS

Calcium Channel Blocker+HMG-CoA Reductase Inhibitor (Statin) Combinations

 amlodipine+atorvastatin (X)(G)

> **Caduet** select according to blood pressure and lipid values; titrate amlodipine over 7-14 days; titrate atorvastatin according to monitored lipid values; max amlodipine 10 mg/day and max atorvastatin 80 mg/day; refer to contraindications and precautions for CCB and statin therapy
>
> *Pediatric:* <10 years: not recommended; ≥10 years (female, post-menarche): same as adult
>
> *Tab:* **Caduet 5/10** amlo 5 mg+ator 10 mg
> **Caduet 5/20** amlo 5 mg+ator 20 mg
> **Caduet 5/40** amlo 5 mg+ator 40 mg
> **Caduet 5/80** amlo 5 mg+ator 80 mg
> **Caduet 10/10** amlo 10 mg+ator 10 mg
> **Caduet 10/20** amlo 10 mg+ator 20 mg
> **Caduet 10/40** amlo 10 mg+ator 40 mg
> **Caduet 10/80** amlo 10 mg+ator 80 mg

DYSMENORRHEA: PRIMARY

NSAIDs *see page* 571
Opioid Analgesics *see Pain page* 354
Combined Oral Contraceptives *see page* 559

BENZENEACETIC ACID DERIVATIVE

▷ *diclofenac* (C) 50-100 mg once; then 50 tid
Pediatric: <14 years: not recommended; ≥14 years: same as adult
> **Cataflam** *Tab:* 50 mg
> **Voltaren** *Tab:* 25, 50, 75 mg ent-coat
> **Voltaren-XR** *Tab:* 100 mg ext-rel

Comment: *diclofenac* is contraindicated with *aspirin* allergy and late (≥30 weeks) pregnancy.

FENAMATE

Comment: Avoid *aspirin* with a fenamate.
▷ *mefenamic acid* (C) 500 mg once; then 250 mg q 6 hours for up to 2-3 days; take with food
Pediatric: <14 years: not recommended; ≥14 years: same as adult
> **Ponstel** *Cap:* 250 mg

COX-2 INHIBITORS

Comment: Cox-2 inhibitors are contraindicated with history of asthma, urticaria, and allergic-type reactions to *aspirin*, other NSAIDs, and sulfonamides, 3rd trimester of pregnancy, and coronary artery bypass graft (CABG) surgery.
▷ *celecoxib* (C)(G) 400 mg x 1 dose; then 200 mg more on 1st day if needed; then 400 mg daily-bid; max 800 mg/day
Pediatric: <18 years: not recommended; ≥18 years: same as adult
> **Celebrex** *Cap:* 50, 100, 200, 400 mg
▷ *meloxicam* (C)(G)
> **Mobic** <2 years, <60 kg: not recommended; ≥2, >60 kg: 0.125 mg/kg; max 7.5 mg once daily; ≥18 years: initially 7.5 mg once daily; max 15 mg once daily; *Hemodialysis:* max 7.5 mg/day
> *Tab:* 7.5, 15 mg; *Oral susp:* 7.5 mg/5 ml (100 ml) (raspberry)
> **Vivlodex** <18 years: not established; ≥18 years: initially 5 mg qd; may increase to max 10 mg/day; *Hemodialysis:* max 5 mg/day
> *Cap:* 5, 10 mg

DYSPAREUNIA (POSTMENOPAUSAL PAINFUL INTERCOURSE)

Oral and Transdermal Hormonal Therapy *see Menopause page* 301

NON-HORMONAL THERAPY

▷ *prasterone (dehydroepiandrosterone [DHEA])* (X) insert 1 tab intravaginally daily at bedtime

   Intrarosa *Vaginal inserts:* 6.5 mg (20 tabs+28 applicators/carton)

   Comment: **Intrarosa** is the first local (intravaginal) non-estrogen drug approved for moderate-to-severe dyspareunia. **prosterone** is an active endogenous steroid converted into active androgens and/or estrogens.

HORMONAL THERAPY

Comment: Estrogen-alone therapy should not be used for the prevention of cardiovascular Disease or dementia. The Women's Health Initiative (WHI) estrogen-alone sub-study reported increased risks of stroke and deep vein thrombosis (DVT). The WHI Memory Study (WHIMS) estrogen-alone ancillary study of WHI reported an increased risk of probable dementia in postmenopausal women 65 years-of-age and older. *Contraindications:* undiagnosed abnormal genital bleeding, known or suspected estrogen-dependent neoplasia (e.g., breast cancer), active DVT, pulmonary embolism (PE), or history of these conditions; active arterial thromoembolic disease (e.g., stroke, myocardial infarction [AMI]), or history of these conditions; known or suspected pregnancy; severe hepatic impairment (Child-Pugh Class C).

▷ *estradiol* (X)(G)

   Imvexxy administer 1 vaginal insert once daily x 2 weeks; then 1 vaginal insert twice weekly x 2 weeks (e.g., mon/thu); consider the addition of a progestin with intact uterus

   Vag inserts: 4, 10 mcg (8, 18/pck) applicator-free

   Comment: **Imvexxy** is the only product in its class that is available in a 4 mcg and 10 mcg dose. The 4-mcg dose is currently the lowest approved dose of vaginal estradiol available. Imvexxy is a bio-identical vaginal estrogen product that offers a fraction of the estrogen contained in the average doses of other products on the market.

   Yuvafem Vaginal Tablet insert one 10 mcg or 25 mcg vaginal tablet once daily x 2 weeks; then twice weekly x 2 weeks (e.g., tues/fri); consider the addition of a progestin with intact uterus

   Vag tab: 10, 25 mcg (8, 18/blister pck with applicator)

ESTROGEN AGONIST-ANTAGONIST

▷ *ospemifene* take 1 tab daily

   Osphena *Tab:* 60 mg

   Comment: *ospemifene* is an estrogen agonist-antagonist with tissue selective effects. In the endometrium, OSPHENA has estrogen agonistic effects. There is an increased risk of endometrial cancer in a woman with a uterus who uses unopposed estrogens. Adding a progestin to estrogen therapy reduces the risk of endometrial hyperplasia, which may be a precursor to endometrial cancer. Estrogen-alone therapy has an increased risk of stroke and deep vein thrombosis (DVT). **Osphena** 60 mg had cerebral thromboembolic and hemorrhagic stroke incidence rates of 0.72 and 1.45 per thousand women, respectively vs. 1.04 and 0 per thousand women, respectively in placebo. For DVT, the incidence rate for **Osphena** 60 mg is 1.45 per thousand women vs. 1.04 per thousand women in placebo. Do not use estrogen or estrogen agonist/antagonist concomitantly with **Osphena**. *fluconazole* increases serum concentration of **Osphena**. *rifampin* decreases serum concentration of **Osphena**).

 EDEMA

THIAZIDE DIURETICS

▷ *chlorthalidone* (B)(G) initially 30-60 mg daily or 60 mg on alternate days; max 90-120 mg/day

   Thalitone *Tab:* 15 mg

▷ *chlorothiazide* (B)(G) 0.5-1 gm/day in a single or divided doses; max 2 gm/day

   Pediatric: <6 months: up to 15 mg/lb/day in 2 divided doses; ≥6 months: 10 mg/lb/day in 2 divided doses; max 375 mg/day

   Diuril *Tab:* 250*, 500*mg; *Oral susp:* 250 mg/5 ml (237 ml)

▷ *hydrochlorothiazide* (B)(G)

   Pediatric: <12 years: not recommended; ≥12 years: same as adult

      Esidrix 25-200 mg daily
        Tab: 25, 50, 100 mg
      Microzide 12.5 mg daily; usual max 50 mg/day
        Cap: 12.5 mg
▷ *hydroflumethiazide* (B) 50-200 mg/day in a single *or* 2 divided doses
    Pediatric: <12 years: not recommended; ≥12 years: same as adult
      Saluron *Tab:* 50 mg
▷ *methyclothiazide+deserpidine* (B) initially 2.5 mg daily; max 5 mg daily
    Pediatric: <12 years: not recommended; ≥12 years: same as adult
      Enduronyl *Tab:* methy 5 mg+deser 0.25 mg*
      Enduronyl Forte *Tab:* methy 5 mg+deser 0.5 mg*
▷ *polythiazide* (C) 1-4 mg daily
    Pediatric: <12 years: not recommended; ≥12 years: same as adult
      Renese *Tab:* 1, 2, 4 mg

POTASSIUM-SPARING DIURETICS

▷ *amiloride* (B)(G) initially 5 mg; may increase to 10 mg; max 20 mg
    Pediatric: <12 years: not recommended; ≥12 years: same as adult
      Tab: 5 mg
▷ *spironolactone* (D) initially 25-200 mg in a single *or* divided doses; titrate at 2-week intervals
    Pediatric: <12 years: not recommended; ≥12 years: same as adult
      Aldactone (G) *Tab:* 25, 50*, 100*mg
      CaroSpir *Oral susp:* 25 mg/5 ml (118, 473 ml) (banana)
▷ *triamterene* (B) 100 mg bid; max 300 mg
    Pediatric: <12 years: not recommended; ≥12 years: same as adult
      Dyrenium *Cap:* 50, 100 mg

LOOP DIURETICS

▷ *bumetanide* (C)(G) 0.5-2 mg daily; *Tab:* 5 mg; may repeat at 4-5 hour intervals; max 10 mg/day
    Pediatric: <18 years: not recommended; ≥18 years: same as adult
      Tab: 1*mg
    Comment: *bumetanide* is contraindicated with sulfa drug allergy.
▷ *ethacrynic acid* (B)(G) initially 50-100 mg once daily-bid; max 400 mg/day
    Pediatric: Infants: not recommended; ≥1 month: initially 25 mg/day; then adjust dose in 25 mg increments
      Edecrin *Tab:* 25, 50 mg
▷ *ethacrynate sodium* for IV injection (B)(G) administer smallest dose required to produce gradual weight loss (about 1-2 pounds per day); onset of diuresis usually occurs at 50-100 mg in children ≥12 years; after diuresis has been achieved, the minimally effective dose (usually 50-200 mg/day) may be administered on a continuous or intermittent dosage schedule; dose titrations are usually in 25-50 mg increments to avoid derangement electrolyte and water excretion; the patient should be weighed under standard conditions before and during administration of *ethacrynate sodium;* the following schedule may be helpful in determining the lowest effective dose: *Day 1:* 50 mg once daily after a meal; *Day 2:* 50 mg bid after meals, if necessary; *Day 3:* 100 mg in the morning and 50-100 mg following the afternoon or evening meal, depending upon response to the morning dose; a few patients may require initial and maintenance doses as high as 200 mg bid; these higher doses, which should be achieved gradually, are most often required in patients with severe, refractory edema
    Pediatric: <1 month: not recommended; ≥1 month-12 years: use the smallest effective dose; initially 25 mg; then careful stepwise increments in dosage of 25 mg to achieve effective maintenance
      Sodium Edecrin *Vial:* 50 mg single-dose
    Comment: *ethacrynate sodium* in is more potent than more commonly used loop and thiazide diuretics. Treatment of the edema associated with congestive heart failure, cirrhosis of the liver, and renal disease, including the nephrotic syndrome, short-term management of ascites due to malignancy, idiopathic edema, and lymphedema, short-term management of hospitalized pediatric patients, other than infants, with congenital heart disease *or* the nephrotic syndrome. IV **Sodium Edecrin** is indicated when a rapid onset of diuresis is desired, e.g., in acute pulmonary edema or when gastrointestinal absorption is impaired or oral medication is not practical.

▷ *furosemide* (C)(G) initially 20-80 mg as a single dose
   Pediatric: <12 years: not recommended; ≥12 years: same as adult
       Lasix *Tab:* 20, 40*, 80 mg; *Oral soln:* 10 mg/ml (2, 4 oz w. dropper)
   Comment: *furosemide* is contraindicated with sulfa drug allergy.
▷ *torsemide* (B) 5 mg daily; may increase to 10 mg daily
   Pediatric: <12 years: not recommended; ≥12 years: same as adult
       Demadex *Tab:* 5*, 10*, 20*, 100*mg

OTHER DIURETICS

▷ *indapamide* (B) initially 1.25 mg daily; may titrate every 4 weeks if needed; max
   5 mg/day
   Pediatric: <12 years: not recommended; ≥12 years: same as adult
       Lozol *Tab:* 1.25, 2.5 mg
   Comment: *indapamide* is contraindicated with sulfa drug allergy.
▷ *metolazone* (B)
   Pediatric: <12 years: not recommended; ≥12 years: same as adult
       Mykrox initially 0.5 mg q AM; max 1 mg/day
           Tab: 0.5 mg
       Zaroxolyn 2.5-5 mg once daily
           Tab: 2.5, 5, 10 mg
   Comment: *metolazone* is contraindicated with sulfa drug allergy.

DIURETIC COMBINATIONS

▷ *amiloride+hydrochlorothiazide* (B)(G) initially 1 tab daily; may increase to 2 tabs/day in a
   single or divided doses
   Pediatric: <12 years: not recommended; ≥12 years: same as adult
       Moduretic *Tab:* amil 5 mg+hctz 50 mg*
▷ *spironolactone+hydrochlorothiazide* (D)(G) usual maintenance is 100 mg each of *spironolactone* and *hydrochlorothiazide* daily, in a single-dose or in divided doses; range 25-200
   mg of each component daily depending on the response to the initial titration
   Pediatric: <12 years: not recommended; ≥12 years: same as adult
       Aldactazide
           Tab: Aldactazide 25 spiro 25 mg+hctz 25 mg
               Aldactazide 50 *Tab:* spiro 50 mg+hctz 50 mg
▷ *triamterene+hydrochlorothiazide* (C)(G)
   Pediatric: <12 years: not recommended; ≥12 years: same as adult
       Dyazide 1-2 caps once daily
           Cap: triam 37.5 mg+hctz 25 mg
       Maxzide 1 tab once daily
           Tab: triam 75 mg+hctz 50 mg*
       Maxzide-25 1-2 tabs once daily
           Tab: triam 37.5 mg+hctz 25 mg*

 EMPHYSEMA

Inhaled Corticosteroids *see Asthma page* 31
Parenteral Corticosteroids *see page* 577
Oral Corticosteroids *see page* 577
Inhaled Beta-2 Agonists (Bronchodilators) *see Asthma page* 30
Oral Beta-2 Agonists (Bronchodilators) *see Asthma page* 36

METHYLXANTHINES

see Asthma page 30

LONG-ACTING INHALED BETA-2 AGONIST (LABA)

▷ *indacaterol* (C)
       Arcapta Neohaler inhale contents of one 75 mcg cap once daily
           Neohaler Device/Cap: 75 mcg (5 blister cards, 6 caps/card)
       Comment: Remove cap from blister cap immediately before use. For oral inhalation
       with neohaler device only. **Arcapta Neohaler** is indicated for the long-term maintenance

treatment of bronchoconstriction in persons with COPD. It is not indicated for treating asthma, for primary treatment of acute symptoms, or for acute deterioration of COPD.

▷ *olodaterol* (C) 12 mcg q 12 hours
Striverdi Respimat *Inhal soln:* 2.5 mcg/cartridge (metered actuation) (40 gm, 60 metered actuations) (benzalkonium chloride)

CORTICOSTEROID+INHALED LONG-ACTING BETA-2 AGONIST (LABA)

▷ *fluticasone furoate/vilanterol* (C) 1 inhalation 100/25 or 200/25 once daily at the same time each day
Breo Ellipta 100/25 *Inhal pwdr:* flu 100 mcg+vil 25 mcg dry pwdr per inhal (30 doses)
Breo Ellipta 200/25 *Inhal pwdr:* flu 200 mcg+vil 25 mcg dry pwdr per inhal (30 doses)
Comment: **Breo Ellipta** is contraindicated with severe hypersensitivity to milk proteins.

INHALED ANTICHOLINERGICS (ANTIMUSCARINICS)

▷ *glycopyrrolate inhalation solution* (C) inhale the contents of 1 capsule twice daily at the same time of day, AM and PM, using the **Neohaler**; do not swallow caps
Pediatric: not indicated
Seebri Neohaler *Inhal cap:* 15.6 mcg (60/blister pck) dry pwdr for inhalation w. 1 **Neohaler** device (lactose)

▷ *ipratropium* (B)(G)
Atrovent 2 inhalations qid; max 12 inhalations/day
Inhaler: 14 gm (200 inh)
Atrovent Inhaled Solution 500 mcg by nebulizer tid to qid
Inhal soln: 0.02%; 500 mcg (2.5 ml)

INHALED LONG-ACTING MUSCARINIC-ANTAGONISITS (LAMAs)

Comment: Inhaled LAMA's are indicated for prophylaxis and chronic treatment, only. Not for primary (rescue) treatment of acute attack. Avoid getting powder/nebulizer solution in the eyes. Caution with narrow-angle glaucoma, BPH, bladder neck obstruction, and pregnancy. Contraindicated with allergy to atropine or its derivatives (e.g., *ipratropium*). Avoid other anticholinergic agents.

▷ *aclidinium bromide* (C) 1 inhalation twice daily using inhaler
Tudorza Pressair *Inhal device:* 400 mcg/actuation (60 doses per inhalation device)

▷ *glycopyrrolate inhalation solution* (C) administer the contents of one vial twice daily at the same times of day, AM and PM, via the **Magnair** neb inhal device; do not swallow solution; do not use **Magnair** with any other medicine; length of treatment is 2-3 minutes; do not use 2 vials/treatment or more than 2 vials/day
Pediatric: <18 years: not indicated
Lonhala Magnair *Vial:* 25 mcg/ml (1 ml) unit dose for use with **Magnair** handset; *Starter Kit:* 60 unit-dose vials w. **Magnair** handset; *Refill Kit:* 60 unit-dose vials (low-density polyethylene [LDPE]) w. **Magnair** handset (preservative-free)
Comment: **Lonhala Magnair** is the first nebulizing long-acting muscarinic antagonist (LAMA) approved for the treatment of COPD in the United States. Its approval was based on data from clinical trials in the Glycopyrrolate for Obstructive Lung Disease via Electronic Nebulizer (GOLDEN) program, including GOLDEN-3 and GOLDEN-4, 2 Phase 3, 12-week, randomized, double-blind, placebo-controlled, parallel-group, multicenter study. Do not initiate **Lonhala Magnair** in acutely deteriorating COPD or to treat acute symptoms. If paradoxical bronchospasm occurs, discontinue **Lonhala Magnair** immediately and institute alternative therapy. Worsening of narrow-angle glaucoma may occur; use with caution in patients with narrow-angle glaucoma and instruct patients to contact a physician immediately if symptoms occur. Worsening of urinary retention may occur. Use with caution in patients with prostatic hyperplasia (BPH) or bladder neck obstruction (BNO) and instruct patients to seek medical care immediately if symptoms occur. Avoid administration with other anticholinergic drugs. Consider risk versus benefit in patients with severe renal impairment. Most common adverse reactions (incidence ≥ 2.0%) have been dyspnea and urinary tract infection. There are no adequate and well-controlled studies in pregnancy. **Lonhala Magnair** should only be used during pregnancy if the expected benefit to the patient outweighs the potential risk to the fetus. There

are no data on the presence of *glycopyrrolate* or its metabolites in human milk or effects on the breastfed infant. The developmental and health benefits of breastfeeding should be considered along with the mother's clinical need for **Lonhala Magnair** and any potential adverse effects on the breastfed infant from **Lonhala Magnair** or from the underlying maternal condition. To report suspected adverse reactions, contact Sunovion Pharmaceuticals at 1 877-737-7226 or FDA at 1-800-FDA-1088 or visit www.fda.gov/medwatch.

▷ *revefenacin inhalation solution* administer the contents of one vial via nebulizer once daily at the same times of day; do not swallow solution; do not use more than 1 vial/day; do not use **Yupelri** with any other medicine
Pediatric: not indicated

Yupelri *Vial:* 175 mcg/3 ml (3 ml) unit-dose solution for nebulizer
Comment: **Yupelri** is the first and only long-acting muscarinic antagonist (LAMA) solution for once daily nebulized administration. **Yupelri** is indicated for maintenance treatment of moderate-to-severe. Do not initiate **Yupelri** in acutely deteriorating COPD or to treat acute symptoms. If paradoxical bronchospasm occurs, discontinue **Yupelri** immediately and institute alternative therapy. Worsening of narrow-angle glaucoma may occur; use with caution in patients with narrow-angle glaucoma and instruct patients to contact a healthcare provider immediately if symptoms occur. Use with caution in patients with prostatic hyperplasia or bladder-neck obstruction and instruct patients to contact a healthcare provider immediately if symptoms occur. May interact additively with other concomitantly used anticholinergic medications; avoid administration of **Yupelri** with other anticholinergic-containing drugs. Co-administration of **Yupelri** with OATP1B1 and OATP1B3 inhibitors (e.g. rifampicin, cyclosporine) may lead to an increase in exposure of the active metabolite; co-administration with **Yupelri** is not recommended. Avoid use of **Yupelri** in patients with hepatic impairment. Most common adverse reactions (incidence ≥2%) include cough, nasopharyngitis, upper respiratory tract infection, headache, and back pain. There are no adequate and well-controlled studies with **Yupelri** in pregnancy and no information regarding the presence of *revefenacin* in human milk or effects on the breastfed infant. To report suspected adverse reactions, contact Mylan at 1-877-446-3679 (1-877-4-INFO-RX) or FDA at 1-800-FDA-1088 or visit www.fda.gov/medwatch.

▷ *tiotropium (as bromide monohydrate)* (C) 2 inhalations once daily using inhalation device; do not swallow caps
Spiriva HandiHaler *Inhal device:* 18 mcg/cap pwdr for inhalation (5, 30, 90 caps w. inhalation device)
Spiriva Respimat *Inhal device:* 1.25, 2.5 mcg/actuation cartridge w. inhalation device (4 gm, 60 metered actuations) (benzylkonian chloride)
Comment: *tiotropium* is for prophylaxis and chronic treatment, only. Not for primary (rescue) treatment of acute attack. Avoid getting powder in eyes. Caution with narrow-angle glaucoma, BPH, bladder neck obstruction, and pregnancy. Contraindicated with allergy to *atropine* or its derivatives (e.g., *ipratropium*).

▷ *umeclidinium* (C) one inhalation once daily at the same time each day
Incruse Ellipta *Inhal pwdr:* 62.5 mcg/inhalation (30 doses) (lactose)
Comment: **Incruse Ellipta** is contraindicated with allergy to atropine or its derivatives.

INHALED BRONCHODILATOR+ANTICHOLINERGIC COMBINATION

▷ *ipratropium/albuterol* (C) 2 inhalations qid; max 12 inhalations/day
Combivent MDI *Inhaler:* 14.7 gm (200 inh)

INHALED ANTICHOLINERGIC+LONG-ACTING BETA-2 AGONIST (LABA) COMBINATIONS

▷ *indacaterol+glycopyrrolate* (C)
Utibron Neohaler inhale the contents of 1 capsule 2 x/day at the same times of day, AM and PM, using the neohaler; do not swallow caps
Inhal cap: indac 27.5 mcg+glycop 15.6 mcg per cap (60/blister pck) dry pwdr for inhalation w. 1 Neohaler device (lactose)

▷ *ipratropium+albuterol* (C) 1 inhalation qid; max 6 inhalations/day
Combivent Respimat *Inhal soln:* ipra 20 mcg+alb 100 mcg per inhal (4 gm, 120 inhal)
Comment: When the labeled number of metered actuations (120) has been dispensed from the **Combivent Respimat** inhaler, the locking mechanism engages and no more actuations can be dispensed. **Combivent Respimat** is contraindicated with atropine allergy.

▷ *tiotropium+olodaterol* (C) 2 inhalations once daily at the same time each day; max 2 inhalations/day

    Stiolto Respimat *Inhal soln:* tio 2.5 mcg+olo 2.5 mcg per actuation (4 gm, 60 inh) (benzalkonium chloride)

    Comment: **Stiolto Respimat** is not for treating asthma, for relief of acute bronchospasm, or acutely deteriorating COPD.

▷ *umeclidinium+vilanterol* (C) 1 inhalation once daily at the same time each day

    Anoro Ellipta *Inhal soln:* ume 62.5 mcg+vila 25 mcg per inhal (30 doses)

    Comment: **Anoro Ellipta** is contraindicated with severe hypersensitivity to milk proteins.

INHALED CORTICOSTEROID+ANTICHOLINERGIC+ LONG-ACTING BETA AGONIST (LABA) COMBINATION

▷ *fluticasone furoate+umeclidinium+vilanterol* one inhalation once daily

    Trelegy Ellipta flutic furo 100 mcg+umec 62.5 mcg+vilan 25 mcg dry pwdr

    Comment: **Trelegy Ellipta** is maintenance therapy for patients with COPD, including chronic bronchitis and emphysema, who are receiving fixed-dose *furoate* and *vilanterol* for airflow obstruction and to reduce exacerbations, or receiving *umeclidinium* and a fixed-dose combination of *fluticasone furoate* and *vilanterol*. **Trelegy Ellipta** is the first FDA-approved once-daily single-dose inhaler that combines *fluticasone furoate*, a corticosteroid, *umeclidinium*, a long-acting muscarinic antagonist, and *vilantero*, a long-acting beta2-adrenergic agonist. Common adverse reactions reported with **Trelegy Ellipta** included headache, back pain, dysgeusia, diarrhea, cough, oropharyngeal pain, and gastroenteritis. **Trelegy Ellipta** has been found to increase the risk of pneumonia in patients with COPD, and increase the risk of asthma-related death in patients with asthma. **Trelegy Ellipta** is not indicated for the treatment of asthma or acute bronchospasm.

METHYLXANTHINES

see Asthma page 30

METHYLXANTHINE+EXPECTORANT COMBINATION

▷ *dyphylline+guaifenesin* (C)

Pediatric: <12 years: not recommended; ≥12 years: same as adult

    Lufyllin GG 1 tab qid

        Tab: dyph 200 mg+guaif 200 mg

    Lufyllin GG Elixir 30 ml qid

        Elix: dyph 100 mg+guaif 100 mg per 15 ml (16 oz)

OTHER METHYLXANTHINE COMBINATION

▷ *theophylline+potassium iodide+ephedrine+phenobarbital* (X)(II) 1 tab tid-qid prn; add an additional dose q HS as needed

Pediatric: <6 years: not recommended; ≥6-12 years: 1/2 tab tid

    Quadrinal *Tab:* theo 130 mg+pot iod 320 mg+ephed 24 mg+phenol 24 mg

 ENCOPRESIS

INITIAL BOWEL EVACUATION

▷ *mineral oil* (C) 1 oz x 1 day

    Comment: Mineral oil can inhibit absorption of the fat-soluble vitamins (A, D, E, and K).

▷ *bisacodyl* (B) 1 suppository daily prn

Pediatric: <12 years: 1/2 suppository daily prn

    Dulcolax *Rectal supp:* 10 mg

▷ *glycerin* suppository (A) 1 adult suppository

Pediatric: <6 years: 1 pediatric suppository; ≥6 years: same as adult

MAINTENANCE

▷ *mineral oil* (C) 5-15 ml once daily

    Comment: Mineral oil can inhibit absorption of the fat-soluble vitamins (A, D, E, and K).

ENDOMETRIOSIS

Acetaminophen for IV Infusion *see Pain page* 352
NSAIDs *see page* 571
Opioid Analgesics *see Pain page* 354
Other Contraceptives *see page* 559
➤ *medroxyprogesterone* (X) 30 mg daily
   Provera *Tab:* 2.5, 5, 10 mg
➤ *medroxyprogesterone acetate* injectable (X) 100-400 mg IM monthly
   Depo-Provera Injectable: 300 mg/ml (2.5, 10 ml)
➤ *norethindrone acetate* (X) initially 5 mg daily x 2 weeks; then increase by 2.5 mg/day every
   2 weeks up to 15 mg/day maintenance dose; then continue for 6 to 9 months unless break-
   through bleeding is intolerable
   Aygestin *Tab:* 5*mg

GONADOTROPIN-RELEASING HORMONE ANALOGS

Comment: GnRHa analogs can have unpleasant side effects (e.g., hot flashes, vaginal dryness,
bone loss, changes in mood).
➤ *goserelin (GnRH analog)* implant (X) implant SC into upper abdominal wall; 1 SC implant
   q 28 days for up to 6 months; re-treatment not recommended
   Pediatric: <18 years: not recommended; ≥18 years: same as adult
   Zoladex SC implant in syringe: 3.6 mg
➤ *leuprolide acetate (GnRH analog)* (X)
   Pediatric: <18 years: not recommended; ≥18 years: same as adult
   Lupron Depot 3.75 mg 3.75 mg SC monthly for up to 6 months; may repeat one
   6-month cycle
      Syringe: 3.75 mg (single-dose depo susp for SC injection)
   Lupron Depot-3 Month 22.5 mg SC q 3 months (84 days); max 2 injections
      Syringe: 22.5 mg (single-dose depo susp for IM injection)
   Comment: Do not split doses.
➤ *nafarelin acetate* (X) 1 spray (200 mcg) into one nostril q AM, then 1 spray (200 mcg) into
   the other nostril q PM x 6 months; if no response after 2 months, may increase to 2 sprays
   (400 mcg) bid
   Pediatric: <18 years: not recommended; ≥18 years: same as adult
   Synarel *Nasal spray:* 2 mg/ml (10 ml)
   Comment: Start *nafarelin acetate* (**Synarel**) on the 3rd or 4th day of the menstrual period or
   after a negative pregnancy test.

GONADOTROPIN-RELEASING HORMONE (GNRH) RECEPTOR ANTAGONIST

➤ *elagolix Normal to mildly impaired hepatic function:* 150 mg once daily for up to 24 months or
   200 mg twice daily for up to 6 months; *Moderate hepatic impairment:* 150 mg once daily for up to
   6 months
   Pediatric: <18 years: not recommended; ≥18 years: same as adult
   Orlissa *Tab:* 150, 200 mg
   Comment: **Orlissa** *(elagolix)* is an orally administered GnRH receptor antagonist
   for the management of moderate-to-severe pain associated with endometriosis.
   Contraindications are severe hepatic impairment, pregnancy, concomitant strong
   organic anion transporting polypeptide (OATP) 1B1 inhibitors, and osteoporosis. Assess
   BMD in women with additional risk factors for bone loss; dose- and duration-dependent
   decreases in bone mineral density (BMD) may occur that may not be completely
   reversible. Due to potential for reduced efficacy with estrogen-containing contraceptives,
   use non-hormonal contraception during treatment and for one week after discontinuing
   Orlissa. Orlissa may alter menstrual bleeding, which may reduce the ability to recognize
   pregnancy. Test if pregnancy is suspected and discontinue if pregnancy is confirmed.
   Dose-dependent elevations in serum alanine aminotransferase (ALT) may occur;
   counsel patients on signs and symptoms of liver injury. Counsel patients about potential
   for suicidal ideation and mood disorders and advise to seek medical attention for
   suicidal ideation, suicidal behavior, new onset or worsening depression, anxiety, or other
   mood changes. The most common adverse reactions (incidence >5%) in clinical trials
   included hot flushes and night sweats, headache, nausea, insomnia, amenorrhea, anxiety,
   arthralgia, depression-related adverse reactions and mood changes.

Gonadotropin-Releasing Hormone Analogs (GnRHa)

Comment: These agonists can have unpleasant side effects (e.g., hot flashes, vaginal dryness, bone loss, changes in mood).

▷ *goserelin (GnRH analog)* implant (X) implant SC into upper abdominal wall; 1 SC implant q 28 days for up to 6 months; re-treatment not recommended
Pediatric: <18 years: not recommended; ≥18 years: same as adult
  Zoladex SC implant in syringe: 3.6 mg

▷ *leuprolide acetate (GnRH analog)* (X)
Pediatric: <18 years: not recommended; ≥18 years: same as adult
  Lupron Depot 3.75 mg 3.75 mg SC monthly for up to 6 months; may repeat one 6-month cycle
    Syringe: 3.75 mg (single-dose depo susp for SC injection)
  Lupron Depot-3 Month 22.5 mg SC q 3 months (84 days); max 2 injections
    Syringe: 22.5 mg (single-dose depo susp for IM injection)
Comment: Do not split doses.

▷ *nafarelin acetate* (X) 1 spray (200 mcg) into one nostril q AM, then 1 spray (200 mcg) into the other nostril q PM x 6 months; if no response after 2 months, may increase to 2 sprays (400 mcg) bid
Pediatric: <18 years: not recommended; ≥18 years: same as adult
  Synarel *Nasal spray:* 2 mg/ml (10 ml)
Comment: Start *nafarelin acetate* (**Synarel**) on the 3rd or 4th day of the menstrual period or after a negative pregnancy test.

Synthetic Steroid Derived From Ethisterone

▷ *danazol* (X) start on 3rd or 4th day of menstrual period or after a negative pregnancy test; initially 400 mg bid; gradual downward titration of dosage may be considered dependent upon patient response; mild cases may respond to 100-200 mg bid
Pediatric: <18 years: not recommended; ≥18 years: same as adult
  Danocrine *Cap:* 50, 100, 200 mg
Comment: *danazol* is a synthetic steroid derived from ethisterone. It suppresses the pituitary-ovarian axis. This suppression is probably a combination of depressed hypothalamic-pituitary response to lowered *estrogen* production, the alteration of sex steroid metabolism, and interaction of *danazol* with sex hormone receptors. The only other demonstrable hormonal effects are weak androgenic activity and depression of both follicle-stimulating hormone (FSH) and luteinizing hormone (LH) output. Recent evidence suggests a direct inhibitory effect at gonadal sites and a binding of **Danocrine** to receptors of gonadal steroids at target organs. In addition, **Danocrine** has been shown to significantly decrease IgG, IgM and IgA levels, as well as phospholipid and IgG isotope autoantibodies in patients with endometriosis and associated elevations of autoantibodies, suggesting this could be another mechanism by which it facilitates regression of endometrial lesions. **Danocrine** alters the normal and ectopic endometrial tissue so that it becomes inactive and atrophic. Complete resolution of endometrial lesions occurs in the majority of cases. Changes in the menstrual pattern may occur. Generally, the pituitary-suppressive action of **Danocrine** is reversible. Ovulation and cyclic bleeding usually return within 60 to 90 days when therapy with **Danocrine** is discontinued. **Danocrine** is also used to treat fibrocystic breast disease (reduces breast tissue nodularity and breast pain) and hereditary angioedema (to prevent attacks). Contraindications include pregnancy, breastfeeding, active or history of thromboembolic disease/event, porphyria, undiagnosed abnormal genital bleeding, androgen-dependent tumor, and markedly impaired hepatic, renal, or cardiac function.

 ENURESIS: PRIMARY, NOCTURNAL

VASOPRESSIN

▷ *desmopressin acetate* (B)
  DDAVP usual dosage 0.2 mg before bedtime
Pediatric: <6 years: not recommended; ≥6 years: same as adult
    Tab: 0.1*, 0.2*mg
  DDAVP Rhinal Tube 10 mcg or 0.1 ml of soln each nostril (20 mcg total dose) before bedtime
Pediatric: <6 years: not recommended; ≥6 years: same as adult
    Nasal spray: 10 mcg/actuation (5 ml, 50 sprays); *Rhinal tube:* 0.1 mg/ml (2.5 ml)

TRICYCLIC ANTIDEPRESSANTS (TCAs)

Comment: Co-administration of SSRIs and TCAs requires extreme caution.

▷ *amitriptyline* (C)(G) initially 10 mg before bedtime; use lowest effective dose
  Pediatric: <12 years: not recommended; ≥12 years: same as adult
    Tab: 10, 25, 50, 75, 100, 150 mg
  Pediatric: <12 years: not recommended; ≥12 years: same as adult
▷ *amoxapine* (C) initially 25 mg before bedtime; use lowest effective dose
    Tab: 25, 50, 100, 150 mg
▷ *clomipramine* (C)(G) initially 25 mg before bedtime; use lowest effective dose
  Pediatric: <10 years: not recommended; ≥10 years: same as adult
    Anafranil *Cap:* 25, 50, 75 mg
▷ *desipramine* (C)(G) initially 25 mg before bedtime; use lowest effective dose
  Pediatric: <12 years: not recommended; ≥12 years: same as adult
    Norpramin *Tab:* 10, 25, 50, 75, 100, 150 mg
▷ *doxepin* (C)(G) initially 10 mg before bedtime; use lowest effective dose
  Pediatric: <12 years: not recommended; ≥12 years: same as adult
    Cap: 10, 25, 50, 75, 100, 150 mg; Oral conc: 10 mg/ml (4 oz w. dropper)
▷ *imipramine* (C)(G) initially 10 mg before bedtime; use lowest effective dose
  Pediatric: <12 years: not recommended; ≥12 years: same as adult
    Tofranil initially 10 at bedtime; use lowest effective dose; if bedtime dose exceeds 75 mg
    daily, may switch to **Tofranil PM**
      Tab: 10, 25, 50 mg
    Tofranil PM initially 75 mg before bedtime; use lowest effective dose
      Cap: 75, 100, 125, 150 mg
▷ *nortriptyline* (D)(G)
  Pediatric: <12 years: not recommended; ≥12 years: initially 10 mg before bedtime; use
  lowest effective dose
    Pamelor *Cap:* 10, 25, 50, 75 mg; *Oral soln:* 10 mg/5 ml (16 oz)
▷ *protriptyline* (C) initially 5 mg before bedtime; use lowest effective dose
  Pediatric: <12 years: not recommended; ≥12 years: same as adult
    Vivactil *Tab:* 5, 10 mg
▷ *trimipramine* (C) initially 25 mg before bedtime; use lowest effective dose
  Pediatric: <12 years: not recommended; ≥12 years: same ad adult
    Surmontil *Cap:* 25, 50, 100 mg

EOSINOPHILIC GRANULOMATOSIS WITH POLYANGITIS (FORMERLY CHURG-STRAUSS SYNDROME)

Comment: Eosinophilic granulomatosis with polyangiitis (EGPA) is a rare autoimmune disease that causes vasculitis, an inflammation in the wall of blood vessels of the body. EGPA is characterized by asthma, high levels of eosinophils, and inflammation of small- to medium-sized blood vessels affecting organ systems including the lungs, GI tract, skin, heart, and nervous system. **Nucala** *(mepolizumab)* is the first FDA-approved therapy specifically to treat EGPA. This expanded indication of **Nucala** meets a critical, and previously unmet need for EGPA patients. It's notable that patients taking **Nucala** in clinical trials reported a significant improvement in their symptoms. The FDA granted this application Priority Review and Orphan Drug designations. Orphan Drug designation provides incentives to assist and encourage the development of drugs for rare diseases.

REFERENCE

https://www.fda.gov/NewsEvents/Newsroom/PressAnnouncements/ucm588594.htm

HUMANIZED INTERLEUKIN-5 ANTAGONIST MONOCLONAL ANTIBODY

▷ *mepolizumab* 100 mg SC once every 4 weeks in upper arm, abdomen, or thigh
  Pediatric: <12 years: not recommended; ≥12 years: same as adult
    Nucala *Vial:* 100 mg pwdr for reconstitution, single-use (preservative-free)
    Comment: **Nucala** is an add-on maintenance treatment for severe asthma. There is a
    pregnancy exposure registry that monitors pregnancy outcomes in women exposed
    to **Nucala** during pregnancy. Healthcare providers can enroll patients or encourage
    patients to enroll themselves by calling 1-877-311-8972 or visiting www.mothertobaby.
    org/asthma.

EPICONDYLITIS

NSAIDs *see page* 571
Opioid Analgesics *see Pain page* 354
Topical & Transdermal Analgesics *see Pain page* 352
Parenteral Corticosteroids *see page* 577
Oral Corticosteroids *see page* 577
Topical Analgesic and Anesthetic Agents *see page* 569

 EPIDIDYMITIS

Comment: The following treatment regimens for epididymitis are published in the **2015 CDC Transmitted Diseases Treatment Guidelines**. Treatment regimens are presented by generic drug name first, followed by information about brands and dose forms. Empiric treatment requires concomitant treatment of chlamydia. Treat all sexual contacts. Patients who are HIV-positive should receive the same treatment as those who are HIV-negative.

RECOMMENDED REGIMEN
Regimen 1
▷ *ceftriaxone* (B)(G) 250 mg IM in a single dose
   plus
▷ *doxycycline* (D)(G) 100 mg bid x 10 days

RECOMMENDED REGIMENS: LIKELY CAUSED BY ENTERIC ORGANISMS
Regimen 1
▷ *levofloxacin* (C) 500 mg daily x 10 days

Regimen 2
▷ *ofloxacin* (C)(G) 300 mg bid x 10 day

DRUG BRANDS AND DOSE FORMS
▷ *ceftriaxone* (B)(G)
   Rocephin *Vial:* 250, 500 mg; 1, 2 gm
▷ *doxycycline* (D)(G)
   Acticlate *Tab:* 75, 150**mg
   Adoxa *Tab:* 50, 75, 100, 150 mg ent-coat
   Doryx *Tab:* 50, 75, 100, 150, 200 mg del-rel
   Doxteric *Tab:* 50 mg del-rel
   Monodox *Cap:* 50, 75, 100 mg
   Oracea *Cap:* 40 mg del-rel
   Vibramycin *Tab:* 100 mg; *Cap:* 50, 100 mg; *Syr:* 50 mg/5 ml (raspberry-apple) (sulfites); *Oral susp:* 25 mg/5 ml (raspberry)
   Vibra-Tab *Tab:* 100 mg film-coat
   Comment: *doxycycline* is contraindicated <8 years-of-age, in pregnancy, and lactation (discolors developing tooth enamel). A side effect may be photo-sensitivity (photophobia). Do <u>not</u> take with antacids, calcium supplements, milk or other dairy, or within 2 hours of taking another drug.
▷ *levofloxacin* (C)
   Levaquin *Tab:* 250, 500, 750 mg; *Oral soln:* 25 mg/ml (480 ml) (benzyl alcohol)
   Comment: *levofloxacin* is contraindicated <18 years-of-age, and during pregnancy, and lactation. Risk of tendonitis or tendon rupture.
▷ *ofloxacin* (C)(G)
   Floxin *Tab:* 200, 300, 400 mg
   Comment: *ofloxacin* is contraindicated <18 years-of-age, and during pregnancy and lactation. Risk of tendonitis or tendon rupture.

 ERECTILE DYSFUNCTION (ED)

Comment: Due to a degree of cardiac risk with sexual activity, consider cardiovascular status of patient before instituting therapeutic measures for erectile dysfunction.

PHOSPHODIESTERASE TYPE 5 (PDE5) INHIBITORS, CGMP-SPECIFIC

Comment: Oral PDE5 inhibitors (**Cialis, Levitra, Staxyn, Viagra**) are contraindicated in patients taking nitrates. Caution with history of recent MI, stroke, life-threatening arrhythmia, hypotension, hypertension, cardiac failure, unstable angina, retinitis pigmentosa, CYP3A4 inhibitors (e.g., *cimetidine*, the azoles, *erythromycin*, grapefruit juice), protease inhibitors (e.g., *ritonavir*), CYP3A4 inducers (e.g., *rifampin*, *carbamazepine*, *phenytoin*, *phenobarbital*), alcohol, antihypertensive agents. Side effects include headache, flushing, nasal congestion, rhinitis, dyspepsia, and diarrhea. Use with caution in patients with anatomical deformation of the penis (e.g., angulation, cavernosal fibrosis, or Peyronie's disease) or in patients who have conditions, which may predispose them to priapism (e.g., sickle cell anemia, multiple myeloma, or leukemia). In the event of an erection that persists longer than 4 hours, the patient should seek immediate medical assistance. If priapism (painful erection greater than 6 hours in duration) is not treated immediately, penile tissue damage and permanent loss of potency could result.

▷ *avanafil* (B) initially 100 mg taken 30 min prior to sexual activity; may decrease to 50 mg or increase to 200 mg based on response; max one administration/day
   Stendra *Tab:* 50, 100, 200 mg

▷ *sildenafil citrate* (B)(G) one dose about 1 hour (range 30 min-4 hrs) before sexual activity; usual initial dose 50 mg; may decrease to 25 mg or increase to max 100 mg/dose based on response; max one administration/day
   Viagra *Tab:* 25, 50, 100 mg

▷ *tadalafil* (B)(G) initially 10 mg prior to sexual activity up to once daily; may decrease to 5 mg or increase to 20 mg based on response; max one administration/day; effect may last 36 hours
   Cialis *Tab:* 2.5, 5, 10, 20 mg

▷ *vardenafil* (B) initially 10 mg taken 60 min prior to sexual activity; may decrease to 5 mg or increase to 20 mg based on response; max one administration/day
   Levitra *Tab:* 2.5, 5, 10, 20 mg film-coat
   Comment: **Levitra** is not interchangeable with **Staxyn**.

▷ *vardenafil (as HCl)* (B)(G) dissolve 1 tab on tongue 60 min prior to sexual activity, max once daily
   Staxyn *Tab:* 10 mg orally disintegrating (peppermint) (phenylalanine)
   Comment: **Staxyn** is not interchangeable with **Levitra**.

▷ *alprostadil* (X) *urethral suppository* initially 125 or 250 mcg inserted in the urethra after urination; adjust dose in stepwise manner on separate occasions; max two administrations/day
   Muse *Urethral supp:* 125, 250, 500, 1000 mcg
   Comment: Contraindicated with urethral stricture, balanitis, severe hypospadias and curvature, urethritis, predisposition to venous thrombosis, hyperviscosity syndrome. Extreme caution with anticoagulant therapy (e.g., warfarin, heparin). Potential for hypotension and/or syncope.

▷ *alprostadil* (X) *injection* inject over 5-10 seconds into the dorsal lateral aspect of the proximal third of the penis; avoid visible veins; rotate injection sites and sides; if no initial response, may give next higher dose within 1 hour; if partial response, give next higher dose after 24 hours; max 60 mcg and 3 self-injections/week; allow at least 24 hours between doses; reduce dose if erection lasts >1 hour.
   Caverject *Vial:* 5, 10, 20, 40 mcg/vial (pwdr for reconstitution w. diluent)
   Caverject Impulse *Cartridge:* 10, 20 mcg (2 cartridge starter and refill pcks)
   Edex *Vial:* 5, 10, 20, 40 mcg (6/pck); *Syringe:* 5, 10, 20, 40 mcg (4/pck); *Cartridge:* 10, 20, 40 mcg (2 cartridge starter and refill pcks)
   Comment: Determine dose of injectable prostaglandins in the office. Contraindicated with predisposition to priapism, penile angulation, cavernosal fibrosis, Peyronies disease, penile implant. Extreme caution with anticoagulant therapy (e.g., *warfarin*, *heparin*).

⊙ ERYSIPELAS

Comment: Erysipelas is most commonly due to GABHS (Group A beta-hemolytic *Streptococcus*).

TREATMENT OF CHOICE

▷ *penicillin v potassium* (B) 250-500 mg q 6 hours x 10 days
   Pediatric: 25-50 mg/kg/day divided q 6 hours x 10 days; *see page 629 for dose by weight*
   Pen-Vee K *Tab:* 250, 500 mg; *Oral soln:* 125 mg/5 ml (100, 200 ml); 250 mg/5 ml (100, 150, 200 ml)

TREATMENT IF PENICILLIN ALLERGIC

▷ *erythromycin base* (B)(G) 250 mg q 6 hours x 10 days
  Pediatric: 30-40 mg/kg/day divided q 6 hours x 10 days; >40 kg: same as adult
    Ery-Tab *Tab:* 250, 333, 500 mg ent-coat
    PCE *Tab:* 333, 500 mg
  Comment: *erythromycin* may increase INR with concomitant *warfarin*, as well as increase serum level of *digoxin*, benzodiazepines, and statins.
▷ *erythromycin ethylsuccinate* (B)(G) 400 mg qid x 7 days
  Pediatric: 30-50 mg/kg/day in 4 divided doses x 7 days; may double dose with severe infection; max 100 mg/kg/day; *see page 626 for dose by weight*
    EryPed *Oral susp:* 200 mg/5 ml (100, 200 ml) (fruit); 400 mg/5 ml (60, 100, 200 ml) (banana); *Oral drops:* 200, 400 mg/5 ml (50 ml) (fruit); *Chew tab:* 200 mg wafer (fruit)
    E.E.S. *Oral susp:* 200, 400 mg/5 ml (100 ml) (fruit)
    E.E.S. Granules *Oral susp:* 200 mg/5 ml (100, 200 ml) (cherry)
    E.E.S. 400 Tablets *Tab:* 400 mg
  Comment: *erythromycin* may increase INR with concomitant *warfarin*, as well as increase serum level of *digoxin*, benzodiazepines, and statins.

ESOPHAGITIS, EROSIVE

Antacids *see GERD page* 170
H2 Antagonists *see GERD page* 172
Proton Pump Inhibitors *see GERD page* 173
▷ *sucralfate* (B)(G) *Active ulcer:* 1 gm qid; *Maintenance:* 1 gm bid
    Carafate *Tab:* 1*g; *Oral susp:* 1 gm/10 ml (14 oz)

EXOCRINE PANCREAS INSUFFICIENCY (EPI)/ PANCREATIC ENZYME DEFICIENCY

Comment: Seen in chronic pancreatitis, post-pancreatectomy, cystic fibrosis, post-GI tract bypass surgery (Whipple procedure), and ductal obstruction from neoplasia. May sprinkle cap; however, do not crush or chew cap or tab. May mix with applesauce or other acidic food; follow with water or juice. Do not let any drug remain in mouth. Take dose with (not before or after) each meal and snack (half dose with snacks). Base dose on lipase units; adjust per diet and clinical response (i.e., steatorrhea). Pancrelipase products are interchangeable. Contraindicated with pork protein hypersensitivity.

PANCRELIPASE PRODUCTS

▷ *pancreatic enzymes* (C)
    Creon 500 units/kg per meal; max 2,500 units/kg per meal or <10,000 units/kg per day or <4,000 units/gm fat ingested per day
    Pediatric: <12 months: 2,000-4,000 units per 120 ml formula or per breast-feeding (do not mix directly into formula or breast milk; 12 months to 4 years: 1,000 units/kg per meal; max 2,500 units/kg per meal <10,000 units/kg per day; >4 years: same as adult
      Cap: **Creon 3000** lip 3,000 units+pro 9,500 units+amyl 15,000 units del-rel
          Creon 6000 lip 6,000 units+pro 19,000 units+amyl 30,000 units del-rel
          Creon 12000 lip 12,000 units+pro 38,000 units+amyl 60,000 units del-rel
          Creon 24000 lip 24,000 units+pro 76,000 units+amyl 120,000 units del-rel
          Creon 36000 lip 36,000 units+pro 114,000 units+amyl 180,000 units del-rel
    Cotazym 1-3 tabs just prior to each meal or snack
    Pediatric: <12 years: not recommended; ≥12 years: same as adult
      Tab: **Cotazym** lip 1,000 units+pro 12,500 units+amyl 12,500 units del-rel
          Cotazym-S lip 5,000 units+pro 20,000 units+amyl 20,000 units del-rel
    Donnazyme 1-3 caps just prior to each meal or snack
    Pediatric: <12 years: not recommended; ≥12 years: same as adult
      Cap: **Donnazyme** lip 5,000 units+pro 20,000 units+amyl 20,000 units del-rel
    Ku-Zyme 1-2 caps just prior to each meal or snack
    Pediatric: <12 years: not recommended; ≥12 years: same as adult
      Cap: **Ku-Zyme** lip 12,000 units+pro 15,000 units+amyl 15,000 units del-rel

Kutrase 1-2 caps just prior to each meal or snack
Pediatric: <12 years: not recommended; ≥12 years: same as adult
> *Cap:* **Kutrase:** lip 12,000 units+pro 30,000 units+amyl 30,000 units del-rel

Pancreaze 2,500 lipase units/kg per meal or <10,000 lipase units/kg per day or <4,000 lipase units/gm fat ingested per day
Pediatric: <12 months: 2,000-4,000 lipase units per 120 ml formula or per breastfeeding; >12 months to <4 years 1,000 lipase units/kg per meal; ≥4 years: 500 lipase units/kg per meal; max: adult dose
> *Cap:* **Pancreaze 4200** lip 4,200 units+pro 10,000 units+amyl 17,500 units ec-micro-tabs
>> **Pancreaze 10500** lip 10,500 units+pro 25,000 units+amyl 43,750 units ec microtabs
>> **Pancreaze 16800** lip 16,800 units+pro 40,000 units+amyl 70,000 units ec-microtabs
>> **Pancreaze 21000** lip 21,000 units+pro 37,000 units+amyl 61,000 units ec-microtabs

Pertyze *12 months to 4 years and ≥8 kg:* initially 1,000 lipase units/kg per meal; *≥4 years and ≥16 kg:* initially 500 lipase units/kg per meal; *Both:* 2,500 lipase units/kg per meal or <10,000 units/kg per day or <4,000 lipase units/gm fat ingested per day
> *Cap:* **Pertyze 8000** lip 8,000 units+pro 28,750 units+amyl 30,250 units del-rel
> **Pertyze 16000** lip 16,000 units+pro 57,500 units+amyl 65,000 units del-rel

Ultrase 1-3 tabs just prior to each meal or snack
Pediatric: same as adult
> *Cap:* **Ultrase** lip 4,500 units+pro 20,000 units+amyl 25,000 units del-rel
> **Ultrase MT** lip 12,000 units+pro 39,000 units+amyl 39,000 units del-rel
> **Ultrase MT 18** lip 18,000 units+pro 58,500 units+amyl 58,500 units del-rel
> **Ultrase MT 20** lip 20,000 units+pro 65,000 units+amyl 65,000 units del-rel

Viokace initially 500 lip units/kg per meal; max 2,500 lipase units/kg per meal, or <10,000 lipase units/kg per meal, or <4,000 units/gm fat ingested per day
Pediatric: same as adult
> *Tab:* **Viokace 8** lip 8,000 units+pro 30,000 units+amyl 30,000 units
> **Viokace 16** lip 16,000 units+pro 60,000 units amyl 60,000 units
> **Viokace 0440** lip 10,440 units+pro 39,150 units amyl 39,150 units
> **Viokace 20880** lip 20,880 units+pro 78,300 units amyl 78,300 units

Comment: **Viokace 10440** and **Viokase 20880** should be taken with a daily proton pump inhibitor.

Viokace Powder 1/4 tsp (0.7 gm) with meals
Viokace Powder lip 16,800 units+pro 70,000 units+amyl 70,000 units per 1/4 tsp (8 oz)

Zenpep initially 500 lipase units/kg per meal; max 2,500 lipase units/kg per meal or <10,000 units/kg per day or <4,000 lipase units/gm fat ingested per day
Pediatric: Infants-12 months: infants may be given 3,000 lipase units (one capsule) per 120 ml of formula or per breast-feeding; do not mix capsule contents directly into formula or breast milk prior to administration; *Children >12 months to <4 Years:* enzyme dosing should begin with 1,000 lipase units/kg of body weight per meal to a maximum of 2,500 lipase units/kg of body weight per meal (or ≤10,000 lipase units/kg/day), or <4,000 lipase units/gm fat ingested per day; *Children >4 Years:* same as adult
> *Cap:* **Zenpep 3000** lip 3,000 units+pro 10,000 units+amyl 14,000 units del-rel
> **Zenpep 5000** lip 5,000 units+pro 17,000 units+amyl 24,000 units del-rel
> **Zenpep 10000** lip 10,000 units+pro 32,000 units+amyl 42,000 units del-rel
> **Zenpep 15000** lip 15,000 units+pro 47,000 units+amyl 63,000 units del-rel
> **Zenpep 20000** lip 20,000 units+pro 63,000 units+amyl 84,000 units del-rel
> **Zenpep 25000** lip 25,000 units+pro 79,000 units+amyl 105,000 units del-rel
> **Zenpep 40000** lip 40,000 units+pro 126,000 units+amyl 168,000 units del-rel

Comment: **Zenpep** is not interchangeable with any other pancrelipase product. Dosing should not exceed the recommended maximum dosage set forth by the Cystic Fibrosis Foundation Consensus Conferences Guidelines. **Zenpep** should be swallowed whole. For infants or patients unable to swallow intact capsules, the contents may be sprinkled on soft acidic food, e.g., applesauce.

Zymase 1-3 caps just prior to each meal or snack
Pediatric: <12 years: not recommended; ≥12 years: same as adult
> *Cap:* **Zymase** lip 12,000 units+prot 24,000 units+amyl 24,000 units del-rel

EXTRAPYRAMIDAL SIDE EFFECTS (EPS)

➤ *amantadine* initial dose 129 mg orally once daily in the morning; may increase dose in weekly intervals; max daily dose 322 mg in the morning; dose frequency reduction and monitoring required for renal impairment; swallow whole; do not chew, crush, or divide

Osmolex ER *Tab:* 129, 193, 258 mg ext-rel

Comment: **Osmolex ER** is not interchangeable with other *amantadine* immediate or extended-release products. Most common adverse reactions (incidence ≥ 5%) are nausea, dizziness/ lightheadedness, and insomnia. **Osmolex ER** is contraindicated in patients with end-stage renal disease (ESRD). Advise patients prior to treatment about potential for falling asleep during activities of daily living (ADLs) and somnolence and discontinue **Osmolex ER** if occurs. Monitor patients for depressed mood, depression, and suicidal ideation or behavior. Patients with major psychotic disorder should ordinarily not be treated with **Osmolex ER**; observe patients throughout treatment for the occurrence of hallucinations, especially at initiation and after dose increases. Monitor patients for dizziness and orthostatic hypotension, especially after starting **Osmolex ER** or increasing the dose. Avoid sudden withdrawal/discontinuation due to risk of Withdrawal-Emergent Hyperpyrexia and confusion: Monitor patient for development of impulse control/compulsive behaviors. Ask patients about increased gambling urges, sexual urges, uncontrolled spending or other urges and consider dose reduction or discontinuation if any occur. Increased risk of anticholinergic effects may require reduction of **Osmolex ER** or dose of the anticholinergic drug(s). Excretion of *amantadine* increases with acidic urine resulting in possible accumulation with urine change towards alkaline. Live Attenuated Influenza Vaccines (LAVs) are not recommended during treatment with **Osmolex ER**. Concomitant use of alcohol is not recommended due to increased potential for CNS effects. There are no adequate data on the developmental risk associated with use of *amantadine* in pregnant women. Animal studies suggest a potential risk for fetal harm with *amantadine*. *Amantadine* is excreted in human milk, but amounts have not been quantified. There is no information on the risk to the breastfed infant. To report suspected reactions, contact Vertical Pharmaceuticals, LLC at 1-877-482-3788 or FDA at 1-800-FDA-1088 or www.fda.gov/medwatch.

 EYE PAIN

OPHTHALMIC NSAIDs

Comment: Concomitant contact lens wear is contraindicated during therapy. Etiology of eye pain must be known prior to use of these agents

➤ *diclofenac* (B) 1 drop affected eye qid

Pediatric: <12 years: not recommended; ≥12 years: same as adult

Voltaren Ophthalmic Solution *Ophth soln:* 0.1% (2.5, 5 ml)

➤ *ketorolac tromethamine* (C) 1 drop affected eye qid for up to 4 days

Pediatric: <3 years: not recommended; ≥3 years: same as adult

Acular *Ophth soln:* 0.5% (3, 5, 10 ml; benzalkonium chloride)

Acular LS *Ophth soln:* 0.4% (5 ml; benzalkonium chloride)

Acular PF *Ophth soln:* 0.5% (0.4 ml; 12 single-use vials/carton) (preservative-free)

➤ *nepafenac* (C) 1 drop affected eye tid

Pediatric: <10 years: not recommended; ≥10 years: same as adult

Nevanac Ophthalmic Suspension *Ophth susp:* 0.1% (3 ml) (benzalkonium chloride)

OPHTHALMIC STEROIDS

Comment: Ophthalmic steroids are contraindicated with mycobacterial, fungal, and viral infection. Effectiveness of treatment should be assessed after 2 days. The corticosteroid should be tapered and treatment concluded within 14 days if possible due to risk of corneal and/or scleral thinning with prolonged use.

➤ *difluprednate* (C) 1 drop affected eye qid; *Post-op Pain:* beginning 24 hours after surgery, 1 drop affected eye qid; continue for 2 weeks post-op; then bid x 1 week; then taper until resolved

Pediatric: <12 years: not recommended; ≥12 years: same as adult

Durezol Ophthalmic Solution *Ophth emul:* 0.05% (5 ml)

➤ *etabonate* (C) 1 drop affected eye qid

Pediatric: <12 years: not recommended; ≥12 years: same as adult

Alrex Ophthalmic Solution *Ophth emul:* 0.2% (5 ml) (benzylkonium chloride)

▷ *eoteprednol etabonate 1%* (C) 1-2 drops affected eye bid
  Pediatric: <12 years: not established; ≥12 years: same as adult
    Inveltys *Ophth soln:* 1% (5 ml) (benzylkonium chloride)
    Comment: Inveltys **is indicated for post-op inflammation and pain following ocular surgery** beginning the day after surgery and continuing throughout the first 2 weeks of the post-operative period.

FACIAL HAIR: EXCESSIVE/UNWANTED

TOPICAL HAIR GROWTH RETARDANT

▷ *eflornithine* 13.9% cream (C) apply a thin layer to affected areas of face and under the chin bid at least 8 hours apart; rub in thoroughly; do not wash treated area for at least 4 hours following application
  Pediatric: <12 years: not recommended; ≥12 years: same as adult
    Vaniqa *Crm:* 13.9% (30, 60 gm)
    Comment: After **Vaniqa** dries, may apply cosmetics or sunscreen. Hair removal techniques may be continued as needed.

FECAL ODOR

▷ *bismuth subgallate powder* (B)(OTC) 1-2 tabs tid with meals
    Devron *Chew tab:* 200 mg; *Cap:* 200 mg
    Comment: **Devron** is an internal (oral) deodorant for control of odors from ileostomy or colostomy drainage or fecal incontinence.

FEVER (PYREXIA)

ACETAMINOPHEN FOR IV INFUSION

▷ *acetaminophen* injectable (B)(G) administer by IV infusion over 15 minutes; 1000 mg q 6 hours prn or 650 mg q 4 hours prn; max 4,000 mg/day
  Pediatric: <2 years: not recommended; 2-13 years <50 kg: 15 mg/kg q 6 hours prn or 12.5 mg/kg q 4 hours prn; max 750 mg/single dose; max 75 mg/kg per day
    Ofirmev *Vial:* 10 mg/ml (100 ml) (preservative-free)
    Comment: The **Ofirmev** vial is intended for single-use. If any portion is withdrawn from the vial, use within 6 hours. Discard the unused portion. For pediatric patients, withdraw the intended dose and administer via syringe pump. Do not ad-mix **Ofirmev** with any other drugs. **Ofirmev** is physically incompatible with diazepam and chlorpromazine hydrochloride.
▷ *acetaminophen* (B)(G)
    Children's Tylenol (OTC) 10-20 mg/kg q 4-6 hours prn
      Oral susp: 80 mg/tsp
        4-11 months (12-17 lb): 1/2 tsp q 4 hours prn; 12-23 months (18-23 lb): 3/4 tsp q 4 hours prn; 2-3 years (24-35 lb): 1 tsp q 4 hours prn; 4-5 years (36-47 lb): 1 tsp q 4 hours prn; 6-8 years (48-59 lb): 2 tsp q 4 hours prn; 9-10 years (60-71 lb): 2 tsp q 4 hours prn; 11 years (72-95 lb): 3 tsp q 4 hours prn; All: max 5 doses/day
      Elix: 160 mg/5 ml (2, 4 oz)
      Chew tab: 80 mg
        2-3 years (24-35 lb): 2 tabs q 4 hours prn; 4-5 years (36-47 lb): 3 tabs q 4 hours prn; 6-8 years (48-59 lb): 4 tabs q 4 hours prn; 9-10 years (60-71 lb): 5 tabs q 4 hours prn; 11 years (72-95 lb): 6 tabs q 4 hours prn; All: max 5 doses/day
      Junior Strength:
        6-8 years: 2 tabs q 4 hours prn; 9-10 years: 2 tabs q 4 hours prn; 11 years: 3 tabs q 4 hours prn; 12 years: 4 tabs q 4 hours prn; All: max 5 doses/day
      Chew tab: 160 mg
      Junior cplt: 160 mg
      Infant's Drops and Suspension: 80 mg/0.8 ml (1/2, 1 oz)
        <3 months: 0.4 ml q 4 hours prn; 4-11 months: 0.8 ml q 4 hours prn; 12-23 months: 1.2 ml q 4 hours prn; 2-3 years (24-35 lb): 1.6 ml q 4 hours prn; 4-5 years (36-47 lb): 2.4 ml q 4 hours prn; All: max 5 doses/day

Extra Strength Tylenol (OTC) 1 gm q 4-6 hours prn; max 4 gm/day
Pediatric: <12 years: not recommended; ≥12 years: same as adult
   Tab/Cplt/Gel tab/Gel cap: 500 mg; *Liq:* 500 mg/15 ml (8 oz)
FeverAll Extra Strength Tylenol (OTC)
Pediatric: <3 months: not recommended; 3-36 months: 80 mg q 4 hours prn; 3-6 years: 120 mg q 4 hours prn; ≥6 years: 325 mg q 4 hours prn; *Rectal supp:* 80, 120, 325 mg (6/carton)
Maximum Strength Tylenol Sore Throat (OTC) 500-1000 mg q 4-6 hours prn
Pediatric: <12 years: not recommended; ≥12 years: same as adult
   Liq: 1000 mg/30 ml (8 oz)
Tylenol (OTC) 650 mg q 4-6 hours; max 4 gm/day
   Pediatric: <6 years: not recommended; 6-11 years: 325 mg q 4-6 hours prn; max 1.625 gm/day; ≥12 years: same as adult
▷ *aspirin* (D)(G)
Bayer (OTC) 325-650 mg q 4 hours prn; max: 5 doses/day
Pediatric: <12 years: not recommended; ≥12 years: same as adult
   Tab/Cplt: 325 mg ext-rel
Extra Strength Bayer (OTC) 500 mg-1 gm q 4-6 hours prn; max 4 gm/day
Pediatric: <12 years: not recommended; ≥12 years: same as adult
   Cplt: 500 mg
Extended-Release Bayer 8 Hour (OTC) 650-1300 mg q 8 hours prn
Pediatric: <12 years: not recommended; ≥12 years: same as adult
   Cplt: 650 mg ext-rel
Comment: *aspirin*-containing medications are contraindicated with history of allergic-type reaction to *aspirin*, children and adolescents with *Varicella* or other viral illness, and 3rd trimester pregnancy.
▷ *aspirin+caffeine* (D)(G)
Anacin (OTC) 800 mg q 4 hours prn; max 4 gm/day
Pediatric: <6 years: not recommended; 6-12 years: 400 mg q 4 hours prn; max 2 gm/day; ≥12 years: same as adult
   Tab/Cplt: 400 mg
Anacin Maximum Strength (OTC) 1 gm tid-qid
Pediatric: <12 years: not recommended; ≥12 years: same as adult
   Tab: 500 mg
Comment: *aspirin*-containing medications are contraindicated with history of allergic-type reaction to *aspirin*, children and adolescents with *Varicella* or other viral illness, and 3rd trimester pregnancy.
▷ *aspirin+antacid* (D)(G)
Extra Strength Bayer Plus (OTC) 500 mg-1 gm q 4-6 hours prn; usual max 4 gm/day
Pediatric: <12 years: not recommended; ≥12 years: same as adult
   Cplt: 500 mg aspirin+calcium carbonate
Bufferin (OTC) 650 mg q 4 hours; max 3.9 mg/day
Pediatric: <12 years: not recommended; ≥12 years: same as adult
   Tab: 325 mg aspirin+calcium carbonate+magnesium carbonate+magnesium oxide
Comment: *aspirin*-containing medications are contraindicated with history of allergic-type reaction to *aspirin*, children and adolescents with *Varicella* or other viral illness, and 3rd trimester of pregnancy.
▷ *ibuprofen* (B; not for use in 3rd)(G)
Comment: *ibuprofen* is contraindicated in children <6 months-of-age.
Children's Advil (OTC), ElixSure IB (OTC), Motrin (OTC), PediaCare (OTC), PediaProfen (OTC)
Pediatric: 5-10 mg/kg q 6-8 hours; max 40 mg/kg/day; <24 lb (<2 years): individualize; 24-35 lb (2-3 years): 5 ml q 6-8 hours prn; 36-47 lb (4-5 years): 7.5 ml q 6-8 hours prn; 48-59 lb (6-8 years): 10 ml or 2 tabs q 6-8 hours prn; 60-71 lb (9-10 years): 12.5 ml or 2 tabs q 6-8 hours prn; 72-95 lb (11 years): 15 ml or 3 tabs q 6-8 hours prn
   Oral susp: 100 mg/5 ml (2, 4 oz) (berry); *Junior tabs:* 100 mg
Children's Motrin Drops (OTC), PediaCare Drops (OTC)
Pediatric: <24 lb (<2 years): individualize; 24-35 lb (2-3 years): 2.5 ml q 6-8 hours prn
   Oral drops: 50 mg/1.25 ml (15 ml; berry)
Children's Motrin Chewables and Caplets (OTC)

Pediatric: 48-59 lb (6-8 years): 200 mg q 6-8 hours prn; 60-71 lb (9-10 years): 250 mg q 6-8 hours prn; 72-95 lb (11 years): 300 mg q 6-8 hours prn; ≥12 years: same as adult
    Chew tab: 100*mg (citrus; phenylalanine); *Cplt:* 100 mg
Motrin (OTC) 400 mg q 6 hours prn
Pediatric: <6 months: not recommended; ≥6 months, fever <102.5: 5 mg/kg q 6-8 hours prn; >6 months, fever >102.5: 10 mg/kg q 6-8 hours prn
All: max 40 mg/kg/day
    Tab: 400 mg; *Cplt:* 100*mg; *Chew tab:* 50*, 100*mg (citrus; phenylalanine); *Oral susp:* 100 mg/5 ml (4, 16 oz) (berry); *Oral drops:* 40 mg/ml (15 ml) (berry)
Advil (OTC), Motrin IB (OTC), Nuprin (OTC) 200-400 mg q 4-6 hours; max 1.2 gm/day
Pediatric: <12 years: not recommended; ≥12 years: same as adult
    Tab/Cplt/Gel cap: 200 mg
▷ *naproxen* (B)(G)
Pediatric: <2 years: not recommended; ≥2 years: 2.5-5 mg/kg bid-tid; max: 15 mg/kg/day
    Aleve (OTC) 400 mg x 1 dose; then 200 mg q 8-12 hours prn; max 10 days
    Tab/Cplt/Gel cap: 200 mg
    Anaprox 550 mg x 1 dose; then 550 mg q 12 hours *or* 275 mg q 6-8 hours prn; max 1.375 gm first day and 1.1 gm/day thereafter
    Tab: 275 mg
    Anaprox DS 1 tab bid
    Tab: 550 mg
    EC-Naprosyn 375 *or* 500 mg bid prn; may increase dose up to max 1500 mg/day as tolerated
    Tab: 375, 500 mg del-rel
    Naprelan 1 gm daily *or* 1.5 gm daily for limited time; max 1 gm/day thereafter
    Tab: 375, 500 mg
    Naprosyn initially 500 mg, then 500 mg q 12 hours *or* 250 mg q 6-8 hours prn; max 1.25 gm first day and 1 gm/day thereafter
    Tab: 250, 375, 500 mg; *Oral susp:* 125 mg/5 ml (473 ml) (pineapple-orange)

FIBROCYSTIC BREAST DISEASE

Contraceptives *see page 559*
▷ *spironolactone* (D) 10 mg bid pre-menstrually
    Aldactone (G) *Tab:* 25, 50*, 100*mg
    CaroSpir *Oral susp:* 25 mg/5 ml (118, 473 ml) (banana)
▷ *vitamin E* (A) 400-600 IU daily
▷ *vitamin B6* (A) 50-100 mg daily

Synthetic Steroid Derived from Ethisterone

▷ *danazol* (X) start on 3rd or 4th day of menstrual period or after a negative pregnancy test; 50-200 mg bid x 2-6 months
Pediatric: <18 years: not recommended; ≥18 years: same as adult
    Danocrine *Cap:* 50, 100, 200 mg
Comment: *danazol* is a synthetic steroid derived from ethisterone. It suppresses the pituitary-ovarian axis. This suppression is probably a combination of depressed hypothalamic-pituitary response to lowered *estrogen* production, the alteration of sex steroid metabolism, and interaction of *danazol* with sex hormone receptors. The only other demonstrable hormonal effects are weak androgenic activity and depression of both follicle-stimulating hormone (FSH) and luteinizing hormone (LH) output. Recent evidence suggests a direct inhibitory effect at gonadal sites and a binding of **Danocrine** to receptors of gonadal steroids at target organs. In addition, **Danocrine** has been shown to significantly decrease IgG, IgM and IgA levels, as well as phospholipid and IgG isotope autoantibodies in patients with endometriosis and associated elevations of autoantibodies, suggesting this could be another mechanism by which it facilitates regression of fibrocystic breast disease. **Danocrine** usually produces partial to complete disappearance of breast tissue nodularity and complete relief of pain and tenderness. Changes in the menstrual pattern may occur. Generally, the pituitary-suppressive action of **Danocrine** is reversible. Ovulation and cyclic bleeding usually return within 60 to 90 days when therapy with **Danocrine** is discontinued. **Danocrine** is also used to treat endometriosis

(to relieve associated abdominal pain) and hereditary angioedema (to prevent attacks). Contraindications include pregnancy, breastfeeding, active or history of thromboembolic disease/event, porphyria, undiagnosed abnormal genital bleeding, androgen-dependent tumor, and markedly impaired hepatic, renal, or cardiac function.

 FIBROMYALGIA

Acetaminophen for IV Infusion *see* **Pain** *page* 352
NSAIDs *see page* 571
Opioid Analgesics *see* **Pain** *page* 354
Topical & Transdermal Analgesics *see* **Pain** *page* 352
Parenteral Corticosteroids *see page* 577
Oral Corticosteroids *see page* 577
Topical Analgesic and Anesthetic Agents *see page* 569

SEROTONIN-NOREPINEPHRINE REUPTAKE INHIBITORS (SNRIs)

▷ *duloxetine* (C)(G) swallow whole; initially 30 mg once daily x 1 week; then increase to 60 mg once daily; max 120 mg/day
   Pediatric: <12 years: not recommended; ≥12 years: same as adult
       Cymbalta *Cap:* 20, 30, 60 mg ent-coat pellets
▷ *milnacipran* (C)(G) *Day 1:* 12.5 mg once; *Days 2-3:* 12.5 mg bid; *Days 4-7:* 25 mg bid; max 100 mg bid
   Pediatric: <17 years: not recommended; ≥17 years: same as adult
       Savella *Tab:* 12.5, 25, 50, 100 mg

GAMMA-AMINOBUTYRIC ACID ANALOG

▷ *gabapentin* (C) initially 300 mg on Day 1; then 600 mg on Day 2; then 900 mg on Days 3-6; then 1200 mg on Days 7-10; then 1500 mg on Days 11-14; titrate up to 1800 mg on Day 15; take entire dose once daily with the evening meal; do not crush, split, or chew
   Pediatric: <3 years: not recommended; 3-12 years: initially 10-15 mg/kg/day in 3 divided doses; max 12 hours between doses; titrate over 3 days; 3-4 years: titrate to 40 mg/kg/day; 5-12 years: titrate to 25-35 mg/kg/day; max 50 mg/kg/day; >12 years: same as adult
       Gralise *Tab:* 300, 600 mg
       Neurontin (G) 100 mg daily x 1 day; then 100 mg bid x 1 day; then 100 mg tid continuously or 300 mg bid; max 900 mg tid
           Tab: 600*, 800*mg; *Cap:* 100, 300, 400 mg; *Oral soln:* 250 mg/5 ml (480 ml) (strawberry-anise)
▷ *gabapentin enacarbil* (C) 600 mg once daily at about 5:00 PM; if dose not taken at recommended time, next dose should be taken the following day; swallow whole; take with food; *CrCl 30-59 mL/min:* 600 mg on Day 1, Day 3, and every day thereafter; *CrCl <30 mL/min:* or on hemodialysis: not recommended
   Pediatric: <12 years: not recommended; ≥12 years: same as adult
       Horizant *Tab:* 300, 600 mg ext-rel
   Comment: Avoid abrupt cessation of *gabapentin* and *gabapentin enacarbil*. To discontinue, withdraw gradually over 1 week or longer.

ALPHA-2 DELTA LIGAND

▷ *pregabalin* (*GABA analog*) (C)(V)
   Pediatric: <18 years: not recommended; ≥18 years: same as adult
       Lyrica initially 50 mg tid; may titrate to 100 mg tid within one week; max 600 mg divided tid; discontinue over 1 week
           Cap: 25, 50, 75, 100, 150, 200, 225, 300 mg; *Oral soln:* 20 mg/ml
       Lyrica CR *Tab:* usual dose: 165 mg once daily; may increase to 330 mg/day within 1 week; max 660 mg/day
           Tab: 82.5, 165, 330 mg ext-rel

OTHER AGENTS

▷ *amitriptyline* (C)(G) 20 mg q HS; may increase gradually to max 50 mg q HS
   Pediatric: <12 years: not recommended; ≥12 years: same as adult
       Tab: 10, 25, 50, 75, 100, 150 mg

▷ *cyclobenzaprine* (B)(G) 10 mg tid; usual range 20-40 mg/day in divided doses; max 60 mg/day x 2-3 weeks <u>or</u> 15 mg ext-rel once daily; max 30 mg ext-rel/day x 2-3 weeks
   Pediatric: <15 years: not recommended; ≥15 years: same as adult
      Amrix *Cap:* 15, 30 mg ext-rel
      Fexmid *Tab:* 7.5 mg
      Flexeril *Tab:* 5, 10 mg
▷ *eszopiclone* (C)(IV)(G) (pyrrolopyrazine) 1-3 mg; max 3 mg/day x 1 month; do not take if unable to sleep for at least 8 hours before required to be active again; delayed effect if taken with a meal
   Pediatric: <18 years: not recommended; ≥18 years: same as adult
      Lunesta *Tab:* 1, 2, 3 mg
▷ *flurazepam* (X)(IV)(G) 15 mg q HS; may increase to 30 mg q HS
   Pediatric: <18 years: not recommended; ≥18 years: same as adult
      Dalmane *Cap:* 15, 30 mg
▷ *trazodone* (C)(G) 50 mg q HS
   Pediatric: <18 years: not recommended; ≥18 years: same as adult
      Desyrel *Tab:* 50, 100, 150, 300 mg
▷ *triazolam* (X)(IV)(G) 0.125 mg q HS, may increase gradually to 0.5 mg
   Pediatric: <18 years: not recommended; ≥18 years: same as adult
      Halcion *Tab:* 0.125, 0.25*mg
▷ *zaleplon* (C)(IV) (imidazopyridine) 5-10 mg at HS <u>or</u> after going to bed if unable to sleep; do not take if unable to sleep for at least 4 hours before required to be active again; max 20 mg/day x 1 month; delayed effect if taken with a meal
   Pediatric: <12 years: not recommended; ≥12 years: same as adult
      Sonata *Cap:* 5, 10 mg (tartrazine)
      Comment: **Sonata** is indicated for the treatment of insomnia when a middle-of-the-night awakening is followed by difficulty returning to sleep.
▷ *zolpidem* oral solution spray (C)(IV)(G) (imidazopyridine hypnotic) 2 actuations (10 mg) immediately before bedtime; *Elderly, debilitated,* <u>or</u> *hepatic impairment:* 2 actuations (5 mg); max 2 actuations (10 mg)
   Pediatric: <18 years: not recommended; ≥18 years: same as adult
      ZolpiMist *Oral soln spray:* 5 mg/actuation (60 metered actuations) (cherry)
      Comment: The lowest dose of *zolpidem* in all forms is recommended for persons >50 years-of-age and women as drug elimination is slower than in men.
▷ *zolpidem* tabs (B)(IV)(G) (pyrazolopyrimidine hypnotic) 5-10 mg <u>or</u> 6.25-12.5 extrel q HS prn; max 12.5 mg/day x 1 month; do not take if unable to sleep for at least 8 hours before required to be active again; delayed effect if taken with a meal
   Pediatric: <18 years: not recommended; ≥18 years: same as adult
      Ambien *Tab:* 5, 10 mg
      Ambien CR *Tab:* 6.25, 12.5 mg ext-rel
      Comment: The lowest dose of *zolpidem* in all forms is recommended for persons >50 years-of-age and women as drug elimination is slower than in men.
▷ *zolpidem* sublingual tabs (imidazopyridine hypnotic) (C)(IV) dissolve 1 tab under the tongue; allow to disintegrate completely before swallowing; take only once per night and only if at least 4 hours of bedtime remain before planned time for awakening
   Pediatric: <18 years: not recommended; ≥18 years: same as adult
      Edluar *SL Tab:* 5, 10 mg
      Intermezzo *SL Tab:* 1.75, 3.5 mg
      Comment: **Intermezzo** is indicated for the treatment of insomnia when a middle-of-the-night awakening is followed by difficulty returning to sleep. The lowest dose of *zolpidem* in all forms is recommended for persons >50 years-of-age and women as drug elimination is slower than in men.

FIFTH DISEASE (*ERYTHEMA INFECTIOSUM*)

Antipyretics *see Fever page 163*

FLATULENCE

▷ *simethicone* (C)(G)
      Gas-X (OTC) 2-4 tabs pc and HS prn
      Tab: 40, 80, 125 mg; *Cap:* 125 mg

Mylicon (OTC) 2-4 tabs pc and HS prn
Tab: 40, 80, 125 mg; *Cap:* 125 mg
Phazyme-95 1-2 tabs with each meal and HS prn
Tab: 95 mg
Phazyme Infant Oral Drops
Pediatric: <2 years: 0.3 ml qid pc and HS prn; 2-12 years: 0.6 ml qid pc and HS prn; >12 years: 1.2 ml qid pc and HS prn
Oral drops: 40 mg/0.6 ml (15, 30 ml w. calibrated dropper) (orange) (alcohol-free)
Maximum Strength Phazyme 1-2 caps with each meal and HS prn
Cap: 125 mg

FLUORIDATION, WATER, <0.6 PPM

▷ *fluoride* (G)
Luride
Pediatric: Water fluoridation 0.3-0.6 ppm: <3 years: use drops; 3-6 years: 0.25 mg daily; 7-16 years: 0.5 mg daily; *Water fluoridation <0.3 ppm:* <3 years: use drops; 6 months-3 years: 0.25 mg daily; 4-6 years: 0.5 mg daily; 7-16 years: 1 mg daily
Chew tab: 0.25, 0.5, 1 mg (sugar-free)
Luride Drops
Pediatric: Water fluoridation 0.3-0.6 ppm: 6 months-3 years: 0.25 ml once daily; 4-6 years: 0.5 ml once daily; 7-16 years: 1 ml once daily; *Water fluoridation <0.3 ppm:* 6 months-3 years: 0.5 ml once daily; 4-6 years: 1 ml once daily; 7-16 years: 2 ml daily
Oral drops: 0.5 mg/ml (50 ml) (sugar-free)

COMBINATION AGENTS

▷ *fluoride+vitamin a+vitamin d+vitamin c* (G)
Pediatric: Water fluoridation 0.3-0.6 ppm: <3 years: not recommended; 3-6 years: 0.25 mg fluoride/day; 7-16 years: 0.5 mg fluoride/day; *Water fluoridation <0.3 ppm:* <6 months: not recommended; 6 months-3 years: 0.25 mg fluoride/day; 4-6 years: 0.5 mg fluoride/day; 7-16 years: 1 mg fluoride/day
Tri-Vi-Flor Drops
Oral drops: fluoride 0.25 mg+vit a 1500 u+vit d 400 u+vit c 35 mg per ml (50 ml)
Oral drops: fluoride 0.5 mg+vit a 1500 u+vit d 400 u+vit c 35 mg per ml (50 ml)
▷ *fluoride+vitamin a+vitamin d+vitamin c+iron*
Pediatric: Water fluoridation 0.3-0.6 ppm: <3 years: not recommended; 3-6 years: 0.25 mg fluoride/day; 7-16 years: 0.5 mg fluoride/day; *Water fluoridation <0.3 ppm:* <6 months: not recommended; 6 months-3 years: 0.25 mg fluoride/day; 4-6 years: 0.5 mg fluoride/day; 7-16 years: 1 mg fluoride/day
Tri-Vi-Flor w. Iron Drops
Oral drops: fluoride 0.25 mg+vit a 1500 u+vit d 400 u+vit c 35 mg+iron 10 mg per ml (50 ml)

FOLLICULITIS BARBAE

Topical Corticosteroids *page 574*

TOPICAL AGENTS

▷ *benzoyl peroxide* (B) apply after shaving; may discolor clothing and linens.
Benzac-W initially apply to affected area once daily; increase to bid-tid as tolerated
Gel: 2.5, 5, 10% (60 gm)
Benzac-W Wash wash affected area bid
Wash: 5% (4, 8 oz); 10% (8 oz)
Benzagel apply to affected area one or more x/day
Gel: 5, 10% (1.5, 3 oz) (alcohol 14%)
Benzagel Wash wash affected area bid
Gel: 10% (6 oz)
Desquam X₅ wash affected area bid
Wash: 5% (5 oz)
Desquam X₁₀ wash affected area bid
Wash: 10% (5 oz)

      Triaz apply to affected area daily bid
        Lotn: 3, 6, 9% (bottle); 3% (tube); *Pads:* 3, 6, 9% (jar)
      ZoDerm apply once or twice daily
        Gel: 4.5, 6.5, 8.5% (125 ml); *Crm:* 4.5, 6.5, 8.5% (125 ml); *Clnsr:* 4.5, 6.5, 8.5%
        (400 ml)

▷ *clindamycin* topical (**B**) apply bid
  Pediatric: same as adult
      Cleocin T *Pad:* 1% (60/pck; alcohol 50%); *Lotn:* 1% (60 ml); *Gel:* 1% (30, 60 gm); *Soln*
      w. applicator: 1% (30, 60 ml) (alcohol 50%)
      Clindagel *Gel:* 1% (42, 77 gm)
      Clindets *Pad:* 1% (60/pck)
      Evoclin *Foam:* 1% (50, 100 gm) (alcohol)

▷ *clindamycin+benzoyl peroxide* topical (**C**)
  Pediatric: <12 years: not recommended; ≥12 years: same as adult
      Acanya (G) apply once daily-bid
        Gel: clin 1.2%+*benz* 2.5% (50 gm)
      BenzaClin apply bid
        Gel: clin 1%+*benz* 5% (25, 50 gm)
      Duac apply daily in the evening
        Gel: clin 1%+*benz* 5% (45 gm)
      Onexton Gel (G) apply once daily
        Gel: clin 1.2%+benz 3.75% (50 gm pump) (alcohol-free) (preservative-free)

▷ *dapsone* topical (**C**)(**G**) apply bid
  Pediatric: <12 years: not recommended; ≥12 years: same as adult
      Aczone *Gel:* 5% (30 gm)

▷ *tazarotene* (**X**)(**G**) apply daily at HS
  Pediatric: <12 years: not recommended; ≥12 years: same as adult
      Avage Cream *Crm:* 0.1% (30 gm)
      Tazorac Cream *Crm:* 0.05, 0.1% (15, 30, 60 gm)
      Tazorac Gel *Gel:* 0.05, 0.1% (30, 100 gm)

▷ *tretinoin* (**C**) apply q HS
  Pediatric: <12 years: not recommended; ≥12 years: same as adult
      Atralin Gel *Gel:* 0.05% (45 gm)
      Avita *Crm:* 0.025% (20, 45 gm); *Gel:* 0.025% (20, 45 gm)
      Renova *Crm:* 0.02% (40 gm); 0.05% (40, 60 gm)
      Retin-A Cream *Crm:* 0.025, 0.05, 0.1% (20, 45 gm)
      Retin-A Gel *Gel:* 0.01, 0.025% (15, 45 gm; alcohol 90%)
      Retin-A Liquid *Soln:* 0.05% (alcohol 55%)
      Retin-A Micro Gel *Gel:* 0.04, 0.08, 0.1% (20, 45 gm)
      Tretin-X Cream *Crm:* 0.075% (35 gm) (parabens-free, alcohol-free, propylene
      glycol-free)
      Retin-A Micro *Microspheres:* 0.04, 0.1% (20, 45 gm)

FOREIGN BODY: ESOPHAGUS

▷ *glucagon* (**B**) 0.02 mg/kg IV or IM with serial x-rays; max 1 mg
      Glucagon (rDNA origin or beef/pork derived)
        Vial: 1 mg/ml w. diluent
Comment: *glucagon* facilitates passage of foreign body from esophagus into stomach.

FOREIGN BODY: EYE

▷ *proparacaine* 1-2 drops to anesthetize surface of eye; then flush with normal saline
      Ophthaine *Ophth soln:* 0.5% (15 ml)
Comment: *proparacaine* facilitates the search, location, and removal of foreign body and
examination of the cornea.

GASTRITIS/DYSPEPSIA

Antacids *see GERD page* 170
H2 Antagonists *see GERD page* 172

GASTRITIS-RELATED NAUSEA/VOMITING

OTC ANTI-EMETIC

▷ *phosphorylated carbohydrate* solution (C)(G) 1-2 tbsp q 15 minutes until nausea subsides; max 5 doses/day
  Pediatric: 1-2 tsp q 15 minutes until nausea subsides; max 5 doses/day
    Emetrol (OTC) *Soln:* dextrose 1.87 gm+fructose 1.87 gm+phosphoric acid 21.5 mg per 5 ml (4, 8, 16 oz)

Rx ANTI-EMETICS

▷ *ondansetron* (C)(G) 8 mg q 8 hours x 2 doses; then 8 mg q 12 hours
  Pediatric: <4 years: not recommended; 4-11 years: 4 mg q 4 hours x 3 doses; then 4 mg q 8 hours
    Zofran *Tab:* 4, 8, 24 mg
    Zofran ODT *ODT:* 4, 8 mg (strawberry) (phenylalanine)
    Zofran Oral Solution *Oral soln:* 4 mg/5 ml (50 ml) (strawberry) (phenylalanine); *Parenteral form:* see mfr pkg insert
    Zofran Injection *Vial:* 2 mg/ml (2 ml single-dose); 2 mg/ml (20 ml multi-dose); 32 mg/50 ml (50 ml multi-dose); *Prefilled syringe:* 4 mg/2 ml, single-use (24/carton)
    Zuplenz Oral Soluble Film: 4, 8 mg oral-dis (10/carton) (peppermint)
  Comment: The FDA has issued an updated warning against *ondansetron* use in pregnancy *ondansetron* is a 5-HT3 receptor antagonist approved by the FDA for preventing nausea and vomiting related to cancer chemotherapy and surgery. However, it has been used "off label" to treat the nausea and vomiting of pregnancy. The FDA has cautioned against the use of *ondansetron* in pregnancy in light of studies of *ondansetron* in early pregnancy and associated with congenital cardiac malformations and oral clefts (i.e., cleft lip and cleft palate). Further, there are potential maternal risks in pregnancy with electrolyte imbalance caused by severe nausea and vomiting (as with hyperemesis gravidarum). These risks include serotonin syndrome (a triad of of cognitive and behavioral changes including confusion, agitation, autonomic instability, and neuromuscular changes). Therefore, *ondansetron* should <u>not</u> be taken during pregnancy.
▷ *promethazine* (C)(G) 25 mg PO <u>or</u> rectally q 4-6 hours prn
  Pediatric: <2 years: not recommended; ≥2 years: 0.5 mg/lb <u>or</u> 6.25-25 mg q 4-6 hours prn
    Phenergan *Tab:* 12.5*, 25*, 50 mg; *Plain syr:* 6.25 mg/5 ml; *Fortis syr:* 25 mg/5 ml; *Rectal supp:* 12.5, 25, 50 mg
  Comment: *promethazine* is contraindicated in children with uncomplicated nausea, dehydration, Reye's syndrome, history of sleep apnea, asthma, and lower respiratory disorders in children. *promethazine* lowers the seizure threshold in children, may cause cholestatic jaundice, anticholinergic effects, extrapyramidal effects, and potentially fatal respiratory depression.

 GASTROESOPHAGEAL REFLUX (GER), GASTROESOPHAGEAL REFLUX DISEASE (GERD), IDIOPATHIC GASTRIC ACID HYPERSECRETION (IGAH)

Comment: Precipitators of gastric reflux include narcotics, benzodiazepines, calcium antagonists, alcohol, nicotine, chocolate, and peppermint. Issues associated with H2 secretion and gastrointestinal health (e.g., chronic remitting gastritis, Barrett's esophagitis, peptic ulcer disease [PUD]), other organ system impairments (e.g., CVD, metabolic syndrome, hepatitis, autoimmune and immune-deficiency disorders, renal insufficiency, iatrogenic consequences of treatments (e.g., steroids, NSAIDs, immune modulators), (advanced age,) and lifestyle (dietary habits and general nutritional health). Risk/benefit discussions with patients can be challenging, but are necessary for informed decision-making and prudent prescribing.

ANTACIDS

Comment: Antacids with *aluminum hydroxide* may potentiate constipation. Antacids with *magnesium hydroxide* may potentiate diarrhea.
▷ *aluminum hydroxide* (C)
    ALTernaGEL (OTC) 5-10 ml between meals and HS prn; max 90 ml/day
    Pediatric: <12 years: not recommended; ≥12 years: same as adult

    Liq: 500 mg/5 ml (5, 12 oz)

Amphojel (OTC) 10 ml 5-6 x/day between meals and HS prn; max 60 ml/day
Pediatric: <12 years: not recommended; ≥12 years: same as adult
    Oral susp: 320 mg/5 ml (12 oz)

Amphojel Tab (OTC) 600 mg 5-6 x/day between meals and HS prn; max 3.6 gm/day
Pediatric: <12 years: not recommended; ≥12 years: same as adult
    Tab: 300, 600 mg

▷ *aluminum hydroxide+magnesium hydroxide* (C)(OTC)(G)

Maalox 10-20 ml qid and HS prn
Pediatric: <12 years: not recommended; ≥12 years: same as adult
    Oral susp: alum 225 mg+mag 200 mg per 5 ml (5, 12, 26 oz) (mint, lemon, cherry)

Maalox Therapeutic Concentrate 10-20 ml qid pc and HS prn
Pediatric: <12 years: not recommended; ≥12 years: same as adult
    Oral susp: alum 600 mg+mag 300 mg per 5 ml (12 oz) (mint)

▷ *aluminum hydroxide+magnesium hydroxide+simethicone* (C)(OTC)(G)

Maalox Plus 10-20 ml qid pc and HS prn
Pediatric: <12 years: not recommended; ≥12 years: same as adult
    Tab: alum 200 mg+mag 200 mg+sim 25 mg

Extra Strength Maalox Plus 10-20 ml qid pc and HS prn
Pediatric: <12 years: not recommended; ≥12 years: same as adult
    Tab: alum 350 mg+mag 350 mg+sim 30 mg
    Oral susp: alum 500 mg+mag 450 mg+sim 40 mg per 5 ml (5, 12, 26 oz)

Extra Strength Maalox Plus Tab 1-3 tabs qid pc and HS prn
Pediatric: <12 years: not recommended; ≥12 years: same as adult
    Tab: alum 350 mg+mag 350 mg+sim 30 mg

Mylanta 10-20 ml between meals and HS prn
Pediatric: <12 years: not recommended; ≥12 years: same as adult
    Liq: alum 200 mg+mag 200 mg+sim 20 mg per 5 ml (5, 12, 24 oz)

Mylanta Double Strength 10-20 ml between meals and HS prn
Pediatric: <12 years: not recommended; ≥12 years: same as adult
    Liq: alum 700 mg+mag 400 mg+sim 40 mg per 5 ml (5, 12, 24 oz)

▷ *aluminum hydroxide+magnesium carbonate* (C)(OTC)(G)

Maalox HRF 10-20 ml qid pc and HS prn
Pediatric: <12 years: not recommended; ≥12 years: same as adults
    Oral susp: alum 280 mg+mag 350 mg per 10 ml (10 oz)

▷ *aluminum hydroxide+magnesium trisilicate* (C)(G)

Gaviscon chew 2-4 tabs qid pc and HS prn
Pediatric: <12 years: not recommended; ≥12 years: same as adult
    Tab: alum 80 mg+mag 20 mg

Gaviscon Liquid 15-30 ml qid pc and HS prn
Pediatric: <12 years: not recommended; ≥12 years: same as adult
    Liq: alum 95 mg+mag 359 mg per 15 ml (6, 12 oz)

Gaviscon Extra Strength 2-4 tabs qid pc and HS prn
Pediatric: <12 years: not recommended; ≥12 years: same as adult
    Tab: alum 160 mg+mag 105 mg

Gaviscon Extra Strength Liquid 10-20 ml qid prn
Pediatric: <12 years: not recommended; ≥12 years: same as adult
    Liq: alum 508 mg+mag 475 mg per 10 ml (12 oz)

▷ *aluminum hydroxide+magnesium hydroxide+simethicone* (C)(OTC)(G)

Maalox Maximum Strength 10-20 ml qid prn; max 60 ml/day
Pediatric: <12 years: not recommended; ≥12 years: same as adult
    Oral susp: alum 500 mg+mag 450 mg+sim 40 mg per 5 ml (5, 12, 26 oz) (mint, cherry)

▷ *calcium carbonate* (C)(OTC)(G)

Children's Mylanta Tab
Pediatric: <2 years: not recommended; 2-5 years (24-47 lb): 1 tab as needed up to tid; 6-11 years (48-95 lb): 2 tabs as needed up to tid
    Tab: 400 mg

Children's Mylanta
Pediatric: <2 years: not recommended; 2-5 years (24-47 lb): 1 tab as needed up to tid; 6-11 years (48-95 lb): 2 tabs as needed up to tid
    Liq: 400 mg/5 ml (4 oz)

Maalox Tab chew 2-4 tabs prn; max 12 tabs/day
Pediatric: <12 years: not recommended; ≥12 years: same as adult
  Chew tab: 600 mg (wild berry, lemon, wintergreen) (phenylalanine)
Maalox Maximum Strength Tab 1-2 tabs prn; max 8 tabs/day
Pediatric: <12 years: not recommended; ≥12 years: same as adult
  Tab: 1 gm (wild berry, lemon, wintergreen; phenylalanine)
Rolaids Extra Strength 1-2 tabs dissolved in mouth <u>or</u> chewed q 1 hour prn; max 8 tabs/day
  Tab: 1000 mg
Tums 1-2 tabs dissolved in mouth <u>or</u> chewed q 1 hour prn; max 16 tabs/day
  Tab: 500 mg
Tums E-X 1-2 tabs dissolved in mouth <u>or</u> chewed q 1 hour prn; max 16 tabs/day
  Tab: 750 mg

▷ *calcium carbonate+magnesium hydroxide* (C)
Mylanta Tab 2-4 tabs between meals and HS prn
Pediatric: <12 years: not recommended; ≥12 years: same as adult
  Tab: calib 350 mg+mag 150 mg
Mylanta DS Tab 2-4 tabs between meals and HS prn
Pediatric: <12 years: not recommended; ≥12 years: same as adult
  Tab: calib 700 mg+mag 300 mg
Rolaids Sodium-Free 1-2 tabs dissolved in mouth <u>or</u> chewed q 1 hour as needed
  Tab: calib 317 mg+mag 64 mg

▷ *calcium carbonate+magnesium carbonate* (C)
Mylanta Gel Caps (OTC) 2-4 caps prn
  Gel cap: calib 550 mg+mag 125 mg

▷ *dihydroxyaluminum*
Rolaids (OTC) 1-2 tabs dissolved in mouth <u>or</u> chewed q 1 hour prn; max 24 tabs/day
  Tab: 334 mg

H2 ANTAGONISTS

▷ *cimetidine* (B)(OTC)(G) 800 mg bid <u>or</u> 400 mg qid; max 12 weeks
Pediatric: <16 years: not recommended; ≥16 years: same as adult
Tagamet 800 mg bid <u>or</u> 400 mg qid; max 12 weeks
  Tab: 200, 300, 400*, 800*mg
Tagamet HB *Prophylaxis:* 1 tab ac; *Treatment:* 1 tab bid
  Tab: 200 mg
Tagamet HB Oral Suspension *Prophylaxis:* 1-3 tsp ac; *Treatment:* 1 tsp bid
  Oral susp: 200 mg/20 ml (12 oz)
Tagamet Liquid *Liq:* 300 mg/5 ml (mint-peach) (alcohol 2.8%)

▷ *famotidine* (B)(OTC)(G)
Pediatric: 0.5 mg/kg/day q HS prn <u>or</u> in 2 divided doses; max 40 mg/day
Maximum Strength Pepcid AC 1 tab ac
  Tab: 20 mg
Pepcid 20-40 mg bid; max 6 weeks
  Tab: 20 mg; *Tab:* 40 mg; *Oral susp:* 40 mg/5 ml (50 ml)
Pepcid AC 1 tab ac; max 2 doses/day
  Tab/Rapid dissolving tab: 10 mg
Pepcid Complete (OTC) 1 tab ac; max 2 doses/day
  Tab: fam 10 mg+$CaCO_2$ 800 mg+mag hydroxide 165 mg
Pepcid RPD *Tab:* 20, 40 mg rapid dissolv

▷ *nizatidine* (B)(OTC)(G) 150 mg bid <u>or</u> 300 mg once daily
Pediatric: <12 years: not recommended; ≥12 years: same as adult
Axid *Cap:* 150, 300 mg; *Oral soln:* 15 mg/ml (480 ml) (bubble gum)

▷ *ranitidine* (B)(OTC)(G)
Pediatric: <1 month: not recommended; 1 month to 16 years: 2-4 mg/kg/day in 2 divided doses; max 300 mg/day; *Duodenal/Gastric Ulcer:* 2-4 mg/kg/day divided bid; max 300 mg/day; *Erosive Esophagitis:* 5-10 mg/kg/day divided bid; max 300 mg/day; 20 lb, 9 kg: 0.6 ml; 30 lb, 13.6 kg: 0.9 ml; 40 lb, 18.2 kg: 1.2 ml; 50 lb, 22.7 kg: 1.5 ml; 60 lb, 27.3 kg: 1.8 ml; 70 lb, 31.8 kg: 2.1 ml
Zantac 150 mg bid <u>or</u> 300 mg q HS
  Tab: 150, 300 mg

Zantac 75 1 tab ac
    Tab: 75 mg
Zantac EFFERdose dissolve 25 mg tab in 5 ml water and dissolve 150 mg tab in 6-8 oz water
    Efferdose: 25, 150 mg effervescent
Zantac Syrup *Syr:* 15 mg/ml (peppermint) (alcohol 7.5%)
▷ *ranitidine bismuth citrate* (C) 400 mg bid
    Pediatric: <12 years: not recommended; ≥12 years: same as adult
        Tritec *Tab:* 400 mg

PROTON PUMP INHIBITORS (PPIs)

Comment: A study of 144,032 incident users of acid suppression therapy, including 125,596 PPI users and 18,436 histamine H2 receptor antagonist users were followed over 5 years. The researchers reported PPI users had an increased risk of having an eGFR <60 mL/min/1.73m^2, incident CKD, eGFR decline over 30%, and ESRD or eGFR decline over 50%, as compared to those taking H2 blockers. They concluded, "reliance on antecedent acute kidney injury (AKI) as a warning sign to guard against the risk of chronic kidney disease (CKD) among PPI users is <u>not</u> sufficient as a sole mitigation strategy." Further, timely PPI discontinuation is warranted if there is a first AKI to avoid progression to CKD.

REFERENCE
Xie, Y., Bowe, B., Li, T., Xian, H., Yan, Y., & Al-Aly, Z. (2017). Long-term kidney outcomes among users of proton pump inhibitors without intervening acute kidney injury. *Kidney International, 91*(6), 1482–1494. doi:10.1016/j.kint.2016.12.021

Comment: Practice guidelines from the American Gastroenterological Association (AGA) address risks and recommendations for prescribing PPI therapy based on an extensive review of the literature. PPI use may increase the risk for fracture, vitamin B12 deficiency, hypomagnesemia, iron-deficiency anemia, small intestinal bacterial overgrowth (SIBO), *C. difficile* infection, kidney disease, cardiovascular disease (CVD), pneumonias, and dementia. Health care providers are advised to discuss the risks/ benefits of PPI therapy with respect to each individual patient's situation.

REFERENCE
Freedberg, D. E., Kim, L. S., & Yang, Y.-X. (2017). The risks and benefits of long-term use of proton pump inhibitors: Expert review and best practice advice from the American Gastroenterological Association. *Gastroenterology, 152*(4), 706–715. doi:10.1053/j.gastro.2017.01.031

▷ *dexlansoprazole* (B)(G) 30-60 mg daily for up to 4 weeks
    Pediatric: <18 years: not recommended; ≥18 years: same as adult
        Dexilant *Cap:* 30, 60 mg ent-coat del-rel granules; may open and sprinkle on apple-sauce; do not crush <u>or</u> chew granules
        Dexilant SoluTab *Tab:* 30 mg del-rel orally disint
▷ *esomeprazole* (B)(OTC)(G) 20-40 mg once daily; max 8 weeks; take 1 hour before food; swallow whole <u>or</u> mix granules with food <u>or</u> juice and take immediately; do not crush <u>or</u> chew granules
    Pediatric: <1 month: not established; 1 month-<1 year, 3-5 kg: 2.5 mg; 5-7.5 kg: 5 mg; 7.5-12 kg: 10 mg; 1-11 years, <20 kg: 10 mg; ≥20 kg: 10-20 mg; 12-17 years: 20 mg; max 8 weeks; >17 years: same as adult
        Nexium *Cap:* 20, 40 mg ent-coat del-rel pellets
        Nexium for Oral Suspension *Oral susp:* 10, 20, 40 mg ent-coat del-rel granules/pkt; mix in 2 tbsp water and drink immediately; 30 pkt/carton
▷ *lansoprazole* (B)(OTC)(G) 15-30 mg daily for up to 8 weeks; may repeat course; take before eating
    Pediatric: <1 year: not recommended; 1-11 years, <30 kg: 15 mg once daily; >11 years: same as adult
        Prevacid *Cap:* 15, 30 mg ent-coat del-rel granules; swallow whole <u>or</u> mix granules with food <u>or</u> juice and take immediately; do not crush <u>or</u> chew granules; follow with water
        Prevacid for Oral Suspension *Oral susp:* 15, 30 mg ent-coat del-rel granules/pkt; mix in 2 tbsp water and drink immediately; 30 pkt/carton (strawberry)
        Prevacid SoluTab *ODT:* 15, 30 mg (strawberry) (phenylalanine)

Prevacid 24HR 15 mg ent-coat del-rel granules; swallow whole or mix granules with food or juice and take immediately; do not crush or chew granules; follow with water

▷ *omeprazole* (C)(OTC)(G) 20-40 mg daily for 14 days; may repeat course in 4 months; take before eating; swallow whole or mix granules with applesauce and take immediately; do not crush or chew granules; follow with water
Pediatric: <18 years: not recommended; ≥18 years: same as adult
Prilosec *Cap:* 10, 20, 40 mg ent-coat del-rel granules
Pediatric: <1 year: not recommended; ≥1 year: 5-<10 kg: 5 mg daily; 10-<20 kg: 10 mg daily; ≥20 kg: same as adult
Prilosec OTC *Tab:* 20 mg del-rel (regular, wildberry, strawberry)
Pediatric: <18 years: not recommended; ≥18 years: same as adult

▷ *pantoprazole* (B)(G) 40 mg daily
Pediatric: <12 years: not recommended; ≥12 years: same as adult
Protonix *Tab:* 40 mg ent-coat del-rel
Protonix for Oral Suspension *Oral susp:* 40 mg ent-coat del-rel granules/pkt; mix in 1 tsp apple juice for 5 seconds or sprinkle on 1 tsp apple sauce, and swallow immediately; do not mix in water or any other liquid or food; take approximately 30 minutes prior to a meal; 30 pkt/carton

▷ *rabeprazole* (B)(OTC)(G) *Tab:* 20 mg daily after breakfast; do not crush or chew; *Cap:* open cap and sprinkle contents on a small amount of soft food or liquid
Pediatric: <1 year: not recommended; 1-11 years, <15 kg: 5 mg once daily for up to 12 weeks; ≥12 years, ≥15 kg: same as adult
AcipHex *Tab:* 20 mg ent-coat del-rel
AcipHex Sprinkle *Cap:* 5, 10 mg del-rel

PROTON PUMP INHIBITORS+SODIUM BICARBONATE COMBINATION

▷ *omeprazole+sodium bicarbonate* (B)(G) 20 mg daily; do not crush or chew; max 8 weeks
Pediatric: <18 years: not recommended; ≥18 years: same as adult
Zegerid *Cap:* omep 20 mg+sod bicarb 1100 mg; omep 40 mg+sod bicarb 1100 mg
Zegerid OTC (OTC) *Cap:* omep 20 mg+sod bicarb 1100 mg
Zegerid for Oral Suspension *Pwdr for oral susp:* omep 20 mg+sod bicarb 1680 mg; omep 40 mg+sod bicarb 1680 mg (30 pkt/carton)

PROMOTILITY AGENT

▷ *metoclopramide* (B)(G) 10-15 mg qid 30 minutes ac and HS prn; up to 20 mg prior to provoking situation; max 12 weeks per therapeutic course
Pediatric: <18 years: not recommended; ≥18 years: same as adult
Metozolv ODT *ODT:* 5, 10 mg (mint)
Reglan *Tab:* 5*, 10 mg; *Syr:* 5 mg/5 ml
Reglan ODT *ODT:* 5, 10 mg (orange)
Comment: *metoclopropamide* is contraindicated when stimulation of GI motility may be dangerous. Observe for tardive dyskinesia and Parkinsonism. Avoid concomitant drugs which may cause an extrapyramidal reaction (e.g., phenothiazines, *haloperidol*).

 GAUCHER DISEASE, TYPE 1

Comment: Gaucher disease, type 1 (GD1) is the most common form of Gaucher disease. Like other types of Gaucher disease, GD1 is caused when insufficient glucocerebrosidase (GBA), an enzyme that breaks down glucocerebroside, is produced. Fat-filled Gaucher cells build up in areas like the spleen, liver, and bone marrow. Unlike type 2 and 3, GD1 does not usually involve the central nervous system. Symptoms of GD1 include enlarged spleen and liver, low blood cell counts, bleeding problems, and bone disease. Symptoms can range from mild to severe and may appear anytime from childhood to adulthood. Gaucher disease is caused by mutations in the GBA gene and is inherited as an autosomal-recessive gene. Treatments may include enzyme replacement therapy or medications that affect the making of fatty molecules (substrate reduction therapy). Patients with GD1 are usually able to live a normal lifespan. GD2 is universally fatal within two years. Patients with GD3 have a 20-40 year life expectancy.

GLUCOSYLCERAMIDE SYNTHASE INHIBITORS

▷ *miglustat* (C)(G) 100 mg 3 x/day at regular intervals; may reduce dose to 100 mg to once daily or twice a day in some patients due to tremor or diarrhea; *CrCl 50-70 mL/min:* start dose at 100 mg bid; *CrCl 30-50 mL/min:* 100 mg once daily; *CrCl <30 mL/min:* not recommended

    Zavesca Cap 100 mg

    Comment: **Zavesca** *(miglustat)* is a glucosylceramide synthase inhibitor indicated as monotherapy for treatment of adult patients with mild/moderate type 1 Gaucher disease for whom enzyme replacement therapy is not a therapeutic option. The most common adverse reactions (incidence ≥5%) diarrhea, weight loss, stomach pain, gas, nausea and vomiting headache including migraine, tremor, leg cramps, dizziness, weakness, vision problems, thrombocytopenia, muscle cramps, back pain, constipation, dry mouth, heaviness in arms and legs, memory loss, unsteady walking, anorexia, indigestion, paresthesia, stomach bloating, stomach pain not related to food, and menstrual changes. Based on animal data, may cause fetal harm. Discontinue **Zavesca** or breastfeeding based on importance of drug to mother. To report suspected adverse reactions, contact Actelion at 1866-228-3546 or FDA at 1-800-FDA-1088 or www.fda.gov/medwatch.

▷ *penicillamine* administer on an empty stomach, at least one hour before meals or two hours after meals, and at least one hour apart from any other drug, food, milk, antacid, zinc or iron-containing preparation; dosage must be individualized, and may require adjustment during the course of treatment; initially, a single daily dose of 125-250 mg; then, increase at 1-3 month intervals by 125-250 mg/day, as patient response and tolerance indicate; if a satisfactory remission of symptoms is achieved, the dose associated with the remission should be continued as the patient's maintenance therapy; if there is no improvement, and there are no signs of potentially serious toxicity after 2-3 months of treatment with doses of 500-750 mg/day, increase by 250 mg/day at 2-3 month intervals until a satisfactory remission occurs or signs of toxicity develop; if there is no discernible improvement after 3-4 months of treatment with 1000-1500 mg/day, discontinue **Cuprimine**; changes in maintenance dosage levels may not be reflected clinically or in the erythrocyte sedimentation rate (ESR) for 2-3 months after each dosage adjustment

    Cuprimine *Cap:* 125, 250 mg

    Depen: 250 mg

Comment: Taking *penicillamine* on an empty stomach permits maximum absorption and reduces the likelihood of inactivation by metal binding in the GI tract. Optimal dosage can be determined by measurement of urinary copper excretion and the determination of free copper in the serum. The urine must be collected in copper-free glassware, and should be quantitatively analyzed for copper before and soon after initiation of therapy with **Cupramine**. Determination of 24-hour urinary copper excretion is of greatest value in the first week of therapy with *penicillamine*. In the absence of any drug reaction, a dose between 0.75 and 1.5 g that results in an initial 24-hour cupriuresis of over 2 mg should be continued for about three months, by which time the most reliable method of monitoring maintenance treatment is the determination of free copper in the serum. This equals the difference between quantitatively determined total copper and ceruloplasmin-copper. Adequately treated patients will usually have less than 10 mcg free copper/dL of serum. It is seldom necessary to exceed a dosage of 2 gm/day. In patients who cannot tolerate as much as 1 g/day initially, initiating dosage with 250 mg/day, and increasing gradually to the requisite amount, gives closer control of the effects of the drug and may help to reduce the incidence of adverse reactions. If the patient is intolerant to therapy with **Cuprimine**, alternative treatment is *trientine* (**Syprine**).

The use of *penicillamine* has been associated with fatalities due to certain diseases such as aplastic anemia, agranulocytosis, thrombocytopenia, Goodpasture's syndrome, and myasthenia gravis. Because of the potential for serious hematological and renal adverse reactions to occur at any time, routine urinalysis, white and differential blood cell count, hemoglobin, and direct platelet count must be checked twice weekly, together with monitoring of the patient's skin, lymph nodes and body temperature, during the first month of therapy, every two weeks for the next five months, and monthly thereafter. Patients should be instructed to report promptly the development of signs and symptoms of granulocytopenia and/or thrombocytopenia such as fever, sore throat, chills, bruising or bleeding; the above laboratory studies should then be promptly repeated.

▷ *trientine* (G) recommended initial dose is 500-750 mg/day for pediatric patients and 750-1250 mg/day for adults given in divided doses two, three or four x/day; may be increased to max 2000 mg/day for adults or 1500 mg/day for patients ≤12 years-of-age; the daily dose of **Syprine** should be increased only when the clinical response is not adequate or the concentration of free serum copper is persistently above 20 mcg/dL; optimal long-term maintenance dose should be determined at 6-12 month intervals; administer on an empty stomach, at least one hour before meals or two hours after meals and at least one hour apart from any other drug, food, or milk; swallow whole with water; do not open the cap or chew the contents

Syprine Cap 250 mg

Comment: **Syprine** is indicated in the treatment of patients with Wilson's disease who are intolerant of *penicillamine*. Clinical experience with **Syprine** is limited and alternate dosing regimens have not been well-characterized; all endpoints in determining an individual patient's dose have not been well defined. **Syprine** and *penicillamine* cannot be considered interchangeable. **Syprine** should be used when continued treatment with *penicillamine* is no longer possible because of intolerable or life endangering side effects. Unlike *penicillamine*, **Syprine** is not recommended in cystinuria or rheumatoid arthritis. The absence of a sulfhydryl moiety renders it incapable of binding cystine and, therefore, it is of no use in cystinuria. In 15 patients with rheumatoid arthritis, **Syprine** was reported not to be effective in improving any clinical or biochemical parameter after 12 weeks of treatment. The most reliable index for monitoring treatment is the determination of free copper in the serum, which equals the difference between quantitatively determined total copper and ceruloplasmin-copper. Adequately treated patients will usually have less than 10 mcg free copper/dL of serum. Therapy may be monitored with a 24-hour urinary copper analysis periodically (i.e., every 6-12 months). Urine must be collected in copper-free glassware. Since a low copper diet should keep copper absorption down to less than one milligram a day, the patient probably will be in the desired state of negative copper balance if 0.5 to 1.0 milligram of copper is present in a 24-hour collection of urine. In general, mineral supplements should not be should not be used since they may block the absorption of **Syprine**. However, iron deficiency may develop, especially in children and menstruating or pregnant women, or as a result of the low copper diet recommended for Wilson's disease. If necessary, iron may be given in short courses, but since iron and **Syprine** each inhibit absorption of the other, two hours should elapse between administration of **Syprine** and iron. *trientine* was teratogenic in animals at doses similar to the human dose. The frequencies of both resorptions and fetal abnormalities, including hemorrhage and edema, increased while fetal copper levels decreased when *trientine* was given in the maternal diets. There are no adequate and well-controlled studies in pregnant women. **Syprine** should be used during pregnancy only if the potential benefit justifies the potential risk to the fetus. It is not known whether this drug is excreted in human milk. Caution should be exercised when **Syprine** is administered to a nursing mother. Clinical studies of **Syprine** did not include sufficient numbers of subjects ≥65 years-of-age to determine whether they respond differently from younger subjects. Other reported clinical experience is insufficient to determine differences in responses between the elderly and younger patients. In general, dose selection should be cautious, usually starting at the low end of the dosing range, reflecting the greater frequency of decreased hepatic, renal, or cardiac function, and of concomitant disease or other drug therapy. Clinical experience with **Syprine** has been limited. The following adverse reactions have been reported in a clinical study in patients with Wilson's disease who were on therapy with *trientine:* iron deficiency, systemic lupus erythematosus. In addition, the following adverse reactions have been reported in marketed use: dystonia, muscular spasm, myasthenia gravis. To report suspected adverse reactions, contact Valeant Pharmaceuticals North America at 1-800-321-4576 or FDA at 1-800-FDA-1088 or www.fda.gov/medwatch.

GIANT CELL ARTERITIS (GCA)/TEMPORAL ARTERITIS

Acetaminophen for IV Infusion *see Pain* page 352
NSAIDs *see page* 571
Opioid Analgesics *see Pain* page 354
Topical & Transdermal Analgesics *see Pain* page 352
Parenteral Corticosteroids *see page* 577
Oral Corticosteroids *see page* 577

Comment: Giant cell arteritis (GCA), or temporal arteritis, is a systemic inflammatory vasculitis of unknown etiology that occurs in persons ≥50 years-of-age (median age of onset is 75 years) and can result in a wide variety of systemic, neurologic, and ophthalmologic complications. GCA is the most common form of systemic vasculitis in adults. Other names for GCA include arteritis cranialis, Horton disease, granulomatous arteritis, and arteritis of the aged. GCA typically affects the superficial temporal arteries—hence the term temporal arteritis. In addition, GCA most commonly affects the ophthalmic, occipital, vertebral, posterior ciliary, and proximal vertebral arteries. It has also been shown to involve medium- and large-sized vessels, including the aorta and the carotid, subclavian, and iliac arteries. Common early symptoms include headache and visual difficulties. Potential consequences include blindness and aortic aneurysms. Newly recognized GCA should be considered a true neuro-ophthalmic emergency. Prompt initiation of treatment may prevent blindness and other potentially irreversible ischemic sequelae. Corticosteroids are the mainstay of therapy. In steroid-resistant cases, drugs such as *cyclosporine*, *azathioprine*, or *methotrexate* may be used as steroid-sparing agents. GCA is the most common systemic vasculitis affecting elderly patients. (http://emedicine.medscape.com/article/332483-overview)

INTERLEUKIN-6 RECEPTOR ANTAGONIST

▷ *tocilizumab* (B) *<100 kg:* 162 mg SC every other week on the same day followed by an increase according to clinical response; *≥100 kg:* 162 mg SC once weekly on the same day; SC injections may be self-administered

Actemra *Vial:* 80 mg/4 ml, 200 mg/10 ml, 400 mg/20 ml, single-use, for IV infusion after dilution; *Prefilled syringe:* 162 mg (0.9 ml, single-dose)

Comment: **Actemra** received FDA approval in May, 2017 to treat GCA. This is the first FDA-approved drug specifically for the treatment of this form of vasculitis. *tocilizumab* is an interleukin-6 receptor-α inhibitor also indicated for use in moderate-to-severe rheumatoid arthritis (RA) that has not responded to conventional therapy, and some subtypes of juvenile idiopathic arthritis (JIA). **Actemra** may be used alone or in combination with *methotrexate* and in RA, other DMARDs may be used. Monitor patient for dose-related laboratory changes including elevated LFTs, neutropenia, and thrombocytopenia. **Actemra** should not be initiated in patients with an absolute neutrophil count (ANC) <2000/mm³, platelet count <100,000/mm³, or who have ALT or AST above 1.5 times the upper limit of normal (ULN). Registration in the Pregnancy Exposure Registry (1-877-311-8972) is encouraged for monitoring pregnancy outcomes in women exposed to **Atemra** during pregnancy. The limited available data with **Actemra** in pregnant women are not sufficient to determine whether there is a drug-associated risk for major birth defects and miscarriage. Monoclonal antibodies, such as *tocilizumab*, are actively transported across the placenta during the third trimester of pregnancy and may affect immune response in the infant exposed *in utero*. It is not known whether *tocilizumab* passes into breast milk; therefore, breastfeeding is not recommended while using **Actemra**.

GIARDIASIS (*GIARDIA LAMBLIA*)

▷ *metronidazole* (not for use in 1st; B in 2nd, 3rd)(G) 250 mg tid x 5-10 days
Pediatric: 35-50 mg/kg/day in 3 divided doses x 10 days
Flagyl *Tab:* 250*, 500*mg
Flagyl 375 *Cap:* 375 mg
Flagyl ER *Tab:* 750 mg ext-rel

▷ *tinidazole* (C) 2 gm in a single dose; take with food
Pediatric: <3 years: not recommended; ≥3 years: 50 mg/kg daily in a single dose; take with food; max 2 gm
Tindamax *Tab:* 250*, 500*mg

Comment: Other than for use in the treatment of *giardiasis* and *amebiasis* in pediatric patients older than three years-of-age, safety and effectiveness of *tinidazole* in pediatric patients have not been established. *tinidazole* is excreted in breast milk in concentrations similar to those seen in serum and can be detected in breast milk for up to 72 hours following administration. Interruption of breast-feeding is recommended during *tinidazole* therapy and for 3 days following the last dose.

▷ *nitazoxanide* (B) 500 mg q 12 hours x 3 days; take with food
  Pediatric: <1 year: not recommended; 1-3 years; 100 mg q 12 hours x 3 days; 4-11 years: 200 mg q 12 hours x 3 days; ≥12 years: same as adult
    Alinia *Tab:* 500 mg; *Oral susp:* 100 mg/5 ml (60 ml)
    Comment: **Alinia** is an antiprotozoal for the treatment of diarrhea due to *G. lamblia* or *C. parvum*.

 GINGIVITIS/PERIODONTITIS

ANTI-INFECTIVE ORAL RINSES
Comment: Oral treatments should be preceded by brushing and flossing the teeth. Avoid foods and liquids for 2-3 hours after a treatment.
▷ *chlorhexidine gluconate* (B)(G) swish 15 ml undiluted for 30 seconds bid; do not swallow; do not rinse mouth after treatment.
    Peridex, PerioGard *Oral soln:* 0.12% (480 ml)

 GLAUCOMA: OPEN ANGLE/OCULAR HYPERTENSION

Comment: Other ophthalmic medications should not be administered within 5-10 minutes of administering an ophthalmic antiglaucoma medication. Contact lenses should be removed prior to instillation of antiglaucoma medications and may be replaced 15 minutes later. Interactions with ophthalmic anti-glaucoma agents include MAOIs, CNS depressants, beta-blockers, tricyclic antidepressants, and hypoglycemics. Choices for medical treatment in progressive cases include *betaxolol* eye drops which have a beneficial effect on optic nerve blood flow in addition to intraocular pressure IOP reduction. Other beta blockers and adrenergic drugs (such as **dipivefrine**) should better be avoided because of the probability of nocturnal systemic hypotension and optic nerve hypoperfusion (e.g., in patients with untreated obstructive sleep apnea). Prostaglandin derivatives tend to have greater IOP-lowering effect which may be of overriding consideration. *dorzolamide-timolol* fixed combination is a safe and effective IOP-lowering agent in patients with normal tension glaucoma (NTG). *brimonidine* significantly improved retinal vascular autoregulation in NTG patients.

REFERENCE
Mallick, J., Devi, L., Malik, P., & Mallick, J. (2016). Update on normal tension glaucoma. *Journal of Ophthalmic and Vision Research, 11*(2), 204. doi:10.4103/2008-322x.183914

OPHTHALMIC ALPHA-2 ADRENERGIC RECEPTOR AGONISTS
Comment: Ophthalmic alpha-2 agonists are contraindicated with concomitant MAOI use. Cautious use with CNS depressants, beta-blockers (ocular and systemic), antihypertensives, cardiac glycosides, and tricyclic antidepressants.
▷ *apraclonidine* ophthalmic solution (C) 1-2 drops affected eye tid
  Pediatric: <12 years: not recommended; ≥12 years: same as adult
    Iopidine *Ophth soln:* 0.5% (5 ml) (benzalkonium chloride)
▷ *brimonidine tartrate* ophthalmic solution (B) 1 drop affected eye q 8 hours
  Pediatric: <2 years: not recommended; ≥2 years: 1 drop affected eye q 8 hours
    Alphagan P *Ophth soln:* 0.1, 0.15% (5, 10, 15 ml) (purite)

OPHTHALMIC CARBONIC ANHYDRASE INHIBITORS
Comment: Ophthalmic carbonic anhydrase inhibitors are contraindicated in patients with sulfa allergy.
▷ *brinzolamide* ophthalmic suspension (C) 1 drop affected eye tid
  Pediatric: <12 years: not recommended; ≥12 years: same as adult
    Azopt *Ophth susp:* 1% (2.5, 5, 10, 15 ml) (benzalkonium chloride)
▷ *dorzolamide* ophthalmic solution (C)(G) 1 drop affected eye tid
  Pediatric: same as adult
    Trusopt *Ophth soln:* 2% (10 ml) (benzalkonium chloride)

OPHTHALMIC ALPHA-2 ADRENERGIC RECEPTOR AGONIST+CARBONIC ANHYDRASE INHIBITOR

▷ *brimonidine+brinzolamide* (C) 1 drop affected eye tid
  Pediatric: <12 years: not recommended; ≥12 years: same as adult
    Simbrinza *Ophth soln:* brim 1% mg+brinz 0.2% per ml (10 ml)

OPHTHALMIC CHOLINERGICS (MIOTICS)

▷ *carbachol+hydroxypropyl methylcellulose* ophthalmic solution (C) 2 drops affected eye tid
  Pediatric: <12 years: not recommended; ≥12 years: same as adult
    Isopto Carbachol *Ophth soln:* carb 0.75% or 2.25%+hydroxy 1% (15 ml); carb 1.5% or 3%+hydroxy 1% (15, 30 ml) (benzalkonium chloride)
▷ *pilocarpine* (C)(G)
  Pediatric: <12 years: not recommended; ≥12 years: same as adult
    Isopto Carpine 2 drops affected eye tid-qid
      Ophth soln: 1, 2, 4% (15 ml) (benzalkonium chloride)
    Ocusert Pilo change ophthalmic insert once weekly
      Ophth inserts: 20 mcg/Hr (8/pck)
    Pilocar Ophthalmic Solution 1-2 drops affected eye 1-6 x/day
      Ophth soln: 0.5, 1, 2, 3, 4, 6, 8% (15 ml)
    Pilopine HS apply 1/2 inch ribbon in lower conjunctival sac q HS
      Opth gel: 4% (4 gm)

OPHTHALMIC CHOLINESTERASE INHIBITORS

▷ *demecarium bromide* ophthalmic solution (X) 1-2 drops affected eye q 12-48 hours
  Pediatric: <12 years: not recommended; ≥12 years: same as adult
    Humorsol Ocumeter *Ophth soln:* 0.125, 0.25% (5 ml)
▷ *echothiophate iodide* ophthalmic solution (C) initially 1 drop of 0.03% affected eye bid; then increase strength as needed
  Pediatric: <12 years: not recommended; ≥12 years: same as adult
    Phospholine Iodide *Ophth soln:* 0.03, 0.06, 0.125, 0.25% (5 ml)

OPHTHALMIC CARDIOSELECTIVE BETA-BLOCKERS

Comment: Ophthalmic beta-blockers are generally contraindicated in severe COPD, history of or current bronchial asthma, sinus bradycardia, 2nd or 3rd degree AV block.
▷ *betaxolol* ophthalmic solution (C)(G) 1-2 drops affected eye bid
  Pediatric: <12 years: not recommended; ≥12 years: same as adult
    Betoptic *Ophth soln:* 0.5% (5, 10, 15 ml) (benzalkonium chloride)
    Betoptic S *Ophth soln:* 0.25% (2.5, 5, 10, 15 ml) (benzalkonium chloride)

OPHTHALMIC BETA-BLOCKERS (NON-CARDIOSELECTIVE)

Comment: Ophthalmic beta-blockers are generally contraindicated in severe COPD, history of or current bronchial asthma, sinus bradycardia, 2nd or 3rd degree AV block.
▷ *carteolol* ophthalmic solution (C)(G) 1 drop affected eye bid
  Pediatric: <12 years: not recommended; ≥12 years: same as adult
    Ocupress *Ophth soln:* 1% (5, 10, 15 ml) (benzalkonium chloride)
▷ *levobunolol* ophthalmic solution (C) 1-2 drops affected eye bid
  Pediatric: <12 years: not recommended; ≥12 years: same as adult
    Betagan *Ophth soln:* 0.5% (5, 10, 15 ml) (benzalkonium chloride)
▷ *metipranolol* ophthalmic solution (C)(G) 1 drop affected eye bid
  Pediatric: <12 years: not recommended; ≥12 years: same as adult
    OptiPranolol *Ophth soln:* 0.3% (5, 10 ml) (benzalkonium chloride)
▷ *timolol* ophthalmic solution and gel (C)(G)
  Pediatric: <12 years: not recommended; ≥12 years: same as adult
    Betimol 1 drop affected eye bid
      Ophth soln: 0.25, 0.5% (5, 10, 15 ml) (benzalkonium chloride)
    Istalol 1 drop affected eye daily
      Ophth soln: 0.5% (2.5, 5 ml) (preservative-free)
    Timoptic 1 drop affected eye bid
      Ophth soln: 0.25, 0.5% (5, 10, 15 ml) (benzalkonium chloride)

Timoptic Ocudose 1 drop bid
Ophth soln: 0.25, 0.5% (0.2 ml/dose, 60 dose) (preservative-free)
Timoptic-XE 1 drop affected eye bid
Ophth gel: 0.25, 0.5% (2.5, 5 ml) (preservative-free)

OPHTHALMIC ALPHA-2 ADRENERGIC RECEPTOR AGONIST+ NON-CARDIOSELECTIVE BETA-BLOCKER COMBINATION

Comment: Generally contraindicated in severe COPD, history of <u>or</u> current bronchial asthma, sinus bradycardia, 2nd <u>or</u> 3rd degree AV block.
▷ *brimonidine tartrate+timolol* ophthalmic solution **(C)** 1 drop affected eye bid
Pediatric: <2 years: not recommended; ≥2 years: same as adult
Combigan *Ophth soln:* brimo 0.2%+timo 0.5% (5, 10, 15 ml) (benzalkonium chloride)

OPHTHALMIC PROSTAMIDE ANALOGS

▷ *bimatoprost* ophthalmic solution **(C)(G)** 1 drop q affected eye HS
Pediatric: <16 years: not recommended; ≥16 years: same as adult
Lumigan *Ophth soln:* 0.01, 0.03% (2.5, 5, 7.5 ml) (benzalkonium chloride)
▷ *latanoprost* ophthalmic solution **(C)** 1 drop affected eye q HS
Pediatric: <12 years: not recommended; ≥12 years: same as adult
Xalatan *Ophth soln:* 0.005% (2.5 ml) (benzalkonium chloride)
▷ *tafluprost* ophthalmic solution **(C)** 1 drop affected eye q HS
Pediatric: <12 years: not recommended; ≥12 years: same as adult
Zioptan *Ophth soln:* 0.0015% (0.3 ml single-use, 30-60/carton) (preservative-free)
▷ *travoprost* ophthalmic solution **(C)(G)** 1 drop affected eye q HS
Pediatric: <16 years: not recommended; ≥16 years: same as adult
Travatan *Ophth soln:* 0.004% (2.5, 5 ml) (benzalkonium chloride)
Travatan Z *Ophth soln:* 0.004% (2.5, 5 ml) (boric acid, propylene glycol, sorbitol, zinc chloride)

PROSTAGLANDIN F$_{2\alpha}$ ANALOG

▷ *latanoprost* I drop in the affected eye(s) in the evening
Xelpros *Ophth emul:* 0.005% (2.5 ml) (potassium sorbate 0.47%)
Comment: *latanoprost* can cause pigmentation of the iris, periorbital tissue (eyelid) and eyelashes (iris pigmentation likely to be permanent) and gradual changes to eyelashes including increased length, thickness and number of lashes (usually reversible).

PROSTAGLANDIN ANALOG (WITH NITRIC OXIDE METABOLITE)

▷ *latanoprostene bunod* ophthalmic solution **(C)** ≤16 years: not recommended (because of potential safety concerns related to increased pigmentation following long-term chronic use); >16 years: 1 drop affected eye once daily
Vyzulta *Ophth soln:* 0.024% (5 ml) (benzalkonium chloride)
Comment: **Vyzulta** is a prostaglandin analog with nitric oxide as one of its metabolites. **Vyzulta** exerts a dual mechanism of action through latanoprost acid and butanediol mononitrate, working in the uveoscleral pathway and Schlemm's canal. Most common ocular adverse reactions with incidence ≥ 2% are conjunctival hyperemia (6%), eye irritation (4%), eye pain (3%), and instillation site pain (2%). There may be increased pigmentation of the iris and periorbital tissue. Iris pigmentation is likely to be permanent. There may be gradual changes to eyelashes including increased length, increased thickness and number of eyelashes, that is usually reversible upon discontinuation of treatment. There are no available human data for the use of **Vyzulta** during pregnancy to inform any drug associated risks. There are no data on the presence of **Vyzulta** in human milk or effects on the breastfed infant.

OPHTHALMIC SYMPATHOMIMETICS

Comment: Contraindicated in narrow-angle glaucoma. Use with caution in cardiovascular disease, hypertension, hyperthyroidism, diabetes, and asthma.

▷ *dipivefrin* ophthalmic solution **(B)** 1 drop affected eye q 12 hours
    Propine *Ophth soln:* 0.1% (5, 10, 15 ml) (benzalkonium chloride)

OPHTHALMIC CARBONIC ANHYDRASE INHIBITOR+NON-CARDIOSELECTIVE BETA-BLOCKER

▷ *dorzolamide+timolol* ophthalmic solution **(C)** 1 drop affected eye bid
    Pediatric: <12 years: not recommended; ≥12 years: same as adult
        Cosopt *Ophth soln:* dorz 2%+tim 0.5% (10 ml) (benzalkonium chloride)
        Cosopt PF *Ophth soln:* dorz 2%+tim 0.5% (10 ml) (preservative-free)

OPHTHALMIC SYNTHETIC DOCOSANOID

▷ *unoprostone isopropyl* ophthalmic solution **(C)** 1 drop affected eye bid
    Pediatric: <12 years: not recommended; ≥12 years: same as adult
        Rescula *Ophth soln:* 0.15% (5 ml) (benzalkonium chloride)

OPHTHALMIC RHO KINASE INHIBITOR

▷ *netarsudil* ophthalmic solution **(C)** 1 drop affected eye once daily in the PM
    Pediatric: <18 years: not established; ≥18 years: same as adult
        Rhopressa *Ophth soln:* 0.02% (0.2 mg/ml, 2.5 ml) (benzalkonium chloride)

OPHTHALMIC ORAL CARBONIC ANHYDRASE INHIBITORS

▷ *acetazolamide* **(C)** 250-1000 mg/day in divided doses <u>or</u> 500 mg bid sust-rel tabs; max 1 gm/day
    Pediatric: <12 years: not recommended; ≥12 years: same as adult
        Diamox *Tab:* 125*, 250*mg
        Diamox Sequels *Tab:* 500 mg sust-rel
▷ *methazolamide* **(C)(G)** 50-100 mg bid-tid times daily
    Pediatric: <12 years: not recommended; ≥12 years: same as adult
        Neptazane *Tab:* 25, 50 mg
    Comment: Administer ophthalmic osmotic and miotic agents concomitantly.

 GONORRHEA (*NEISSERIA GONORRHOEAE*)

Comment: The following treatment regimens for *N. gonorrhoeae* are published in the **2015 CDC Transmitted Diseases Treatment Guidelines**. Treatment regimens are presented by generic drug name first, followed by information about brands and dose forms. Empiric treatment requires concomitant treatment of chlamydia. Treat all sexual contacts. Patients who are HIV-positive should receive the same treatment as those who are HIV-negative. Sexual abuse must be considered a cause of gonococcal infection in preadolescent children.

RECOMMENDED REGIMENS, ≥12 YEARS: UNCOMPLICATED INFECTIONS OF THE CERVIX, URETHRA, AND RECTUM
Regimen 1

▷ *ceftriaxone* 250 mg IM in a single dose
    plus
▷ *azithromycin* 1 gm in a single dose

Regimen 2

▷ *ceftriaxone* 250 mg IM in a single dose
    plus
▷ *doxycycline* 100 mg bid x 7 days

RECOMMENDED REGIMENS, ≥12 YEARS: UNCOMPLICATED INFECTIONS OF THE PHARYNX
Regimen 1

▷ *ceftriaxone* 250 mg IM in a single dose
    plus
▷ *azithromycin* 1 gm in a single dose

Regimen 2

▷ *ceftriaxone* 250 mg IM in a single dose
    plus
▷ *doxycycline* 100 mg bid x 7 days

RECOMMENDED REGIMENS, CHILDREN ≥45 KG, ≥8 YEARS; UNCOMPLICATED INFECTIONS OF THE CERVIX, URETHRA, AND RECTUM

Regimen 1

▷ *ceftriaxone* 250 mg IM in a single dose
    plus
▷ *azithromycin* 1 gm in a single dose

RECOMMENDED REGIMEN: CHILDREN >45 KG

Regimen 1

▷ *ceftriaxone* 250 mg IM in a single dose

RECOMMENDED REGIMEN: CHILDREN >45 KG WHO HAVE GONOCOCCAL BACTEREMIA OR GONOCOCCAL ARTHRITIS

Regimen 1

▷ *ceftriaxone* 50 mg/kg IM or IV in a single dose daily x 7 days

RECOMMENDED REGIMENS, CHILDREN <45 KG, <8 YEARS: UNCOMPLICATED GONOCOCCAL VULVOVAGINITIS, CERVICITIS, URETHRITIS, PHARYNGITIS, OR PROCTITIS

Regimen 1

▷ *ceftriaxone* 250 mg IM in a single dose

RECOMMENDED REGIMEN, CHILDREN <45 KG, <8 YEARS: GONOCOCCAL BACTEREMIA OR ARTHRITIS

Regimen 1

▷ *ceftriaxone* 50 mg/kg (max dose 1 gm) IM or IV in a single dose daily x 7 days

DRUG BRANDS AND DOSE FORMS

▷ *azithromycin* (B)(G)
    Zithromax *Tab:* 250, 500, 600 mg; *Oral susp:* 100 mg/5 ml (15 ml); 200 mg/5 ml (15, 22.5, 30 ml) (cherry); *Pkt:* 1 gm for reconstitution (cherry-banana)
    Zithromax Tri-pak *Tab:* 3 x 500 mg tabs/pck
    Zithromax Z-pak *Tab:* 6 x 250 mg tabs/pck
    Zmax *Oral susp:* 2 gm ext-rel for reconstitution (cherry-banana) (148 mg Na$^+$)
▷ *ceftriaxone* (B)(G)
    Rocephin *Vial:* 250, 500 mg; 1, 2 gm
▷ *doxycycline* (D)(G)
    Acticlate *Tab:* 75, 150**mg
    Adoxa *Tab:* 50, 75, 100, 150 mg ent-coat
    Doryx *Tab:* 50, 75, 100, 150, 200 mg del-rel
    Doxteric *Tab:* 50 mg del-rel
    Monodox *Cap:* 50, 75, 100 mg
    Oracea *Cap:* 40 mg del-rel
    Vibramycin *Tab:* 100 mg; *Cap:* 50, 100 mg; *Syr:* 50 mg/5 ml (raspberry-apple) (sulfites); *Oral susp:* 25 mg/5 ml (raspberry)
    Vibra-Tab *Tab:* 100 mg film-coat
    Comment: *doxycycline* is contraindicated <8 years-of-age, in pregnancy, and lactation (discolors developing tooth enamel). A side effect may be photosensitivity (photophobia). Do **not** take with antacids, calcium supplements, milk or other dairy, or within 2 hours of taking another drug.

ALTERNATE THERAPY

▷ *azithromycin* (B)(G) 2 gm x 1 dose
    Pediatric: not recommended for treatment of gonorrhea in children

Zithromax *Tab:* 250, 500, 600 mg; *Oral susp:* 100 mg/5 ml (15 ml); 200 mg/5 ml (15, 22.5, 30 ml) (cherry); *Pkt:* 1 gm for reconstitution (cherry-banana)

Zithromax Tri-pak *Tab:* 3 x 500 mg tabs/pck

Zithromax Z-pak *Tab:* 6 x 250 mg tabs/pck

Zmax *Oral susp:* 2 gm ext-rel for reconstitution (cherry-banana) (148 mg Na⁺)

➤ *cefotaxime* 500 mg IM x 1 dose

Claforan *Vial:* 500 mg; 1, 2 gm

➤ *cefotetan* 1 gm IM x 1 dose

Pediatric: <12 years: not recommended; ≥12 years: same as adult

Cefotan *Vial:* 1, 2 gm

➤ *cefoxitin* (B) 2 gm IM x 1 dose

Pediatric: <3 months: not recommended; ≥3 months: same as adult

Mefoxin *Vial:* 1, 2 gm

plus

➤ *probenecid* (B)(G)

Benemid 1 gm 30 minutes before *cefoxitin*

Pediatric: <2 years: not recommended; 2-14 years: 25 mg/kg 30 minutes before *cefoxitin*; ≥14 years: same as adult

Tab: 500*mg; *Cap:* 500 mg

➤ *cefpodoxime proxetil* (B) 200 mg x 1 dose

Pediatric: <2 months: not recommended; 2 months-12 years: 10 mg/kg/day (max 400 mg/ dose) or 5 mg/kg/day bid (max 200 mg/dose)

Vantin *Tab:* 100, 200 mg; *Oral susp:* 50, 100 mg/5 ml (50, 75, 100 mg) (lemon creme)

➤ *ceftizoxime* (B) 1 gm IM x 1 dose

Pediatric: <6 months: not recommended; ≥6 months: same as adult

Cefizox *Vial:* 500 mg; 1, 2, 10 g

➤ *demeclocycline* (X) 600 mg initially, followed by 300 mg q 12 hours x 4 days (total 3 gm)

Pediatric: <8 years: not recommended; ≥8 years: same as adult

Declomycin *Tab:* 300 mg

Comment: *demeclocycline* is contraindicated <8 years-of-age, in pregnancy, and lactation (discolors developing tooth enamel). A side effect may be photo-sensitivity (photophobia). Do not give with antacids, calcium supplements, milk or other dairy, or within two hours of taking another drug.

➤ *enoxacin* (C) 400 mg x 1 dose

Pediatric: <18 years: not recommended; ≥18 years: same as adult

Penetrex *Tab:* 200, 400 mg

➤ *imipramine* (C) 400 mg x 1 dose

Pediatric: <18 years: not recommended; ≥18 years: same as adult

Maxaquin *Tab:* 400 mg

➤ *norfloxacin* (C) 800 mg x 1 dose

Pediatric: <18 years: not recommended; ≥18 years: same as adult

Noroxin *Tab:* 400 mg

➤ *spectinomycin* (B) 2 gm IM x 1 dose

Pediatric: 40 mg/kg IM x 1 dose

Trobicin *Vial:* 2 g

 GOUT (HYPERURICEMIA)

Pseudogout *see page 415*
Acetaminophen for IV Infusion *see page 352*
NSAIDs *see page 571*
Opioid Analgesics *see Pain page 354*
Topical & Transdermal Analgesics *see Pain page 352*
Parenteral Corticosteroids *see page 577*
Oral Corticosteroids *see page 577*

XANTHINE OXIDASE INHIBITORS (PROPHYLAXIS)

➤ *allopurinol* (C)(G) initially 100 mg daily; increase by 100 mg weekly; max 800 mg/day and 300 mg/dose; usual range for mild symptoms 200-300 mg/day; for severe symptoms 400-600 mg/day; take with food

Pediatric: <6 years: max 150 mg/day; 6-10 years: max 400 mg/day; max single dose 300 mg;
>10 years: same as adult
    Zyloprim *Tab:* 100*, 300*mg
Comment: Do not take *allopurinol* concurrent with *colchicine*. Gout flares may occur
after initiation of urate lowering therapy, such as allopurinol, due to changing serum uric
acid concentrations resulting in mobilization of urate from tissue deposits. If a gout flare
occurs during treatment, allopurinol does not need to be discontinued. Manage the flare
concurrently, as appropriate for the individual patient. The correct dose and frequency
of dosage for maintaining the serum uric acid concentration within the normal range are
best determined by using the serum uric acid concentration as an index. Allopurinol is not
recommended for the treatment of asymptomatic hyperuricemia. Discontinue allopurinol
when the potential for overproduction of uric acid is no longer present.

ACUTE ATTACK

▷ *colchicine* (C)(G) 0.6-1.2 mg at first sign of attack; then 0.6 mg every hour or 1.2 mg every 2
hours until pain relief; then consider 0.6 mg/day or every other day for maintenance
Pediatric: <12 years: not recommended; ≥12 years: same as adult
    Colcrys *Tab:* 0.6 mg
    Mitigare *Cap:* 0.6 mg
Comment: Do not take *colchicine* concurrently with *allopurinol*.

▷ *febuxostat* (C)(G) initially 40 mg daily; after 2 weeks, may increase to 80 mg daily.
Pediatric: <18 years: not recommended; ≥18 years: same as adult
    Uloric *Tab:* 40, 80 mg
Comment: Gout flare prophylaxis with *colchicine* or NSAID is recommended on initiation
of *febuxostat* (**Uloric**) and up to 6 months. In a recent report of research, gout patients
with established cardiovascular (CV) disease treated with **Uloric** had a higher rate of CV
death as compared to those treated with *allopurinol*. Therefore, the FDA issued a new BBW
(black box warning) to consider the risks and benefits of **Uloric** when deciding to prescribe
or continue patients on **Uloric**. Further, **Uloric** should only be used in patients who have
an inadequate response to a maximally titrated dose of *allopurinol*, who are intolerant to
allopurinol, or for whom treatment with *allopurinol* is not advisable.

PEGYLATED URIC ACID SPECIFIC ENZYME

▷ *pegloticase* (C) pre-medicate with antihistamine and corticosteroid; 8 mg once every 2
weeks; administer IV infusion after dilution over at least 2 hours; observe at least 1 hour
post-infusion
Pediatric: <18 years: not recommended; ≥18 years: same as adult
    Krystexxa *Vial:* 8 mg/ml (1 ml) single-use pwdr for IV infusion after dilution
    Comment: Slow rate, or stop and restart at lower rate, if infusion reaction occurs
(e.g., **Krystexxa** is contraindicated with G6PD deficiency; screen patients of African
or Mediterranean descent). **Krystexxa** is not for the treatment of asymptomatic
hyperuricemia.

URICOSURIC AGENT

▷ *probenecid* (C)(G) 250 mg bid x 1 week; maintenance 500 mg bid
Pediatric: <18 years: not recommended; ≥18 years: same as adult
    Tab: 500*mg; *Cap:* 500 mg
Comment: Avoid concomitant use of *probenecid* and salicylates.

URICOSURIC+ANTI-INFLAMMATORY COMBINATIONS

▷ *probenecid+colchicine* (G) 1 tab once daily x 1 week; then, 1 tab bid thereafter
Pediatric: <18 years: not recommended; ≥18 years: same as adult
    Tab: prob 500 mg+colch 0.5 mg
Comment: *probenecid+colchicine* is contraindicated in the treatment of acute gout attack,
patients with blood dyscrasias, and patients with uric acid kidney stones. Concomitant
salicylates antagonize the uricosuric effects.

▷ *sulfinpyrazone* (C) initially 200-400 mg bid; may gradually increase to 800 mg bid
Pediatric: <18 years: not recommended; ≥18 years: same as adult
    Anturane *Cap:* 100, 200 mg
Comment: Goal is serum uric acid <6.5 mg/dL.

XANTHINE OXIDASE INHIBITOR

▷ *febuxostat* (C) 40 mg once daily x 2 weeks; if serum uric acid is not <6 mg/dL, may increase to 80 mg once daily

Pediatric: <18 years: not established; ≥18 years: same as adult

   Uloric *Tab:* 40, 80 mg

   Comment: Gout flare prophylaxis with *colchicine* or NSAID is recommended on initiation of *febuxostat* Uloric and up to 6 months. In a recent report of research, gout patients with established cardiovascular (CV) disease treated with *feboxostat* Uloric had a higher rate of CV death as compared to those treated with *allopurinol*. Therefore, the FDA issued a new BBW (black box warning) to consider the risks and benefits of Uloric when deciding to prescribe or continue patients on Uloric. Further, Uloric should only be used in patients who have an inadequate response to a maximally titrated dose of *allopurinol*, who are intolerant to *allopurinol*, or for whom treatment with *allopurinol* is not advisable.

XANTHINE OXIDASE INHIBITOR+URATI INHIBITOR COMBINATION

▷ *allopurinol+lesinurad* take 1 tab once daily

Pediatric: <18 years: not established; ≥18 years: same as adult

   Duzallo *Tab:* 200/200, 300/200 mg

   Comment: The US Food and Drug Administration recently approved Duzallo for the treatment of hyperuricemia associated with gout in patients who have not achieved target serum uric acid (sUA) levels with *allopurinol* alone. Duzallo is the first drug to combine *allopurinol*, the current standard of care for hyperuricemia associated with gout, and *lesinurad*, the most recent FDA-approved treatment for this condition. The fixed-dose combination addresses the overproduction and underexcretion of serum uric acid. Patients with asymptomatic hyperuricemia are not recommended to receive Duzallo. Common adverse reactions associated with Duzallo include headache, influenza, higher levels of blood creatinine, and heart burn. In addition, Duzallo has a boxed warning for the risk of acute renal failure associated with *lesinurad*. There are no available human data on use of Duzallo or *lesinurad* in pregnancy to inform a drug-associated risk of adverse developmental outcomes. Limited published data on *allopurinol* use in pregnancy do not demonstrate a clear pattern or increase in frequency of adverse development outcomes. There is no information regarding the presence of Duzallo or *lesinurad* in human milk or the effects on the breastfed infant. Based on information from a single case report, *allopurinol* and its active metabolite, *oxypurinol*, were detected in the milk of a mother at five weeks postpartum. The effect of *allopurinol* on the breastfed infant is unknown. CrCl 45-< 60 mL/min: adjust the allopurinol to a medically appropriate dose (200 mg). CrCl <45, *allopurinol* not recommended. Max *lesinurad* 200 mg/day. In clinical trials evaluating the safety and efficacy of this combined therapy among adult patients with gout who failed to achieve target sUA levels on *allopurinol* alone, Duzallo was found to nearly double the number of patients who achieved target sUA at 6 months, mean sUA was reduced to less than 6 mg/dL by 1 month, and this level was maintained through 12 months.

SELECTIVE URIC ACID REABSORPTION INHIBITOR (SURI)

▷ *lesinurad* (C) 200 mg once daily in combination with a xanthine oxidase inhibitor (XOI)

Pediatric: <18 years: not established; ≥18 years: same as adult

   Zurampic *Tab:* 200 mg

   Comment: Zurampic inhibits URATI, a urate transporter, which is responsible for the majority of renal absorption of uric acid and (OAT) 4, organic anion transporter, a uric acid transporter involved in diuretic-induced hyperuricemia. Do not use as monotherapy. Use in combination with an XOI, such as *allopurinol* or *febuxostat*, (to reduce the production of uric acid). Do not initiate if CrCl <45 mL/min, ESRD, dialysis, or kidney transplant.

 GOUTY ARTHRITIS

See **Gout (Hyperuricemia)** for gout management drugs page 183
Acetaminophen for IV Infusion *see Pain page* 352
NSAIDs *see page* 571
Opioid Analgesics *see Pain page* 354
Topical & Transdermal Analgesics *see Pain page* 352

Parenteral Corticosteroids *see page* 577
Oral Corticosteroids *see page* 577
Topical Analgesic and Anesthetic Agents *see page* 569

TOPICAL & TRANSDERMAL ANALGESICS

▷ *capsaicin* (B)(G) apply tid-qid prn to intact skin
   Pediatric: <2 years: not recommended; ≥2 years: same as adult
      Axsain *Crm:* 0.075% (1, 2 oz)
      Capsin *Lotn:* 0.025, 0.075% (59 ml)
      Capzasin-HP (OTC) *Crm:* 0.075% (1.5 oz), 0.025% (45, 90 gm); *Lotn:* 0.075% (2 oz);
      0.025% (45, 90 gm)
      Capzasin-P (OTC) *Crm:* 0.025% (1.5 oz); *Lotn:* 0.025% (2 oz)
      Dolorac *Crm:* 0.025% (28 gm)
      Double Cap (OTC) *Crm:* 0.05% (2 oz)
      R-Gel *Gel:* 0.025% (15, 30 gm)
      Zostrix (OTC) *Crm:* 0.025% (0.7, 1.5, 3 oz)
      Zostrix HP (OTC) *Emol crm:* 0.075% (1, 2 oz)
▷ *capsaicin* 8% patch (B) apply up to 4 patches for one 60-minute application to clean dry
skin; may prep area with topical anesthetic; wear non-latex gloves; patches may be cut to
size/shape; treatment may be repeated every 3 months
   Pediatric: <18 years: not recommended; ≥18 years: same as adult
      Qutenza *Patch:* 8% 1640 mcg/cm (179 mg) (1 or 2 patches w. 1-50 gm tube cleansing
      gel/carton)
▷ *diclofenac sodium* (C; D ≥30 wks)(G) apply qid prn to intact skin
   Pediatric: <12 years: not established; ≥12 years: same as adult
      Pennsaid 1.5% in 10 drop increments, dispense and rub into front, side, and back of
      knee: usually; 40 drops (40 mg) qid
        Topical soln: 1.5% (150 ml)
      Pennsaid 2% apply 2 pump actuations (40 mg) and rub into front, side, and back of
      knee bid
        Topical soln: 2% (20 mg/pump actuation, 112 gm)
      Solaraze Gel massage in to clean skin bid prn
        Gel: 3% (50 gm) (benzyl alcohol)
      Voltaren Gel (G) apply qid prn to intact skin
        Gel: 1% (100 gm)
   Comment: *diclofenac* is contraindicated with *aspirin* allergy. As with other NSAIDs, should
be avoided in late pregnancy (≥30 weeks) because it may cause premature closure of the
ductus arteriosus.
▷ *doxepin* (B) cream apply to affected area qid at intervals of at least 3-4 hours; max 8 days
   Pediatric: <12 years: not recommended; >12 years: same as adult
      Prudoxin *Crm:* 5% (45 gm)
      Zonalon *Crm:* 5% (30, 45 gm)
▷ *pimecrolimus* 1% cream (C)(G) <2 years: not recommended; ≥2 years: apply to affected
area bid; do not apply an occlusive dressing
      Elidel *Crm:* 1% (30, 60, 100 gm)
   Comment: *pimecrolimus* is indicated for short-term and intermittent long-term use.
Discontinue use when resolution occurs. Contraindicated if the patient is immunosuppressed. Change to the 0.1% preparation or if secondary bacterial infection is present.
▷ *trolamine salicylate* apply tid-qid
   Pediatric: <2 years: not recommended; ≥2 years: same as adult
      Mobisyl Creme *Crm:* 10% (100 gm)

TOPICAL AND TRANSDERMAL ANESTHETICS

Comment: *lidocaine* should not be applied to non-intact skin.
▷ *lidocaine* cream (B) apply to affected area bid prn
   Pediatric: <12 years: not recommended; ≥12 years: same as adult
      LidaMantle *Crm:* 3% (1, 2 oz)
      Lidoderm *Crm:* 3% (85 gm)
      ZTlido *lidocaine* topical system 1% (30/carton)
      Comment: Compared to **Lidoderm** (*lidocaine* patch 5%) which contains 700 mg/patch,
      ZTlido only requires 35 mg per topical system to achieve the same therapeutic dose.

➤ *lidocaine* lotion (B) apply to affected area bid prn
Pediatric: <12 years: not recommended; ≥12 years: same as adult
    LidaMantle *Lotn:* 3% (177 ml)

➤ *lidocaine* 5% patch (B)(G) apply up to 3 patches at one time for up to 12 hours/24-hour period (12 hours on/12 hours off); patches may be cut into smaller sizes before removal of the release liner; do <u>not</u> re-use
Pediatric: <12 years: not recommended; ≥12 years: same as adult
    Lidoderm *Patch:* 5% (10x14 cm; 30/carton)

➤ *lidocaine+dexamethasone* (B)
Pediatric: <12 years: not recommended; ≥12 years: same as adult
    Decadron Phosphate with Xylocaine *Lotn:* dexa 4 mg+lido 10 mg per ml (5 ml)

➤ *lidocaine+hydrocortisone* (B)(G) apply to affected area bid prn
Pediatric: <12 years: not recommended; ≥12 years: same as adult
    LidaMantle HC *Crm:* lido 3%+hydro 0.5% (1, 3 oz); *Lotn:* (177 ml)

➤ *lidocaine 2.5%+prilocaine 2.5%* apply sparingly to the burn bid-tid prn
Pediatric: <12 years: not recommended; ≥12 years: same as adult
    Emla Cream (B) 5, 30 gm/tube

ORAL SALICYLATE

➤ *indomethacin* (C) initially 25 mg bid-tid; increase as needed at weekly intervals by 25-50 mg/day; max 200 mg/day
Pediatric: <14 years: usually not recommended; ≤2-14 years, if risk warranted: 1-2 mg/kg/day in divided doses; max 3-4 mg/kg/day (or 150-200 mg/day, whichever is less); ≤14 years: ER cap not recommended; >14 years: same as adult
Cap: 25, 50 mg; *Susp:* 25 mg/5 ml (pineapple-coconut, mint; alcohol 1%); *Supp:* 50 mg; *ER Cap:* 75 mg ext-rel
Comment: *indomethacin* is indicated only for acute painful flares. Administer with food and/or antacids. Use lowest effective dose for shortest duration.

NSAID PLUS PPI

➤ *esomeprazole+naproxen* (C; not for use in 3rd)(G) 1 tab bid; use lowest effective dose for the shortest duration; swallow whole; take at least 30 minutes before a meal
Pediatric: <18 years: not recommended; ≥18 years: same as adult
    Vimovo *Tab:* nap 375 mg+eso 20 mg ext-rel; nap 500 mg+eso 20 mg ext-rel

COX-2 INHIBITORS

Comment: Cox-2 inhibitors are contraindicated with history of asthma, urticaria, and allergic-type reactions to *aspirin*, other NSAIDs, and sulfonamides, 3rd trimester of pregnancy, and coronary artery bypass graft (CABG) surgery.

➤ *celecoxib* (C)(G) 100-400 mg bid; max 800 mg/day
Pediatric: <18 years: not recommended; ≥18 years: same as adult
    Celebrex *Cap:* 50, 100, 200, 400 mg

➤ *meloxicam* (C)(G)
    Mobic initially 7.5 mg once daily; max 15 mg once daily; Hemodialysis: max 7.5 mg/day
    Pediatric: <2 years, <60 kg: not recommended; ≥2 years, >60 kg-12 years: 0.125 mg/kg; max 7.5 mg once daily; ≥12 years: same as adult
      Tab: 7.5, 15 mg; *Oral susp:* 7.5 mg/5 ml (100 ml) (raspberry)
    Vivlodex initially 5 mg qd; may increase to max 10 mg/day; Hemodialysis: max 5 mg/day
      Cap: 5, 10 mg

⬤ GRANULOMA INGUINALE (DONOVANOSIS)

Comment: The following treatment regimens are published in the **2015 CDC Sexually Transmitted Diseases Treatment Guidelines**. Treatment regimens are for adults only; consult a specialist for treatment of patients less than 18 years-of-age. Treatment regimens are presented by generic drug name first, followed by information about brands and dose forms. Persons who have sexual contact with a patient who has had granuloma inguinale within the past 60 days before onset of the patient's symptoms should be examined and offered therapy. Patients who are HIV-positive should receive the same treatment as those who are HIV-negative; however, the addition of a parenteral aminoglycoside (e.g., *gentamicin*) can also be considered.

RECOMMENDED REGIMEN

➤ *doxycycline* 100 mg bid x at least 3 weeks and until all lesions have completely healed

ALTERNATE REGIMENS

➤ *azithromycin* 1 gm once weekly for at least 3 weeks and until all lesions have completely healed
➤ *ciprofloxacin* 750 mg bid x at least 3 weeks and until all lesions have completely healed
➤ *erythromycin base* 500 mg qid x 14 days or *erythromycin ethylsuccinate* 400 mg qid x 14 days
➤ *trimethoprim+sulfamethoxazole* take 1 double-strength (160/800) dose bid x at least 3 weeks and until all lesions have completely healed

DRUG BRANDS AND DOSE FORMS

➤ *azithromycin* (B)(G)
> **Zithromax** *Tab:* 250, 500, 600 mg; *Oral susp:* 100 mg/5 ml (15 ml); 200 mg/5 ml (15, 22.5, 30 ml) (cherry); *Pkt:* 1 gm for reconstitution (cherry-banana)
> **Zithromax Tri-pak** *Tab:* 3 x 500 mg tabs/pck
> **Zithromax Z-pak** *Tab:* 6 x 250 mg tabs/pck
> **Zmax** *Oral susp:* 2 gm ext-rel for reconstitution (cherry-banana) (148 mg Na$^+$)
➤ *ciprofloxacin* (C)
> **Cipro (G)** *Tab:* 250, 500, 750 mg; *Oral susp:* 250, 500 mg/5 ml (100 ml) (strawberry)
> **Cipro XR** *Tab:* 500, 1000 mg ext-rel
> **ProQuin XR** *Tab:* 500 mg ext-rel
> Comment: *ciprofloxacin* is contraindicated <18 years-of-age, and during pregnancy and lactation. Risk of tendonitis or tendon rupture.
➤ *doxycycline* (D)(G)
> **Acticlate** *Tab:* 75, 150**mg
> **Adoxa** *Tab:* 50, 75, 100, 150 mg ent-coat
> **Doryx** *Tab:* 50, 75, 100, 150, 200 mg del-rel
> **Doxteric** *Tab:* 50 mg del-rel
> **Monodox** *Cap:* 50, 75, 100 mg
> **Oracea** *Cap:* 40 mg del-rel
> **Vibramycin** *Tab:* 100 mg; *Cap:* 50, 100 mg; *Syr:* 50 mg/5 ml (raspberry-apple) (sulfites); *Oral susp:* 25 mg/5 ml (raspberry)
> **Vibra-Tab** *Tab:* 100 mg film-coat
> Comment: *doxycycline* is contraindicated <8 years-of-age, in pregnancy, and lactation (discolors developing tooth enamel). A side effect may be photosensitivity (photophobia). Do not take with antacids, calcium supplements, milk or other dairy, or within 2 hours of taking another drug.
➤ *erythromycin base* (B)(G)
> **Ery-Tab** *Tab:* 250, 333, 500 mg ent-coat
> **PCE** *Tab:* 333, 500 mg
> Comment: *erythromycin* may increase INR with concomitant *warfarin*, as well as increase serum level of *digoxin*, benzodiazepines, and statins.
➤ *erythromycin ethylsuccinate* (B)(G)
> **EryPed** *Oral susp:* 200 mg/5 ml (100, 200 ml) (fruit); 400 mg/5 ml (60, 100, 200 ml) (banana); *Oral drops:* 200, 400 mg/5 ml (50 ml) (fruit); *Chew tab:* 200 mg wafer (fruit)
> **E.E.S.** *Oral susp:* 200, 400 mg/5 ml (100 ml) (fruit)
> **E.E.S. Granules** *Oral susp:* 200 mg/5 ml (100, 200 ml) (cherry)
> **E.E.S. 400 Tablets** *Tab:* 400 mg
> Comment: *erythromycin* may increase INR with concomitant *warfarin*, as well as increase serum level of *digoxin*, benzodiazepines, and statins.
➤ *trimethoprim+sulfamethoxazole (TMP-SMX)*(C)(G)
> **Bactrim, Septra**
> > *Tab:* trim 80 mg+sulfa 400 mg*
> **Bactrim DS, Septra DS**
> > *Tab:* trim 160 mg+sulfa 800 mg*
> **Bactrim Pediatric Suspension, Septra Pediatric Suspension**
> > *Oral susp:* trim 40 mg+sulfa 200 mg per 5 ml (100 ml) (cherry) (alcohol 0.3%)

Comment: Sulfonamides are contraindicated in the first trimester of pregnancy, the final month of pregnancy, and infants <8 weeks-of-age. *CrCl 15-30 mL/min:* reduce dose by 1/2; *CrCl <15 mL/min:* not recommended. Contraindicated with G6PD deficiency. A high fluid intake is indicated during sulfonamide therapy to avoid crystallization in the kidneys.

GROWTH FAILURE

Comment: Administer growth hormones by SC injection into thigh, buttocks, or abdomen. Rotate sites with each dose. Contraindicated in children with fused epiphyses or evidence of neoplasia.

▷ *mecasermin* (recombinant human insulin-like growth factor-1 [rhIGF-1])

Increlex (B) see mfr pkg insert
Vial: 10 mg/ml (benzyl alcohol)
Comment: Increlex is indicated for growth failure in children with severe primary IGF-1 deficiency (primary IGFD) or in those with growth hormone (GH) gene deletion who have developed neutralizing antibodies to GH.

▷ *somatropin* (rDNA origin)

Genotropin (B) initially not more than 0.04 mg/kg/week divided into 6-7 doses; may increase at 4-8 week intervals; max 0.08 mg/kg/week divided into 6-7 doses
Pediatric: usually 0.16-0.024 mg/kg/week divided into 6-7 doses
  Intra-Mix Device: 1.5 mg (1.3 mg/ml after reconstitution), 5.8 mg (5 mg/ml after reconstitution) (two-chamber cartridge w. diluent); *Pen or Intra-Mix Device:* 5.8 mg (5 mg/ml after reconstitution), 13.8 mg (512 mg/ml after reconstitution) (2-chamber cartridge w. diluent)

Genotropin Miniquick (B) initially not more than 0.04 mg/kg/week divided into 6-7 doses; may increase at 4-8-week intervals; max 0.08 mg/kg/week divided into 6-7 doses
Pediatric: usually 0.16-0.024 mg/kg/week divided into 6-7 doses
  MiniQuick: 0.2, 0.4, 0.6, 0.8, 1, 1.2, 1.4, 1.6, 1.8, 2 mg/0.25 ml (pwdr for SC injection after reconstitution) (2-chamber cartridge w. diluent)

Humatrope (C)
Pediatric: initially 0.18 mg/kg/week IM or SC divided into equal doses given either on 3 alternate days or 6 x/week; max 0.3 mg/kg/week
  Vial: 5 mg w. 5 ml diluent

Norditropin (C)
Pediatric: 0.024-0.034 mg/kg SC 6-7 x/week
  Vial: 4 mg (12 IU), 8 mg (24 IU); *Cartridge for inj:* 5, 10, 15 mg/1.5 ml; *FlexPro prefilled pen:* 5, 10, 15 mg/1.5 ml
  NordiFlex prefilled pen: 5, 10, 15 mg/1.5 ml; 30 mg/3 ml

Nutropin (C)
Pediatric: 0.7 mg/kg/week SC in divided daily doses
  Vial: 5, 10 mg/vial w. diluent

Nutropin AQ (C)
<35 years: initially not more than 0.006 mg/kg SC daily; may increase to max 0.025 mg/kg SC daily; ≥35 years: initially not more than 0.006 mg/kg SC daily; may increase to max 0.0125 mg/kg SC daily
Pediatric: Prepubertal: up to 0.043 mg/kg SC daily; *Pubertal:* up to 0.1 mg/kg SC daily; *Turner Syndrome:* up to 0.0375 mg/kg/week divided into equal doses 3-7 x/week
  Vial: 5 mg/ml (2 ml)

Nutropin Depot (C) 1.5 mg/kg SC monthly on same day each month; max 22.5 mg/inj; divide injection if >22.5 mg
Pediatric: same as adult
  Vial: 13.5, 18, 22.5 mg/vial (pwdr for injection after reconstitution; single-use w. diluent and needle)

Omnitrope (B) 0.16-0.24 mg/kg/week SC divided 3-7 x/week
  Vial: 5.8 mg

Omnitrope Pen 5 (B) 0.16-0.24 mg/kg/week SC divided 3-7 x/week
  Cartridge for inj: 5 mg/1.5 ml

Omnitrope Pen 10 (B) 0.16-0.24 mg/kg/week SC divided 3-7 x/week
  Cartridge for inj: 10 mg/1.5 ml

Saizen (B)(G) 0.18 mg/kg/week IM or SC divided 3-7 x/week
  Vial: 5 mg (pwdr for SC injection w. diluent)

Serostim (B) 0.1 mg/kg SC once daily at HS; max 6 mg
Vial: 5, 4, 6, 8.8 mg (pwdr for SC injection w. diluent) (benzyl alcohol)

HAND, FOOT, AND MOUTH DISEASE (*COXSACKIEVIRUS*)

NSAIDs *see page* 571
Opioid Analgesics *see Pain* page 354
OTC Throat Lozenges
OTC Cough Drops and Cough Syrup

Comment: The hand, foot, and mouth disease occurs most commonly in children <10 years-of-age. Although adults are susceptible, most have built up natural immunity. The causative organism, *Coxsackievirus*, is transmitted via droplet spread (coughing and/or sneezing) and contact with contaminated objects and surfaces (same as influenza). Clinical signs and symptoms are typically relatively mild and include fever, sore throat, feeling generally unwell, malaise, headache, and poor appetite. Red spots, some painful blister-like lesions, most often appear on the tongue and roof of the mouth, palms of the hands, and soles of the feet (but not necessarily all three), and are often faint or sparse. Lesions, which are not pruritic, may also be noted on the dorsal surfaces of the hands/fingers and feet/ toes. Medical treatment, per se, is not required. Treatment in the home with age/ weight-dosed ibuprofen or acetaminophen for relief of sore throat, lesion pain, and fever. Other comfort measures include salt water gargles, throat lozenges, cough drops or cough syrup, and fluids. The disease typically resolves in 7 to 10 days.

HANSEN'S DISEASE (LEPROMATOUS LEPROSY, *MYCOBACTERIUM LEPRAE*)

Comment: Hansen's disease is treated with a combination of antibiotics. Typically, 2 or 3 antibiotics are used at the same time. These are *dapsone* with *rifampicin*, and *clofazimine* is added for some types of the disease. These drugs must never be used alone as monotherapy for leprosy. *Paucibacillary form:* 2 antibiotics are used at the same time, daily *dapsone* and *rifampicin* once per month. *Multibacillary form:* daily *clofazimine* is added to *rifampicin* and *dapsone*. This multi-drug treatment (MDT) strategy helps prevent the development of antibiotic resistance by the bacteria, which may otherwise occur due to length of the treatment. Treatment usually lasts between one to two years. The illness can be cured if treatment is completed as prescribed. A single dose of combination therapy has been used to cure single lesion paucibacillary leprosy: *rifampicin* 600 mg, *ofloxacin* 400 mg, and *minocycline* 100 mg. The child with a single lesion takes half the adult dose of the 3 medications. WHO has designed blister pack medication kits for both paucibacillary leprosy and for multibacillary leprosy. Each kit contains medication for 28 days. The blister pack medication kit for single lesion paucibacillary leprosy contains the necessary medication for the one-time administration of the 3 medications.

ANTIMYCOBACTERIALS

▷ *clofazimine* (G) should be administered with meals or milk
Dapsone-Sensitive Lepromatous Leprosy: 100 mg daily as a part of a combination regimen for at least 2 years
Dapsone-Resistant Lepromatous Leprosy: 100 mg daily in combination with one or more other agents for 3 years
Leprosy Complicated by Erythema Nodosum Leprosum: 100-200 mg daily for up to 3 months; taper dose to 100 mg as quickly as possible
Pediatric: Safety and effectiveness in pediatric patients have not been established
Soft gelcap: 50 mg
Comment: *clofazimine* is sometimes given with other medicines for leprosy. When *clofazimine* is used to treat disease flares, it may be given with a cortisone-like medicine. *clofazimine* may deposit in intestinal mucosa causing intestinal disturbances, including abdominal obstruction, bleeding, splenic infarction and death. Reduce dose or discontinue *clofazimine* if patient complains of pain in abdomen or other gastrointestinal symptoms. QT prolongation and Torsade de Pointes may occur with *clofazimine*. Concomitant use with other QT-prolonging drugs or *bedaquiline* may cause additive

QT prolongation. Monitor ECGs and discontinue *clofazimine* if significant ventricular arrhythmia or QTcF interval ≥500 ms develop. Advise patients that skin and body
fluid discoloration frequently occur. Depression and suicide due to skin discoloration
may occur; monitor patients for psychological effects of skin discoloration. The most
common adverse reactions reported in 40% to 50% of patients are skin and body fluid
discoloration, abdominal and epigastric pain, diarrhea, nausea, vomiting, gastrointestinal intolerance. No dose adjustment of *clofazimine* is needed for HIV-infected patients.
Severe Renal Impairment: use with caution. *Hepatic Impairment:* avoid. Monitor for
toxicities when used concomitantly with substrates of CYP3A4/5. It may take up to 6
months before the full benefit of *clofazimine* is seen. Sexually-active females of reproductive potential should have a pregnancy test prior to starting treatment. There are no
studies of *clofazimine* use in pregnant women and few cases of *clofazimine* use during
pregnancy have been reported in the literature. These reports indicate that the skin of
infants born to women who had received *clofazimine* during pregnancy was deeply
pigmented at birth; therefore, *clofazimine* should be used during pregnancy only if the
potential benefit justifies the risk to the fetus. *clofazimine* is excreted in human milk.
Skin discoloration has been observed in breastfed infants of mothers receiving *clofazimine*. There are no adequate studies in women for determining infant risk when using
this medication during breastfeeding.; therefore, weigh the potential benefits against
the potential risks before taking this medication while breastfeeding. In some areas,
clofazimine is considered an investigational new drug (IND) that must be prescribed by a
registered investigator; providers are encouraged to request investigator status by calling
the NDHP at 1-800-642-2477.

SULFONE

▷ *dapsone* topical (C)(G) apply to affected area bid
   Pediatric: <12 years: not recommended; ≥12 years: same as adult
      Aczone *Gel:* 5, 7.5% (30, 60, 90 gm pump)
▷ *rifampin* (C)(G) 600 mg orally once daily x 12 months
   Pediatric: <12 years: not recommended; ≥12 years: same as adult
      Rifadin, Rimactane *Cap:* 150, 300 mg

ALTERNATE DRUGS

Comment: *ofloxacin* may be substituted for *clofazimine*. *clarithromycin* may be substituted for
any of the drugs. *minocycline* may be substituted for *dapsone* in patients intolerant of *dapsone*,
and may also be used to substitute *clofazimine*; however, anti-inflammatory activity is not as
substantial as with *clofazimine*.

▷ *clarithromycin* (C)(G) 500 mg/day
      Biaxin *Tab:* 250, 500 mg
      Biaxin Oral Suspension *Oral susp:* 125, 250 mg/5 ml (50, 100 ml) (fruit-punch)
      Biaxin XL *Tab:* 500 mg ext-rel
   Comment: The FDA is advising caution before prescribing *clarithromycin* to patients with
   heart disease because of a potential increased risk of heart problems or death that can occur
   years later. This recommendation is based on a review of the results of a 10-year follow-up
   study of patients with coronary heart disease from a large clinical trial that first observed
   this safety issue. Consider risk benefit and the use of other antibiotics in such patients.
▷ *ofloxacin* (C)(G) 400 mg/day
   Pediatric: <18 years: not recommended; ≥18 years: same as adult
      Floxin *Tab:* 200, 300, 400 mg
   Comment: *ofloxacin* is contraindicated <18 years-of-age and during pregnancy and lactation. Risk of tendonitis or tendon rupture.
▷ *minocycline* (D)(G) 100 mg/day
   Pediatric: <8 years: not recommended; ≥8 years: same as adult
      Dynacin *Cap:* 50, 100 mg
      Minocin *Cap:* 50, 75, 100 mg; *Oral susp:* 50 mg/5 ml (60 ml) (custard) (sulfites, alcohol
      5%)
   Comment: *minocycline* is contraindicated <8 years-of-age, in pregnancy, and lactation
   (discolors developing tooth enamel). A side effect may be photo-sensitivity (photophobia).
   Do not take with antacids, calcium supplements, milk or other dairy, or within two hours of
   taking another drug.

HEADACHE: MIGRAINE, CLUSTER, VASCULAR

ERGOTAMINE AGENTS

Comment: Do not use an ergotamine-type drug within 24 hours of any triptan or other 5-HT agonist.

▷ *dihydroergotamine mesylate* (X)
> **DHE 45** 1 mg SC, IM, or IV; may repeat at 1 hour intervals; max 3 mg/day SC or IM/ day; max 2 mg IV/day; max 6 mg/week
> *Pediatric:* <12 years: not recommended; ≥12 years: same as adult
> > *Amp:* 1 mg/ml (1 ml)
> **Migranal** 1 spray in each nostril; may repeat 15 minutes later; max 6 sprays/day and 8 sprays/week
> *Pediatric:* <12 years: not recommended; ≥12 years: same as adult
> > *Nasal spray:* 4 mg/ml; 0.5 mg/spray (caffeine)

▷ *ergotamine* (X)(G) 1 tab SL at onset of attack; then q 30 minutes as needed; max 3 tabs/day and 5 tabs/week
> *Tab:* 2 mg

▷ *ergotamine+caffeine* (X)(G)
> *Pediatric:* <12 years: not recommended; ≥12 years: same as adult
> **Cafergot** 2 tabs at onset of attack; then 1 tab every 1/2 hour if needed; max 6 tabs/attack and 10 tabs/week
> > *Tab:* ergot 1 mg+caf 100 mg
> **Cafergot Suppository** 1 suppository rectally at onset of headache; may repeat x 1 after 1 hour; max 2/attack, 5/week
> > *Rectal supp:* ergot 2 mg+caf 100 mg

5-HT RECEPTOR AGONISTS

Comment: Contraindications to 5-HT receptor agonists include cardiovascular disease, ischemic heart disease, cerebral vascular syndromes, peripheral vascular disease, uncontrolled hypertension, hemiplegic or basilar migraine. Do not use any triptan within 24 hours of ergot-type drugs or other 5-HT1A agonists, or within 2 weeks of taking an MAOI.

▷ *almotriptan* (C)(G) 6.25 or 12.5 mg; may repeat once after 2 hours; max 2 doses/day
> *Pediatric:* <12 years: not recommended; ≥12 years: same as adult
> **Axert** *Tab:* 6.25 mg (6/card), 12.5 mg (12/card)
> **Comment:** *almotriptan* is indicated for patients 12-17 years-of-age with PMHx migraine headache lasting ≥4 hours untreated.

▷ *eletriptan* (C)(G) 20 or 40 mg; may repeat once after 2 hours; max 80 mg/day
> *Pediatric:* <18 years: not recommended; ≥18 years: same as adult
> **Relpax** *Tab:* 20, 40 mg

▷ *frovatriptan* (C)(G) 2.5 mg with fluids; may repeat once after 2 hours; max 7.5 mg/day
> *Pediatric:* <18 years: not recommended; ≥18 years: same as adult
> **Frova** *Tab:* 2.5 mg

▷ *naratriptan* (C) 1 or 2.5 mg with fluids; may repeat once after 4 hours; max 5 mg/day
> *Pediatric:* <18 years: not recommended; ≥18 years: same as adult
> **Amerge** *Tab:* 1, 2.5 mg

▷ *rizatriptan* (C) initially 5 or 10 mg; may repeat in 2 hours if needed; max 30 mg/day
> *Pediatric:* <18 years: not recommended; ≥18 years: same as adult
> **Maxalt** *Tab:* 5, 10 mg
> **Maxalt-MLT** *ODT:* 5, 10 mg (peppermint) (phenylalanine)

▷ *sumatriptan* (C)(G)
> *Pediatric:* <18 years: not recommended; ≥18 years: same as adult
> **Alsuma** 6 mg SC to the upper arm or lateral thigh only; may repeat after 1 hour if needed; max 2 doses/day
> > *Prefilled syringe:* 6 mg/0.5 ml (2/pck with auto injector)
> **Imitrex Injectable** 4-6 mg SC; may repeat after 1 hour if needed; max 2 doses/day
> > *Prefilled syringe:* 4, 6 mg/0.5 ml (2/pck with or without autoinjector)
> **Imitrex Nasal Spray** (G) 5-20 mg intranasally; may repeat once after 2 hours if needed; max 40 mg/day
> > *Nasal spray:* 5, 20 mg/spray (single-dose)
> **Imitrex Tab** 25-200 mg x 1 dose; may be repeated at intervals of at least 2 hours if needed; max 200 mg/day
> > *Tab:* 25, 50, 100 mg rapid-rel

Imitrex STATdose Pen 6 mg/0.5 mg SC; may repeat once after 2 hours if needed; max 2 doses/day

> *Prefilled needle-free autoinjector delivery system:* 6 mg/0.5 ml (6/pck)

Onzetra Xsail each disposable white nosepiece contains half a dose of medication (11 mg of sumatriptan). A full dose is 22 mg. Do not use more than 2 nosepieces per dose; attach the mouthpiece and one nasal piece; then press the white button on the delivery device to pierce the capsule in the nasal piece, then insert the nasal piece into one nostril and blow into the mouth piece to deliver the nasal powder in the contents of one capsule (11 mg); repeat in the opposite nostril for a total single 22 mg dose

> *Cap:* 11 mg nasal pwdr; *Kit:* nosepieces (2), capsules (2), reusable breath powered delivery device (1)

Sumavel DosePro 6 mg SC to the upper arm or lateral thigh only; may repeat after 1 hour if needed; max 2 doses/day

> *Prefilled needle-free delivery system:* 6 mg/0.5 ml (6/pck)

Tosymra 10 mg (1 nasal spray); max 3 nasal sprays (30 mg)/24 hours; separate doses by at least one hour

> *Nasal spray:* 10 mg/spray ready-to-use, single-dose, disposable unit (6 units/carton)

Zembrace SymTouch administer 3 mg SC at onset of headache; may repeat hourly; max 12 mg/24 hours

Pediatric: <18 years: not recommended; ≥18 years: same as adult

> *Autoinjector:* 3 mg/0.5 ml (prefilled single-dose disposable autoinjector)

▷ *zolmitriptan* (C)(G) initially 2.5 mg; may repeat after 2 hours if needed; max 10 mg/day
Pediatric: <18 years: not recommended; ≥18 years: same as adult

Zomig *Tab:* 2.5*, 5 mg

Zomig Nasal Spray *Nasal spray:* 5 mg/spray single-dose (6/carton)

Zomig-ZMT *ODT:* 2.5 mg (6 tabs), 5*mg (3 tabs) (orange) (phenylalanine)

Comment: Do not use any *triptan* within 24 hours of ergotamine-type drugs or other 5-HT agonists, or within 2 weeks of taking an MAOI.

5-HT IB+ID RECEPTOR AGONIST+NSAID COMBINATION

▷ *sumatriptan+naproxen* (C; D in 3rd)(G)
Pediatric: <18 years: not recommended; ≥18 years: same as adult

Treximet initially 1 tab; may repeat after 2 hours; max 2 doses/day

> *Tab:* suma 85 mg+naprox 500 mg (9/blister card)

Comment: Do not use *sumatriptan* within 24 hours of ergot-type drugs or other 5-HT agonists, or within 2 weeks of taking an MAOI.

OTHER ANALGESICS

▷ *acetaminophen+aspirin+caffeine* (D)(G)
Comment: *aspirin*-containing medications are contraindicated with history of allergic-type reaction to *aspirin*, children and adolescents with *Varicella* or other viral illness, and 3rd trimester of pregnancy.

Excedrin Migraine (OTC) 2 tabs q 6 hours prn; max 8 tabs/day x 2 days

Pediatric: <18 years: not recommended; ≥18 years: same as adult

> *Tab:* acet 250 mg+asp 250 mg+caf 65 mg

▷ *diclofenac potassium powder for oral solution* (C; D ≥30 weeks)(G) empty the contents of one pkt into a cup containing 1-2 oz or 2-4 tbsp (30-60 ml) of water, mix well, and drink immediately; water only, no other liquids; take on an empty stomach; use the closest effective dose for the shortest duration of time; safety and effectiveness of a 2nd dose has not been established

Pediatric: <18 years: not established; ≥18 years: same as adult

Cambia *Pwdr for oral soln:* 50 mg/pkt (3 pkts/set, conjoined with a perforated border

Comment: **Cambia** is not indicated for migraine prophylaxis. May not be bioequivalent with other *diclofenac* forms (e.g., *diclofenac sodium* ent-coat tabs, *diclofenac sodium* ext-rel tabs, *diclofenac potassium* immed-rel tabs) even of the mg strength is the same, therefore, it is not possible to convert dosing from any other diclofenac formulation to **Cambia**. **Cambia** is contraindicated in the setting of coronary artery bypass graft. Use of **Cambia** should not be considered with hepatic impairment, gastric/duodenal ulcer, starting at 30 weeks gestation (risk of premature closure of the ductus arteriosus in the fetus), concomitant NSAIDs, SSRIs, anticoagulants/antiplatelets, any risk factor for potential bleeding.

▷ *isometheptene mucate+dichloralphenazone+acetaminophen* (C)(IV)
   Midrin 2 caps initially; then 1 cap q 1 hour until relieved; max 5 caps/12 hours
   Pediatric: <12 years: not recommended; ≥12 years: same as adult
      Cap: iso 65 mg+dichlor 100 mg+acet 325 mg

CALCITONIN GENE-RELATED PEPTIDE (CGRP) RECEPTOR ANTAGONIST

Comment: The CGRP receptor antagonists are a class of drugs that block a the activity of calcitonin gene-related peptide as prophylaxis against migraine attacks.

▷ *erenumab-aooe* administer by SC injection only in the upper arm, abdomen, or thigh; recommended dose is 70 mg SC once monthly; some patients may benefit from a dosage of 140 mg SC once monthly (i.e., two consecutive injections of 70 mg each); the needle shield within the white cap of the prefilled autoinjector and the gray needle cap of the prefilled syringe contain dry natural rubber (a derivative of latex), which may cause allergic reactions in individuals sensitive to latex
   Pediatric: <18 years: not recommended; ≥18 years: same as adult
      Aimovig *Autoinjector:* 70 mg/ml (1 ml), prefilled single-dose, SureClick
      Comment: The most common adverse side effects are injection site reaction and constipation. There are no adequate data on the developmental risk associated with the use of **Aimovig** in pregnant females. There are no data on the presence of *erenumab-aooe* in human milk or effects on the breastfed infant. Safety and effectiveness in pediatric patients have not been established.
▷ *fremanezumab-vfrm* administer by SC injection only in the upper arm, abdomen, or thigh; recommended dose is 225 mg SC once monthly or 675 mg SC once every 3 months (3 x 225 mg SC doses once quarterly)
   Pediatric: <18 years: not recommended; ≥18 years: same as adult
      Ajovy *Prefilled syringe:* 225 mg/1.5 ml (1.5 ml) solution single-dose
      Comment: The most common adverse side effects are injection site reaction and constipation. There are no adequate data on the developmental risk associated with the use of **Ajovy** in pregnant females. There are no data on the presence of *erenumab-vfrm* in human milk or effects on the breastfed infant. Safety and effectiveness in pediatric patients have not been established.
▷ *galcanezumab-gnlm* administer by SC injection only in the back of the upper arm, abdomen, thigh or buttocks; *Loading Dose:* 240 mg (2 x 120 mg) SC; *Maintenance:* 120 mg SC once monthly
   Pediatric: <18 years: not recommended; ≥18 years: same as adult
      Emgality *Prefilled pen/Prefilled syringe:* 120 mg/ml (1 ml) solution single-dose
      Comment: The most common adverse side effect (incidence ≥2%) is injection site reaction. There are no adequate data on the developmental risk associated with the use of **Emgality** in pregnant females. There are no data on the presence of *erenumab-vfrm* in human milk or effects on the breastfed infant. Safety and effectiveness in pediatric patients have not been established.

ANTICONVULSANTS

▷ *divalproex sodium* (D) *Delayed-release*: initially 250 mg bid; titrate weekly to usual max 500 mg bid; *Extended-release*: initially 500 mg once daily; may increase after one week to 1 gm once daily
   Pediatric: <10 years: not recommended; ≥10 years: same as adult
      Depakene *Cap:* 250 mg del-rel; syr: 250 mg/5 ml (16 oz)
      Depakote *Tab:* 125, 250, 500 mg del-rel
      Depakote ER *Tab:* 250, 500 mg ext-rel
      Depakote Sprinkle *Cap:* 125 mg del-rel
▷ *topiramate* (D)(G) initially 25 mg daily in the PM and titrate up daily as tolerated; then 25 mg bid; then, 25 mg in the AM and 50 mg in the PM; then, 50 mg bid
   Pediatric: <12 years: not recommended; ≥12 years: same as adult
      Topamax *Tab:* 25, 50, 100, 200 mg
      Topamax Sprinkle Caps *Cap:* 15, 25 mg
      Trokendi XR *Cap:* 25, 50, 100, 200 mg ext-rel
      Quedexy XR *Cap:* 25, 50, 100, 150, 200 mg ext-rel

BETA-BLOCKERS

▷ *atenolol* (D)(G) initially 25 mg bid; max 150 mg/day in divided doses
  Pediatric: <12 years: not recommended; ≥12 years: same as adult
    Tenormin *Tab:* 25, 50, 100 mg
▷ *metoprolol succinate* (C)
  Pediatric: <12 years: not recommended; ≥12 years: same as adult
    ToprolR-XL initially 25-100 mg in a single dose daily; increase weekly if needed; max 400 mg/day
      Tab: 25*, 50*, 100*, 200*mg ext-rel
▷ *metoprolol tartrate* (C)
  Pediatric: <12 years: not recommended; ≥12 years: same as adult
    Lopressor (G) initially 25-50 mg bid; increase weekly if needed; max 400 mg/day
      Tab: 25, 37.5, 50, 75, 100 mg
▷ *nadolol* (C)(G) initially 20 mg daily; max 240 mg/day in divided doses
  Pediatric: <12 years: not recommended; ≥12 years: same as adult
    Corgard *Tab:* 20*, 40*, 80*, 120*, 160*mg
▷ *propranolol* (C)(G)
  Pediatric: <12 years: not recommended; ≥12 years: same as adult
    Inderal initially 10 mg bid; usual range 160-320 mg/day in divided doses
      Tab: 10*, 20*, 40*, 60*, 80*mg
    Inderal LA initially 80 mg daily in a single dose; increase q 3-7 days; usual range 120-160 mg/day; max 320 mg/day in a single dose
      Cap: 60, 80, 120, 160 mg sust-rel
    InnoPran XL initially 80 mg q HS; max 120 mg/day
      Cap: 80, 120 mg ext-rel
▷ *timolol* (C)(G) initially 5 mg bid; max 60 mg/day in divided doses
  Pediatric: <12 years: not recommended; ≥12 years: same as adult
    Blocadren *Tab:* 5, 10*, 20*mg

CALCIUM ANTAGONISTS

▷ *diltiazem* (C)(G)
  Pediatric: <12 years: not recommended; ≥12 years: same as adult
    Cardizem initially 30 mg qid; may increase gradually every 1-2 days; max 360 mg/day in divided doses
      Tab: 30, 60, 90, 120 mg
    Cardizem CD initially 120-180 mg once daily; adjust at 1- to 2-week intervals; max 480 mg/day
      Cap: 120, 180, 240, 300, 360 mg ext-rel
    Cardizem LA initially 180-240 mg once daily; titrate at 2-week intervals; max 540 mg/day
      Tab: 120, 180, 240, 300, 360, 420 mg ext-rel
    Cardizem SR initially 60-120 mg bid; adjust at 2-week intervals; max 360 mg/day
      Cap: 60, 90, 120 mg sust-rel
▷ *nifedipine* (C)(G)
  Pediatric: <12 years: not recommended; ≥12 years: same as adult
    Adalat initially 10 mg tid; usual range 10-20 mg tid; max 180 mg/day
      Cap: 10, 20 mg
    Procardia initially 10 mg tid; titrate over 7-14 days: max 30 mg/dose and 180 mg/day in divided doses
      Cap: 10, 20 mg
    Procardia XL initially 30-60 mg daily; titrate over 7-14 days; max 90 mg/day in divided doses
▷ *verapamil* (C)(G)
  Pediatric: <12 years: not recommended; ≥12 years: same as adult
    Calan 80-120 mg tid; increase daily <u>or</u> weekly if needed
      Tab: 40, 80*, 120*mg
    Covera HS initially 180 mg q HS; titrate in steps to 240 mg; then to 360 mg; then to 480 mg if needed
      Tab: 180, 240 mg ext-rel
    Isoptin initially 80-120 mg tid
      Tab: 40, 80, 120 mg

Isoptin SR initially 120-180 mg in the AM; may increase to 240 mg in the AM; then, 180 mg q 12 hours or 240 mg in the AM and 120 mg in the PM; then, 240 mg q 12 hours
> *Tab:* 120, 180*, 240*mg sust-rel

TRICYCLIC ANTIDEPRESSANTS (TCAs)

Comment: Co-administration of TCAs with SSRIs requires extreme caution.
▷ *amitriptyline* (C)(G) 10-20 mg q HS
   Pediatric: <12 years: not recommended; ≥12 years: same as adult
      Tab: 10, 25, 50, 75, 100, 150 mg
▷ *doxepin* (C)(G) 10-200 mg q HS
   Pediatric: <12 years: not recommended; ≥12 years: same as adult
      Cap: 10, 25, 50, 75, 100, 150 mg; *Oral conc:* 10 mg/ml (4 oz w. dropper)
▷ *imipramine* (C)(G) 10-200 mg q HS
      Tofranil 25-50 mg; max 200 mg/day; if maintenance dose exceeds 75 mg daily, may switch to **Tofranil PM**
      Pediatric: <6 years: not recommended; 6-12 years: initially 25 mg; >12 years: 50 mg max 2.5 mg/kg/day
         Tab: 10, 25, 50 mg
      Tofranil PM initially 75 mg once daily 1 hour before HS; max 200 mg
         Cap: 75, 100, 125, 150 mg
▷ *nortriptyline* (D)(G) 10-150 mg q HS
   Pediatric: <12 years: not recommended; ≥12 years: same as adult
      Pamelor *Cap:* 10, 25, 50, 75 mg; *Oral soln:* 10 mg/5 ml (16 oz)

SELECTIVE SEROTONIN REUPTAKE INHIBITORS (SSRIs)

Comment: Co-administration of SSRIs with TCAs requires extreme caution. Concomitant use of MAOIs and SSRIs is absolutely contraindicated. Avoid other serotonergic drugs. A potentially fatal adverse event is Serotonin Syndrome, caused by serotonin excess. Milder symptoms require HCP intervention to avert severe symptoms which can be rapidly fatal without urgent/emergent medical care. Symptoms include restlessness, agitation, confusion, hallucinations, tachycardia, hypertension, dilated pupils, muscle twitching, muscle rigidity, loss of muscle coordination, diaphoresis, diarrhea, headache, shivering, piloerection, hyperpyrexia, cardiac arrhythmias, seizures, loss of consciousness, coma, death. Abrupt withdrawal or interruption of treatment with an antidepressant medication is sometimes associated with an Antidepressant Discontinuation Syndrome which may be mediated by gradually tapering the drug over a period of two weeks or longer, depending on the dose strength and length of treatment. Common symptoms of the Serotonin Discontinuation Syndrome include flu-like symptoms (nausea, vomiting, diarrhea, headaches, sweating), sleep disturbances (insomnia, nightmares, constant sleepiness), mood disturbances (dysphoria, anxiety, agitation), cognitive disturbances (mental confusion, hyperarousal), sensory and movement disturbances (imbalance, tremors, vertigo, dizziness, electric-shock-like sensations in the brain, often described by sufferers as "brain zaps."
▷ *fluoxetine* (C)(G)
      Prozac initially 20 mg daily; may increase after 1 week; doses >20 mg/day may be divided into AM and noon doses; max 80 mg/day
      Pediatric: <8 years: not recommended; 8-17 years: initially 10-20 mg/day; start lower weight children at 10 mg/day; if starting at 10 mg daily, may increase after 1 week to 20 mg once daily
         Cap: 10, 20, 40 mg; *Tab:* 30*, 60*mg; *Oral soln:* 20 mg/5 ml (4 oz) (mint)
      Prozac Weekly following daily fluoxetine therapy at 20 mg/day for 13 weeks, may initiate **Prozac Weekly** 7 days after the last 20 mg fluoxetine dose
      Pediatric: <12 years: not recommended; ≥12 years: same as adult
         Cap: 90 mg ent-coat del-rel pellets

OTHER AGENT

▷ *methysergide maleate* (X) 4-8 mg daily in divided doses with food; max 8 mg/day; max 6 month treatment course; wean off over last 2-3 weeks of treatment course; separate treatment courses by 3-4 week drug-free interval
   Pediatric: <18 years: not recommended; ≥18 years: same as adult
      Sansert *Tab:* 2 mg

Comment: *methysergide maleate* is indicated for the prevention or reduction of intensity and frequency of vascular headaches. It is contraindicated in pregnancy due to its oxytocic actions. *methysergide maleate* is a semi-synthetic compound structurally related to ergotamine, and thus it may appear in breast milk. Ergot alkaloids have been reported to cause nausea, vomiting, diarrhea and weakness in the nursing infant and suppression of prolactin secretion and lactation in the mother.

MAGNESIUM SUPPLEMENTS

▷ *magnesium* (B)
    Slow-Mag 2 tabs daily
      Tab: 64 mg (as chloride)+110 mg (as carbonate)
▷ *magnesium oxide* (B)
    Mag-Ox 400 1-2 tabs daily
      Tab: 400 mg

 HEADACHE: TENSION (MUSCLE CONTRACTION)

Acetaminophen for IV Infusion *see Pain page* 352
NSAIDs *see page* 571
Opioid Analgesics *see Pain page* 354
Topical and Transdermal Analgesics *see Pain page* 352
Parenteral Corticosteroids *see page* 577
Oral Corticosteroids *see page* 577
Topical Analgesic and Anesthetic Agents *see page* 569

ORAL ANALGESICS COMBINATIONS

Other Oral Analgesics *see Pain page* 352
▷ *butalbital+acetaminophen* (C)(G)
    Pediatric: <12 years: not recommended; ≥12 years: same as adult
      Phrenilin 1-2 tabs q 4 hours prn; max 6 tabs/day
        Tab: but 50 mg+acet 325 mg
      Phrenilin Forte 1 tab <u>or</u> cap q 4 hours prn; max 6 caps/day
        Cap/Tab: but 50 mg+acet 650 mg
▷*butalbital+acetaminophen+caffeine* (C)(G)
    Pediatric: <12 years: not recommended; ≥12 years: same as adult
      Fioricet 1-2 tabs q 4 hours prn; max 6/day
        Tab: but 50 mg+acet 325 mg+caf 40 mg
      Zebutal 1 cap q 4 hours prn; max 5/day
        Cap: but 50 mg+acet 500 mg+caf 40 mg
▷ *butalbital+acetaminophen+codeine+caffeine* (C)(III)(G)
    Pediatric: <18 years: not recommended; ≥18 years: same as adult
      Fioricet with Codeine 1-2 tabs at onset q 4 hours prn; max 6 tabs/day
        Tab: but 50 mg+acet 325 mg+cod 30 mg+caf 40 mg
Comment: *Codeine* is known to be excreted in breast milk. <12 years: not recommended; 12-<18 years: use extreme caution; not recommended for children and adolescents with asthma <u>or</u> other chronic breathing problem. The FDA and the European Medicines Agency (EMA) are investigating the safety of using *codeine* containing medications to treat pain, cough and colds, in children 12-<18 years because of the potential for serious side effects, including slowed <u>or</u> difficult breathing.
▷ *butalbital+aspirin+caffeine* (C)(III)(G)
    Pediatric: <12 years: not recommended; ≥12 years: same as adult
      Fiorinal 1-2 tabs <u>or</u> caps q 4 hours prn; max 6 caps/tabs/day
        Tab/Cap: but 50 mg+asa 325 mg+caf 40 mg
Comment: *aspirin*-containing medications are contraindicated with history of allergic-type reaction to *aspirin*, children and adolescents with *Varicella* or other viral illness, and 3rd trimester of pregnancy.
▷ *butalbital+aspirin+codeine+caffeine* (C)(III)(G)
    Pediatric: 18 years: not recommended; ≥18 years: same as adult
      Fiorinal with Codeine 1-2 caps q 4 hours prn; max 6 caps/day
        Cap: but 50 mg+asp 325 mg+cod 30 mg+caf 40 mg

Comment: *Codeine* is known to be excreted in breast milk. <12 years: not recommended; 12-<18: use extreme caution; not recommended for children and adolescents with asthma or other chronic breathing problem. The FDA and the European Medicines Agency (EMA) are investigating the safety of using *codeine* containing medications to treat pain, cough and colds, in children 12-<18 years because of the potential for serious side effects, including slowed or difficult breathing. *aspirin*-containing medications are contraindicated with history of allergic-type reaction to *aspirin*, children and adolescents with *Varicella* or other viral illness, and 3rd trimester of pregnancy.

▷ *butorphanol tartrate* (C)(IV)(G) initially 1 spray (1 mg) in one nostril and may repeat after 60-90 minutes (*Elderly* 90-120 minutes) in opposite nostril if needed or 1 spray in each nostril and may repeat q 3-4 hours prn
   Pediatric: <18 years: not recommended; ≥18 years: same as adult
      Butorphanol Nasal Spray *Nasal spray:* 1 mg/actuation (10 mg/ml, 2.5 ml)
      Stadol Nasal Spray *Nasal spray:* 10 mg/ml, 1 mg/actuation (10 mg/ml, 2.5 ml)

▷ *tramadol* (C)(IV)(G) initially 100 mg once daily; may increase by 100 mg every 5 days; max 300 mg/day; *CrCl <30 mL/min or severe hepatic impairment*: not recommended; *Cirrhosis:* max 50 mg q 12 hours
   Pediatric: <18 years: not recommended; ≥18 years: same as adult
      Rybix ODT *ODT:* 50 mg (mint) (phenylalanine)
      Ryzolt *Tab:* 100, 200, 300 mg ext-rel
      Ultram *Tab:* 50*mg
      Ultram ER *Tab:* 100, 200, 300 mg ext-rel
   Comment: *tramadol* is known to be excreted in breast milk. The FDA and the European Medicines Agency (EMA) are investigating the safety of using *tramadol*-containing medications to treat pain in children 12-18 years because of the potential for serious side effects, including slowed or difficult breathing.

▷ *tramadol+acetaminophen* (C)(IV)(G) 2 tabs q 4-6 hours prn; max 8 tabs/day; 5 days; *CrCl <30 mL/min:* max 2 tabs q 12 hours; max 4 tabs/day x 5 days; *Cirrhosis or other liver disease:* contraindicated
   Pediatric: <18 years: not recommended; ≥18 years: same as adult
      Ultracet *Tab:* tram 37.5+acet 325 mg
   Comment: *tramadol* is known to be excreted in breast milk. The FDA and the European Medicines Agency (EMA) are investigating the safety of using *tramadol*-containing medications to treat pain in children 12-18 years because of the potential for serious side effects, including slowed or difficult breathing.

TRICYCLIC ANTIDEPRESSANTS (TCAs)

Comment: Co-administration of TCAs with SSRIs requires extreme caution.
▷ *amitriptyline* (C)(G) 50-100 mg/day
   Pediatric: <12 years: not recommended; ≥12 years: same as adult
      Tab: 10, 25, 50, 75, 100, 150 mg
▷ *desipramine* (C)(G) 50-100 mg bid
   Pediatric: <12 years: not recommended; ≥12 years: same as adult
      Norpramin *Tab:* 10, 25, 50, 75, 100, 150 mg
▷ *imipramine* (C)(G)
   Pediatric: <12 years: not recommended; ≥12 years: same as adult
      Tofranil initially 75 mg daily (max 200 mg); adolescents initially 30-40 mg daily (max 100 mg/day); if maintenance dose exceeds 75 mg daily, may switch to **Tofranil PM** for divided or bedtime dosing
         Tab: 10, 25, 50 mg
      Tofranil PM initially 75 mg once daily 1 hour before HS; max 200 mg
         Cap: 75, 100, 125, 150 mg
      Tofranil Injection 50 mg IM; lower dose for adolescents; switch to oral form as soon as possible
         Amp: 25 mg/2 ml (2 ml)
▷ *nortriptyline* (D)(G) 25-50 mg/day
   Pediatric: <12 years: not recommended; ≥12 years: same as adult
      Pamelor *Cap:* 10, 25, 50, 75 mg; *Oral soln:* 10 mg/5 ml (16 oz)

MAGNESIUM SUPPLEMENTS

➤ *magnesium* (B)
    Slow-Mag 2 tabs daily
        Tab: 64 mg (as chloride)/110 mg (as carbonate)
➤ *magnesium oxide* (B)
    Mag-Ox 400 1-2 tabs daily
        Tab: 400 mg

 HEART FAILURE (HF)

HEART FAILURE AND DIABETES

Comment: Heart failure (**HF**) in the presence of type 2 diabetes (**T2DM**) has a 5-year survival rate on par with some of the worst diseases, such as lung cancer, because diabetes makes the pathophysiology of heart failure worse. Diabetes amplifies the neurohormonal response to heart failure, so it drives progressive heart failure and increases the risk for sudden death. **As left ventricular function decreases, patients with diabetes have heightened activation of the renin angiotensin system (RAS).** They have increased left ventricular hypertrophy, and they have increased sympathetic nervous system activation. A "four Ds" framework that clinicians can use to improve prognosis in these patients: (1) *Loop diuretics* to get the patient out of congestive cardiac syndrome as quickly as possible; (2) *Disease modification* with beta-blockers (β and ACE inhibitors, to the maximal dose tolerated, the mainstays of treatment for patients with heart failure (ACEI's protect these patients against cardiac myocyte cell death and vasoconstriction and beta-blockers protect against the activation of the sympathetic nervous system [SNS]); (3) Consider *device therapy* (including defibrillators and resynchronization therapy); and (4) *Optimize diabetes management*.

REFERENCE

Reported by Mark Kearney, MD, Director of the Leeds Institute of Cardiovascular & Metabolic Medicine at Leeds (England) University, the World Congress on Insulin Resistance, Diabetes & Cardiovascular Disease [published online January 28, 2018]. https://www.mdedge.com/clinicalendocrinologynews/article/157198/diabetes/learn-four-ds-approach-heart-failure-diabetes

ACE INHIBITORS (ACEIs)

➤ *captopril* (C; D in 2nd, 3rd)(G) initially 25 mg tid; after 1-2 weeks may increase to 50 mg tid; max 450 mg/day
    Pediatric: <12 years: not recommended; ≥12 years: same as adult
        Capoten *Tab:* 12.5*, 25*, 50*, 100*mg
➤ *enalapril* (D) initially 5 mg daily; usual dosage range 10-40 mg/day; max 40 mg/day
    Pediatric: <12 years: not recommended; ≥12 years: same as adult
        Epaned Oral Solution *Oral soln:* 1 mg/ml (150 ml) (mixed berry)
        Vasotec (G) *Tab:* 2.5*, 5*, 10, 20 mg
➤ *fosinopril* (C; D in 2nd, 3rd) initially 10 mg daily, usual maintenance 20-40 mg/day in a single or divided doses
    Pediatric: <6 years, <50 kg: not recommended; 6-12 years, ≥50 kg: 5-10 mg daily; ≥12 years: same as adult
        Monopril *Tab:* 10*, 20, 40 mg
➤ *lisinopril* (D) initially 5 mg daily
    Prinivil initially 10 mg daily; usual range 20-40 mg/day
    Pediatric: <12 years: not recommended; ≥12 years: same as adult
        Tab: 5*, 10*, 20*, 40 mg
    Qbrelis Oral Solution administer as a single dose once daily
    Pediatric: <6 years, GFR <30 mL/min: not recommended; ≥6 years, GFR >30 mL/min: initially 0.07 mg/kg, max 5 mg; adjust according to BP up to a max 0.61 mg/kg (40 mg) once daily
        Oral soln: 1 mg/ml (150 ml)
    Zestril initially 10 mg daily; usual range 20-40 mg/day
    Pediatric: <12 years: not recommended; ≥12 years: same as adult
        Tab: 2.5, 5*, 10, 20, 30, 40 mg

➤ *quinapril* (C; D in 2nd, 3rd) initially 5 mg bid; increase weekly to 10-20 mg bid
  Pediatric: <12 years: not recommended; ≥12 years: same as adult
    Accupril *Tab:* 5*, 10, 20, 40 mg
➤ *ramipril* (C; D in 2nd, 3rd) initially 2.5 mg bid; usual maintenance 5 mg bid
  Pediatric: <12 years: not recommended; ≥12 years: same as adult
    Altace *Tab/Cap:* 1.25, 2.5, 5, 10 mg
➤ *trandolapril* (C; D in 2nd, 3rd) initially 1 mg daily; titrate to dose of 4 mg daily as tolerated
  Pediatric: <12 years: not recommended; ≥12 years: same as adult
    Mavik *Tab:* 1*, 2, 4 mg

BETA-BLOCKERS (CARDIOSELECTIVE)

➤ *carvedilol* (C)(G)
    Coreg initially 3.125 mg bid; may increase at 1-2 week intervals to 12.5 mg bid; usual max 50 mg bid
    Pediatric: <18 years: not recommended; ≥18 years: same as adult
      Tab: 3.125, 6.25, 12.5, 25 mg
    Coreg CR initially 10 mg once daily x 2 weeks; may double dose at 2 week intervals; max 80 mg once daily; may open caps and sprinkle on food
      Pediatric: <18 years: not recommended; ≥18 years: same as adult
      Cap: 10, 20, 40, 80 mg cont-rel
➤ *metoprolol succinate* (C)
  Pediatric: <12 years: not recommended; ≥12 years: same as adult
    Toprol-XL initially 12.5-25 mg in a single dose daily; increase weekly if needed; reduce if symptomatic bradycardia occurs; max 400 mg/day
      Tab: 25*, 50*, 100*, 200*mg ext-rel
➤ *metoprolol tartrate* (C)
  Pediatric: <12 years: not recommended; ≥12 years: same as adult
    Lopressor (G) initially 25-50 mg bid; increase weekly if needed; max 400 mg/day
      Tab: 25, 37.5, 50, 75, 100 mg

ANGIOTENSIN II RECEPTOR BLOCKERS (ARBs)

➤ *valsartan* (C; D in 2nd, 3rd) initially 40 mg bid; increase to 160 mg bid as tolerated or 320 mg daily after 2-4 weeks; usual range 80-320 mg/day
  Pediatric: <12 years: not recommended; ≥12 years: same as adult
    Diovan *Tab:* 40*, 80, 160, 320 mg
    Prexxartan Oral Solution *Oral soln:* 20 mg/5 ml, 80 mg/20 ml (120, 473 ml; 20 ml unit-dose cup)

NEPRILYSIN INHIBITOR+ARB COMBINATION

➤ *sacubitril+valsartan* (D)(G) initially 49/51 bid; double dose after 2-4 weeks; maintenance 97/103 bid; *GFR <30 mL/min or moderate hepatic impairment:* initially 24/26 bid; double dose every 2-4 weeks to target maintenance 97/103 bid
  Pediatric: <12 years: not established; ≥12 years: same as adult
    Entresto
      Tab: **Entresto 24/26:** sacu 24 mg+val 26 mg
        Entresto 49/51: sacu 49 mg+val 51 mg
        Entresto 97/103: sacu 97 mg+val 103 mg

ALDOSTERONE RECEPTOR BLOCKER

➤ *eplerenone* (B) initially 25 mg once daily; titrate within 4 weeks to 50 mg once daily; adjust dose based on serum K^+
  Pediatric: <12 years: not recommended; ≥12 years: same as adult
    Inspra *Tab:* 25, 50 mg
    Comment: **Inspra** is contraindicated with concomitant potent CYP3A4 inhibitors. Risk of hyperkalemia with concomitant ACEI or ARB. Monitor serum potassium at baseline, 1 week, and 1 month. Caution with serum Cr >2 mg/dL (male) or >1.8 mg/dL (female) and/or CrCl <50 mL/min, and DM with proteinuria.

THIAZIDE DIURETICS

Comment: Monitor hydration status, blood pressure, urine output, serum K^+.

➤ *chlorothiazide* (C)(G) 0.5-1 gm/day in single or divided doses; max 2 gm/day
  Pediatric: <6 months: up to 15 mg/lb/day in 2 divided doses; ≥6 months: 10 mg/lb/day in 2 divided doses
    Diuril *Tab:* 250*, 500*mg; *Oral susp:* 250 mg/5 ml (237 ml)
➤ *hydrochlorothiazide* (B)(G)
  Pediatric: <12 years: not recommended; ≥12 years: same as adult
    Esidrix 25-100 mg once daily
      Tab: 25, 50, 100 mg
    Microzide 12.5 mg daily; usual max 50 mg/day
      Cap: 12.5 mg
➤ *methyclothiazide+deserpidine* (B) initially 2.5 mg once daily; max 5 mg once daily
  Pediatric: <12 years: not recommended; ≥12 years: same as adult
    Enduronyl *Tab:* methy 5 mg+deser 0.25 mg*
    Enduronyl Forte *Tab:* methy 5 mg+deser 0.5 mg*
➤ *polythiazide* (C) 2-4 mg once daily
  Pediatric: <12 years: not recommended; ≥12 years: same as adult
    Renese *Tab:* 1, 2, 4 mg

POTASSIUM-SPARING DIURETICS

Comment: Monitor hydration status, blood pressure, urine output, serum K^+.
➤ *amiloride* (B) initially 5 mg once daily; may increase to 10 mg; max 20 mg
  Pediatric: <12 years: not recommended; ≥12 years: same as adult
    Midamor *Tab:* 5 mg
➤ *spironolactone* (D) initially 50-100 mg in a single or divided doses; titrate at 2 week intervals
  Pediatric: <12 years: not established; ≥12 years: same as adult
    Aldactone (G) *Tab:* 25, 50*, 100*mg
    CaroSpir *Oral susp:* 25 mg/5 ml (118, 473 ml) (banana)

LOOP DIURETICS

Comment: Monitor hydration status, blood pressure, urine output, serum K^+.
➤ *bumetanide* (C)(G) 0.5-2 mg as a single dose; may repeat at 4-5 hour intervals; max 10 mg/day
  Pediatric: <18 years: not recommended; ≥18 years: same as adult
    Bumex *Tab:* 0.5*, 1*, 2*mg
  Comment: *bumetanide* is contraindicated with sulfa drug allergy.
➤ *ethacrynic acid* (B)(G) initially 50-200 mg once daily
  Pediatric: infants: not recommended; >1 month: initially 25 mg/day; then adjust dose in 25 mg increments
    Edecrin *Tab:* 25, 50 mg
➤ *ethacrynate sodium* (B)(G) for IV injection
    Sodium Edecrin *Vial:* 50 mg single-dose
    Comment: **Sodium Edecrin** is more potent than more commonly used loop and thiazide diuretics.
➤ *furosemide* (C)(G) initially 40 mg bid
  Pediatric: <12 years: not recommended; ≥12 years: same as adult
    Lasix *Tab:* 20, 40*, 80 mg; *Oral soln:* 10 mg/ml (2, 4 oz w. dropper)
  Comment: *furosemide* is contraindicated with sulfa drug allergy.
➤ *torsemide* (B) 5 mg once daily; may increase to 10 mg daily
  Pediatric: <12 years: not recommended; ≥12 years: same as adult
    Demadex *Tab:* 5*, 10*, 20*, 100*mg

OTHER DIURETICS

Comment: Monitor hydration status, blood pressure, urine output, serum K^+.
➤ *indapamide* (B) initially 1.25 mg once daily; may titrate dosage upward every 4 weeks if needed; max 5 mg/day
    Lozol *Tab:* 1.25, 2.5 mg
  Comment: *indapamide* is contraindicated with sulfa drug allergy.
➤ *metolazone* (B) 2.5-5 mg once daily
  Pediatric: <12 years: not recommended; ≥12 years: same as adult
    Zaroxolyn *Tab:* 2.5, 5, 10 mg
  Comment: *metolazone* is contraindicated with sulfa drug allergy.

DIURETIC COMBINATIONS

Comment: Monitor hydration status, blood pressure, urine output, serum K⁺.

▷ *amiloride+hydrochlorothiazide* (B)(G) initially 1 tab once daily; may increase to 2 tabs/day in a single or divided doses
    Pediatric: <12 years: not recommended; ≥12 years: same as adult
        Moduretic *Tab:* amil 5 mg+hctz 50 mg*

▷ *spironolactone+hydrochlorothiazide* (D)(G)
    Pediatric: <12 years: not recommended; ≥12 years: same as adult
        Aldactazide 25 usual maintenance 50-100 mg in a single or divided doses
            Tab: spiro 25 mg+hctz 25 mg
        Aldactazide 50 usual maintenance 50-100 mg in a single or divided doses
            Tab: spiro 50 mg+hctz 50 mg

▷ *triamterene+hydrochlorothiazide* (C)(G)
    Pediatric: <12 years: not recommended; ≥12 years: same as adult
        Dyazide 1-2 caps daily
            Cap: triam 37.5 mg+hctz 25 mg
        Maxzide 1 tab once daily
            Tab: triam 75 mg+hctz 50 mg*
        Maxzide-25 1-2 tabs once daily
            Tab: triam 37.5 mg+hctz 25 mg*

NITRATE+PERIPHERAL VASODILATOR COMBINATION

▷ *isosorbide dinitrate+hydralazine* (C) initially 1 tab tid; may reduce to 1/2 tab tid if not tolerated; titrate as tolerated after 3-5 days; max 2 tabs tid
    Pediatric: <12 years: not recommended; ≥12 years: same as adult
        BiDil *Tab:* isosor 20 mg+hydral 37.5 mg
        Comment: **BiDil** is an adjunct to standard therapy in self-identified black persons to improve survival, to prolong time to hospitalization for heart failure, and to improve patient-reported functional status.

CARDIAC GLYCOSIDES

Comment: In selecting a digoxin dosing regimen, it is important to consider factors that affect digoxin blood levels (e.g., body weight, age, renal function, concomitant drugs) since digoxin has a very narrow therapeutic index (i.e., toxic levels of digoxin are only slightly higher than therapeutic levels). Therapeutic serum level of digoxin is 0.8-2 mcg/mL. Dosing can be initiated either with a loading dose followed by maintenance dosing if rapid titration is desired or initiated with maintenance dosing without a loading dose. Parenteral administration of digoxin should be used only when the need for rapid digitalization is urgent or when the drug cannot be taken orally. Intramuscular injection can lead to severe pain at the injection site, thus intravenous administration is preferred. If the drug must be administered by the intramuscular route, it should be injected deep into the muscle followed by massage. For adults, no more than 500 mcg of parenteral digoxin (Lanoxin Injection) should be injected into a single site. For pediatric patients, no more than 200 mcg of digoxin (Lanoxin Injection Pediatric) should be injected into a single site.

Administer IV digoxin dose over a period of 5 minutes or longer and avoid bolus administration to prevent systemic and coronary vasoconstriction. Mixing of Lanoxin Injection and Lanoxin Injection Pediatric with other drugs in the same container or simultaneous administration in the same intravenous line is not recommended. Lanoxin Injection and Lanoxin Injection Pediatric can be administered undiluted or diluted with a 4-fold or greater volume of Sterile Water for Injection, 0.9% Sodium Chloride for Injection, or D5W. The use of less than a 4-fold volume of diluent could lead to precipitation of the digoxin. Immediate use of the diluted product is recommended.

Lanoxin (digoxin) is a positive inotrope, negative chronotrope, and negative dromatrope. Therefore, monitor the patient for bradycardia and hypotension.

The classic features of digitalis toxicity are nausea, vomiting, abdominal pain, headache, dizziness, confusion, delirium, visual disturbance (blurred or yellow vision), and symptomatic/unstable bradycardia and/or hypotension.

For more information on the use of digoxin in pediatric heart failure, see Jain, S & Vaidyanathan, B. Digoxin in management of heart failure in children: Should it be continued or relegated to the history books? *Ann Pediatr Cardiol.* Jul-Dec 2009: 2(2):149–152.

▷ *digoxin* (C)(G) Loading Dose: 1-1.5 mg IM, IV, or PO in divided doses over1-3 days; Maintenance: 0.125-0.5 mg/day

Pediatric: Total oral pediatric digitalizing dose (in 24 hours): <2 years: 40-50 mcg/kg; 2-10 years: 30-40 mcg/kg; >10 years: 0.75-1.5 mg; Daily Oral Pediatric Maintenance (single dose once daily): <2 years: 10-12 mcg/kg; 2-10 years: 8-10 mcg/kg; >10 years: 0.125–0.5 mg; Max: 0.125-0.5 mg; <10 years: use elixir or parenteral form

> **Lanoxicap** *Cap:* 0.05, 0.1, 0.2 mg soln-filled (alcohol)
> **Lanoxin** *Tab:* 0.0625, 0.125*, 0.1875, 0.25*mg; Elix: 0.05 mg/ml (2 oz w. dropper) (lime) (alcohol 10%)
> **Lanoxin Injection** *Amp:* 0.25 mg/ml (2 ml)
> **Lanoxin Injection Pediatric** *Amp:* 0.1 mg/ml (1 ml)

HYPERPOLARIZATION-ACTIVATED CYCLIC NUCLEOTIDE-GATED CHANNEL BLOCKER

▷ **ivabradine** (D) initially 5 mg bid with food; assess after 2 weeks and adjust dose to achieve a resting heart rate 50-60 bpm; thereafter, adjust dose as needed based on resting heart rate and tolerability; max 7.5 mg bid; in patients with a history of conduction defects, or for whom bradycardia could lead to hemodynamic compromise, initiate at 2.5 mg bid before increasing the dose based on heart rate

Pediatric: <18 years: not established; ≥18 years: same as adult

> **Corlanor** *Tab:* 5, 7.5 mg
> **Comment:** **Corlanor** is indicated to reduce the risk of hospitalization for worsening heart failure in patients with stable, symptomatic, chronic heart failure with left ventricular ejection fraction (LVEF) ≤35%, who are in sinus rhythm with resting heart rate ≤70 bpm and either are on maximally tolerated doses of beta-blockers or have a contraindication to beta-blocker use. **Corlanor** is contraindicated with acute decompensated heart failure, BP <90/50, sick sinus syndrome (SSS), sinoatrial block, and 3rd degree AV block (unless patient has a functioning demand pacemaker). **Corlanor** may cause fetal toxicity when administered pregnant women based on embryo-fetal toxicity and cardiac teratogenic to effects observed in animal studies. Therefore, females should be advised to use effective contraception when taking this drug.

HELICOBACTER PYLORI (H. PYLORI) INFECTION

ERADICATION REGIMENS

Comment: There are many H2 receptor blocker-based and PPI-based treatment regimens suggested in the professional literature for the eradication of the *H. pylori* organism and subsequent ulcer healing. Generally, regimens range from 10-14 days for eradication and 2-6 more weeks of continued gastric acid suppression. A three- or four-antibiotic combination may increase treatment effectiveness and decrease the likelihood of resistant strain emergence. Empirical treatment is not recommended. Diagnosis should be confirmed before treatment is started. Antibiotic choices include ***doxycycline, tetracycline, amoxicillin, amoxicillin+clavulanate, clarithromycin, clindamycin,*** and ***metronidazole.*** Follow-up visits are recommended at 2 and 6 weeks to evaluate treatment outcomes.

▷ **Regimen 1:** Helidac Therapy (D)(G) ***bismuth subsalicylate*** 525 mg qid + ***tetracycline*** 500 mg qid + ***metronidazole*** 250 mg qid x 14 days

Pediatric: <12 years: not recommended; ≥12 years: same as adult

Pack: **bismuth subsalicylate** *chew tab:* 262.4 mg (112/pck); **tetracycline** *cap:* 500 mg (56/pck); **metronidazole** *Tab:* 250 mg (56/pck)

▷ **Regimen 2:** PrevPac (D)(G) ***amoxicillin*** 500 mg 2 caps bid + ***lansoprazole*** 30 mg bid + ***clarithromycin*** 500 mg bid x 14 days (one card per day)

Pediatric: <12 years: not recommended; ≥12 years: same as adult

Kit: **lansoprazole** *cap:* 30 mg (2/card); **amoxicillin** *cap:* 500 mg (4/card); **clarithromycin** *tab:* 500 mg (2/card) (14 daily cards/carton)

▷ **Regimen 3:** Pylera (D) take 3 caps qid after meals and at bedtime x 10 days; take with 8 oz water plus ***omeprazole*** 20 mg bid, with breakfast and dinner, for 10 days

Pediatric: <12 years: not recommended; ≥12 years: same as adult

Cap: **bismuth subsalicylate** 140 mg+**tetracycline** 125 mg+**metronidazole** 125 mg (120 caps)

Comment: *omeprazole* not included with Pylera.

▷ **Regimen 4:** Omeclamox-Pak (C) ***omeprazole*** 20 mg bid + ***amoxicillin*** 1000 mg bid + ***clarithromycin*** 500 mg bid x 10 days

Kit: **omeprazole** *cap:* 20 mg (2/pck); **amoxicillin** *cap:* 500 mg (4/pck); **clarithromycin** *tab:* 500 mg (2/pck) (10 pcks/carton)

▷ **Regimen 5:** (C) *omeprazole* 40 mg daily + *clarithromycin* 500 mg tid x 2 weeks; then continue *omeprazole* 10-40 mg daily x 6 more weeks

▷ **Regimen 6:** (B) *lansoprazole* 30 mg tid + *amoxicillin* 1 gm tid x 10 days; then continue *lansoprazole* 15-30 mg daily x 6 more weeks

▷ **Regimen 7:** (C) *omeprazole* 40 mg daily + *amoxicillin* 1 gm bid + *clarithromycin* 500 mg bid x 10 days; then continue *omeprazole* 10-40 mg daily x 6 more weeks

▷ **Regimen 8:** (D) *bismuth subsalicylate* 525 mg qid + *metronidazole* 250 mg qid + *tetracycline* 500 mg qid + H$_2$ receptor agonist x 2 weeks; then continue H$_2$ receptor agonist x 6 more weeks

▷ **Regimen 9:** (not for use in 1st; B in 2nd, 3rd) *bismuth subsalicylate* 525 mg qid + *metronidazole* 250 mg qid + *amoxicillin* 500 mg qid + H$_2$ receptor agonist x 2 weeks; then continue H$_2$ receptor agonist x 6 more weeks

▷ **Regimen 10:** (C) *ranitidine bismuth citrate* 400 mg bid + *clarithromycin* 500 mg bid x 2 weeks; then continue *ranitidine bismuth citrate* 400 mg bid x 2 more weeks

▷ **Regimen 11:** (D) *omeprazole* 20 mg or *lansoprazole* 30 mg q AM + *bismuth subsalicylate* 524 mg qid + *metronidazole* 500 mg tid + *tetracycline* 500 mg qid x 2 weeks; then continue *omeprazole* 20 mg or *lansoprazole* 30 mg q AM for 6 more weeks

( ) HEMOLYTIC UREMIC SYNDROME: ATYPICAL (aHUS)

COMPLEMENT INHIBITORS

▷ *eculizumab* (C) dilute to a final admixture concentration of 5 mg/ml using the following steps: (1) withdraw the required amount of **Soliris** from the vial into a sterile syringe; (2) transfer the dose to an infusion bag; (3) add IV fluid equal to the drug volume (0.9% NaCl or 0.45% NaCl or D5W or Ringer's Lactate); the final admixed **Soliris** 5 mg/ml infusion volume is: 300 mg dose (60 ml), 600 mg dose (120 ml), 900 mg dose (180 ml), 1200 mg dose (240 ml); administer a 900 mg IV infusion once weekly for the first 4 weeks; then, 1200 mg IV infusion for the 5th dose 1 week after the 4th dose; then, 1200 mg IV infusion once every 2 weeks thereafter

Pediatric: <18 years: >40 kg: 900 mg IV infusion once weekly x 4 doses; then, 1200 mg at week 5; then, 1200 mg once every 2 weeks thereafter;30-<40 kg: 600 mg IV infusion once weekly x 2 doses; then, 900 mg IV infusion at week 3; then, 900 mg IV infusion once every 2 weeks thereafter; 20-<30 kg: 600 mg IV infusion once weekly x 2 doses; then, 600 mg IV infusion at week 3; then, 600 mg IV infusion once every 2 weeks thereafter; 5-<10 kg: 300 mg IV infusion x 1 dose; then, 300 mg IV infusion at week 2; then, 300 mg IV infusion once every 3 weeks thereafter; <5 kg: not established

   Soliris *Vial:* 300 mg (10 mg/ml, 30 ml), single-use, concentrated solution for intravenous infusion (preservative-free)

   Comment: **Soliris** *(eculizumab)* is a complement inhibitor indicated for the treatment of patients with paroxysmal nocturnal hemoglobinuria (PNH) to reduce hemolysis, patients with atypical hemolytic uremic syndrome (aHUS) to inhibit complement-mediated thrombotic acetylcholine receptor (AchR) antibody positive. **Soliris** should be administered at the above recommended dosage regimen time points or within 2 days of each time point. Supplemental dosing of **Soliris** is required in the setting of concomitant support with plasmapheresis (PI) or plasma exchange (PE) or fresh frozen plasma (FFP) infusion (see mfr pkg insert for supplemental dosing). **Soliris** is not indicated for the treatment of patients with Shiga toxin *E. coli*-related hemolytic uremic syndrome (STEC-HUS). **Soliris** is contraindicated in patients with unresolved *Neisseria meningitides* infection and patients who are not currently vaccinated against *Neisseria meningitides*, unless the risks of delaying **Soliris** treatment outweigh the risks of developing meningococcal infection. Prescribers must enroll in the **Soliris** REMS Program (1-888-SOLIRIS, 1-888-765-4747), counsel patients about the risk of meningococcal infection, provide patients with **Soliris** REMS Educational materials, and ensure that patients are vaccinated with meningococcal vaccine. The most frequently reported adverse reactions in the PNH randomized trial (incidence ≥10%) are headache, nasopharyngitis, back pain, and nausea. There are no adequate and well-controlled human studies of **Soliris** in pregnancy or effects on the breastfed infant. Based on animal studies, **Soliris** may cause fetal harm. It is not known whether **Soliris** is excreted in human milk. IgG is excreted in human milk, so it is expected that **Soliris** will be present in human milk. However, published data suggest that antibodies in human milk do not enter the neonatal and infant circulation in

substantial amounts. Caution should be exercised when **Soliris** is administered to a breast-feeding patient. To report suspected adverse reactions, contact Alexion Pharmaceuticals at 1-888-SOLIRIS
(1-888-765-4747 or FDA at 1-800-FDA-1088 or visit www.fda.gov/medwatch.

HEMOPHILIA A (CONGENITAL FACTOR VIII DEFICIENCY)

BI-SPECIFIC FACTOR IXA- AND FACTOR X-DIRECTED ANTIBODY

▶ *emicizumab-kxwh* initially 3 mg/kg by SC injection once weekly for the first 4 weeks; followed by 1.5 mg/kg once weekly
Pediatric: same as adult

Hemlibra *Vial:* 30 mg/ml (single-dose); 60 mg/0.4 ml (single-dose); 105 mg 0.7 ml (single-dose); 150 mg/ml (single-dose)

Comment: **Hemlibra** is a bi-specific factor IXa- and factor X-directed antibody indicated for routine prophylaxis to prevent or reduce the frequency of bleeding episodes in adult and pediatric patients with hemophilia A (congenital factor VIII deficiency) with factor VIII inhibitors. *Laboratory Coagulation Test Interference:* **Hemlibra** interferes with activated clotting time (ACT), activated partial thromboplastin time (aPTT), and coagulation laboratory tests based on aPTT, including one stage aPTT-based single-factor assays, aPTT-based Activated Protein C Resistance (APC-R), and Bethesda assays (clotting-based) for factor VIII (FVIII) inhibitor titers. Intrinsic pathway clotting-based laboratory tests should not be used. Black Box Warning (BBW): Cases of thrombotic microangiopathy and thrombotic events were reported when on average a cumulative amount of >100 U/kg/24 hours of activated prothrombin complex concentrate (aPCC) was administered for 24 hours or more to patients receiving Hemlibra prophylaxis. Monitor for the development of thrombotic microangiopathy and thrombotic events if aPCC is administered. Discontinue aPCC and suspend dosing of Hemlibra if symptoms occur. Most common adverse reactions (incidence are injection site reactions, headache, and arthralgia. There are no available data on **Hemlibra** use in pregnant women to inform a drug-associated risk of major birth defects and miscarriage. Women of childbearing potential should use contraception while receiving **Hemlibra** and **Hemlibra** should be used during pregnancy only if the potential benefit for the mother outweighs the risk to the fetus. There is no information regarding the presence of *emicizumab-kxwh* in human milk or effects on the breastfed infant. To report suspected adverse reactions, contact Genentech at 1-888-835-2555 or FDA at 1-800-FDA-1088 or www.fda.gov/medwatch.

HEMORRHOIDS

▶ *dibucaine* (C)(OTC)(G) 1 applicatorful or suppository bid and after each stool; max 6/day
Pediatric: <12 years: not recommended; ≥12 years: same as adult
Nupercainal (OTC) *Rectal oint:* 1% (30, 60 gm); *Rectal supp:* 1% (12, 14/pck)
▶ *hydrocortisone* (C)(OTC)(G)
Pediatric: <12 years: not recommended; ≥12 years: same as adult
Anusol-HC 1 suppository rectally bid-tid or 2 suppositories bid x 2 weeks
Rectal supp: 25 mg (12, 24/pck)
Anusol-HC Cream 2.5% apply bid-qid prn
Rectal crm: 2.5% (30 gm)
Anusol HC-1 apply tid-qid prn; max 7 days
Rectal crm: 1% (0.7 oz)
Hydrocortisone Rectal Cream
Rectal crm: 1, 2.5% (30 gm)
Nupercainal apply tid-qid prn
Rectal crm: 1% (30 gm)
Proctocort 1 suppository rectally bid-tid prn or 2 suppositories bid x 2 weeks
Rectal supp: 30 mg (12/pck)
Proctocream HC 2.5% apply rectally bid-qid prn
Rectal crm: 2.5% (30 gm)
Proctofoam HC 1% apply rectally tid-qid prn
Rectal foam: 1% (14 applications/10 gm)

▷ *hydrocortisone+pramoxine* (C) 1 applicatorful tid-qid and after each stool; max 2 weeks
  Pediatric: <12 years: not recommended; ≥12 years: same as adult
    Procort *Rectal crm:* hydrocort 1.85%+pramox 1.15% (30 gm)
▷ *hydrocortisone+lidocaine* (B) apply bid-tid prn
  Pediatric: <12 years: not recommended; ≥12 years: same as adult
    AnaMantle HC, LidaMantle HC *Crm/Lotn:* hydrocort 5%+lido 3% (1 oz)
▷ *petrolatum+mineral oil+shark liver oil+phenylephrine* (C)(OTC)(G)
    Preparation H Ointment apply up to qid prn
      Rectal oint: 1, 2 oz
▷ *petrolatum+glycerin+shark liver oil+phenylephrine* (C)(OTC)(G)
    Preparation H Cream apply up to qid prn
      Rectal crm: 0.9, 1.8 oz
▷ *phenylephrine+cocoa butter+shark liver oil* (C)(OTC)(G)
    Preparation H Suppositories 1 suppository or 1 application of rectal ointment or
    cream, up to qid
      Rectal supp: phenyle 0.25%+cocoa 85.5%+shark 3% (12, 24, 45/pck); *Rectal oint:*
      phenyle 0.25%+petro 1.9%+mineral oil 14%+shark liv 3% (1, 2 oz); *Rectal crm:*
      phenyle 0.25%+petro 18%+gly 12%+shark liv 3% (0.9, 1.8 oz)
▷ *witch hazel* topical soln/gel (OTC)
    Tucks apply up to 6 x/day; leave on x 5-15 minutes
      Pad: 12, 40, 100/pck; *Gel:* 19.8 g

TOPICAL AND TRANSDERMAL ANALGESICS

▷ *capsaicin* 8% patch (B) apply up to 4 patches for one 60-minute application to clean dry
  skin; may prep area with topical anesthetic; wear non-latex gloves; patches may be cut to
  size/shape; treatment may be repeated every 3 months
  Pediatric: <18 years: not recommended; ≥18 years: same as adult
    Qutenza *Patch:* 8% 1640 mcg/cm (179 mg) (1 or 2 patches w. 1-50 gm tube cleansing
    gel/carton)
▷ *diclofenac sodium* (C; D ≥30 wks)(G) apply qid prn to intact skin
  Pediatric: <12 years: not established; ≥12 years: same as adult
    Pennsaid 1.5% in 10 drop increments, dispense and rub into front, side, and back of
    knee: usually; 40 drops (40 mg) qid
      Topical soln: 1.5% (150 ml)
    Pennsaid 2% apply 2 pump actuations (40 mg) and rub into front, side, and back of
    knee bid
      Topical soln: 2% (20 mg/pump actuation, 112 gm)
    Solaraze Gel massage in to clean skin bid prn
      Gel: 3% (50 gm) (benzyl alcohol)
    Voltaren Gel (G) apply qid prn to intact skin
      Gel: 1% (100 gm)
  Comment: *diclofenac* is contraindicated with *aspirin* allergy. As with other NSAIDs, should
  be avoided in late pregnancy (≥30 weeks) because it may cause premature closure of the
  ductus arteriosus.
▷ *doxepin* (B) cream apply to affected area qid at intervals of at least 3-4 hours; max 8 days
  Pediatric: <12 years: not recommended; >12 years: same as adult
    Prudoxin *Crm:* 5% (45 gm)
    Zonalon *Crm:* 5% (30, 45 gm)
▷ *pimecrolimus* 1% cream (C)(G) <2 years: not recommended; ≥2 years: apply to affected area
  bid; do not apply an occlusive dressing
    Elidel *Crm:* 1% (30, 60, 100 gm)
  Comment: *pimecrolimus* is indicated for short-term and intermittent long-term use.
  Discontinue use when resolution occurs. Contraindicated if the patient is immunosuppressed. Change to the 0.1% preparation or if secondary bacterial infection is present.
▷ *trolamine salicylate* apply tid-qid
  Pediatric: <2 years: not recommended; ≥2 years: same as adult
    Mobisyl Creme *Crm:* 10% (100 gm)

TOPICAL AND TRANSDERMAL ANESTHETICS

Comment: *lidocaine* should not be applied to non-intact skin.

▷ *lidocaine* cream **(B)** apply to affected area bid prn
  Pediatric: <12 years: not recommended; ≥12 years: same as adult
      LidaMantle *Crm:* 3% (1, 2 oz)
      Lidoderm *Crm:* 3% (85 gm)
      ZTlido *lidocaine* topical system 1% (30/carton)
  Comment: Compared to **Lidoderm** (*lidocaine* patch 5%) which contains 700 mg/patch,
  ZTlido only requires 35 mg per topical system to achieve the same therapeutic dose.
▷ *lidocaine* lotion **(B)** apply to affected area bid prn
  Pediatric: <12 years: not recommended; ≥12 years: same as adult
      LidaMantle *Lotn:* 3% (177 ml)
▷ *lidocaine* 5% patch **(B)(G)** apply up to 3 patches at one time for up to 12 hours/24-hour
  period (12 hours on/12 hours off); patches may be cut into smaller sizes before removal of
  the release liner; do not re-use
  Pediatric: <12 years: not recommended; ≥12 years: same as adult
      Lidoderm *Patch:* 5% (10x14 cm; 30/carton)
▷ *lidocaine+dexamethasone* **(B)**
  Pediatric: <12 years: not recommended; ≥12 years: same as adult
      Decadron Phosphate with Xylocaine *Lotn:* dexa 4 mg+lido 10 mg per ml (5 ml)
▷ *lidocaine+hydrocortisone* **(B)(G)** apply to affected area bid prn
  Pediatric: <12 years: not recommended; ≥12 years: same as adult
      LidaMantle HC *Crm:* lido 3%+hydro 0.5% (1, 3 oz); *Lotn:* (177 ml)
▷ *lidocaine 2.5%+prilocaine 2.5%* apply sparingly to the burn bid-tid prn
  Pediatric: <12 years: not recommended; ≥12 years: same as adult
      Emla Cream (B) 5, 30 gm/tube

Bulk-Forming Agents, Stool Softeners, and Stimulant Laxatives *see **Constipation** page* 106

HEPATITIS A (HAV)

Comment: Administer a 2-dose series. Schedule first immunization at least 2 weeks before
expected exposure. Booster dose recommended 6-12 months later. Under 1 year-of-age
administer in the vastus lateralis; over 1 year-of-age administer in the deltoid.

PROPHYLAXIS (HEPATITIS A)

▷ *hepatitis A vaccine, inactivated* **(C)**
  Pediatric: <12 years: not approved; ≥12 years: same as adult
      Havrix 1,440 El.U IM; repeat in 6-12 months
      Pediatric: <2 years: not recommended; 2-18 years: 720 El.U IM; repeat in 6-12 months
      or 360 El.U IM; repeat in 1 month
      Vaqta 25 U (1 ml) IM; repeat in 6 months
      Pediatric: <2 years: not recommended; 2-18 years: 0.5 ml IM; repeat in 6-18 months
          Vial: 25 U/ml single-dose (preservative-free); *Prefilled syringe:* 25 U/ml, (0.5, 1 ml,
          single-dose)

PROPHYLAXIS VACCINE (HAV+HBV COMBINATION)

▷ *hepatitis A inactivated+hepatitis b surface antigen (recombinant vaccine)* **(C)**
  Pediatric: <18 years: not approved; ≥18 years: same as adult
      Twinrix 1 ml IM in deltoid; repeat in 1 month and 6 months
          Vial (soln): hepatitis a inactivated 720 IU+*hepatitis b* surface antigen (recombinant)
          20 mcg/ml (1, 10 ml); *Prefilled syringe: hepatitis a* inactivated 720 IU+*hepatitis b*
          surface antigen (recombinant) 20 mcg/ml

PRE- AND POST-EXPOSURE PROPHYLAXIS
Immune Globulin (Human)

▷ *immune globulin* **(human)** administer via intramuscular injection only (never intravenously); ensure adequate hydration prior to administration Household and Institutional
  HAV Case Contacts: 0.1 ml/kg IM as a single dose Planned Travel to HAV Endemic Area:
  administer as a single dose at least 2 weeks prior to travel
  Pediatric: 0.25 ml/kg IM (0.5 mg/kg in immunocompromised children)

Length of Stay	Prior Dose	Dose
Up to 1 month	--------	0.1 ml/kg
Up to 2 months	--------	0.2 ml/kg
More than 2 months	--------	repeat dose of 0.2 ml/kg every 2 months
Less than 3 months	0.02 mL/kg	--------
3 months or longer	0.06 mL/kg	repeat every 4-6 months

GamaSTAN S/D *Vial:* 2, 10 ml single-dose

Comment: **GamaSTAN S/D** is the only gammaglobulin product FDA-approved for measles and HAV post-exposure prophylaxis (PEP). **GamaSTAN S/D** is also FDA-approved for varicella post-exposure prophylaxis (PEP). Other **GamaSTAN S/D** indications: to prevent or modify measles in a susceptible person exposed fewer than 6 days previously; to modify varicella; to modify rubella in exposed women who will not consider a therapeutic abortion. **GamaSTAN S/D** is not indicated for routine prophylaxis or treatment of viral hepatitis B, rubella, poliomyelitis, mumps or varicella. Contraindications to **GamaSTAN S/D** include persons with cancer, chronic liver disease, and persons allergic to gammaglobulin, the HAV vaccine, or a component of the HAV vaccine. Dosage is higher for HAV PEP than for measles and varicella PEP based on recently observed decreasing concentrations of HAV antibodies in **GamaSTAN S/D**, attributed to the decreasing prevalence of previous HAV infection among plasma donors. Defer live vaccines for at least 6 months.

HEPATITIS B (HBV)

PROPHYLAXIS VACCINE (HBV)

Comment: Administer IM; under 1 year-of-age, administer in vastus lateralis. Over 1 year-of-age, administer in the deltoid. Administer a 3-dose series; *First dose:* newborn (or now); *Second dose:* 1-2 months after first dose; *Third dose:* 6 months after first dose.

 hepatitis B recombinant vaccine (C)

Engerix-B Adult 20 mcg (1 ml) IM; repeat in 1 and 6 months
Pediatric: infant-19 years: 10 mcg (1/2 ml) IM; repeat in 1 and 6 months
   Vial: 20 mcg/ml single-dose (preservative-free, thimerosal); *Prefilled syringe:* 20 mcg/ml

Engerix-B Pediatric/Adolescent
Pediatric: infant-19 years: 10 mcg IM; repeat in 1 and 6 months; *Vial:* 10 mcg/0.5 ml single-dose (preservative-free, thimerosal)
   Prefilled syringe: 10 mcg/0.5 ml

Recombivax HB Adult 10 mcg (1 ml) IM in deltoid; repeat in 1 and 6 months
   Vial: 10 mcg/ml single-dose; *Vial:* 10 mcg/3 ml multi-dose

Recombivax HB Pediatric/Adolescent 5 mcg (0.5 ml) IM; repeat in 1 and 6 months
Pediatric: birth-19 years: 5 mcg (0.5 ml) IM; repeat in 1 and 6 months; >19 years: use adult formulation or 10 mcg (1 ml) pediatric/adolescent formulation
   Vial: 5 mcg/0.5 ml single-dose

PROPHYLAXIS VACCINE (HAV+HBV COMBINATION)

Comment: Administer IM; under 1 year-of-age, administer in vastus lateralis. Over 1 year-of-age, administer in the deltoid. Administer a 3-dose series; *First dose:* newborn (or now); *Second dose:* 1-2 months after first dose; *Third dose:* 6 months after first dose.

▷ *hepatitis A inactivated+hepatitis b surface antigen (recombinant) vaccine* (C)
Pediatric: <18 years: not approved; ≥18 years: same as adult
   Twinrix 1 ml IM in deltoid; repeat in 1 months and 6 months
      Vial (soln): hepatitis A inactivated 720 IU+*hepatitis b* surface antigen (recombinant) 20 mcg/ml (1, 10 ml); *Prefilled syringe:* hepatitis A inactivated 720 IU+*hepatitis b* surface antigen (recombinant) 20 mcg/ml

CHRONIC HBV INFECTION TREATMENT

Nucleoside Analogs (Reverse Transcriptase Inhibitors and HBV Polymerase Inhibitors)

Comment: Nucleoside analogs are indicated for chronic hepatitis infection with viral replication and either elevated ALT/AST or histologically active disease.

▷ *adefovir dipivoxil* (C)(G) 10 mg daily; *CrCl 20-49 mL/min:* 10 mg q 48 hours; *CrCl 10-19 mL/min:* 10 mg q 72 hours
  Pediatric: <12 years: not recommended; ≥12 years: same as adult
  Hepsera *Tab:* 10 mg

▷ *entecavir* (C)(G) take on an empty stomach;
  Nucleoside naïve: 0.5 mg daily; *Nucleoside naïve, CrCl 30-49 mL/min:* 0.25 mg daily;
  Nucleoside naïve, CrCl 10-29 mL/min: 0.15 mg daily; *Nucleoside naïve, CrCl <10 mL/min:*
  0.05 mg daily; *lamivudine-refractory:* 1 mg daily; *lamivudine-refractory, renal impairment:*
  see mfr pkg insert
  Pediatric: <18 years: not recommended; ≥18 years: same as adult
  Baraclude *Tab:* 0.5, 1 mg; *Oral Soln:* 0.05 mg/ml (orange; parabens)

▷ *lamivudine* (C)(G) 100 mg daily; *CrCl <5 mL/min:* 35 mg for 1st dose, then 10 mg once
  daily; *CrCl 5-14 mL/min:* 35 mg for 1st dose, then 15 mg once daily; *CrCl 15-29 mL/min:*
  100 mg for 1st dose, then 25 mg once daily; *CrCl 30-49 mL/min:* 100 mg for 1st dose, then
  50 mg once daily
  Pediatric: <2 years: not recommended; 2-17 years: 3 mg/kg (max 100 mg) once daily
  Epivir-HBV *Tab:* 100 mg
  Epivir-HBV Oral Solution *Oral Soln:* 5 mg/ml (240 ml) (strawberry-banana)

▷ *telbivudine* (C) 600 mg daily; *CrCl <40 mL/min:* 600 mg q 72 hours; *CrCl 30-49 mL/min:*
  600 mg q 48 hours
  Pediatric: <16 years: not recommended; ≥16 years: same as adult
  Tyzeka *Tab:* 600 mg

▷ *tenofovir alafenamide (TAF)* (C) take with food; take 1 tab once daily with concomitant
  carbamazepine 2 tablets
  Pediatric: <18 years: not established; ≥18 years: same as adult
  Vemlidy *Tab:* 25 mg
  Comment: No dosage adjustment of **Vemlidy** is required in patients with mild hepatic
  impairment (Child-Pugh Class A). The safety and efficacy of **Vemlidy** in patients
  with decompensated cirrhosis (Child-Pugh Class B or C) have not been established;
  therefore **Vemlidy** is not recommended in patients with decompensated (Child-Pugh
  Class B or C) hepatic impairment, Healthcare providers are encouraged to register
  patients by calling the Antiretroviral Pregnancy Registry (APR) at 1-800-258-4263.

Interferon Alpha

▷ *interferon alfa-2b* (C) 5 million IU SC or IM daily or 10 million IU SC or IM 3 x/week x 16
  weeks; reduce dose by half or interrupt dose if WBCs, granulocyte count, or platelet count
  decreases
  Pediatric: <1 year: not recommended; ≥1 year: 3 million IU/m², 3 x/week x 1 week; then
  increase to 6 million IU/m², 3 x/week to 16-24 weeks; max 10 million IU/dose; reduce dose
  by half or interrupt dose if WBCs, granulocyte count, or platelet count decreases
  Intron A *Vial (pwdr):* 5, 10, 18, 25, 50 million IU/vial (pwdr+diluent; single-dose) (benzoyl alcohol); *Vial (soln):* 3, 5, 10 million IU/vial (single-dose); *Multi-dose vials (soln):* 18,
  25 million IU/vial soln; *Multi-dose pens (soln):* 3, 5, 10 million IU/0.2 ml (6 doses/pen)

Integrase Strand Transfer Inhibitor (INSTI)

▷ *tenofovir disoproxil fumarate* (C)(G) 300 mg once daily; *CrCl 30-49 mL/min:* 300 mg q 48
  hours; *CrCl 10-29:* 300 mg q 72-96 hours; *Hemodialysis:* 300 mg once every 7 days or after a
  total of 12 hours of dialysis; *CrCl <10 mL/min:* not recommended
  Pediatric: <12 years: not recommended; ≥12 years, 35 kg: 300 mg once daily; mix oral pwdr
  with 2-4 oz soft food
  Viread *Tab:* 150, 200, 250, 300 mg; *Oral pwdr:* 40 mg/gm (60 gm w. dosing scoop)

 HEPATITIS C (HCV)

CHRONIC HCV INFECTION TREATMENT

Nucleoside Analogs (Reverse Transcriptase Inhibitors)

Comment: Nucleoside analogs are indicated for patients with compensated liver disease
previously untreated with *alpha interferon* or who have relapsed after *alpha interferon*
therapy. Primary toxicity is hemolytic anemia. Contraindicated in male partners of pregnant
women; use 2 forms of contraception during therapy and for 6 months after discontinuation.

▷ **ribavirin** (X)(G) take with food in 2 divided doses; *Genotype 2, 3:* 800 mg/day x 24 weeks; *Genotype 1, 4, <75 kg:* 1 gm/day x 48 weeks; *≥75 km* 1.2 gm/day x 48 weeks; *HIV co-infection:* 800 mg/day x 48 weeks; *CrCl 30-50 mL/min:* alternate 200 mg and 400 mg every other day; *CrCl <30 mL/min or hemodialysis:* reduce dose or discontinue if hematologic abnormalities occur
Pediatric: <5 years: not established; ≥5-<18 years: 23-33 kg: 400 mg/day; 34-46 kg: 600 mg/day; 47-59 kg: 800 mg/day; 60-75 kg: 1 gm/day; 1.2 gm/day; ≥75 kg: *Genotype 2, 3:* treat for 24 weeks; *Genotype 1, 4:* treat for 48 weeks; reduce dose or discontinue if hematologic abnormalities occur; ≥18 years: same as adult
    Copegus *Tab:* 200 mg
    Rebetol *Cap:* 200 mg
    Rebetol Oral Solution *Oral soln:* 40 mg/ml (120 ml) (bubble gum)
    Ribasphere RibaPak 600 mg *Tab:* 600 mg (14/pck)
    Virazole *Vial:* 6 gm for inhalation

Interferon Alpha

▷ **interferon alfacon-1** (C)
Pediatric: <18 years: not recommended; ≥18 years: same as adult
    Infergen 9 mcg SC 3 x/week x 24 weeks, then 15 mcg SC 3 x/week x 6 months; allow at least 48 hours between doses
        Vial (soln): 9, 15 mcg/vial soln (6 single-dose/pck) (preservative-free)
▷ **interferon alfa-2b** (C)
    Intron A *Vial (pwdr):* 5, 10, 18, 25, 50 million IU/vial (pwdr w. diluent; single-dose) (benzoyl alcohol); *Vial (soln):* 3, 5, 10 million IU/vial (single-dose); *Multi-dose vials (soln):* 18, 25 million IU/vial; *Multi-dose pens (soln):* 3, 5, 10 million IU/0.2 ml (6 doses/pen)
▷ **peginterferon alfa-2a** (C) administer 180 mcg SC once weekly (on the same day of the week); treat for 48 weeks; consider discontinuing if adequate response after 12-24 weeks
Pediatric: <18 years: not recommended; ≥18 years: same as adult
    PEGasys *Vial:* 180 mcg/ml (single-dose); *Monthly pck (vials):* 180 mcg/ml (1 ml, 4/pck)
▷ **peginterferon alfa-2b** (C) administer SC once weekly (on the same day of the week); treat for 1 year; consider discontinuing if inadequate response after 24 weeks; 37-45 kg: 40 mcg (100 mg/ml, 0.4 ml); 46-56 kg: 50 mcg (100 mg/ml, 0.5 ml); 57-72 kg: 64 mcg (160 mg/ml, 0.4 ml); 73-88 kg: 80 mcg (160 mg/ml, 0.5 ml); 89-106 kg: 96 mcg (240 mg/ml, 0.4 ml); 107-136 kg: 120 mcg (240 mg/ml, 0.5 ml); 137-160 kg: 150 mcg (300 mg/ml, 0.5 ml)
Pediatric: <18 years: not recommended; ≥18 years: same as adult
    PEG-Intron *Vial:* 50, 80, 120, 150 mcg/ml (single-dose)
    PEG-Intron Redipen *Pen:* 50, 80, 120, 150 mcg/ml (disposable pens)

HCV NS5A Inhibitor

▷ **daclatasvir** (X) 60 mg once daily for 12 weeks (with *sofosbuvir*); if *sofosbuvir* is discontinued, daclatasvir should also be discontinued; with concomitant CY3P inhibitors, reduce dose to 30 mg once daily; with concomitant CY3P inducers, increase dose to 90 mg once daily
    Daklinza *Tab:* 30, 60 mg
    Comment: **Daklinza** is indicated in combination with *sofosbuvir* with or without *ribavirin*, for the treatment of HCV genotypes 1 and 3, and in patients with co-morbid HIV-1 infection, advanced cirrhosis, or post-liver transplant recurrence of HCV.

HCV NS5A Inhibitor+HCV NS3+4A Protease Inhibitor Combinations

▷ **elbasvir+grazoprevir** 1 tab as a single dose once daily; see mfr pkg insert for length of treatment
Pediatric: <18 years: not recommended; ≥18 years: same as adult
    Zepatier *Tab:* elba 50 mg+grazo 100 mg
    Comment: **Zepatier** is contraindicated with moderate or severe hepatic impairment, concomitant *atazanavir, carbamazepine, cyclosporine, darunavir, efavirenz, lopinavir, phenytoin, rifampin, saquinavir,* St. John's wort, *tipranavir.* When co-administered with *ribavirin,* pregnancy category (X)
▷ **glecaprevir+pibrentasvir** take 3 tablets (total daily dose: *glecaprevir* 300 mg and *pibrentasvir* 120 mg) once daily with food
Pediatric: <18 years: not recommended; ≥18 years: same as adult
    Mavyret *Tab:* gleca 100 mg+pibre 40 mg

Comment: **Mavyret** is a drug for the treatment of adults who have chronic Hepatitis C virus genotypes 1, 2, 3, 4, 5 or 6 infection and who do not have cirrhosis or who have early stage cirrhosis. **Mavyret** may cause serious liver problems including liver failure and death in patients who had hepatitis B virus infection. This is because the hepatitis B virus could become active again (i.e., reactivated) during or after treatment with **Mavyret**. Test all patients for HBV infection by measuring HBsAg and anti-HBc prior to initiating therapy with **Mavyret**. The most common side effects of **Mavyret** are headache and tiredness. See mfr insert for table of recommended duration of treatment based on patient characteristics. No adequate human data are available to establish whether or not **Mavyret** poses a risk to pregnancy outcomes. It is not known whether the components of **Mavyret** are excreted in human breast milk or have effects on the breastfed infant.

HCV NS5A Inhibitor+HCV NS3/4A Protease Inhibitor+ CYP3A Inhibitor Combinations

▷ *ombitasvir+paritaprevir+ritonavir* (B) take 2 tabs once daily in the AM x 12 weeks
   Pediatric: <18 years: not established; ≥18 years: same as adult
   Technivie *Tab:* omvi 25 mg+pari 75 mg+rito 50 mg (4 x 7 daily dose pcks/carton)
   Comment: **Technivie** is indicated for use in chronic HCV genotype 4 without cirrhosis. **Technivie** is not for use with moderate hepatic impairment.

HCV NS3/4A Protease Inhibitor

▷ *simeprevir* (C) 150 mg once daily; swallow whole; take with food, not for monotherapy; do not reduce dose or interrupt therapy; if discontinued, do not reinitiate; discontinue if HCV-RNA levels indicate futility; discontinue if *peginterferon, ribavirin,* or *sofosbuvir* is permanently discontinued; *Treatment naïve, treatment relapses, with* or *without cirrhosis:* treat x 12 weeks (*simeprevir + peginterferon + ribavirin*) followed by additional 12 weeks *peginterferon + ribavirin* (total = 24 weeks). *Partial and non-responders, with* or *without cirrhosis:* treat x 12 weeks (*simeprevir + peginterferon + ribavirin*) followed by additional 36 weeks *peginterferon + ribavirin* (total = 48 weeks); *Treatment naïve* or *treatment experienced without cirrhosis:* treat x 12 weeks (*simeprevir + sofosbuvir*); *Treatment naïve* or *treatment experienced with cirrhosis:* treat x 24 weeks (*simeprevir + sofosbuvir*)
   Olysio *Cap:* 150 mg

HCV NS5A Inhibitor+HCV NS5B Polymerase Inhibitor Combinations

▷ *ledipasvir+sofosbuvir Treatment naïve, without cirrhosis, with pretreatment HCV RNA <6 million IU/ml:* 1 tab daily x 8 weeks; *Treatment naïve with* or *without cirrhosis* or *treatment-experienced without cirrhosis:* 1 tab daily x 12 weeks; *Treatment-experienced with cirrhosis:* 1 tab daily x 24 weeks; *In combination with ribavirin:* 1 tab daily x 12 weeks
   Pediatric: <18 years: not established; ≥18 years: same as adult
   Harvoni *Tab:* ledi 90 mg+sofo 400 mg
   Comment: **Harvoni** is indicated for patients with advanced liver disease, genotype 1, 4, 5, or 6 infection: chronic HCV genotype 1- or 4-infected liver transplant recipients with or without cirrhosis or with compensated cirrhosis (Child-Pugh Class A), and for HCV genotype 1-infected patients with decompensated cirrhosis (Child-Pugh Class B or C), including those who have undergone liver transplantation. No adequate human data are available to establish whether or not **Harvoni** poses a risk to pregnancy outcomes; the background risk of major birth defects and miscarriage for the indicated population is unknown. If **Harvoni** is administered with *ribavirin*, the combination regimen is contraindicated (X) in pregnant women and in men whose female partners are pregnant. It is not known whether **Harvoni** and its metabolites are present in human breast milk, affect human milk production or have effects on the breastfed infant. If **Harvoni** is administered with *ribavirin*, the nursing mother's information for *ribavirin* also applies to this combination regimen.
▷ *sofosbuvir+velpatasvir Without cirrhosis* or *compensated cirrhosis (Child-Pug A):* 1 tablet daily x 12 weeks; *Decompensated cirrhosis (Child Pugh Class B* or *C):* 1 tablet daily plus *ribavirin* (RBV)
   Pediatric: <18 years: not established; ≥18 years: same as adult
   Epclusa *Tab:* sofo 400 mg+velpa 100 mg
   Comment: **Epclusa** is indicated for patients with chronic HCV with genotype 1, 2, 3, 4, 5, or 6 infection.

HCV NS5A Inhibitor+HCV NS3/4A Protease Inhibitor+CYP3A Inhibitor Combination

▷ *sofosbuvir+velpatasvir* (B) 1 tab daily

Pediatric: <12 years: not established; ≥12 years: same as adult

Viekira XR *Tab:* dasa 200 mg+omvi 8.33 mg+pari 50 mg+rito 33.33 mg ext-rel (4 weekly cartons, each containing 7 daily dose pcks/carton)

Comment: **Viekira XR** is indicated for HCV genotype 1 with mild liver dysfunction (Child-Pugh Class A). **Viekira XR** is contraindicated for moderate (Child-Pugh Class B) to severe (Child-Pugh Class C) liver dysfunction. No adjustment is recommended with mild, moderate, or severe renal dysfunction.

HCV NS5A Inhibitor+HCV NS3/4A Protease Inhibitor+CYP3A Inhibitor PLUS HCV NS5B Polymerase Inhibitor Combination

▷ *ombitasvir+paritaprevir+ritonavir* plus *dasabuvir* (B)

Pediatric: <12 years: not established; ≥12 years: same as adult

Viekira Pak *ombitasvir+paritaprevir+ritonavir* fixed-dose combination tablet: 2 tablets orally once a day (in the morning); *dasabuvir:* 250 mg orally twice a day (morning and evening)

Tab: omvi 12.5 mg+pari 75 mg+rito 50 mg plus *Tab:* dasa 250 mg (28 day supply/pck)

Comment: **Viekira Pak** is indicated for mild liver dysfunction (Child-Pugh Class A). **Viekira Pak** is contraindicated for moderate (Child-Pugh Class B) to severe (Child-Pugh Class C) liver dysfunction. No adjustment is recommended with mild, moderate, or severe renal dysfunction.

HCV NS5B Polymerase Inhibitor+HCV NS5A Inhibitor+HCV NS3/4A Protease Inhibitor Combination

▷ *sofosbuvir+velpatasvir+voxilaprevir* 1 tablet once daily with food x 12 weeks; pre-test for HBV infection by measuring HBsAg and anti-HBc prior to the initiation of therapy

Pediatric: <12 years: not established; ≥12 years: same as adult

Vosevi *Tab:* sofo 400 mg+velpa 100 mg+voxil 100 mg fixed-dose combination

Comment: **Vosevi** is not recommended in patients with moderate or severe hepatic impairment (Child-Pugh Class B or C). A dosage recommendation cannot be made for patients with severe renal impairment or end stage renal disease. **Vosevi** is contraindicated while taking any medicines containing *rifampin* (**Rifater, Rifamate, Rimactane, Rifadin**). **Vosevi** is indicated for the treatment of adult patients with chronic HCV infection without cirrhosis or with compensated cirrhosis (Child-Pugh Class A) who have: (1) genotype 1, 2, 3, 4, 5, or 6 infection and have previously been treated with an HCV regimen containing an NS5A inhibitor or (2) genotype 1a or 3 infection and have previously been treated with an HCV regimen containing *sofosbuvir* without an NS5A inhibitor. Duration of treatment is 12 weeks. Additional benefit of **Vosevi** over *sofosbuvir+velpatasvir* has not been demonstrated with genotype 1b, 2, 4, 5, or 6 infection previously treated with *sofosbuvir* without an NS5A inhibitor. Because there is risk of Hepatitis B virus reactivation, test all patients for evidence of current or prior HBV infection before initiation of HCV treatment. Monitor HCV/HBV co-infected patients for HBV reactivation and hepatitis flare during HCV treatment and post-treatment follow-up. Initiate appropriate patient management for HBV infection as clinically indicated. The most common adverse reactions are headache, fatigue, diarrhea, and nausea. To report a suspected adverse reaction, contact Gilead Sciences at 1-800-GILEAD-5 or FDA at 1-800-FDA-1088 or www.fda.gov/medwatch.

DUAL TREATMENT REGIMEN

Harvoni+Sovaldi

Comment: Patients who are co-infected with hepatitis B are at risk for HBV reactivation during or after treatment with HCV direct-acting retrovirals. Therefore, patients should be screened for current or past HBV infection before starting this treatment protocol.

TRIPLE TREATMENT REGIMEN

Sovaldi+Harvoni+Ribavirin

Comment: For this FDA-approved triple therapy regimen, follow the recommended regimen for each individual drug. Patients who are co-infected with hepatitis B are at risk for HBV reactivation during or after treatment with HCV direct-acting retrovirals. Therefore, patients should be screened for current or past HBV infection before starting this triple therapy regimen.

 **HEREDITARY ANGIOEDEMA (HAE)/
C1 ESTERASE INHIBITOR DEFICIENCY**

Comment: Agents administered for the treatment of hereditary angioedema carry a risk of hypersensitivity reactions, which are similar to HAE attacks, and the patient should be monitored closely for signs and symptoms accordingly (e.g., hives, urticaria, tightness of the chest, wheezing, hypotension and/or anaphylaxis).

HAE PROPHYLAXIS
Synthetic Steroid

▶ *danazol* (X) *Females:* start on 3rd or 4th day of menstrual period or after a negative pregnancy test; *Males/Females:* dosage requirements for continuous treatment of hereditary angioedema should be adjusted based on individual clinical response; initially 200 mg bid-tid; after a favorable initial response is achieved (prevention of episodes of edematous attacks), continuing dosage should be determined by decreasing the dosage by 50% or less at intervals of 1 to 3 months or longer if frequency of attacks prior to treatment dictates; if an attack occurs, daily dosage may be increased by up to 200 mg. During the dose adjusting phase, close monitoring of the patient's response is indicated, particularly if the patient has a history of airway involvement.
Pediatric: <18 years: not recommended; ≥18 years: same as adult
  Danocrine *Cap:* 50, 100, 200 mg
Comment: *danazol* is a synthetic steroid derived from ethisterone. It suppresses the pituitary-ovarian axis. This suppression is probably a combination of depressed hypothalamic-pituitary response to lowered *estrogen* production, the alteration of sex steroid metabolism, and interaction of *danazol* with sex hormone receptors. The only other demonstrable hormonal effects are weak androgenic activity and depression of both follicle-stimulating hormone (FSH) and luteinizing hormone (LH) output. Recent evidence suggests a direct inhibitory effect at gonadal sites and a binding of **Danocrine** to receptors of gonadal steroids at target organs. In addition, **Danocrine** has been shown to significantly decrease IgG, IgM and IgA levels, as well as phospholipid and IgG isotope autoantibodies in patients with endometriosis and associated elevations of autoantibodies, suggesting this could be another mechanism by which it facilitates regression of fibrocystic breast disease. Changes in the menstrual pattern may occur. Generally, the pituitary-suppressive action of **Danocrine** is reversible. Ovulation and cyclic bleeding usually return within 60 to 90 days when therapy with **Danocrine** is discontinued. In the treatment of hereditary angioedema, **Danocrine** at effective doses prevents attacks of the disease characterized by episodic edema of the abdominal viscera, extremities, face, and airway which may be disabling and, if the airway is involved, fatal. In addition, **Danocrine** corrects partially or completely the primary biochemical abnormality of hereditary angioedema by increasing the levels of the deficient C1 esterase inhibitor (C1EI). As a result of this action the serum levels of the C4 component of the complement system are also increased. **Danocrine** is also used to treat endometriosis (to relieve associated abdominal pain) and fibrocystic breast disease (to reduce breast tissue nodularity and breast pain/tenderness). Contraindications include pregnancy, breastfeeding, active or history of thromboembolic disease/event, porphyria, undiagnosed abnormal genital bleeding, androgen-dependent tumor, and markedly impaired hepatic, renal, or cardiac function.

C1 Esterase Inhibitor [Human]

▶ *C1 esterase inhibitor (human)* administer 60 International Units per kg body weight SC in the abdomen twice weekly (every 3 or 4 days); administer at room temperature within 8 hours after reconstitution; use a silicone-free syringe for reconstitution and administration; use either the Mix2Vial transfer set provided with **Haegarda** or a commercially available 566 double-ended needle and vented filter spike
Pediatric: <12 years: not recommended; ≥12 years: same as adult
  Haegarda *Vial:* 2000, 3000 IU C1 INH pwdr for reconstitution, single-use
Comment: **Haegarda** is a plasma-derived concentrate of C1 esterase inhibitor [human], a serine proteinase inhibitor. Indicated for routine prophylaxis to prevent

HAE attacks in adults and adolescents. It is not indicated for treating acute attacks of HAE. **Haegarda** is the first C1 esterase inhibitor (human) SC injection approved for self-administration by the patient or caregiver after healthcare provider instruction. An international consensus panel states that human plasma-derived C1 esterase inhibitor is considered to be the therapy of choice for both treatment and prophylaxis of maternal hereditary angioedema during lactation. There are no prospective clinical data from **Haegarda** use in pregnant women. C1-INH is a normal component of human plasma. There is no information regarding the excretion of **Haegarda** in human milk or effect the breastfed infant. The developmental and health benefits of breastfeeding should be considered along with the mother's clinical need for **Haegarda** and any potential adverse effects on the breastfed infant from **Haegarda** or from the underlying maternal condition.

Plasma Kallikrein Inhibitor (Monoclonal Antibody)

▶ *lanadelumab-flyo* initially administer 300 mg SC every 2 weeks into the upper arm, abdomen, or thigh; dosing interval of 300 mg every 4 weeks is also effective and may be considered if the patient is well-controlled (i.e., attack free) for more than 6 months; with appropriate health care provider instruction, patients may self-administer
Pediatric: <12 years: not established; ≥12 years: same as adult
   Takhzyro *Vial:* 300 mg/2 ml (2 ml) soln single-dose (preservative-free)
   COMMENT: Takhzyro *(lanadelumab-flyo)* is a plasma kallikrein inhibitor (monoclonal antibody) indicated for prophylaxis to prevent attacks of hereditary angioedema (HAE). No dedicated drug interaction studies have been conducted. There are no available data on **Takhzyro** use in pregnant women to inform any drug associated risks. Monoclonal antibodies such as *lanadelumab-flyo* are transported across the placenta during the third trimester of pregnancy; therefore, potential effects on a fetus are likely to be greater during the third trimester of pregnancy. Animal studies have revealed no evidence of harm to the developing fetus. There are no data on the presence of *lanadelumab-flyo* in human milk or effects on the breastfed infant. To report suspected adverse reactions, contact Dyax at 1-800-828-2088 or FDA at 1-800-FDA-1088 or www.fda.gov/medwatch.

HAE ACUTE ATTACK

C1 Esterase Inhibitors [Human]

▶ *C1 esterase inhibitor [human]* (C)
   Berinert reconstitute pwdr using the sterile water provided; administer 20 IU/kg body weight via IVP injection at approximately 4 ml/min, at room temperature within 8 hours of reconstitution; store the vial at room temperature in the original carton to protect from light; appropriately trained patients may self-administer upon recognition of an HAE attack; hypersensitivity reactions may occur, therefore, have epinephrine immediately available for treatment of acute severe hypersensitivity reaction
Pediatric: <12 years: not established; ≥12 years: same as adult
   Vial: 500 Units/10 ml vial, single-use, pwdr for reconstitution with the 10 ml sterile water diluent (provided)
   COMMENT: To report suspected adverse reactions, contact the CSL Behring Pharmacovigilance Department at 1-866-915-6958 or to the FDA at 1-800-FDA-1088 or www.fda.gov/medwatch.
   Cinryze administer 1,000 Units (2 x 500 U vials) via IVP injection, after reconstitution with 5 ml sterile H2O/vial; reconstitute 1,000 U pwdr in a 10 ml syringe with 10 ml sterile water; administer over 10 minutes (1 ml/min) at room temperature within 3 hours of reconstitution; each 1,000 Unit treatment is administered every 3-4 days; hypersensitivity reactions may occur, therefore, have epinephrine immediately available for treatment of acute severe hypersensitivity reaction
Pediatric: <16 years: not established; ≥16 years: same as adult
   Vial: 500 Units/8 ml vial pwdr for reconstitution (sterile water diluent not provided)
   COMMENT: No adequate and well-controlled studies have been conducted in pregnant women. It is not known whether **Cinryze** can cause fetal harm when administered to a pregnant woman or can affect reproduction capacity. **Cinryze** should be administered to a pregnant woman only if clearly needed. It is not known whether **Cinryze** is excreted in human milk. **Cinryze** Pharmacovigilance Department at 1-866-915-6958 or to the FDA at 1-800-FDA-1088 or www.fda.gov/medwatch.

C1 Esterase Inhibitor [Recombinant]

▷ *C1 esterase inhibitor [recombinant]* (B) reconstitute 2.100 IU pwdr (1 vial) with 14 ml sterile H2O; administer reconstituted solution at room temperature, slow IVP injection over approximately 5 minutes; appropriately trained patients may self-administer upon recognition of HAE attack; Weight-based dose: <84 kg: 50 IU /kg [wt in kg ÷ 3 = vol (ml) reconst soln for administration]; ≥84 kg: 4,200 IU (28 ml, 2 vials); if the attack symptoms persist, an additional (second) dose can be administered at the recommended dose level; do not exceed 4200 IU per dose; max two doses within a 24 hour period; hypersensitivity reactions may occur, therefore, have epinephrine immediately available for treatment of acute severe hypersensitivity reaction
Pediatric: <13 years: not established; ≥13 years: same as adult
   Ruconest *Vial:* 2,100 IU, pwdr, single-use for IVP injection after reconstitution (sterile water diluent not provided)
   Comment: To report **Ruconest** suspected adverse reactions, contact Salix Pharmaceuticals at 1-800-508-0024 or FDA at 1-800-FDA-1088 or www.fda.gov/medwatch.

Bradykinen B2 Receptor Antagonist

▷ *icatibant* (C) administer 30 mg SC injection in the abdominal area; if response is inade-quate or symptoms recur, additional injections of 30 mg may be administered at intervals of at least 6 hours; max 3 injections/24 hours; patients may self-administer upon recognition of an HAE attack
Pediatric: <18 years: not established; ≥18 years: same as adult
   Firazyr *Prefilled syringe:* 10 mg/ml (3 ml) single-dose w. 25 gauge luer lock needle (1/carton, 3 cartons/pck)
   Comment: **Firazyr**, as a bradykinin B2 receptor antagonist, may attenuate the antihypertensive effect of ACE inhibitors. The most commonly reported adverse reaction is injection site reaction (97% in clinical trials). To report suspected adverse reactions, contact Shire Human Genetic Therapies OnePath at 1-800-828-2088 or FDA at 1-800-FDA-1088 or www.fda.gov/medwatch.

Plasma Kallikrein Inhibitor

▷ *ecallantide* (C) administer 30 mg (3 ml) SC in three 10 mg (I ml) injections; if an attack persists, an additional dose of 30 mg may be administered within a 24 hour period; should only be administered by a healthcare professional with appropriate medical support to manage anaphylaxis and hereditary angioedema
Pediatric: <12 years: not established; ≥12 years: same as adult
   Kalbitor *Vial:* 10 mg/ml (1/carton, 3 vials/pkg) single-use
   Comment: Anaphylaxis has occurred in 3.9% of patients treated with **Kalbitor**. Therefore, **Kalbitor** should only be administered in a setting equipped to manage anaphylaxis and hereditary angioedema. Given the similarity in hyper sensitivity symptoms and acute HAE symptoms, monitor patients closely for hypersensitivity reactions. To report suspected adverse reactions, contact Dyax Corp at 1-888-452-5248 or FDA at 1-800-FDA-1088 or ww.fda.gov/medwatch.

 HERPANGINA

Other Oral Analgesics *see Pain page* 352

ORAL ANALGESICS

▷ *acetaminophen* (B) *see Fever page* 163
▷ *tramadol* (C)(IV)(G)
Comment: *tramadol* is known to be excreted in breast milk. The FDA and the European Medicines Agency (EMA) are investigating the safety of using *tramadol*-containing medications to treat pain in children 12-18 years because of the potential for serious side effects, including slowed or difficult breathing.
   Rybix ODT initially 100 mg once daily; may increase by 100 mg every 5 days; max 300 mg/day; *CrCl <30 mL/min or severe hepatic impairment:* not recommended; *Cirrhosis:* max 50 mg q 12 hours
   Pediatric: <18 years: not recommended; ≥18 years: same as adult
      ODT: 50 mg (mint) (phenylalanine)

Ryzolt initially 100 mg once daily; may increase by 100 mg every 5 days; max 300 mg/day; *CrCl <40 mL/min or severe hepatic impairment:* not recommended
Pediatric: <18 years: not recommended; ≥18 years: same as adult
   Tab: 100, 200, 300 mg ext-rel
Ultram 50-100 mg q 4-6 hours prn; max 400 mg/day; *CrCl <40 mL/min:* max 100 mg q 12 hours; *Cirrhosis:* max 50 mg q 12 hours
Pediatric: <18 years: not recommended; ≥18 years: same as adult
   Tab: 50*mg
Ultram ER initially 100 mg once daily; may increase by 100 mg every 5 days; max 300 mg/day; *CrCl <40 mL/min or severe hepatic impairment:* not recommended
Pediatric: <18 years: not recommended; ≥18 years: same as adult
   Tab: 100, 200, 300 mg ext-rel

Comment: *tramadol* is known to be excreted in breast milk. The FDA and the European Medicines Agency (EMA) are investigating the safety of using *tramadol*-containing medications to treat pain in children 12-18 years because of the potential for serious side effects, including slowed or difficult breathing.

▷ *tramadol+acetaminophen* (C)(IV)(G) 2 tabs q 4-6 hours; max 8 tabs/day; 5 days; *CrCl <40 mL/min:* max 2 tabs q 12 hours; max 4 tabs/day x 5 days
Pediatric: <18 years: not recommended; ≥18 years: same as adult
   Ultracet *Tab:* tram 37.5+acet 325 mg

Comment: *tramadol* is known to be excreted in breast milk. The FDA and the European Medicines Agency (EMA) are investigating the safety of using *tramadol*-containing medications to treat pain in children 12-18 years because of the potential for serious side effects, including slowed or difficult breathing.

TOPICAL AND TRANSDERMAL ANESTHETICS

Comment: *lidocaine* should not be applied to non-intact skin.
▷ *lidocaine* cream (B) apply to affected area bid prn
Pediatric: <12 years: not recommended; ≥12 years: same as adult
   LidaMantle *Crm:* 3% (1, 2 oz)
   Lidoderm *Crm:* 3% (85 gm)
   ZTlido *lidocaine* topical system 1% (30/carton)
   Comment: Compared to **Lidoderm** (*lidocaine* patch 5%) which contains 700 mg/patch, **ZTlido** only requires 35 mg per topical system to achieve the same therapeutic dose.
▷ *lidocaine* lotion (B) apply to affected area bid prn
Pediatric: <12 years: not recommended; ≥12 years: same as adult
   LidaMantle *Lotn:* 3% (177 ml)
▷ *lidocaine* 5% patch (B)(G) apply up to 3 patches at one time for up to 12 hours/24-hour period (12 hours on/12 hours off); patches may be cut into smaller sizes before removal of the release liner; do not re-use
Pediatric: <12 years: not recommended; ≥12 years: same as adult
   Lidoderm *Patch:* 5% (10x14 cm; 30/carton)
▷ *lidocaine+dexamethasone* (B)
Pediatric: <12 years: not recommended; ≥12 years: same as adult
   Decadron Phosphate with Xylocaine *Lotn:* dexa 4 mg+lido 10 mg per ml (5 ml)
▷ *lidocaine+hydrocortisone* (B)(G) apply to affected area bid prn
Pediatric: <12 years: not recommended; ≥12 years: same as adult
   LidaMantle HC *Crm:* lido 3%+hydro 0.5% (1, 3 oz); *Lotn:* (177 ml)
▷ *lidocaine* 2.5%+*prilocaine* 2.5% apply sparingly to the burn bid-tid prn
Pediatric: <12 years: not recommended; ≥12 years: same as adult
   Emla Cream (B) 5, 30 gm/tube

HERPES GENITALIS (HSV TYPE II)

Comment: The following treatment regimens are published in the **2015 CDC Sexually Transmitted Diseases Treatment Guidelines**. Treatment regimens are for adults only; consult a specialist for treatment of patients less than 18 years-of-age. Treatment regimens are presented in alphabetical order by generic drug name, followed by brands and dose forms.

RECOMMENDED REGIMENS: FIRST CLINICAL EPISODE
Regimen 1
▷ *acyclovir* 400 mg tid x 7-10 days <u>or</u> 200 mg 5 x/day x 10 days <u>or</u> until clinically resolved

Regimen 2
▷ *acyclovir* cream apply q 3 hours 6 x/day x 7 days

Regimen 3
▷ *famciclovir* 250 mg tid x 7-10 days <u>or</u> until clinically resolved

Regimen 4
▷ *valacyclovir* 1 gm bid x 10 days <u>or</u> until clinically resolved

RECOMMENDED RECURRENT/EPISODIC REGIMENS
Comment: Initiate treatment of recurrent episodes within 1 day of onset of lesions.

Regimen 1
▷ *acyclovir* 200 mg 5 x/day x 5 days

Regimen 2
▷ *famciclovir* 125 mg bid x 5 days

Regimen 3
▷ *valacyclovir* 500 mg bid x 3-5 days <u>or</u> until clinically resolved

SUPPRESSION THERAPY REGIMENS
Regimen 1
▷ *acyclovir* 400 mg bid x 1 year

Regimen 2
▷ *famciclovir* 250 mg bid x 1 year

Regimen 3
▷ *valacyclovir* 500 mg daily x 1 year (for ≤9 recurrences/year) <u>or</u> 1 gm daily x 1 year (for ≥10 recurrences/year)

DAILY SUPPRESSIVE REGIMENS FOR PERSONS WITH HIV
Regimen 1
▷ *acyclovir* 400-800 mg bid-tid

Regimen 2
▷ *famciclovir* 500 mg bid

Regimen 3
▷ *valacyclovir* 500 mg bid

RECURRENT/EPISODIC REGIMENS FOR PERSONS WITH HIV
Regimen 1
▷ *acyclovir* 400 mg tid x 5-10 days

Regimen 2
▷ *famciclovir* 500 mg bid x 5-10 days

Regimen 3
▷ *valacyclovir* 1 gm bid x 5-10 days

DRUG BRANDS AND DOSE FORMS
▷ *acyclovir* (B)(G)
   Zovirax *Cap:* 200 mg; *Tab:* 400, 800 mg

        Zovirax Oral Suspension *Oral susp:* 200 mg/5 ml (banana)
        Zovirax Cream *Crm:* 5% (3, 15 gm); *Oint:* 5% (3, 15 gm)
▷ *famciclovir* (B)
        Famvir *Tab:* 125, 250, 500 mg
▷ *valacyclovir* (B)
        Valtrex *Cplt:* 500, 1 gm

 HERPES LABIALIS/HERPES FACIALIS (HSV TYPE I, COLD SORE, FEVER BLISTER)

PRIMARY INFECTION

▷ *acyclovir* (B)(G) do not chew, crush, or swallow the buccal tab; apply within 1 hour of symptom onset and before appearance of lesion; apply a single buccal tab to the upper gum region on the affected side and hold in place for 30 seconds
        Sitavig *Buccal tab:* 50 mg
            Pediatric: see page 616 for dose by weight
        Comment: **Sitavig** is contraindicated with allergy to milk protein concentrate.
▷ *valacyclovir* (B) 2 gm q 12 hours x 1 day
    Pediatric: <12 years: not recommended; ≥12 years: same as adult
        Valtrex *Cplt:* 500, 1,000 mg

SUPPRESSION THERAPY (≥6 OUTBREAKS/YEAR)

▷ *acyclovir* (B)(G) 200 mg 2-5 x/day x 1 year
    Pediatric: <2 years: not recommended; ≥2 years, <40 kg: 20 mg/kg 2-5 x/day x 1 year; ≥2 years, >40 kg: 200 mg 2-5 x/day x 1 year; *see page 616 for dose by weight*
        Zovirax *Cap:* 200 mg; *Tab:* 400, 800 mg
        Zovirax Oral Suspension *Oral susp:* 200 mg/5 ml (banana)

TOPICAL ANTIVIRAL THERAPY

▷ *acyclovir* (B)(G) apply q 3 hours 6 x/day x 7 days
    Pediatric: <2 years: not recommended; ≥2 years: same as adult
        Zovirax Cream *Crm:* 5% (3, 15 gm); *Oint:* 5% (3, 15 gm)
▷ *docosanol* (B)(G) apply and gently rub in 5 x daily until healed
    Pediatric: <12 years: not recommended; ≥12 years: same as adult
        Abreva (OTC) *Crm:* 10% (2 gm)
▷ *penciclovir* (B) apply q 2 hours while awake x 4 days
    Pediatric: <12 years: not recommended; ≥12 years: same as adult
        Denavir *Crm:* 1% (2 gm)

TOPICAL ANTIVIRAL+CORTICOSTEROID THERAPY

▷ *acyclovir+hydrocortisone* (B)(G) cream apply to affected area 5 x/day x 5 days
    Pediatric: <12 years: not recommended; ≥12 years: same as adult
        Crm: 1% (2, 5 gm)

 HERPES ZOSTER (HZ, SHINGLES)

Post-Herpetic Neuralgia *see page 402*

PROPHYLAXIS VACCINES

Comment: *Herpes zoster* (shingles) vaccine is indicated for adults ≥50 years-of-age (<50 years: not recommended). The vaccine is not for preventing primary infection (chickenpox) or treatment of shingles. Contraindications to herpes zoster vaccine are: history of anaphylactic/anaphylactoid reaction to gelatin, *neomycin*, or any other component of the vaccine, immunosuppression or immunodeficiency, and pregnancy. Pregnancy should be avoided for 3 months following *Varicella zoster* vaccine administration.
▷ *zoster vaccine live* administer 0.65ml dose SC as a single dose
        Zostavax *Vial:* 0.65 ml single-dose susp for IM injection after reconstitution with diluent (10/carton) (preservative-free)
        Comment: In a randomized clinical study, a reduced immune response to **Zostavax**, as measured by gpELISA, was observed in individuals who received concurrent

administration of **Pneumovax 23** and **Zostavax** compared with individuals who received these vaccines 4 weeks apart. Therefore, consider administration of **Pneumovax 23** and **Zostavax** separated by at least 4 weeks. The most frequent adverse reactions to **Zostavax** by subjects (1%) have been headache and injection site reactions. To report suspected adverse reactions, contact Merck Sharp & Dohme at 1-877-888-4231 or VAERS at 1-800-822-7967 or visit www.vaers.hhs.gov.

▷ *zoster vaccine recombinant, adjuvanted* administer one 0.5 ml dose at month 0 followed by second dose anytime between 2–6 months later; administer immediately upon reconstitution or store refrigerated and use within 6 hours
Pediatric: <18 years: not established
    Shingrix *Vial:* 0.5 ml single-dose susp for IM injection after reconstitution with diluent (10/carton) (preservative-free)
    Comment: Local adverse reactions to **Shringrix** include injection site pain (78%), redness (38.1%), and swelling (25.9%). Generalized adverse reactions include myalgia (44.7%), fatigue (44.5%), headache (37.7%), shivering (26.8%), fever (20.5%), and gastrointestinal symptoms (17.3%). There are no available human data to inform whether there is vaccine-associated risk with **Shingrix** in pregnancy. It is not known whether **Shingrix** is excreted in human milk or effects on the breastfed infant. To report suspected adverse reactions contact Glaxo/Smith/Kline at 1-888-825-5249 or VAERS at 1-800-822-7967 or visit www.vaers.hhs.gov.

ORAL ANTIVIRALS

▷ *acyclovir* (B)(G) 800 mg 5 x/day x 7-10 or 14 days
Pediatric: <2 years: not recommended; ≥2 years, <40 kg: 20 mg/kg 5 x/day x 7-10 days; *see page 616 for dose by weight;* >2 years, >40 kg: 800 mg 5 x/day x 7-10 days;
    Zovirax *Cap:* 200 mg; *Tab:* 400, 800 mg
    Zovirax Oral Suspension *Oral susp:* 200 mg/5 ml (banana)
▷ *famciclovir* (B) 500 mg tid x 7-10 days
Pediatric: <18 years: not recommended; ≥18 years: same as adult
    Famvir *Tab:* 125, 250, 500 mg
▷ *valacyclovir* (B) 1 gm tid x 7-10 days
Pediatric: <12 years: not recommended; ≥12 years: same as adult
    Valtrex *Cplt:* 500, 1,000 mg

PROPHYLAXIS AGAINST SECONDARY INFECTION

▷ *silver sulfadiazine* (B) apply qid
Pediatric: <12 years: not recommended; ≥12 years: same as adult
    Silvadene *Crm:* 1% (20, 50, 85, 400, 1,000 gm jar; 20 gm tube)

ORAL ANALGESICS

Other Oral Analgesics *see Pain page 352*

▷ *acetaminophen* (B) *see Fever page 163*
▷ *aspirin* (D)(G) *see Fever page 164*
    Comment: *aspirin*-containing medications are contraindicated with history of allergic-type reaction to *aspirin*, children and adolescents with *varicella* or other viral illness, and 3rd trimester pregnancy.
▷ *tramadol* (C)(IV)(G)
    Comment: *tramadol* is known to be excreted in breast milk. The FDA and the European Medicines Agency (EMA) are investigating the safety of using *tramadol*-containing medications to treat pain in children 12-18 years because of the potential for serious side effects, including slowed or difficult breathing.
    Rybix ODT initially 100 mg once daily; may increase by 100 mg every 5 days; max 300 mg/day; *CrCl <30 mL/min or severe hepatic impairment:* not recommended; *Cirrhosis:* max 50 mg q 12 hours
Pediatric: <18 years: not recommended; ≥18 years: same as adult
    ODT: 50 mg (mint) (phenylalanine)
    Ryzolt initially 100 mg once daily; may increase by 100 mg every 5 days; max 300 mg/day; *CrCl <30 mL/min or severe hepatic impairment,* not recommended
Pediatric: <18 years: not recommended; ≥18 years: same as adult
    Tab: 100, 200, 300 mg ext-rel

Ultram 50-100 mg q 4-6 hours prn; max 400 mg/day; *CrCl <40 mL/min:* max 100 mg q 12 hours; *Cirrhosis:* max 50 mg q 12 hours
Pediatric: <18 years: not recommended; ≥18 years: same as adult
   Tab: 50*mg
Ultram ER initially 100 mg once daily; may increase by 100 mg every 5 days; max 300 mg/day; *CrCl <30 mL/min* or *severe hepatic impairment:* not recommended
Pediatric: <18 years: not recommended; ≥18 years: same as adult
   Tab: 100, 200, 300 mg ext-rel
▷ *tramadol+acetaminophen* **(C)(IV)(G)** 2 tabs q 4-6 hours; max 8 tabs/day x 5 days; *CrCl <40 mL/min:* max 2 tabs q 12 hours; max 4 tabs/day x 5 days
Pediatric: <18 years: not recommended; ≥18 years: same as adult
   Ultracet *Tab:* tram 37.5+acet 325 mg

Comment: *tramadol* is known to be excreted in breast milk. The FDA and the European Medicines Agency (EMA) are investigating the safety of using *tramadol*-containing medications to treat pain in children 12-18 years because of the potential for serious side effects, including slowed or difficult breathing.

TOPICAL AND TRANSDERMAL ANESTHETICS

Comment: *lidocaine* should not be applied to non-intact skin.
▷ *lidocaine* cream **(B)** apply to affected area bid prn
Pediatric: <12 years: not recommended; ≥12 years: same as adult
   LidaMantle *Crm:* 3% (1, 2 oz)
   Lidoderm *Crm:* 3% (85 gm)
   ZTlido *lidocaine* topical system 1% (30/carton)
   Comment: Compared to **Lidoderm** (*lidocaine* patch 5%) which contains 700 mg/patch, ZTlido only requires 35 mg per topical system to achieve the same therapeutic dose.
▷ *lidocaine* lotion **(B)** apply to affected area bid prn
Pediatric: <12 years: not recommended; ≥12 years: same as adult
   LidaMantle *Lotn:* 3% (177 ml)
▷ *lidocaine* 5% patch **(B)(G)** apply up to 3 patches at one time for up to 12 hours/24-hour period (12 hours on/12 hours off); patches may be cut into smaller sizes before removal of the release liner; do not re-use
Pediatric: <12 years: not recommended; ≥12 years: same as adult
   Lidoderm *Patch:* 5% (10x14 cm; 30/carton)
▷ *lidocaine+dexamethasone* **(B)**
Pediatric: <12 years: not recommended; ≥12 years: same as adult
   Decadron Phosphate with Xylocaine *Lotn:* dexa 4 mg+lido 10 mg per ml (5 ml)
▷ *lidocaine+hydrocortisone* **(B)(G)** apply to affected area bid prn
Pediatric: <12 years: not recommended; ≥12 years: same as adult
   LidaMantle HC *Crm:* lido 3%+hydro 0.5% (1, 3 oz); *Lotn:* (177 ml)
▷ *lidocaine* 2.5%+*prilocaine* 2.5% apply sparingly to the burn bid-tid prn
Pediatric: <12 years: not recommended; ≥12 years: same as adult
   Emla Cream (B) 5, 30 gm/tube

SECONDARY INFECTION PROPHYLAXIS

▷ *silver sulfadiazine* **(B)** apply qid
Pediatric: <12 years: not recommended; ≥12 years: same as adult
   Silvadene *Crm:* 1% (20, 50, 85, 400, 1,000 gm/jar; 20 gm tube)

 HERPES ZOSTER OPHTHALMICUS (HZO)

Comment: Herpes Zoster ophthalmicus (HZO) is an ophthalmologic emergency. Standard therapy involves initiating systemic (oral or intravenous) antiviral therapy as soon as possible. Pharmacotherapy options include *acyclovir*, *valacyclovir*, and *famciclovir*. IV acyclovir is recommended for immunocompromised persons. Duration of treatment is 7-10 or 14 days, depending on severity. Ocular complications include conjunctivitis with or without superimposed bacterial infections, episcleritis, scleritis, keratitis, and uveitis, involvement of the 3rd, 4th, and 5th cranial nerves, acute optic neuritis, and necrotizing retinopathy (that often leads to permanent vision loss). Corticosteroids reduce the duration of pain during the acute phase, however, they have not been shown to decrease the incidence of postherpetic neuralgia and can exacerbate some ocular complications. Ophthalmology consultation is mandatory before initiating corticosteroid therapy.

REFERENCES

Anderson, E., Fantus, R. J., & Haddadin, R. I. (2017). Diagnosis and management of herpes zoster ophthalmicus. *Disease-a-Month, 63*(2), 38–44. doi:10.1016/j.disamonth.2016.09.004

Vrcek, I., Choudhury, E., & Durairaj, V. (2017). Herpes zoster ophthalmicus: A review for the internist. *The American Journal of Medicine, 130*(1), 21–26. doi:10.1016/j.amjmed.2016.08.039

ORAL ANTIVIRALS

➤ *acyclovir* (B)(G) 800 mg 5 x/day x 7-10 days
  Pediatric: <2 years: not recommended; 2 years, ≤40 kg: 20 mg/kg 5 x/day x 7-10 days; 2 years, >40 kg: 800 mg 5 x/day x 7-10 days; *see page 616 for dose by weight*
    Zovirax *Cap:* 200 mg; *Tab:* 400, 800 mg; *IVF bag:* 500 mg, 1 gm pre-mixed in 0.9% NS
    Zovirax Oral Suspension *Oral susp:* 200 mg/5 ml (banana)
➤ *famciclovir* (B) 500 mg tid x 7-10 days
  Pediatric: <18 years: not recommended; ≥18 years: same as adult
    Famvir *Tab:* 125, 250, 500 mg
➤ *valacyclovir* (B) 1 gm tid x 7-10 days
  Pediatric: <12 years: not recommended; ≥12 years: same as adult
    Valtrex *Cplt:* 500, 1 gm

HICCUPS: INTRACTABLE

➤ *chlorpromazine* (C) 25-50 mg tid-qid
  Pediatric: <6 months: not recommended; ≥6 months: 0.25 mg/lb orally q 4-6 hours prn or 0.5 mg/lb rectally q 6-8 hours prn
    Thorazine *Tab:* 10, 25, 50, 100, 200 mg; *Spansule:* 30, 75, 150 mg sust-rel; *Syr:* 10 mg/5 ml (4 oz; orange custard); *Oral conc:* 30 mg/ml (4 oz); 100 mg/ml (2, 8 oz); *Supp:* 25, 100 mg

HIDRADENITIS SUPPURATIVA

ORAL ANTI-INFECTIVES

➤ *doxycycline* (D)(G) 100 mg bid x 7-14 days
  Pediatric: <8 years: not recommended; ≥8 years, <100 lb: 2 mg/lb on first day in 2 divided doses, followed by 1 mg/lb/day in 1-2 divided doses; ≥8 years, ≥100 lb: same as adult; *see page 625 for dose by weight*
    Acticlate *Tab:* 75, 150**mg
    Adoxa *Tab:* 50, 75, 100, 150 mg ent-coat
    Doryx *Tab:* 50, 75, 100, 150, 200 mg del-rel
    Doxteric *Tab:* 50 mg del-rel
    Monodox *Cap:* 50, 75, 100 mg
    Oracea *Cap:* 40 mg del-rel
    Vibramycin *Tab:* 100 mg; *Cap:* 50, 100 mg; *Syr:* 50 mg/5 ml (raspberry-apple); (sulfites); *Oral susp:* 25 mg/5 ml (raspberry)
    Vibra-Tab *Tab:* 100 mg film-coat
  Comment: *doxycycline* is contraindicated <8 years-of-age, in pregnancy, and lactation (discolors developing tooth enamel). A side effect may be photo-sensitivity (photophobia). Do not take with antacids, calcium supplements, milk or other dairy, or within 2 hours of taking another drug.
➤ *erythromycin base* (B)(G) 1-1.5 gm divided qid x 7-14 days
  Pediatric: <45 kg: 30-50 mg in 2-4 divided doses x 7-14 days; ≥45 kg: same as adult
    Ery-Tab *Tab:* 250, 333, 500 mg ent-coat
    PCE *Tab:* 333, 500 mg
  Comment: *erythromycin* may increase INR with concomitant *warfarin*, as well as increase serum level of *digoxin*, benzodiazepines, and statins.
➤ *erythromycin ethylsuccinate* (B)(G) 1200-1600 mg divided qid x 7-14 days
  Pediatric: 30-50 mg/kg/day in 4 divided doses x 7 days; may double dose with severe infection; max 100 mg/kg/day; *see page 626 for dose by weight*

EryPed *Oral susp:* 200 mg/5 ml (100, 200 ml) (fruit); 400 mg/5 ml (60, 100, 200 ml) (banana); *Oral drops:* 200, 400 mg/5 ml (50 ml) (fruit); *Chew tab:* 200 mg wafer (fruit)
E.E.S. *Oral susp:* 200, 400 mg/5 ml (100 ml) (fruit)
E.E.S. Granules *Oral susp:* 200 mg/5 ml (100, 200 ml) (cherry)
E.E.S. 400 Tablets *Tab:* 400 mg
Comment: *erythromycin* may increase INR with concomitant *warfarin*, as well as increase serum level of *digoxin*, benzodiazepines, and statins.

▷ *minocycline* (D)(G) 100 mg bid x 7-14 days
Pediatric: <8 years: not recommended, ≥8 years: same as adult
Dynacin *Cap:* 50, 100 mg
Minocin *Cap:* 50, 75, 100 mg; *Oral susp:* 50 mg/5 ml (60 ml) (custard) (sulfites, alcohol 5%)
Comment: *minocycline* is contraindicated <8 years-of-age, in pregnancy, and lactation (discolors developing tooth enamel). A side effect may be photo-sensitivity (photophobia). Do not take with antacids, calcium supplements, milk or other dairy, or within two hours of taking another drug.

▷ *tetracycline* (D)(G) 250 mg qid or 500 mg tid x 7-14 days
Pediatric: <8 years: not recommended; ≥8 years, <100 lb: 25-50 mg/kg/day in 2-4 divided doses x 7-14 days; ≥8 years, ≥100 lb: same as adult; *see page 630 for dose by weight*
Achromycin V *Cap:* 250, 500 mg
Sumycin *Tab:* 250, 500 mg; *Cap:* 250, 500 mg; *Oral susp:* 125 mg/5 ml (100, 200 ml) (fruit, sulfites)
Comment: *tetracycline* is contraindicated <8 years-of-age, in pregnancy, and lactation (discolors developing tooth enamel). A side effect may be photo-sensitivity (photophobia). Do not take with antacids, calcium supplements, milk or other dairy, or within two hours of taking another drug.

TOPICAL ANTI-INFECTIVES

▷ *clindamycin* (B) topical apply bid x 7-14 days
Cleocin T *Pad:* 1% (60/pck; alcohol 50%); *Lotn:* 1% (60 ml); *Gel:* 1% (30, 60 gm); *Soln w. applicator:* 1% (30, 60 ml; alcohol 50%)

HOOKWORM (UNCINARIASIS, CUTANEOUS LARVAE MIGRANS)

ANTHELMINTICS

▷ *albendazole* (C) 400 mg as a single dose; may repeat in 3 weeks
Pediatric: <2 years: 200 mg daily x 3 days; may repeat in 3 weeks; ≥2-12 years: 400 mg daily x 3 days; may repeat in 3 weeks
Albenza *Tab:* 200 mg

▷ *ivermectin* (C) take with water; chew or crush and mix with food; may repeat in 3 months if needed; <15 kg: not recommended; ≥15 kg: 200 mcg/kg as a single dose
Pediatric: <15 kg: not recommended; ≥15 kg: same as adult
Stromectol *Tab:* 3, 6*mg

▷ *mebendazole* (C)(G) chew, swallow, or mix with food; 100 mg bid x 3 days; may repeat in 3 weeks if needed; take with a meal
Pediatric: <2 years: not recommended; ≥2 years: same as adult
Emverm *Chew tab:* 100 mg
Vermox *Chew tab:* 100 mg

▷ *pyrantel pamoate* (C) 11 mg/kg x 1 dose; max 1 gm/dose
Pediatric: 25-37 lb: 1/2 tsp x 1 dose; 38-62 lb: 1 tsp x 1 dose; 63-87 lb: 1 tsp x 1 dose; 88-112 lb: 2 tsp x 1 dose; 113-137 lb: 2 tsp x 1 dose; 138-162 lb: 3 tsp x 1 dose; 163-187 lb: 3 tsp x 1 dose; >187 lb: 4 tsp x 1 dose
Antiminth *Cap:* 180 mg; *Liq:* 50 mg/ml (30 ml); 144 mg/ml (30 ml); *Oral susp:* 50 mg/ml (60 ml)
Pin-X (OTC) *Cap:* 180 mg; *Liq:* 50 mg/ml (30 ml); 144 mg/ml (30 ml); *Oral susp:* 50 mg/ml (30 ml)

▷ *thiabendazole* (C) take with a meal; may crush and mix with food; treat x 7 days; <30 lb: consult mfr pkg insert; ≥30 lb: 25 mg/kg/dose bid with meals; 30-50 lb: 250 mg bid with meals; >50 lb: 10 mg/lb/dose bid with meals; max 1.5 gm/dose; max 3 gm/day
Pediatric: same as adult

Mintezol *Chew tab:* 500*mg (orange); *Oral susp:* 500 mg/5 ml (120 ml) (orange)
Comment: *thiabendazole* is not for prophylaxis. May impair mental alertness. May not be available in the US.

HUMAN IMMUNODEFICIENCY VIRUS (HIV) INFECTION, HIV PRE-EXPOSURE PROPHYLAXIS (PrEP), HIV OCCUPATIONAL POST-EXPOSURE PROPHYLAXIS (oPEP), HIV NON-OCCUPATIONAL POST-EXPOSURE PROPHYLAXIS (nPEP)

ANTIRETROVIRAL HIV POST-EXPOSURE PROPHYLAXIS (oPEP and nPEP)

Comment: Antiretroviral prophylactic treatment regimens for occupational HIV post-exposure prophylaxis (oPEP) and non-occupational HIV post-exposure prophylaxis (nPEP) are referenced from the **2015 CDC Sexually Transmitted Diseases Treatment Guidelines, MMWR,** and **NIH** available at: https://www.cdc.gov/hiv/pdf/programresources/cdc-hiv-npep-guidelines.pdf.

In this section, the 2015 CDC-recommended highly active antiretroviral treatment (HAART) regimens are followed by a listing of the single and combination drugs with dosing regimens and dose forms. Appendix S is an alphabetical listing of the HIV drugs and dose forms. For more information on the management of HIV infection in adults and adolescents, see *Guidelines for the Use of Antiretroviral Agents in HIV-1-Infected Adults and Adolescents:* https://aidsinfo.nih.gov/contentfiles/lvguidelines/adultandadolescentgl.pdf.

For specific dosing information in the management of HIV infection in children, see *Guidelines for Use of Antiretroviral Agents in Pediatric HIV Infection:* www.aidsinfo.nih. gov/contentfiles/lvguidelines/pediatricguidelines.pdf. Providers should consult, and/or refer HIV-infected patients to, a specialist and/or specialty community services for age-appropriate dosing regimens and other patient-specific needs.

Initiation of oPEP/nPEP with ART as soon as possible increases the likelihood of prophylactic benefit. Treatment regimens must be initiated ≥72 hours following exposure. A 28-day course of ART is recommended for persons with *substantial risk for HIV exposure* (i.e., exposure of vagina, rectum, eye, mouth, or other mucous membrane, non-intact skin, or percutaneous contact with blood, semen, vaginal secretions, breast milk, or any body fluid that is visibly contaminated with blood, when the source is known to be infected with HIV). ART is not recommended for persons with *negligible risk for HIV exposure* (i.e., exposure of vagina, rectum, eye, mouth, or other mucus membrane, intact or non-intact skin, or percutaneous contact with urine, nasal secretions, saliva, sweat, or tears, if not visibly contaminated with blood, regardless of the known or suspected HIV status of the source). There is no evidence indicating any specific antiretroviral medication, or combination of medications is optimal for suppressing local viral replication. There is no evidence to indicate that a 3-drug ART regimen is any more beneficial than a 2-drug regimen. When the source person is available for interview and testing, his or her history of retroviral medication use and most recent/current viral load measurement should be considered when selecting an ART treatment regimen (e.g., to help avoid prescribing an antiretroviral medication to which the source virus is likely to be resistant). Register pregnant patients exposed to antiretroviral agents to the Antiretroviral Pregnancy Registry (APR) at 800-258-4263. The CDC recommends that HIV-infected mothers not breastfeed their infants to avoid risking postnatal transmission of HIV infection.

ANTIRETROVIRAL HIV POST-EXPOSURE PROPHYLAXIS (PEP)

Comment: **Truvada** is indicated for treatment of HIV-1 infection and pre-exposure prophylaxis (PrEP) to reduce the risk of sexually acquired HIV-1 in persons at high risk for exposure, ≥35 kg, in combination with safe sex practices.

▷ Truvada (B)(G) *emtricitabine+tenofovir disoproxil fumarate*
   Pediatric: <17 kg: not established; 17-<22 kg: 100/150 once daily; 22-<28 kg: 133/200 once daily; 28-35 kg: 167/250 once daily; ≥35 kg: 200/300 once daily
      Tab: **Truvada 100/150** emt 100 mg+teno 150 mg
         Truvada 133/200 emt 133 mg+teno 200 mg
         Truvada 167/250 emt 167 mg+teno 250 mg
         Truvada 200/300 emt 200 mg+teno 300 mg

HIV INFECTION ANTIRETROVIRAL TREATMENT REGIMENS

Comment: Immune Reconstitution Syndrome (IRS) has been reported in patients treated with combination antiretroviral therapy. During the initial phase of combination antiretroviral treatment, patients whose immune system responds may develop an inflammatory response to indolent or residual opportunistic infections (such as *Mycobacterium avium* infection, cytomegalovirus, *Pneumocystis jirovecii* pneumonia (PCP), or tuberculosis), which may necessitate further evaluation and treatment. Autoimmune disorders (such as Graves' disease, polymyositis, and Guillain-Barré syndrome) have also been reported to occur in the setting of immune reconstitution; however, the time to onset is more variable and can occur many months after initiation of treatment. Patients with HIV-1 should be tested for the presence of chronic hepatitis B virus (HBV) before initiating antiretroviral therapy.

NONNUCLEOSIDE REVERSE TRANSCRIPTASE INHIBITOR (NNRTI)-BASED REGIMEN

▷ *efavirenz* plus (*lamivudine* or *emtricitabine*) plus (*zidovudine* or *tenofovir*)

PROTEASE INHIBITOR (PI)-BASED REGIMENS

▷ *lopinavir+ritonavir* (co-formulated as **Kaletra**) plus (*lamivudine* or *emtricitabine*) plus *zidovudine*
▷ *darunavir+cobicistat* (co-formulated as **Prezcobix**) plus *other retroviral agents*

ALTERNATIVE REGIMENS

NNRTI-Based Regimen

▷ *efavirenz* plus (*lamivudine* or *emtricitabine*) plus (*abacavir* or *didanosine* or *stavudine*)
  Comment: *efavirenz* should be avoided in pregnant women and women of child-bearing potential.

Protease Inhibitor-Based Regimens

Regimen 1

▷ *atazanavir* plus (*lamivudine* or *emtricitabine*) plus (*zidovudine* or *stavudine* or *abacavir* or *didanosine*) or (*tenofovir* plus *ritonavir* (100 mg/day)

Regimen 2

▷ *fosamprenavir* plus (*lamivudine* or *emtricitabine*) plus (*zidovudine* or *stavudine*) or (*abacavir* or *tenofovir* or *didanosine*)

Regimen 3

▷ *fosamprenavir+ritonavir* plus (*lamivudine* or *emtricitabine*) plus (*zidovudine* or *stavudine* or *abacavir* or *tenofovir* or *didanosine*)

Regimen 4

▷ *indinavir+ritonavir* plus (*lamivudine* or *emtricitabine*) plus (*zidovudine* or *stavudine* or *abacavir* or *tenofovir* or *didanosine*)
  Comment: Using *ritonavir* with *indinavir* may increase risk for renal adverse events.

Regimen 5

▷ *lopinavir+ritonavir* (co-formulated as **Kaletra**) plus (*lamivudine* or *emtricitabine*) plus (*stavudine* or *abacavir* or *tenofovir* or *didanosine*)

Regimen 6

▷ *nelfinavir* plus (*lamivudine* or *emtricitabine*) plus (*zidovudine* or *stavudine* or *abacavir* or *tenofovir* or *didanosine*)

Regimen 7

▷ *saquinavir+ritonavir* plus (*lamivudine* or *emtricitabine*) plus (*zidovudine* or *stavudine* or *abacavir* or *tenofovir* or *didanosine*)

Triple Nucleoside Reverse Transcriptase Inhibitor (NRTI)-Based Regimen

abacavir plus *lamivudine* plus *zidovudine*
Comment: Triple NRTI therapy should be used only when an NNRTI- or PI-based regimen cannot or should not be used.

BRAND NAMES, DOSING AND DOSE FORMS: SINGLE AGENTS

Integrase Strand Transfer Inhibitors (INSTIs)

▷ *dolutegravir* (C) *Treatment naïve* or *treatment experienced but INSTI naïve:* 50 mg once daily; *Treatment experienced* or *naïve and co-administered with efavirenz, FPV/r, TPV/r,* or *rifampin:* 50 mg bid; *INSTI experienced with certain INSTI-associated resistance substitutions:* 50 mg bid
  Pediatric: <12 years, <40 kg: not established; ≥12 years, ≥40 kg: same as adult
  Tivicay *Tab:* 10, 25, 50 mg

▷ *raltegravir (as potassium)* (C) 400 mg (one film-coat tab) bid; take with concomitant *rifampin* 800 mg bid; swallow whole; do not crush or chew
  Pediatric: ≥4 weeks, 3-11 kg [oral susp] 3-<4 kg: 20 mg bid; 4-<6 kg: 30 mg bid; 6-<8 kg: 40 mg bid; 8-<11 kg: 60 mg bid; ≥11-<25 kg [oral susp/chew tab]; 6 mg/kg/dose bid; see mfr pkg insert for dose by weight; ≥25 kg and unable to swallow tablet use chewable tab; 25-<28 kg: 150 mg bid; 28-<40 kg: 200 mg bid; ≥40 kg: 300 mg bid; 6 years, ≥25 kg, and able to swallow tablets use film-coat tab; 400 mg bid
  Isentress *Tab:* 400 mg film-coat; *Chew tab:* 25, 100*mg (orange banana) (phenylalanine)
  Isentress HD *Tab:* 600 mg film-coat
  Isentress Oral Suspension *Oral susp:* 100 mg/pkt pwdr for oral susp (banana)
  Comment: Oral suspension, chewable tablets and film-coat *raltegravir* tablets are not bioequivalent. Maximum dose for chewable tablets is 300 mg twice daily. Previously, the maximum dose for film-coat tablets was 400 mg twice daily. However, the US Food and Drug Administration has recently approved a new 1200 mg daily dosage of **Isentress HD** (*raltegravir*) for the treatment of HIV-1 infection in adults, and pediatric patients who weigh ≥ 40 kg and are treatment-naïve or whose virus has been suppressed on an initial regimen of 400 mg twice-daily dose of **Isentress HD**. **Isentress HD** is administered as two 600 mg film-coat oral tablets in combination with other antiretroviral agents, and can be taken with or without food. Co-administration of **Isentress HD** can include a wide range of antiretroviral agents and non-antiretroviral agents, however aluminum and/or magnesium-containing antacids, calcium carbonate antacids, *rifampin*, *tipranavir+ritonavir, etravirine,* and other strong inducers of drug metabolizing enzymes are not recommended to be combined with **Isentress HD**. Health care providers should consider the potential for drug-drug interactions prior to and during treatment with **Isentress HD** and any other recommended agents. Adverse effects associated with treatment included abdominal pain, diarrhea, vomiting and decreased appetite. In addition, severe, potentially life-threatening and fatal skin reactions can occur, including Stevens-Johnson syndrome, hypersensitivity reaction, and toxic epidermal necrolysis. Treatment should be immediately discontinued if severe hypersensitivity, severe rash, or rash with systemic symptoms or liver aminotransferase elevations develop.

Nucleoside Reverse Transcriptase Inhibitors (NRTIs)

▷ *abacavir sulfate* (C)(G) 600 mg once daily or 300 mg bid; *Mild hepatic impairment:* use oral solution for titration
  Pediatric: 3 months-16 years: [tab/oral soln] 16 mg/kg qd or 8 mg/kg bid; max 300 mg bid; >14 kg: see mfr pkg insert for tablet dosing by weight band
  Ziagen (as sulfate) *Tab:* 300*mg
  Ziagen Oral Solution *Oral soln:* 20 mg/ml (240 ml) (strawberry-banana) (parabens, propylene glycol)

▷ *didanosine* (C)
  Videx EC take once daily on an empty stomach; swallow whole; <20 kg: use oral solution; 20-<25 kg: 200 mg; 25-<60 kg: 250 mg; ≥60 kg: 400 mg; *CrCl 30-59 mL/min:* <60 kg: 125 mg; ≥60 kg: 200 mg; *CrCl 10-29 mL/min:* 125 mg; *CrCl<10 mL/min* or *dialysis:*<60 kg: use oral solution ≥60 kg: 125 mg
  Pediatric: same as adult
      Cap: 125, 200, 250, 400 mg ent-coat del-rel; *Chew tab:* 25, 50, 100, 150, 200 mg (mandarin orange) (buffered with calcium carbonate and magnesium hydroxide, phenylalanine)
  Videx Pediatric Pwdr for Solution <60 kg: 125 mg bid; ≥60 kg: 200 mg bid; *If once daily dosing required:* <60 kg: 250 mg once daily; ≥60 kg: 400 mg once daily; *CrCl 30-59 mL/min:* <60 kg: 150 mg once daily or 75 mg bid; ≥60 kg: 200 mg once daily or 100 mg bid; *CrCl 10-29 mL/min:* <60 kg: 100 mg once daily; ≥60 kg: 150 mg once daily; *CrCl <10*

mL/min or *dialysis:* <60 kg: 75 mg once daily; ≥60 kg: 100 mg once daily; take on an empty stomach *Pediatric:* <2 weeks: not recommended; 2 weeks-8 months: 100 mg/m² bid; >8 months: 120 mg/m² bid; *Renal impairment:* consider reducing dose or increasing dosing interval; take on an empty stomach

  Pwdr for oral soln: 2, 4 gm (120, 240 ml)

Comment: *didanosine* is contraindicated with concomitant *allopurinal* or *ribavirin*.

▷ *emtricitabine* (B)(G) 200 mg once daily; *CrCl 30-49 mL/min:* 200 mg q 48 hours; *CrCl 15-29 mL/min:* 200 mg q 72 hours; *CrCl <15 mL/min* or *dialysis:* 200 mg q 96 hours
Pediatric: <3 months: 3 mg/kg oral soln once daily; 3 months-17 years, 6 mg/kg once daily; ≤33 kg: use oral soln, max 240 mg (24 ml); >33 kg: 200 mg cap once daily; max 240 mg/day; ≥18 years: same as adult
    Emtriva *Cap:* 200 mg
    Emtriva Oral Solution *Oral soln:* 10 mg/ml (170 ml) (cotton candy)

▷ *lamivudine* (C)(G) *CrCl ≤50 mL/min:* 300 mg qd or 150 mg bid; *CrCl >30-50 mL/min:* 150 mg qd; *CrCl 15-29:* first dose 150 mg, then 100 mg once daily; *CrCl 5-14 mL/min:* first dose 150 mg, then 50 mg qd; *CrCl <5 mL/min:* first dose 50 mg, the 25 mg once daily; max 8 mg/kg once daily or 150 mg bid
Pediatric: <3 months: not established; 3 months-16 years: 4 mg/kg oral soln or tab bid; [tab] 14-<20 kg: 150 mg once daily or 75 mg bid; ≥20-<25 kg: 225 mg once daily or 75 mg in the AM and 150 mg in the PM; ≥25 kg: 300 mg once daily or 150 mg bid; max 8 mg/kg once daily or 150 mg bid or 300 mg once daily
    Epivir *Tab:* 150*, 300 mg
    Epivir Oral Solution *Oral soln:* 10 mg/ml (240 ml) (strawberry-banana) (sucrose 3 gm/15 ml)

Comment: With renal impairment reduce *lamivudine* dose or extend dosing interval.

▷ *stavudine* (C)(G) ≥60 kg: 40 mg q 12 hours; ≤60 kg: 30 mg q 12 hours; *If peripheral neuropathy develops:* discontinue; *After resolution, ≥60 kg:* may re-start at 20 mg q 12 hours; *After resolution, ≤60 kg:* may restart at 15 mg q 12 hours; *if neuropathy returns:* consider permanent discontinuation; *CrCl 10-50 mL/min, ≥60 kg:* 20 mg q 12 hours; *CrCl 10-50 mL/min, ≥60 kg:* 15 mg q 12 hours; *Hemodialysis, ≥60 kg:* 20 mg q 24 hours; *Hemodialysis, ≤60 kg:* 15 mg q 24 hours; administer at the same time of day; *Hemodialysis:* administer at the end of dialysis
Pediatric: birth-13 days: [tab/oral soln] 0.5 mg/kg q 12 hours; >14 days, <30 kg: [tab/oral soln] 1 mg/kg q 12 hours; ≥30-<60 kg: 30 mg q 12 hours; ≥60 kg: 40 mg q 12 hours
    Zerit *Cap:* 15, 20, 30, 40 mg
    Zerit for Oral Solution *Oral soln:* 1 mg/ml pwdr for reconstitution (fruit) (dye-free)
Comment: Withdraw *stavudine* if peripheral neuropathy occurs. After complete resolution, may restart at half the recommended dose. If peripheral neuropathy recurs consider permanent discontinuation.

▷ *tenofovir disoproxil fumarate* (C)(G) 300 mg once daily; *CrCl 30-49 mL/min:* 300 mg q 48 hours; *CrCl 10-29:* 300 mg q 72-96 hours; *Hemodialysis:* 300 mg once every 7 days or after a total of 12 hours of dialysis; *CrCl <10 mL/min:* not recommended
Pediatric: <2 years: not established; 2-12 years: 8 mg/kg once daily; >12 years, 35 kg: 300 mg once daily; mix oral pwdr with 2-4 oz soft food
    Viread *Tab:* 150, 200, 250, 300 mg; *Oral pwdr:* 40 mg/gm (60 gm w. dosing scoop)

▷ *zidovudine* (C)(G) 600 mg daily divided bid-tid; *ESRD/dialysis:* 100 mg q 6-8 hours; *Vertical transmission, severe anemia, or neutropenia:* see mfr pkg insert
Pediatric: Treatment of HIV-1 infection: 4-<9 kg: 24 mg/kg/day divided bid or tid; ≥9-<30 kg: 18 mg/kg/day divided bid or tid; ≥30 kg: 600 mg/day divided bid or tid; *Prevention of maternal-fetal neonatal transmission:* <12 hours after birth until 6 weeks of age: [Soln] 2 mg/kg q 6 hours until 6 weeks-of-age; [IV] 1.5 mg/kg infused over 30 minutes q 6 hours until 6 weeks-of-age; max 200 mg q 8 hours
    Retrovir Tablets *Tab:* 300 mg
    Retrovir Capsules *Cap:* 100 mg
    Retrovir Syrup *Syrup:* 50 mg/5 ml (strawberry)
    Retrovir IV *Vial:* 10 mg/ml after dilution (20 ml) (preservative-free)

Nonnucleoside Reverse Transcriptase Inhibitors (NNRTIs)

▷ *delavirdine mesylate* (C) 400 mg (4 x 100-mg or 2 x 200 mg) tablets tid in combination with other antiretroviral agents
Pediatric: <16 years: not established; ≥16 years: same as adult
    Rescriptor *Tab:* 100, 200 mg

Comment: The 100 mg **Rescriptor** tablets may be dispersed in water prior to consumption. To prepare a dispersion, add four 100 mg Rescriptor tablets to at least 3 ounces of water, allow to stand for a few minutes, and then stir until a uniform dispersion occurs. The dispersion should be consumed promptly. The glass should be rinsed with water and the rinse swallowed to insure the entire dose is consumed. The 200 mg tablets should be taken as intact tablets, because they are not readily dispersed in water.

▷ *doravirine* 100 mg once daily in combination with other antiretroviral agents; as a dosage adjustment when taking *rifabutin* with *Delstrigo*, administer 100 mg of *doravirine* (**Pifeltro**) approximately 12 hours after the dose of **Delstrigo**
Pediatric: <18 years: not established; ≥18 years: same as adult
   Pifeltro *Tab*: 100 mg

▷ *efavirenz* (D)(G) 600 mg once daily
Pediatric: >3 months, 3.5 kg: [tab/cap] 3.5-< 5 kg: 100 mg once daily 5-<7.5 kg: 150 mg once daily; 7.5-<15 kg: 200 mg once daily; 15-<20 kg: 250 mg once daily; 20-<25 kg: 300 mg once daily; 25-<32.5 kg: 350 once daily; 32.5-<40 kg: 400 mg once daily; >40 kg: 600 mg once daily; max 600 mg once daily
Comment: For children who cannot swallow capsules, the capsule contents can be administered with a small amount of food or infant formula using the capsule sprinkle method of administration. See mfr pkg insert for instructions. Tablets should not be crushed or chewed. Administer at bedtime to limit CNS effects.
   Sustiva *Tab*: 75, 150, 600, 800 mg; *Cap*: 50, 200 mg

▷ *etravirine* (B) 200 mg (1 x 200 mg tablet or 2 x 100 mg tablets) bid following a meal
Pediatric: <3 year: not recommended; **≥3 years,** >16 kg: 16-< 20 kg: 100 mg bid; **20-<25 kg:** 125 mg bid; **25-<30 kg:** 150 mg bid; ≥30 kg: 200 mg bid; max 200 mg bid; take following a mail
   Intelence *Tab*: 25*, 100, 200 mg

▷ *nevirapine* (B)(G) initially one 200 mg tablet of immediate-release **Viramune** once daily for the first 14 days in combination with other antiretroviral agents; then, one 400 mg tablet of **Viramune XR** once daily
Comment: The 14-day lead-in period has been found to lessen the frequency of rash.
Pediatric: <6 years: not recommended; 6-<18 years: BSA 0.58-0.83 kg/m²: 200 mg once daily; BSA 0.84-1.16 kg/m²: 300 mg once daily; BSA ≥1.17 kg/m²: 400 mg; once daily; max 400 mg once daily
Comment: Children must initiate therapy with immediate-release **Viramune** for the first 14 days; ≥15 days: [oral susp/tab]: 150 mg/m² once daily for 14 days, then 150 mg/m² bid
   Viramune *Tab*: 200*mg
   Viramune Oral Suspension *Oral susp*: 50 mg/5 ml (240 ml)
   Viramune XR *Tab*: 100, 400 mg ext-rel

▷ *rilpivirine* (D) 25 mg once daily; *If concomitant rifabutin*: 50 mg once daily; *If concomitant rifabutin stopped*: 25 mg once daily
Pediatric: <12 years: not recommended; ≥12 years, >35 kg: same adult
   Edurant *Tab*: 25 mg

Nucleoside and Nonnucleoside Reverse Transcriptase Inhibitor (NRTI/NNRTI) Combinations

▷ **Atripla** (B)(G) *efavirenz+emtricitabine+tenofovir disoproxil fumarate* 1 tab once daily preferably at HS; take on an empty stomach; *Concomitant rifabutin*: >50 kg: take additional *efavirenz* 200 mg/day
Pediatric: <12 years: not recommended; ≥12 years, 40 kg: same as adult
   Tab: efa 600 mg+emtri 200 mg+teno dis fum 300 mg

▷ **Complera** (B) *emtricitabine+tenofovir disoproxil fumarate+rilpivirine* 1 tab once daily; *CrCl <50 mL/min*: not recommended; *Concomitant rifabutin*: take additional *ribavirin* 25 mg qd
Pediatric: <12 years, <35 kg: not established; ≥12 years, ≥35 kg: same as adult
   Tab: emtri 200 mg+teno dis 300 mg+rilpiv 25 mg

Protease Inhibitors (PIs)

▷ *atazanavir* (B)(G) *Treatment naive: Recommended regimen*: 300 mg plus **ritonavir** 100 mg once daily; *Unable to tolerate ritonavir*: 400 mg once daily; *In combination with efavirenz*: 400 mg plus *ritonavir* 100 mg once daily; *Treatment experienced: Recommended regimen*: 300 mg plus *ritonavir* 100 mg once daily; *In combination with both an H2-blocker or PPI and tenofovir*: 400 mg plus *ritonavir* 100 mg once daily; take with food

Pediatric: <3 months: not recommended; ≥3 months, 5 kg: [oral pwdr] 5-<15 kg: 200 mg (4 packets) plus *ritonavir* 80 mg once daily; 15-<25 kg: 250 mg (5 packets) plus *ritonavir* 80 mg once daily; ≥25 kg, unable to swallow capsules: 300 mg (6 packets) plus *ritonavir* once daily; 6 years, <15 kg: [cap] 15-<20 kg: 150 mg plus *ritonavir* 100 mg once daily; 20-<40 kg: 200 mg plus *ritonavir* 100 mg once daily; ≥40 kg: 300 mg plus *ritonavir* 100 mg once daily; [capsule]15-<20 kg: 150 mg plus *ritonavir* 100 mg once daily; 20-<40 kg: 200 mg plus *ritonavir* 100 mg once daily; ≥40 kg: 300 mg plus *ritonavir* 100 mg once daily; max dose 400 mg once daily; take with food

    Reyataz *Cap:* 100, 150, 200, 300 mg; *Oral pwdr:* 50 mg/pkt (30/carton) (phenylalanine)

Comment: Administration of *atazanavir* with *ritonavir* is preferred. Dose for treatment-naïve children ≥13 years of age and ≥40 kg unable to tolerate *ritonavir*, administer 400 mg once daily. See mfr pkg insert for special dosing considerations when combining *atazanavir* with other retrovirals.

▷ *darunavir* (C)(G) *Treatment naïve and treatment experienced with no darunavir resistance associated substitutions:* 800 mg once daily with *ritonavir* 100 mg once daily; *Treatment-experienced with at least one darunavir resistance associated substitution:* 600 mg bid with ritonavir 100 mg bid; *Severe hepatic impairment:* not recommended
    Pediatric: ≥3 years, 10 kg [oral soln/tab/cap] *Treatment naïve or experienced without darunavir-associated substitutions:* 10-<15 kg: 35 mg/kg once daily plus *ritonavir* 7 mg/kg once daily; 15-<30 kg: 600 mg plus *ritonavir* 100 mg once daily; 30-<40 kg: 675 mg plus *ritonavir* 100 mg once daily; >40 kg: 800 mg plus *ritonavir* 100 mg once daily; *Treatment experienced with ≥1 darunavir-associated substitution(s):* 10-15 kg: 20 mg/kg bid plus *ritonavir* 3 mg/kg bid; 15-<30 kg: 375 mg plus *ritonavir* 48 mg bid; 30-<40 kg: 450 mg plus *ritonavir* 60 mg bid; >40 kg: 600 mg plus *ritonavir* 100 mg bid

    Prezista *Tab:* 75, 150, 600, 800 mg film-coat

    Prezista Oral Suspension *Susp:* 100 mg/ml (strawberry cream)

Comment: **Prezista** is FDA approved for treatment of HIV-1-infected pregnant women and for the treatment of children >3 years-of-age in combination with *ritonavir* and other antiretrovirals.

▷ *fosamprenavir* (C)(G) *Treatment-naïve:* 1,400 mg bid or 1,400 mg once daily plus *ritonavir* 200 mg once daily or 1,400 mg once daily plus *ritonavir* 100 mg once daily or 700 mg bid plus *ritonavir* 100 mg bid; *Protease inhibitor-experienced:* 700 mg bid plus *ritonavir* 100 mg bid
    Pediatric: <4 weeks: not recommended; *Protease inhibitor-naïve, ≥4 weeks or protease inhibitor-experienced:* ≥6 Months, <11 kg: 45 mg/kg plus *ritonavir* 7 mg/kg bid; 11-<15 kg: 30 mg/kg plus *ritonavir* 3 mg/kg bid; 15 kg-<20 kg: 23 mg/kg plus *ritonavir* 3 mg/kg bid; ≥20 kg: 18 mg/kg plus *ritonavir* 3 mg/kg bid; *Protease-inhibitor naïve, ≥2 years:* 30 mg/kg bid without *ritonavir*: max dose 700 mg plus *ritonavir* 100 mg bid

    Lexiva: *Tab:* 700 mg film-coat

    Lexiva Oral Suspension *Oral susp:* 50 mg/ml (225 ml) (grape-bubble gum-peppermint)

Comment: *fosamprenavir* 1 ml is equivalent to approximately 43 mg of *amprenavir* 1 ml.

▷ *indinavir sulfate* (C) 800 mg q 8 hours; *Concomitant rifabutin:* 1 gm q 8 hours and reduce *rifabutin* dose by half; *Hepatic insufficiency or concomitant ketoconazole, itraconazole, or delavirdine:* 600 mg q 8 hours; take with water on an empty stomach or with a light meal
    Pediatric: <3 years: not established ≥3-18 years, doses of 500 mg/m² every 8 hours have been used; see mfr pkg insert)

    Crixivan *Cap:* 100, 200, 333, 400 mg

▷ *nelfinavir mesylate* (B) 1250 mg (5 x 250 mg tablets or 2 x 625 mg tablets) bid or 750 mg (3 x 250 mg tablets) tid; take with a meal; may dissolve tablets in a small amount of water; max 2500 mg/day
    Pediatric: <2 years: not established; 2-13 years: 45-55 mg/kg bid or 25-35 mg/kg tid; take with a meal; max 2500 mg/day; ≥13 years: same as adult

    Viracept *Tab:* 250, 625 mg

    Viracept Oral Powder *Oral pwdr:* 50 mg/gm (144 gm) (phenylalanine)

Comment: The 250 mg **Viracept** tabs are interchangeable with oral powder, the 625 mg tabs are not.

▷ *raltegravir (as potassium)* (C) 400 mg bid
    Pediatric: ≥4 weeks, 3-11 kg: [oral susp] 3-<4 kg: 20 mg bid; 4-<6 kg: 30 mg bid; 6-<8 kg: 40 mg bid; 8-<11 kg: 60 mg bid; ≥11-<25 kg: [oral susp/chew tab] 6 mg/kg/dose bid; see mfr pkg insert for dosage by weight; ≥25 kg and unable to swallow tablet: [chew tab] 25-<28 kg: 150 mg bid; 28-<40 kg: 200 mg bid; ≥40 kg: 300 mg bid; ≥6 years, ≥25 kg, able to swallow tablets: 400 mg film-coat tablet bid

Comment: Oral suspension, chewable tablets, and film-coat tablets are not bioequivalent. Chewable tablet max dose 300 mg bid. Film-coat tablets max dose 400 mg bid. Oral suspension max dose 100 mg bid

Isentress *Tab:* 400 mg film-coat; *Chew tab:* 25, 100*mg (orange-banana) (phenylalanine)

Isentress Oral Suspension *Oral susp:* 100 mg/pkt pwdr for oral susp (banana)

▷ *ritonavir* (B)(G) initially 300 mg bid; increase at 2-3 day intervals by 100 mg bid; max 600 mg bid

Pediatric: <1 month: not recommended; ≥1 month: 350-400 mg/m² bid; initiate at 250 mg/m² bid and titrate upward every 2-3 days by 50 mg/m² bid; max dose 600 mg bid

Comment: Lower doses of *ritonavir* have been used to boost other protease inhibitors but the *ritonavir* doses used for boosting have not been specifically approved in children.

Norvir *Tab:* 100 mg film-coat; *Gel cap:* 100 mg (alcohol)

Norvir Oral Solution *Oral soln:* 80 mg/ml, 600 mg/7.5 ml (8 oz) (peppermint-caramel) (alcohol)

Comment: Norvir tablets should be swallowed whole. Take Norvir with meals. Patients may improve the taste of Norvir Oral Solution by mixing with chocolate milk, Ensure, or Advera within one hour of dosing. Dose reduction of Norvir is necessary when used with other protease inhibitors (*atazanavir, darunavir, fosamprenavir, saquinavir,* and *tipranavir.* Patients who take the 600 mg gel cap bid may experience more gastrointestinal side effects such as nausea, vomiting, abdominal pain or diarrhea when switching from the gel cap to the tablet because of greater maximum plasma concentration (Cmax) achieved with the tablet. These adverse events (gastrointestinal or paresthesias) may diminish as treatment is continued.

▷ *saquinavir mesylate* (B)

Pediatric: <16 years: not established; ≥16 years: same as adult

Fortovase *Tab/Cap:* 200 mg

Invirase *Tab:* 500 mg; *Cap:* 200 mg

▷ *tipranavir* (C) 500 mg bid plus ritonavir 200 mg bid

Pediatric: <2 years: not recommended; 2-18 years: [cap/oral soln] 14 mg/kg plus *ritonavir* 6 mg/kg bid or 375 mg/m² plus *ritonavir* 150 mg/m² bid; max 500 mg plus *ritonavir* 200 mg bid

Aptivus *Gel cap:* 250 mg (alcohol)

Aptivus Oral Solution *Oral soln:* 100 mg/ml (buttermint-butter toffee) (Vit E 116 IU/ml)

FUSION INHIBITORS—CCR5 CO-RECEPTOR ANTAGONISTS

▷ *enfuvirtide* (B) 90 mg (1 ml) SC bid; administer in upper arm, abdomen, or anterior thigh; rotate injection sites

Pediatric: <6 years: not established; 6-16 years: administer 2 mg/kg SC bid; max 90 mg SC bid; >16 years: same as adult; rotate injection sites

Fuzeon *Vial:* 90 mg/ml pwdr for SC inj after reconstitution (1 ml, 60 vials/kit) (preservative-free)

▷ *maraviroc* (B) must be administered concomitant with other retrovirals; *Concomitant potent CYP3A inhibitors (with or without a potent CYP3A inducer) including protease inhibitors (*except *tipranavir+ritonavir), delavirdine, ketoconazole, itraconazole, clarithromycin, other potent CYP3A inhibitors (e.g., nefazodone, telithromycin): CrCl ≥30 mL/min:* 150 mg bid; *<30 mL/min, dialysis:* not recommended; *Potent CYP3A inducers (without a potent CYP3A inhibitor) including efavirenz, rifampin, etravirine, carbamazepine, phenobarbital, and phenytoin:* 300 mg bid; *CrCl ≥30 mL/min:* 600 mg bid; *<30 mL/min:* not recommended; *Other concomitant agents, including tipranavir+ritonavir, nevirapine, raltegravir, all NRTIs, and enfuvirtide:* 300 mg bid

Pediatric: <16 years: not established; ≥16 years: same as adult

Selzentry *Tab:* 150, 300 mg film-coat

CD4-DIRECTED POST-ATTACHMENT HIV-1 INHIBITOR

▷ *ibalizumab-uiyk* administer as an IV injection once every 14 days

Pediatric: <18 years: not established; ≥18 years: same as adult

Trogarzo *Vial:* 200 mg/1.33 ml (1.33 ml) single-dose

Comment: Trogarzo *(ibalizumab)* is indicated for the treatment of patients with HIV infection who are heavily treatment-experienced and multi-drug resistant infection. It is intended for use in combination with other anti-retroviral medications.

BRAND NAMES, DOSING, AND DOSE FORMS: COMBINATION AGENTS

▷ Atripla (B)(G) *efavirenz+emtricitabine+tenofovir disoproxil fumarate* 1 tablet once daily on an empty stomach; bedtime dosing may improve the tolerability of nervous system symptoms; *CrCl <50 mL/min:* not recommended
Pediatric: <12 years, <40 kg: not established; ≥12 years, ≥40 kg: same as adult
   Tab: efa 600 mg+emtri 200 mg+teno dis fum 300 mg film-coat

▷ Biktarvy *bictegravir+emtricitabine+tenofovir alafenamide* take 1 tablet once daily with or without food
Pediatric: <18 years: not established; ≥18 years: same as adult
   Tab: bict 50 mg+emtri 200 mg+teno alaf 25 mg

Comment: **Biktarvy** is a three-drug combination of *bictegravir*, a human immunodeficiency virus type 1 (HIV-1) integrase strand transfer inhibitor (INSTI), and *emtricitabine* and *tenofovir alafenamide* , both HIV-1 nucleoside analog reverse transcriptase inhibitors (NRTIs) indicated as a complete regimen for the treatment of HIV-1 infection in adults who have no antiretroviral treatment history or to replace the current antiretroviral regimen in those who are virologically suppressed (HIV-1 RNA less than 50 copies per mL) on a stable antiretroviral regimen for at least 3 months with no history of treatment failure and no known substitutions associated with resistance to the individual components of **Biktarvy**. **Biktarvy** is not recommended in patients with estimated CrCl <30 mL/min and/or with severe hepatic impairment.

▷ Cimduo *lamivudine+tenofovir disoproxil fumarate* 1 tablet once daily with or without food
Pediatric: <35 kg: not recommended; ≥35 kg: same as adult
   Tab: lami 300 mg+teno teno diso 300 mg

Comment: **Cimduo** is a two-drug fixed-dose combination of *lamivudine* and *tenofovir disoproxil fumarate*, both nucleoside reverse transcriptase inhibitors (NRTIs) and is indicated for the treatment of HIV-1 infection in in combination with other antiretroviral agents. Prior to initiation and during treatment with **Cimduo**, patients should be tested for hepatitis B virus (HBV) infection, and estimated CrCl, serum phosphorus, urine glucose, and urine protein should be obtained. **Cimduo** is not recommended in patients with CrCL < 50 mL/min or patients with end-stage renal disease (ESRD) requiring hemodialysis. Discontinue treatment in patients who develop symptoms or laboratory findings suggestive of lactic acidosis or pronounced hepatotoxicity.

▷ Combivir (C)(G) *lamivudine+zidovudine*
Pediatric: <12 years: not recommended; ≥12 years, ≥30 kg: 1 tablet bid with food
   Tab: lami 150 mg+zido 300 mg

▷ Complera (B) *emtricitabine+tenofovir disoproxil fumarate+rilpivirine* 1 tablet once daily; *CrCl <50 mL/min:* not recommended
Pediatric: <12 years, <40 kg: not recommended; ≥12 years, ≥40 kg: same as adult
   Tab: emtri 200 mg+teno dis 300 mg+rilpiv 25 mg

▷ Delstrigo *doravirine+lamivudine+tenofovir disoproxil fumarate* 1 tablet once daily with or without food; *CrCl <50 mL/min:* not recommended
Pediatric: <18 years: not established; ≥18 years: same as adult
   Tab: dora 100 mg+lami ala 300 mg+teno dis 300 mg

Comment: *Delstrigo is approved as a complete 3-drug fixed-dose once daily regimen for patients with no prior antiretroviral treatment experience.* Monitor for new onset or worsening renal impairment. Prior to or when initiating **Delstrigo**, and during treatment on a clinically appropriate schedule, assess serum creatinine, estimated creatinine clearance, urine glucose, and urine protein in all patients. Avoid administering **Delstrigo** with concurrent or recent use of nephrotoxic drugs. In patients with chronic kidney disease (CKD), also assess serum phosphorus. Severe acute exacerbations of hepatitis B (HBV) have been reported in patients co-infected with HIV-1 and HBV who have discontinued *lamivudine* or *tenofovir disoproxil fumarate* (TDF), two of the components of **Delstrigo**. Closely monitor hepatic function in these patients. If appropriate, initiation of anti-hepatitis B therapy may be warranted. Dosage adjustment with *rifabutin:* Take one tablet of **Delstrigo** once daily, followed by one tablet of *doravirine* 100 mg (**Pifeltro**) approximately 12 hours after the dose of **Delstrigo**. There is a pregnancy exposure registry that monitors pregnancy outcomes in individuals exposed to **Delstrigo** during pregnancy. Healthcare providers are encouraged to register patients by calling the Antiretroviral Pregnancy Registry (APR) at 1-800-258-4263.

▷ Descovy (D) *emtricitabine+tenofovir alafenamide* 1 tablet once daily with or without food; *CrCl <30 mL/min:* not recommended

Pediatric: <12 years, <35 kg: not recommended; ≥12 years, ≥35 kg: same as adult
   Tab: emtri 200 mg+teno ala 25 mg

Comment: Patients with HIV-1 should be tested for the presence of chronic hepatitis B virus (HBV) before initiating antiretroviral therapy. **Descovy** is not approved for the treatment of chronic HBV infection, and the safety and efficacy of **Descovy** have not been established in patients co-infected with HIV-1 and HBV.

▷ **Epzicom (B)(G)** *abacavir sulfate+lamivudine* 1 tab daily; *Mild hepatic impairment* <u>or</u> *CrCl<50 mL/min:* not recommended
Pediatric: <25 kg: use individual components; ≥25 kg: one tablet once daily; *Mild hepatic impairment* <u>or</u> *CrCl<50 mL/min:* not recommended
   Tab: aba 600 mg/lami 300 mg

▷ **Evotaz (B)** *atazanavir+cobicistat* 1 tab once daily
Pediatric: <12 years, <35 kg: not established; ≥12 years, ≥35 kg: same as adult
   Tab: ataz 600 mg+cobi 300 mg

▷ **Genvoya (B)** *elvitegravir+cobicistat+emtricitabine+tenofovir alafenamide* 1 tab once daily; *Severe hepatic impairment* <u>or</u> *CrCl <30 mL/min:* not recommended; take with food
Pediatric: <12 years, <35 kg: not established; ≥12 years, ≥35 kg: same as adult
   Tab: elvi 150 mg+cobi 150 mg+emtri 200 mg+teno 10 mg

▷ **Juluca** *dolutegravir+rilpivirine* take one tablet once daily with <u>or</u> without food
Pediatric: <18 years: not established; ≥18 years: same as adult
   Tab: dolu 50 mg+rilp 25 mg film-coat

Comment: **Juluca** is a complete two-drug fixed-dose combination of *dolute gravir*, a human immunodeficiency virus type 1 (HIV-1) integrase strand transfer inhibitor (INSTI) and *rilpivirine*, a HIV-1 non-nucleoside reverse transcriptase inhibitor (NNRTI), indicated for treatment of HIV infection to replace the current antiretroviral regimen in those who are virologically suppressed (HIV-1 RNA <50 copies per mL) on a stable antiretroviral regimen for at least 6 months, with no history of treatment failure, and no known substitutions associated with resistance to the individual components of **Juluca**. Pregnancy testing and contraception are recommended before initiation of **Juluca** in females of childbearing potential. Avoid use of **Juluca** at the time of conception through the first trimester due to the risk of neural tube defects.

▷ **Kaletra, Kaletra Oral Solution (C)(G)** *lopinavir+ritonavir* 800+200 mg (4 tablets <u>or</u> 10 ml) once daily <u>or</u> 400/100 (2 tablets <u>or</u> 5 ml) bid; *May administer once daily <u>or</u> bid:* patients with <3 *lopinavir* resistance-associated substitutions; *May dose bid only:* patients with ≥3 resistance-associated substitutions; *Dose must be increased:* when administered in combination with *efavirenz, nevirapine,* <u>or</u> *nelfinavir* (500 mg/125 mg (2 x 200/50 tab <u>plus</u> 1 x 100/25 tab) bid <u>or</u> 520/130 (6.5 ml) bid; *Once daily dosing regimen not recommended:* in combination with ≥3 *lopinavir* resistance-associated substitutions <u>or</u> in combination with: *carbamazepine, phenobarbital,* <u>or</u> *phenytoin*; Patients receiving *nevirapine* <u>or</u> *efavirenz* with **Kaletra** should have their **Kaletra** dose increased; swallow whole with <u>or</u> without food
Pediatric: dose calculation is based on the *lopinavir* component; 14 days-6 months: 16 mg/kg bid; 6 months-12 years: [tab/cap/soln] 7-<15 kg: 12 mg/kg bid (13 mg/kg <u>plus</u> *nevirapine*); 15-40 kg: 10 mg/kg bid (11 mg/kg <u>plus</u> *nevirapine*), ≥40 kg, >12 years: *lopinavir* 400 mg bid (533 mg <u>plus</u> *nevirapine*); max *lopinavir* 400 mg bid for patients who are not receiving *nevirapine* <u>or</u> *efavirenz*; Kaletra should not be used in combination with NNRTIs in children <6 months-of-age; see mfr pkg insert for BSA-based dosing
   Tab: **Kaletra 100/25** lopin 100 mg+riton 25 mg
      Kaletra 200/50 lopin 200 mg+riton 50 mg
   Oral Soln: lopin 80 mg+riton 20 mg per ml; lopin 400 mg+riton 500 mg per 5 ml (160 ml) (cotton candy) (alcohol 42.4%)

▷ **Odefsey (D)** *emtricitabine+rilpivirine+tenofovir alafenamide* 1 tab once daily with food; *CrCl <30 mL/min:* not recommended
Pediatric: <12 years, <35 kg: not established; ≥12 years, >35 kg: same as adult
   Tab: emtri 200 mg+rilpi 25 mg+teno alafen 25 mg

▷ **Prezcobix (C)** *darunavir+cobicistat* 1 tab once daily; *Treatment naïve and treatment experienced with no darunavir resistance-associated substitution:* 800 mg once daily <u>plus</u> *ritonavir* 100 mg once daily; *Treatment experienced with at least one darunavir resistance associated substitution:* 600 mg bid <u>plus</u> *ritonavir* 100 mg bid; take with food; *CrCl <70 mL/min:* not recommended
Pediatric: not recommended
   Tab: darun 800 mg+cobi 150 mg

▷ **Stribild (B)(G)** *elvitegravir+cobicistat+emtricitabine+tenofovir disoproxil fumarate* 1 tab once daily; *CrCl <70 mL/min:* not recommended; *if CrCl declines to <50 mL/min during treatment:* discontinue; *Severe hepatic impairment:* not recommended
Pediatric: <12 years: not recommended; ≥12 years: same as adult
    Tab: elvi 150 mg+cobi 150 mg+emtri 200 mg+teno dis fum 300 mg

▷ **Symfi** *efavirenz+lamivudine+tenofovir disoproxil fumarate* take 1 tablet once daily with or without food
Pediatric: <40 kg: not studied; ≥40 kg: same as adult
    Tab: efav 600 mg+lami 300 mg+teno diso fum 300 mg

Comment: **Symfi** is a complete three-drug fixed-dose regimen for the treatment HIV-1 infection in adults and children weighing >40 kg. It contains the same triple combination ingredients found in **Symfi Lo** but with a 600 mg dose of *efavirenzvs* vs the 400 mg in **Symfi Lo**. Safety and effectiveness of **Symfi** as a fixed-dose tablet in pediatric patients weighing ≥40 kg have been established based on clinical studies using the individual components.

▷ **Symfi Lo** *efavirenz+lamivudine+tenofovir disoproxil fumarate* 1 tablet once daily with or without food
Pediatric: <35 kg: not studied; ≥35 kg: same as adult
    Tab: efav 400 mg+lami 300 mg+teno diso fum 300 mg

Comment: **Symfi Lo** is a complete three-drug fixed-dose regimen for the treatment HIV-1 infection in adults and children weighing ≥45 kg. It contains the same triple combination ingredients found in **Symfi** but with a 400 mg dose of *efavirenz* vs the 600 mg in **Symfi Lo**. Safety and effectiveness of **Symfi** as a fixed-dose tablet in pediatric patients weighing ≥40 kg have been established based on clinical studies using the individual components.

▷ **Symtuza** *darunavir+cobicistat+emtricitabine+tenofovir alafenamide* 1 tablet once daily with food
Pediatric: <18 years: not recommended; ≥18 years: same as adult
    Tab: daru 800 mg+cobic 150 mg+emtri 200 mg+tenofo alafen 10 mg

Comment: **Symtuza** is indicated as a complete regimen for the treatment of HIV infection in adults who have no prior antiretroviral treatment history or who are virologically suppressed (HIV-1 RNA less than 50 copies per ml) on a stable antiretroviral regimen for at least 6 months and have no known substitutions associated with resistance to *darunavir* or *tenofovir*. Assess serum creatinine, estimated creatinine clearance, urine glucose, and urine protein on a clinically appropriate schedule. In patients with chronic kidney disease, also assess serum phosphorus. **Symtuza** is not recommended in patients with estimated CrCl <30 mL/min and patients with severe hepatic impairment. **Symtuza** is not recommended during pregnancy due to substantially lower exposures of *darunavir* and *cobicistat* during pregnancy. Breastfeeding is not recommended. Co-administration of **Symtuza** with other drugs can alter the concentration of other drugs and other drugs may alter the concentrations of **Symtuza** components. Consult the mfr pkg insert prior to and during treatment for potential drug interactions.

▷ **Temixys** *lamivudine+tenofovir disoproxil fumarate* 1 tab once daily with or without food
Pediatric: <35 kg: not recommended; ≥35 kg: same as adult
    Tab: lami 300 mg+teno diso fum 300mg

Comment: **Temixys**, a fixed-dose combination of two nucleoside reverse transcriptase inhibitors is indicated in combination with other antiretroviral agents. Discontinue treatment in patients who develop symptoms or laboratory findings suggestive of lactic acidosis or pronounced hepatotoxicity including severe hepatomegaly with steatosis. In patients at risk for renal dysfunction, assess estimated creatinine clearance, serum phosphorus, urine glucose, and urine protein before initiating treatment with **Temixys** and periodically during treatment. Avoid administering **Temixys** with concurrent or recent use of nephrotoxic drugs. Healthcare providers are encouraged to register patients exposed to **Temexis** by calling the Antiretroviral Pregnancy Registry (APR) at 1-800-258-4263. Instruct mothers not to breastfeed if they are receiving **Temixys**.

▷ **Triumeq (C)(G)** *abacavir sulfate+dolutegravir+lamivudine* 1 tab once daily
Pediatric: <12 years: not recommended; ≥12 years: same as adult
    Tab: aba 600 mg+dolu 50 mg+lami 300 mg

▷ **Trizivir (C)(G)** *abacavir sulfate+lamivudine+zidovudine* 1 tab bid
Pediatric: <40 kg: not recommended; ≥40 kg: same as adult
    Tab: aba 300 mg+lami 150 mg+zido 300 mg

HUMAN PAPILLOMAVIRUS (HPV, VENEREAL WART)

TREATMENT
see Wart: Venereal page 533

PROPHYLAXIS
▶ *human papillomavirus 9-valent (types 6, 11, 16, 18, 31, 33, 45, 52, and 58) vaccine, recombinant, aluminum adsorbed* (B)
Males and Females 9 to 45 Years-of-Age: administer IM in the deltoid <u>or</u> thigh *9-14 years (2-dose regimen):* 0.5 ml IM at 0 and 6-12 months; (if the second dose is administered earlier than 5 months after the first dose, administer a third dose at least 4 months after the second dose) *9-14 years: (3-dose regimen):* administer 0.5 ml IM at 0, 2, and 6 months *15-45 years (3-dose regimen):* administer 0.5 ml IM at 0, 2, and 6 months
    Gardasil 9 *Vial:* 0.5 ml (single-dose); *Prefilled syringe w. needles <u>or</u> tip caps:* 0.5 ml (single-dose) (preservative-free)
Comment: **Gardasil 9** is indicated for prevention of genital warts *(condyloma acuminata)* caused by HPV types 6 and11 and prevention of cervical, vulvar, vaginal, and anal cancer caused by HPV types 16, 18, 31, 33, 45, 52, and 58. There are no adequate and well-controlled studies of **Gardasil 9** in pregnancy. Available human data do not demonstrate vaccine-associated increase in risk of major birth defects and miscarriages when **Gardasil 9** is administered during pregnancy. Register pregnant patients exposed to **Gardasil 9** by calling 1-800-986-8999. Available data are not sufficient to assess the effects of **Gardasil 9** on the breastfed infant.

 HUNTINGTON DISEASE-ASSOCIATED CHOREA

VESICULAR MONOAMINE TRANSPORTER 2 (VMAT2) INHIBITOR
▶ *deutetrabenazine* take with food; initially 6 mg once daily; titrate up at weekly intervals by 6 mg per day to a tolerated dose that reduces chorea; administer total daily dosages ≥12 mg in two divided doses; max recommended daily dose 36 mg/day divided bid (18 mg twice daily); swallow whole; do not chew, crush, <u>or</u> break; if switching from *tetrabenazine,* discontinue *tetrabenazine* and initiate **Austedo** the following day; see mfr pkg insert for full prescribing information and for a recommended conversion table
Pediatric: <12 years: not established; ≥12 years: same as adult
    Austedo *Tab:* 6, 9, 12 mg
Comment: The most common adverse effects of *deutetrabenazine* are somnolence, diarrhea, dry mouth, fatigue, and sedation, as well as an increased risk of depression and suicidal thoughts and behaviors. **Austedo** is contraindicated for patients with untreated or inadequately treated depression, who are suicidal, have hepatic impairment, are taking MAOIs, *reserpine,* <u>or</u> *tetrabenazine.* **Austedo** may increase the risk of akathisia, agitation and restlessness, and may cause parkinsonism in patients with Huntington disease. There are no adequate data on the developmental risk associated with the use of **Austedo** in pregnant women <u>or</u> lactation.
▶ *trabenazine* individualization of dose with careful weekly titration is required. *Week 1:* starting dose is 12.5 mg daily; *Week 2:* 25 mg (12.5 mg twice daily); then slowly titrate dose by 12.5 mg/day at weekly intervals as tolerated to a dose that reduces chorea; doses of 37.5 mg and up to 50 mg per day should be administered in three divided doses per day with a maximum recommended single dose not to exceed 25 mg; patients requiring doses above 50 mg per day should be genotyped for the drug metabolizing enzyme CYP2D6 to determine if the patient is a poor metabolizer (PM) <u>or</u> an extensive metabolizer (EM); max daily dose in PMs is 50 mg with a max single dose of 25 mg
Pediatric: <12 years: not established; ≥12 years: same as adult
    Xenazine *Tab:* 12.5, 25*mg
Comment: Most common adverse reactions are sedation/somnolence, fatigue, insomnia, depression, akathisia, anxiety/anxiety aggravated, nausea. BBW: **Xenazine** increases the risk of depression and suicidal thoughts and behavior (suicidality) in patients with Huntington's disease. Balance risks of depression and suicidality with the clinical need for control of chorea when considering the use of **Xenazine**. Monitor patients for the emergence <u>or</u> worsening of depression, suicidality, <u>or</u> unusual changes

in behavior. Inform patients, caregivers and families of the risk of depression and suicidality and instruct to report behaviors of concern promptly to the treating health care provider. Exercise caution when treating patients with a history of depression or prior suicide attempts or ideation.

Xenazine is contraindicated in patients who are actively suicidal, and in patients with untreated or inadequately treated depression, hepatic impairment, concomitant an MAOI or reserpine, taking **deutetrabenazine** or **valbenazine**.

▶ **valbenazine** initially 40 mg once daily; after one week, increase to the recommended 80 mg once daily; take with or without food; recommended dose for patients with moderate or severe hepatic impairment is 40 mg once daily; consider dose reduction based on tolerability in known CYP2D6 poor metabolizers; concomitant use of strong CYP3A4 inducers is not recommended; avoid concomitant use of MAOIs
Pediatric: <18 years: not established; ≥18 years: same as adult

    Ingrezza *Cap:* 40 mg

    Comment: Safety and effectiveness of **Ingrezza** have not been established in pediatric patients. No dose adjustment is required for elderly patients. The limited available data on **Ingrezza** use in pregnant women are insufficient to inform a drug-associated risk. There is no information regarding the presence of **Ingrezza** or its metabolites in human milk, the effects on the breastfed infant, or the effects on milk production. However, women are advised not to breastfeed during treatment and for 5 days after the final dose. To report suspected adverse reactions, contact Neurocrine Biosciences, Inc. at 877-641-3461 or FDA at 1-800-FDA-1088 or www.fda.gov/medwatch.

HYPERCALCEMIA

CALCIUM-SENSING RECEPTOR AGONIST

See page 238 for *cinacalcet* dosing in adult patients with secondary hyperparathyroidism (HPT) due to chronic kidney disease CKD.

▶ **cinacalcet** (C)(G) take tabs whole; with food or shortly after a meal; *Hypercalcemia, including hypercalcemia in patients with primary HPT:* initially 30 mg 2 x/day; titrate dose every 2 to 4 weeks through sequential doses of 30 mg 2 x/day, 60 mg 2 x/day, 90 mg 2 x/day, and 90 mg 3 or 4 x/day as necessary to normalize serum calcium levels; once the maintenance dose has been established, monitor serum calcium approximately every 2 months; iPTH levels should be measured no earlier than 12 hours after most recent dose
Pediatric: <18 years: not indicated; ≥18 years: same as adult

    Sensipar *Tab:* 30, 60, 90 mg

    Comment: **Sensipar** is indicated for the treatment of hypercalcemia in adult patients with parathyroid carcinoma and patients with primary HPT for whom parathyroidectomy would be indicated on the basis of serum calcium levels, but who are unable to undergo parathyroidectomy. Co-administration with a strong CYP3A4 inhibitor may increase serum levels of *cinacalcet*; dose adjustment and monitoring of iPTH serum phosphorus and serum calcium may be required. *cinacalcet* is a strong inhibitor of CYP2D6. Dose adjustments may be required for concomitant medications that are predominantly metabolized by CYP2D6. **Sensipar** has been shown to cross the placental barrier in animal studies. There are no adequate and well-controlled studies of *Sensipar* in pregnancy. **Sensipar** should be used during pregnancy only if the potential benefit justifies the potential risk to the fetus. Animal studies have shown that **Sensipar** is excreted in milk with a high milk-to-plasma ratio. It is not known whether **Sensipar** is excreted in human milk. Because of the potential for clinically significant adverse reactions in infants from **Sensipar**, risk/benefit should be discussed and a decision should be made whether to discontinue breast-feeding or to discontinue the drug. No differences in the safety and efficacy of **Sensipar** were observed in patients > or < than 65 years-of-age.

HYPEREMESIS GRAVIDARUM/NAUSEA AND VOMITING OF PREGNANCY

ANTIHISTAMINE+VITAMIN B ANALOG

Comment: **Bonjesta** and **Diclegis** are indicated for nausea/vomiting of pregnancy in women who do not respond to conservative management. Somnolence (severe drowsiness) can occur when used in combination with alcohol or other sedating medications. Use with caution in patients with asthma, increased intraocular pressure, narrow angle glaucoma, stenosing peptic ulcer, pyloroduodenal obstruction and urinary bladder-neck obstruction. Concomitant monoamine oxidase inhibitors (MAOIs) are contraindicated because MAOIs prolong and intensify the anticholinergic effects of antihistamines, especially long-acting formulations. *doxylamine* is secreted in breast milk; therefore, breastfeeding is not recommended.

➤ *doxylamine* succinate+*pyridoxine* **hydrochloride** one tab at HS prn; if symptoms are not adequately controlled, the dose can be increased to max one tablet in the AM and one tab at HS
Pediatric: <18 years: not established; ≥18 years: same as adult
    Bonjesta *Tab:* doxy 20 mg+pyri 20 mg ext-rel
    Diclegis *Tab:* doxy 10 mg+pyri 10 mg ext-rel

 HYPERHIDROSIS (PERSPIRATION, EXCESSIVE)

Comment: Hyperhidrosis is a common, self-limiting problem that affects 2% to3% of the US population. Patients may complain of localized sweating of the hands, feet, face, or underarms, or more systemic, generalized sweating in multiple locations and report a significant impact on their quality of life.

REFERENCE

Varella, A. Y., Fukuda, J. M., Telvelis, M. P., Campos, J. R., Kauffman, P., Cucato, G. G., . . . Wolosker, N. (2016). Translation and validation of hyperhidrosis disease severity scale. *Revista da Associação Médica Brasileira, 62*(9), 843–847. doi:10.1590/1806-9282.62.09.843

➤ *aluminum chloride* 20% solution apply q HS; wash treated area the following morning; after 1-2 treatments, may reduce frequency to 1-2 x/week
    Drysol *Soln:* 35, 60 ml (alcohol 93%) cont-rel
Comment: Apply to clean dry skin (e.g., underarms). Do not apply to broken, irritated, or recently shaved skin.

TOPICAL ANTICHOLINERGIC

➤ *glycopyrronium* unfold one **Qbrexza** cloth and apply by wiping across one entire underarm one time; using the same cloth, wipe across the other under arm one time; discard used cloth; wash hands immediately; repeat once every 24 hours
Pediatric: <9 years: not recommended; ≥9 years:
    Qbrexza Pre-moistened cloth (single-use pouch)
    Comment: Qbrexza (*glycopyrronium*) is the first FDA-approved, once-daily, topical treatment indicated for patients ≥9 years-of-age with primary axillary hyperhidrosis. *glycopyrronium* is anticholinergic; it is important to wash hands after **Qbrexza** cloths are used because it can cause blurred vision if the eyes are touched. Do not re-use **Qbrexza** cloths. **Qbrexza** is flammable. Avoid heat and flame while applying **Qbrexza**. **Qbrexza** is contraindicated in patients with medical conditions that can be exacerbated by the anticholinergic effect of *glycopyrronium* (e.g., glaucoma, paralytic ileus, unstable cardiovascular status in acute hemorrhage, severe ulcerative colitis, toxic megacolon complicating ulcerative colitis, myasthenia gravis, Sjogren's syndrome). The most common adverse reactions (incidence ≥2%) have been dry mouth (24.2%), mydriasis (6.8%), oropharyngeal pain (5.7%), headache (5.0%), urinary hesitation (3.5%), vision blurred (3.5%), nasal dryness (2.6%), dry throat (2.6%), dry eye (2.4%), dry skin (2.2%) and constipation (2.0%). Local skin reactions, including erythema (17.0%), burning/stinging (14.1%), and pruritus (8.1%). Co-administration of Qbrexza with anticholinergic medications may result in additive interaction; therefore, avoid co-administration of **Qbrexza** with other anticholinergic drugs. There are no available data on Qbrexza use in pregnancy to inform a drug-associated risk for adverse developmental outcomes. There are no data on the presence of *glycopyrrolate* or its metabolites in human milk or effects on the breastfed infant.

ORAL ANTICHOLINERGIC

Comment: *oxybutynin*, a cholinergic antagonist commonly prescribed for overactive bladder, is the first oral agent to emerge as a treatment option for hyperhidrosis.

REFERENCES

Scholhammer, M., Brenaut, E., Menard-Andivot, N., Pillette-Delarue, M., Zagnoli, A., Chassain-Le Lay, M., . . . Le Gal, G. (2015). Oxybutynin as a treatment for generalized hyperhidrosis: A randomized, placebo-controlled trial. *British Journal of Dermatology*, *173*(5), 1163–1168. doi:10.1111/bjd.13973

Wolosker, N., de Campos, J. R., Kauffman, P., & Puech-Leão, P. (2012). A randomized placebo-controlled trial of oxybutynin for the initial treatment of palmer and axillary hyperhidrosis. *Journal of Vascular Surgery*, *55*(6), 1696–1700. doi:10.1016/j.jvs.2011.12.039

▷ *oxybutynin chloride* (B)(G)

> **Ditropan** 5 mg bid-tid; max 20 mg/day
> *Pediatric:* <5 years: not recommended; 5-12 years: 5 mg bid; max 15 mg/day; ≥16 years: same as adult
>> *Tab:* 5*mg; *Syr:* 5 mg/5 ml
> **Ditropan XL** initially 5 mg daily; may increase weekly in 5-mg increments as needed; max 30 mg/day
> *Pediatric:* <6 years: not recommended; ≥6 years: initially 5 mg once daily; may increase weekly in 5-mg increments as needed; max 20 mg/day
>> *Tab:* 5, 10, 15 mg ext-rel
> **GelniQUE 3 mg Pump:** apply 3 pumps (84 mg) once daily to clean dry intact skin on the abdomen, upper arm, shoulders, <u>or</u> thighs; rotate sites; wash hands; avoid washing application site for 1 hour after application
> *Pediatric:* <12 years: not recommended; ≥12 years: same as adult
>> *Gel:* 3% (92 gm, metered pump dispenser) (alcohol)
> **GelniQUE 1 gm Sachet:** apply 1 gm gel (1 sachet) once daily to dry intact skin on abdomen, upper arms/shoulders, <u>or</u> thighs; rotate sites; wash hands; avoid washing application site for 1 hour after application
> *Pediatric:* <12 years: not recommended; ≥12 years: same as adult
>> *Gel:* 10%, 1 gm/sachet (30/carton) (alcohol)
> **Oxytrol Transdermal Patch (OTC):** apply patch to clean dry area of the abdomen, hip, <u>or</u> buttock; one patch twice weekly; rotate sites
> *Pediatric:* <12 years: not recommended; ≥12 years: same as adult
>> *Transdermal patch:* 3.9 mg/day

HYPERHOMOCYSTEINEMIA

Comment: Elevated homocysteine is associated with cognitive impairment, vascular dementia, and dementia of the Alzheimer's type.

HOMOCYSTEINE-LOWERING NUTRITIONAL SUPPLEMENTS

▷ *L-methylfolate calcium (as metafolin)+pyridoxyl 5-phosphate+methylcobalamin* take 1 cap daily
Pediatric: <12 years: not recommended; ≥12 years: same as adult
> **Metanx** *Cap:* metafo 3 mg+pyrid 35 mg+methyl 2 mg (gluten-free, yeast-free, lactose-free)
> **Comment:** Metanx is indicated as adjunct treatment of endothelial dysfunction <u>and/or</u> hyperhomocysteinemia in patients who have lower extremity ulceration.

▷ *L-methylfolate calcium (as metafolin)+methylcobalamin+n-acetylcysteine* take 1 cap daily
Pediatric: <12 years: not recommended; ≥12 years: same as adult
> **Cerefolin** *Cap:* metafo 5.6 mg+methyl 2 mg+N-ace 600 mg (gluten-free, yeast-free, lactose-free)
> **Comment:** Cerefolin is indicated in the dietary management of patients treated for early memory loss, with emphasis on those at risk for neurovascular oxidative stress, hyperhomocysteinemia, mild to moderate cognitive impairment with <u>or</u> without vitamin B12 deficiency, vascular dementia, <u>or</u> Alzheimer's disease.

HYPERKALEMIA

POTASSIUM BINDERS

Comment: Normal serum K^+ range is approximately 3.5-5.5 mEq/L. Hyperkalemia is associated with cardiac dysrhythmias and metabolic acidosis. Risk factors include kidney disease, heart failure, and drugs that inhibit the renin-angiotensin-aldosterone system (RAAS) including ACEIs, ARBs, direct renin inhibitors, and aldosterone antagonists. Cation exchange resins are not for emergency treatment of life-threatening hyperkalemia, severe constipation, bowel obstruction or impaction. May cause GI irritability, ulceration, necrosis, sodium retention, hypocalcemia, hypomagnesemia, fecal impaction, ischemic colitis. Avoid non-absorbable cation-donating antacids and laxatives (e.g., *magnesium hydroxide, aluminum hydroxide*). Concomitant sorbitol should be avoided because it may cause intestinal necrosis.

▷ *patiromer sorbitex calcium* (B) initially 8.4 gm once daily; adjust dosage as prescribed based on potassium concentration and target range; may increase dosage at 1-week (or longer) intervals in increments of 8.4 gm; max dose 25.2 gm once daily; prepare immediately prior to administration; do not take in dry form; administer with food; measure 1/3 cup of water and pour half into a glass; then add **Veltassa** and stir; add the remaining water and stir well; the powder will not dissolve and the mixture will look cloudy; add more water as needed for desired consistency; take with or without food; do not heat or mix with heated food or fluids; take other oral drugs at least 6 hours before or 6 hours after taking **Veltassa**
Pediatric: <18 years: not recommended; ≥18 years: same as adult

    Veltassa *Pkt:* 8, 4, 16.8, 25.2 gm pwdr for oral susp, 30 single-use pkts/carton

    Comment: Store packets in the refrigerator. It stored at room temperature, product must be used within 3 months.

▷ *sodium polystyrene sulfonate* (C)(G) *Oral:* average total daily adult dose is 15 gm to 60 gm, administered as a 15-gm dose (four level teaspoons), one to four times daily; *Rectal:* average adult dose is 30 gm to 50 gm every six hours
Pediatrics: Use 1 gm/1 mEq of K+ as basis of calculation; in pediatric patients, as in adults, **Kayexalate** is expected to bind potassium at the practical exchange ratio of 1mEq potassium per 1 gm of resin; in neonates, **Kayexalate** should not be given by the oral route; in both children and neonates, excessive dosage or inadequate dilution could result in impaction of the resin; premature infants or low birth weight infants may have an increased risk for gastrointestinal adverse effects

    Kayexalate *Jar:* 1 lb (453.6 gm) pwdr for dilution

    Comment: **Kayexalate** should not be used an emergency treatment for life-threatening hyperkalemia because of its delayed onset of action. Contraindications are hypersensitivity to polystyrene sulfonate resins, obstructive bowel disease, and neonates with reduced gut motility. Take other orally administered drugs at least 3 hours before or 3 hours after **Kayexalate**. Cation-donating antacids may reduce the resin's potassium exchange capability and increase risk of systemic alkalosis. Concomitant use of sorbitol may contribute to the risk of intestinal necrosis and is not recommended. **Kayexalate** is not absorbed systemically so breastfeeding is not expected to result in risk to the infant.

▷ *sodium zirconium cyclosilicate* *Starting dose:* 10 gm administered 3 x/day for up to 48 hours; *Maintenance treatment:* 10 gm once daily; adjust dose at one-week intervals by 5 g daily, as needed, to obtain desired serum potassium target range; in general, other oral medications should be administered at least 2 hours before or 2 hours after a **Lokelma** dose
Pediatric: <18 years: not established; >18 years: same as adult

    Lokelma for Oral Suspension *Pwdr for oral susp:* 5, 10 gm/pkt (30 pkts/box)

    Comment: **Lokelma** (*sodium zirconium cyclosilicate*) is a potassium binder. ≥18 years-of-age. *In vitro*, **Lokelma** has a high affinity for potassium ions, even in the presence of other cations such as calcium and magnesium. **Lokelma** increases fecal potassium excretion through binding of potassium in the lumen of the GI tract. **Lokelma** should not be used as an emergency treatment for life-threatening hyperkalemia because of its delayed onset of action. The most common adverse reaction with **Lokelma** is mild-to-moderate edema. Patients with motility disorders may experience gastrointestinal adverse reactions. As **Lokelma** is not absorbed systemically, maternal use is not expected to result in fetal exposure and breastfeeding is not expected to result in infant exposure.

HYPERPARATHYROIDISM (HPT)

▷ *calcifediol* (C)(G) 1 cap daily
Pediatric: <18 years: not established; ≥18 years: same as adult

    Rayaldee *Cap:* 30 mcg ext-rel

Comment: Rayaldee is indicated for the prevention and treatment of secondary hyperparathyroidism associated with chronic kidney disease (CKD), stage 3 or 4 and serum total 25-hydroxyvitamin D levels <30 mg/mL.

▷ *paricalcitol* (C)(G) administer 0.04-1 mcg/kg (2.8-7 mcg) IV bolus, during dialysis, no more than every other day; may be increased by 2-4 mcg every 2-4 weeks; monitor serum calcium and phosphorus during dose adjustment periods; if Ca x P ≥75, immediately reduce dose or discontinue until these levels normalize; discard unused portion of sin-gle-use vials immediately

Pediatric: <18 years: not established; ≥18 years: same as adult

Zemplar *Vial:* 2, 5 mcg/ml soln for inj

Comment: Zemplar is indicated for the prevention and treatment of secondary hyper-parathyroidism associated with chronic kidney disease (CKD), stage 5.

CALCIUM-SENSING RECEPTOR AGONIST

▷ *cinacalcet* (C) *Initial Dose:* 30 mg bid; titrate every 2 to 4 weeks through sequential doses of 30 mg bid, then 60 mg bid, then 90 mg bid, then 90 mg tid-qid as needed to normalize serum calcium levels; swallow whole, do not break; take with food or shortly after a meal; *Maintenance:* serum calcium and serum phosphorus should be measured approximately monthly, and PTH every 1 to 3 months

Sensipar Tab 30, 60, 90 mg

Comment: Sensipar (*cinacalet*) is indicated (1) for the treatment of hypercalcemia in adult patients with primary hyperparathyroidism (pHPT) for whom parathyroidectomy would be indicated on the basis of serum calcium levels, but who are unable to undergo parathyroidectomy, (2) for the treatment of secondary hyperparathyroidism in patients with Chronic Kidney Disease (CKD) on dialysis (see HYPERCALCEMIA), and (3) for the treatment of hypercalcemia in patients with parathyroid carcinoma. Sensipar can be used as monotherapy or in combination with vitamin D sterols and/or phosphate binders. Secondary hyperparathyroidism (sHPT) in patients with chronic kidney disease (CKD) is a progressive disease, associated with increases in parathyroid hormone (PTH) levels and derangements in calcium and phosphorus metabolism. Increased PTH stimulates osteoclastic activity resulting in cortical bone resorption and marrow fibrosis. The goals of treatment of secondary hyperparathyroidism are to lower levels of PTH, calcium, and phosphorus in the blood, in order to prevent progressive bone disease and the systemic consequences of disordered mineral metabolism. In CKD patients on dialysis with uncontrolled secondary HPT, reductions in PTH are associated with a favorable impact on bone-specific alkaline phosphatase (BALP), bone turnover and bone fibrosis. The calcium-sensing receptor on the surface of the chief cell of the parathyroid gland is the principal regulator of PTH secretion. Sensipar directly lowers PTH levels by increasing the sensitivity of the calcium-sensing receptor to extracellular calcium. The reduction in PTH is associated with a concomitant decrease in serum calcium levels. Patients should be aware of potential manifestations of hypocalcemia including paresthesias, myalgias, cramping, tetany, and convulsions. Sensipar treatment should not be initiated if serum calcium is less than the lower limit of the normal range (8.4 mg/dL). Serum calcium should be measured within 1 week after any Sensipar dose adjustment. If serum calcium falls below 8.4 mg/dL but remains above 7.5 mg/dL, or if symptoms of hypocalcemia occur, calcium-containing phosphate binders and/or vitamin D sterols can be used to raise serum calcium. If serum calcium falls below 7.5 mg/dL, or if symptoms of hypocalcemia persist and the dose of vitamin D cannot be increased, withhold administration of Sensipar until serum calcium levels reach 8.0 mg/dL, and/or symptoms of hypocalcemia have resolved. Treatment should be re-initiated using the next lowest dose of Sensipar. Adynamic bone disease may develop if iPTH levels are suppressed below 100 pg/mL. Sensipar is metabolized in part by the enzyme CYP3A4. Co-administration of *ketoconazole*, a strong inhibitor of CYP3A4, can cause an approximate 2-fold increase in *cinacalcet* exposure. Dose adjustment of Sensipar may be required and PTH and serum calcium concentrations should be closely monitored if a patient initiates or discontinues therapy with a strong CYP3A4 inhibitor (e.g., *ketoconazole, erythromycin, itraconazole*). Patients with congenital long QT syndrome, history of QT interval prolongation, family history of long QT syndrome or sudden cardiac death, and other conditions that predispose to QT interval prolongation and ventricular arrhythmia may be at increased risk for QT interval prolongation and ventricular arrhythmias if they develop hypocalcemia due to **Sensipar**. Closely monitor corrected serum calcium and QT interval in patients at risk receiving **Sensipar**. Seizure threshold is lowered by significant reductions in serum calcium levels. Monitor patients with seizure disorders receiving **Sensipar**. Patients with risk factors for upper GI bleeding (e.g., known gastritis, esophagitis, ulcers or severe vomiting) may be at increased risk for GI bleeding when receiving **Sensipar** treatment. In post-marketing safety surveillance, isolated, idiosyncratic cases of hypotension, worsening heart failure, and/or arrhythmia have been reported in patients with impaired cardiac function.

 HYPERPHOSPHATEMIA

FERRIC CITRATE

▶ **ferric citrate** *Hyperphosphatemia in Chronic Kidney Disease on Dialysis:* starting dose is 2 tabs orally 3 x/day with meals; adjust dose by 1 to 2 tabs as needed to maintain serum phosphorus at target levels, up to max 12 tabs/day; dose can be titrated at 1 week or longer intervals; *Iron Deficiency Anemia in Chronic Kidney Disease Not on Dialysis:* starting dose is 1 tablet 3 x/day with meals; adjust dose as needed to achieve and maintain hemoglobin goal, up to max 12 tabs/day
Pediatric: <18 years: not recommended; ≥18 years: same as adult
   Aurexia *Tab:* 210 mg *ferric iron* (equivalent to 1 gm *ferric citrate*)
   Comment: **Auryxia** is a phosphate binder indicated for the control of serum phosphorus levels in patients ≥18 years-of-age with chronic kidney disease (CKD) on dialysis. Ferric iron binds dietary phosphate in the GI tract and precipitates as ferric phosphate. This compound is insoluble and is excreted in the stool. **Auryxia** is also an iron replacement product indicated for the treatment of iron deficiency anemia in patients >18 years-of-age with chronic kidney (CKD) not on dialysis. Ferric iron is reduced from the ferric to the ferrous form by ferric reductase in the GI tract. After transport through the enterocytes into the blood, oxidized ferric iron circulates bound to the plasma protein transferrin, for incorporation into hemoglobin. **Auryxia** is contraindicated in iron overload syndromes (e.g., hemochromatosis). Monitor ferritin and TSAT. When clinically significant drug interactions are expected, consider separation of the timing of administration. Consider monitoring clinical responses or blood levels of the concomitant medication. The most common adverse reactions (incidence ≥5%) are discolored feces, diarrhea, constipation, nausea, vomiting, cough, abdominal pain, and hyperkalemia. There are no available data on **Auryxia** use in pregnancy to inform a drug-associated risk of major birth defects and miscarriage; however, an overdose of iron may carry a risk for spontaneous abortion, gestational diabetes and fetal malformation. There are no human data regarding effects of **Auryxia** on the breastfed infant. Accidental overdose of iron-containing products is a leading cause of fatal poisoning in children under 6 years-of-age. Keep this product out of reach of children. In case of accidental overdose, contact poison control center immediately and transfer to emergency care.

PHOSPHATE BINDERS

Comment: Monitor for development of hypercalcemia. Normal serum PO_4^- is 2.5-4.5 mg/dL and normal serum calcium is 8.5-10.5 mg/dL.
▶ *calcium acetate* (C)(G) initially 2 tabs or caps with each meal; then titrate gradually to keep serum phosphate at <6 mg/dL; usual maintenance is 3-4 tabs or caps with each meal
Pediatric: <12 years: not recommended; ≥12 years: same as adult
   PhosLo *Tab:* 667 mg; *Cap:* 667 mg
▶ *lanthanum carbonate* (C)(G) initially 750 mg to 1.5 gm per day in divided doses; take with meals; titrate at 2-3-week intervals in increments of 750 mg/day based on serum phosphate; usual range 1.5-3 gm/day; usual max 3,750 mg/day
Pediatric: <12 years: not recommended; ≥12 years: same as adult
   Fosrenol *Chew tab:* 250, 500, 750 mg; 1 gm
▶ *sevelamer* (C)(G) for patients not taking a phosphate binder, take tid with meals; swallow whole; titrate by 1 tab per meal at 1-week intervals to keep serum phosphorus 3.5-5.5 mg/

dL; switching from calcium acetate to *sevelamer*, see mfr pkg insert. *Serum phosphorus* ≥5.5 to ≤7.5 mg/dL: 800 mg tid; *Serum phosphorus* 7.5-9: 1.2-1.6 gm tid
Pediatric: <12 years: not recommended; ≥12 years: same as adult

    Renagel *Tab:* 400, 800 mg
    Renvela *Tab:* 800 mg

HYPERPIGMENTATION

Comment: Depigmenting agents may be used for hyperpigmented skin conditions including chloasma, melasma, freckles, senile lentigines. Limit treatments to small areas at one time. Sunscreen ≥30 SPF recommended.

▶ *hydroquinone* (C)(G) apply sparingly to affected area and rub in bid
    Lustra *Crm:* 4% (1, 2 oz) (sulfites)
    Lustra AF *Crm:* 4% (1, 2 oz) (sunscreen, sulfites)

▶ *monobenzone* (C) apply sparingly to affected area and rub in bid-tid; depigmentation occurs in 1-4 months
    Benoquin *Crm:* 20% (1.25 oz)

▶ *tazarotene* (X)(G) apply daily at HS
    Pediatric: <12 years: not recommended; ≥12 years: same as adult
        Avage Cream *Crm:* 0.1% (30 gm)
        Tazorac Cream *Crm:* 0.05, 0.1% (15, 30, 60 gm)
        Tazorac Gel *Gel:* 0.05, 0.1% (30, 100 gm)

▶ *tretinoin* (C) apply daily at HS
    Pediatric: <12 years: not recommended; ≥12 years: same as adult
        Avita *Crm/Gel:* 0.025% (20, 45 gm)
        Renova *Crm:* 0.02% (40 gm); 0.05% (40, 60 gm)
        Retin-A Cream *Crm:* 0.025, 0.05, 0.1% (20, 45 gm)
        Retin-A Gel *Gel:* 0.01, 0.025% (15, 45 gm) (alcohol 90%)
        Retin-A Liquid *Liq:* 0.05% (28 ml) (alcohol 55%)
        Retin-A Micro *Microspheres:* 0.04, 0.1% (20, 45 gm)

COMBINATION AGENTS

▶ *hydroquinone+fluocinolone+tretinoin* (C) apply sparingly to affected area and rub in daily at HS
    Pediatric: <12 years: not recommended; ≥12 years: same as adult
        Tri-Luma *Crm:* hydroquin 4%+fluo 0.01%+tretin 0.05% (30 gm) (parabens, sulfites)

▶ *hydroquinone+padimate o+oxybenzone+octyl methoxycinnamate* (C) apply sparingly to affected area and rub in bid
    Pediatric: <12 years: not recommended; ≥16 years: same as adult
        Glyquin *Crm:* 4% (1 oz jar)

▶ *hydroquinone+ethyl dihydroxypropyl PABA+dioxybenzone+oxybenzone* (C) apply sparingly to affected area and rub in bid; max 2 months
    Pediatric: <12 years: not recommended; ≥12 years: same as adult
        Solaquin *Crm:* hydroquin 2%+PABA 5%+dioxy 3%+oxy 2% (1 oz) (sulfites)

▶ *hydroquinone+padimate+dioxybenzone+oxybenzone* (C) apply sparingly to affected area and rub in bid; max 2 months
    Pediatric: <12 years: not recommended; ≥12 years: same as adult
        Solaquin Forte *Crm:* hydroquin 4%+pad 0.5%+dioxy 3%+oxy 2% (1oz) (sunscreen, sulfites)

▶ *hydroquinone+padimate+dioxybenzone* (C) apply sparingly to affected area and rub in bid; max 2 months
    Pediatric: <12 years: not recommended; ≥12 years: same as adult
        Solaquin Forte Gel: hydroquin 4%+pad 0.5%+dioxy 3% (1 oz) (alcohol, sulfites)

HYPERPROLACTINEMIA

DOPAMINE RECEPTOR AGONIST

▶ *dostinex* (B)(G) initial therapy is 0.25 mg twice a week; may increase by 0.25 mg twice weekly up to 1 mg twice a week according to the patient's serum prolactin level; dose increases should not occur more than every 4 weeks; after a normal serum prolactin level has been maintained for 6 months, may be discontinued, with periodic monitoring of serum prolactin level to determine if/when treatment should be reinstituted

Pediatric: <12 years: not established; ≥12 years: same as adult
  Cabergoline *Tab:* 0.5 mg
  Comment: **Cabergoline** is indicated to treat hyperprolactinemia disorders due to idiopathic or pituitary adenoma.

HYPERTENSION: PRIMARY, ESSENTIAL

see JNC-8 Recommendations page 549

BETA-BLOCKERS (CARDIOSELECTIVE)
Comment: Cardioselective beta-blockers are less likely to cause bronchospasm, peripheral vasoconstriction, or hypoglycemia than non-cardioselective beta-blockers.
▶ *acebutolol* (B)(G) initially 400 mg in 1-2 divided doses; usual range 200-800 mg/day; max 1.2 gm/day in 2 divided doses
  Pediatric: <12 years: not recommended; ≥12 years: same as adult
    Sectral *Cap:* 200, 400 mg
▶ *atenolol* (D)(G) initially 50 mg daily; may increase after 1-2 weeks to 100 mg daily; max 100 mg/day
  Pediatric: <12 years: not recommended; ≥12 years: same as adult
    Tenormin *Tab:* 25, 50, 100 mg
▶ *betaxolol* (C) initially 10 mg daily; may increase to 20 mg/day after 7-14 days; usual max 20 mg/day
  Pediatric: <12 years: not recommended; ≥12 years: same as adult
    Kerlone *Tab:* 10*, 20 mg
▶ *bisoprolol* (C) 5 mg daily; max 20 mg daily
  Pediatric: <12 years: not recommended; ≥12 years: same as adult
    Zebeta *Tab:* 5*, 10 mg
▶ *metoprolol succinate* (C)
  Pediatric: <12 years: not recommended; ≥12 years: same as adult
    Toprol-XL initially 25-100 mg in a single dose once daily; increase weekly if needed; max 400 mg/day; as monotherapy or with a diuretic
      Tab: 25*, 50*, 100*, 200*mg ext-rel
▶ *metoprolol tartrate* (C) initially 25-50 mg bid; increase weekly if needed; max 400 mg/day; as monotherapy or with a diuretic
  Pediatric: <12 years: not recommended; ≥12 years: same as adult
    Lopressor (G) *Tab:* 25, 37.5, 50, 75, 100 mg
▶ *nebivolol* (C)(G) initially 5 mg once daily; may increase at 2 week intervals; max 40 mg/day
  Pediatric: <12 years: not recommended; ≥12 years: same as adult
    Bystolic *Tab:* 2.5, 5, 10, 20 mg

BETA-BLOCKERS (NON-CARDIOSELECTIVE)
Comment: Non-cardioselective beta-blockers are more likely to cause bronchospasm, peripheral vasoconstriction, and/or hypoglycemia than cardioselective beta-blockers.
▶ *nadolol* (C)(G) initially 40 mg daily; usual maintenance 40-80 mg daily; max 320 mg/day
  Pediatric: <12 years: not recommended; ≥12 years: same as adult
    Corgard *Tab:* 20*, 40*, 80*, 120*, 160*mg
▶ *penbutolol* (C) 10-20 mg once daily
  Pediatric: <12 years: not recommended; ≥12 years: same as adult
    Levatol *Tab:* 20*mg
▶ *pindolol* (B)(G) initially 5 mg bid; may increase after 3-4 weeks in 10 mg increments; max 60 mg/day
  Pediatric: <12 years: not recommended; ≥12 years: same as adult
    Pindolol *Tab:* 5, 10 mg
    Visken *Tab:* 5, 10 mg
▶ *propranolol* (C)(G)
    Inderal initially 40 mg bid; usual maintenance 120-240 mg/day; max 640 mg/day
    Pediatric: initially 1 mg/kg/day; usual range 2-4 mg/kg/day in 2 divided doses; max 16 mg/kg/day
      Tab: 10*, 20*, 40*, 60*, 80*mg
    Inderal LA initially 80 mg daily in a single dose; increase q 3-7 days; usual range 120-160 mg/day; max 320 mg/day in a single dose

Pediatric: <12 years: not recommended; ≥12 years: same as adult
  Cap: 60, 80, 120, 160 mg sust-rel
  InnoPran XL initially 80 mg q HS; max 120 mg/day
Pediatric: <12 years: not recommended; ≥12 years: same as adult
  Cap: 80, 120 mg ext-rel
▷ *timolol* (C)(G) initially 10 mg bid, increase weekly if needed; usual maintenance 20-40 mg/day; max 60 mg/day in 2 divided doses
Pediatric: <12 years: not recommended; ≥12 years: same as adult
  Blocadren *Tab:* 5, 10*, 20*mg

BETA-BLOCKER (NON-CARDIOSELECTIVE)+ALPHA-1 BLOCKER COMBINATIONS

▷ *carvedilol* (C)(G)
Pediatric: <12 years: not recommended; ≥12 years: same as adult
  Coreg initially 6.25 mg bid; may increase at 1-2-week intervals to 12.5 mg bid; max 25 mg bid
    Tab: 3.125, 6.25, 12.5, 25 mg
  Coreg CR initially 20 mg once daily for 2 weeks; may increase at 1-2-week intervals; max 80 mg once daily
    Tab: 10, 20, 40, 80 mg cont-rel
▷ *carteolol* (C) initially 2.5 mg daily, gradually increase to 5 or 10 mg once daily; usual maintenance 2.5-5 mg once daily
Pediatric: <12 years: not recommended; ≥12 years: same as adult
  Cartrol *Tab:* 2.5, 5 mg
▷ *labetalol* (C)(G) initially 100 mg bid; increase after 2-3 days if needed; usual maintenance 200-400 mg bid; max 2.4 gm/day
Pediatric: <12 years: not recommended; ≥12 years: same as adult
  Normodyne *Tab:* 100*, 200*, 300 mg
  Trandate *Tab:* 100*, 200*, 300*mg

DIURETICS
Thiazide Diuretics

▷ *chlorthalidone* (B)(G) initially 15 mg daily; may increase to 30 mg once daily based on clinical response; max 45-60 mg/day
Pediatric: <12 years: not established; ≥12 years: same as adult
  Chlorthalidone *Tab:* 25, 50 mg
  Thalitone *Tab:* 15 mg
▷ *chlorothiazide* (B)(G) 0.5-1 gm/day in a single or divided doses; max 2 gm/day
Pediatric: <6 months: up to 15 mg/lb/day in 2 divided doses; ≥6 months: 10 mg/lb/day in 2 divided doses
  Diuril *Tab:* 250*, 500*mg; *Oral susp:* 250 mg/5 ml (237 ml)
▷ *hydrochlorothiazide* (B)(G)
Pediatric: <12 years: not recommended; ≥12 years: same as adult
  Esidrix 25-100 mg once daily
    Tab: 25, 50, 100 mg
  Hydrochlorothiazide 12.5 mg once daily; usual max 50 mg/day
    Tab: 25*, 50*mg
  Microzide 12.5 mg once daily; usual max 50 mg/day
    Cap: 12.5 mg
▷ *methyclothiazide+deserpidine* (B) initially 5/0.25 mg once daily; titrate individual components
Pediatric: <12 years: not recommended; ≥12 years: same as adult
  Enduronyl *Tab:* methy 5 mg+deser 0.25 mg*
  Enduronyl Forte *Tab:* methy 5 mg+deser 0.5 mg*
▷ *polythiazide* (C) 2-4 mg once daily
Pediatric: <12 years: not recommended; ≥12 years: same as adult
  Renese *Tab:* 1, 2, 4 mg

Potassium-Sparing Diuretics

▷ *amiloride* (B)(C) initially 5 mg; may increase to 10 mg; max 20 mg
Pediatric: <12 years: not recommended; ≥12 years: same as adult
  Midamor *Tab:* 5 mg

▷ *spironolactone* (D)(G) initially 50-100 mg in a single or divided doses; titrate at 2-week intervals
   Pediatric: <12 years: not established; ≥12 years: same as adult
      Aldactone *Tab:* 25, 50*, 100*mg
      CaroSpir *Oral susp:* 25 mg/5 ml (118, 473 ml) (banana)
▷ *triamterene* (B) 100 mg bid; max 300 mg
   Pediatric: <12 years: not recommended; ≥12 years: same as adult
      Dyrenium *Cap:* 50, 100 mg

Loop Diuretics

▷ *bumetanide* (C)(G) 0.5-2 mg daily; may repeat at 4-5-hour intervals; max 10 mg/day
   Pediatric: <18 years: not recommended; ≥18 years: same as adult
   Tab: 1*mg
   Comment: *bumetanide* is contraindicated with sulfa drug allergy.
▷ *ethacrynic acid* (B)(G) initially 50-200 mg/day
   Pediatric: <1 month: not recommended; ≥1 month: initially 25 mg/day; then adjust dose in 25-mg increments
      Edecrin *Tab:* 25, 50 mg
▷ *ethacrynate sodium* (B)(G) <1 month: not recommended; ≥1 month-12 years: use the smallest effective dose; initially 25 mg; then careful stepwise increments in dosage of 25 mg to achieve effective maintenance; ≥12 years: administer smallest dose required to produce gradual weight loss (about 1-2 pounds per day); onset of diuresis usually occurs at 50-100 mg in children ≥12 years; after diuresis has been achieved, the minimally effective dose (usually 50-200 mg/day) may be administered on a continuous or intermittent dosage schedule; dose titrations are usually in 25-50 mg increments to avoid derangement electrolyte and water excretion; the patient should be weighed under standard conditions before and during administration of *ethacrynate sodium;* the following schedule may be helpful in determining the lowest effective dose; *Day 1:* 50 mg once daily after a meal; *Day 2:* 50 mg bid after meals, if necessary; *Day 3:* 100 mg in the morning and 50-100 mg following the afternoon or evening meal, depending upon response to the morning dose; a few patients may require initial and maintenance doses as high as 200 mg bid; these higher doses, which should be achieved gradually, are most often required in patients with severe, refractory edema
      Sodium Edecrin *Vial:* 50 mg single-dose
      Comment: **Sodium Edecrin** is more potent than more commonly used loop and thiazide diuretics. Treatment of the edema associated with congestive heart failure, cirrhosis of the liver, and renal disease, including the nephrotic syndrome, short-term management of ascites due to malignancy, idiopathic edema, and lymphedema, short-term management of hospitalized pediatric patients, other than infants, with congenital heart disease or the nephrotic syndrome. IV **Sodium Edecrin** is indicated when a rapid onset of diuresis is desired, for example, in acute pulmonary edema or when gastrointestinal absorption is impaired or oral medication is not practical.
▷ *furosemide* (C)(G) initially 40 mg bid
   Pediatric: <12 years: not recommended; ≥12 years: same as adult
      Lasix *Tab:* 20, 40*, 80 mg; *Oral Soln:* 10 mg/ml (2, 4 oz w. dropper)
   Comment: *furosemide* is contraindicated with sulfa drug allergy.
▷ *torsemide* (B) 5 mg once daily; may increase to 10 mg once daily
   Pediatric: <12 years: not recommended; ≥12 years: same as adult
      Demadex *Tab:* 5*, 10*, 20*, 100*mg

Indoline Diuretic

▷ *indapamide* (B) initially 1.25 mg daily; may titrate dosage upward q 4 weeks if needed; max 5 mg/day
   Pediatric: <12 years: not recommended; ≥12 years: same as adult
      Lozol *Tab:* 1.25, 2.5 mg
   Comment: *indapamide* is contraindicated with sulfa drug allergy.

Quinazoline Diuretic

▷ *metolazone* (B) 2.5-5 mg daily
   Pediatric: <12 years: not recommended; ≥12 years: same as adult

Zaroxolyn 2.5-5 mg daily
Tab: 2.5, 5, 10 mg
Comment: *metolazone* is contraindicated with sulfa drug allergy.

DIURETIC COMBINATIONS

▷ *amiloride+hydrochlorothiazide* (B)(G) initially 1 tab daily; may increase to 2 tabs/day in a single or divided doses
Pediatric: <12 years: not recommended; ≥12 years: same as adult
Moduretic *Tab:* amil 5 mg+hctz 50 mg*

▷ *methyclothiazide+deserpidine* (C) initially 5/0.25 mg once daily; titrate individual components
Pediatric: Safety and effectiveness in children have not been established; therefore, age at which this drug may be initially prescribed is not specified
Enduronyl *Tab:* methyl 5 mg+deser 0.25 mg*
Enduronyl Forte *Tab:* methyl 5 mg+deser 0.5 mg*

Comment: **Enduronyl** (*methyclothiazide* and *deserpidine*) is indicated in the treatment of mild to moderately severe hypertension. The combined antihypertensive actions of *methyclothiazide* and *deserpidine* result in a total clinical antihypertensive effect which is greater than can ordinarily be achieved by either drug given individually and more potent agents can be administered at reduced dosage. *methylchlorothiazide* (**Enduron**) is a thiazide (benzothiadiazine) diuretic-antihypertensive. *deserpidine* is a purified rauwolfia alkaloid. The pharmacologic actions of *deserpidine* are essentially the same as those of other active rauwolfia alkaloids. *deserpidine* probably produces its antihypertensive effects through depletion of tissue stores of catecholamines (epinephrine and norepinephrine) from peripheral sites. By contrast, its sedative and tranquilizing properties are thought to be related to depletion of 5-hydroxytryptamine from the brain. The antihypertensive effect is often accompanied by bradycardia. There is no significant alteration in cardiac output or renal blood flow. The carotid sinus reflex is inhibited, but postural hypotension is rarely seen with the use of conventional doses of **deserpidine** alone. *methyclothiazide* is contraindicated in patients with anuria and in patients with a history of hypersensitivity to this or other sulfonamide-derived drugs. *deserpidine* is contraindicated in patients with known hypersensitivity, active peptic ulcer, history of mental depression, especially with suicidal tendencies and patients receiving electroconvulsive therapy. Animal reproduction studies have not been conducted with methyclothiazide or deserpidine. It is also not known whether *methyclothiazide* or *deserpidine* can cause fetal harm when administered to a pregnant woman. *methyclothiazide* and *deserpidine* should be given to a pregnant woman only if clearly needed. *methyclothiazide* and *deserpidine* are excreted in human milk. Effects on the breastfed infant are unknown; therefore, assess maternal need/benefit as against potential fetal risk.

▷ *spironolactone+hydrochlorothiazide* (D)(G)
Pediatric: <12 years: not recommended; ≥12 years: same as adult
Aldactazide 25 usual maintenance 1-4 tabs in a single or divided doses
Tab: spiro 25 mg+hctz 25 mg
Aldactazide 50 usual maintenance 1-2 tabs in a single or divided doses
Tab: spiro 50 mg+hctz 50 mg

▷ *triamterene+hydrochlorothiazide* (C)(G)
Pediatric: <12 years: not recommended; ≥12 years: same as adult
Dyazide 1-2 caps once daily
Cap: triam 37.5 mg/hctz 25 mg
Maxzide 1 tab once daily
Tab: triam 75 mg/hctz 50 mg*
Maxzide-25 1-2 tabs once daily
Tab: triam 37.5 mg/hctz 25 mg*

ANGIOTENSIN CONVERTING ENZYME INHIBITORS (ACEIs)

Comment: Black patients receiving ACEI monotherapy have been reported to have a higher incidence of angioedema compared to non-Blacks. Non-Blacks have a greater decrease in BP when ACEIs are used compared to Black patients.

▷ *benazepril* (D)(G) initially 10 mg daily; usual maintenance 20-40 mg/day in 1-2 divided doses; usual max 80 mg/day

Pediatric: <12 years: not recommended; ≥12 years: same as adult
Lotensin *Tab:* 5, 10, 20, 40 mg
▶ *captopril* (D)(G) initially 25 mg bid-tid; after 1-2 weeks increase to 50 mg bid-tid
Pediatric: <12 years: not recommended; ≥12 years: same as adult
Capoten *Tab:* 12.5*, 25*, 50*, 100*mg
▶ *enalapril* (D) initially 5 mg daily; usual dosage range 10-40 mg/day; max 40 mg/day
Pediatric: <12 years: not recommended; ≥12 years: same as adult
Epaned Oral Solution *Oral soln:* 1 mg/ml (150 ml) (mixed berry)
Vasotec (G) *Tab:* 2.5*, 5*, 10, 20 mg
▶ *fosinopril* (D) initially 10 mg daily; usual maintenance 20-40 mg/day in a single or divided doses; max 80 mg/day
Pediatric: <6 years, <50 kg: not recommended; ≥6-12 years, ≥50 kg: 5-10 mg once daily
Monopril *Tab:* 10*, 20, 40 mg
▶ *lisinopril* (D)
Prinivil initially 10 mg daily; usual range 20-40 mg/day
Pediatric: <12 years: not recommended; ≥12 years: same as adult
Tab: 5*, 10*, 20*, 40 mg
Qbrelis Oral Solution administer as a single dose once daily
Pediatric: <6 years, GFR <30 mL/min: not recommended; ≥6 years, GFR >30 mL/min: initially 0.07 mg/kg, max 5 mg; adjust according to BP up to a max 0.61 mg/kg (40 mg) once daily
Oral soln: 1 mg/ml (150 ml)
Zestril initially 10 mg daily; usual range 20-40 mg/day
Pediatric: <12 years: not recommended; ≥12 years: same as adult
Tab: 2.5, 5*, 10, 20, 30, 40 mg
▶ *moexipril* (D) initially 7.5 mg daily; usual range 15-30 mg/day in 1-2 divided doses; max 30 mg/day
Pediatric: <12 years: not recommended; ≥12 years: same as adult
Univasc *Tab:* 7.5*, 15*mg
▶ *perindopril* (D) initially 2-8 mg daily-bid; max 16 mg/day
Pediatric: <12 years: not recommended; ≥12 years: same as adult
Aceon *Tab:* 2*, 4*, 8*mg
▶ *quinapril* (D) initially 10 mg once daily; usual maintenance 20-80 mg daily in 1-2 divided doses
Pediatric: <12 years: not recommended; ≥12 years: same as adult
Accupril *Tab:* 5*, 10, 20, 40 mg
▶ *ramipril* (D)(G) initially 2.5 mg bid; usual maintenance 2.5-20 mg in 1-2 divided doses
Pediatric: <12 years: not established; ≥12 years: same as adult
Altace *Tab/Cap:* 1.25, 2.5, 5, 10 mg
▶ *trandolapril* (C; D in 2nd, 3rd) initially 1-2 mg once daily; adjust at 1-week intervals; usual range 2-4 mg in 1-2 divided doses; max 8 mg/day
Pediatric: <12 years: not recommended; ≥12 years: same as adult
Mavik *Tab:* 1*, 2, 4 mg

ANGIOTENSIN II RECEPTOR BLOCKERS (ARBs)

▶ *azilsartan medoxomil* (D) *Monotherapy, not volume depleted:* 80 mg once daily; *Volume-depleted (concomitant high-dose diuretic):* initially 40 mg once daily
Pediatric: <12 years: not recommended; ≥12 years: same as adult
Edarbi *Tab:* 40, 80 mg
▶ *candesartan* (D)(G) initially 16 mg daily; range 8-32 mg in 1-2 divided doses
Pediatric: <12 years: not recommended; ≥12 years: same as adult
Atacand *Tab:* 4, 8, 16, 32 mg
▶ *eprosartan* (D)(G) initially 400 mg bid or 600 mg once daily; max 800 mg/day
Pediatric: <12 years: not established; ≥12 years: same as adult
Teveten *Tab:* 400, 600 mg
▶ *irbesartan* (D)(G) initially 150 mg daily; titrate up to 300 mg
Pediatric: <12 years: not recommended; ≥12 years: same as adult
Avapro *Tab:* 75, 150, 300 mg
▶ *losartan* (D)(G) initially 50 mg daily; max 100 mg/day
Pediatric: <12 years: not recommended; ≥12 years: same as adult
Cozaar *Tab:* 25, 50, 100 mg

▷ *olmesartan medoxomil* (D)(G) initially 20 mg once daily; after 2 weeks, may increase to 40 mg daily
   Pediatric: <6 years: not recommended; ≥6-16 years: 20-35 kg: initially 10 mg once daily; after 2 weeks, may increase to max 20 mg once daily; ≥6-16 years: >35 kg: initially 20 mg once daily; after 2 weeks, may increase to max 40 mg once daily
      Benicar *Tab:* 5, 20, 40 mg
▷ *valsartan* (D)(G) initially 80 mg once daily; may increase to 160 or 320 mg once daily after 2-4 weeks; usual range 80-320 mg/day
   Pediatric: <12 years: not recommended; ≥12 years: same as adult
      Diovan *Tab:* 40*, 80, 160, 320 mg
      Prexxartan Oral Solution *Oral soln:* 20 mg/5 ml, 80 mg/20 ml (120, 473 ml; 20 ml unit dose cup)

CALCIUM CHANNEL BLOCKERS (CCBs)

Benzothiazepines

▷ *diltiazem* (C)(G)
   Pediatric: <12 years: not established; ≥12 years: same as adult
      Cardizem initially 30 mg qid; may increase gradually every 1-2 days; max 360 mg/day in divided doses
         Tab: 30, 60, 90, 120 mg
      Cardizem CD initially 120-180 mg daily; adjust at 1-2-week intervals; max 480 mg/day
         Cap: 120, 180, 240, 300, 360 mg ext-rel
      Cardizem LA initially 180-240 mg daily; titrate at 2-week intervals; max 540 mg/day
         Tab: 120, 180, 240, 300, 360, 420 mg ext-rel
      Cardizem SR initially 60-120 mg bid; adjust at 2-week intervals; max 360 mg/day
         Cap: 60, 90, 120 mg sust-rel
      Cartia XT initially 180 or 240 mg once daily; max 540 mg once daily
         Cap: 120, 180, 240, 300 mg ext-rel
      Dilacor XR initially 180 or 240 mg in AM; usual range 180-480 mg/day; max 540 mg/day
         Cap: 120, 180, 240 mg ext-rel
      Tiazac (G) initially 120-240 mg daily; adjust at 2-week intervals; usual max 540 mg/day
         Cap: 120, 180, 240, 300, 360, 420 mg ext-rel
▷ *diltiazem maleate* (C) initially 120-180 mg daily; adjust at 2-week intervals; usual range 120-480 mg daily
   Pediatric: <12 years: not recommended; ≥12 years: same as adult
      Tiamate *Cap:* 120, 180, 240 mg ext-rel

Dihydropyridines

▷ *amlodipine* (C) initially 5 mg once daily; max 10 mg/day
   Pediatric: <12 years: not recommended; ≥12 years: same as adult
      Norvasc *Tab:* 2.5, 5, 10 mg
▷ *clevidipine butyrate* (C) administer by IV infusion; initially 1-2 mg/hour; double dose at 90-second intervals until BP approaches goal; then titrate slower; adjust at 5-10-minute intervals; maintenance 4-6 mg/hour; usual max, 16-32 mg/hour; do not exceed 1,000 ml (21 mg/hour for 24 hours) due to lipid load
   Pediatric: <18 years: not recommended; ≥18 years: same as adult
      Cleviprex *Vial:* 0.5 mg/ml soln for IV infusion (single-use, 50, 100 ml) (lipids)
      Comment: Cleviprex is indicated to reduce blood pressure when oral therapy is not feasible or desirable. Cleviprex is contraindicated with egg or soy allergy.
▷ *felodipine* (C)(G) initially 5 mg daily; usual range 2.5-10 mg daily; adjust at 2-week intervals; max 10 mg/day
   Pediatric: <12 years: not recommended; ≥12 years: same as adult
      Plendil *Tab:* 2.5, 5, 10 mg ext-rel
▷ *isradipine* (C)
   Pediatric: <12 years: not recommended; ≥12 years: same as adult
      DynaCirc initially 2.5 mg bid; adjust in increments of 5 mg/day at 2-4-week intervals; max 20 mg/day
         Cap: 2.5, 5 mg
      DynaCirc CR initially 5 mg daily; adjust in increments of 5 mg/day at 2-4-week intervals; max 20 mg/day
         Tab: 5, 10 mg cont-rel

▷ *nicardipine* (C)(G)
  Pediatric: <18 years: not recommended; ≥18 years: same as adult
      Cardene initially 10-20 mg tid; adjust at intervals of at least 3 days; max 120 mg/day
        Cap: 20, 30 mg
      Cardene SR 30-60 mg bid
        Cap: 30, 45, 60 mg sust-rel
▷ *nifedipine* (C)(G)
  Pediatric: <12 years: not recommended; ≥12 years: same as adult
      Adalat initially 10 mg tid; usual range 10-20 mg tid; max 180 mg/day
        Cap: 10, 20 mg
      Adalat CC initially 10 mg tid; usual range 10-20 mg tid; max 180 mg/day
        Cap: 30, 60, 90 mg ext-rel
      Afeditab CR initially 30 mg once daily; titrate over 7-14 days; max 90 mg/day
        Cap: 30, 60 mg ext-rel
      Procardia initially 10 mg tid; titrate over 7-14 days: max 30 mg/dose and 180 mg/day in divided doses
        Cap: 10, 20 mg
      Procardia XL initially 30-60 mg daily; titrate over 7-14 days; max dose 90 mg/day
        Tab: 30, 60, 90 mg ext-rel
▷ *nisoldipine* (C) initially 20 mg daily; may increase by 10 mg weekly; usual maintenance 20-40 mg/day; max 60 mg/day
  Pediatric: <12 years: not recommended; ≥12 years: same as adult
      Sular *Tab:* 10, 20, 30, 40 mg ext-rel

Diphenylalkylamines

▷ *verapamil* (C)(G)
  Pediatric: <12 years: not recommended; ≥12 years: same as adult
      Calan 80-120 mg tid; may titrate up; usual max 360 mg in divided doses
        Tab: 40, 80*, 120*mg
      Calan SR initially 120 mg in the AM; may titrate up; max 480 mg/day in divided doses
        Cplt: 120, 180*, 240*mg sust-rel
      Covera HS initially 180 mg q HS; titrate to 240 mg; then to 360 mg; then to 480 mg if needed
        Tab: 180, 240 mg ext-rel
      Isoptin initially 80-120 mg tid
        Tab: 40, 80, 120 mg
      Isoptin SR initially 120-180 mg in the AM; may increase to 240 mg in the AM; then 180 mg q 12 hours <u>or</u> 240 mg in the AM and 120 mg in the PM; then 240 mg q 12 hours
        Tab: 120, 180*, 240*mg sust-rel
      Verelan initially 240 mg once daily; adjust in 120 mg increments; max 480 mg/day
        Cap: 120, 180, 240, 360 mg sust-rel
      Verelan PM initially 200 mg q HS; may titrate upward to 300 mg; then 400 mg if needed
        Cap: 100, 200, 300 mg ext-rel

ALPHA-1 ANTAGONISTS

Comment: Educate the patient regarding potential side effects of hypotension when taking an alpha-1 antagonist, especially with first dose ("first dose effect"). Start at lowest dose and titrate upward.

▷ *doxazosin* (C)(G) initially 1 mg once daily at HS; increase dose slowly every 2 weeks if needed; max 16 mg/day
  Pediatric: <12 years: not recommended; ≥12 years: same as adult
      Cardura *Tab:* 1*, 2*, 4*, 8*mg
      Cardura XL *Tab:* 4, 8 mg
▷ *prazosin* (C)(G) first dose at HS, 1 mg bid-tid; increase dose slowly; usual range 6-15 mg/day in divided doses; max 20-40 mg/day
  Pediatric: <12 years: not recommended; ≥12 years: same as adult
      Minipress *Cap:* 1, 2, 5 mg
▷ *terazosin* (C) 1 mg q HS, then increase dose slowly; usual range 1-5 mg q HS; max 20 mg/day
  Pediatric: <12 years: not recommended; ≥12 years: same as adult
      Hytrin *Cap:* 1, 2, 5, 10 mg

CENTRAL ALPHA-AGONISTS

▷ *clonidine* (C)
   Pediatric: <12 years: not recommended; ≥12 years: same as adult
      Catapres initially 0.1 mg bid; usual range 0.2-0.6 mg/day in divided doses; max 2.4 mg/day
         Tab: 0.1*, 0.2*, 0.3*mg
      Catapres-TTS initially 0.1 mg patch weekly; increase after 1-2 weeks if needed; max 0.6 mg/day
         Patch: 0.1, 0.2 mg/day (12/carton); 0.3 mg/day (4/carton)
      Kapvay (G) initially 0.1 mg bid; usual range 0.2-0.6 mg/day in divided doses; max 2.4 mg/day
         Tab: 0.1, 0.2 mg
      Nexiclon XR initially 0.18 mg (2 ml) suspension or 0.17 mg tab once daily; usual max 0.52 mg (6 ml suspension) once daily
         Tab: 0.17, 0.26 mg ext-rel; *Oral susp:* 0.09 mg/ml ext-rel (4 oz)
▷ *guanabenz* (C)(G) initially 4 mg bid; may increase by 4-8 mg/day every 1-2 weeks; max 32 mg/day
   Pediatric: <12 years: not recommended; ≥12 years: same as adult
      Tab: 4, 8 mg
▷ *guanfacine* (B)(G) initially 1 mg/day q HS; may increase to 2 mg/day q HS; usual max 3 mg/day
   Pediatric: <12 years: not recommended; ≥12 years: same as adult
      Tenex *Tab:* 1, 2 mg
▷ *methyldopa* (B)(G) initially 250 mg bid-tid; titrate at 2-day intervals; usual maintenance 500 mg/day to 2 gm/day; max 3 gm/day
   Pediatric: initially 10 mg/kg/day in 2-4 divided doses; max 65 mg/kg/day or 3 gm/day, whichever is less
      Aldomet *Tab:* 125, 250, 500 mg; *Oral susp:* 250 mg/5 ml (473 ml)

ALDOSTERONE RECEPTOR BLOCKER

▷ *eplerenone* (B) initially 25-50 mg daily; may increase to 50 mg bid; max 100 mg/day
   Pediatric: <12 years: not recommended; ≥12 years: same as adult
      Inspra *Tab:* 25, 50 mg
   Comment: Contraindicated with concomitant potent CYP3A4 inhibitors. Risk of hyperkalemia with concomitant ACE-I or ARB. Monitor serum potassium at baseline, 1 week, and 1 month. Caution with serum Cr >2 mg/dL (male) or >1.8 mg/dL (female) and/or CrCl <50 mL/min, and DM with proteinuria.

PERIPHERAL ADRENERGIC BLOCKER

▷ *guanethidine* (C) initially 10 mg daily; may adjust dose at 5-7 day intervals; usual range 25-50 mg/day
   Pediatric: <12 years: not recommended; ≥12 years: same as adult
      Ismelin *Tab:* 10, 25 mg

DIRECT RENIN INHIBITOR

▷ *aliskiren* (D) initially 150 mg once daily; max 300 mg/day
   Pediatric: <18 years: not recommended; ≥18 years: same as adult
      Tekturna *Tab:* 150, 300 mg

PERIPHERAL VASODILATORS

▷ *hydralazine* (C)(G) initially 10 mg qid x 2-4 days; then increase to 25 mg qid for remainder of 1st week; then increase to 50 mg qid; max 300 mg/day
   Pediatric: initially 0.75 mg/kg/day in 4 divided doses; increase gradually over 3-4 weeks; max 7.5 mg/kg/day or 2,000 mg/day
      Tab: 10, 25, 50, 100 mg
▷ *minoxidil* (C) initially 5 mg daily; may increase at 3-day intervals to 10 mg/day, then 20 mg/day, then 40 mg/day; usual range 10-40 mg/day; max 100 mg/day
   Pediatric: initially 0.2 mg/kg daily; may increase in 50%-100% increments every 3 days; usual range 0.25-1 gm/kg/day; max 50 mg/day
      Loniten *Tab:* 2.5*, 10*mg

ACEI+DIURETIC COMBINATIONS

▷ *benazepril+hydrochlorothiazide* (D)
    Pediatric: <12 years: not recommended; ≥12 years: same as adult
        Lotensin HCT
          Tab: Lotensin HCT 5/6.25 benaz 5 mg+hctz 6.25 mg*
              Lotensin HCT 10/12.5 benaz 10 mg+hctz 12.5 mg*
              Lotensin HCT 20/12.5 benaz 20 mg+hctz 12.5 mg*
              Lotensin HCT 20/25 benaz 20 mg+hctz 25 mg*

▷ *captopril+hydrochlorothiazide* (D)(G)
    Pediatric: <12 years: not recommended; ≥12 years: same as adult
        Capozide 1 tab once daily; titrate individual components
          Tab: Capozide 25/15 capt 25 mg+hctz 15 mg*
              Capozide 25/25 capt 25 mg+hctz 25 mg*
              Capozide 50/15 capt 50 mg+hctz 15 mg*
              Capozide 50/25 capt 50 mg+hctz 25 mg*

▷ *enalapril+hydrochlorothiazide* (D)
    Pediatric: <12 years: not recommended; ≥12 years: same as adult
        Vaseretic 1 tab once daily; titrate individual components
          Tab: Vaseretic 5/12.5 enal 5 mg+hctz 12.5 mg
              Vaseretic 10/25 enal 10 mg+hctz 25 mg

▷ *lisinopril+hydrochlorothiazide* (D)
    Pediatric: <12 years: not recommended; ≥12 years: same as adult
        Prinzide 1 tab once daily; titrate individual components
          Tab: Prinzide 10/12.5 lis 10 mg+hctz 12.5 mg
              Prinzide 20/12.5 lis 20 mg+hctz 12.5 mg
              Prinzide 20/25 lis 20 mg+hctz 25 mg
        Zestoretic 1 tab once daily; titrate individual components; *CrCl <40 mL/min:* not recommended
          Tab: Zestoretic 10/12.5 lis 10 mg+hctz 12.5 mg
              Zestoretic 20/12.5 lis 20 mg+hctz 12.5 mg*
              Zestoretic 20/25 lis 20 mg+hctz 25 mg

▷ *moexipril+hydrochlorothiazide* (D)
    Pediatric: <12 years: not recommended; ≥12 years: same as adult
        Uniretic 1 tab once daily; titrate individual components
          Tab: Uniretic 7.5/12.5 moex 7.5 mg+hctz 12.5 mg*
              Uniretic 15/12.5 moex 15 mg+hctz 12.5 mg*
              Uniretic 15/25 moex 15 mg+hctz 25 mg*

▷ *quinapril+hydrochlorothiazide* (D)
    Pediatric: <12 years: not recommended; ≥12 years: same as adult
        Accuretic 1 tab once daily; titrate individual components
          Tab: Accuretic 10/12.5 quin 10 mg+hctz 12.5 mg*
              Accuretic 20/12.5 quin 20 mg+hctz 12.5 mg*
              Accuretic 20/25 quin 20 mg+hctz 25 mg*

ARB+DIURETIC COMBINATIONS

▷ *azilsartan+chlorthalidone* (D)
    Pediatric: <18 years: not recommended; ≥18 years: same as adult
        Edarbyclor 1 tab once daily; titrate individual components
          Tab: Edarbyclor 40/12.5 azil 40 mg+chlor 12.5 mg
              Edarbyclor 40/25 azil 40 mg+chlor 25 mg

▷ *candesartan+hydrochlorothiazide* (D)
    Pediatric: <12 years: not recommended; ≥12 years: same as adult
        Atacand HCT
          Tab: Atacand HCT 16/12.5 cande 16 mg+hctz 12.5 mg
              Atacand HCT 32/12.5 cande 32 mg+hctz 12.5 mg

▷ *eprosartan+hydrochlorothiazide* (D)
    Pediatric: <12 years: not recommended; ≥12 years: same as adult
        Teveten HCT 1 tab once daily; titrate individual components
          Tab: Teveten HCT 600/12.5 epro 600 mg+hctz 12.5 mg
              Teveten HCT 600/25 epro 600 mg+hctz 25 mg

▷ *irbesartan+hydrochlorothiazide* (D)
  Pediatric: <12 years: not recommended; ≥12 years: same as adult
      Avalide 1 tab once daily; titrate individual components
        Tab: **Avalide 150/12.5** irbes 150 mg+hctz 12.5 mg
               Avalide 300/12.5 irbes 300 mg+hctz 12.5 mg
▷ *losartan+hydrochlorothiazide* (D)(G)
  Pediatric: <12 years: not recommended; ≥12 years: same as adult
      Hyzaar 1 tab once daily; titrate individual components
        Tab: **Hyzaar 50/12.5** losar 50 mg+hctz 12.5 mg
               Hyzaar 100/12.5 losar 100 mg+hctz 12.5 mg
               Hyzaar 100/25 losar 100 mg+hctz 25 mg
▷ *olmesartan medoxomil+hydrochlorothiazide* (D)(G)
  Pediatric: <12 years: not recommended; ≥12 years: same as adult
      Benicar HCT 1 tab once daily; titrate individual components
        Tab: **Benicar HCT 20/12.5** olmi 20 mg+hctz 12.5 mg
               Benicar HCT 40/12.5 olmi 40 mg+hctz 12.5 mg
               Benicar HCT 40/25 olmi 40 mg+hctz 25 mg
▷ *telmisartan+hydrochlorothiazide* (D)(G)
  Pediatric: <12 years: not recommended; ≥12 years: same as adult
      Micardis HCT 1 tab once daily; titrate individual components
        Tab: **Micardis HCT 40/12.5** telmi 40 mg+hctz 12.5 mg
               Micardis HCT 80/12.5 telmi 80 mg+hctz 12.5 mg
               Micardis HCT 80/25 telmi 80 mg+hctz 25 mg
▷ *valsartan+hydrochlorothiazide* (D)
  Pediatric: <12 years: not recommended; ≥12 years: same as adult
      Diovan HCT 1 tab once daily; titrate individual components
        Tab: **Diovan HCT 80/12.5** vals 80 mg+hctz 12.5 mg
               Diovan HCT 160/12.5 vals 160 mg+hctz 12.5 mg
               Diovan HCT 160/25 vals 160 mg+hctz 25 mg
               Diovan HCT 320/12.5 vals 320 mg+hctz 12.5 mg
               Diovan HCT 320/25 vals 320 mg+hctz 25 mg

CENTRAL ALPHA-AGONIST+DIURETIC COMBINATIONS

▷ *clonidine+chlorthalidone* (C)
  Pediatric: <12 years: not recommended; ≥12 years: same as adult
      Combipres 1 tab daily-bid
        Tab: **Combipres 0.1** clon 0.1 mg+chlor 15 mg*
               Combipres 0.2 clon 0.2 mg+chlor 15 mg*
               Combipres 0.3 clon 0.3 mg+chlor 15 mg*
▷ *methyldopa+hydrochlorothiazide* (C)(G)
  Pediatric: <12 years: not recommended; ≥12 years: same as adult
      Aldoril initially **Aldoril 15** bid-tid or **Aldoril 25** bid; titrate individual components
        Tab: **Aldoril 15** meth 250 mg+hctz 15 mg
               Aldoril 25 meth 250 mg+hctz 25 mg
               Aldoril D30 meth 500 mg+hctz 30 mg
               Aldoril D50 meth 500 mg+hctz 50 mg

BETA-BLOCKER (CARDIOSELECTIVE)+DIURETIC COMBINATIONS

▷ *atenolol+chlorthalidone* (D)(G)
  Pediatric: <12 years: not recommended; ≥12 years: same as adult
      Tenoretic initially *tenoretic* 50 mg once daily; may increase to *tenoretic* 100 mg once
      daily
        Tab: **Tenoretic 50/25** aten 50 mg+chlor 25 mg*
               Tenoretic 100/25 aten 100 mg+chlor 25 mg
▷ *bisoprolol+hydrochlorothiazide* (C)
  Pediatric: <12 years: not recommended; ≥12 years: same as adult
      Ziac initially one 2.5/6.25 mg tab daily; adjust at 2 week intervals; max two 10/6.25 mg
      tabs daily
        Tab: **Ziac 2.5** biso 2.5 mg+hctz 6.25 mg
               Ziac 5 biso 5 mg+hctz 6.25 mg
               Ziac 10 biso 10 mg+hctz 6.25 mg

▷ *metoprolol succinate+hydrochlorothiazide* (C)
    Pediatric: <12 years: not recommended; ≥12 years: same as adult
        Lopressor HCT titrate individual components
           Tab: Lopressor HCT 50/25 meto succ 50 mg+hctz 25 mg*
                Lopressor HCT 100/25 meto succ 100 mg+hctz 25 mg*
                Lopressor HCT 100/50 meto succ 100 mg+hctz 50 mg*
▷ *metoprolol succinate+ext-rel hydrochlorothiazide* (C)
    Pediatric: <12 years: not established; ≥12 years: same as adult
        Dutoprol titrate individual components; may titrate to max 200/25 mg once daily
           Tab: Dutoprol 25/12.5 meto succ 25 mg+hctz 12.5 mg *ext-rel*
                Dutoprol 50/12.5 meto succ 50 mg+hctz 12.5 mg *ext-rel*
                Dutoprol 100/12.5 meto succ 100 mg+hctz 12.5 mg *ext-rel*

BETA-BLOCKER (NON-CARDIOSELECTIVE)+DIURETIC COMBINATIONS

▷ *nadolol+bendroflumethiazide* (C)
    Pediatric: <12 years: not recommended; ≥12 years: same as adult
        Corzide titrate individual components
           Tab: Corzide 40/5 nado 40 mg+bend 5 mg*
                Corzide 80/5 nado 80 mg+bend 5 mg*
▷ *propranolol+hydrochlorothiazide* (C)(G)
    Pediatric: <12 years: not recommended; ≥12 years: same as adult
        Inderide titrate individual components
           Tab: Inderide 40/25 prop 40 mg+hctz 25 mg*
                Inderide 80/25 prop 80 mg+hctz 25 mg*
        Inderide LA titrate individual components
           Cap: Inderide LA 80/50 prop 80 mg+hctz 50 mg sust-rel
                Inderide LA 120/50 prop 120 mg+hctz 50 mg sust-rel
                Inderide LA 160/50 prop 160 mg+hctz 50 mg sust-rel
▷ *timolol+hydrochlorothiazide* (C)
    Pediatric: <12 years: not recommended; ≥12 years: same as adult
        Timolide usual maintenance 2 tabs/day in a single or 2 divided doses
           Tab: timo 10 mg+hctz 25 mg

BETA-BLOCKER (CARDIOSELECTIVE)+ARB COMBINATION

▷ *nebivolol+valsartan* (X)(G) 1 tab daily; may initiate when inadequately controlled on
   nebivolol 10 mg or *valsartan* 80 mg
    Pediatric: <12 years: not established; ≥12 years: same as adult
        Byvalson *Tab:* nebi 5 mg+val 80 mg

ALPHA-1 ANTAGONIST+DIURETIC COMBINATIONS

▷ *prazosin+polythiazide* (C)
    Pediatric: <12 years: not recommended; ≥12 years: same as adult
        Minizide titrate individual components
           Cap: Minizide 1 praz 1 mg+poly 0.5 mg
                Minizide 2 praz 2 mg+poly 0.5 mg
                Minizide 5 praz 5 mg+poly 0.5 mg

PERIPHERAL ADRENERGIC BLOCKER+HCTZ COMBINATION

▷ *guanethidine+hydrochlorothiazide* (C)
    Pediatric: <12 years: not recommended; ≥12 years: same as adult
        Esimil titrate individual components
           Tab: Esimil 10/25 guan 10 mg+hctz 25 mg

ACEI+CCB COMBINATIONS

▷ *amlodipine+benazepril* (D)
    Pediatric: <12 years: not recommended; ≥12 years: same as adult
        Lotrel titrate individual components
           Cap: Lotrel 2.5/10 amlo 2.5 mg+benaz 10 mg
                Lotrel 5/10 amlo 5 mg+benaz 10 mg
                Lotrel 5/20 amlo 5 mg+benaz 20 mg
                Lotrel 10/20 amlo 10 mg+benaz 20 mg

        Lotrel 5/40 amlo 5 mg+benaz 40 mg
        Lotrel 10/40 amlo 10 mg+benaz 40 mg

▷ *amlodipine+perindopril* (D)
  Pediatric: <12 years: not recommended; ≥12 years: same as adult
    Prestalia titrate individual components
      Cap: **Prestalia 2.5/3.5** amlo 2.5 mg+peri 3.5 mg
        Prestalia 5/7 amlo 5 mg+peri 7 mg
        Prestalia 5/14 amlo 5 mg+peri 14 mg

▷ *enalapril+diltiazem* (D)
  Pediatric: <12 years: not recommended; ≥12 years: same as adult
    Teczem titrate individual components
      Tab: enal 5 mg+dil 180 mg ext-rel

▷ *enalapril+felodipine* (D)
  Pediatric: <18 years: not recommended; ≥18 years: same as adult
    Lexxel titrate individual components
      Tab: **Lexxel 5/2.5** enal 5 mg+felo 2.5 mg ext-rel
        Lexxel 5/5 enal 5 mg+felo 5 mg ext-rel

▷ *perindopril+amlodipine* (D)
  Pediatric: <12 years: not established; ≥12 years: same as adult
    Prestalia titrate individual components; max 14/10 once daily
      Tab: **Prestalia 3.5/2.5** peri 3.5 mg+amlo 2.5 mg
        Prestalia 7/5 peri 7 mg+amlo 5 mg
        Prestalia 14/10 peri 14 mg+amlo 10 mg

▷ *trandolapril+verapamil* (D)
  Pediatric: <12 years: not established; ≥12 years: same as adult
    Tarka titrate individual components
      Tab: **Tarka 1/240** tran 1 mg+ver 240 mg ext-rel
        Tarka 2/180 tran 2 mg+ver 180 mg ext-rel
        Tarka 2/240 tran 2 mg+ver 240 mg ext-rel
        Tarka 4/240 tran 4 mg+ver 240 mg ext-rel

DRI+HCTZ COMBINATIONS

▷ *aliskiren+hydrochlorothiazide* (D) initially *aliskiren* 150 mg once daily; max *aliskiren* 300 mg/day
  Pediatric: <18 years: not recommended; ≥18 years: same as adult
    Tekturna HCT
      Tab: **Tekturna HCT 150/12.5** alisk 150 mg+hctz 12.5 mg
        Tekturna HCT 150/25 alisk 150 mg+hctz 25 mg
        Tekturna HCT 300/12.5 alisk 300 mg+hctz 12.5 mg
        Tekturna HCT 300/25 alisk 300 mg+hctz 25 mg

DRI+ARB COMBINATION

▷ *aliskiren+valsartan* (D)
  Pediatric: <12 years: not recommended; ≥12 years: same as adult
    Valturna initially 150/160 once daily; may increase to max 300/320 once daily
      Tab: **Valturna 150/160** alisk 150 mg+vals 160 mg
        Valturna 300/320 alisk 300 mg+vals 320 mg

DRI+CCB COMBINATION

▷ *aliskiren+amlodipine* (D)
  Pediatric: <12 years: not recommended; ≥12 years: same as adult
    Tekamlo initially 150/5 once daily; may increase to max 300/10 once daily
      Tab: **Tekamlo 150/5** alisk 150 mg+amlo 5 mg
        Tekamlo 150/10 alisk 150 mg+amlo 10 mg
        Tekamlo 300/5 alisk 300 mg+amlo 5 mg
        Tekamlo 300/10 alisk 300 mg+amlo 10 mg

DRI+CCB+HCTZ COMBINATIONS

▷ *aliskiren+amlodipine+hydrochlorothiazide* (D)
  Pediatric: <12 years: not established; ≥12 years: same as adult

Amturnide initially 150/5/12.5 once daily; may increase to max 300/10/25 once daily
Tab: **Amturnide 150/5/12.5** alisk 150 mg+amlo 5 mg+hctz 12.5 mg
Amturnide 300/5/12.5 alisk 300 mg+amlo 5 mg+hctz 12.5 mg
Amturnide 300/5/25 alisk 300 mg+amlo 5 mg+hctz 25 mg

ARB+CCB COMBINATIONS

➤ *amlodipine+valsartan medoxomil* (D)(G)
Pediatric: <12 years: not recommended; ≥12 years: same as adult
Exforge 1 tab daily; titrate individual components at 1-week intervals; max 10/320 once daily
Tab: **Exforge 5/160** amlo 5 mg+vals 160 mg
Exforge 5/320 amlo 5 mg+vals 320 mg
Exforge 10/160 amlo 10 mg+vals 160 mg
Exforge 10/320 amlo 10 mg+vals 320 mg
➤ *amlodipine+olmesartan medoxomil* (D)(G)
Pediatric: <12 years: not established; ≥12 years: same as adult
Azor titrate individual components
Tab: **Azor 5/20** amlo 5 mg+olme 20 mg
Azor 10/20 amlo 10 mg+olme 20 mg
Azor 5/40 amlo 5 mg+olme 40 mg
Azor 10/40 amlo 10 mg+olme 40 mg
➤ *telmisartan+amlodipine* (D)(G)
Pediatric: <12 years: not established; ≥12 years: same as adult
Twynsta initially 40/5 once daily; titrate at 1 week intervals; max 80/10 once daily
Tab: **Twynsta 40/5** telmi 40 mg+amlo 5 mg
Twynsta 40/10 telmi 40 mg+amlo 10 mg
Twynsta 80/5 telmi 80 mg+amlo 5 mg
Twynsta 80/10 telmi 80 mg+amlo 10 mg

ARB+CCB+HCTZ COMBINATIONS

➤ *amlodipine+valsartan medoxomil+hydrochlorothiazide* (D)(G)
Pediatric: <12 years: not recommended; ≥12 years: same as adult
Exforge HCT: initially 5/160/12.5 once daily; may titrate at 1-week intervals to max 10/320/25 once daily
Tab: **Exforge HCT 5/160/12.5** amlo 5 mg+vals 160 mg+hctz 12.5 mg
Exforge HCT 5/160/25 amlo 5 mg+vals 160 mg+hctz 25 mg
Exforge HCT 10/160/12.5 amlo 10 mg+vals 160 mg+hctz 12.5 mg
Exforge HCT 10/160/25 amlo 10 mg+vals 160 mg+hctz 25 mg
Exforge HCT 10/320/25 amlo 10 mg+vals 320 mg+hctz 25 mg
➤ *olmesartan medoxomil+amlodipine+hydrochlorothiazide* (D)(G)
Pediatric: <12 years: not recommended; ≥12 years: same as adult
Tribenzor: initially 20/5/12.5 once daily; may titrate at 1-week intervals to max 40/10/25 daily
Tab: **Tribenzor 20/5/12.5** olme 20 mg+amlo 5 mg+hctz 12.5 mg
Tribenzor 40/5/12.5 olme 40 mg+amlo 5 mg+hctz 12.5 mg
Tribenzor 40/5/25 olme 40 mg+amlo 5 mg+hctz 25 mg
Tribenzor 40/10/12.5 olme 40 mg+amlo 10 mg+hctz 12.5 mg
Tribenzor 40/10/25 olme 40 mg+amlo 10 mg+hctz 25 mg

OTHER COMBINATION AGENTS

➤ *clonidine+chlorthalidone* (C)
Pediatric: <12 years: not recommended; ≥12 years: same as adult
Clorpres initially 0.1/15 once daily; may titrate to max 0.3/15 bid
Tab: **Clorpres 0.1/15** clon 0.1 mg+chlor 15 mg
Clorpres 0.2/15 clon 0.2 mg+chlor 15 mg
Clorpres 0.3/15 clon 0.3 mg+chlor 15 mg
➤ *reserpine+hydroflumethiazide* (C)
Pediatric: <12 years: not recommended; ≥12 years: same as adult
Salutensin initially 1.25/25 once daily; may titrate to 1.25/25 bid or 1.25/50 once daily
Tab: **Salutensin 1.25/25** enal 1.25 mg+hydro 25 mg
Salutensin 1.25/50: enal 1.25 mg+hydro 50 mg

ANTIHYPERTENSION+ANTILIPID COMBINATIONS

CCB+Statin Combinations

▷ *amlodipine+atorvastatin* (X)
  Pediatric: <10 years: not established; ≥10 years (female postmenarche): same as adult
    Caduet select according to blood pressure and lipid values; titrate *amlodipine* over 7-14 days; titrate *atorvastatin* according to monitored lipid values; max *amlodipine* 10 mg/day and max *atorvastatin* 80 mg/day; refer to contraindications and precautions for CCB and statin therapy
      Tab: **Caduet 2.5/10** amlo 2.5 mg+ator 10 mg
        Caduet 2.5/20 amlo 2.5 mg+ator 20 mg
        Caduet 5/10 amlo 5 mg+ator 10 mg
        Caduet 5/20 amlo 5 mg+ator 20 mg
        Caduet 5/40 amlo 5 mg+ator 40 mg
        Caduet 5/80 amlo 5 mg+ator 80 mg
        Caduet 10/10 amlo 10 mg+ator 10 mg
        Caduet 10/20 amlo 10 mg+ator 20 mg
        Caduet 10/40 amlo 10 mg+ator 40 mg
        Caduet 10/80 amlo 10 mg+ator 80 mg

ANTIHYPERTENSION+ANTI-OSTEOARTHRITIS COMBINATION

CCB + Cox-2 Inhibitor

▷ *amlodipine+celecoxib*
  Pediatric: not established
    Cosensi take as a single dose once daily; max *amlodipine* 10 mg and max *celecoxib* 200 mg per day
      Tab: **Consensi 2.5/200** *Tab:* amlo 2.5 mg + celecox 200 mg
        Consensi 5/200 *Tab:* amlo 5 mg + celecox 200 mg
        Consensi 10/200 *Tab:* amlo 10 mg + celecox 200 mg

  Comment: **Consensi** is a combination of *amlodipine besylate* (calcium channel blocker) and *celecoxib* (Cox-2 inhibitor) indicated for patients for whom treatment with are appropriate. Lowering blood pressure reduces the risk of fatal and nonfatal CV events, primarily stroke and myocardial infarction.

HYPERTHYROIDISM

▷ *methimazole* (D) initially 15-60 mg/day in 3 divided doses; maintenance 5-15 mg/day
  Pediatric: initially 0.4 mg/kg/day in 3 divided doses; maintenance 0.2 mg/kg/day or 1/2 initial dose
    Tapazole *Tab:* 5*, 10* mg

  Comment: *methimazole* potentiates anticoagulants. Contraindicated in nursing mothers.

▷ *propylthiouracil (ptu)* (D)(G)
    Propyl-Thyracil initially 100-900 mg/day in 3 divided doses; maintenance usually 50-600 mg/day in 2 divided doses
      Pediatric: <6 years: not recommended; ≥6-10 years: initially 50-150 mg/day or 5-7 mg/kg/day in 3 divided doses; ≥10 years: initially 150-300 mg/day or 5-7 mg/kg/day in 3 divided doses; *maintenance:* 0.2 mg/kg/day or 1/2-2/3 of initial dose
        Tab: 50* mg

  Comment: Preferred agent in pregnancy. Side effects include dermatitis, nausea, agranulocytosis, and hypothyroidism. Should be taken regularly for 2 years. Do not discontinue abruptly.

BETA-ADRENERGIC BLOCKER

▷ *propranolol* (C)(G) 40-240 mg daily
  Pediatric: <12 years: not recommended; ≥12 years: same as adult
    Inderal *Tab:* 10*, 20*, 40*, 60*, 80* mg
    Inderal LA initially 80 mg daily in a single dose; increase q 3-7 days; usual range 120-160 mg/day; max 320 mg/day in a single dose
      Cap: 60, 80, 120, 160 mg sust-rel
    InnoPran XL initially 80 mg q HS; max 120 mg/day
      Cap: 80, 120 mg ext-rel

HYPERTRIGLYCERIDEMIA

OMEGA 3-FATTY ACID ETHYL ESTERS

Comment: Vascepa, Lovaza, and Epanova are indicated for the treatment of TG ≥500 mg/dL.
➤ *icosapent ethyl (omega 3-fatty acid ethyl ester of EPA)* (C) 2 caps bid with food; max 4 gm/day; swallow whole, do not crush or chew
  Pediatric: <18 years: not recommended; ≥18 years: same as adult
    Vascepa sgc: 0.5, 1 gm (α-tocopherol 4 mg/cap)
➤ *omega 3-fatty acid ethyl esters* (C)(G) 2 gm bid or 4 gm daily; swallow whole, do not crush or chew
  Pediatric: <18 years: not recommended; ≥18 years: same as adult
    Lovaza *Gelcap*: 1 gm (α-tocopherol 4 mg/cap) *omega 3-carcartonyl acids* (C) take 2-4 gel aps (2-4 gm) daily without regard to meals
    Epanova *Gelcap*: 1 gm

ISOBUTYRIC ACID DERIVATIVE

➤ *gemfibrozil* (C)(G)
  Pediatric: <12 years: not recommended; ≥12 years: same as adult
    Lopid 600 mg bid 30 minutes before AM and PM meals
      Tab: 600*mg

FIBRATES (FIBRIC ACID DERIVATIVES)

➤ *fenofibrate* (C) take with meals; adjust at 4-8-week intervals; discontinue if inadequate response after 2 months; lowest dose or contraindicated with renal impairment and the elderly
  Pediatric: <12 years: not recommended; ≥12 years: same as adult
    Antara 43-130 mg once daily; max 130 mg/day
      Cap: 43, 87, 130 mg
    FibriCor 30-105 mg once daily; max 105 mg/day
      Tab: 30, 105 mg
    TriCor (G) 48-145 mg once daily; max 145 mg/day
      Tab: 48, 145 mg
    TriLipix (G) 45-135 mg once daily; max 135 mg/day
      Cap: 45, 135 mg del-rel
    Lipofen (G) 50-150 mg once daily; max 150 mg/day
      Cap: 50, 150 mg
    Lofibra 67-200 mg daily; max 200 mg/day
      Tab: 67, 134, 200 mg

NICOTINIC ACID DERIVATIVES

Comment: Contraindicated in liver disease. Decrease total cholesterol, LDL-C, and TG; increase HDL-C. Before initiating and at 4-6 weeks, 3 months, and 6 months of therapy, check fasting lipid profile or as indicated by manufacturer, LFT, glucose, and uric acid. Significant side effect of transient skin flushing. Take with food and take *aspirin* 325 mg 30 minutes before *niacin* dose to decrease flushing.
➤ *niacin* (C)
    Niaspan 375 mg daily for 1st week, then 500 mg daily for 2nd week, then 750 mg daily for 3rd week, then 1 gm daily for weeks 4-7; may increase by 500 mg q 4 weeks; usual range 1-3 gm/day
    Pediatric: <12 years: not recommended; ≥12 years: same as adult
      Tab: 500, 750, 1,000 mg ext-rel
    Slo-Niacin 250 mg or 500 mg or 750 mg q AM or HS
    Pediatric: <12 years: not recommended; ≥12 years: same as adult
      Tab: 250, 500, 750 mg cont-rel

HMG-COA REDUCTASE INHIBITORS (STATINS)

➤ *atorvastatin* (X)(G) initially 10 mg daily; usual range 10-80 mg daily
  Pediatric: <10 years: not recommended; ≥10 years (female post-menarche): same as adult
    Lipitor *Tab*: 10, 20, 40, 80 mg
➤ *fluvastatin* (X)(G) initially 20-40 mg q HS; usual range 20-80 mg/day
  Pediatric: <18 years: not established; ≥18 years: same as adult

      Lescol *Cap:* 20, 40 mg
      Lescol XL *Tab:* 80 mg ext-rel
▷ *lovastatin* (X) initially 20 mg daily at evening meal; may increase at 4 week intervals; max 80 mg/day in a single or divided doses; *Concomitant fibrates,* **niacin,** *or CrCl <40 mL/min:* usual max 20 mg/day
    Pediatric: <10 years: not recommended; 10-17 years: initially 10-20 mg daily at evening meal; may increase at 4 week intervals; max 40 mg daily; *Concomitant fibrates,* **niacin,** *or CrCl <40 mL/min:* usual max 20 mg/day
      Mevacor *Tab:* 10, 20, 40 mg
▷ *pravastatin* (X)(G) initially 10-20 mg q HS; usual range 10-80 mg/day; may start at 40 mg/day
    Pediatric: <8 years: not recommended; 8-13 years: 20 mg q HS; 14-17 years: 40 mg q HS; >17 years: same as adult
      Pravachol *Tab:* 10, 20, 40, 80 mg
▷ *rosuvastatin* (X) initially 20 mg q HS; usual range 5-40 mg/day; adjust at 4 week intervals
    Pediatric: <10 years: not recommended; 10-17 years: 5-20 mg q HS; max 20 mg q HS; >17 years: same as adult
      Crestor *Tab:* 5, 10, 20, 40 mg
▷ *simvastatin* (X)(G) initially 20 mg q HS; usual range 5-80 mg/day; adjust at 4 week intervals
    Pediatric: <10 years: not recommended; 10-17 years: initially 10 mg q HS; may increase at 4 week intervals; max 40 mg q HS; >17 years: same as adult
      Zocor *Tab:* 5, 10, 20, 40, 80 mg

NICOTINIC ACID DERIVATIVE+HMG-COA REDUCTASE INHIBITOR COMBINATION

Comment: Nicotinic acid derivatives decrease total cholesterol, LDL-C, and TG; increase HDL-C. Before initiating and at 4-6 weeks, 3 months, and 6 months of therapy, check fasting lipid profile, LFT, glucose, and uric acid. Side effects include hyperglycemia, upper GI distress, hyperuricemia, hepatotoxicity, and significant transient skin flushing. Take with food and take **aspirin** 325 mg 30 minutes before **niacin** dose to decrease flushing. *Relative contraindications:* diabetes, hyperuricemia (gout), and PUD. *Absolute contraindications:* severe gout and chronic liver disease.

▷ *niacin+lovastatin* (X)
    Pediatric: <18 years: not recommended; ≥18 years: same as adult
      Advicor monitor lab values; may titrate up to max 1,000/20 once daily
      Tab: **Advicor 500/20** niac 500 mg ext-rel+lova 20 mg
          Advicor 750/20 niac 750 mg ext-rel+lova 20 mg
          Advicor 1,000/20 niac 1,000 mg ext-rel+lova 20 mg

⬤ HYPOCALCEMIA

Comment: Hypocalcemia resulting in metabolic bone disease may be secondary to hyperparathyroidism, pseudoparathyroidism, and chronic renal disease. Normal serum Ca++ range is approximately 8.5-12 mg/dL. Signs and symptoms of hypocalcemia include confusion, increased neuromuscular excitability, muscle spasms, paresthesias, hyperphosphatemia, positive Chvostek's sign, and positive Trousseau's sign. Signs and symptoms of hypercalcemia include fatigue, lethargy, decreased concentration and attention span, frank psychosis, anorexia, nausea, vomiting, constipation, bradycardia, heart block, shortened QT interval. Foods high in calcium include almonds, broccoli, baked beans, salmon, sardines, buttermilk, turnip greens, collard greens, spinach, pumpkin, rhubarb, and bran. Recommended daily calcium intake: 1-3 years: 700 mg; 4-8 years: 1,000 mg; 9-18 years: 1,300 mg; 19-50 years: 1,000 mg: 51-70 years (males): 1,000 mg; ≥51 years (females): 1,200 mg; pregnancy or nursing: 1,000-1,300 mg. Recommended daily vitamin D intake: >1 year: 600 IU; 50+ years: 800-1,000 IU. The American Academy of Rheumatology (AAR) recommends the following daily doses for anyone on a chronic oral corticosteroid regimen: Calcium 1,200-1,500 mg/day and vitamin D 800-1,000 IU/day.

CALCIUM SUPPLEMENTS

Comment: Take *calcium* supplements after meals to avoid gastric upset. Dosages of *calcium* over 2,000 mg/day have not been shown to have any additional benefit. *Calcium* decreases *tetracycline* absorption. *Calcium* absorption is decreased by corticosteroids.

➤ *calcitonin-salmon* (C)

    Miacalcin 200 units (1 spray intranasally) once daily; alternate nostrils each day
        Nasal spray: 14 dose (2 ml)

    Miacalcin injection 100 units/day SC <u>or</u> IM
        Vial: 2 ml

➤ *calcium carbonate* (C)(OTC)(G)

    Rolaids chew 2 tabs bid; max 14 tabs/day
        Tab: calcium carbonate: 550 mg

    Rolaids Extra Strength chew 2 tabs bid; max 8 tabs/day
        Tab: 1,000 mg

    Tums chew 2 tabs bid; max 16 tabs/day
        Tab: 500 mg

    Tums Extra Strength chew 2 tabs bid; max 10 tabs/day
        Tab: 750 mg

    Tums Ultra chew 2 tabs bid; max 8 tabs/day
        Tab: 1,000 mg

    Os-Cal 500 (OTC) 1-2 tab bid-tid
        Tab: elemental calcium carbonate 500 mg

➤ *calcium carbonate+vitamin D* (C)(G)

    Os-Cal 250+D (OTC) 1-2 tabs tid
        Tab: elemental calcium carbonate 250 mg+vit d 125 IU

    Os-Cal 500+D (OTC) 1-2 tabs bid-tid
        Tab: elemental calcium carbonate 500 mg+vit d 125 IU

    Viactiv (OTC) 1 tab tid
        Chew tab: elemental calcium 500 mg+vit d and vit a100 IU+Vit k 40 mEq

➤ *calcium citrate*

    Citracal (OTC) 1-2 tabs bid
        Tab: elemental calcium citrate 200 mg

➤ *calcium citrate+vitamin D* (C)(G)

    Citracal+D (OTC) 1-2 cplts bid
        Cplt: elemental calcium citrate 315 mg+vit d 200 IU

    Citracal 250+D (OTC) 1-2 tabs bid
        Tab: elemental calcium citrate 250 mg+vit d 62.3 IU

VITAMIN D ANALOGS

Comment: Concurrent *vitamin D* supplementation is contraindicated for patients taking *calcitriol* <u>or</u> *doxercalciferol* due to the risk of *vitamin D* toxicity. Symptoms of hypervitaminosis D: hypercalcemia, hypercalciuria, elevated creatinine, erythema multiforme, hyperphosphatemia. Maintain adequate daily calcium and fluid intake. Keep serum calcium times phosphate (Ca x P) product below 70. Monitor serum calcium (esp. during dose titration), phosphorus, other lab values (see literature for frequency).

➤ *calcitriol* (C)(G) *Predialysis:* initially 0.25 mcg daily; may increase to 0.5 mcg daily; *Dialysis:* initially 0.25 mcg daily; may increase by 0.25 mcg/day at 4-8-week intervals; usual maintenance 0.5-1 mcg/day; *Hypoparathyroidism:* initially 0.25 mcg q AM; may increase by 0.25 mcg/day at 4-8 week intervals; usual maintenance 0.5-2 mcg/day
Pediatric: <12 years: *Predialysis:* <3 years: 10-15 ng/kg per day; ≥3 years: initially 0.25 mcg daily; may increase to 0.5 mcg daily; *Dialysis:* not recommended; *Hypoparathyroidism:* initially 0.25 mcg daily in the AM; may increase by 0.25 mcg/day at 2-4 week intervals; usual maintenance: (1-5 years): 0.25-0.75 mcg daily; (≥6 years): 0.5-2 mcg daily; *Pseudo-hypoparathyroidism:* (<6 years): insufficient data, see mfr pkg insert; ≥12 years: *Predialysis:* initially 0.25 mcg daily; may increase to 0.5 mcg daily *Dialysis:* initially 0.25 mcg daily; may increase by 0.25 mcg daily at 4-8 week intervals; usual maintenance: 0.5-1 mcg daily.

    Rocaltrol *Cap:* 0.25, 0.5 mcg

    Rocaltrol Solution *Soln:* 1 mcg/ml (15 ml, single-use dispensers)

Comment: *calcitriol* is indicated for the treatment of secondary hyperparathyroidism and resultant metabolic bone disease in predialysis patients (CrCl 15-55 mL/min), hypocalcemia and resultant metabolic bone disease in patients on chronic renal dialysis, hypocalcemia in hypoparathyroidism, and pseudohypoparathyroidism.

➤ *doxecalciferol* (C)(G) *Dialysis:* initially 10 mcg 3 x/week at dialysis; adjust to maintain intact parathyroid hormone (iPTH) between 150-300 pg/mL; if iPTH is not lowered by 50% and fails to reach target range, may increase by 2.5 mcg at 8-week intervals; max 20 mcg 3 x/week; if iPTH <100 pg/mL, suspend for 1 week, then resume at a dose that is at least 2.5 mcg lower; *Predialysis:* initially 1 mcg once daily; may increase by 0.5 mcg at 2 week intervals to target iPTH levels; max 3.5 mcg/day

Pediatric: <12 years: not established; ≥12 years: same as adult

> Hectorol *Cap:* 0.25, 0.5, 1, 2.5 mcg

Comment: Oral **Hectorol** is indicated for the treatment of secondary hyperparathyroidism in patients with chronic kidney disease (CKD) on dialysis; Predialysis stage 3 or 4 CKD: use oral form only.

Hectoral Injection <12 years: not recommended; ≥12 years: 4 mcg 3 x weekly after dialysis; adjust dose to maintain intact parathyroid hormone (iPTH) between 150-300 pg/mL; if iPTH is not lowered by 50% and fails to reach target range, may increase by 1-2 mcg at 8 week intervals; max 18 mcg/week; if iPTH <100 pg/mL, suspend for 1 week, then resume at a dose that is at least 1 mcg lower

> *Vial:* 2 mcg/ml (1, 2 ml single-dose; 2 ml multi-dose)

Comment: **Hectorol Injection** is indicated for the treatment of secondary hyperparathyroidism in patients with chronic kidney disease (CKD) on dialysis.

▷ *paricalcitol* (C)(G) administer 0.04-1 mcg/kg (2.8-7 mcg) IV bolus, during dialysis, no more than every other day; may be increased by 2-4 mcg/dose every 2-4 weeks; monitor serum calcium and phosphorus during dose adjustment periods; if Ca x P >75, immediately reduce dose or discontinue until these levels normalize; discard unused portion of single-use vials immediately

Pediatric: <18 years: not established; ≥18 years: same as adult

> Zemplar *Vial:* 2, 5 mcg/ml soln for inj

Comment: *paricalcitol* is indicated for the prevention and treatment of secondary hyperparathyroidism associated with chronic kidney disease (CKD) stage 5.

BIOENGINEERED REPLICA OF HUMAN PARATHYROID HORMONE

▷ *bioengineered replica of human parathyroid hormone* (C) before starting, confirm 25-hydroxyvitamin D stores are sufficient; if insufficient, replace to sufficient levels per standard of care; confirm serum calcium is above 7.5 mg/dL; the goal of treatment is to achieve serum calcium within the lower half of the normal range; administer SC into the thigh once daily; alternate thighs; initially, 50 mcg/day; when initiating, decrease dose of active vitamin D by 50%, if serum calcium is above 7.5 mg/dL; monitor serum calcium levels every 3 to 7 days after starting or adjusting dose and when adjusting either active vitamin D or calcium supplements dose. Abrupt interruption or discontinuation of **Natpara** can result in severe hypocalcemia. Resume treatment with, or increase the dose of, an active form of vitamin D and calcium supplements. Monitor for signs and symptoms of hypocalcemia and monitor serum calcium levels, In the case of a missed dose, the next **Natpara** dose should be administered as soon as reasonably feasible and additional exogenous calcium should be taken in the event of hypocalcemia.

> Natpara *Soln for inj:* 25, 50, 75, 100 mcg (2/pkg) multiple dose, dual-chamber glass cartridge containing a sterile powder and diluent

Comment: **Natpara** is indicated as an adjunct to calcium and vitamin D in patients with hypoparathyroidism. Because of a potential risk of osteosarcoma, use **Natpara** only in patients who cannot be well-controlled on calcium and active forms of vitamin D alone and for whom the potential benefits are considered to outweigh the potential risk. Avoid use of **Natpara** in patients who are at increased baseline risk for osteosarcoma, such as patients with Paget's disease of bone or unexplained elevations of alkaline phosphatase, pediatric and young adult patients with open epiphyses, patients with hereditary disorders predisposing to osteosarcoma or patients with a prior history of external beam or implant radiation therapy involving the skeleton. Because of the risk of osteosarcoma, **Natpara** is available only through a restricted program under a Risk Evaluation and Mitigation Strategy (REMS) (www.natparaREMS.com).

 HYPOKALEMIA

Comment: Normal serum K⁺ range is approximately 3.5-5.5 mEq/L. Signs and symptoms of hypokalemia include neuromuscular weakness, muscle twitching and cramping, hyporeflexia, postural hypotension, anorexia, nausea and vomiting, depressed ST segments, flattened T waves, and cardiac tachyarrhythmias. Signs and symptoms of hyperkalemia include peaked T waves, elevated ST segment, and widened QRS complexes.

PROPHYLAXIS

Comment: Usual dose range is 8-10 mEq/day.

TREATMENT OF HYPOKALEMIA: NON-EMERGENCY (K⁺ <3.5 mEq/L)

Comment: Usual dose range 40-120 mEq/day in divided doses. Solutions are preferred; potentially serious GI side effects may occur with tablet formulations or when taken on an empty stomach.

POTASSIUM SUPPLEMENTS

Comment: Potassium supplements should be taken with food. Solutions are the preferred form. Extended-release and sustained-release forms should be swallowed whole; do not crush or chew. Potassium supplementation is indicated for hypokalemia including that caused by diuretic use, and digitalis intoxication without atrioventricular (AV) block.

▷ *potassium* (C)(G)
   Pediatric: <12 years: not established; ≥12 years: same as adult
      KCL Solution Oral soln: 10% (30 ml unit dose, 50/case)
      K-Dur (as chloride) *Tab:* 10, 20* mEq sust-rel
      K-Lor for Oral Solution (as chloride) *Pkts* for reconstitution: 20 mEq/pkt (fruit)
      Klor-Con/25 (as chloride) *Pkts* for reconstitution: 25 mEq/pkt
      Klor-Con/EF 25 (as bicarbonate) *Pkts* for reconstitution: 25 mEq/pkt (effervescent) (fruit)
      Klor-Con Extended-Release (as chloride) *Tab:* 8, 10 mEq ext-rel
      Klor-Con M (as chloride) *Tab:* 10, 15*, 20* mEq ext-rel
      Klor-Con Powder (as chloride) 20, 25 mEq *Pkts* for reconstitution: (30/carton) (fruit)
      Klorvess (as bicarbonate and citrate) *Tab:* 20 mEq effervescent for solution; *Granules:* 20 mEq/pkt effervescent for solution; *Oral liq:* 20 mEq/15 ml (16 oz)
      Klotrix (as chloride) *Tab:* 10 mEq sust-rel
      K-Lyte (as bicarbonate and citrate) *Tab:* 25 mEq effervescent for solution (lime, orange)
      K-Lyte/CL (as chloride) *Tab:* 25 mEq effervescent for solution (citrus, fruit)
      K-Lyte/CL 50 (as chloride) *Tab:* 50 mEq effervescent for solution (citrus, fruit)
      K-Lyte/DS (as bicarbonate and citrate) *Tab:* 50 mEq effervescent for solution (lime, orange)
      K-Tab (as chloride) *Tab:* 10 mEq sust-rel
      Micro-K (as chloride) *Cap:* 8, 10 mEq sust-rel
      Potassium Chloride Extended Release Caps *Cap:* 8, 10 mEq ext-rel
      Potassium Chloride Sust-Rel Tabs *Tab/Cap:* 10 mEq sust-rel
      Potassium Chloride ER *Tab:* 8 mEq (600 mg), 10 mEq (750 mg)

 HYPOMAGNESEMIA

Comment: Normal serum Mg⁺⁺ range is approximately 1.2-2.6 mEq/L. Signs and symptoms of hypomagnesemia include confusion, disorientation, hallucinations, hyperreflexia, tetany, convulsions, tachyarrhythmia, positive Chvostek's sign, and positive Trousseau's sign. Signs and symptoms of hypermagnesemia include drowsiness, lethargy, muscle weakness, hypoactive reflexes, slurred speech, bradycardia, hypotension, convulsions, and cardiac arrhythmias.

MAGNESIUM SUPPLEMENTS

▷ *magnesium* (B) 2 tabs daily
      Slow-Mag
         Tab: 64 mg (as chloride)+110 mg (as carbonate)
▷ *magnesium oxide* (B) 1-2 tabs daily
      Mag-Ox 400
         Tab: 400 mg

HYPOPARATHYROIDISM

VITAMIN D ANALOGS

Comment: Concurrent vitamin D supplementation is contraindicated for patients taking *calcitriol* or *doxecalciferol* owing to the risk of vitamin D toxicity.

➤ *calcitriol* (**C**) initially 0.25 mcg q AM; may increase by 0.25 mcg/day at 4-8-week intervals; usual maintenance 0.5-2 mcg/day
Pediatric: initially 0.25 mcg daily; may increase by 0.25 mcg/day at 2-4-week intervals; usual maintenance (1-5 years) 0.25-0.75 mcg/day, (≥6 years) 0.5-2 mcg/day
   Rocaltrol *Cap:* 0.25, 0.5 mcg
   Rocaltrol Solution *Soln:* 1 mcg/ml (15 ml, single-use dispensers)
➤ *doxecalciferol* (**C**) initially 0.25 mcg q AM; may increase by 0.25 mcg/day at 4-8-week intervals; usual maintenance 0.5-2 mcg/day
Pediatric: initially 0.25 mcg daily; may increase by 0.25 mcg/day at 2-4-week intervals; usual maintenance (1-5 years) 0.25-0.75 mcg/day, (≥6 years) 0.5-2 mcg/day
   Hectorol *Cap:* 0.25, 0.5 mcg

HUMAN PARATHYROID HORMONE

➤ *teriparatide* (**C**) 20 mcg SC daily in the thigh or abdomen; may treat for up to 2 years
   Forteo *Multi-dose pen:* 250 mcg/ml (3 ml)
   Comment: **Forteo** is indicated for the treatment of postmenopausal osteoporosis in women who are at high risk for fracture and to increase bone mass in men with primary or hypogonadal osteoporosis who are at high risk for fracture.

HUMAN PARATHYROID HORMONE-RELATED PEPTIDE (PTHrP) ANALOG

➤ *abaloparatide* (**C**) Administer 80 mcg SC once daily into the periumbilical region of the abdomen; sit or lie down in case of orthostatic hypotension, especially for first dose; patients should receive supplemental calcium and vitamin D if dietary intake is inadequate
   Tymlos *Multi-dose pen:* 3120 mcg/1.56 ml (2000 mcg/ml, 30 daily doses) disposable
   Comment: **Tymlos** is indicated for the treatment of postmenopausal osteoporosis in women who are at high risk for fracture (defined as a history of osteoporotic fracture, or multiple risk factors for fracture, or patients who have failed or are intolerant to other available osteoporosis therapy. **Tymlos** is not recommended in patients who are at risk for osteosarcoma (boxed warning). Cumulative use of **Tymlos** or other parathyroid analogs (e.g., *teriparatide*) for >2 years during a patient's lifetime is not recommended (boxed warning). Avoid use in patients with pre-existing hypercalcemia and those known to have an underlying hypercalcemic disorder, such as primary hyperparathyroidism. Monitor urine calcium if preexisting hypercalciuria or active urolithiasis are suspected.

BIOENGINEERED REPLICA OF HUMAN PARATHYROID HORMONE

➤ *bioengineered replica of human parathyroid hormone* (**C**) initially inject mg IM into the thigh once daily; when initiating, decrease dose of active vitamin D by 50% if serum calcium is above 7.5 mg/dL; monitor serum calcium levels every 3-7 days after starting or adjusting dose and when adjusting either active vitamin D or calcium supplements dose
   Natpara *Soln for inj:* 25, 50, 75, 100 mcg (2/pkg) multiple dose, dual-chamber glass cartridge containing a sterile powder and diluent
   Comment: **Natpara** is indicated as an adjunct to calcium and vitamin D in patients with parathyroidism.

 HYPOPHOSPHATASIA (OSTEOMALACIA, RICKETS)

Comment: Hypophosphatasia (HPP) is an inborn error of metabolism marked by abnormally low serum alkaline phosphatase activity and phosphoethanolamine in the urine. It is manifested by osteomalacia in adults and rickets in infants and children. It is most severe in infants under 6 months-of-age. With congenital absence of alkaline phosphatase, an enzyme essential to the calcification of bone tissue, complications include vomiting, growth retardation, and often death in infancy. Surviving children have numerous skeletal abnormalities and dwarfism.
➤ *asfotase alfa* 6 mg/kg/week SC, administered as 2 mg/kg or 1 mg/kg 6 x/week; max 9 mg/kg/week SC administered as 3 mg/kg 3 x/week
Pediatric: same as adult
   Strensiq *Vial:* 18 mg/0.45 ml, 28 mg/0.7 ml, 40 mg/ml, 80 mg/0.8 ml for SC inj, single-use (1, 12/carton) (preservative-free)
   Comment: **Strensiq** is the first FDA-approved (2015) treatment for perinatal, infantile, and juvenile onset HPP. Prior to the availability of **Strensiq**, there was no effective treatment and patient prognosis was very poor.

HYPOPHOSPHATEMIA, X-LINKED (XLH)

FIBROBLAST GROWTH FACTOR (FGF23) BLOCKING ANTIBODY

▷ *burosumab-twza* (C) 1 mg/kg body weight rounded to the nearest 10 mg up to max dose of 90 mg administered every four weeks
Pediatric: <1 year: not recommended; ≥1-17 years: starting dose 0.8 mg/kg rounded to the nearest 10 mg; min starting dose 10 mg; max dose 90 mg; administer SC every 2 weeks; dose may be increased up to approximately 2 mg/kg (max 90 mg), administered every two weeks to achieve normal serum phosphorus; ≥18 years: same as adult
   Crysvita *Vial:* 10, 20, 30 mg/ml (1 ml) single-dose
   Comment: The most common adverse side effects associated with **Crysvita** in pediatric XLH patients are headache, injection site reaction, vomiting, pyrexia, pain in extremity, and decreased serum vitamin D. The most common adverse side effects associated with **Crysvita** in patients with XLH ≥18 years-of-age are back pain, headache, tooth infection, restless leg syndrome, dizziness, constipation, decreased serum vitamin D, and increased serum phosphorus. There are no available data on *burosumab-twza* use to inform a drug-associated risk of adverse developmental outcomes in pregnancy. There are no data to inform the presence of *burosumab-twza* in human milk or effects on the breastfed infant.

HYPOTENSION: NEUROGENIC, ORTHOSTATIC

ALPHA-1 AGONIST

▷ *midodrine* (C)(G) 10 mg tid at 3-4-hour intervals; take while upright; take last dose at least 4 hours before bedtime
Pediatric: <12 years: not recommended; ≥12 years: same as adult
   ProAmatine *Tab:* 2.5*, 5*, 10*mg

SYNTHETIC AMINO ACID PRECURSOR OF NOREPINEPHRINE

▷ *droxidopa* (C) initially 100 mg, taken 3 x/day (upon arising in the morning, at midday, and in the late afternoon at least 3 hours prior to bedtime (to reduce the potential for supine hypertension during sleep); administer with or without; swallow whole; titrate to symptomatic response, in increments of 100 mg tid every 24-48 hours; max 600 mg tid (max total 1,800 mg/day)
Pediatric: <12 years: not recommended; ≥12 years: same as adult
   Northera *Cap:* 100, 200, 300 mg
   Comment: **Northera** is indicated for the treatment of orthostatic dizziness, lightheadedness, or feeling about to black out in adult patients with symptomatic neurogenic orthostatic hypotension (NOH) caused by primary autonomic failure [Parkinson's disease (PD), multiple system atrophy (MSA) and pure autonomic failure], dopamine beta-hydroxylase deficiency, and nondiabetic autonomic neuropathy. Effectiveness beyond 2 weeks of treatment has not been established. The continued effectiveness of **Northera** should be assessed. Administering **Northera** in combination with other agents that increase blood pressure (e.g., norepinephrine, ephedrine, midodrine, triptans) would be expected to increase the risk for supine hypertension.

HYPOTHYROIDISM

Comment: Take thyroid replacement hormone in the morning on an empty stomach. For the elderly, start thyroid hormone replacement at 25 mcg/day. Target TSH is 0.4-5.5 mIU/L; target T4 is 4.5-12.5 ng/L. Signs and symptoms of thyroid toxicity include tachycardia, palpitations, nervousness, chest pain, heat intolerance, and weight loss.

ORAL THYROID HORMONE SUPPLEMENTS
T3

▷ *liothyronine* (A) initially 25 mcg daily; may increase by 25 mcg every 1-2 weeks as needed; usual maintenance 25-75 mcg/day

Pediatric: initially 5 mcg/day; may increase by 5 mcg/day every 3-4 days; *Cretinism:* maintenance dose: <1 year: 20 mcg/day; 1-3 years: 50 mcg/day; >3 years: same as adult
> Cytomel *Tab:* 5, 25, 50 mcg

T4

▷ *levothyroxine* (A)(G)
> Levoxyl initially 25-100 mcg/day; increase by 25 mcg/day q 2-3 weeks as needed; main-
tenance 100-200 mcg/day
Pediatric: <6 months: 8-10 mcg/kg/day; 6-12 months: 6-8 mcg/kg/day; >1-5 years: 5-6
mcg/kg/day; 6-12 years: 4-5 mcg/kg/day; >12 years: same as adult
> *Tab:* 25*, 50* (dye-free), 75*, 88*, 100*, 112*, 125*, 137*, 150*, 175*, 200*, 300*mcg
> Synthroid initially 50 mcg/day; increase by 25 mcg/day q 2-3 weeks as needed; max 300
mcg/day
Pediatric: <6 months: 8-10 mcg/kg/day; 6-12 months: 6-8 mcg/kg/day; >1-5 years: 5-6
mcg/kg/day; 6-12 years: 4-5 mcg/kg/day; >12 years: same as adult
> *Tab:* 25*, 50* (dye-free), 75*, 88*, 100*, 112*, 125*, 137*, 150*, 175*, 200*, 300*mcg
> Unithroid initially 50 mcg/day; increase by 25 mcg/day q 2-3 weeks as needed; max 300
mcg/day
Pediatric: 0-3 months: 10-15 mcg/kg/day; 3-6 months: 8-10 mcg/kg/day; 6-12 months:
6-8 mcg/kg/day; 1-5 years: 5-6 mcg/kg/day; 6-12 years: 4-5 mcg/kg/day; >12 years: 2-3
mcg/kg/day; *Growth and puberty complete:* same as adult
> *Tab:* 25*, 50* (dye-free), 75*, 88*, 100*, 112*, 125*, 150*, 175*, 200*, 300*mcg

T3+T4 Combination

▷ *liothyronine+levothyroxine* (A) initially 15-30 mg/day; increase by 15 mg/day q 2-3 weeks
to target goal; usual maintenance 60-120 mg/day
Pediatric: <6 months: 4.6-6 mcg/kg/day; 6-12 months: 3.6-4.8 mcg/kg/day; >1-5 years:
3-3.6 mcg/kg/day; 6-12 years: 2.4-3 mcg/kg/day; >12 years: 1.2-1.8 mcg/kg/day; *Growth
and puberty complete:* same as adult
> Armour Thyroid Tab *Tab:* per grain: T3 9 mcg+T4 38 mcg: 1/4, 1/2, 1, 1, 2, 3*, 4*, 5*
gr; 15, 30, 60, 90, 120, 180*, 240*, 300*mg
> Thyrolar *Tab:* per grain: T3 12.5 mcg+T4 50 mcg: 1/4, 1/5, 1, 2, 3 gr

PARENTERAL THYROID HORMONE SUPPLEMENT

▷ *levothyroxine sodium* (A)(G) 1/2 oral dose by IV or IM and titrate; *Myxedema Coma:* 200-
500 mcg IV x 1 dose; may administer 100-300 mcg (or more) IV on second day if needed;
then 50-100 mcg IV daily; switch to oral form as soon as possible
Pediatric: <12 years: not recommended; ≥12 years: same as adult
> T4 *Vial:* 100, 200, 500 mcg (pwdr for IM or IV administration after reconstitution)

ⓞ HYPOTRICHOSIS (THIN/SPARSE EYELASHES)

PROSTAGLANDIN ANALOG

▷ *bimatoprost* ophthalmic solution (C)(G) apply one drop nightly directly to the skin of
the upper eyelid margin at the base of the eyelashes using the accompanying applicators;
blot any excess solution beyond the eyelid margin; dispose of the applicator after one use;
repeat for the opposite eyelid margin using a new sterile applicator. Repeat treatment of the
opposite eye using a new applicator
Pediatric: <16 years: not recommended; ≥16 years: same as adult
> Latisse *Ophth soln:* 0.03% (3 ml in 5 ml bottle w. 70 disposable sterile applicators; 5 ml
in 5 ml bottle w. 140 disposable sterile applicators)
> Comment: Latisse is indicated to treat hypotrichosis of the eyelashes by increasing their
growth including length, thickness and darkness. Ensure the face is clean, all makeup is
removed, and contact lenses removed. Place one drop of Latisse on the disposable sterile
applicator and brush cautiously along the skin of the upper eyelid margin at the base of
the eyelashes. Do not to apply to the lower eyelash line. If eyelid skin darkening occurs,
it may be reversible after discontinuation of Latisse. If any Latisse solution gets into the
eye proper, it will not cause harm; the eye should not be rinsed. Any excess solution
outside the upper eyelid margin should be blotted with a tissue or other absorbent
material. Onset of effect is gradual but is not significant in the majority of patients until 2
months. The effect is not permanent and can be expected to gradually return to previous.
Additional applications of Latisse will not increase the growth of eyelashes.

IDIOPATHIC (IMMUNE) THROMBOCYTOPENIA PURPURA (ITP)

SPLEEN TYROSINEKINASE (SYK) INHIBITOR

➤ *fostamatinib disodium hexahydrate* initially 100mg twice daily; increase to 150 mg twice daily if platelet count not at ≥50x10⁹/L after 4 weeks; discontinue if insufficient increase in platelet count after 12 weeks; for dose modifications, see mfr pkg insert
Pediatric: <18 years: not recommended; ≥18yrs: same as adult
  Tavalisse *Tab:* 100, 150mg
  Comment: Tavalisse *(fostamatinib)* is an oral spleen tyrosine kinase (SYK) inhibitor for the treatment of patients with chronic immune thrombocytopenia (ITP). Monitor CBCs, including platelets, monthly until stable count (≥50 x 10⁹/L) achieved, then periodically thereafter. Monitor LFTs monthly. Discontinue if AST/ALT >5XULN for ≥2 weeks or ≥3XULN and total bilirubin >2XULN. Monitor blood pressure every 2 weeks until stable dose established, then monthly thereafter. Interrupt or discontinue dose if hypertensive crisis (>180/120 mm Hg) occurs; discontinue if repeat BP >160/100 mmHg for >4 weeks. Temporarily interrupt if severe diarrhea (Grade ≥3) occurs; resume at next lower daily dose if improved to Grade 1. Monitor ANC monthly and for infection. Temporarily interrupt if ANC <1 x 10⁹/L occurs and remains low after 72 hours until resolved; resume at next lower daily dose. Use lowest effective dose. Due to potential for embryo-fetal toxicity, use effective contraception during and for ≥1 month after last dose. Confirm negative pregnancy status prior to initiation. Breastfeeding not recommended (during and for ≥1 month after last dose). Concomitant strong CYP3A4 inducers not recommended. Concomitant strong CYP3A4 inhibitors or substrates; monitor for toxicity. May potentiate concomitant BCRP (eg, *rosuvastatin*) or P-gp (e.g., *digoxin*) substrates; monitor for toxicity. Adverse reactions include diarrhea, hypertension, nausea, respiratory infection, dizziness, ALT/AST increase, rash, abdominal pain, fatigue, chest pain, neutropenia.

IMMUNODEFICIENCY: PRIMARY HUMORAL (PHI)

Comment: Primary Humoral Immunodeficiency (PHI) includes, but is not limited to, Congenital or X-linked Agammaglobulinemia, Common Variable Immunodeficiency, Wiskott-Aldrich Syndrome, Severe Combined Immuno deficiencies.

IMMUNE GLOBULIN, HUMAN

➤ *immune globulin subcutaneous [human] 20% liquid* administer via SC Infusion only; up to 8 infusion sites are allowed simultaneously, with at least 2 inches between sites; *Infusion volume:* for the first infusion, up to 15 ml per injection site; may increase to 20 ml per site after the fourth infusion; max 25 ml per site as tolerated; *Infusion rate:* first infusion, up to 15 ml/hr per site; may increase, to max 25 ml/hr per site as tolerated; however, maximum flow rate is not to exceed a total of 50 ml/hr for all sites combined before switching to **Hizentra**, obtain the patient's serum IgG trough level to guide subsequent dose adjustments; adjust the dose based on clinical response and serum IgG trough levels; administer at regular intervals from daily up to every 2 week. *Weekly dosing:* start **Hizentra** 1 week after last Immune Globulin Intravenous, Human (IGIV) infusion; initial weekly dose: [previous IGIV dose (in grams) x 1.37] divided by # of weeks between IGIV doses *Biweekly dosing (every 2 weeks):* start **Hizentra** 1 or 2 weeks after the last IGIV infusion or 1 week after the last weekly IGSC infusion; administer twice the calculated weekly dose *Frequent dosing (2 to 7 times per week):* start **Hizentra** 1 week after the last IGIV or IGSC infusion; divide the calculated weekly dose by the desired number of times per week
Pediatric: <12 years: not established; ≥12 years: same as adult
  Hizentra *Vial:* 0.2 mg/ml (20%; 5, 10, 20, 50 ml)
  Comment: IgA-deficient patients with anti-IgA antibodies are at greater risk of severe hypersensitivity and anaphylactic reactions. Thrombosis may occur following treatment with immune globulin products, including **Hizentra**. Aseptic meningitis syndrome has been reported with IGIV and IGSC, including **Hizentra**. Monitor renal function in patients at risk of acute renal failure (ARF). Monitor for clinical signs and symptoms of hemolysis. Monitor for pulmonary adverse reactions (transfusion-related acute lung injury [TRALI]). **Hizentra** is made from human blood and may contain infectious agents (e.g., viruses, the variant Creutzfeldt-Jakob disease [vCJD] agent and, theoretically, the Creutzfeldt-Jakob disease [CJD] agent). Monitor for clinical signs and symptoms

of hemolysis. The most common adverse reactions observed in ≥5% of study subjects were local infusion site reactions, headache, diarrhea, fatigue, back pain, nausea, pain in extremity, cough, upper respiratory tract infection, rash, pruritus, vomiting, abdominal pain (upper), migraine, arthralgia, pain, fall and nasopharyngitis. No human or animal reproduction studies have not been conducted with **Hizentra**. It is not known whether **Hizentra** can cause fetal harm when administered during pregnancy. No human data are available to inform maternal use of **Hizentra** on the breastfed infant. Safety and effectiveness of weekly **Hizentra** administration have not been established in children <2 years-of-age. To report suspected adverse reactions, contact CSL Behring Pharmacovigilance at 1-866-915-6958 or FDA at 1-800-FDA-1088 or www.fda.gov/medwatch.

Hizentra *Vial:* 0.2 mg/ml (20%; 5, 10, 20, 50 ml)

Comment: IgA-deficient patients with anti-IgA antibodies are at greater risk of severe hypersensitivity and anaphylactic reactions. Thrombosis may occur following treatment with immune globulin products, including **Hizentra**. Aseptic meningitis syndrome has been reported with IGIV and IGSC, including **Hizentra**. Monitor renal function in patients at risk of acute renal failure ARF). Monitor for clinical signs and symptoms of hemolysis. Monitor for pulmonary adverse reactions (transfusion-related acute lung injury [TRALI]). **Hizentra** is made from human blood and may contain infectious agents (e.g., viruses, the variant Creutzfeldt-Jakob disease (vCJD) agent and, theoretically, the Creutzfeldt-Jakob disease (CJD) agent). Monitor for clinical signs and symptoms of hemolysis. The most common adverse reactions observed in ≥5% of study subjects were local infusion site reactions, headache, diarrhea, fatigue, back pain, nausea, pain in extremity, cough, upper respiratory tract infection, rash, pruritus, vomiting, abdominal pain (upper), migraine, arthralgia, pain, fall and nasopharyngitis. No human or animal reproduction studies have not been conducted with **Hizentra**. It is not known whether **Hizentra** can cause fetal harm when administered during pregnancy. No human data are available to inform maternal use of **Hizentra** on the breastfed infant. Safety and effectiveness of weekly **Hizentra** administration have not been established in children <2 years of age. To report suspected adverse reactions, contact CSL Behring Pharmacovigilance at 1-866-915-6958 or FDA at 1-800-FDA-1088 or www.fda.gov/medwatch.

IMPETIGO CONTAGIOSA (INDIAN FIRE)

Comment: The most common infectious organisms are *Staphylococcus aureus* and *Streptococcus pyogenes*.

TOPICAL ANTI-INFECTIVES

▷ *mupirocin* (B)(G) apply to lesions bid; apply to walls of nares bid
  Pediatric: same as adult
    Bactroban *Oint:* 2% (22 gm); *Crm:* 2% (15, 30 gm)
    Centany *Oint:* 2% (15, 30 gm)

ORAL ANTI-INFECTIVES

▷ *amoxicillin* (B)(G) 500-875 mg bid or 250-500 mg tid x 10 days
  Pediatric: <40 kg (88 lb): 20-40 mg/kg/day in 3 divided doses x 10 days or 25-45 mg/kg/day in 2 divided doses x 10 days; ≥40 kg: same as adult; *see page 617 for dose by weight*
    Amoxil *Cap:* 250, 500 mg; *Tab:* 875*mg; *Chew tab:* 125, 200, 250, 400 mg (cherry-banana-peppermint) (phenylalanine); *Oral susp:* 125, 250 mg/5 ml (80, 100, 150 ml) (strawberry); 200, 400 mg/5 ml (50, 75, 100 ml) (bubble gum); Oral drops: 50 mg/ml (30 ml) (bubble gum)
    Moxatag *Tab:* 775 mg ext-rel
    Trimox *Tab:* 125, 250 mg; *Cap:* 250, 500 mg; *Oral susp:* 125, 250 mg/5 ml (80, 100, 150 ml) (raspberry-strawberry)
▷ *amoxicillin+clavulanate* (B)(G)
    Augmentin 500 mg tid or 875 mg bid x 7-10 days
    Pediatric: 40-45 mg/kg/day divided tid x 10 days or 90 mg/kg/day divided bid x 10 days *see pages 618 for dose by weight*
      Tab: 250, 500, 875 mg; *Chew tab:* 125, 250 mg (lemon-lime); 200, 400 mg (cherry-banana) (phenylalanine); *Oral susp:* 125 mg/5 ml (banana), 250 mg/5 ml (75, 100, 150 ml) (orange); 200, 400 mg/5 ml (50, 75, 100 ml) (orange) (phenylalanine)
    Augmentin ES-600 not recommended for adults

Pediatric: <3 months: not recommended; ≥3 months, <40 kg: 90 mg/kg/day in 2 divided doses x 7-10 days; ≥40 kg: not recommended
> *Oral susp:* 42.9 mg/5 ml (50, 75, 100, 125, 150, 200 ml) (strawberry cream) (phenyl-alanine)

Augmentin XR 2 tabs q 12 hours x 7-10 days
Pediatric: <16 years: use other forms; ≥16 years: same as adult
> *Tab:* 1000*mg ext-rel

▶ *azithromycin* (B)(G) 500 mg x 1 dose on day 1, then 250 mg daily on days 2-5 or 500 mg daily x 3 days or 2 gm in a single dose
> **Zithromax** *Tab:* 250, 500, 600 mg; *Oral susp:* 100 mg/5 ml (15 ml); 200 mg/5 ml (15, 22.5, 30 ml) (cherry); *Pkt:* 1 gm for reconstitution (cherry-banana)
> **Zithromax Tri-pak** *Tab:* 3 x 500 mg tabs/pck
> **Zithromax Z-pak** *Tab:* 6 x 250 mg tabs/pck
> **Zmax** *Oral susp:* 2 gm ext-rel for reconstitution (cherry-banana) (148 mg Na⁺)

▶ *cefaclor* (B)(G) 250-500 mg q 8 hours x 10 days; max 2 gm/day
Pediatric: <1 month: not recommended; 20-40 mg/kg/day or q 12 hours x 10 days; max 1 gm/day; *see page 620 for dose by weight*
> *Tab:* 500 mg; *Cap:* 250, 500 mg; *Susp:* 125 mg/5 ml (75, 150 ml) (strawberry); 187 mg/5 ml (50, 100 ml) (strawberry); 250 mg/5 ml (75, 150 ml) (strawberry); 375 mg/5 ml (50, 100 ml) (strawberry)
> **Cefaclor Extended Release** *Tab:* 375, 500 mg ext-rel
Pediatric: <16 years: ext-rel not recommended; ≥16 years: same as adult

▶ *cefadroxil* (B) 1-2 gm in 1-2 divided doses x 10 days
Pediatric: 30 mg/kg/day in 2 divided doses x 10 days; *see page 620 for dose by weight*
> **Duricef** *Cap:* 500 mg; *Tab:* 1 gm; *Oral susp:* 250 mg/5 ml (100 ml); 500 mg/5 ml (75, 100 ml) (orange-pineapple)

▶ *cefpodoxime proxetil* (B) 200 mg bid x 10 days
Pediatric: <2 months: not recommended; 2 months-12 years: 10 mg/kg/day (max 400 mg/dose) or 5 mg/kg/day bid (max 200 mg/dose) x 10 days; *see page 622 for dose by weight*
> **Vantin** *Tab:* 100, 200 mg; *Oral susp:* 50, 100 mg/5 ml (50, 75, 100 mg) (lemon creme)

▶ *cefprozil* (B) 500 mg bid x 10 days
Pediatric: ≤6 months: not recommended; 6 months-12 years: *see page 622 for dose by weight*
> **Cefzil** *Tab:* 250, 500 mg; *Oral susp:* 125, 250 mg/5 ml (50, 75, 100 ml) (bubble gum) (phenylalanine)

▶ *ceftaroline fosamil* (B) administer by IV infusion after reconstitution every 12 hours x 5-14 days; *CrCl >50 mL/min:* 600 mg; *CrCl >30-<50 mL/min:* 400 mg; *CrCl >1 5-<30 mL/min:* 300 mg; ESRD: 200 mg
> **Teflaro** *Vial:* 400, 600 mg

▶ *cephalexin* (B) (G) 250-500 mg qid or 500 mg bid x 10 days
Pediatric: 25-50 mg/kg/day in 4 divided doses x 10 days; *see page 623 for dose by weight*
> **Keflex** *Cap:* 250, 333, 500, 750 mg; *Oral susp:* 125, 250 mg/5 ml (100, 200 ml) (strawberry)

▶ *clarithromycin* (C)(G) 500 mg bid or 500 mg ext-rel once daily x 7 days
Pediatric: <6 months: not recommended; ≥6 months: 7.5 mg/kg bid x 7 days; *see page 624 for dose by weight*
> **Biaxin** *Tab:* 250, 500 mg
> **Biaxin Oral Suspension** *Oral susp:* 125, 250 mg/5 ml (50, 100 ml) (fruit punch)
> **Biaxin XL** *Tab:* 500 mg ext-rel

Comment: The FDA is advising caution before prescribing *clarithromycin* to patients with heart disease because of a potential increased risk of heart problems or death that can occur years later. This recommendation is based on a review of the results of a 10-year follow-up study of patients with coronary heart disease from a large clinical trial that first observed this safety issue. Consider risk benefit and the use of other antibiotics in such patients.

▶ *dicloxacillin* (B) (G) 500 mg q 6 hours x 10 days
Pediatric: 12.5-25 mg/kg/day in 4 divided doses x 10 days; *see page 624 for dose by weight*
> **Dynapen** *Cap:* 125, 250, 500 mg; *Oral susp:* 62.5 mg/5 ml (80, 100, 200 ml)

▶ *erythromycin base* (B)(G) 250 mg qid, or 333 mg tid, or 500 mg bid x 7-10 days
Pediatric: ≤45 kg: 30-50 mg in 2-4 divided doses x 7-10 days; ≥45 kg: same as adult
> **Ery-Tab** *Tab:* 250, 333, 500 mg ent-coat
> **PCE** *Tab:* 333, 500 mg

Comment: *erythromycin* may increase INR with concomitant *warfarin*, as well as increase serum level of *digoxin*, benzodiazepines, and statins.

▷ *erythromycin ethylsuccinate* (B)(G) 400 mg tid x 7-10 days
  Pediatric: 30-50 mg/kg/day in 4 divided doses x 7-10 days; may double dose with severe infection; max 100 mg/kg/day; *see page 626 for dose by weight*
      EryPed *Oral susp:* 200 mg/5 ml (100, 200 ml) (fruit); 400 mg/5 ml (60, 100, 200 ml) (banana); *Oral drops:* 200, 400 mg/5 ml (50 ml) (fruit); *Chew tab:* 200 mg wafer (fruit)
      E.E.S. *Oral susp:* 200, 400 mg/5 ml (100 ml) (fruit)
      E.E.S. Granules *Oral susp:* 200 mg/5 ml (100, 200 ml) (cherry)
      E.E.S. 400 Tablets *Tab:* 400 mg
  Comment: *erythromycin* may increase INR with concomitant *warfarin*, as well as increase serum level of *digoxin*, benzodiazepines, and statins.
▷ *loracarbef* (B) 200 mg bid x 10 days
  Pediatric: 15 mg/kg/day in 2 divided doses x 10 days; *see page 628 for dose by weight*
  Pediatric: 30 mg/kg/day in 2 divided doses x 7 days
      Lorabid *Pulvule:* 200, 400 mg; *Oral susp:* 100 mg/5 ml (50, 100 ml); 200 mg/5 ml (50, 75, 100 ml) (strawberry bubble gum)
▷ *ozenoxacin* <2 months: not recommended; ≥2 months: apply a thin layer topically to the affected area bid x 5 days; affected area may be up to 100 cm² in patients ≥12 years-of-age or 2% of the total BSA and not exceeding 100 cm² in patients <12 years-of-age
      Xepi *Crm:* 1% 10 mg/gm (45 gm)
      Comment: Xepi (azenoxacin) is indicated for the topical treatment of impetigo due to *Staphylococcus aureus* or *Streptococcus pyogenes*. There are no available data on the use of Xepi in pregnancy to inform a drug associated risk; however, systemic absorption of *ozenoxacin* in humans is negligible following topical administration. No data are available regarding the presence of *ozenoxacin* in human milk or effects on the breastfed infant; however; however, breastfeeding is not expected to result in infant exposure due to the negligible systemic absorption. There are no available data on the use of Xepi in pregnancy to inform a drug associated risk; however, systemic absorption of *ozenoxacin* in humans is negligible following topical administration. No data are available regarding the presence of *ozenoxacin* in human milk or effects on the breastfed infant; however, breastfeeding is not expected to result in infant exposure due to the negligible systemic absorption.
▷ *penicillin g (benzathine)* (B)(G) 1.2 million units IM x 1 dose
  Pediatric: <60 lb: 300,000-600,000 units IM x 1 dose; ≥60 lb: 900,000 units x 1 dose
      Bicillin L-A *Cartridge-needle unit:* 600,000 units (1 ml); 1.2 million units (2 ml)
▷ *penicillin g (benzathine procaine)* (B)(G) 2.4 million units IM x 1 dose
  Pediatric: <30 lb: 600,000 units IM x 1 dose; 30-60 lb: 900,000-1.2 million units IM x 1 dose
      Bicillin C-R *Cartridge-needle unit:* 600,000 units (1 ml); 1.2 million units (2 ml); 2.4 million units (4 ml)
▷ *penicillin v potassium* (B) 250-500 mg q 6 hours x 10 days
  Pediatric: 50 mg/kg/day in 4 divided doses x 3 days; ≥12 years: same as adult; *see page 629 for dose by weight*
      Pen-Vee K *Tab:* 250, 500 mg; *Oral soln:* 125 mg/5 ml (100, 200 ml); 250 mg/5 ml (100, 150, 200 ml)

◯ INCONTINENCE: FECAL

Comment: Treatment of fecal incontinence in patients who have failed conservative therapy (e.g., diet, fiber therapy, antimotility agents).
▷ *dextranomer microspheres+sodium hyaluronate*
  Pediatric: <18 years: not recommended; ≥18 years: same as adult
      Pretreatment: bowel preparation using enema (required) and prophylactic antibiotics (recommended) prior to injection
      Treatment: inject slowly into the deep submucosal layer in the proximal part of the high pressure zone of the anal canal about 5 mm above the dentate line; four 1-ml injections in the following order: posterior, left lateral, anterior, right lateral; keep needle in place 15-30 seconds to minimize leakage; use a new needle for each syringe and injection site
      Posttreatment: avoid hot baths and physical activity during first 24 hours; avoid antidiarrheal drugs, sexual intercourse, and strenuous activity for 1 week; avoid anal manipulation for 1 month
      Retreatment: may repeat if needed with max 4 ml, no sooner than 4 weeks after the first injection; point of injection should be made in between initial injection sites (i.e., shifted 1/8 of a turn)

Solesta dex micro 50 mg+sod hyal 15 mg per ml
    Syringe: 1 ml (4 w. needles)

INCONTINENCE: URINARY OVERACTIVE BLADDER, STRESS INCONTINENCE, URGE INCONTINENCE

See **Enuresis** *page* 156
➤ *estrogen* replacement (X) *see Menopause page* 301
➤ *pseudoephedrine* (C)(G) 30-60 mg tid
    Sudafed (OTC) *Tab:* 30 mg; *Liq:* 15 mg/5 ml (1, 4 oz)

VASOPRESSIN

➤ *desmopressin acetate (DDAVP)* (B)(G)
    DDAVP usual dosage 0.1-1.2 mg/day in 2-3 divided doses; 0.2 mg q HS prn for nocturnal enuresis
    Pediatric: <6 years: not recommended; ≥6 years: 0.5 mg daily or q HS prn
        Tab: 0.1*, 0.2*mg
    DDAVP Rhinal Tube
    Pediatric: <6 years: not recommended; ≥6 years: 10 mcg or 0.1 ml of soln each nostril (20 mcg total dose) q HS prn; max 40 mcg total dose
        Rhinal tube: 0.1 mg/ml (2.5 ml)

BETA-3 ADRENERGIC AGONIST

➤ *mirabegron* (C) initially 25 mg once daily; max 50 mg once daily; severe renal impairment, 25 mg once daily
    Myrbetriq *Tab:* 25, 50 mg ext-rel
    Comment: **Myrbetriq** *(mirabegron)* is FDA-approved to be taken in combination with **VESIcare** *(solifenacin succinate)* for the treatment of overactive bladder (OAB) with symptoms of frequency, urgency, and urge urinary incontinence.

MUSCARINIC RECEPTOR ANTAGONISTS

➤ *fesoterodine* (C)(G) 4 mg daily; max 8 mg/day
    Pediatric: <12 years: not recommended; ≥12 years: same as adult
        Toviaz *Tab:* 4, 8 mg ext-rel
➤ *tolterodine tartrate* (C)(G) **Detrol** 1-2 mg bid or **Detrol LA** 2-4 mg once daily or **Detrol XL** one tab daily
    Pediatric: <12 years: not recommended; ≥12 years: same as adult
        Detrol *Tab:* 1, 2 mg
        Detrol *Cap:* 2, 4 mg ext-rel
        Detrol XL *Tab:* 5, 10, 15 mg ext-rel

ANTISPASMODIC/ANTICHOLINERGICS AGENTS

➤ *darifenacin* (C) 7.5-15 mg daily with liquid; max 15 mg/day
    Pediatric: <12 years: not recommended; ≥12 years: same as adult
        Enablex 7.5-15 mg daily with liquid; max 15 mg/day
        Tab: 7.5, 15 mg ext-rel
➤ *dicyclomine* (B)(G) 10-20 mg qid
    Pediatric: <12 years: not recommended; ≥12 years: same as adult
        Bentyl *Tab:* 20 mg; *Cap:* 10 mg; *Syr:* 10 mg/5 ml (16 oz)
➤ *flavoxate* (B) 100-200 mg tid-qid
    Pediatric: <12 years: not recommended; ≥12 years: same as adult
        Urispas *Tab:* 100 mg
➤ *hyoscyamine* (C)(G)
    Anaspaz 1-2 tabs q 4 hours prn; max 12 tabs/day
    Pediatric: <2 years: not recommended; 2-12 years: 0.0625-0.125 mg q 4 hours prn; max 0.75 mg/day
        Tab: 0.125*mg
    Levbid 1-2 tabs q 12 hours prn; max 4 tabs/day
    Pediatric: <12 years: not recommended; ≥12 years: same as adult
        Tab: 0.375*mg ext-rel

Levsin 1-2 tabs q 4 hours prn; max 12 tabs/day
Pediatric: <6 years: not recommended; 6-12 years: 1 tab q 4 hours prn
  Tab: 0.125*mg
Levsin Drops 1-2 ml q 4 hours prn; max 60 ml/day
Pediatric: 3.4 kg: 4 drops q 4 hours prn; max 24 drops/day; 5 kg: 5 drops q 4 hours prn; max 30 drops/day; 7 kg: 6 drops q 4 hours prn; max 36 drops/day; 10 kg: 8 drops q 4 hours prn; max 40 drops/day; 2-12 years: 0.25-1 ml; max 6 ml/day
  Oral drops: 0.125 mg/ml (15 ml) (orange) (alcohol 5%)
Levsin Elixir 5-10 ml q 4 hours prn
Pediatric: <10 kg: use drops; 10-19 kg: 1.25 ml q 4 hours prn; 20-39 kg: 2.5 ml q 4 hours prn; 40-49 kg: 3.75 ml q 4 hours prn; ≥50 kg: 5 ml q 4 hours prn
  Elix: 0.125 mg/5 ml (16 oz) (orange) (alcohol 20%)
Levsinex SL 1-2 tabs q 4 hours SL or PO; max 12 tabs/day
Pediatric: <2 years: not recommended; 2-12 years: 1 tab q 4 hours; max 6 tabs/day; >12 years: same as adult
  Tab: 0.125 mg sublingual
Levsinex Timecaps 1-2 caps q 12 hours; may adjust to 1 cap q 8 hours
Pediatric: 2-12 years: 1 cap q 12 hours; max 2 caps/day; >12 years: same as adult
  Cap: 0.375 mg time-rel
NuLev dissolve 1-2 tabs on tongue, with or without water, q 4 hours prn; max 12 tabs/day
Pediatric: <2 years: not recommended; 2-12 years: dissolve 1 tab on tongue, with or without water, q 4 hours prn; max 6 tabs/day; ≥12 years: same as adult
  ODT: 0.125 mg (mint) (phenylalanine)

▷ *oxybutynin chloride* (B)
Ditropan 5 mg bid-tid; max 20 mg/day
Pediatric: <5 years: not recommended; 5-12 years: 5 mg bid; max 15 mg/day; ≥16 years: same as adult
  Tab: 5*mg; *Syr:* 5 mg/5 ml
Ditropan XL initially 5 mg daily; may increase weekly in 5-mg increments as needed; max 30 mg/day
Pediatric: <6 years: not recommended; ≥6 years: initially 5 mg once daily; may increase weekly in 5-mg increments as needed; max 20 mg/day
  Tab: 5, 10, 15 mg ext-rel
GelniQUE 3 mg Pump: apply 3 pumps (84 mg) once daily to clean dry intact skin on the abdomen, upper arm, shoulders, or thighs; rotate sites; wash hands; avoid washing application site for 1 hour after application
Pediatric: <12 years: not recommended; ≥12 years: same as adult
  Gel: 3% (92 gm, metered pump dispenser) (alcohol)
GelniQUE 1 gm Sachet: apply 1 gm gel (1 sachet) once daily to dry intact skin on abdomen, upper arms/shoulders, or thighs; rotate sites; wash hands; avoid washing application site for 1 hour after application
Pediatric: <12 years: not recommended; ≥12 years: same as adult
  Gel: 10%, 1 gm/sachet (30/carton) (alcohol)
Oxytrol Transdermal Patch (OTC): apply patch to clean dry area of the abdomen, hip, or buttock; one patch twice weekly; rotate sites
Pediatric: <12 years: not recommended; ≥12 years: same as adult
  Transdermal patch: 3.9 mg/day

▷ *propantheline* (C) 15-30 mg tid
Pediatric: <12 years: not recommended; ≥12 years: same as adult
  Pro-Banthine *Tab:* 7.5, 15 mg

▷ *solifenacin* (C)(G) 5-10 mg daily
Pediatric: <12 years: not recommended; ≥12 years: same as adult
  VESIcare *Tab:* 5, 10 mg
  Comment: VESIcare *(solifenacin succinate)* is FDA-approved to be taken in combination with **Myrbetriq** *(mirabegron)* for the treatment of overactive bladder (OAB) with symptoms of frequency, urgency, and urge urinary incontinence.

▷ *trospium chloride* (C)(G)
Pediatric: <12 years: not recommended; ≥12 years: same as adult
  Sanctura 20 mg twice daily; ≥75 years: *CrCl ≤30 mL/min:* 20 mg once daily
  Tab: 20 mg

Sanctura XR 60 mg daily in the morning
  Cap: 60 mg ext-rel
Comment: Take *trospium chloride* on an empty stomach.

OVERFLOW INCONTINENCE: ATONIC BLADDER
▷ *bethanechol* (C) 10-30 mg tid
   Urecholine *Tab:* 5, 10, 25, 50 mg

OVERFLOW INCONTINENCE: PROSTATIC ENLARGEMENT
Alpha-1 Blockers

Comment: Educate the patient regarding the potential side effect of hypotension when taking an alpha-1 blocker, especially with first dose. Start at lowest dose and titrate upward.
▷ *terazosin* (C) initially 1 mg q HS; titrate to 10 mg q HS; max 20 mg/day
   Hytrin *Cap:* 1, 2, 5, 10 mg
▷ *doxazosin* (C) initially 1 mg q HS; may double dose every 1-2 weeks; max 8 mg/day
   Cardura *Tab:* 1*, 2*, 4*, 8*mg
   Cardura XL *Tab:* 4, 8 mg
▷ *prazosin* (C)(G) 1-15 mg q HS; max 15 mg/day
   Minipress *Tab:* 1, 2, 5 mg
▷ *tamsulosin* (C) initially 0.4 mg daily; may increase to 0.8 mg daily after 2-4 weeks if needed
   Flomax *Cap:* 0.4 mg

5-ALPHA REDUCTASE INHIBITOR
▷ *finasteride* (X)(G) 5 mg daily
   Proscar *Tab:* 5 mg

ALPHA 1A-BLOCKER
▷ *silodosin* (B)(G) take 8 mg with food once daily; *CrCl 30-50 mL/min:* take 4 mg
   Rapaflo *Cap:* 4, 8 mg

INFLUENZA, SEASONAL (FLU)

Comment: Egg allergy affects as many as 2% of children in the US. New data have affirmed what the American College of Allergy, Asthma and Immunology said has been known for several years: there are no special precautions needed to dispense the influenza vaccine in people with egg allergy. Based on recommendations from the clinical immunization safety assessment hypersensitivity working group of the ACIP, the members voted during the meeting this week to recommend administration of trivalent inactivated influenza vaccine to patients with a history of egg allergy. The consensus of the working group: egg allergy of any severity, including anaphylaxis, should not be a contraindication of the administration of the influenza vaccine, but rather a precaution. Both the single-dose and two-dose methods are appropriate for administering influenza vaccine to those who are allergic to eggs. No special precautions beyond those recommended for providing any vaccine to any patient are necessary for administration of influenza vaccine to persons allergic to eggs. The recommendation will be included in the ACIP draft guidelines for use of influenza vaccines for the upcoming season.

REFERENCES
Greenhawt, M., Turner, P. J., & Kelso, J. M. (2017). Allergy experts set the record straight on flu shots for patients with egg sensitivity. *Annals of Allergy, Asthma & Immunology, 120*(1), 49–52. doi:10.1016/j.anai.2017.10.020
Turner, P. J., Southern, J., Andrews, N. J., Miller, E., & Erlewyn-Lajeunesse, M. (2015). Safety of live attenuated influenza vaccine in atopic children with egg allergy. *Journal of Allergy and Clinical Immunology, 136*(2), 376–381. doi:10.1016/j.jaci.2014.12.1925

Comment: Until official guidelines are available, provider discretion should be used with appropriate precautions with individual patient consideration and informed consent. Refer to mfr's pkg insert for product maker's recommendations and precautions. With the exception of **Flucelvax**, current flu vaccine mfr pkg inserts report that flu vaccine is contraindicated with allergy to egg or chicken proteins, or egg products, and all flu vaccines are contraindicated with allergy to latex, active infection, acute respiratory disease, active neurological disorder; history of Guillain-Barre syndrome. Have epinephrine 1:1,000 on hand. Flu vaccine is contraindicated for children under 18 years-of-age who are taking *aspirin* and/or an *aspirin*-containing product due to the risk of developing Reye's syndrome. Under 1 year-of-age, administer flu vaccine in the vastus lateralis in two split doses one month apart. Over 1 year-of-age, administer flu vaccine in the deltoid. Flu vaccine formulations change annually. Administer flu vaccine 1 month before flu season. Flu vaccine delivered via nasal spray may be administered earlier.

PROPHYLAXIS (NASAL SPRAY)

▷ *trivalent, live attenuated influenza* vaccine, types A and B **(C)** 1 spray each nostril; ≥50 years not recommended
Pediatric: ≤5 years: not recommended; ≥5 years: same as adult
    Never vaccinated with FluMist: 5-8 years: 2 divided doses 46-74 days apart. *Previously vaccinated with FluMist:* 5-8 years: same as adult
    FluMist Nasal Spray 0.5 ml spray annually
        Nasal spray: 0.5 ml (0.25 ml/spray) (10/carton) (preservative-free)

PROPHYLAXIS (INJECTABLE)

▷ *quadrivalent inactivated influenza subvirion vaccine, types a and b* **(C)**

▷ **Afluria Quadrivalent (B)** <6 months: not recommended; 6 months-18 years: 1-2 doses/ season at least 4 weeks apart; >9 years: 1 dose/season
    Vial/Prefilled Pen/PharmaJet Stratis Needle-Free Injection System: 0.5 ml single-dose (preservative-free); Vial: 5 ml multi-dose (thimerosol)
Comment: Contraindicated with allergy to egg or chicken protein, neoeomycin, polymyxin, or history of life-threatening reaction to any previous flu vaccine. PharmaJet Stratis Needle-Free Injection System is only approved as a method of administration for patients 18-64 years-of-age.
    Fluad 0.5 ml IM annually
    Comment: **Fluad** is the first seasonal influenza vaccine with adjuvant, indicated for persona ≥65 years-of-age. Adjuvants are incorporated into some vaccine formulations to enhance or direct the immune response.
    Fluarix Quadrivalent 0.5 ml IM annually
    Pediatric: <3 years: not recommended; ≥3 years: same as adult
        Prefilled syringe: 0.5 ml (10/carton) (preservative-free, latex-free)
▷ *trivalent inactivated influenza subvirion vaccine, types a and b*
    Fluarix (B) 0.5 ml IM annually
    Pediatric: <3 years: not recommended; 3-9 years (previously unvaccinated or vaccinated for the first time last season with one dose of flu vaccine): 2 doses per season at least 1 month apart; 3-9 years (previously vaccinated with two doses of flu vaccine); and >9 years: 1 dose per season
        Prefilled syringe: 0.5 ml single-dose (5/carton) (may contain trace amounts of hydro-cortisone, gentamicin; preservative-free)
    Flublok 0.5 ml IM annually; ≥49 years, not recommended
    Pediatric: <18 years: not recommended; ≥18 years: same as adult
        Vial: 0.5 ml single-dose (10/carton) (preservative-free, egg protein-free, antibiot-ic-free, latex-free)
    Comment: **Flublok** is a cell culture-derived vaccine and, therefore, is an alternative to the traditional egg-based vaccines. Contains 3 times the amount of active ingredient in traditional flu vaccines **Flucelvax** 0.5 ml IM annually
    Pediatric: <18 years: not recommended; ≥18 years: same as adult
        Prefilled syringes: 0.5 ml (10/carton; preservative-free, latex-free)
    Comment: **Flucelvax** is a cell culture-derived vaccine and, therefore, is an alternative to the traditional egg-based vaccines.
    FluLaval (C) 0.5 ml IM annually
    Pediatric: <6 months: not recommended; ≥6 years: same as adult
        Vial: (5 ml)
    FluShield 0.5 ml IM annually

Pediatric: <6 months: not recommended; *Never vaccinated:* <9 years: 2 doses at least 4 weeks apart; 9-12 years: same as adult; *Previously vaccinated:* 6-35 months: 0.25 ml IM x 1 dose; 3-8 years: same as adult

Fluzone 0.5 ml IM annually
> *Vial:* 5 ml (thimerosal)

Fluzone Preservative-Free: Adult Dose 0.5 ml IM annually
Pediatric: <6 months: not recommended; *Not previously vaccinated:* 6 months-8 years: 0.25 ml IM; repeat in 1 month; *Previously vaccinated:* 6-35 months: 0.25 ml IM x 1 dose; >3 years: same as adult
> *Prefilled syringe:* 0.5 ml (10/carton) (preservative-free, trace thimerosal)

Fluzone Preservative-Free: Pediatric Dose
Pediatric: <6 months: not recommended; *Not previously vaccinated:* 6 months-8 years: 0.25 ml IM; repeat in 1 month; *Previously vaccinated:* 6-35 months: 0.25 ml IM x 1 dose; ≥3 years: 0.5 ml IM (use **Fluzone for Adult**)
> *Prefilled syringe:* 0.5 ml (10/carton; preservative-free; trace thimerosal)

Comment: Contraindicated with allergy to egg protein, or history of life-threatening reaction to any previous flu vaccine.

PROPHYLAXIS AND TREATMENTS
Neuraminidase Inhibitors

Comment: Effective for influenza type A and B. Indicated for treatment of uncomplicated acute illness in patients who have been symptomatic for no more than 2 days; therefore, start within 2 days of symptom onset or exposure. Indicated for influenza prophylaxis in patients ≥3 months of age.

▷ *oseltamivir* phosphate (C)(G)
Prophylaxis: 75 mg daily for at least 7 days and up to 6 weeks for community outbreak
> *Pediatric:* <1 year: not recommended; 1-12 years: <15 kg: 30 mg once daily x 10 days; 16-23 kg: 45 mg once daily x 10 days; 24-40 kg: 60 mg once daily x 10 days; >40 kg: same as adult
Treatment: 75 mg bid x 5 days; initiate treatment only if symptomatic <2 days
> *Pediatric:* <1 year: not recommended; 1-12 years: <15 kg: 30 mg bid x 5 days; 16-23 kg: 45 mg bid x 5 days; 24-40 kg: 60 mg bid x 5 days; >40 kg: same as adult
>> **Tamiflu** *Cap:* 30, 45, 75 mg; *Oral susp:* 6 mg/ml pwdr for reconstitution (60 ml w. oral dispenser) (tutti-frutti)
>> Comment: **Tamiflu** is effective for influenza type A and B.

▷ *peramivir* start within 2 days of symptom onset; administer via IV infusion over 15-30 minutes; 600 mg as a single dose; *CrCl 30-49 mL/min:* 200 mg; *CrCl 10-29 mL/min:* 100 mg; *Hemodialysis:* administer after dialysis
Pediatric: start within 2 days of symptom onset; administer via IV infusion over 15-30 minutes; <2 years: not established; 2-12 years: 12 mg/kg as a single dose; max 600 mg; ≥13 years: same as adult; *CrCl 30-49 mL/min:* 4 mg/kg; *CrCl 10-29 mL/min:* 2 mg/kg; *Hemodialysis:* administer after dialysis
>> **Rapivab** *Vial:* 10 mg/ml (20 ml) single-use soln for IV administration after dilution (preservative-free)
>> Comment: avoid live attenuated influenza vaccine 2 weeks prior and 48 hours after treatment with **Rapivab** (*peramivir).*

▷ *zanamivir* (C) 2 inhalations (10 mg) bid x 5 days
Pediatric: <7 years: not recommended; ≥7 years: same as adult
>> **Relenza Inhaler** *Inhaler:* 5 mg/inh blister; 4 blisters/Rotadisk (5 Rotadisks/carton w. 1 inhaler)
>> Comment: **Relenza Inhaler** is effective for influenza type A and B. Use caution with asthma and COPD.s

Polymerase Acidic (PA) Endonuclease Inhibitor

▷ *baloxavir marboxil* take as a single dose within 48 hours of symptom onset; *40-<80 kg:* 40 mg; *≥80 kg:* 80 mg; take with or without food; do not take with dairy products, calcium-fortified beverages, laxatives, antacids or oral supplements containing iron, zinc, selenium, calcium or magnesium (polyvalent cations)
Pediatric: <12 years, <88 lb (40 kg): not established; ≥12 years, ≥88 lb (40 kg): same as adult

Xofluza *Tab:* 20, 40 mg

Comment: **Xofluza** *(baloxavir marboxil)* is a first-in-class, single-dose, oral antiviral drug with a novel mechanism of action designed to target the influenza A and B viruses, including *oseltamivir*-resistant strains and avian strains (e.g., H7N9, H5N1). Unlike other currently available antiviral treatments, *baloxavir marboxil* is the first polymerase acidic [PA] endonuclease inhibitor designed to inhibit the cap-dependent endonuclease protein within the flu virus, which is essential for viral replication, thereby reducing symptoms and duration of the illness. This is the first new antiviral flu treatment with a novel mechanism of action approved by the FDA in nearly 20 years. Safety and efficacy of **Xofluza** was demonstrated in two randomized controlled clinical trials of 1,832 patients where participants were randomly assigned to receive a single dose of 40 mg or 80 mg of *baloxavir marboxil* (according to body weight), placebo, or 75 mg of *oseltamivir* twice a day for five days, within 48 hours of experiencing flu symptoms. **Xofluza** was granted priority review (FDA action on an application within an expedited time frame where the agency determines that the drug, if approved, would significantly improve the safety or effectiveness of treating, diagnosing or preventing a serious condition). Co-administration with polyvalent cation-containing products may decrease plasma concentrations of *baloxavir* which may reduce **Xofluza** efficacy. Therefore avoid co-administration of **Xofluza** with polyvalent cation-containing laxatives, antacids, or oral supplements (e.g., calcium, iron, magnesium, selenium, or zinc). The concurrent use of **Xofluza** with intranasal live attenuated influenza vaccine (LAIV) has not been evaluated. Concurrent administration of antiviral drugs may inhibit viral replication of LAIV and thereby decrease the effectiveness of LAIV vaccination. Interactions between inactivated influenza vaccines and **Xofluza** have not been evaluated. It is not known if **Xofluza** is safe and effective in children younger than 12 years-of-age or weighing less than 88 pounds (40 kg). Safety in pregnancy is unknown. It is not known whether **Xofluza** is present in breastmilk or effects on the breastfed infant. To report suspected adverse reactions, contact Genentech at 1-888-835-2555 or FDA at 1-800-FDA-1088 or www.fda.gov/medwatch.

 INSECT BITE/STING

Topical Corticosteroids *see page* 574
Parenteral Corticosteroids *see page* 577
Oral Corticosteroids *see page* 577

TOPICAL AND TRANSDERMAL ANESTHETICS

Comment: *lidocaine* should not be applied to non-intact skin.

▶ *lidocaine* cream (B) apply to affected area bid prn
Pediatric: <12 years: not recommended; ≥12 years: same as adult
   LidaMantle *Crm:* 3% (1, 2 oz)
   Lidoderm *Crm:* 3% (85 gm)
   ZTlido *lidocaine* topical system 1% (30/carton)
   Comment: Compared to **Lidoderm** (*lidocaine* patch 5%) which contains 700 mg/patch, **ZTlido** only requires 35 mg per topical system to achieve the same therapeutic dose.

▶ *lidocaine* lotion (B) apply to affected area bid prn
Pediatric: <12 years: not recommended; ≥12 years: same as adult
   LidaMantle *Lotn:* 3% (177 ml)

▶ *lidocaine* 5% patch (B)(G) apply up to 3 patches at one time for up to 12 hours/24-hour period (12 hours on/12 hours off); patches may be cut into smaller sizes before removal of the release liner; do not re-use
Pediatric: <12 years: not recommended; ≥12 years: same as adult
   Lidoderm *Patch:* 5% (10x14 cm; 30/carton)

▶ *lidocaine+dexamethasone* (B)
Pediatric: <12 years: not recommended; ≥12 years: same as adult
   Decadron Phosphate with Xylocaine *Lotn:* dexa 4 mg+lido 10 mg per ml (5 ml)

▶ *lidocaine+hydrocortisone* (B)(G) apply to affected area bid prn
Pediatric: <12 years: not recommended; ≥12 years: same as adult
   LidaMantle HC *Crm:* lido 3%+hydro 0.5% (1, 3 oz); *Lotn:* (177 ml)

▷ *lidocaine* 2.5%+prilocaine 2.5% apply sparingly to the burn bid-tid prn
   Pediatric: <12 years: not recommended; ≥12 years: same as adult
      Emla Cream (B) 5, 30 gm/tube

EPINEPHRINE

▷ *epinephrine* **(C)(G)** 1:1,000 0.3-0.5 ml SC
   Pediatric: 0.01 ml/kg SC

TETANUS PROPHYLAXIS

▷ *tetanus toxoid* vaccine **(C)(G)** 0.5 ml IM x 1 dose if previously immunized
   Vial: 5 Lf units/0.5 ml (0.5, 5 ml); *Prefilled syringe:* 5 Lf units/0.5 ml (0.5 ml) (For patients
   not previously immunized *see Tetanus page* 478)

 INSOMNIA

Tricyclic Antidepressants *see Depression page* 119

MELATONIN RECEPTOR AGONIST

▷ *ramelteon* **(C)(IV)** 8 mg within 30 minutes of bedtime; delayed effect if taken with a meal
   Pediatric: <12 years: not recommended; ≥12 years: same as adult
      Rozerem *Tab:* 8 mg

NON-BENZODIAZEPINES

▷ *eszopiclone* **(C)(IV)(G)** (pyrrolopyrazine) 1-3 mg; max 3 mg/day x 1 month; do not take if
   unable to sleep for at least 8 hours before required to be active again; delayed effect if taken
   with a meal
   Pediatric: <18 years: not recommended; ≥18 years: same as adult
      Lunesta *Tab:* 1, 2, 3 mg
▷ *zaleplon* **(C)(IV)** (imidazopyridine) 5-10 mg at HS or after going to bed if unable to sleep;
   do not take if unable to sleep for at least 4 hours before required to be active again; max 20
   mg/day x 1 month; delayed effect if taken with a meal
   Pediatric: <12 years: not recommended; ≥12 years: same as adult
      Sonata *Cap:* 5, 10 mg (tartrazine)
      Comment: **Sonata** is indicated for the treatment of insomnia when a middle-of-the-
      night awakening is followed by difficulty returning to sleep.
▷ *zolpidem* oral solution spray **(C)(IV)** (imidazopyridine hypnotic) 2 actuations (10 mg)
   immediately before bedtime; *Elderly, debilitated,* or *hepatic impairment:* 2 actuations (5
   mg); max 2 actuations (10 mg)
   Pediatric: <18 years: not recommended; ≥18 years: same as adult
      ZolpiMist *Oral soln spray:* 5 mg/actuation (60 metered actuations) (cherry)
      Comment: The lowest dose of *zolpidem* in all forms is recommended for persons >50 years-
      of-age and women as drug elimination is slower than in men.
▷ *zolpidem* tabs **(B)(IV)(G)** (pyrazolopyrimidine hypnotic) 5-10 mg or 6.25-12.5 ext-rel
   q HS prn; max 12.5 mg/day x 1 month; do not take if unable to sleep for at least 8 hours
   before required to be active again; delayed effect if taken with a meal
   Pediatric: <18 years: not recommended; ≥18 years: same as adult
      Ambien *Tab:* 5, 10 mg
      Ambien CR *Tab:* 6.25, 12.5 mg ext-rel
      Comment: The lowest dose of *zolpidem* in all forms is recommended for persons >50 years-
      of-age and women as drug elimination is slower than in men.
▷ *zolpidem* sublingual tabs **(C)(IV)(G)** (imidazopyridine hypnotic) dissolve 1 tab under the
   tongue; allow to disintegrate completely before swallowing; take only once per night and
   only if at least 4 hours of bedtime remain before planned time for awakening
   Pediatric: <18 years: not recommended; ≥18 years: same as adult
      Edluar *SL Tab:* 5, 10 mg
      Intermezzo *SL Tab:* 1.75, 3.5 mg
      Comment: **Intermezzo** is indicated for the treatment of insomnia when a middle-of-
      the-night awakening is followed by difficulty returning to sleep. The lowest dose of
      zolpidem in all forms is recommended for persons >50 years-of-age and women as drug
      elimination is slower than in men.

OREXIN RECEPTOR ANTAGONIST

▷ *suvorexant* (C)(IV) use lowest effective dose; take 30 minutes before bedtime; do not take if unable to sleep for ≥7 hours, max 20 mg
  Pediatric: <12 years: not recommended; ≥12 years: same as adult
    Belsomra *Tab:* 5, 10, 15, 20 mg (30/blister pck)

BENZODIAZEPINES

▷ *estazolam* (X)(IV)(G) initially 1 mg q HS prn; may increase to 2 mg q HS
  Pediatric: <18 years: not recommended; ≥18 years: same as adult
    ProSom *Tab:* 1*, 2*mg
▷ *flurazepam* (X)(IV)(G) 30 mg q HS prn; elderly or debilitated, 15 mg
  Pediatric: <15 years: not recommended; ≥15 years: same as adult
    Dalmane *Cap:* 15, 30 mg
▷ *temazepam* (X)(IV)(G) 7.5-30 mg q HS prn; short term, 7-10 days; max 30 mg; max 1 month
  Pediatric: <18 years: not recommended; ≥18 years: same as adult
    Restoril *Cap:* 7.5, 15, 22.5, 30 mg
▷ *triazolam* (X)(IV) 0.125-0.25 mg q HS prn; short term, 7-10 days; max 0.5 mg; max 1 month
  Pediatric: <18 years: not recommended; ≥18 years: same as adult
    Halcion *Tab:* 0.125, 0.25*mg
    Barbiturates
▷ *pentobarbital* (D)(II)(G)
    Nembutal 100 mg q HS prn
      Cap: 50, 100 mg
    Nembutal Suppository 120 or 200 mg suppository rectally q HS prn
    Pediatric: 2-12 months (10-20 lb): 30 mg supp; 1-4 years (21-40 lb): 30 or 60 mg supp; 5-12 years (41-80 lb): 60 mg supp; 12-14 years (81-110 lb): 60 or 120 mg sup
      Rectal supp: 30, 60, 120, 200 mg

ORAL H1 RECEPTOR AGONIST (FIRST GENERATION ANTIHISTAMINE)

▷ *doxepin* (C)
    Silenor 3-6 mg q HS prn; *Elderly, hepatic impairment, tendency to urinary retention:* initially 3 mg
      Tab: 3, 6 mg
Other Oral 1st Generation Antihistamines *see page 603*

ANALGESIC+FIRST GENERATION ANTIHISTAMINE COMBINATIONS

▷ *acetaminophen+diphenhydramine* (B)
    Excedrin PM (OTC) 2 tabs q HS prn
      Pediatric: <12 years: not recommended; ≥12 years: same as adult
      Tab/Geltab: acet 500 mg+diphen 38 mg
    Tylenol PM (OTC) 2 caps q HS prn
      Pediatric: <12 years: not recommended; ≥12 years: same as adult
      Tab/Cap/Gel cap: acet 500 mg+diphen 25 mg

 INTERSTITIAL CYSTITIS

Acetaminophen for IV Infusion *see Pain page 352*
Oral Prescription NSAIDs *see page 571*
Comment: Avoid peppers and spicy food, citrus, vinegar, caffeine (e.g., coffee, tea, colas), alcohol, carbonated beverages, and other GU tract irritants.

MANAGEMENT OF PAIN AND URINARY URGENCY

▷ *phenazopyridine* (B)(G) 95-200 mg q 6 hours prn; max 2 days
  Pediatric: <12 years: not recommended; ≥12 years: same as adult
    AZO Standard, Prodium, Uristat (OTC) *Tab:* 95 mg
    AZO Standard Maximum Strength (OTC) *Tab:* 97.5 mg
    Pyridium, Urogesic *Tab:* 100, 200 mg *phenazopyridine* (B)(G) 190-200 mg tid; max 2 days

Azo Standard (OTC) *Tab:* 95 mg
Azo Standard Maximum Strength (OTC) *Tab:* 97.5 mg
Pyridium *Tab:* 100, 200 mg ent-coat
Uristat (OTC) *Tab:* 95 mg
Urogesic *Tab:* 100, 200 mg

▷ *hyoscyamine* (C)(G)

Anaspaz 1-2 tabs q 4 hours prn; max 12 tabs/day
Pediatric: <2 years: not recommended; 2-12 years: 0.0625-0.125 mg q 4 hours prn; max 0.75 mg/day; ≥12 years: same as adult
   Tab: 0.125*mg
Levbid 1-2 tabs q 12 hours prn; max 4 tabs/day
Pediatric: <12 years: not recommended; ≥12 years: same as adult
   Tab: 0.375*mg ext-rel
Levsin 1-2 tabs q 4 hours prn; max 12 tabs/day
Pediatric: <6 years: not recommended; 6-12 years: 1 tab q 4 hours prn; ≥12 years: same as adult
   Tab: 0.125*mg
Levsin Drops 1-2 ml q 4 hours prn; max 60 ml/day
Pediatric: 3.4 kg: 4 drops q 4 hours prn; max 24 drops/day; 5 kg: 5 drops q 4 hours prn; max 30 drops/day; 7 kg: 6 drops q 4 hours prn; max 36 drops/day; 10 kg: 8 drops q 4 hours prn; max 40 drops/day
   Oral drops: 0.125 mg/ml (15 ml) (orange) (alcohol 5%)
Levsin Elixir 5-10 ml q 4 hours prn
Pediatric: <10 kg: use drops; 10-19 kg: 1.25 ml q 4 hours prn; 20-39 kg: 2.5 ml q 4 hours prn; 40-49 kg: 3.75 ml q 4 hours prn; ≥50 kg: 5 ml q 4 hours prn;
   Elix: 0.125 mg/5 ml (16 oz) (orange) (alcohol 20%)
Levsinex SL 1-2 tabs q 4 hours SL or PO; max 12 tabs/day
Pediatric: <2 years: not recommended; 2-12 years: 1 tab q 4 hours; max 6 tabs/day; ≥12 years: same as adult
   SL tab: 0.125 mg
Levsinex Timecaps 1-2 caps q 12 hours; may adjust to 1 cap q 8 hours
Pediatric: <2 years: not recommended; 2-12 years: 1 cap q 12 hours; max 2 caps/day; ≥12 years: same as adult
   Cap: 0.375 mg time-rel
NuLev dissolve 1-2 tabs on tongue, with or without water, q 4 hours prn; max 12 tabs/day
Pediatric: <2 years: not recommended; 2-12 years: dissolve 1 tab on tongue, with or without water, q 4 hours prn; max 6 tabs/day; ≥12 years: same as adult
   ODT: 0.125 mg (mint) (phenylalanine)

▷ *methenamine+sod phosphate monobasic+phenyl salicylate+methylene blue+hyoscyamine sulfate* (C) 1 cap qid
Pediatric: <6 years: not recommended; ≥6 years: individualize dose
   Uribel *Cap:* meth 118 mg+sod phos 40.8 mg+phenyl sal 36 mg+meth blue 10 mg+hyoscy 0.12 mg

▷ *methenamine+phenyl salicylate+methylene blue+benzoic acid+atropine sulfate+-hyoscyamine sulfate* (C)(G) 2 tabs qid
Pediatric: <6 years: not recommended; ≥6 years: same as adult
   Urised *Tab:* meth 40.8 mg+phenyl sal 18.1 mg+meth blue 5.4 mg+benz acid 4.5 mg+atro sul 0.03 mg+hyoscy 0.03 mg
   Comment: Urised imparts a blue-green color to urine which may stain fabrics.

▷ *oxybutynin chloride* (B)

Ditropan 5 mg bid-tid; max 20 mg/day
Pediatric: <5 years: not recommended; 5-12 years: 5 mg bid; max 15 mg/day; ≥12 years: same as adult
   Tab: 5*mg; *Syr:* 5 mg/5 ml
Ditropan XL initially 5 mg daily; may increase weekly in 5-mg increments as needed; max 30 mg/day
Pediatric: <5 years: not recommended; ≥5 years: same as adult
   Tab: 5, 10, 15 mg ext-rel

▷ *pentosan* (B) 100 mg tid; reevaluate at 3 and 6 months
Pediatric: <16 years: not recommended; ≥16 years: same as adult
   Elmiron *Cap:* 100 mg

URINARY TRACT ANALGESIA

▷ *phenazopyridine* (B)(G) 95-200 mg q 6 hours prn; max 2 days

    Pediatric: <12 years: not recommended; ≥12 years: same as adult

        AZO Standard, Prodium, Uristat (OTC) *Tab:* 95 mg

        AZO Standard Maximum Strength (OTC) *Tab:* 97.5 mg

        Pyridium, Urogesic *Tab:* 100, 200 mg

        Azo Standard (OTC) *Tab:* 95 mg

        Azo Standard Maximum Strength (OTC) *Tab:* 97.5 mg

        Pyridium *Tab:* 100, 200 mg ent-coat

        Uristat (OTC) *Tab:* 95 mg

        Urogesic *Tab:* 100, 200 mg

    Comment: *Phenazopyridine* imparts an orange-red color to urine which may stain fabrics.

▷ *propantheline* (C) 15-30 mg tid

        Pro-Banthine *Tab:* 7.5, 15 mg

▷ *tolterodine tartrate* (C)(G) **Detrol** 1-2 mg bid <u>or</u> **Detrol LA** 2-4 mg once daily <u>or</u> **Detrol XL** one tab daily

    Pediatric: <12 years: not recommended; ≥12 years: same as adult

        Detrol *Tab:* 1, 2 mg

        Detrol *Cap:* 2, 4 mg ext-rel

        Detrol XL *Tab:* 5, 10, 15 mg ext-rel

ANTICHOLINERGIC+SEDATIVE COMBINATION

▷ *chlordiazepoxide+clidinium* (D)(IV) 1-2 caps ac and HS; max 8 caps/day

    Pediatric: <12 years: not recommended; ≥12 years: same as adult

        Librax *Cap:* chlor 5 mg+clid 2.5 mg

TRICYCLIC ANTIDEPRESSANTS (TCAs)

▷ *amitriptyline* (C)(G) 25-50 mg q HS

    Pediatric: <12 years: not recommended; ≥12 years: same as adult

        Tab: 10, 25, 50, 75, 100, 150 mg

▷ *imipramine* (C)(G)

    Pediatric: <12 years: not recommended; ≥12 years: same as adult

        Tofranil initially 75 mg daily (max 200 mg); adolescents initially 30-40 mg daily (max 100 mg/day); if maintenance dose exceeds 75 mg daily, may switch to **Tofranil PM** for divided <u>or</u> bedtime dose

            Tab: 10, 25, 50 mg

        Tofranil PM initially 75 mg daily 1 hour before HS; max 200 mg

            Cap: 75, 100, 125, 150

 INTERTRIGO

See **Candidiasis: Skin** *page* 70

Topical Antifungals *see* **Tinea Corporis** *page* 482

Topical Anti-infectives *see* **Skin Infection: Bacterial** *page* 461

Topical Corticosteroids *see page* 574

OTC hydrocortisone 1% paste or ointment

OTC Zinc Oxide paste or ointment

OTC A&D Ointment

Comment: Intertrigo is an irritant dermatitis in the intertriginous zones (skin creases and folds) characterized by inflammation and excoriation caused by skin-to-skin friction, moisture, and heat and may be itching, stinging, burning with a musty odor. Common areas at risk include breast folds, axillae, groin folds, buttocks folds, and the abdominal panniculus in obese persons, finger and toe webs. Treatment includes keeping the areas clean, moisture-free, application of a steroid cream and a protective lubricant barrier. Intertrigo may be complicated by a superimposed infection such as yeast (*Candida albicans*), dermatophytic fungi, <u>or</u> bacteria. Oral agents may be required based on severity of the skin breakdown and invasive infectious process. Apply appropriate topical anti-infective first and barrier product last. Non-medicated powders (e.g., corn starch) are contraindicated in the affected areas as they trap moisture. Exposure to light and air when possible and as appropriate facilitates integumentary healing.

INTRA-ABDOMINAL INFECTION: COMPLICATED (cIAI)

PARENTERAL CEPHALOSPORIN ANTIBACTERIAL+BETA-LACTAMASE INHIBITOR

▶ *ceftazidime+avibactam* (B) infuse dose over 2 hours; recommended duration of treatment: 5 to 4 days; *CrCl 31-50 mL/min:* 1.25 gm every 8 hours; *CrCl 16-30 mL/min:* 0.94 gm every 12 hours; *CrCl 6-15 mL/min:* 0.94 gm every 24 hours; *CrCl ≤5 mL/min:* 0.94 gm every 48 hours; both *ceftazidime* and *avibactam* are hemodialyzable; thus, administer Avycaz after hemodialysis on hemodialysis days

Pediatric: <18 years: not recommended; ≥18 years: same as adult

Avycaz *Vial:* 2.5 gm, single-dose, pwdr for reconstitution and IV infusion

Comment: Avycaz 2.5 gm contains *ceftazidime* (a cephalosporin) 2 grams (equivalent to 2.635 grams of *ceftazidime pentahydrate/sodium carbonate powder*) and *avibactam* (a beta lactam inhibitor) 0.5 grams (equivalent to 0.551 grams of *avibactam sodium*). As only limited clinical safety and efficacy data for Avycaz are currently available, reserve Avycaz for use in patients who have limited or no alternative treatment options. To reduce the development of drug-resistant bacteria and maintain the effectiveness of Avycaz and other antibacterial drugs, Avycaz should be used only to treat infections that are proven or strongly suspected to be caused by susceptible bacteria. Seizures and other neurologic events may occur, especially in patients with renal impairment. Adjust dose in patients with renal impairment. Decreased efficacy in patients with baseline CrCl 30--≤50 mL/min. Monitor CrCl at least daily in patients with changing renal function and adjust the dose of Avycaz accordingly. Monitor for hypersensitivity reactions, including anaphylaxis and serious skin reactions. Cross-hypersensitivity may occur in patients with a history of penicillin allergy. If an allergic reaction occurs, discontinue Avycaz. *Clostridium difficile*-associated diarrhea CDAD) has been reported with nearly all systemic antibacterial agents, including Avycaz. There are no adequate and well-controlled studies of Avycaz, *ceftazidime*, or *avibactam* in pregnant females. *ceftazidime* is excreted in human milk in low concentrations. It is not known whether *avibactam* is excreted into human milk. There are no studies to inform effects on the breastfed infant.

PARENTERAL TETRACYCLINE-CLASS (FLUOROCYCLINE) ANTIBACTERIAL

▶ *eravacycline* 1 mg/kg by intravenous infusion over approximately 60 minutes every 12 hours x 4-14 days; *Severe Hepatic Impairment (Child Pugh C):* 1 mg/kg every 12 hours on Day 1, then 1 mg/kg every 24 hours starting on Day 2 for a total duration of 4-14 days; *Concomitant Use of a Strong Cytochrome P450 Isoenzymes (CYP)3A Inducer:* 1.5 mg/kg every 12 hours x 4-14 days

Pediatric: <18 years: not established; ≥18 years: same as adult

Xerava *Vial:* 50 mg pwdr for IV reconstitution and further dilution for IV infusion, single use

Comment: Xerava *(eravacycline)* is a tetracycline-class (fluorocycline) antibacterial indicated for the treatment of complicated intra-abdominal infections in patients ≥18 years-of-age. Xerava is <u>not</u> indicated for the treatment of complicated urinary tract infections (cUTI). Patients who are on anticoagulant therapy may require downward adjustment of their anticoagulant dosage. Most common adverse reactions (incidence ≥ 3%) have been infusion site reactions, nausea, and vomiting. The use of Xerava during tooth development (last half of pregnancy, infancy and childhood up to 8 years-of-age) may cause permanent discoloration of the teeth (yellow-gray-brown) and enamel hypoplasia. The use of Xerava during the second and third trimester of pregnancy, infancy and childhood up to 8 years-of-age may cause reversible inhibition of bone growth. *erevacycline* and its metabolites are excreted in breast milk. Breastfeeding is <u>not</u> recommended; consider fetal risk and maternal benefit.

IRITIS: ACUTE

▶ *loteprednol etabonate* (C) 1-2 drops qid; may increase to 1 drop hourly as needed
Pediatric: <12 years: not recommended; ≥12 years: same as adult
Lotemax Ophthalmic Solution *Ophth soln:* 0.3% (2.5, 5, 10, 15 ml)
▶ *prednisone acetate* (C) 1 drop q 1 hour x 24-48 hours, then 1 drop q 2 hours while awake x 24-48 hours, then 1 drop bid-qid until resolved
Pediatric: <12 years: not recommended; ≥12 years: same as adult
Pred Forte *Ophth soln:* 1% (1, 5, 10, 15 ml)

IRON OVERLOAD

IRON CHELATING AGENTS

▷ *deferasirox (tridentate ligand)* (C)(G) initially 20 mg/kg/day; titrate; may increase 5-10 mg/kg q 3-6 months based on serum ferritin trends; max 30 mg/kg/day
Pediatric: <2 years: not recommended; ≥2 years: same as adult
    Exjade *Tab for oral soln:* 125, 250, 500 mg
    Jadenu *Tab:* 90, 180, 360 mg film-coat
    Jadenu Sprinkle *Sachet:* 90, 180, 360 mg (30/carton)
    Comment: *deferasirox* is an orally active chelator selective for iron. It is indicated for the treatment of chronic iron overload due to blood transfusions (transfusional hemosiderosis). Monitor serum ferritin monthly. Consider interrupting therapy if serum ferritin falls below 500 mcg/L. Take *deferasirox* (**Exjade, Jadenu, Jadenu Sprinkle**) on an empty stomach. Completely disperse tablet(s) or granules in 3.5 oz liquid if dose is ≤1 gm or 7 oz liquid if dose is ≥1 gm.

▷ *Succimer* (C) initially 10 mg/kg q 8 hours x 5 days; then, reduce frequency to every 12 hours x 14 more days; allow at least 14 days between courses unless blood lead levels indicate need for prompt treatment
Pediatric: <12 months: not recommended; ≥12 months: same as adult
    Chemet Cap: 100 mg
    Comment: *Chemet is* indicated for the treatment of lead poisoning when blood lead level 45 mcg/dL. Treatment for more than 3 consecutive weeks is not recommended. Monitor hydration, renal, and hepatic function.

 IRRITABLE BOWEL SYNDROME WITH CONSTIPATION (IBS-C)

Bulk-Producing Agents, Laxatives, Stool Softeners *see Constipation* page 103

GUANYLATE CYCLASE-C AGONIST

Comment: Guanylate cyclase-c agonists increase intestinal fluid and intestinal transit time may induce diarrhea and bloating and therefore, are contraindicated with known or suspected mechanical GI obstruction.

▷ *linaclotide* (C) 290 mcg once daily; take on an empty stomach at least 30 minutes before the first meal of the day; swallow whole or may open cap and sprinkle on applesauce or in water for administration
    Pediatric: <6 years: not recommended; 6-17 years: avoid; >17 years: same as adult
        Linzess *Cap:* 145, 290 mcg
    Comment: *linaclotide* and its active metabolite are negligibly absorbed systemically following oral administration and maternal use is not expected to result in fetal exposure to the drug. There is no information regarding the presence of *plecanatide* in human milk or its effects on the breastfed infant.

CHLORIDE CHANNEL ACTIVATOR

▷ *lubiprostone* (C) 8 mcg bid; take with food and water; *Severe hepatic impairment (Child-Pugh Class C):* 8 mcg once daily
Pediatric: <18 years: not recommended; ≥18 years: same as adult
    Amitiza *Cap:* 8, 24 mcg
    Comment: **Amitiza** increases intestinal fluid and intestinal transit time. Suspend dosing and rehydrate if severe diarrhea occurs. **Amitiza** is contraindicated with known or suspected mechanical GI obstruction. Most common adverse reactions in CIC are nausea, diarrhea, headache, abdominal pain, abdominal distension, and flatulence.

 IRRITABLE BOWEL SYNDROME WITH DIARRHEA (IBS-D)

Bulk-Producing Agents *see Constipation* page 103

CONSTIPATING AGENTS

▷ *difenoxin+atropine* (C) 2 tabs, then 1 tab after each loose stool <u>or</u> 1 tab q 3-4 hours as needed; max 8 tab/day x 2 days
Pediatric: <12 years: not recommended; ≥12 years: same as adult
   Motofen *Tab:* difen 1 mg+atro 0.025 mg

▷ *diphenoxylate+atropine* (C)(G) 2 tabs <u>or</u> 10 ml qid
Pediatric: <2 years: not recommended; 2-12 years: initially 0.3-0.4 mg/kg/day in 4 divided doses; ≥12 years: same as adult
   Lomotil *Tab:* difen 2.5 mg+atro 0.025 mg; *Liq:* difen 2.5 mg+atro 0.025 mg per 5 ml (2 oz)

▷ *eluxadoline* (NA)(IV) 100 mg bid; 75 mg bid if unable to tolerate 100 mg, <u>or</u> without a gall bladder, <u>or</u> mild-to-moderate hepatic impairment, <u>or</u> receiving concomitant OATP1B1 inhibitors
Pediatric: <12 years: not established; ≥12 years: same as adult
   Viberzi 4 mg initially, then 2 mg after each loose stool; max 16 mg/day
    Tab: 75, 100 mg film-coat

Comment: *Eluxadoline* is a mu-opioid receptor agonist. It is contraindicated with biliary obstruction, Sphincter of Oddi disease <u>or</u> dysfunction, alcohol abuse <u>or</u> addiction, pancreatitis, pancreatic duct obstruction, severe hepatic impairment, and mechanical GI obstruction.

▷ *loperamide* (B)(G)
   Imodium (OTC) 4 mg initially, then 2 mg after each loose stool; max 16 mg/day
   Pediatric: <5 years: not recommended; ≥5 years: same as adult
    Cap: 2 mg
   Imodium A-D (OTC) 4 mg initially, then 2 mg after each loose stool; usual max 8 mg/day x 2 days
   Pediatric: <2 years: not recommended; 2-5 years (24-47 lb): 1 mg up to tid x 2 days; 6-8 years (48-59 lb): 2 mg initially, then 1 mg after each loose stool; max 4 mg/day x 2 days; 9-11 years (60-95 lb): 2 mg initially, then 1 mg after each loose stool; max 6 mg/day x 2 days; ≥12 years: same as adult
    Cplt: 2 mg; *Liq:* 1 mg/5 ml (2, 4 oz)

▷ *loperamide+simethicone* (B)(G)
   Imodium Advanced (OTC) 2 tabs chewed after loose stool, then 1 after the next loose stool; max 4 tabs/day
    Pediatric: <6 years: not recommended; 6-8 years: 1 tab chewed after loose stool, then 1/2 after next loose stool; max 2 tabs/day; 9-11 years: 1 tab chewed after loose stool, then 1/2 after next loose stool; max 3 tabs/day; ≥12 years: same as adult
    Chew tab: lop 2 mg+sim 125 mg

SEROTONIN (5-HT3) RECEPTOR ANTAGONIST

▷ *alosetron* (B)(G) initially 0.5 mg bid; may increase to 1 mg bid after 4 weeks if starting dose is tolerated but inadequate
Pediatric: <12 years: not recommended; ≥12 years: same as adult
   Lotronex *Tab:* 0.5, 1 mg

ANTISPASMODIC+ANTICHOLINERGIC COMBINATIONS

▷ *dicyclomine* (B)(G) initially 20 mg bid-qid; may increase to 40 mg qid PO; usual IM dose 80 mg/day divided qid; do not use IM route for more than 1-2 days
Pediatric: <12 years: not recommended; ≥12 years: same as adult
   Bentyl *Tab:* 20 mg; *Cap:* 10 mg; *Syr:* 10 mg/5 ml (16 oz); *Vial:* 10 mg/ml (10 ml); *Amp:* 10 mg/ml (2 ml)

▷ *methscopolamine bromide* (B) 1 tab q 6 hours prn
Pediatric: <12 years: not recommended; ≥12 years: same as adult
   Pamine *Tab:* 2.5 mg
   Pamine Forte *Tab:* 5 mg

ANTICHOLINERGICS

▷ *hyoscyamine* (C)(G)
   Anaspaz 1-2 tabs q 4 hours prn; max 12 tabs/day

Pediatric: <2 years: not recommended; 2-12 years: 0.0625-0.125 mg q 4 hours prn; max 0.75 mg/day; ≥12 years: same as adult

    Tab: 0.125*mg

Levbid 1-2 tabs q 12 hours prn; max 4 tabs/day

Pediatric: <12 years: not recommended; ≥12 years: same as adult

    Tab: 0.375*mg ext-rel

Levsin 1-2 tabs q 4 hours prn; max 12 tabs/day

Pediatric: <6 years: not recommended; 6-12 years: 1 tab q 4 hours prn; >12 years: same as adult

    Tab: 0.125*mg

Levsinex SL 1-2 tabs q 4 hours SL <u>or</u> PO; max 12 tabs/day

Pediatric: <2 years: not recommended; 2-12 years: 1 tab q 4 hours; max 6 tabs/day; >12 years: same as adult

    Tab: 0.125 mg sublingual

Levsinex Timecaps 1-2 caps q 12 hours; may adjust to 1 cap q 8 hours

Pediatric: <2 years: not recommended; 2-12 years: 1 cap q 12 hours; max 2 caps/day; >12 years: same as adult

    Cap: 0.375 mg time-rel

NuLev dissolve 1-2 tabs on tongue, with <u>or</u> without water, q 4 hours prn; max 12 tabs/day

Pediatric: <2 years: not recommended; 2-12 years: dissolve 1 tab on tongue, with <u>or</u> without water, q 4 hours prn; max 6 tabs/day; >12 years: same as adult

    ODT: 0.125 mg (mint; phenylalanine)

▷ *simethicone* (C)(G) 0.3 ml qid pc and HS

    Mylicon Drops (OTC) *Oral drops:* 40 mg/0.6 ml (30 ml)

▷ *phenobarbital+hyoscyamine+atropine+scopolamine* (C)(IV)(G)

    Donnatal 1-2 tabs ac and HS

Pediatric: <12 years: not recommended; ≥12 years: same as adult

    Tab: pheno 16.2 mg+hyo 0.1037 mg+atro 0.0194 mg+scop 0.0065 mg

    Donnatal Elixir 1-2 tsp ac and HS

Pediatric: 20 lb: 1 ml q 4 hours <u>or</u> 1.5 ml q 6 hours; 30 lb: 1.5 ml q 4 hours <u>or</u> 2 ml q 6 hours; 50 lb: 1/2 tsp q 4 hours <u>or</u> 3/4 tsp q 6 hours; 75 lb: 3/4 tsp q 4 hours <u>or</u> 1 tsp q 6 hours; 100 lb: 1 tsp q 4 hours <u>or</u> 1 tsp q 6 hours

    Elix: pheno 16.2 mg+hyo 0.1037 mg+atro 0.0194 mg+scop 0.0065 mg per 5 ml (4, 16 oz)

    Donnatal Extentabs 1 tab q 12 hours

Pediatric: <12 years: not recommended; ≥12 years: same as adult

    Tab: pheno 48.6 mg+hyo 0.3111 mg+atro 0.0582 mg+scop 0.0195 mg ext-rel

ANTICHOLINERGIC+SEDATIVE COMBINATION

▷ *chlordiazepoxide+clidinium* (D)(IV) 1-2 caps ac and HS: max 8 caps/day

Pediatric: <12 years: not recommended; ≥12 years: same as adult

    Librax *Cap:* chlor 5 mg+clid 2.5 mg

TRICYCLIC ANTIDEPRESSANTS (TCAs)

▷ *amitriptyline* (C)(G) 25-50 mg q HS

Pediatric: <12 years: not recommended; ≥12 years: same as adult

    Tab: 10, 25, 50, 75, 100, 150 mg

▷ *imipramine* (C)(G) 25-50 mg tid

Pediatric: <12 years: not recommended; ≥12 years: same as adult

    Tofranil initially 75 mg daily (max 200 mg); adolescents initially 30-40 mg daily (max 100 mg/day); if maintenance dose exceeds 75 mg daily, may switch to **Tofranil PM** for divided <u>or</u> bedtime dose

    Tab: 10, 25, 50 mg

    Tofranil PM initially 75 mg daily 1 hour before HS; max 200 mg

    Cap: 75, 100, 125, 150

    Tofranil Injection 50 mg IM; lower dose for adolescents; switch to oral form as soon as possible

    Amp: 25 mg/2 ml (2 ml)

▷ *nortriptyline* (D)(G) initially 25 mg tid-qid; max 150 mg/day

Pediatric: <12 years: not recommended; ≥12 years: same as adult

    Pamelor *Cap:* 10, 25, 50, 75 mg; *Oral soln:* 10 mg/5 ml (16 oz)

➤ *protriptyline* (C) initially 5 mg tid; usual dose 15-40 mg/day in 3-4 divided doses; max 60 mg/day

    Pediatric: <12 years: not recommended; ≥12 years: same as adult

      Vivactil *Tab:* 5, 10 mg

➤ *trimipramine* (C) initially 75 mg/day in divided doses; max 200 mg/day

    Pediatric: <12 years: not recommended; ≥12 years: same as adult

      Surmontil *Cap:* 25, 50, 100 mg

JAPANESE ENCEPHALITIS VIRUS (JEV)

Comment: Japanese encephalitis is a viral disease spread by the bite of an infected mosquito. It is not spread from person-to-person. Currently there is no cure. A person with encephalitis can experience fever, neck stiffness, seizures, and coma. About 1 person in 4 with encephalitis dies. Up to half of those who don't die have permanent disability. There is one vaccine for Japanese encephalitis, currently licensed in the UK, for use in adults and children >2 months-of-age. The **live** attenuated vaccine is administered in two doses for full protection, with the second dose administered 28 days after the first. The second dose should be given at least a week before travel. Children younger than 3 years of age get a smaller dose than patients who are 3 <u>or</u> older. A booster dose might be recommended for anyone 17 <u>or</u> older who was vaccinated more than a year ago and is still at risk of exposure. There is no information yet on the need for a booster dose for children. The (JEV) vaccine is usually available through the local health department.

➤ *Japanese encephalitis vaccine (JEV), inactivated, adsorbed* (B) shake the prefilled syringe containing 0.5 ml to obtain a homogeneous suspension; *18-65 years:* 0.5 ml IM x 2 doses 7-28 days apart; *>65 years:* 0.5 ml IM x 2 doses 28 days apart

    Pediatric: shake the prefilled syringe containing 0.5 ml to obtain a homogeneous suspension; <2 months: not recommended; 2 months to <3 years: 0.25 ml IM x 2 doses 28 days apart; 3 to <18 years: 0.5 ml IM x 2 doses 28 days apart

      Ixiaro *Prefilled syringe:* 0.5 ml (protamine sulfate)

      Comment: Administer **Ixiaro** intramuscularly <u>only</u>. Preferred injection sites are the anterolateral aspect of the thigh (LAT) in infants 2 to 11 months-of-age, the anterolateral aspect of the thigh (LAT) <u>or</u> the deltoid muscle if muscle mass is adequate) in children 1 to <3 years-of-age, and the deltoid muscle in patients ≥3 years-of-age. To administer a 0.25 ml JEV dose, expel and discard half of the volume from the 0.5 ml prefilled syringe by pushing the plunger stopper up to the edge of the red line on the syringe barrel prior to injection. Complete the primary immunization series at least 1 week prior to potential exposure to JEV. A booster dose (third dose) may be administered at least 11 months after completion of the primary immunization series if ongoing exposure <u>or</u> re-exposure to JEV is expected. Embryo-fetal effects of JEV exposure in pregnancy and effects on the breastfed infant have not been studied. To report use in pregnant women, contact Valneva USA at 844-349-4276 (8443-IXIARO).

JUVENILE IDIOPATHIC ARTHRITIS (JIA), POLYARTICULAR JUVENILE IDIOPATHIC ARTHRITIS (PJIA), SYSTEMIC JUVENILE IDIOPATHIC ARTHRITIS (SJIA)

Acetaminophen for IV Infusion *see Pain page* 352
NSAIDs *see page* 571
Opioid Analgesics *see Pain page* 354
Topical & Transdermal Analgesics *see Pain page* 352
Parenteral Corticosteroids *see page* 577
Oral Corticosteroids *see page* 577
Topical Analgesic and Anesthetic Agents *see page* 569

TOPICAL & TRANSDERMAL ANALGESICS

➤ *capsaicin* (B)(G) apply tid <u>or</u> qid prn to intact skin

    Pediatric: <2 years: not recommended; ≥2 years: same as adult

      Axsain *Crm:* 0.075% (1, 2 oz)

      Capsin *Lotn:* 0.025, 0.075% (59 ml)

      Capzasin-HP (OTC) *Crm:* 0.075% (1.5 oz), 0.025% (45, 90 gm); *Lotn:* 0.075% (2 oz); 0.025% (45, 90 gm)

Capzasin-P (OTC) *Crm:* 0.025% (1.5 oz); *Lotn:* 0.025% (2 oz)
Dolorac *Crm:* 0.025% (28 gm)
Double Cap (OTC) *Crm:* 0.05% (2 oz)
R-Gel *Gel:* 0.025% (15, 30 gm)
Zostrix (OTC) *Crm:* 0.025% (0.7, 1.5, 3 oz)
Zostrix HP (OTC) *Emol crm:* 0.075% (1, 2 oz)

▷ *capsaicin* 8% patch (B) apply up to 4 patches for one 60-minute application to clean dry skin; may prep area with topical anesthetic; wear non-latex gloves; patches may be cut to size/shape; treatment may be repeated every 3 months
Pediatric: <18 years: not recommended; ≥18 years: same as adult
Qutenza *Patch:* 8% 1640 mcg/cm (179 mg) (1 or 2 patches w. 1-50 gm tube cleansing gel/carton)

▷ *diclofenac sodium* (C; D ≥30 wks)(G) apply qid prn to intact skin
Pediatric: <12 years: not established; ≥12 years: same as adult
Pennsaid 1.5% in 10 drop increments, dispense and rub into front, side, and back of knee: usually; 40 drops (40 mg) qid
Topical soln: 1.5% (150 ml)
Pennsaid 2% apply 2 pump actuations (40 mg) and rub into front, side, and back of knee bid
Topical soln: 2% (20 mg/pump actuation, 112 gm)
Solaraze Gel massage in to clean skin bid prn
Gel: 3% (50 gm) (benzyl alcohol)
Voltaren Gel (G) apply qid prn to intact skin
Gel: 1% (100 gm)

Comment: *diclofenac* is contraindicated with *aspirin* allergy. As with other NSAIDs, should be avoided in late pregnancy (≥30 weeks) because it may cause premature closure of the ductus arteriosus.

▷ *doxepin* (B) cream apply to affected area qid at intervals of at least 3-4 hours; max 8 days
Pediatric: <12 years: not recommended; >12 years: same as adult
Prudoxin *Crm:* 5% (45 gm)
Zonalon *Crm:* 5% (30, 45 gm)

▷ *pimecrolimus* 1% cream (C)(G) <2 years: not recommended; ≥2 years: apply to affected area bid; do not apply an occlusive dressing
Elidel *Crm:* 1% (30, 60, 100 gm)

Comment: *pimecrolimus* is indicated for short-term and intermittent long-term use. Discontinue use when resolution occurs. Contraindicated if the patient is immunosuppressed. Change to the 0.1% preparation or if secondary bacterial infection is present.

▷ *trolamine salicylate* apply tid-qid
Pediatric: <2 years: not recommended; ≥2 years: same as adult
Mobisyl Creme *Crm:* 10% (100 gm)

TOPICAL AND TRANSDERMAL ANESTHETICS

Comment: *lidocaine* should not be applied to non-intact skin.

▷ *lidocaine* cream (B) apply to affected area bid prn
Pediatric: <12 years: not recommended; ≥12 years: same as adult
LidaMantle *Crm:* 3% (1, 2 oz)
Lidoderm *Crm:* 3% (85 gm)
ZTlido *lidocaine* topical system 1% (30/carton)

Comment: Compared to Lidoderm (*lidocaine* patch 5%) which contains 700 mg/patch, ZTlido only requires 35 mg per topical system to achieve the same therapeutic dose.

▷ *lidocaine* lotion (B) apply to affected area bid prn
Pediatric: <12 years: not recommended; ≥12 years: same as adult
LidaMantle *Lotn:* 3% (177 ml)

▷ *lidocaine* 5% patch (B)(G) apply up to 3 patches at one time for up to 12 hours/24-hour period (12 hours on/12 hours off); patches may be cut into smaller sizes before removal of the release liner; do not re-use
Pediatric: <12 years: not recommended; ≥12 years: same as adult
Lidoderm *Patch:* 5% (10x14 cm; 30/carton)

▷ *lidocaine+dexamethasone* (B)
Pediatric: <12 years: not recommended; ≥12 years: same as adult
Decadron Phosphate with Xylocaine *Lotn:* dexa 4 mg+lido 10 mg per ml (5 ml)

▶ *lidocaine+hydrocortisone* (B)(G) apply to affected area bid prn
  Pediatric: <12 years: not recommended; ≥12 years: same as adult
    LidaMantle HC *Crm:* lido 3%+hydro 0.5% (1, 3 oz); *Lotn:* (177 ml)
▶ *lidocaine 2.5%+prilocaine 2.5%* apply sparingly to the burn bid-tid prn
  Pediatric: <12 years: not recommended; ≥12 years: same as adult
    Emla Cream (B) 5, 30 gm/tube

ORAL SALICYLATES

▶ *indomethacin* (C) initially 25 mg bid <u>or</u> tid, increase as needed at weekly intervals by 25-50 mg/day; max 200 mg/day
  Pediatric: <14 years: usually not recommended; >2 years, if risk warranted: 1-2 mg/kg/day in divided doses; max 3-4 mg/kg/day (<u>or</u> 150-200 mg/day, whichever is less; <14 years: ER cap not recommended
    Cap: 25, 50 mg; *Susp:* 25 mg/5 ml (pineapple-coconut, mint) (alcohol 1%); *Supp:* 50 mg; *ER Cap:* 75 mg ext-rel
  Comment: *indomethacin* is indicated only for acute painful flares. Administer with food and/or antacids. Use lowest effective dose for shortest duration.
▶ *methotrexate* (X) 7.5 mg x 1 dose per week <u>or</u> 2.5 mg x 3 at 12 hour intervals once a week; max 20 mg/week; therapeutic response begins in 3-6 weeks; administer *methotrexate* injection SC only into the abdomen <u>or</u> thigh
  Pediatric: <2 years: not recommended; ≥2 years: 10 mg/m^2 once weekly; max 20 mg/m^2
    Rasuvo *Autoinjector:* 7.5 mg/0.15 ml, 10 mg/0.20 ml, 12.5 mg/0.25 ml, 15 mg/0.30 ml, 17.5 mg/0.35 ml, 20 mg/0.40 ml, 22.5 mg/0.45 ml, 25 mg/0.50 ml, 27.5 mg/0.55 ml, 30 mg/0.60 ml (solution concentration for SC injection is 50 mg/ml)
    Rheumatrex *Tab:* 2.5*mg (5, 7.5, 10, 12.5, 15 mg/week, 4/card unit dose pack)
    Trexall *Tab:* 5*, 7.5*, 10*, 15*mg (5, 7.5, 10, 12.5, 15 mg/week, 4/card unit dose pack)
  Comment: *methotrexate* (MTX) is contraindicated with immunodeficiency, blood dyscrasias, alcoholism, and chronic liver disease.

INTERLEUKIN-6 RECEPTOR ANTAGONIST

▶ *tocilizumab* (B) *IV Infusion:* administer over 1 hour; do not administer as bolus <u>or</u> IV push; *Adults, PJIA, and SJIA,* ≥30 kg: dilute to 100 mL in 0.9% <u>or</u> 0.45% NaCl. *PJIA and SJIA,* <30 kg: dilute to 50 mL in 0.9% <u>or</u> 0.45% NaCl.
  Pediatric: <2 years: not recommended; ≥2 years: same as adult
    Adults: IV Infusion: Whether used in combination with DMARDs <u>or</u> as monotherapy, the recommended IV infusion starting dose is 4 mg/kg IV every 4 weeks followed by an increase to 8 mg/kg IV every 4 weeks based on clinical response; Max 800 mg per infusion in RA patients; *SC Administration:* ≥100 kg: 162 mg SC once weekly on the same day; <100 kg: 162 mg SC every other week on the same day followed by an increase according to clinical response
    Pediatric: <2 years: not recommended; ≥2 years: weight-based dosing according to diagnosis: *PJIA:* ≥30 kg: 8 mg/kg SC every 4 weeks; <30 kg: 10 mg/kg SC every 4 weeks; *SJIA:* ≥30 kg: 8 mg/kg SC every 2 weeks; <30 kg: 12 mg/kg SC every 2 weeks
      Actemra *Vial:* 80 mg/4 ml, 200 mg/10 ml, 400 mg/20 ml, single-use, for IV infusion after dilution; *Prefilled syringe:* 162 mg (0.9 ml, single-dose)
  Comment: *tocilizumab* is an interleukin-6 receptor-α inhibitor indicated for use in moderate-to-severe rheumatoid arthritis (RA) that has not responded to conventional therapy, and also for some subtypes of juvenile idiopathic arthritis (JIA). **Actemra** may be used alone <u>or</u> in combination with *methotrexate* and in RA, other DMARDs may be used. Monitor patient for dose related laboratory changes including elevated LFTs, neutropenia, and thrombocytopenia. **Actemra** should not be initiated in patients with an absolute neutrophil count (ANC) below 2000 per mm^3, platelet count below 100,000 per mm^3, <u>or</u> who have ALT <u>or</u> AST above 1.5 times the upper limit of normal (ULN). Registration in the Pregnancy Exposure Registry (1-877-311-8972) is encouraged for monitoring pregnancy outcomes in women exposed to **Actemra** during pregnancy. The limited available data with **Actemra** in pregnant women are not sufficient to determine whether there is a drug-associated risk for major birth defects and miscarriage. Monoclonal antibodies, such as *tocilizumab*, are actively transported across the placenta during the third trimester of pregnancy and may affect immune response in the infant exposed in *utero*. It is not known whether *tocilizumab* passes into breast milk; therefore, breastfeeding is not recommended while using **Actemra**.

Selective Co-stimulation Modulator

▶ *abatacept* (C) <2 years: not recommended; 2- 17 years: administer as an IV Infusion over 30 minutes at weeks 0, 2, and 4; then every 4 weeks thereafter; <75 kg, administer 10 mg/ kg; same as adult (max 1 gm); administer as an IV infusion over 30 minutes at weeks 0, 2, and 4; then every 4 weeks thereafter; <60 kg, administer 500 mg/dose; 60-100 kg, administer 750 mg/dose; >100 kg, administer 1 gm/dose

Orencia *Vial:* 250 mg pwdr for IV infusion after reconstitution (silicone-free) (preservative-free); *Prefilled syringe:* 125 mg/ml soln for SC injection (preservative-free); *ClickJect Autoinjector:* 125 mg/ml soln for SC injection

Comment: **Orencia** is indicated to reduce signs/symptoms of moderate-to-severe active polyarticular juvenile idiopathic arthritis (PJIA) in patients >2 years-of-age as monotherapy or with *methotrexate*. **Orencia** is also indicated to reduce signs/ symptoms, induce major clinical response, inhibit progression of structural damage, and improve physical function in adult patients with moderate-to-severe active RA. **Orencia** may be used as monotherapy or with DMARDs other than TNF antagonists.

TUMOR NECROSIS FACTOR (TNF) BLOCKER

▶ *adalimumab* (B) <2 years, <10 kg: not recommended; 10-<15 kg: 10 mg every other week; 15-<30 kg: 20 mg every other week; ≥30 kg: 40 mg every other week; 2-17 years, supervise first dose; ≥12 years: 40 mg SC once every other week; may increase to once weekly without MTX; administer in abdomen or thigh; rotate sites

Humira *Prefilled syringe:* 20 mg/0.4 ml; 40 mg/0.8 ml single-dose (2/pck; 2, 6/starter pck) (preservative-free)

Comment: May use with *methotrexate* (MTX), DMARDs, corticosteroids, salicylates, NSAIDs, or analgesics.

▶ *adalimumab-adaz* (B) ≥*30 kg (66 lbs):* 40 mg every other week; inject into thigh or abdomen; rotate sites
Pediatric: <4 years, <30 kg (<66 lbs): not recommended; ≥4 years, ≥30 kg (≥66 lbs): same as adult

Hyrimoz *Prefilled syringe:* 40 mg/0.8 ml single-dose (preservative-free)

Comment: **Hyrimox** is biosimilar to **Humira** (*adalimumab*).

▶ *adalimumab-adbm* (B) ≥*30 kg (66 lbs):* 40 mg every other week; inject into thigh or abdomen; rotate sites
Pediatric: <30 kg, <66 lbs: not recommended; ≥30 kg, ≥66 lbs: same as adult

Cyltezo *Prefilled syringe:* 40 mg/0.8 ml single-dose (preservative-free)

Comment: **Cyltezo** is biosimilar to **Humira** (*adalimumab*).

 JUVENILE RHEUMATOID ARTHRITIS (JRA)

Juvenile Idiopathic Arthritis (JIA), Polyarticular Juvenile Idiopathic Arthritis (PJIA), Systemic Juvenile Idiopathic Arthritis (SJIA) *see page* 281
Acetaminophen for IV Infusion *see Pain page* 352
NSAIDs *see page* 571
Opioid Analgesics *see Pain page* 354
Topical & Transdermal Analgesics *see Pain page* 352
Parenteral Corticosteroids *see page* 577
Oral Corticosteroids *see page* 577

TOPICAL & TRANSDERMAL ANALGESICS

▶ *capsaicin* (B)(G) apply tid-qid prn to intact skin
Pediatric: <2 years: not recommended; ≥2 years: same as adult

Axsain *Crm:* 0.075% (1, 2 oz)
Capsin *Lotn:* 0.025, 0.075% (59 ml)
Capzasin-HP (OTC) *Crm:* 0.075% (1.5 oz), 0.025% (45, 90 gm); *Lotn:* 0.075% (2 oz); 0.025% (45, 90 gm)
Capzasin-P (OTC) *Crm:* 0.025% (1.5 oz); *Lotn:* 0.025% (2 oz)
Dolorac *Crm:* 0.025% (28 gm)
Double Cap (OTC) *Crm:* 0.05% (2 oz)
R-Gel *Gel:* 0.025% (15, 30 gm)

Zostrix (OTC) *Crm:* 0.025% (0.7, 1.5, 3 oz)
Zostrix HP (OTC) *Emol crm:* 0.075% (1, 2 oz)
▷ *capsaicin* 8% patch **(B)** apply up to 4 patches for one 60-minute application to clean dry skin; may prep area with topical anesthetic; wear non-latex gloves; patches may be cut to size/shape; treatment may be repeated every 3 months
Pediatric: <18 years: not recommended; ≥18 years: same as adult
Qutenza *Patch:* 8% 1640 mcg/cm (179 mg) (1 *or* 2 patches w. 1-50 gm tube cleansing gel/carton)
▷ *diclofenac sodium* **(C; D ≥30 wks)(G)** apply qid prn to intact skin
Pediatric: <12 years: not established; ≥12 years: same as adult
Pennsaid 1.5% in 10 drop increments, dispense and rub into front, side, and back of knee: usually; 40 drops (40 mg) qid
Topical soln: 1.5% (150 ml)
Pennsaid 2% apply 2 pump actuations (40 mg) and rub into front, side, and back of knee bid
Topical soln: 2% (20 mg/pump actuation, 112 gm)
Solaraze Gel massage in to clean skin bid prn
Gel: 3% (50 gm) (benzyl alcohol)
Voltaren Gel **(G)** apply qid prn to intact skin
Gel: 1% (100 gm)
Comment: *diclofenac* is contraindicated with *aspirin* allergy. As with other NSAIDs, should be avoided in late pregnancy (≥30 weeks) because it may cause premature closure of the ductus arteriosus.
▷ *doxepin* **(B)** cream apply to affected area qid at intervals of at least 3-4 hours; max 8 days
Pediatric: <12 years: not recommended; >12 years: same as adult
Prudoxin *Crm:* 5% (45 gm)
Zonalon *Crm:* 5% (30, 45 gm)
▷ *pimecrolimus* 1% cream **(C)(G)** <2 years: not recommended; ≥2 years: apply to affected area bid; do not apply an occlusive dressing
Elidel *Crm:* 1% (30, 60, 100 gm)
Comment: *pimecrolimus* is indicated for short-term and intermittent long-term use. Discontinue use when resolution occurs. Contraindicated if the patient is immunosuppressed. Change to the 0.1% preparation *or* if secondary bacterial infection is present.
▷ *trolamine salicylate* apply tid-qid
Pediatric: <2 years: not recommended; ≥2 years: same as adult
Mobisyl Creme *Crm:* 10% (100 gm)

TOPICAL & TRANSDERMAL ANESTHETICS

Comment: *lidocaine* should not be applied to non-intact skin.
▷ *lidocaine* cream **(B)** apply to affected area bid prn
Pediatric: <12 years: not recommended; ≥12 years: same as adult
LidaMantle *Crm:* 3% (1, 2 oz)
Lidoderm *Crm:* 3% (85 gm)
ZTlido *lidocaine* topical system 1% (30/carton)
Comment: Compared to Lidoderm (*lidocaine* patch 5%) which contains 700 mg/patch, ZTlido only requires 35 mg per topical system to achieve the same therapeutic dose.
▷ *lidocaine* lotion **(B)** apply to affected area bid prn
Pediatric: <12 years: not recommended; ≥12 years: same as adult
LidaMantle *Lotn:* 3% (177 ml)
▷ *lidocaine* 5% patch **(B)(G)** apply up to 3 patches at one time for up to 12 hours/24-hour period (12 hours on/12 hours off); patches may be cut into smaller sizes before removal of the release liner; do not re-use
Pediatric: <12 years: not recommended; ≥12 years: same as adult
Lidoderm *Patch:* 5% (10x14 cm; 30/carton)
▷ *lidocaine+dexamethasone* **(B)**
Pediatric: <12 years: not recommended; ≥12 years: same as adult
Decadron Phosphate with Xylocaine *Lotn:* dexa 4 mg+lido 10 mg per ml (5 ml)
▷ *lidocaine+hydrocortisone* **(B)(G)** apply to affected area bid prn
Pediatric: <12 years: not recommended; ≥12 years: same as adult
LidaMantle HC *Crm:* lido 3%+hydro 0.5% (1, 3 oz); *Lotn:* (177 ml)

286 ■ Juvenile Rheumatoid Arthritis (JRA)

lidocaine 2.5%+prilocaine 2.5% apply sparingly to the burn bid-tid prn
Pediatric: <12 years: not recommended; ≥12 years: same as adult
  Emla Cream (B) 5, 30 gm/tube

ORAL SALICYLATE

▷ *indomethacin* (C) initially 25 mg bid-tid, increase as needed at weekly intervals by 25-50 mg/day; max 200 mg/day
Pediatric: <14 years: usually not recommended; ≥2 years, if risk warranted: 1-2 mg/kg/day in divided doses; max 3-4 mg/kg/day (or total 150-200 mg/day, whichever is less); ≤14 years: ER cap not recommended
  Cap: 25, 50 mg; Susp: 25 mg/5 ml (pineapple-coconut, mint; alcohol 1%); Supp: 50 mg; ER Cap: 75 mg ext-rel
  Comment: *Indomethacin* is indicated only for acute painful flares. Administer with food and/or antacids. Use lowest effective dose for shortest duration.
▷ *methotrexate* (X) 7.5 mg x 1 dose per week or 2.5 mg x 3 at 12-hour intervals once a week; max 20 mg/week; therapeutic response begins in 3-6 weeks; administer methotrexate injection SC only into the abdomen or thigh
Pediatric: <2 years: not recommended; ≥2 years: 10 mg/m² once weekly; max 20 mg/m²
  Rasuvo *Autoinjector:* 7.5 mg/0.15 ml, 10 mg/0.20 ml, 12.5 mg/0.25 ml, 15 mg/0.30 ml, 17.5 mg/0.35 ml, 20 mg/0.40 ml, 22.5 mg/0.45 ml, 25 mg/0.50 ml, 27.5 mg/0.55 ml, 30 mg/0.60 ml (solution concentration for SC injection is 50 mg/ml)
  Rheumatrex *Tab:* 2.5*mg (5, 7.5, 10, 12.5, 15 mg/week, 4/card unit-of-use dose pack)
  Trexall *Tab:* 5*, 7.5*, 10*, 15*mg (5, 7.5, 10, 12.5, 15 mg/week, 4/card unit-of-use dose pack)
  Comment: *methotrexate* (MTX) is contraindicated with immunodeficiency, blood dyscrasias, alcoholism, and chronic liver disease.

INTERLEUKIN-6 RECEPTOR ANTAGONIST

▷ *tocilizumab* (B) <2 years: not recommended; ≥2 years: weight-based dosing ≥*30 kg:* 8 mg/kg SC every 2 weeks; <*30 kg:* 12 mg/kg SC every 2 weeks; *IV Infusion:* administer over 1 hour; do not administer as bolus or IV push; ≥*30 kg:* dilute to 100 mL in 0.9% or 0.45% NaCl. <*30 kg:* dilute to 50 mL in 0.9% or 0.45% NaCl; ≥*18 years:* whether used in combination with DMARDs or as monotherapy, the recommended IV infusion starting dose is 4 mg/kg IV every 4 weeks followed by an increase to 8 mg/kg IV every 4 weeks based on clinical response; Max 800 mg per infusion in RA patients; *SC Administration:* ≥*100 kg:* 162 mg SC once weekly on the same day; <*100 kg:* 162 mg SC every other week on the same day followed by an increase according to clinical response
  Actemra *Vial:* 80 mg/4 ml, 200 mg/10 ml, 400 mg/20 ml, single-use, for IV Infusion after dilution; *Prefilled syringe:* 162 mg (0.9 ml, single-dose)
  Comment: *tocilizumab* is an interleukin-6 receptor-α inhibitor indicated for use in moderate-to-severe rheumatoid arthritis (RA) that has not responded to conventional therapy, and also for some subtypes of JRA. **Actemra** may be used alone or in combination with *methotrexate* and in RA, other DMARDs may be used. Monitor patient for dose related laboratory changes including elevated LFTs, neutropenia, and thrombocytopenia. **Actemra** should not be initiated in patients with an absolute neutrophil count (ANC) below 2000 per mm3, platelet count below 100,000 per mm3, or who have ALT or AST above 1.5 times the upper limit of normal (ULN). Registration in the Pregnancy Exposure Registry (1-877-311-8972) is encouraged for monitoring pregnancy outcomes in women exposed to **Actemra** during pregnancy. The limited available data-associated risk for major birth defects and miscarriage. Monoclonal antibodies, such as *tocilizumab*, are actively transported across the placenta during the third trimester of pregnancy and may affect immune response in the infant exposed *in utero*. It is not known whether *tocilizumab* passes into breast milk; therefore, breastfeeding is not recommended while using **Actemra**.

Selective Co-stimulation Modulator

▷ *abatacept* (C) <2 years: not recommended; 2-17 years: administer as an IV infusion over 30 minutes at weeks 0, 2, and 4; then every 4 weeks thereafter; <75 kg, administer 10 mg/kg; same as adult (max 1 gm); administer as an IV infusion over 30 minutes at weeks 0, 2, and 4; then every 4 weeks thereafter; <60 kg, administer 500 mg/dose; 60-100 kg, administer 750 mg/dose; >100 kg, administer 1 gm/dose

Orencia *Vial:* 250 mg pwdr for IV infusion after reconstitution (silicone-free) (preservative-free); *Prefilled syringe:* 125 mg/ml soln for SC injection (preservative-free); *ClickJect Autoinjector:* 125 mg/ml soln for SC injection

Comment: **Orencia** is also indicated to reduce signs/symptoms, induce major clinical response, inhibit progression of structural damage, and improve physical function in adult patients with moderate-to-severe active RA. **Orencia** may be used as monotherapy or with DMARDs other than TNF antagonists. **Orencia** is also indicated to reduce signs/symptoms of moderate-to-severe active polyarticular juvenile idiopathic arthritis (PJIA) in patients >2 years-of-age as monotherapy or with *methotrexate*.

alpha insert new diagnosis:

KERATITIS/KERATOCONJUNCTIVITIS SICCA/DRY EYE SYNDROME

➤ *cyclosporine* (C) using 1 single-use disposable vial, instill 1 drop in each eye twice daily q 12 hours

Pediatric: <16 years: not recommended; ≥16 years: same as adult

Cequa *Ophth soln:* 0.09% single-use vials (0.25 ml, 6 pouches, 10 vials/pouch per carton) (preservative-free)

Comment: **Cequa** ophthalmic solution is a calcineurin inhibitor immune-suppressant indicated to increase tear production in patients with keratoconjunctivitis sicca. It is the first cyclosporine product to utilize nanomicellar technology, facilitating the drug molecule to penetrate the eye's aqueous layer, and preventing the release of active lipophilic molecule prior to penetration.

Restasis *Ophth emul:* 0.05% (0.4 ml) (preservative-free)

KERATITIS/KERATOCONJUNCTIVITIS: HERPES SIMPLEX

➤ *ganciclovir* (C) instill 1 drop 5 x/day (every 3 hours) while awake until corneal ulcer heals; then 1 drop tid x 7 days

Pediatric: <2 years: not recommended; ≥2 years: same as adult

Zirgan *Ophth gel:* 0.15% (5 gm) (benzalkonium chloride)

➤ *idoxuridine* (C) instill 1 drop q 1 hour during day and every other hour at night or 1 drop every minute for 5 minutes and repeat q 4 hours during day and night

Herplex *Ophth soln:* 0.1% (15 ml)

➤ *trifluridine* (C) instill 1 drop q 2 hours while awake (max 9 drops/day until reepithelialization; then 1 drop q 4 hours x 7 more days (at least 5 drops/day); max 21 days

Pediatric: <6 years: not recommended; ≥6 years: same as adult

Viroptic *Ophth soln:* 1% (7.5 ml) (thimerosal)

➤ *vidarabine* (C) apply 1/2 inch in lower conjunctival sac 5 x/day q 3 hours until reepithelialization occurs, then bid x 7 more days

Pediatric: <2 years: not recommended; ≥2 years: same as adult

Vira-A *Ophth oint:* 3% (3.5 gm)

KERATITIS: NEUROTROPHIC

Comment: **Oxervate** is a recombinant form of human nerve growth factor (hNGF) structurally similar to endogenous NGF protein. NGF is an endogenous protein involved in the differentiation and maintenance of neurons, which acts through specific high-affinity (i.e., TrkA) and low-affinity (i.e. p75NTR) nerve growth factor receptors in the anterior segment of the eye to support corneal innervation and integrity. Prior to FDA- approval of **Oxervate**, treatment was limited to symptomatic relief such as artificial tears, antibiotics, autologous serum-derived eye drops, tarsorrhaphy, and botulinum-induced ptosis, or surgical intervention.

➤ *cenegermin-bkbj* 1 drop in affected eye(s) 6 x/ day at 2-hour intervals x 8 weeks; pharmacy storage of the weekly carton in the freezer at or below -4°F (-20°C) until dispensed in the insulated pack in the Delivery System Kit; within 5 hours of leaving the pharmacy, store the weekly carton in the refrigerator between 36°F to 46°F (2°C to 8°C) for up to 14 days; opened vials may be stored in the original weekly carton in the refrigerator between 36°F to 46°F (2°C to 8°C) or at room temperature up to 77°F (25°C) for up to 12 hours; do not re-freeze; do not shake the vial; discard any unused portion after 12 hours

Pediatric: <2 years: not recommended; ≥2 years: same as adult
    Oxervate *Vial:* 0.002% multi-dose (7/carton; Delivery System Kit contains, insulated pack, 8 vial adapters, 45 pipettes, 45 sterile disinfectant wipes, dose card) (preservative-free)

KERATITIS/KERATOCONJUNCTIVITIS: VERNAL

OPHTHALMIC MAST CELL STABILIZERS

Comment: Contact lens wear is contraindicated
▷ *cromolyn sodium* (B) 1-2 drops 4-6 x/day
    Pediatric: <4 years: not recommended; ≥4 years: same as adult
        Crolom, Opticrom *Ophth soln:* 4% (10 ml) (benzalkonium chloride)
▷ *lodoxamide tromethamine* (B) 1-2 drops qid; max 3 months
    Pediatric: <2 years: not recommended; ≥2 years: same as adult
        Alomide *Ophth susp:* 0.1% (10 ml)

LABYRINTHITIS

▷ *meclizine* (B) 25 mg tid
    Pediatric: <12 years: not recommended; ≥12 years: same as adult
        Antivert *Tab:* 12.5, 25, 50*mg
        Bonine (OTC) *Cap:* 15, 25, 30 mg; *Tab:* 12.5, 25, 50 mg; *Chew tab/Film-coat tab:* 25 mg
        Dramamine II (OTC) *Tab:* 25*mg
        Zentrip *Strip:* 25 mg orally disintegrating
▷ *promethazine* (C)(G) 25 mg tid
    Pediatric: <2 years: not recommended; ≥2 years: 0.5 mg/lb or 6.25-25 mg tid
        Phenergan *Tab:* 12.5*, 25*, 50 mg; *Plain syr:* 6.25 mg/5 ml; *Fortis syr:* 25 mg/5 ml; *Rectal supp:* 12.5, 25, 50 mg
    Comment: *promethazine* is contraindicated in children with uncomplicated nausea, dehydration, Reye's syndrome, history of sleep apnea, asthma, and lower respiratory disorders in children. *promethazine* lowers the seizure threshold in children, may cause cholestatic jaundice, anticholinergic effects, extrapyramidal effects, and potentially fatal respiratory depression.
▷ *scopolamine* (C)
        Transderm Scop 1 patch behind ear at least 4 hours before travel; each patch is effective for 3 days
        Transdermal patch: 1.5 mg (4/carton)

LACTOSE INTOLERANCE

▷ *lactase* enzyme 9,000 FCC units taken with dairy food; adjust based on abatement of symptoms; usual max 18,000 units/dose
    Pediatric: same as adult
        Lactaid Drops (OTC) 5-7 drops to each quart of milk and shake gently; may increase to 10-15 drops if needed; hydrolyzes 70%-99% of lactose at refrigerator temperature in 24 hours
            Oral drops: 1,250 units/5 gtts (7 ml w. dropper)
        Lactaid Extra (OTC) *Cplt:* 4,500 FCC units
        Lactaid Fast ACT (OTC) *Cplt:* 9,000 FCC units; *Chew tab:* 9,000 FCC units (vanilla twist)
        Lactaid Original (OTC) *Cplt:* 3,000 FCC units
        Lactaid Ultra (OTC) *Cplt:* 9,000 FCC units; *Chew tab:* 9,000 FCC units (vanilla twist)

LARVA MIGRANS: CUTANEOUS, VISCERAL

▷ *thiabendazole* (C) Adult and pediatric dosing schedules are the same; dosing is bid, is based on weight in pounds, and must be taken with meals.
    Cutaneous Larva Migrans: treat bid x 2 days
    Visceral Larva Migrans: treat bid x 7 days

<30 lbs: consult mfr pkg insert; 30 lbs: 250 mg bid; 50 lbs: 500 mg bid; 75 lbs: 750 mg bid; 100 lbs: 1000 mg bid; 125 lbs: 1250 mg bid; ≥150 lbs: 1500 mg bid; max 3000 mg/day.

Mintezol *Chew tab:* 500*mg (orange); *Oral susp:* 500 mg/5 ml (120 ml) (orange)

Comment: **thiabendazole** is not for prophylaxis. May impair mental alertness. May not be available in the US.

LEAD POISONING

Comment: Chelation therapy for lead poisoning requires maintenance of adequate hydration, close monitoring of renal and hepatic function, and monitoring for neutropenia; discontinue therapy at first sign of toxicity. Contraindicated with severe renal disease <u>or</u> anuria.

CHELATING AGENTS

➤ *deferoxamine mesylate* (C) initially 1 gm IM, followed by 500 mg IM every 4 hours x 2 doses; then repeat every 4-12 hours if needed; max 6 gm/day
Pediatric: <3 months: not recommended; ≥3 months: same as adult
Desferal *Vial:* 250 mg/ml after reconstitution (500 mg)

➤ *edetate calcium disodium (EDTA)* (B) administer IM <u>or</u> IV; use IM route of administration for children and overt lead encephalopathy
Pediatric: same as adult; *Serum lead level:* 20-70 mcg/dL: 1 gm/m² per day; *IV:* infuse over 8-12 hours; *IM:* divided doses q 8-12 hours; Treat for 5 days; then stop for 2-4 days; may repeat if serum lead level is ≥70 mcg/dL
Calcium Disodium Versenate *Amp:* 200 mg/ml (5 ml)

➤ *succimer* (C) may swallow caps whole <u>or</u> put contents onto a small amount of soft food <u>or</u> a spoon and swallow, followed by a fruit drink
Pediatric: <12 months: not recommended; ≥12 months: same as adult; *Serum lead level:* >45 mcg/dL: initially 10 mg/kg (<u>or</u> 350 mg/m²) every 8 hours for 5 days; then reduce frequency to every 12 hours for 14 more days; allow at least 14 days between courses unless serum lead levels indicate a need for more prompt treatment; for more than 3 consecutive weeks not recommended
Chemet *Cap:* 100 mg

LEG CRAMPS: NOCTURNAL, RECUMBENCY

➤ *quinine sulfate* (C)(G) 1 tab <u>or</u> cap q HS
Pediatric: <16 years: not recommended; ≥16 years: same as adult
Qualaquin *Tab:* 260 mg; *Cap:* 260, 300, 325 mg
Comment: If **hypokalemia** is the cause of leg cramps, treat with potassium supplementation (*see page 258*).

LEISHMANIASIS: CUTANEOUS, MUCOSAL, VISCERAL

Comment: The leishmanial parasite species addressed in this section are: **cutaneous leishmaniasis** (due to *Leishmania braziliensis, Leishmania guyanensis, Leishmania panamensis*), **mucosal leishmaniasis** (due to *Leishmania braziliensis*), and **visceral leishmaniasis** (due to *Leishmania donovani*). The weight-based treatment for adults and adolescents is the same for each of the species, the anti-leishmanial drug *miltefosone* (**Impavido**). Contraindications to this drug include pregnancy, lactation, and Sjogren-Larsson-Syndrome. The contraindication in pregnancy is due to embryo-fetal toxicity, teratogenicity, and fetal death. Obtain a serum <u>or</u> urine pregnancy test for females of reproductive potential and advise females to use effective contraception during therapy and for 5 months following treatment. Breastfeeding is contraindicated while taking this drug and for 5 months following termination of breastfeeding. Potential ASEs include loss of appetite, abdominal pain, nausea, vomiting, diarrhea, headache, dizziness, pruritis, somnolence, elevated liver transaminases, bilirubin, and serum creatinine and thrombocytopenia. *miltefosine* is associated with impaired fertility in females and males in animal studies. To report a suspected adverse reaction to this drug, call 888-550-6060 <u>or</u> the FDA at 800-FDA-1088 <u>or</u> visit www.fda.gov/medwatch.

➤ *miltefosine* (D)(G) 30-44 kg: one cap bid x 28 consecutive days; ≥45 kg: one cap tid x 28 consecutive days; take with a full meal

Pediatric: <12 years, <30 kg (60 lbs): not established; ≥12 years, ≥30 kg (≥60 lbs): same as adult

Impavido *Cap:* 50 mg

 LENNOX-GASTAUT SYNDROME (LGS)/DRAVET SYNDROME

CANNABINOID-DERIVED TREATMENT

Comment: The FDA Peripheral and Central Nervous System Drugs Advisory Committee's **Epidiolex** (*cannabidiol*) recommendation was based on three randomized, double-blind, placebo-controlled clinical trials. These trials showed a 50% reduction of drop seizure frequency in 40%-44% of patients with Lennox-Gastaut syndrome, and a 39% decrease in convulsive seizure frequency for trial participants with Dravet Syndrome. A total of 516 patients with one of the two seizure disorders participated in the clinical trials. The FDA Advisory Committee judged that CBD-OS, derived from a non-psychoactive chemical found in marijuana, was very unlikely to have potential for abuse.

▷ *cannibidiol* initially 2.5mg/kg 2 x/day (5mg/kg/day); after one week, may be increased to a maintenance dose of 5 mg/kg 2 x/day (10 mg/kg/day); max 10 mg/kg 2 x/day (20 mg/kg/day); titration based on effectiveness and tolerability; dose adjustment is recommended for patients with moderate or severe hepatic impairment.

Epidiolex *Oral soln:* 100 mg/ml (100 ml) (strawberry)

Comment: **Epidiolex** (*cannibidiol*) is indicated for the treatment of seizures associated with Lennox-Gastaut syndrome or Dravet syndrome in patients ≥2 years-of-age. Obtain serum transaminases (ALT and AST) and total bilirubin levels in all patients prior to starting treatment. Concomitant use of *valproate* and higher doses of **Epidiolex** increase the risk of transaminase elevations. Consider dose reduction of **Epidiolex** with concomitant moderate or strong inhibitors of CYP3A4 or CYP2C19. Consider dose increase of **Epidiolex** with strong inducers of CYP3A4 or CYP2C19. Consider dose reduction of substrates of UGT1A9, UGT2B7, CYP2C8, CYP2C9, and CYP2C19 (e.g., *clobazam*). Substrates of CYP1A2 and CYP2B6 may also require dose adjustment. Monitor for somnolence and sedation and advise patients not to drive or operate machinery until they have gained sufficient experience on **Epidiolex**. Monitor patients for suicidal behavior and thoughts. Advise patients to seek immediate medical care for any hypersensitivity reaction. Discontinue and do not restart **Epidiolex** if hypersensitivity occurs. **Epidiolex** should be gradually withdrawn to minimize the risk of increased seizure frequency and status epilepticus. The most common adverse reactions (incidence ≥10%) include somnolence, decreased appetite, diarrhea, transaminase elevations, fatigue, malaise, and asthenia, rash, insomnia, sleep disorder, and poor quality sleep, and infections. There are no adequate data on the developmental risks associated with the use of **Epidiolex** in pregnant females. However, animal studies have demonstrated **Epidiolex** may cause fetal harm. There are no data on the presence of *cannabidiol* or its metabolites in human milk or effects on the breastfed infant. Encourage females who take **Epidiolex** during pregnancy to enroll in the North American Antiepileptic Drug (NAAED) Pregnancy Registry by calling 1-888-233-2334 or visiting www.aedpregnancyregistry.org/. To report suspected adverse reactions, contact Greenwich Biosciences at 1-833-424-6724 (1-833-GBIOSCI) or FDA at 1-800-FDA1088 or www.fda.gov/medwatch.

OTHER ANTICONVULSANTS

▷ *clobazam* (C)(IV)(G) take with or without food; for doses above 5 mg/day, administer in two divided doses; *≤30 kg body weight:* initiate at 5 mg daily and titrate as tolerated up to 20 mg daily; *>30 kg body weight:* initiate at 10 mg daily and titrate as tolerated up to 40 mg daily; *Tablets:* administer whole, broken in half along the score line, or crushed and mixed in applesauce; *Suspension:* measure prescribed amount using provided adapter and dosing syringe; *Mild-to-Moderate Hepatic Impairment:* reduce dose or discontinue gradually; *Severe Hepatic Impairment:* no information; *Geriatric Patients and CYP2C19 poor metabolizers:* adjust dose

Pediatric: <2 years: not recommended; ≥2 years: same as adult

Onfi *Tab:* 10*, 20*mg

Onfi Oral Suspension *Oral susp:* 2.5 mg/ml (120 ml w. adapter and 2 dosing syringes) (berry)

Sympaza Oral Film *Oral film:* 5, 10, 20 mg single-dose (60/pkg) (berry)

Comment: *clobazam* is a benzodiazepine indicated for adjunctive treatment of seizures associated with Lennox-Gastaut syndrome (LGS) in patients ≥2 years-of-age. Monitor for central nervous system (CNS) depression (somnolence, sedation), caution with concomitant CNS depressants, avoid rapid dose reduction or discontinuation. Monitor for potential Stevens-Johnson syndrome and toxic epidermal necrolysis. Discontinue *clobazam* at first sign of rash unless the rash is clearly not drug-related. Monitor patients with a history of substance abuse for signs of habituation and dependence. Monitor for suicidal thoughts or behaviors. Adverse reactions which have occurred (incidence ≥ 10%) with any *clobazam* dose included constipation, somnolence or sedation, pyrexia, lethargy, and drooling. *clobazam* is excreted in human milk. Breastfed infants of mothers taking benzodiazepines, such as *clobazam*, may have effects of lethargy, somnolence and poor sucking. *clobazam* is excreted in human milk. Breastfed infants of mothers taking benzodiazepines, such as *clobazam*, may have effects of lethargy, somnolence and poor sucking. There is insufficient evidence to assess the effect of benzodiazepine pregnancy exposure on neurodevelopment. Prescribers are advised to recommend pregnant patients taking **Onfi** or **Sympaza** self-enroll in the North American Antiepileptic Drug (NAAED) Pregnancy Registry by calling 1-888-233-2334 or visiting www.aedpregnancyregistry.org

▷ *stiripentol* 50 mg/kg/day in 2 or 3 divided doses; reduce dose or discontinue dose gradually; capsules must be swallowed whole with a glass of water during a meal; do not break or open capsules; mix contents of one packet in a glass of water and take immediately after mixing during a meal

Pediatric: <2 years: not recommended; ≥2 years: same as adult

Diacomit *Cap:* 250, 500 mg; *Pwdr for Oral Susp:* 250, 500 mg (60 pkts/carton)(fruit)

Comment: **Diacomit** is indicated for the treatment of seizures associated with Dravet syndrome in patients ≥2 years-of-age taking *clobazam*. There are no clinical data to support the use of **Diacomit** as monotherapy in Dravet syndrome.

 LENTIGINES: BENIGN, SENILE

Comment: Wash affected area with a soap-free cleanser; pat dry and wait 20-30 minutes; then apply agent sparingly to affected area; use only once daily in PM. Avoid eyes, ears, nostrils, mouth, and healthy skin. Avoid sun exposure. Cautious use of concomitant astringents, alcohol-based products, sulfur-containing products, salicylic acid-containing products, soap, and other topical agents.

TOPICAL RETINOIDS

▷ *tazarotene* (X)(G) apply daily at HS
Pediatric: <12 years: not recommended; ≥12 years: same as adult
Avage Cream *Crm:* 0.1% (30 gm)
Tazorac Cream *Crm:* 0.05, 0.1% (15, 30, 60 gm)
Tazorac Gel *Gel:* 0.05, 0.1% (30, 100 gm)

▷ *tretinoin* (C)(G) apply daily at HS
Pediatric: <12 years: not recommended; ≥12 years: same as adult
Avita *Crm:* 0.025% (20, 45 gm); *Gel:* 0.025% (20, 45 gm)
Renova *Crm:* 0.02% (40 gm); 0.05% (40, 60 gm)
Retin-A Cream *Crm:* 0.025, 0.05, 0.1% (20, 45 gm)
Retin-A Gel *Gel:* 0.01, 0.025% (15, 45 gm) (alcohol 90%)
Retin-A Liquid *Liq:* 0.05% (28 ml; alcohol 55%)
Retin-A Micro *Microspheres:* 0.04, 0.1% (20, 45 gm)
Retin-A Micro Gel *Gel:* 0.04, 0.1% (20, 45 gm)

 LISTERIOSIS *(LISTERIA MONOCYTOGENES)*

Comment: *L. monocytogenes* is a potentially lethal foodborne pathogen that is a common contaminant of food and food preparation equipment, and has been isolated in soil, farm environments, produce, raw foods, dairy products, and the feces of asymptomatic people. IV *ampicillin* is the mainstay of treatment, but penicillin may be as effective. Some experts recommend combination antibiotic therapy for neuro-invasive *L. monocytogenes*. The most common antimicrobial combination is IV *ampicillin* and IV *gentamycin* (which is usually discontinued when the patient shows signs of improvement to limit the potential for toxicity). If the patient is penicillin-allergic, IV *trimethoprim-sulfamethoxazole* (TMP-SMX) as mono therapy x 28 days. Patients with bacteremia but without CNS involvement may be treated with combination (*ampicillin+gentamycin*) therapy for 14 days, but patients with meningitis require a full 21 day combination course of antibiotics. Endocarditis, encephalitis, and brain abscesses may require a longer duration of high dose antimicrobials. Cephalosporins are ineffective. Supportive care and standard isolation precautions are required.

REFERENCES

Kasper, D. L., & Fauci, A. S. (2017). Listeria monocytogenes infections. In: *Harrison's Infectious Diseases (3rd ed.).* New York: McGraw Hill Education.

McNeill, C., Sisson, W., & Jarrett, A. (2017). Listeriosis: A resurfacing menace. *The Journal for Nurse Practitioners, 13*(10), 647–654. doi:10.1016/j.nurpra.2017.09.014

▶ *ampicillin* **(B)(G)** 2 gm IV infusion q 4 hours (in combination with IV gentamycin q 8 hours)
  Pediatric: 50-100 mg/kg (max 3 gm) IV infusion q 6 hours
    Unasyn *Vial:* 1.5, 3 gm
▶ *gentamicin* **(C)(G)** 1-2 mg/kg q 8 hours (in combination with IV ampicillin q 4 hours; monitor plasma levels; dilution not less than 1 mg/ml in D5W or NS; administer dose over 30 min-2 hours
  Pediatric: 2 mg/kg/dose q 8 hours; monitor plasma levels; dilution not less than 1 mg/ml in D5W or NS; administer dose over 30 min-2 hours
    Geramycin *Vial:* 20, 80 mg/2 ml (2 ml) for dilution (not less than 1 mg/ml) and IV infusion (over 30 min-2 hours
▶ *penicillin g potassium* **(B)(G)** 4 million units via IV infusion q 4 hours
  Pediatric: 65,000 units/kg/dose via IV infusion q 4 hours; max 4 million units/dose; infuse dose over 1-2 hours
    Vial: 5, 20 MU pwdr for reconstitution (in D5W or NS) and IV infusion; *Pre-mixed bag:* 1, 2, 3 MU (50 ml); infuse dose over 1-2 hours
▶ *trimethoprim-sulfamethoxazole (TMP-SMX)* **(C)(G)** TMP 5 mg/kg IV infusion q 6 hours; max TMP 160 mg/dose
  Pediatric: <2 months: contraindicated: ≥2 months: 2-5 mg/kg/dose q 8 hours; max TMP 160 mg/dose
  Comment: Sulfonamides are contraindicated in the first trimester of pregnancy, the final month of pregnancy, and infants <8 weeks-of-age. *CrCl 15-30 mL/min:* reduce dose by 1/2; *CrCl <15 mL/min:* not recommended. Contra-indicated with G6PD deficiency. A high fluid intake is indicated during sulfonamide therapy to avoid crystallization in the kidneys.

LIVER FLUKES

TREMATODICIDE

Comment: *praziquantel* is a trematodicide indicated for the treatment of infections due to all species of Schistosoma (e.g., *Schistosoma mekongi, Schistosoma japonicum, Schistosoma mansoni,* and *Schistosoma hematobium*) and infections due to liver flukes (i.e., *Clonorchis sinensis, Opisthorchis viverrini*). *praziquantel* induces a rapid contraction of schistosomes by a specific effect on the permeability of the cell membrane. The drug further causes vacuolization and disintegration of the schistosome tegument.

▶ *praziquantel* **(B)** 25 mg/kg tid as a one-day treatment; take the 3 doses at intervals of not less than 4 hours and not more than 6 hours; swallow whole with water during meals; holding the tablets in the mouth leaves a bitter taste which can trigger gagging or vomiting.
  Pediatric: <4 years: not established; >4 years: same as adult
    Biltricide *Tab:* 600mg*** film-coat (3 scores, 4 segments, 150 mg/segment)
  Comment: Concomitant administration with strong Cytochrome P450 (P450) inducers, such as *rifampin*, is contraindicated since therapeutically effective blood levels of *praziquantel* may not be achieved. In patients receiving *rifampin* who need immediate treatment for schistosomiasis, alternative agents for schistosomiasis should be considered. However, if treatment with *praziquantel* is necessary, *rifampin* should be discontinued 4 weeks before administration of *praziquantel*. Treatment with *rifampin* can then be restarted one day after completion of *praziquantel* treatment. Concomitant administration

of other P450 inducers (e.g., antiepileptic drugs such as *phenytoin, phenobarbital, carbamazepine*) and *dexamethasone*, may also reduce plasma levels of *praziquantel*. Concomitant administration of P450 inhibitors (e.g., *cimetidine, ketoconazole, itraconazole, erythromycin*) may increase plasma levels of *praziquantel*. Patients should be warned not to drive a car or operate machinery on the day of **Biltricide** treatment and the following day. There are no adequate or well-controlled studies in pregnant women. This drug should be used during pregnancy only if clearly needed. *praziquantel* appears in the milk of nursing women at a concentration of about 1/4 that of maternal serum. It is not known whether a pharmacological effect is likely to occur in children. Women should not nurse on the day of **Biltricide** treatment and during the subsequent 72 hours.

LOW BACK STRAIN (LBS)

Acetaminophen for IV Infusion *see Pain page* 352
NSAIDs *see page* 571
Opioid Analgesics *see Pain page* 354
Topical & Transdermal Analgesics *see Pain page* 352
Muscle Relaxants *see page* 311
Parenteral Corticosteroids *see page* 577
Oral Corticosteroids *see page* 577
Topical Analgesic and Anesthetic Agents *see page* 569

LOW LIBIDO, HYPOACTIVE SEXUAL DESIRE DISORDER (HSDD)

5-HT1A AGONIST/5-HT2A

➤ *flibanserin* 1 tab once daily at bedtime; discontinue if no improvement in 8 weeks
  Pediatric: <18 years: not recommended; ≥18 years: same as adult
    Addyi *Tab:* 100 mg
    Comment: **Addyi** is for use in premenopausal women. **Addyi** is not for use in men, postmenopausal women, and is not recommended in pregnancy, or lactation. Potential ASEs include dry mouth, nausea, hypotension, dizziness, syncope, fatigue, somnolence, and insomnia.

LYME DISEASE (*ERYTHEMA CHRONICUM MIGRANS*)

Comment: The bite of the deer tick (*Ioxodes scapularis*) carries the *Borrelia burgdorferi* organism causing Lyme disease. Proper removal of the tick, and early diagnosis and treatment are essential to effective management of this disease.

STAGE 1

➤ *amoxicillin* (B)(G) 500-875 mg bid or 250-500 mg tid x 10 days
  Pediatric: <40 kg (88 lb): 20-40 mg/kg/day in 3 divided doses x 10 days or 25-45 mg/kg/day in 2 divided doses x 10 days; ≥40 kg: same as adult; *see page* 617 *for dose by weight*
    Amoxil *Cap:* 250, 500 mg; *Tab:* 875*mg; *Chew tab:* 125, 200, 250, 400 mg (cherry-banana-peppermint) (phenylalanine); *Oral susp:* 125, 250 mg/5 ml (80, 100, 150 ml) (strawberry); 200, 400 mg/5 ml (50, 75, 100 ml) (bubble gum); *Oral drops:* 50 mg/ml (30 ml) (bubble gum)
    Moxatag *Tab:* 775 mg ext-rel
    Trimox *Tab:* 125, 250 mg; *Cap:* 250, 500 mg; *Oral susp:* 125, 250 mg/5 ml (80, 100, 150 ml) (raspberry-strawberry)
➤ *clarithromycin* (C)(G) 500 mg bid or 500 mg ext-rel once daily x 14-21 days
  Pediatric: <6 months: not recommended; ≥6 months: 7.5 mg/kg bid x 7 days; *see page* 624 *for dose by weight*
    Biaxin *Tab:* 250, 500 mg
    Biaxin Oral Suspension *Oral susp:* 125, 250 mg/5 ml (50, 100 ml)
    Biaxin XL *Tab:* 500 mg ext-rel
    Comment: The FDA is advising caution before prescribing *clarithromycin* to patients with heart disease because of a potential increased risk of heart problems or death that can occur years later. This recommendation is based on a review of the results of a 10-year follow-up

study of patients with coronary heart disease from a large clinical trial that first observed this safety issue. Consider risk benefit and the use of other antibiotics in such patients.

➤ *doxycycline* (D)(G) 100 mg bid x 14-21 days
Pediatric: <8 years: not recommended; ≥8 years, ≤100 lb: 2 mg/lb on first day in 2 divided doses, followed by 1 mg/lb/day in 1-2 divided doses; ≥8 years, >100 lb: same as adult; *see page 625 for dose by weight*

> Acticlate *Tab:* 75, 150**mg
> Adoxa *Tab:* 50, 75, 100, 150 mg ent-coat
> Doryx *Tab:* 50, 75, 100, 150, 200 mg del-rel
> Doxteric *Tab:* 50 mg del-rel
> Monodox *Cap:* 50, 75, 100 mg
> Oracea *Cap:* 40 mg del-rel
> Vibramycin *Tab:* 100 mg; *Cap:* 50, 100 mg; *Syr:* 50 mg/5 ml (raspberry-apple) (sulfites); *Oral susp:* 25 mg/5 ml (raspberry)
> Vibra-Tab *Tab:* 100 mg film-coat

Comment: *doxycycline* is contraindicated <8 years-of-age, in pregnancy, and lactation (discolors developing tooth enamel). A side effect may be photosensitivity (photophobia). Do <u>not</u> take with antacids, calcium supplements, milk or other dairy, or within 2 hours of taking another drug.

➤ *minocycline* (D)(G) 200 mg on first day; then 100 mg q 12 hours x 9 more days
Pediatric: ≤8 years: not recommended; ≥8 years, <100 lb: 2 mg/lb on first day in 2 divided doses, followed by 1 mg/lb q 12 hours x 9 more days; ≥8 years, >100 lb: same as adult

> Dynacin *Cap:* 50, 100 mg
> Minocin *Cap:* 50, 75, 100 mg; *Oral susp:* 50 mg/5 ml (60 ml) (custard) (sulfites, alcohol 5%)

Comment: *minocycline* is contraindicated <8 years-of-age, in pregnancy, and lactation (discolors developing tooth enamel). A side effect may be photo-sensitivity (photophobia). Do <u>not</u> take with antacids, calcium supplements, milk or other dairy, or within two hours of taking another drug.

➤ *tetracycline* (D)(G) 250-500 mg qid ac x 21 days
Pediatric: <8 years: not recommended; ≥8 years, ≤100 lb: 25-50 mg/kg/day in 2-4 divided doses x 7 days; ≥8 years, >100 lb: same as adult; *see page 630 for dose by weight*

> Achromycin V *Cap:* 250, 500 mg
> Sumycin *Tab:* 250, 500 mg; *Cap:* 250, 500 mg; *Oral susp:* 125 mg/5 ml (100, 200 ml) (fruit) (sulfites)

Comment: *tetracycline* is contraindicated <8 years-of-age, in pregnancy, and lactation (discolors developing tooth enamel). A side effect may be photo-sensitivity (photophobia). Do <u>not</u> take with antacids, calcium supplements, milk or other dairy, or within two hours of taking another drug.

⬤ LYMPHADENITIS

Comment: Therapy should continue for no less than 5 days after resolution of symptoms.

➤ *amoxicillin+clavulanate* (B)(G)

> Augmentin 500 mg tid <u>or</u> 875 mg bid x 7-10 days
> *Pediatric:* 40-45 mg/kg/day divided tid x 10 days <u>or</u> 90 mg/kg/day divided bid x 10 days *see pages 618 for dose by weight*
> *Tab:* 250, 500, 875 mg; *Chew tab:* 125, 250 mg (lemon-lime); 200, 400 mg (cherry-banana) (phenylalanine); *Oral susp:* 125 mg/5 ml (banana), 250 mg/5 ml (75, 100, 150 ml) (orange); 200, 400 mg/5 ml (50, 75, 100 ml) (orange) (phenylalanine)
> Augmentin ES-600 not recommended for adults
> *Pediatric:* <3 months: not recommended; ≥3 months, <40 kg: 90 mg/kg/day in 2 divided doses x 7-10 days; ≥40 kg: not recommended
> *Oral susp:* 42.9 mg/5 ml (50, 75, 100, 125, 150, 200 ml) (strawberry cream) (phenylalanine)
> Augmentin XR 2 tabs q 12 hours x 7-10 days
> *Pediatric:* <16 years: use other forms; ≥16 years: same as adult
> *Tab:* 1000*mg ext-rel

➤ *cephalexin* (B)(G) 500 mg bid x 10 days
Pediatric: 25-50 mg/kg/day in 4 divided doses x 10 days; *see page 623 for dose by weight*

Keflex *Cap:* 250, 333, 500, 750 mg; *Oral susp:* 125, 250 mg/5 ml (100, 200 ml) (strawberry)
▷ **dicloxacillin** (B) 500 mg qid x 10 days
  Pediatric: 12.5-25 mg/kg/day in 4 divided doses x 10 days; *see page 624 for dose by weight*
    Dynapen *Cap:* 125, 250, 500 mg; *Oral susp:* 62.5 mg/5 ml (80, 100, 200 ml)

 LYMPHOGRANULOMA VENEREUM

Comment: The following treatment regimens are published in the **2015 CDC Sexually Transmitted Diseases Treatment Guidelines**. This section contains treatment regimens for adults only; consult a specialist for treatment of patients less than 18 years of age. Treatment regimens are presented in alphabetical order by generic drug name, followed by brands and dose forms. Treat all sexual contacts. Persons with both LGV and HIV infection should receive the same treatment regimens as those who are HIV-negative; however, prolonged treatment may be required and delay in resolution of symptoms may occur.

RECOMMENDED REGIMEN
Regimen 1
▷ **doxycycline** 100 mg bid x 21 days

ALTERNATIVE REGIMEN
Regimen 1
▷ **erythromycin base** 500 mg qid x 21 days *or* **erythromycin ethylsuccinate** 400 mg qid x 21 days

RECOMMENDED REGIMENS FOR THE MANAGEMENT OF SEXUAL CONTACTS
Comment: LGV is caused by *C. trachomatis* serovars L1, L2, *or* L3. Persons who have had sexual contact with a patient who has LGV within 60 days before onset of the patient's symptoms should be examined, tested for urethral *or* cervical chlamydial infection, and treated with a chlamydia regimen.

Regimen 1
▷ **azithromycin** 1 gm in a single dose

Regimen 2
▷ **doxycycline** 100 mg bid x 7 days

DRUG BRANDS AND DOSE FORMS
▷ **azithromycin** (B)(G)
    Zithromax *Tab:* 250, 500, 600 mg; *Oral susp:* 100 mg/5 ml (15 ml); 200 mg/5 ml (15, 22.5, 30 ml) (cherry); *Pkt:* 1 gm for reconstitution (cherry-banana)
    Zithromax Tri-pak *Tab:* 3 x 500 mg tabs/pck
    Zithromax Z-pak *Tab:* 6 x 250 mg tabs/pck
    Zmax *Oral susp:* 2 gm ext-rel for reconstitution (cherry-banana) (148 mg Na$^+$)
▷ **doxycycline** (D)(G)
    Acticlate *Tab:* 75, 150**mg
    Adoxa *Tab:* 50, 75, 100, 150 mg ent-coat
    Doryx *Tab:* 50, 75, 100, 150, 200 mg del-rel
    Doxteric *Tab:* 50 mg del-rel
    Monodox *Cap:* 50, 75, 100 mg
    Oracea *Cap:* 40 mg del-rel
    Vibramycin *Tab:* 100 mg; *Cap:* 50, 100 mg; *Syr:* 50 mg/5 ml (raspberry-apple) (sulfites); *Oral susp:* 25 mg/5 ml (raspberry)
    Vibra-Tab *Tab:* 100 mg film-coat
Comment: *doxycycline* is contraindicated <8 years-of-age, in pregnancy, and lactation (discolors developing tooth enamel). A side effect may be photo-sensitivity (photophobia). Do <u>not</u> take with antacids, calcium supplements, milk or other dairy, or within 2 hours of taking another drug.

▷ *erythromycin base* (B)(G)

> **Ery-Tab** *Tab:* 250, 333, 500 mg ent-coat
> **PCE** *Tab:* 333, 500 mg

Comment: *erythromycin* may increase INR with concomitant *warfarin*, as well as increase serum level of *digoxin*, benzodiazepines, and statins.

▷ *erythromycin ethylsuccinate* (B)(G)

> **EryPed** *Oral susp:* 200 mg/5 ml (100, 200 ml) (fruit); 400 mg/5 ml (60, 100, 200 ml) (banana); *Oral drops:* 200, 400 mg/5 ml (50 ml) (fruit); *Chew tab:* 200 mg wafer (fruit)
> **E.E.S.** *Oral susp:* 200, 400 mg/5 ml (100 ml) (fruit)
> **E.E.S. Granules** *Oral susp:* 200 mg/5 ml (100, 200 ml) (cherry)
> **E.E.S. 400 Tablets** *Tab:* 400 mg

Comment: *erythromycin* may increase INR with concomitant *warfarin*, as well as increase serum level of *digoxin*, benzodiazepines, and statins.

MALARIA (*PLASMODIUM FALCIPARUM, PLASMODIUM VIVAX*)

▷ *doxycycline* (D)(G) 100 mg daily; initiate 1-2 days prior to travel; take during travel; continue for 4 weeks after leaving the endemic area
Pediatric: ≤8 years: not recommended; ≥8 years, ≤100 lb: 1 mg/lb/day prior to travel; take during travel; continue for 4 weeks after leaving the endemic area; ≥8 years, ≥100 lb: same as adult; *see page 625 for dose by weight*

> **Acticlate** *Tab:* 75, 150**mg
> **Adoxa** *Tab:* 50, 75, 100, 150 mg ent-coat
> **Doryx** *Tab:* 50, 75, 100, 150, 200 mg del-rel
> **Doxteric** *Tab:* 50 mg del-rel
> **Monodox** *Cap:* 50, 75, 100 mg
> **Oracea** *Cap:* 40 mg del-rel
> **Vibramycin** *Tab:* 100 mg; *Cap:* 50, 100 mg; *Syr:* 50 mg/5 ml (raspberry-apple) (sulfites); *Oral susp:* 25 mg/5 ml (raspberry)
> **Vibra-Tab** *Tab:* 100 mg film-coat

Comment: *doxycycline* is contraindicated <8 years-of-age, in pregnancy, and lactation (discolors developing tooth enamel). A side effect may be photosensitivity (photophobia). Do not take with antacids, calcium supplements, milk or other dairy, or within 2 hours of taking another drug.

▷ *minocycline* (D)(G) 100 mg daily; initiate 1-2 days prior to travel; take during travel; continue for 4 weeks after leaving the endemic area
Pediatric: <8 years: not recommended; ≥8 years, ≤100 lb: 2 mg/lb on first day in 2 divided doses, followed by 1 mg/lb q 12 hours x 9 more days; ≥8 years, >100 lb: same as adult

> **Dynacin** *Cap:* 50, 100 mg
> **Minocin** *Cap:* 50, 75, 100 mg; *Oral susp:* 50 mg/5 ml (60 ml) (custard) (sulfites, alcohol 5%)

Comment: *minocycline* is contraindicated <8 years-of-age, in pregnancy, and lactation (discolors developing tooth enamel). A side effect may be photosensitivity (photophobia). Do not take with antacids, calcium supplements, milk or other dairy, or within 2 hours of taking another drug.

▷ *tetracycline* (D) 250 mg daily; initiate 1-2 days prior to travel; take during travel; continue for 4 weeks after leaving the endemic area
Pediatric: <8 years: not recommended; ≥8 years, ≤100 lb: 25-50 mg/kg/day in 4 divided doses x 10 days; ≥8 years, >100 lb: same as adult; *see page 630 for dose by weight*

> **Achromycin V** *Cap:* 250, 500 mg
> **Sumycin** *Tab:* 250, 500 mg; *Cap:* 250, 500 mg; *Oral susp:* 125 mg/5 ml (100, 200 ml) (fruit) (sulfites)

Comment: *tetracycline* is contraindicated <8 years-of-age, in pregnancy, and lactation (discolors developing tooth enamel). A side effect may be photosensitivity (photophobia). Do not take with antacids, calcium supplements, milk or other dairy, or within 2 hours of taking another drug.

ANTIMALARIALS

▷ *atovaquone* (C)(G) take as a single dose with food or a milky drink at the same time each day; repeat dose if vomited within 1 hour; *Prophylaxis:* 1,500 mg once daily; *Treatment:* 750 mg bid x 21 days

> **Mepron** *Susp:* 750 mg/5 ml

▷ *atovaquone+proguanil* (C)(G) take as a single dose with food <u>or</u> a milky drink at the same time each day; repeat dose if vomited within 1 hour; *Prophylaxis:* 1 tab daily starting 1-2 days before entering endemic area, during stay, and for 7 days after return; *Treatment (acute, uncomplicated):* 4 tabs daily x 3 days
Pediatric: <5 kg: not recommended; 5-40 kg:
Prophylaxis: daily dose starting 1-2 days before entering endemic area, during stay, and for 7 days after return; 5-20 kg: 1 ped tab; 21-30 kg: 2 ped tabs; 31-40 kg: 3 ped tabs; ≥40 kg: same as adult; *Treatment (acute, uncomplicated):* daily dose x 3 days; 5-8 kg: 2 ped tabs; 9-10 kg: 3 ped tabs; 11-20 kg: 1 adult tab; 21-30 kg: 2 adult tabs; 31-40 kg: 3 adult tabs; >40 kg: same as adult
    Malarone *Tab:* atov 250 mg+prog 100 mg
    Malarone Pediatric *Tab:* atov 62.5 mg+prog 25 mg
  Comment: *atovaquone* is antagonized by *tetracycline* and *metoclopramide*. Concomitant *rifampin* is not recommended (may elevate LFTs).

▷ *chloroquine* (C)(G) *Prophylaxis:* 500 mg once weekly (on the same day of each week); start 2 weeks prior to exposure, continue while in the endemic area, and continue 4 weeks after departure; *Treatment:* initially 1 gm; then 500 mg 6 hours, 24 hours, and 48 hours after initial dose <u>or</u> initially 200-250 mg IM; may repeat in 6 hours; max 1 gm in first 24 hours; continue to 1.875 gm in 3 days
Pediatric: Suppression: 8.35 mg/kg (max 500 mg) weekly (on the same day of each week); *Treatment:* initially 16.7 mg/kg (max 1 gm); then 8.35 mg/kg (max 500 mg) 6 hours, 24 hours, and 48 hours after initial dose, <u>or</u> initially 6.25 mg/kg IM; may repeat in 6 hours; max 12.5 mg/kg/day
    Aralen *Tab:* 500 mg; *Amp:* 50 mg/ml (5 ml)

▷ *hydroxychloroquine* (C)(G) *Prophylaxis:* 400 mg once weekly (on the same day of each week); start 2 weeks prior to exposure, continue while in the endemic area, and continue 8 weeks after departure; *Treatment:* initially 800 mg; then 400 mg 6 hours, 24 hours, and 48 hours after initial dose
Pediatric: Suppression: 6.45 mg/kg (max 400 mg) weekly (on the same day of each week) beginning 2 weeks prior to arrival, continuing while in endemic area, and continuing 4 weeks after departure; *Treatment:* initially 12.9 mg/kg (max 800 mg); then 6.45 mg/kg (max 400 mg) 6 hours, 24 hours, and 48 hours after initial dose hours after initial dose
    Plaquenil *Tab:* 200 mg

▷ *mefloquine* (C) *Prophylaxis:* 250 mg once weekly (on the same day of each week); start 1 week prior to exposure, continue while in the endemic area, and continue for 4 weeks after departure; *Treatment:* 1,250 mg as a single dose
Pediatric: <6 months: not recommended; *Prophylaxis:* ≥6 months: 3-5 mg/kg (max 250 mg) weekly (on the same day of each week); start 1 week prior to exposure, continue while in the endemic area, and continue for 4 weeks after departure; *Treatment:* ≥6 months: 25-50 mg/kg as a single dose; max 250 mg
    Lariam *Tab:* 250*mg
  Comment: *mefloquine* is contraindicated with active <u>or</u> recent history of depression, generalized anxiety disorder, psychosis, schizophrenia <u>or</u> any other psychiatric disorder <u>or</u> history of convulsions.

▷ *quinine sulfate* (C)(G) 1 tab <u>or</u> cap every 8 hours x 7 days
Pediatric: <16 years: not recommended; ≥16 years: same as adult
    Tab: 260 mg; *Cap:* 260, 300, 325 mg
    Qualaquin *Cap:* 324 mg
  Comment: **Qualaquin** is indicated in the treatment of uncomplicated *P. falciparum* malaria (including chloroquine-resistant strains).

▷ *tafenoquine* (C)(G) *Loading Regimen:* take 200 mg (2 x 100 mg tabs) once daily x 3 days before travel to endemic area; *Maintenance:* take 200 mg (2 x 100 mg tabs) once weekly beginning 7 days after the last loading regimen dose; maintenance dose may be continued for up to 6 months; take with food
Pediatric: <18 years: not recommended; ≥18 years: same as adult
    Arakoda *Tab:* 100 mg
  Comment: **Arakoda** *(tafenoquine)* is an 8-aminoquinoline antimalarial drug indicated for the prophylaxis of malaria. **Arakoda** provides effective protection against both of the major types of malaria (*P. vivax* and *P. falciparum*), killing the parasites in both the blood and liver. **Arakoda** is <u>not</u> recommended for with a history of psychosis or current psychotic symptoms. **Arakoda** is not recommended for patients with G6PD deficiency

or unknown G6PD status. Because **Arakoda** may cause fetal harm when administered to a pregnant female with a G6PD-deficient fetus, **Arakoda** is not recommended during pregnancy, breastfeeding when the infant is found to be G6PD deficient or if G6PD status is unknown and during treatment and for 3 months after the last dose of **Arakoda**. All patients must be tested for glucose-6-phosphate dehydrogenase (G6PD) deficiency prior to prescribing **Arakoda** and pregnancy testing is recommended for females of reproductive potential prior to initiating treatment. Due to the long half-life of **Arakoda** (approximately 17 days), psychiatric effects, hemolytic anemia, methemoglobinemia, and hypersensitivity reactions may be delayed in onset and/or duration. Avoid co-administration with drugs that are substrates of organic cation transporter-2 (OCT2) or multidrug and toxin extrusion (MATE) transporters. The most common adverse reactions (incidence ≥1%) have been headache, dizziness, back pain, diarrhea, nausea, vomiting, increased alanine, aminotransferase (ALT), motion sickness, insomnia, depression, abnormal dreams, and anxiety. To report suspected adverse reactions, contact 60 Degrees Pharmaceuticals at 1-888-834-0225 or FDA at 1-800-FDA-1088 or www.fda.gov/medwatch.

RADICAL CURE (PREVENTION OF RELAPSE)
8-AMINOQUINOLINE DERIVATIVE
▷ *tafenoquine* take 300 mg (2 x 150 mg tabs) as a single dose with food; co-administer on the first or second day of the appropriate antimalarial therapy for acute *P. vivax* malaria
Pediatric: <16 years: not recommended; ≥16 years: same as adult
Krintafel *Tab:* 150 mg
Comment: **Krintafel** *(tafenoquine)* is an 8-aminoquinoline derivative antimalarial for the radical cure (prevention of relapse) of *Plasmodium vivax* malaria in patients who are receiving appropriate antimalarial therapy for acute *P. vivax* infection. **Krintafel** is not indicated for the treatment of acute *P. vivax* malaria. Contraindications are glucose-6-phosphate dehydrogenase (G6PD) deficiency or unknown G6PD status and breastfeeding by a lactating woman when the infant is found to be G6PD deficient or if G6PD status is unknown (due to the risk of hemolytic anemia in patients with G6PD deficiency). All patients must be tested for G6PD deficiency prior to prescribing **Krintafel** and pregnancy testing is recommended for females of reproductive potential prior to initiating treatment with **Krintafel**. Also, the G6PD-deficient infant may be at risk for hemolytic anemia from exposure to **Krintafel** through breast milk; check infant's G6PD status before breastfeeding begins. Asymptomatic elevations in blood methemoglobin have been observed; initiate appropriate therapy if signs or symptoms of methemoglobinemia occur. Serious psychiatric adverse reactions have been observed in patients with a previous history of psychiatric conditions at doses higher than the approved dose. Therefore, benefit of treatment with **Krintafel** must be weighed against the potential risk for psychiatric adverse reactions in patients with a history of psychiatric illness. Due to the long half-life of **Krintafel** (15 days), psychiatric effects and hypersensitivity reactions may be delayed in onset and/or duration. Common adverse reactions (incidence ≥5%) have been dizziness, nausea, vomiting, headache, and decreased hemoglobin. To report suspected adverse reactions, contact GlaxoSmithKline at 1-888-825-5249 or FDA at 1-800-FDA-1088 or www.fda.gov/medwatch.

◯ MASTITIS (BREAST ABSCESS)

ANTI-INFECTIVES
▷ *amoxicillin+clavulanate* (B)(G)
Augmentin 500 mg tid or 875 mg bid x 7-10 days
Pediatric: 40-45 mg/kg/day divided tid x 10 days or 90 mg/kg/day divided bid x 10 days
see pages 618 for dose by weight
Tab: 250, 500, 875 mg; *Chew tab:* 125, 250 mg (lemon-lime); 200, 400 mg (cherry-banana) (phenylalanine); *Oral susp:* 125 mg/5 ml (banana), 250 mg/5 ml (75, 100, 150 ml) (orange); 200, 400 mg/5 ml (50, 75, 100 ml) (orange) (phenylalanine)
Augmentin ES-600 not recommended for adults
Pediatric: <3 months: not recommended; ≥3 months, <40 kg: 90 mg/kg/day in 2 divided doses x 7-10 days; ≥40 kg: not recommended

Oral susp: 42.9 mg/5 ml (50, 75, 100, 125, 150, 200 ml) (strawberry cream) (phenyl-alanine)

Augmentin XR 2 tabs q 12 hours x 7-10 days
Pediatric: <16 years: use other forms; ≥16 years: same as adult
Tab: 1000*mg ext-rel

▷ *cefaclor* (B)(G) 250-500 mg q 8 hours x 10 days; max 2 gm/day
Pediatric: <1 month: not recommended; 20-40 mg/kg bid or q 12 hours x 10 days; max 1 gm/day; *see page 620 for dose by weight*
Tab: 500 mg; *Cap:* 250, 500 mg; *Susp:* 125 mg/5 ml (75, 150 ml) (strawberry); 187 mg/5 ml (50, 100 ml) (strawberry); 250 mg/5 ml (75, 150 ml) (strawberry); 375 mg/5 ml (50, 100 ml) (strawberry)
Pediatric: <16 years: ext-rel not recommended; ≥12 years: same as adult
Cefaclor Extended Release *Tab:* 375, 500 mg ext-rel

▷ *ceftriaxone* (B)(G) 1-2 gm IM daily continued 2 days after signs of infection have disap-peared; max 4 gm/day
Pediatric: 50 mg/kg IM daily continued 2 days after signs of infection have disappeared
Rocephin *Vial:* 250, 500 mg; 1, 2 gm

▷ *cephalexin* (B)(G) 500 mg bid x 10 days
Pediatric: 25-50 mg/kg/day in 4 divided doses x 10 days; *see page 623 for dose by weight*
Keflex *Cap:* 250, 333, 500, 750 mg; *Oral susp:* 125, 250 mg/5 ml (100, 200 ml) (straw-berry)

▷ *clindamycin* (B)(G) 300 mg tid x 10 days
Pediatric: <12 years: not recommended; ≥12 years: same as adult
Cleocin *Cap:* 75 (tartrazine), 150 (tartrazine), 300 mg
Cleocin Pediatric Granules *Oral susp:* 75 mg/5 ml (100 ml) (cherry)

▷ *erythromycin base* (B)(G) 250-500 mg qid x 10 days
Pediatric: <45 kg: 30-40 mg/kg/day in 4 divided doses x 10 days; ≥45 kg: same as adult
Ery-Tab *Tab:* 250, 333, 500 mg ent-coat
PCE *Tab:* 333, 500 mg

Comment: *erythromycin* may increase INR with concomitant *warfarin*, as well as increase serum level of *digoxin,* benzodiazepines, and statins.

MELASMA/CHLOASMA

SKIN DEPIGMENTING AGENTS

▷ *hydroquinone* (C) apply a thin film to clean dry affected areas bid; discontinue if lightening does not occur after 2 months
Pediatric: <12 years: not recommended; ≥12 years: same as adult
Lustra *Crm:* hydro 4% (1, 2 oz) (sulfites)
Lustra AF *Crm:* hydro 4% (1, 2 oz) (sunscreens, sulfites)

▷ *hydroquinone+fluocinolone acetonide+tretinoin* (C) apply a thin film to clean dry affected areas once daily at least 30 minutes before bedtime
Pediatric: <12 years: not recommended; ≥12 years: same as adult
Tri-Luma *Crm:* hydro 4%+fluo acet 0.01%+tret 0.05% (30 gm) (sulfites, parabens)

MÉNIÈRE'S DISEASE

▷ *diazepam* (D)(IV)(G) initially 1-2.5 mg tid-qid; may increase gradually
Pediatric: <6 months: not recommended; ≥6 months: same as adult
Diastat *Rectal gel delivery system:* 2.5 mg
Diastat AcuDial *Rectal gel delivery system:* 10, 20 mg
Valium *Tab:* 2*, 5*, 10*mg
Valium Intensol Oral Solution *Conc oral soln:* 5 mg/ml (30 ml w. dropper) (alcohol 19%)
Valium Oral Solution *Oral soln:* 5 mg/5 ml (500 ml) (wintergreen-spice)

▷ *dimenhydrinate* (B) 50 mg q 4-6 hours
Pediatric: <2 years: not recommended; 2-6 years: 12.5-25 mg q 6-8 hours; max 75 mg/day; >6-11 years: 25-50 mg q 6-8 hours; max 150 mg/day; >11 years: same as adult
Dramamine (OTC) *Tab:* 50*mg; *Chew tab:* 50 mg (phenylalanine, tartrazine); *Liq:* 12.5 mg/5 ml (4 oz)

▷ *diphenhydramine* **(B)(OTC)(G)** 25-50 mg q 6-8 hours; max 100 mg/day
  Pediatric: <2 years: not recommended; 2-6 years: 6.25 mg q 4-6 hours; max 37.5 mg/day;
  >6-12 years: 12.5-25 mg q 4-6 hours; max 150 mg/day; >12 years: same as adult
    Benadryl (OTC) *Chew tab:* 12.5 mg (grape; phenylalanine); *Liq:* 12.5 mg/5 ml (4, 8 oz);
    Cap: 25 mg; *Tab:* 25 mg; *dye-free softgel:* 25 mg; Dye-free liq: 12.5 mg/5 ml (4, 8 oz)
▷ *meclizine* **(B)(G)** 25-100/day in divided doses
  Pediatric: <12 years: not recommended; ≥12 years: same as adult
    Antivert *Tab:* 12.5, 25, 50*mg; *Amp:* 50 mg/ml (1 ml); *Vial:* 50 mg/ml (1 ml single-use);
    50 mg/ml (10 ml multi-dose)
    Bonine (OTC) *Cap:* 15, 25, 30 mg; *Tab:* 12.5, 25, 50 mg; *Chew tab/Film-coat tab:* 25 mg
    Dramamine II 25 mg bid; max 50 mg/day
      Tab: 25*mg
    Zentrip *Strip:* 25 mg orally disintegrating
▷ *promethazine* **(C)** 12.5-25 q 4-6 hours PO or rectally
  Pediatric: <2 years: not recommended; ≥2 years: 0.5 mg/lb or 6.25-25 mg q 4-6 hours PO
  or rectally
    Phenergan *Tab:* 12.5*, 25*, 50 mg; *Plain syr:* 6.25 mg/5 ml; *Fortis syr:* 25 mg/5 ml;
    Rectal supp: 12.5, 25, 50 mg
  Comment: *promethazine* is contraindicated in children with uncomplicated nausea,
  dehydration, Reye's syndrome, history of sleep apnea, asthma, and lower respiratory
  disorders in children. *promethazine* lowers the seizure threshold in children, may cause
  cholestatic jaundice, anticholinergic effects, extrapyramidal effects, and potentially fatal
  respiratory depression.
▷ *scopolamine* transdermal patch **(C)** 1 patch behind ear; each patch is effective for 3 days;
  change patch every 4th day; alternate sites
  Pediatric: <12 years: not recommended; ≥12 years: same as adult
    Transderm Scop *Patch:* 1.5 mg (4/carton)

⬤ MENINGITIS (*NEISSERIA MENINGITIDIS*)

PROPHYLAXIS

Comment: Meningitis vaccine is a 3-dose series (0, 2, 6 month schedule) indicated for persons
age ≥10-25 years. Have epinephrine 1:1,000 readily available and monitor for 15 minutes post-
dose of meningitis vaccine.
▷ *Meningococcal group b vaccine [recombinant, absorbed]* administer first dose IM in the
  deltoid; administer second dose 2 months later; administer the third dose 6 months from
  the first dose;
  Pediatric: <10 years: not established; ≥10 years: same as adult
    Bexsero *Susp for IM inj:* 0.5 ml single-dose prefilled syringes (1, 10/carton)
    Trumenba *Susp for IM inj:* 0.5 ml single-dose prefilled syringes (5, 10/carton)
▷ *Neisseria meningitides oligosaccharide conjugate* quadrivalent meningococcal vaccine **(B)**
  contains *Corynebacterium diphtheria* CRM197 protein; 10 mcg of Group A + 5 mcg each of
  Group C, Y, and W-135 + 32.7-64.1 mcg of diphtheria CRM 197 protein per 0.5 m.
  Pediatric: <11 years: not recommended; ≥11-55 years: 0.5 ml IM x 1 dose in the deltoid
    Menveo *Vial multi-dose:* 5 doses/vial (MenA conjugate component pwdr for reconsti-
    tution + 1 vial liquid MenCWY conjugate component for reconstitution) (preserva-
    tive-free)
▷ *Neisseria meningitidis polysaccharides* vaccine **(C)** 0.5 ml SC x 1 dose; if at high risk, may
  revaccinate after 3-5 years; age ≥55 years contact mfr
    Menactra (A/C/Y/W-135)
  Pediatric: <2 years: see mfr pkg insert; ≥2 years: same as adult; if at high risk, may
  revaccinate children first vaccinated ≤4 years-of-age after 2-3 years
    Vial (single-dose): 4 mcg each of group A, C, Y, and W-135 per 0.5 ml (pwdr for SC
    inj after reconstitution) (preservative-free diluent); *Vial (multi-dose):* 4 mcg each of
    group A, C, Y, and W-130 per 0.5 ml [pwdr for SC inj after reconstitution (5 doses/
    vial) (preservative-free)]
  Comment: Latex allergy is a contraindication to **Menactra**.
    Menomune-A/C/Y/W-135
  Pediatric: <2 years: not recommended (except ≥3 months of age as short-term
  protection against group A); ≥2 years: same as adult; if at high risk, may revaccinate

children first vaccinated ≤4 years of age after 2-3 years (older children after 3-5 years)

Vial *(single-dose):* 50 mcg each of group A, C, Y, and W-135 per 0.5 ml (pwdr for SC inj after reconstitution; preservative-free diluent); *Vial (multi-dose):* 50 mcg each of group A, C, Y, and W-130 per 0.5 ml [pwdr for SC inj after reconstitution (10 doses/vial) (thimerosal-preserved diluent)]

Comment: Use precaution with latex allergy.

MENOMETRORRHAGIA: IRREGULAR HEAVY MENSTRUAL BLEEDING, MENORRHAGIA: HEAVY CYCLICAL MENSTRUAL BLEEDING

ANTIFIBROLYTIC AGENT

▶ *tranexamic acid* (B)(G) 1,300 mg tid; treat for up to 5 days during menses; *Normal renal function (SCr ≤1.4 mg/dL):* 1,300 mg tid; *SCr ≥1.4-2.8 mg/dL:* 1,300 mg bid; *SCr ≥2.8-5.7 mg/dL:* 1,300 mg once daily; *SCr ≥5.7 mg/dL:* 650 mg once daily
Pediatric: <18 years: not recommended; ≥18 years: same as adult
Lysteda *Tab:* 650 mg

Injectible Progesterone Only Contraceptives

▶ *medroxyprogesterone* (X)(G)
Depo-Provera 150 mg deep IM q 3 months
Vial: 150 mg/ml (1 ml)
Prefilled syringe: 150 mg/ml
Depo-SubQ 104 mg SC q 3 months
Prefilled syringe: 104 mg/ml (0.65 ml; parabens)
Comment: Administer first dose within 5 days of onset of normal menses, within 5 days postpartum if not breastfeeding, or at 6 weeks postpartum if breastfeeding exclusively. Do not use for >2 years unless other methods are inadequate.
Combined Oral Contraceptives *see page 560*
Intrauterine Contraceptives *see page 569*

MENOPAUSE

Comment: *Estrogen* replacement lowers LDL and raises HDL. *Estrogen* replacement is indicated for osteoporosis prevention. However, exogenous *estrogen* administration increases risk for endometrial cancer, MI, stroke, invasive breast cancer, pulmonary embolism, and DVT. *estrogen* replacement is contraindicated in known or suspected pregnancy, known or suspected cancer of the breast, known or suspected *estrogen*-dependent neoplasia, undiagnosed genital bleeding, and active thrombophlebitis or thromboembolic disorders. HRT should be used with extreme caution, and only after a thorough risk/benefit assessment, in patients with cardiovascular or peripheral vascular disease. The US Preventive Services Task Force (USPSTF) recommends against using hormone replacement therapy (HRT) for primary prevention of chronic conditions among postmenopausal women. The harms associated with combined use of estrogen and a progestin, such as increased risks of invasive breast cancer, venous thromboembolism and coronary heart disease, far outweigh the benefits.

However, In an update of their 2012 Hormone Therapy Position Statement, the North American Menopause Society (NAMS) suggests the benefits of hormone therapy, particularly for vasomotor symptoms, outweigh the risks among women under age 60, within a decade of the onset of menopause without other contraindications, who also have an increased risk of fracture or bone loss. Current FDA-approved indications for hormone therapy include the treatment of vasomotor symptoms, prevention of bone loss, genitourinary symptoms, and premature hypoestrogenism caused by castration, hypogonadism, or primary ovarian insufficiency. The work group suggested there are notably higher risks with initiation of hormone therapy after a decade of the onset of menopause, or among women who are over the age of 60, citing an increased absolute risk for cardiovascular harms including stroke, coronary heart disease, venous thromboembolism, and dementia. The statement also noted that for women who exclusively have genitourinary syndrome symptoms, such as urinary, vulvar, and vaginal-related symptoms alone, low-dose vaginal estrogen therapy, such as creams, rings, and tablets that contain estradiol or conjugated equine estrogens are considered "generally safe," but should be more closely considered among women with breast cancer. Patients who require longer durations of hormone therapy, such as to treat persistent vasomotor symptoms or continued bone loss, should determine the benefit-risk profile with her healthcare provider in addition to reassessment during treatment, the statement recommended. The full 2017 position statement appears in *Menopause: The Journal of the North American Menopause Society*.

REFERENCES

Langer, R. D., Simon, J. A., Pines, A., Lobo, R. A., Hodis, H. N., Pickar, J. H., . . . Utian, W. H. (2017). Menopausal hormone therapy for primary prevention: Why the USPSTF is wrong. *Menopause, 24*(10), 1101–1112. doi:10.1097/gme.0000000000000983

Monaco, K. (2017). HRT benefits outweigh risks for certain menopausal women—Menopause Society statement aims to clear up confusion. Retrieved from https://www.medpagetoday.com/Endocrinology/Menopause/66158?xid=NL_MPT_IRXHealthWomen_2017-12-27&eun=g766320d0r

The 2017 hormone therapy position statement of The North American Menopause Society. (2017). *Menopause, 24*(7), 728–753. doi:10.1097/gme.0000000000000921

VAGINAL RINGS

▷ *estradiol, acetate* (X)

  Femring Vaginal Ring insert high into vagina; replace every 90 days

▷ *estradiol, micronized* (X)

  Estring Vaginal Ring insert high into vagina; replace every 90 days

  Vag ring: 7.5 mcg/24 hours (1/pck)

REGIMENS FOR PATIENTS WITH INTACT UTERUS

Vaginal Preparations (With Uterus)

Comment: Vaginal preparations provide relief from vaginal and urinary symptoms only (i.e., atrophic vaginitis, dyspareunia, dysuria, and urinary frequency).

▷ *estradiol* (X)(G)

  Vagifem Tabs insert one 10 mcg or 25 mcg vaginal tablet once daily x 2 weeks; then twice weekly for 2 weeks (e.g., tues/fri); consider the addition of a progestin

  Vag tab: 10, 25 mcg (8, 18/blister pck with applicator)

  Yuvafem Vaginal Tablet 1 tab intravaginally daily x 2 weeks; then 1 tab intravaginally twice weekly

  Vag tab: 10 mcg (15 tabs w. applicators)

▷ *estradiol, micronized* (X)(G)

  Estrace Vaginal Cream 2-4 gm daily x 1-2 weeks, then gradually reduced to 1/2 initial dose x 1-2 weeks, then maintenance dose of 1 gm 1-3 x/week

  Vag crm: 0.01% (12, 42.5 gm w. calib applicator)

▷ *estrogen, conjugated equine* (X)

  Premarin Vaginal Cream 0.5-2 gm/day intravaginally; cyclically (3 weeks on, 1 week off)

  Vag crm: 1.5 oz w. applicator marked in 1/2 gm increments to max of 2 gm

Transdermal Systems (With Uterus)

Comment: Alternate sites. Do not apply patches on or near breasts.

▷ *estradiol* (X)(G)

  Climara initially 0.025 mg/day patch once/week to trunk (3 weeks on and 1 week off)

  Transdermal patch: 0.025, 0.0375, 0.05, 0.075, 0.1 mg/day (4/pck)

  Esclim apply twice weekly x 3 weeks, then 1 week off; use with an oral progestin to prevent endometrial hyperplasia

  Transdermal patch: 0.025, 0.0375, 0.05, 0.075, 0.1 mg/day (8, 48/pck)

  Vivelle initially one 0.0375 mg/day patch twice weekly to trunk area; use with an oral progestin to prevent endometrial hyperplasia

  Transdermal patch: 0.025, 0.0375, 0.05, 0.075, 0.1 mg/day (8, 48/pck)

  Vivelle-Dot initially one 0.05 mg/day patch twice weekly to lower-abdomen, below the waist; use with an oral progestin to prevent endometrial-hyperplasia

  Transdermal patch: 0.025, 0.0375, 0.05, 0.075, 0.1 mg/day (8, 24/pck)

▷ *estradiol+levonorgestrel* (X) apply 1 patch weekly to lower abdomen; avoid waistline; alternate sites

    Climara Pro *Transdermal patch:* estra 0.045 mg+levo 0.015 mg per day (4/pck)

▷ *estradiol+norethindrone* (X)

    CombiPatch apply twice weekly or q 3-4 days

        Transdermal patch: 9 cm²: estra 0.05 mg+noreth 0.14 mg; 16 cm²: estra 0.05 mg+*noreth* 0.25 mg

Comment: May cause irregular bleeding in first 6 months of therapy, but usually decreases over time (often to amenorrhea).

ORAL AGENTS (WITH UTERUS)

▷ *estradiol* (X)(G)

    Estrace 1-2 mg daily cyclically (3 weeks on and 1 week off)

        Tab: 0.5, 1, 2*mg (tartrazine)

▷ *estradiol+drospirenone* (X)

    Angeliq 1 tab daily

        Tab: **Angeliq 0.5/0.25** estra 0.5 mg+dros 0.25 mg

            Angeliq 1/0.5 estra 1 mg+dros 0.5 mg

▷ *estradiol+norethindrone* (X) 1 tab daily

    Activella (G) *Tab:* estra 1 mg+noreth 0.5 mg

    FemHRT (G) **1/5** *Tab:* estra 5 mcg+noreth 1 mg

    Fyavolv (G) *Tab:* estra 0.25 mg+noreth 1 mg; *Tab:* estra 0.5 mg+noreth 1 mg

    Mimvey LO *Tab:* estra 0.5 mg+noreth 0.1 mg

▷ *estradiol+norgestimate* (X) 1 x estradiol 1 mg tab once daily x 3 days, then 1 x estradiol 1 mg+norgestimate 0.09 mg tab daily x 3 days; repeat this pattern continuously

    Ortho-Prefest *Tab:* estra 1 mg+norgest 0.09 mg (30/blister pck)

▷ *estrogen, conjugated+medroxyprogesterone* (X)

    Prempro 1 tab daily

        Tab: **Prempro 0.3/1.5** estro, conj 0.3 mg+medroxy 1.5 mg

            Prempro 0.45/1.5 estro, conj 0.45 mg+medroxy 1.5 mg

            Prempro 0.625/2.5 estro, conj 0.625 mg+medroxy 2.5 mg

            Prempro 0.625/5 estro, conj 0.625 mg+medroxy 5 mg

    Premphase 0.625 *estrogen* on days 1-14, then 0.625 mg *estrogen*+5 mg *medroxyprogesterone* on days 15-28

        Tab (in dial dispenser): estro, conj 0.625 mg (14 maroon tabs) + medroxy 5 mg (14 blue tabs)

▷ *estrogen, esterified (plant derived)* (X)

    Menest 0.3-2.5 mg daily cyclically, 3 weeks on and 1 week off (with progestins in the latter part of the cycle to prevent endometrial hyperplasia)

        Tab: 0.3, 0.625, 1.25, 2.5 mg

▷ *estrogen, esterified+methyltestosterone* (X)

    Estratest 1 tab daily cyclically, 3 weeks on and 1 week off

        Tab: estro ester 1.25 mg+meth 2.5 mg

    Estratest HS 1-2 tabs daily cyclically, 3 weeks on and 1 week off

        Tab: estro ester 0.625 mg+meth 1.25 mg

▷ *ethinyl estradiol* (X) 0.02-0.05 mg q 1-2 days cyclically, 3 weeks on and 1 week off (with progestins in the latter part of the cycle to prevent endometrial hyperplasia)

    Estinyl *Tab:* 0.02 (tartrazine), 0.05 mg

▷ *estropipate, piperazine estrone sulfate* (X)(G)

    Ogen 0.625-1.25 mg daily cyclically (3 weeks on and 1 week off)

        Tab: 0.625, 1.25, 2.5 mg

    Ortho-Est 0.75-6 mg daily cyclically (3 weeks on and 1 week off)

        Tab: 0.625, 1.25 mg

▷ *medroxyprogesterone* (X) 5-10 mg daily for 12 sequential days of each 28-day cycle to prevent endometrial hyperplasia in the postmenopausal women with an intact uterus receiving conjugated estrogens

    Provera 2.5, 5, 10 mg

▷ *norethindrone acetate* (X) 2.5-10 mg daily x 5-10 days during second half of menstrual cycle

    Aygestin *Tab:* 5*mg

▷ *progesterone, micronized* (X)(G)

    Prometrium 200 mg daily in the PM for 12 sequential days of each 28-day cycle to prevent endometrial hyperplasia in the postmenopausal woman with an intact uterus receiving conjugated estrogens

      Cap: 100, 200 mg (peanut oil)

BIO-IDENTICAL ESTRADIOL+PROGESTERONE

▷ *estradiol+projesterone (bio-identical)* take 1 gelcap once daily

    Bijuvia *Gelap:* estro 1 mg+progest 100 mg

    Comment: **Bijuvia** is the first and only bio-identical estradiol and bio-identical progesterone product offering women an alternative to the available FDA-approved synthetic (non-bio-identical) hormones, the separate FDA-approved bio-identical estrogen and progesterone products that are used together but are not approved for combination use, and the unapproved compounded bio-identical hormone products.

ESTROGENS, CONJUGATED+ESTROGEN AGONIST-ANTAGONIST

▷ *estrogen, conjugated+bazedoxifene* (X)

    Duavee 1 tab daily

      Tab: conj estra 0.45 mg+baze 20 mg

REGIMENS FOR PATIENTS WITHOUT UTERUS
Oral Agents (Without Uterus)

▷ *estradiol* (X)(G)

    Estrace 1-2 mg daily

      Tab: 0.5*, 1*, 2*mg (tartrazine)

▷ *estrogen, conjugated (equine)* (X)

    Premarin 1 tab daily

      Tab: 0.3, 0.45, 0.625, 0.9, 1.25, 2.5 mg

▷ *estrogen, conjugated (synthetic)* (X) 1 tab daily; may titrate up to max 1.25 mg/day

    Cenestin *Tab:* 0.3, 0.625, 0.9, 1.25 mg

    Enjuvia *Tab:* 0.3, 0.45, 0.625 mg

▷ *estrogen, esterified (plant derived)* (X) 1 tab daily

    Estratab *Tab:* 0.3, 0.625, 2.5 mg

    Menest *Tab:* 0.3, 0.625, 1.25, 2.5 mg

▷ *ethinyl estradiol* (X) 0.02-0.05 mg q 1-2 days

    Estinyl *Tab:* 0.02 (tartrazine), 0.05 mg

Vaginal Preparations (Without Uterus)

Comment: Vaginal preparations provide relief from vaginal and urinary symptoms only (i.e., atrophic vaginitis, dyspareunia, dysuria, and urinary frequency).

▷ *estradiol* (X)(G)

    Vagifem Tabs insert one 10 mcg or 25 mcg vaginal tablet once daily x 2 weeks; then twice weekly for 2 weeks (e.g., tues/fri); consider the addition of a progestin

      Vag tab: 10, 25 mcg (8, 18/blister pck with applicator)

    Yuvafem Vaginal Tablet 1 tab intravaginally daily x 2 weeks; then 1 tab intravaginally twice weekly

      Vag tab: 10 mcg (15 tabs w. applicators)

Topical Agents (Without Uterus)

▷ *estradiol* (X)

    Estrasorb apply 3.48 gm (2 pouches) every morning; apply one pouch to each leg from the upper thigh to the calf; rub in for 3 minutes; rub excess on hands onto buttocks

      Emul: 0.025 mg/day/pouch (2.5 mg/gm; 1.74 gm/pouch)

    EstroGel apply 1.25 gm (one compression) to one arm from wrist to shoulder once daily at the same time each day

      Gel: 0.06% per compression (93 gm)

Transdermal Systems (Without Uterus)

Comment: Do not apply patches on or near breasts. Alternate sites.

estradiol (X)

    Alora initially 0.05 mg/day apply patch twice weekly to lower abdomen, upper quadrant of buttocks <u>or</u> outer aspect of hip

       Transdermal patch: 0.025, 0.05, 0.075, 0.1 mg/day (8, 24/pck)

    Climara initially 0.025 mg/day patch once/week to trunk

       Transdermal patch: 0.025, 0.0375, 0.05, 0.075, 0.1 mg/day (4, 8, 24/pck)

    Esclim initially 0.025 mg/day apply patch twice weekly to buttocks, femoral triangle, <u>or</u> upper arm

       Transdermal patch: 0.025, 0.0375, 0.05, 0.075, 0.1 mg/day (8/pck)

    Estraderm initially apply one 0.05 mg/day patch twice weekly to trunk

       Transdermal patch: 0.05, 0.1 mg/day (8, 24/pck)

    Menostar apply one patch weekly to lower abdomen, below the waist; avoid the breasts; alternate sites

       Transdermal patch: 14 mcg/day (4/pck)

    Minivelle initially one 0.0375 mg/day patch twice weekly to trunk area; adjust after one month of therapy

       Transdermal patch: 0.025, 0.0375, 0.05, 0.075, 0.1 mg/day (8/pck)

    Vivelle initially one 0.0375 mg/day patch twice weekly to trunk area; adjust after one month of therapy

       Transdermal patch: 0.025, 0.0375, 0.05, 0.075, 0.1 mg/day (8, 48/pck)

    Vivelle-Dot initially apply one 0.05 mg/day patch twice weekly to lower abdomen, below the waist; adjust after one month of therapy

       Transdermal patch: 0.025, 0.0375, 0.05, 0.075, 0.1 mg/day (8, 24/pck)

    Comment: The *estrogens* in **Alora**, **Climara**, **Estraderm**, and **Vivelle-Dot** are plant derived.

⦿ METHAMPHETAMINE-INDUCED PSYCHOSIS

ANTIPSYCHOSIS AGENTS

For more antipsychotics, see **Appendix Q: Antipsychosis Drugs** *pages* 589–591
Tardive Dyskinesia *see page* 473

Comment: First-generation antipsychotics (e.g., *haloperidol* <u>or</u> *fluphenazine*) should be used sparingly and cautiously in patients with methamphetamine-induced psychosis because of the risk of developing extrapyramidal symptoms (EPS) and because these patients are prone to develop motor complications as a result of methamphetamine abuse. Second-generation antipsychotics (e.g., *risperidone* and *olanzapine*) may be more appropriate because of the lower risks of EPS. The presence of high norepinephrine levels in some patients with recurrent methamphetamine psychosis suggests that drugs that block norepinephrine receptors (e.g., *prazosin* <u>or</u> *propranolol*) might be of therapeutic benefit although they have not been studied in controlled trials.

REFERENCE

Zarrabi, H., Khalkhali, M., Hamidi, A., Ahmadi, R., & Zavarmousavi, M. (2016). Clinical features, course and treatment of methamphetamine-induced psychosis in psychiatric inpatients. *BMC Psychiatry, 16*, 44. doi:10.1186/s12888-016-0745-5

▷ *aripiprazole* (C)(G) initially 15 mg once daily; may increase to max 30 mg/day

    Pediatric: <10 years: not recommended; ≥10-17 years: initially 2 mg/day in a single dose for 2 days; then increase to 5 mg/day in a single dose for 2 days; then increase to target dose of 10 mg/day in a single dose; may increase by 5 mg/day at weekly intervals as needed to max 30 mg/day

    Abilify *Tab:* 2, 5, 10, 15, 20, 30 mg

    Abilify Discmelt *Tab:* 15 mg orally-disint (vanilla) (phenylalanine)

    Abilify Maintena *Vial:* 300, 400 mg ext-rel pwdr for IM injection after reconstitution; 300, 400 mg single-dose prefilled dual-chamber syringes w. supplies

▷ *aripiprazole lauroxil* (C) administer by IM injection in the deltoid (441 mg dose only) <u>or</u> gluteal (441 mg, 662 mg, 882 mg <u>or</u> 1064 mg) muscle by a qualified healthcare professional; initiate at a dose of 441 mg, 662 mg <u>or</u> 882 mg administered monthly, <u>or</u> 882 mg every 6 weeks, <u>or</u> 1064 mg every 2 months

    Pediatric: <18 years: not recommended; ≥18 years: same as adult

    Aristada *Prefilled syringe:* 441, 662, 882, 1064 mg single-use, ext-rel susp

Comment: **Aristada** (*aripiprazole*) is an atypical antipsychotic available in 4 doses with 3 dosing duration options for flexible dosing. For patients naïve to *aripiprazole*, establish tolerability with oral *aripiprazole* prior to initiating treatment with **Aristada**. **Aristada** can be initiated at any of the 4 doses at the appropriate dosing duration option. In conjunction with the first injection, administer treatment with oral *aripiprazole* for 21 consecutive days for all 4 dose sizes. The most common adverse event associated with **Aristada** is akathisia. Patients are also at increased risk for developing neuroleptic malignant syndrome, tardive dyskinesia, pathological gambling or other compulsive behaviors, orthostatic hypotension, hyperglycemic, dyslipidemia, and weight gain. Hypersensitive reactions can occur and range from pruritus or urticaria to anaphylaxis. Stroke, transient ischemic attacks, and falls have been reported in elderly patients with dementia-related psychosis who were treated with *aripiprazole*. **Aristada** is not for treatment of people who have lost touch with reality (psychosis) due to confusion and memory loss (dementia). May cause extrapyramidal and/or withdrawal symptoms in neonates exposed in utero in the third trimester of pregnancy. aripiprazole is present in human breast milk; however, there are insufficient data to assess the amount in human milk or the effects on the breast-fed infant. The development and health benefits of breastfeeding should be considered along with the mother's clinical need for **Aristada** and any potential adverse effects on the breastfed infant from **Aristada** or from the underlying maternal condition. For more information or to report ASEs, contact the National Pregnancy Registry for Atypical Antipsychotics at 1-866-961-2388 or visit http://womensmentalhealth.org/clinical-and-research-programs/pregnancyregistry. Limited published data on aripiprazole use in pregnant women are not sufficient to inform any drug-associated risks for birth defects or miscarriage. To report suspected adverse reactions, contact Alkermes at 1-866-274-7823 or FDA at 1-800-FDA-1088 or www.fda.gov/medwatch.

Aristada Initio administer a single 675 mg **Aristada Initio** injection plus a single 30 mg dose of oral *aripiprazole*; administer the IM injection into the deltoid or gluteal muscle; must be administered only by a qualified healthcare professional; Aristada Initio is only to be used as a single dose and is not for repeated dosing

   Prefilled pen: 675 mg/2.4 ml ext-rel single-dose

Comment: **Aristada Initio** (*aripiprazole lauroxil*) is a smaller particle-size version of extended-release injectable (*aripiprazole*) for adults with schizophrenia. It is the first and only long-acting atypical antipsychotic that can be initiated on day one. Combining **Aristada Initio** with a single 30 mg dose of oral *aripiprazole* provides an alternative regimen to initiate patients onto any dose of **Aristada** on day one. Previously, the initiation process for the older *aripiprazole* product was to give the first dose and to then give oral *aripiprazole* for 21 consecutive days. **Aristada Initio** releases relevant levels of *aripiprazole* within 4 days of initiation. **Aristada Initio** carries a warning that it is not approved for use by older patients with dementia-related psychosis, as this patient population is at risk for increased mortality when treated with antipsychotics. For patients naïve to *aripiprazole*, establish tolerability with oral *aripiprazole* prior to initiating treatment with **Aristada Initio**. Avoid use in known CYP2D6 poor metabolizers. Avoid use with strong CYP2D6 or CYP 3A4 inhibitors and strong CYP3A4 inducers. **Aristada Initio** is not interchangeable with **Aristada**. Most commonly observed adverse reaction (incidence ≥5%) has been akathisia. May cause extrapyramidal and/or withdrawal symptoms in neonates in females exposed during the third trimester of pregnancy. There is a pregnancy exposure registry that monitors pregnancy outcomes in women exposed to **Aristada Initio** during pregnancy. aripiprazole is present in human breast milk; however, there are insufficient data to assess the amount in human milk, the effects on the breastfed infant. For more information, contact the National Pregnancy Registry for Atypical Antipsychotics at 1-866-961-2388 or visit http://womensmentalhealth.org/clinical-and-research-programs/pregnancyregistry

▷ *fluphenazine hcl* [**Prolixin**] (C)(G)
   Pediatric: <18 years: not studied
      Tab: 1, 2.5, 5, 10 mg; *Elixer:* 2.5 mg/5 ml; *Conc:* 5 mg/ml; *Vial:* 2.5 mg/ml for injection

▷ *fluphenazine decanoate* [**Prolixin Decanoate**] (C)(G)
   Pediatric: <18 years: not studied
      Vial: 2.5 mg/ml (5 ml)

Comment: Previously, *fluphenazine* was marketed as **Prolixin**, but is currently only available in generic form. Optimal dose and frequency of administration of *fluphenazine* must be determined for each patient, since dosage requirements have been found to vary with clinical circumstances as well as with individual response; dosage should not exceed 100 mg; if doses > 50 mg are deemed necessary, the next dose and succeeding doses should be increased cautiously in increments of 12.5 mg. *fluphenazine decanoate injection* and *fluphenazine enanthate injection* are long-acting parenteral antipsychotic forms intended for use in the management of patients requiring prolonged parenteral neuroleptic therapy. *fluphenazine* has activity at all levels of the central nervous system (CNS) as well as on multiple organ systems. The mechanism whereby its therapeutic action is exerted is unknown. *fluphenazine* differs from other phenothiazine derivatives in several respects: it is more potent on a milligram basis, it has less potentiating effect on CNS depressants and anesthetics than do some of the phenothiazines and appears to be less sedating, and it is less likely than some of the older phenothiazines to produce hypotension (nevertheless, appropriate cautions should be observed. Neuroleptic Malignant Syndrome (NMS), a potentially fatal symptom complex, is associated with all antipsychotic drugs. Clinical manifestations of NMS are hyperpyrexia, muscle rigidity, altered mental status and evidence of autonomic instability (irregular pulse or blood pressure, tachycardia, diaphoresis, and cardiac dysrhythmias). Anticholinergic effects may be potentiated with concomitant *atropine* and *fluphenazine.* Safety and efficacy in children have not been established. Safety during pregnancy has not been established; therefore, the possible hazards should be weighed against the potential benefits when administering this drug to pregnant patients.

▶ *haloperidol* (C)(G)
Oral Route of Administration: Moderate Symptomology: 0.5 to 2 mg orally 2 to 3 times a day; *Severe symptomology:* 3 to 5 mg orally 2 to 3 times a day; initial doses of up to 100 mg/day have been necessary in some severely resistant cases; *Maintenance:* after achieving a satisfactory response, the dose should be adjusted as practical to achieve optimum control
Parenteral Route of Administration: Prompt Control of Acute Agitation: 2 to 5 mg IM every 4 to 8 hours; *Maintenance:* frequency of IM administration should be determined by patient response and may be given as often as every hour; max: 20 mg/day
    Haldol *Tab:* 0.5*, 1*, 2*, 5*, 10*, 20*mg
    Haldol Lactate *Vial:* 5 mg for IM injection, single-dose
▶ *mesoridazine* (C) initially 25 mg tid; max 300 mg/day
    Serentil *Tab:* 10, 25, 50, 100 mg; *Conc:* 25 mg/ml (118 ml)
▶ *olanzapine* (C) initially 2.5-10 mg daily; increase to 10 mg/day within a few days; then by 5 mg/day at weekly intervals; max 20 mg/day
    Zyprexa *Tab:* 2.5, 5, 7.5, 10 mg
    Zyprexa Zydis *ODT:* 5, 10, 15, 20 mg (phenylalanine)
▶ *quetiapine fumarate* (C)(G)
    SeroQUEL initially 25 mg bid, titrate q 2nd or 3rd day in increments of 25-50 mg bid-tid; usual maintenance 400-600 mg/day in 2-3 divided doses
      Tab: 25, 50, 100, 200, 300, 400 mg
    SeroQUEL XR administer once daily in the PM; *Day 1:* 50 mg; *Day 2:* 100 mg; *Day 3:* 200 mg; *Day 4:* 300 mg; usual range 400-600 mg/day
      Tab: 50, 150, 200, 300, 400 mg ext-rel
▶ *risperidone* (C) 0.5 mg bid x 1 day; adjust in increments of 0.5 mg bid; usual range 0.5-5 mg/day
    Risperdal *Tab:* 1, 2, 3, 4 mg; *Oral soln:* 1 mg/ml (100 ml)
    Risperdal M-Tab *Tab:* 0.5, 1, 2 mg
▶ *thioridazine* (C)(G) 10-25 mg bid
    Mellaril *Tab:* 10, 15, 25, 50, 100, 150, 200 mg; *Oral susp:* 25 mg/5 ml, 100 mg/5 ml; *Oral conc:* 30 mg/ml, 100 mg/ml (4 oz)

MITRAL VALVE PROLAPSE (MVP)

▶ *propranolol* (C)(G)
    Inderal 10-30 mg tid-qid
      Tab: 10*, 20*, 40*, 60*, 80*mg
    Inderal LA initially 80 mg daily in a single dose; increase q 3-7 days; usual range 120-160 mg/day; max 320 mg/day in a single dose
      Cap: 60, 80, 120, 160 mg sust-rel
    InnoPran XL initially 80 mg q HS; max 120 mg/day
      Cap: 80, 120 mg ext-rel

MONONUCLEOSIS (MONO)

Opioid Analgesics *see Pain page 354*
Parenteral Corticosteroids *see page 577*
Oral Corticosteroids *see page 577*

▷ *prednisone* (C) initially 40-80 mg/day, then taper off over 5-7 days
Comment: Corticosteroids are recommended in patients with significant pharyngeal edema.

MOTION SICKNESS

▷ *dimenhydrinate* (B)(OTC) 50-100 mg q 4-6 hours; start 1 hour before travel; max 400 mg/day
Pediatric: <2 years: not recommended; 2-6 years: 12.5-25 mg; max 75 mg/day; start 1 hour before travel; may repeat q 6-8 hours; 6-11 years: 25-50 mg; max 150 mg/day; start 1 hour before travel; may repeat q 6-8 hours; ≥12 years: same as adult
   Dramamine *Tab:* 50*mg; *Chew tab:* 50 mg (phenylalanine, tartrazine); *Liq:* 12.5 mg/5 ml (4 oz)

▷ *meclizine* (B)(G) 25-50 mg 1 hour before travel; may repeat q 24 hours as needed; max 50 mg/day
Pediatric: <12 years: not recommended; ≥12 years: same as adult
   Antivert *Tab:* 12.5, 25, 50*mg
   Bonine (OTC) *Cap:* 15, 25, 50 mg; *Tab:* 12.5, 25, 50 mg;
   Chew tab/Film-coat tab: 25 mg
   Dramamine II (OTC) *Tab:* 25 mg
   Zentrip *Strip:* 25 mg orally-disint

▷ *prochlorperazine* (C)(G)
Pediatric: <12 years: not recommended; ≥12 years: same as adult
   Compazine 5-10 mg q 4 hours as needed
      Tab: 5 mg; *Syr:* 5 mg/5 ml (4 oz; fruit); *Rectal supp:* 2.5, 5, 25 mg
   Compazine Spansule 15 mg q AM or 10 mg q 12 hours
      Spansules: 10, 15 mg sust-rel

▷ *promethazine* (C)(G) 25 mg 30-60 minutes before travel; may repeat in 8-12 hours
Pediatric: <2 years: not recommended; ≥2 years: 12.5-25 mg 30-60 minutes before travel; may repeat in 8-12 hours
   Phenergan *Tab:* 12.5*, 25*, 50 mg; *Plain syr:* 6.25 mg/5 ml; *Fortis syr:* 25 mg/5 ml;
   Rectal supp: 12.5, 25, 50 mg
Comment: *promethazine* is contraindicated in children with uncomplicated nausea, dehydration, Reye's syndrome, history of sleep apnea, asthma, and lower respiratory disorders in children. *promethazine* lowers the seizure threshold in children, may cause cholestatic jaundice, anticholinergic effects, extrapyramidal effects, and potentially fatal respiratory depression.

▷ *scopolamine* (C)
Pediatric: <12 years: not recommended; ≥12 years: same as adult
   Scopace 0.4-0.8 mg 1 hour before travel; may repeat in 8 hours
      Tab: 0.4 mg
   Transderm Scop 1 patch behind ear at least 4 hours before travel; each patch is effective for 3 days
      Transdermal patch: 1.5 mg (4/carton)

MULTIPLE SCLEROSIS (MS)

NICOTINIC ACID RECEPTOR AGONIST

▷ *dimethyl fumarate* (C) initially 120 mg bid x 7 days; then maintenance 240 mg bid
Pediatric: <18 years: not recommended; ≥18 years: same as adult
   Tecfidera *Cap:* 120, 240 mg del-rel; *Starter Pack:* 14 x 120 mg, 46 x 240 mg
Comment: The mechanism by which *dimethyl fumarate* (DMF) exerts its therapeutic effect in multiple sclerosis is unknown. DMF and the metabolite, *mono-methyl fumarate* (MMF), have been shown to activate the nuclear factor (erythroid-derived 2)-like 2 (Nrf2) pathway in vitro and in vivo in animals and humans. The Nrf2 pathway is involved in the cellular response to oxidative stress. MMF has been identified as a nicotinic acid receptor agonist in vitro.

POTASSIUM CHANNEL BLOCKER

▷ *dalfampridine* (C)(G) 10 mg q 12 hours
  Pediatric: <18 years: not recommended; ≥18 years: same as adult
    Ampyra *Tab:* 10 mg ext-rel
  Comment: *dalfampridine* is indicated to improve walking speed.

PYRIMIDINE SYNTHESIS INHIBITOR (DMARD)

▷ *teriflunomide* (X) 7 mg or 14 mg once daily
  Pediatric: <12 years: not recommended; ≥12 years: same as adult
    Aubagio *Tab:* 7, 14 mg
  Comment: Contraindicated with severe hepatic impairment and women of childbearing
  potential not using reliable contraception. Co-administer *teriflunomide* with the DMARD
  leflunomide (**Arava**).

IMMUNOMODULATORS

Comment: The role of immunomodulators in the treatment of MS is to slow the progression of
physical disability and to decrease frequency of clinical exacerbations.

▷ *alemtuzumab* (C) administer two treatment courses:
  First treatment course: 12 mg/day x 5 days (total 60 mg); *Second treatment course:* 12
  months later, administer 12 mg/day x 3 days (total 36 mg); complete all immunizations
  6 weeks prior to the first treatment; pre-medicate with 1000 mg methylprednisolone or
  equivalent immediately prior to the first 3 treatment days in each treatment course
  Pediatric: <18 years: not recommended; ≥18 years: same as adult
    Lemtrada *Vial:* 12 mg/1.2 ml soln for IV infusion, single-use vial
    Comment: **Lemtrada** is indicated for the treatment of patients with relapsing forms
    of MS. Because of its safety profile, the use of **Lemtrada** should generally be reserved
    for patients who have had an inadequate response to two or more drugs indicated
    for the treatment of MS. **Lemtrada REMS** is a restricted distribution program, which
    allows early detection and management of some of the serious risks associated with
    its use.
▷ *fingolimod* (C) 0.5 mg once daily
  Pediatric: <10 years: not recommended; ≥10 years: same as adult
    Gilenya *Cap:* 0.5 mg
  Comment: First-dose monitoring for bradycardia. In the first 2 weeks, first-dose
  monitoring is recommended after an interruption of 1 day or more. During weeks 3 and
  4, first-dose monitoring is recommended after an interruption of more than 7 days. FDA
  warning: when **Gilenya** (*fingolimod*) is stopped, the MS disability can become much worse
  than before the medicine was started or while it was being taken. This MS worsening
  is rare but can result in permanent disability. Before starting treatment with **Gilenya**,
  patient's should be warned about the potential risk of severe increase in disability after
  stopping **Gilenya**.
▷ *glatiramer acetate* (B)(G)
  Copaxone 20-40 mg SC once daily
  Pediatric: <18 years: not recommended; ≥18 years: same as adult
    Prefilled syringe: 20, 40 mg/ml (1 ml) single-dose (mannitol 40 mg; preservative-free)
  Glatopa 20 mg SC once daily or 40 mg SC 3 x/weekly at least 48 hours apart
  Pediatric: <18 years: not recommended; ≥18 years: same as adult
    Prefilled syringe: 20, 40 mg/ml (1 ml) single dose (mannitol 40 mg; preservative-free)
  Comment: *glatiramer acetate* injection *(Copaxone, Glatopa)* is indicated for the
  treatment of patients with relapsing forms of multiple sclerosis. Mechanism(s) by
  which *glatiramer acetate* exerts its effects in patients with MS are not fully understood.
  However, *glatiramer acetate* is thought to act by modifying immune processes that are
  believed to be responsible for the pathogenesis of MS. The biological activity of *glatiramer
  acetate* is informed by its ability to block the induction of experimental autoimmune
  encephalomyelitis (EAE) in animal studies. Further, studies in animals and in vitro
  systems suggest that upon its administration, *glatiramer acetate*-specific suppressor
  T-cells are induced and activated in the periphery. **Glatopa** is a fully-substitutable, AP-
  rated generic version of **Copaxone**.
▷ *interferon beta-1a* (C)
  Pediatric: <18 years: not recommended; ≥18 years: same as adult

Avonex 30 mcg IM weekly; rotate sites; may titrate to reduce flu-like symptoms; may use concurrent analgesics/antipyretics on treatment days; *Titration Schedule:* 7.5 mcg week 1; 15 mcg week 2; 22.5 mcg week 3; 30 mcg week 4 and ongoing

Vial: 30 mcg/vial pwdr for reconstitution (single-dose w. diluent, 4 vials/kit) (albumin [human], preservative-free); *Prefilled syringe:* 30 mcg single-dose (0.5 ml) (4/dose pck)

Rebif, administer SC 3x/week (at least 48 hours apart and preferably in the late afternoon or evening); increase over 4 weeks to usual dose 22-44 mcg 3x/week; *Titration Schedule (22 mcg prescribed dose):* 4.4 mcg week 1 and 2; 11 mcg week 3 and 4; 22 mcg week 5 and ongoing; *Titration Schedule (44 mcg prescribed dose):* 8.8 mcg week 1 and 2; 22 mcg week 3 and 4; 44 mcg week 5 and ongoing

Prefilled syringe: 22, 44 mcg/0.5 ml w. needle (12/carton) (albumin [human], preservative-free); (titration pack, 6 doses of 8.8 mcg [0.2 ml] w. needle per carton) (albumin [human], preservative-free)

Comment: Only prefilled syringes (**Rebif**) can be used to titrate to the 22 mcg prescribed dose. Prefilled syringes or autoinjectors (**Rebif Rebidose**) can be used to titrate to the 44 mcg prescribed dose.

Rebif Rebidose administer SC 3x/week (at least 48 hours apart and preferably in the late afternoon or evening) after titration to 22 mcg or 44 mcg

Titration Schedule: *see* **Rebif**.

Prefilled autoinjector: 22, 44 mcg/0.5 ml (0.5 ml, 12/carton) (titration pack, 6 doses of 8.8 mcg [0.2 ml] per carton (albumin [human], preservative-free)

Comment: Only prefilled syringes (**Rebif**) can be used to titrate to the 22 mcg prescribed dose. Prefilled syringes or autoinjectors (**Rebif Rebidose**) can be used to titrate to the 44 mcg prescribed dose.

▷ *interferon beta-1b* (C)
Pediatric: <18 years: not recommended; ≥18 years: same as adult

Actimmune *BSA ≤0.5m²:* 1.5 mcg/kg SC in a single dose 3x weekly; *BSA ≥0.5m²:* 50 mcg/m² SC in a single dose 3x weekly *Vial:* 100 mcg/0.5 ml single-dose for SC injection

Betaseron, Extavia 0.0625 mg (0.25 ml) SC every other day; increase over 6 weeks to 0.25 mg (1 ml) SC every other day

Vial: 0.3 mg/vial pwdr for reconstitution (single-dose w. prefilled diluents syringes) (albumin [human], mannitol, preservative-free)

▷ *natalizumab* (C) administer 300 mg by IV infusion over 1 hour every 4 weeks; monitor during infusion and for 1 hour postinfusion
Pediatric: <18 years: not recommended; ≥18 years: same as adult

Tysabri *Vial:* 300 mg/15 ml (15 ml)

CD20-DIRECTED CYTOLYTIC MONOCLONAL ANTIBODY

▷ *ocrelizumab* pre-medicate with corticosteroid and antihistamine, and consider antipyretic, prior to each infusion; initially administer 300 mg by IV infusion followed by another 300 mg infusion 2 weeks later; then administer 600 mg every 6 months; see mfr lit for infusion rates and dose modifications
Pediatric: <18 years: not recommended; ≥18 years: same as adult

Ocrevus *Vial:* 30 mg/ml (10 ml, single-dose) for dilution (preservative-free)

Comment: The precise mechanism of action is unknown; however, it is thought to involve binding to CD20, a cell surface antigen present on pre-B and mature B lymphocytes which results in antibody-dependent cellular cytolysis and complement-mediated lysis. **Ocrevus** is contraindicated with active HBV infection. Screen for HBV infection (HBsAg/anti-HB) prior to initiation. Concomitant live or attenuated vaccine not recommended during treatment and until B-cell repletion. Administer these at least 6 weeks prior to initiation of treatment. Additive immunosuppressive effects with other immunosupressants. Monitor for infusion reaction (pruritis, rash, urticaria, erythema, throat irritation, bronchospasm). Delay treatment with active infection. Withhold at first sign/symptom of progressive multifocal leukoencephalopathy (PMI) or HBV reactivation. Females of reproductive potential should use effective contraception during treatment and for 6 months after the last dose of **Ocrevus**. It is not known whether *ocrelizumab* is excreted in human breast milk or has any effect on the breastfed infant.

PSEUDOBULBAR AFFECT (PBA)

Comment: Pseudobulbar affect (PBA), emotional lability, labile affect, or emotional incontinence refers by to a neurologic disorder characterized by involuntary crying or uncontrollable episodes of crying and/or laughing, or other emotional outbursts. PBA occurs secondary to a neurologic disease or brain injury such as traumatic brain injury (TBI), stroke, Parkinson's disease, multiple sclerosis, and amyotrophic lateral sclerosis (ALS, or Lou Gehrig's disease).

▷ *dextromethorphan+quinidine* (C)(G) 1 cap once daily x 7 days; then starting on day 8, 1 cap bid
  Pediatric: <12 years: not recommended; ≥12 years: same as adult
    Nuedexta *Cap:* dextro 20 mg+quini 10 mg
  Comment: *dextromethorphan hydrobromide* is an uncompetitive NMDA receptor antagonist and sigma-1 agonist. *quinidine sulfate* is a CYP450 2D6 inhibitor. **Nuedexta** is contraindicated with an MAOI or within 14 days of stopping an MAOI, with prolonged QT interval, congenital long QT syndrome, history suggestive of torsades de pointes, or heart failure, complete atrioventricular (AV) block without implanted pacemaker or patients at high risk of complete AV block, and concomitant drugs that both prolong QT interval and are metabolized by CYP2D6 (e.g., *thioridazine* or *pimozide*). Discontinue **Nuedexta** if the following occurs: hepatitis or thrombocytopenia or any other hypersensitivity reaction. Monitor ECG in patients with left ventricular hypertrophy (LVH) or left ventricular dysfunction (LVD). *desipramine* exposure increases **Nuedexta** 8-fold; reduce *desipramine* dose and adjust based on clinical response. Use of **Nuedexta** with selective serotonin reuptake inhibitors (SSRIs) or tricyclic antidepressants (TCAs) increases the risk of serotonin syndrome. *paroxetine* exposure increases **Nuedexta** 2-fold; therefore, reduce *paroxetine* dose and adjust based on clinical response (*digoxin* exposure may increase *digoxin* substrate plasma concentration. **Nuedexta** is not recommended in pregnancy or breastfeeding. Safety and effectiveness of **Nuedexta** in children have not been established. To report suspected adverse reactions, contact Avanir Pharmaceuticals at 1-866-388-5041 or FDA at 1-800-FDA-1088 or www.fda.gov/medwatch.

 MUMPS (INFECTIOUS PAROTITIS, *PARAMYXOVIRUS*)

see **Childhood Immunizations** *page 558*
Parenteral Corticosteroids *see page 577*
Oral Corticosteroids *see page 577*
Antipyretics *see Fever page 163*

PROPHYLAXIS VACCINE

▷ *measles, mumps, rubella, live, attenuated, neomycin vaccine* (C)
    MMR II 25 mcg SC (preservative-free)
  Comment: Contraindications: hypersensitivity to *neomycin* or eggs, primary or acquired immune deficiency, immunosuppressant therapy, bone marrow or lymphatic malignancy, and pregnancy (within 3 months after vaccination).

 MUSCLE STRAIN

Acetaminophen for IV Infusion *see Pain page 352*
Parenteral Corticosteroids *see page 577*
Oral Corticosteroids *see page 577*
Opioid Analgesics *see Pain page 354*

Comment: Usual length of treatment for acute injury is approximately 5 days.

SKELETAL MUSCLE RELAXANTS

▷ *baclofen* (C)(G) 5 mg tid; titrate up by 5 mg every 3 days to 20 mg tid; max 80 mg/day
  Pediatric: <12 years: not recommended; ≥12 years: same as adult
    Lioresal *Tab:* 10*, 20*mg

Comment: *baclofen* is indicated for muscle spasm pain and chronic spasticity associated with multiple sclerosis and spinal cord injury <u>or</u> disease. Potential for seizures <u>or</u> hallucinations on abrupt withdrawal.

▷ *carisoprodol* (C)(G) 1 tab tid <u>or</u> qid
  Pediatric: <12 years: not recommended; ≥12 years: same as adult
    Soma *Tab:* 350 mg
▷ *chlorzoxazone* (G) 1 caplet qid; max 750 mg qid
  Pediatric: <12 years: not recommended; ≥12 years: same as adult
    Parafon Forte DSC *Cplt:* 500*mg
▷ *cyclobenzaprine* (B)(G) 10 mg tid; usual range 20-40 mg/day in divided doses; max 60 mg/day x 2-3 weeks <u>or</u> 15 mg ext-rel once daily; max 30 mg ext-rel/day x 2-3 weeks
  Pediatric: <15 years: not recommended; ≥15 years: same as adult
    Amrix *Cap:* 15, 30 mg ext-rel
    Fexmid *Tab:* 7.5 mg
    Flexeril *Tab:* 5, 10 mg
▷ *dantrolene* (C) 25md daily x 7 days; then 25 mg tid x 7 days; then 50 mg tid x 7 days; max 100 mg qid
  Pediatric: 0.5 mg/kg daily x 7 days; then 0.5 mg/kg tid x 7 days; then 1 mg/kg tid x 7 days; then 2 mg/kg tid; max 100 mg qid
    Dantrium *Tab:* 25, 50, 100 mg

Comment: *dantrolene* is indicated for chronic spasticity associated with multiple sclerosis and spinal cord injury <u>or</u> disease.

▷ *diazepam* (C)(IV) 2-10 mg bid-qid; may increase gradually
  Pediatric: <6 months: not recommended; ≥6 months: initially 1-2.5 mg bid-qid; may increase gradually
    Diastat *Rectal gel delivery system:* 2.5 mg
    Diastat AcuDial *Rectal gel delivery system:* 10, 20 mg
    Valium *Tab:* 2, 5, 10 mg
    Valium Intensol Oral Solution *Conc oral soln:* 5 mg/ml (30 ml w. dropper)(alcohol 19%)
    Valium Oral Solution *Oral soln:* 5 mg/5 ml (500 ml) (wintergreen spice)
▷ *metaxalone* (B) 1 tab tid-qid
  Pediatric: <12 years: not recommended; ≥12 years: same as adult
    Skelaxin *Tab:* 800*mg
▷ *methocarbamol* (C)(G) initially 1.5 gm qid x 2-3 days; maintenance, 750 mg every 4 hours <u>or</u> 1.5 gm 3x daily; max 8 gm/day
  Pediatric: <16 years: not recommended; ≥16 years: same as adult
    Robaxin *Tab:* 500 mg
    Robaxin 750 *Tab:* 750 mg
    Robaxin Injection 10 ml IM <u>or</u> IV; max 30 ml/day; max 3 days; max 5 ml/gluteal injection q 8 hours; max IV rate 3 ml/min
      Vial: 100 mg/ml (10 ml)
▷ *nabumetone* (C)
  Pediatric: <12 years: not recommended; ≥12 years: same as adult
    Relafen *Tab:* 500, 750 mg
    Relafen 500 *Tab:* 500 mg
▷ *orphenadrine citrate* (C)(G) 1 tab bid
  Pediatric: <12 years: not recommended; ≥12 years: same as adult
    Norflex *Tab:* 100 mg sust-rel
▷ *tizanidine* (C) 1-4 mg q 6-8 hours; max 36 mg/day
  Pediatric: <12 years: not recommended; ≥12 years: same as adult
    Zanaflex *Tab:* 2*, 4**mg; *Cap:* 2, 4, 6 mg

SKELETAL MUSCLE RELAXANT+NSAID COMBINATIONS

Comment: *aspirin*-containing medications are contraindicated with history of allergic-type reaction to *aspirin*, children and adolescents with *Varicella* <u>or</u> other viral illness, and 3rd trimester of pregnancy.

▷ *carisoprodol+aspirin* (C)(III)(G) 1-2 tabs qid
  Pediatric: <12 years: not recommended; ≥12 years: same as adult
    Soma Compound *Tab:* caris 200 mg+asp 325 mg (sulfites)
▷ *meprobamate+aspirin* (D)(IV) 1-2 tabs tid <u>or</u> qid
  Pediatric: <12 years: not recommended; ≥12 years: same as adult

Equagesic *Tab:* mepro 200 mg+asp 325*mg
Comment: *aspirin*-containing medications are contraindicated with history of allergic-type reaction to *aspirin*, children and adolescents with *varicella* or other viral illness, and 3rd trimester of pregnancy.

SKELETAL MUSCLE RELAXANT+NSAID+CAFFEINE COMBINATIONS
▷ *orphenadrine+aspirin+caffeine* (D)(G)
  Pediatric: <12 years: not recommended; ≥12 years: same as adult
    Norgesic 1-2 tabs tid-qid
      Tab: orphen 25 mg+asp 385 mg+caf 30 mg
    Norgesic Forte 1 tab tid or qid; max 4 tabs/day
      Tab: orphen 50 mg+asp 770 mg+caf 60 mg*
  Comment: *aspirin*-containing medications are contraindicated with history of allergic-type reaction to *aspirin*, children and adolescents with *Varicella* or other viral illness, and 3rd trimester of pregnancy.

SKELETAL MUSCLE RELAXANT+NSAID+CODEINE COMBINATIONS
▷ *carisoprodol+aspirin+codeine* (D)(III)(G) 1-2 tabs qid prn
  Pediatric: <12 years: contraindicated; 12-<18: use extreme caution; not recommended for children and adolescents with obesity, asthma, obstructive sleep apnea, or other chronic breathing problem, or for post-tonsillectomy/adenoidectomy pain; ≥18 years: same as adult
    Soma Compound w. Codeine
      Tab: caris 200 mg+asp 325 mg+cod 16 mg (sulfites)
  Comment: *codeine* is known to be excreted in breast milk. <12 years: not recommended; 12-<18: use extreme caution; not recommended for children and adolescents with asthma or other chronic breathing problem. The FDA and the European Medicines Agency (EMA) are investigating the safety of using *codeine* containing medications to treat pain, cough and colds, in children 12-<18 years because of the potential for serious side effects, including slowed or difficult breathing. *aspirin*-containing medications are contraindicated with history of allergic-type reaction to *aspirin*, children and adolescents with *Varicella* or other viral illness, and 3rd trimester of pregnancy.

TOPICAL & TRANSDERMAL ANALGESICS
▷ *capsaicin* (B)(G) apply tid-qid prn to intact skin
  Pediatric: <2 years: not recommended; ≥2 years: apply sparingly tid-qid prn
    Axsain *Crm:* 0.075% (1, 2 oz)
    Capsin *Lotn:* 0.025, 0.075% (59 ml)
    Capzasin-HP (OTC) *Crm:* 0.075% (1.5 oz), 0.025% (45, 90 gm); *Lotn:* 0.075% (2 oz); 0.025% (45, 90 gm)
    Capzasin-P (OTC) *Crm:* 0.025% (1.5 oz); *Lotn:* 0.025% (2 oz)
    Dolorac *Crm:* 0.025% (28 gm)
    Double Cap (OTC) *Crm:* 0.05% (2 oz)
    R-Gel *Gel:* 0.025% (15, 30 gm)
    Zostrix (OTC) *Crm:* 0.025% (0.7, 1.5, 3 oz)
    Zostrix HP (OTC) *Emol crm:* 0.075% (1, 2 oz)
▷ *capsaicin* 8% patch (B) apply up to 4 patches for one 60-minute application to clean dry skin; may prep area with topical anesthetic; wear non-latex gloves; patches may be cut to size/shape; treatment may be repeated every 3 months
  Pediatric: <18 years: not recommended; ≥18 years: same as adult
    Qutenza *Patch:* 8% 1640 mcg/cm (179 mg) (1 or 2 patches w. 1-50 gm tube cleansing gel/carton)
▷ *diclofenac sodium* (C; D ≥30 wks)(G) apply qid prn to intact skin
  Pediatric: <12 years: not established; ≥12 years: same as adult
    Pennsaid 1.5% in 10 drop increments, dispense and rub into front, side, and back of knee: usually; 40 drops (40 mg) qid
      Topical soln: 1.5% (150 ml)
    Pennsaid 2% apply 2 pump actuations (40 mg) and rub into front, side, and back of knee bid
      Topical soln: 2% (20 mg/pump actuation, 112 gm)
    Solaraze Gel massage in to clean skin bid prn
      Gel: 3% (50 gm) (benzyl alcohol)

Voltaren Gel (G) apply qid prn to intact skin
> *Gel:* 1% (100 gm)

Comment: *diclofenac* is contraindicated with **aspirin** allergy. As with other NSAIDs, should be avoided in late pregnancy (≥30 weeks) because it may cause premature closure of the ductus arteriosus.

▷ *doxepin* (B) cream apply to affected area qid at intervals of at least 3-4 hours; max 8 days
Pediatric: <12 years: not recommended; >12 years: same as adult
> **Prudoxin** *Crm:* 5% (45 gm)
> **Zonalon** *Crm:* 5% (30, 45 gm)

▷ *pimecrolimus* 1% cream (C)(G) <2 years: not recommended; ≥2 years: apply to affected area bid; do not apply an occlusive dressing
> **Elidel** *Crm:* 1% (30, 60, 100 gm)

Comment: *pimecrolimus* is indicated for short-term and intermittent long-term use. Discontinue use when resolution occurs. Contraindicated if the patient is immunosuppressed. Change to the 0.1% preparation or if secondary bacterial infection is present.

▷ *trolamine salicylate* apply tid-qid
Pediatric: <2 years: not recommended; ≥2 years: same as adult
> **Mobisyl Creme** *Crm:* 10% (100 gm)

TOPICAL AND TRANSDERMAL ANESTHETICS

Comment: *lidocaine* should not be applied to non-intact skin.

▷ *lidocaine* cream (B) apply to affected area bid prn
Pediatric: <12 years: not recommended; ≥12 years: same as adult
> **LidaMantle** *Crm:* 3% (1, 2 oz)
> **Lidoderm** *Crm:* 3% (85 gm)
> **ZTlido** *lidocaine* topical system 1% (30/carton)
> Comment: Compared to **Lidoderm** (*lidocaine* patch 5%) which contains 700 mg/patch, **ZTlido** only requires 35 mg per topical system to achieve the same therapeutic dose.

▷ *lidocaine* lotion (B) apply to affected area bid prn
Pediatric: <12 years: not recommended; ≥12 years: same as adult
> **LidaMantle** *Lotn:* 3% (177 ml)

▷ *lidocaine* 5% patch (B)(G) apply up to 3 patches at one time for up to 12 hours/24-hour period (12 hours on/12 hours off); patches may be cut into smaller sizes before removal of the release liner; do not re-use
Pediatric: <12 years: not recommended; ≥12 years: same as adult
> **Lidoderm** *Patch:* 5% (10x14 cm; 30/carton)

▷ *lidocaine+dexamethasone* (B)
Pediatric: <12 years: not recommended; ≥12 years: same as adult
> **Decadron Phosphate with Xylocaine** *Lotn:* dexa 4 mg+lido 10 mg per ml (5 ml)

▷ *lidocaine+hydrocortisone* (B)(G) apply to affected area bid prn
Pediatric: <12 years: not recommended; ≥12 years: same as adult
> **LidaMantle HC** *Crm:* lido 3%+hydro 0.5% (1, 3 oz); *Lotn:* (177 ml)

▷ *lidocaine* 2.5%+*prilocaine* 2.5% apply sparingly to the burn bid-tid prn
Pediatric: <12 years: not recommended; ≥12 years: same as adult
> **Emla Cream** (B) 5, 30 gm/tube

ORAL NSAIDs

For an expanded list of NSAIDs *see page 571*

▷ *diclofenac* (C) take on empty stomach; 35 mg tid; *Hepatic impairment:* use lowest dose
Pediatric: <18 years: not recommended; ≥18 years: same as adult
> **Zorvolex** *Gelcap:* 18, 35 mg

▷ *diclofenac sodium* (C)
Pediatric: <18 years: not recommended; ≥18 years: same as adult
> **Voltaren** 50 mg bid-qid or 75 mg bid or 25 mg qid with an additional 25 mg at HS if necessary
> *Tab:* 25, 50, 75 mg ent-coat
> **Voltaren XR** 100 mg once daily; rarely, 100 mg bid may be used
> *Tab:* 100 mg ext-rel

ORAL NSAIDs+PPI COMBINATIONS

▷ *esomeprazole+naproxen* (C)(G) 1 tab bid; use lowest effective dose for the shortest duration swallow whole; take at least 30 minutes before a meal
Pediatric: <18 years: not recommended; ≥18 years: same as adult
 Vimovo *Tab:* nap 375 mg+eso 20 mg ext-rel; nap 500 mg+eso 20 mg ext-rel
 Comment: **Vimovo** is indicated to improve signs/symptoms, and risk of gastric ulcer in patients at risk of developing NSAID-associated gastric ulcer.

COX-2 INHIBITORS

Comment: Cox-2 inhibitors are contraindicated with history of asthma, urticaria, and allergic-type reactions to *aspirin*, other NSAIDs, and sulfonamides, 3rd trimester of pregnancy, and coronary artery bypass graft (CABG) surgery.
▷ *celecoxib* (C)(G) 100-400 mg daily bid; max 800 mg/day
Pediatric: <18 years: not recommended; ≥18 years: same as adult
 Celebrex *Cap:* 50, 100, 200, 400 mg
▷ *meloxicam* (C)(G)
 Mobic <2 years, <60 kg: not recommended; ≥2, >60 kg: 0.125 mg/kg; max 7.5 mg once daily; ≥18 years: initially 7.5 mg once daily; max 15 mg once daily; *Hemodialysis:* max 7.5 mg/day
  Tab: 7.5, 15 mg; *Oral susp:* 7.5 mg/5 ml (100 ml) (raspberry)
 Vivlodex <18 years: not established; ≥18 years: initially 5 mg qd; may increase to max 10 mg/day; *Hemodialysis:* max 5 mg/day
  Cap: 5, 10 mg

TOPICAL & TRANSDERMAL LIDOCAINE

▷ *lidocaine* transdermal patch (C)(G) apply one patch to affected area for 12 hours (then off for 12 hours); remove during bathing; avoid non-intact skin
Pediatric: <12 years: not recommended; ≥12 years: same as adult
 Lidoderm *Patch:* 5% (10 cm x 14 cm; 30/carton)

 MYASTHENIA GRAVIS (MG)

COMPLEMENT INHIBITORS

▷ *eculizumab* (C) dilute to a final admixture concentration of 5 mg/ml using the following steps: (1) withdraw the required amount of **Soliris** from the vial into a sterile syringe; (2) transfer the dose to an infusion bag; (3) add IV fluid equal to the drug volume (0.9% NaCl or 0.45% NaCl or D5W or Ringer's Lactate); the final admixed **Soliris** 5 mg/ml infusion volume is: 300 mg dose (60 ml), 600 mg dose (120 ml), 900 mg dose (180 ml), 1200 mg dose (240 ml); administer 900 mg IV infusion once weekly for the first 4 weeks; then, 1200 mg IV infusion for the 5th dose 1 week after the 4th dose; then, 1200 mg IV infusion once every 2 weeks thereafter
Pediatric: <18 years: safety and effectiveness not established; ≥18 years: same as adult
 Soliris *Vial:* 300 mg (10 mg/ml, 30 ml), single-use, concentrated solution for intravenous infusion (preservative-free)
Comment: **Soliris** *(eculizumab)* is a complement inhibitor indicated for the treatment of patients with paroxysmal nocturnal hemoglobinuria (PNH) to reduce hemolysis, patients with atypical hemolytic uremic syndrome (aHUS) to inhibit complement-mediated thrombotic microangiopathy (TMA), and adult patients with generalized myasthenia gravis (gMG) who are anti-acetylcholine receptor (AchR) antibody positive. **Soliris** should be administered for generalized MG at the above recommended dosage regimen time points or within 2 days of each time point. Supplemental dosing of **Soliris** is required in the setting of concomitant support with plasmapheresis (PI) or plasma exchange (PE) or fresh frozen plasma (FFP) infusion (see mfr pkg insert for supplemental dosing). **Soliris** is not indicated for the treatment of patients with Shiga toxin *E. coli*-related hemolytic uremic syndrome (STEC-HUS). **Soliris** is contraindicated in patients with unresolved *Neisseria meningitides* infection and patients who are not currently vaccinated against *Neisseria meningitides,* unless the risks of delaying **Soliris** treatment outweigh the risks of

developing meningococcal infection. Prescribers must enroll in the **Soliris** REMS Program (1-888-SOLIRIS, 1-888-765-4747), counsel patients about the risk of meningococcal infection, provide patients with **Soliris** REMS educational materials, and ensure that patients are vaccinated with a meningococcal vaccine. There are no adequate and well-controlled human studies of **Soliris** in pregnancy or effects on the breastfed infant. Based on animal studies, **Soliris** may cause fetal harm. It is not known whether **Soliris** is excreted in human milk. IgG is excreted in human milk, so it is expected that **Soliris** will be present in human milk. However, published data suggest that antibodies in human milk do not enter the neonatal and infant circulation in substantial amounts. Caution should be exercised when **Soliris** is administered to a breast-feeding patient. To report suspected adverse reactions, contact Alexion Pharmaceuticals at 1-888-SOLIRIS (1-888-765-4747 or FDA at 1-800-FDA-1088 or visit www.fda.gov/medwatch.

NARCOLEPSY, CATAPLEXY

STIMULANTS

▷ *amphetamine sulfate* (C)(II) administer first dose on awakening, and additional doses at 4- to 6-hour intervals; usual range 5-60 mg/day
Pediatric: <6 years: not recommended; 6-12 years: 5 mg daily in the AM; may increase by 5 mg/day at weekly intervals; ≥12-18 years: initially 10 mg in the AM; may increase by 10 mg daily at weekly intervals; >18 years: same as adult
  Evekeo initially 10 mg once or twice daily at the same time(s) each day; may increase by 10 mg/day at weekly intervals; max 40 mg/day
  Tab: 5, 10 mg

▷ *armodafinil* (C)(IV)(G) *OSAHS:* 50-250 mg once daily in the AM; *SWSD:* 150 mg 1 hour before starting shift; reduce dose with severe hepatic impairment
Pediatric: <17 years: not recommended; ≥17 years: same as adult
  Nuvigil *Tab:* 50, 150, 200, 250 mg

▷ *modafinil* (C)(IV)(G) 100-200 mg q AM; max 400 mg/day
Pediatric: <17 years: not recommended; ≥17 years: same as adult
  Provigil *Tab:* 100, 200*mg
  Comment: Provigil also promotes wakefulness in patients with shift work sleep disorder and excessive sleepiness due to obstructive sleep apnea/hypopnea syndrome.

▷ *sodium oxybate* (B)(G) initiate dosage at 4.5 gm per night orally divided into two doses; titrate to effect in increments of 1.5 gm per night at weekly intervals (0.75 gm at bedtime and 0.75 gm taken 2½ to 4 hours later)

Total Nightly Dose (gm)	4.5 gm	6 gm	7.5 gm	9 gm
Bedtime (gm)	2.25 gm	3 gm	3.75 gm	4.5 gm
2½ to 4 hours later (gm)	2.25 gm	3 gm	3.75 gm	4.5 gm

Pediatric: <7 years: not recommended; ≥7-17 years: see mfr pkg insert for weight-based (in kilograms) dosing table; ≥18 years: same as adult
  Xyrem *Oral soln:* 500 mg/ml
  Comment: Xyrem is used to reduce the number of cataplexy attacks (sudden and transient episode of muscle weakness coupled with full conscious awareness, typically triggered by emotions such as laughing, crying, or terror) and reduce daytime sleepiness in patients with narcolepsy. The rapid onset of sedation coupled with amnesia, particularly when combined with alcohol, has posed risks for voluntary and involuntary users (e.g., assault victims). Contraindicated with *alcohol* and CNS depressants (may impair consciousness; may lead to respiratory depression, coma, or death), and in patients with succinic semialdehyde dehydrogenase deficiency (an inborn error of metabolism). Prepare both doses prior to bedtime and do not attempt to get out of bed after taking the first dose. Place both doses within reach at the bedside. Set the bedside clock to awaken for the second dose. Dilute each dose in 60 ml (1/4 cup, 4 tbsp) water in child resistant dosing containers. Food significantly reduces the bioavailability of *sodium oxybate*; take at least 2 hours after ingesting food. There are no adequate data on the fetal developmental risk associated with the use of *sodium oxybate* in pregnant women. GHB is excreted in human milk. There is insufficient information on risk to the breastfed infant Comment: Xyrem is a Schedule III controlled substance. The active ingredient of **Xyrem**, sodium oxybate or gamma-hydroxy-butyrate (GHB), is a Schedule I controlled substance. **Xyrem** is available

only through a restricted distribution **Xyrem** REMS Program because of the risks of CNS depression and abuse and misuse, healthcare providers who prescribe **Xyrem** are specially certified, **Xyrem** is dispensed only by the central pharmacy that is specially certified, and **Xyrem** is dispensed and shipped only to patients who are enrolled in the **Xyrem** REMS Program with documentation of safe use (www.XYREMREMS.com or 1-866-XYREM88 [1-866-997-3688]).

STIMULANTS

▷ *dextroamphetamine sulfate* (C)(II)(G) initially start with 10 mg daily; increase by 10 mg at weekly intervals if needed; may switch to daily dose with sust-rel spansules when titrated
Pediatric: <3 years: not recommended; 3-5 years: 2.5 mg daily; may increase by 2.5 mg daily at weekly intervals if needed; 6-12 years: initially 5 mg daily-bid; may increase by 5 mg/day at weekly intervals; usual max 40 mg/day; >12 years: initially 10 mg daily; may increase by mg/day at weekly intervals; max 40 mg/day 10
    Dexedrine *Tab:* 5*mg (tartrazine)
    Dexedrine Spansule *Cap:* 5, 10, 15 mg sust-rel
    Dextrostat *Tab:* 5, 10 mg (tartrazine)

▷ *dextroamphetamine saccharate+dextroamphetamine sulfate+amphetamine aspartate+am-phetamine sulfate* (C)(II)(G)
    Adderall initially 10 mg daily; may increase weekly by 10 mg/day; usual max 60 mg/day in 2-3 divided doses; first dose on awakening and then q 4-6 hours prn
    Pediatric: <6 years: not indicated; 6-12 years: initially 5 mg daily; may increase weekly by 5 mg/day; usual max 40 mg/day in 2-3 divided doses; >12 years: same as adult
        Tab: 5**, 7.5**, 10**, 12.5**, 15**, 20**, 30**mg
    Adderall XR
    Pediatric: <6 years: not recommended; 6-12 years: initially 10 mg daily in the AM; may increase by 10 mg weekly; max 30 mg/day; 13-17 years: initially 10 mg daily; may in-crease to 20 mg/day after 1 week; max 30 mg/day; Do not crush or chew; may sprinkle on apple sauce
        Cap: 5, 10, 15, 20, 25, 30 mg ext-rel
    Comment: **Adderall** is also indicated to improve wakefulness in patients with shift-work sleep disorder and excessive sleepiness due to obstructive sleep apnea/hypopnea syndrome.

▷ *dexmethylphenidate* (C)(II)(G) take once daily in the AM
Pediatric: <6 years: not recommended; ≥6 years: same as adult
    Focalin initially 2.5 mg bid; allow at least 4 hours between doses; may increase at 1 week intervals; max 40 mg/day
        Tab: 2.5, 5, 10*mg (dye-free)
    Focalin XR 20-40 mg q AM; max 40 mg/day
        Tab: 5, 10, 15, 20, 30, 40 mg ext-rel (dye-free)

▷ *methylphenidate (regular-acting)* (C)(II)(G)
Pediatric: <6 years: not recommended; ≥6 years: initially 5 mg bid ac (before breakfast and lunch); may gradually increase by 5-10 mg at weekly intervals as needed; max 60 mg/day
    Methylin, Methylin Chewable, Methylin Oral Solution usual dose 20-30 mg/day in 2-3 divided doses 30-45 minutes before a meal; may increase to 60 mg/day
    Ritalin 10-60 mg/day in 2-3 divided doses 30-45 minutes ac; max 60 mg/day
        Tab: 5, 10*, 20*mg

▷ *methylphenidate (long-acting)* (C)(II)
    Concerta initially 18 mg q AM; may increase in 18 mg increments as needed; max 54 mg/day; do not crush or chew
        Tab: 18, 27, 36, 54 mg sust-rel
    Metadate CD (G) 1 cap daily in the AM; may sprinkle on food; do not crush or chew
    Pediatric: <6 years: not recommended; ≥6 years: initially 20 mg daily; may gradually increase by 20 mg/day at weekly intervals as needed; max 60 mg/day
        Cap: 10, 20, 30, 40, 50, 60 mg immed- and ext-rel beads
    Metadate ER 1 tab daily in the AM; do not crush or chew
    Pediatric: <6 years: not recommended; ≥6 years: use in place of regular-acting *meth-ylphenidate* when the 8-hour dose of **Metadate-ER** corresponds to the titrated 8-hour dose of regular-acting *methylphenidate*
        Tab: 10, 20 mg ext-rel (dye-free)
    Ritalin LA 1 cap daily in the AM

Pediatric: <6 years: not recommended; ≥6 years: use in place of regular-acting ***methyl-phenidate*** when the 8-hour dose of **Ritalin LA** corresponds to the titrated 8-hour dose of regular-acting ***methylphenidate***; max 60 mg/day

    Cap: 10, 20, 30, 40 mg ext-rel (immed- and ext-rel beads)

Ritalin SR 1 cap daily in the AM

Pediatric: <6 years: not recommended; ≥6 years: use in place of regular-acting ***methyl-phenidate*** when the 8-hour dose of **Ritalin SR** corresponds to the titrated 8-hour dose of regular-acting ***methylphenidate***; max 60 mg/day

    Tab: 20 mg sust-rel (dye-free)

▷ ***methylphenidate (transdermal patch)*** **(C)(II)(G)** 1 patch daily in the AM

Pediatric: <6 years: not recommended; ≥6 years: initially 10 mg patch daily in the AM; may increase by 5-10 mg/week; max 60 mg/day

    Transdermal patch: 10, 15, 20, 30 mg

▷ ***pemoline*** **(B)(IV)** 18.75-112.5 mg/day; usually start with 37.5 mg in AM; increase weekly by 18.75 mg/day if needed; max 112.5 gm/day

Pediatric: <6 years: not recommended; ≥6 years: same as adult

    Cylert *Tab:* 18.75*, 37.5*, 75*mg

    Cylert Chewable *Chew tab:* 37.5*mg

Comment: Monitor baseline serum ALT and repeat every 2 weeks thereafter.

NAUSEA/VOMITING: CHEMOTHERAPY-INDUCED (CINV)

SUBSTANCE P/NEUROKININ-1 (NK-1) RECEPTOR ANTAGONIST AND SEROTONIN-3 (5-HT3) RECEPTOR ANTAGONIST COMBINATION

▷ ***fosnetupitant*** and ***palonosetron***

Akynzeo capsule: one cap administered approximately 1 hour prior to the start of chemo-therapy, with *or* without food

Akynzeo for injection: one vial reconstituted in 50 ml of D5W *or* 0.9% NS administered as 30-minute IV infusion starting approximately 30 minutes prior to the start of chemotherapy.

Pediatric: <18 years: not established; ≥18 years: same as adult

    Akynzeo *Cap:* 300 mg netu+palo 0.5 mg

    Akynzeo for injection *Vial:* fosnetu 235 mg+palo 0.25 mg, single-dose, pwdr for recon-stitution and IV infusion

    Comment: **Akynzeo for Injection** is indicated in combination with ***dexamethasone*** for the prevention of acute and delayed nausea and vomiting associated with initial and repeat courses of highly emetogenic cancer chemotherapy. **Akynzeo for injection** has not been studied for the prevention of nausea and vomiting associated with ***anthracycline*** plus ***cyclophosphamide*** chemotherapy. **Akynzeo** capsules are indicated in combination with ***dexamethasone*** for prevention of acute and delayed nausea and vomiting associated with initial and repeat courses of cancer chemotherapy, including, but not limited to, highly emetogenic chemotherapy. Avoid in patients with severe hepatic impairment and patients with severe renal disease and end stage renal disease (ESRD). May cause fetal harm.

NAUSEA/VOMITING: POST-ANESTHESIA

Rx ANTIEMETICS

▷ ***ondansetron*** **(C)(G)** 8 mg q 8 hours x 2 doses; then 8 mg q 12 hours

Pediatric: <4 years: not recommended; 4-11 years: 4 mg q 4 hours x 3 doses; then 4 mg q 8 hours

    Zofran *Tab:* 4, 8, 24 mg

    Zofran ODT *ODT:* 4, 8 mg (strawberry) (phenylalanine)

    Zofran Oral Solution *Oral soln:* 4 mg/5 ml (50 ml) (strawberry) (phenyl-alanine); *Parenteral form:* see mfr pkg insert

    Zofran Injection *Vial:* 2 mg/ml (2 ml single-dose); 2 mg/ml (20 ml multi-dose); 32 mg/50 ml (50 ml multi-dose); *Prefilled syringe:* 4 mg/2 ml, single-use (24/carton)

    Zuplenz Oral Soluble Film: 4, 8 mg oral-dis (10/carton) (peppermint)

Comment: The FDA has issued an updated warning against ***ondansetron*** use in pregnancy ***ondansetron*** is a 5-HT3 receptor antagonist approved by the FDA for preventing nausea and vomiting related to cancer chemotherapy and surgery. However, it has been used "off label" to treat the nausea and vomiting of pregnancy. The FDA has cautioned against the use of *ondansetron* in pregnancy in light of studies of *ondansetron* in early pregnancy and associated with congenital cardiac malformations and oral clefts (i.e., cleft lip and cleft palate). Further, there are potential maternal risks in pregnancy with electrolyte imbalance caused by severe nausea and vomiting (as with hyperemesis gravidarum). These risks include serotonin syndrome (a triad of of cognitive and behavioral changes including confusion, agitation, autonomic instability, and neuromuscular changes). Therefore, *ondansetron* should <u>not</u> be taken during pregnancy.

➤ *palonosetron* (B)(G) administer 0.25 mg IV over 30 seconds; max 1 dose/week
  Pediatric: <1 month: not recommended; 1 month to 17 years: 20 mcg/kg; max 1.5 mg/single dose; infuse over 15 minutes beginning 30 minutes
   Aloxi *Vial (single-use):* 0.075 mg/1.5 ml; 0.25 mg/5 ml (mannitol)

➤ *promethazine* (C)(G) 25 mg PO <u>or</u> rectally q 4-6 hours prn
  Pediatric: <2 years: not recommended; ≥2 years: 0.5 mg/lb <u>or</u> 6.25-25 mg q 4-6 hours prn
   Phenergan *Tab:* 12.5*, 25*, 50 mg; *Plain syr:* 6.25 mg/5 ml; *Fortis syr:* 25 mg/5 ml; *Rectal supp:* 12.5, 25, 50 mg

Comment: *promethazine* is contraindicated in children with uncomplicated nausea, dehydration, Reye's syndrome, history of sleep apnea, asthma, and lower respiratory disorders in children. *promethazine* lowers the seizure threshold in children, may cause cholestatic jaundice, anticholinergic effects, extrapyramidal effects, and potentially fatal respiratory depression.

NERVE AGENT POISONING

➤ *atropine sulfate* (G) 2 mg IM
  Pediatric: <15 lb: not recommended; ≥15-40 lb: 0.5 mg IM; ≥40-90 lb: 1 mg IM; >90 lb: same as adult
   AtroPen *Pen (single-use):* 0.5, 1, 2 mg (0.5 ml)

NEUTROPENIA: CHEMOTHERAPY-ASSOCIATED, NEUTROPENIA: FEBRILE, NEUTROPENIA: MYELOSUPPRESSION-ASSOCIATED

LEUKOCYTE GROWTH FACTOR

➤ *pegfilgrastim* <45 kg: see mfr pkg insert for weight-based dosing Table 1; ≥45 kg: *Patients with Cancer receiving Myelosuppressive Chemotherapy:* 6 mg SC once per chemotherapy cycle; do not administer between 14 days before and 24 hours after administration of cytotoxic chemotherapy; *Patients Acutely Exposed to Myelosuppressive Doses of Radiation.* <45 kg: see mfr pkg insert for weight-based dosing table 1; ≥45 kg: 6 mg SC x 2 doses one week apart; administer the first dose as soon as possible after suspected <u>or</u> confirmed exposure to myelosuppressive doses of radiation
   Neulasta *Prefilled syringe:* 6 mg/0.6 ml, single-dose, for manual use only; 6 mg/0.6 ml, single-dose, co-packaged with the on-body *Neulasta Auto-injector*

Comment: *pegfilgrastim* is a leukocyte growth factor, to help reduce the risk/incidence of infection, as manifested by febrile neutropenia, in patients with non-myeloid malignancies receiving myelosuppressive anti-cancer drugs and to increase survival in patients acutely exposed to myelosuppressive doses of radiation (i.e., Hematopoietic Subsyndrome of Acute Radiation Syndrome). **Neulasta** is not indicated for the mobilization of peripheral blood progenitor cells for hematopoietic stem cell transplantation. Warnings and precautions associated with **Neulasta** include fatal splenic rupture, acute respiratory distress syndrome (ARDS), serious allergic reaction/anaphylaxis, allergic reaction to acrylic adhesive (used to attach the autoinjector), fatal sickle cell crisis, glomerulonephritis, on-body injector failure. There are no adequate <u>or</u> well-controlled studies of **Neulasta** use in pregnancy. Based on animal data, may cause fetal harm. It is not known whether *pegfilgrastim* is secreted in human milk. Other recombinant G-CSF products are poorly secreted in breast milk and G-CSF is not orally absorbed by neonates. Caution should be exercised when administered to a nursing female. To report suspected adverse reactions, contact Amgen at 1-800-77-AMGEN (1-800-772-6436) <u>or</u> FDA at 1-800-FDA-1088 <u>or</u> visit www.fda.gov/medwatch.

➤ *pegfilgrastim-jmdb*
   Fulphila *Prefilled syringe:* 6 mg/0.6 ml, single-dose, for manual use only

Comment: **Fulphila** (*pegfilgrastim-jmdb*) is the first biosimilar to **Neulasta** (*pegfilgrastim*). **Fulphila** was approved under the FDA category for biosimilars and demonstrated no clinically meaningful differences for use, dosing regimens, strengths, dosage forms, and routes of administration from the FDA-approved biological product **Neulasta**. See *pegfilgastrim* (**Neulasta**) above for full prescribing information. To report suspected adverse reactions, contact Mylan at 1-877-446-3679 (1-877-4-INFO-RX) or FDA at 1-800-FDA-1088 or visit www.fda.gov/" www.fda.gov/medwatch.

FILGRASTIM PRODUCTS

Comment: *filgrastim* (**Neupogen**) and *filgrastim* biosimilar products (**Nivestym, Zarxio, Granix**) are contraindicated in patients with a prior history of serious allergic reactions to human granulocyte colony-stimulating factors (e.g., *filgrastim*, *pegfilgrastim*). Administration to patients <18 years is not recommended. Direct administration of less than 0.3 ml is not recommended due to potential for dosing errors. Use during pregnancy only if the potential benefit justifies the potential risk to the fetus. It is not known whether *filgrastim* or biosimilar products are excreted in human milk or effects on the breastfed infant. Prior to using *filgrastim* or a *filgrastim* biosimilar product, remove the vial or prefilled syringe from the refrigerator and allow to reach room temperature for a minimum of 30 minutes and a maximum of 24 hours. Discard any vial or prefilled syringe left at room temperature for greater than 24 hours. Visually inspect for particulate matter and discoloration prior to administration (the solution is clear and colorless). Do not administer if particulates or discoloration are observed. Discard any unused portion. Do not re-enter a vial. Inject subcutaneously in the outer area of upper arms, abdomen, thighs, or upper outer areas of the buttock. Patients or caregivers may administer the SC dose after appropriate education and supervised training by a qualified health care provider. For IV infusion, may be diluted in D5%W USP from a concentration of 300 mcg/ml to 5 mcg/ml (do not dilute to a final concentration < 5 mcg/mL). Dilution to concentrations from 5 mcg/ml to 15 mcg/ml should be protected from adsorption to plastic materials by the addition of Albumin (Human) to a final concentration of 2 mg/ml. When diluted in D5%W USP or D5%W plus Albumin (Human), *filgrastim* and *filgrastim* biosimilar products are compatible with glass bottles, polyvinyl chloride (PVC) and polyolefin intravenous bags, and polypropylene syringes. Do not dilute with saline at any time because the product may precipitate. Warnings and precautions include: splenic rupture, acute respiratory distress syndrome (ARDS), serious allergic reaction, sickle cell disorders, glomerulonephritis, alveolar hemorrhage and hemoptysis, capillary leak syndrome (CLS), thrombocytopenia, leukocytosis, cutaneous vasculitis (see mfr pkg insert for detailed discussion of potential ASEs and complications).

▷ *filgrastim*

  Patients with cancer receiving myelosuppressive chemotherapy or induction and/or consol-idation chemotherapy for AML: recommended starting dose is 5 mcg/kg/day via SC injection, short intravenous infusion (over 15-30 minutes), or continuous intravenous infusion; see mfr pkg insert for recommended dosage adjustments and timing of ad-ministration; obtain a complete blood count (CBC) and platelet count before instituting *filgrastim* therapy and monitor twice weekly during therapy; consider dose escalation in increments of 5 mcg/kg for each chemotherapy cycle, according to the duration and severity of the absolute neutrophil count (ANC) nadir; recommend stopping *filgrastim* if the ANC increases beyond 10,000/mm³

  Patients with cancer undergoing bone marrow transplantation: 10 mcg/kg/day via IV infusion over ≤24 hour; see mfr pkg insert for recommended dosage adjustments and timing of administration based on ANC

  Patients undergoing autologous peripheral blood progenitor cell collection and therapy: 10 mcg/kg/day via SC injection; administer for at least 4 days before first leukapheresis procedure and continue until last leukapheresis

  Patients with severe chronic congenital neutropenia: recommended starting dose is 6 mcg/kg via SC injection twice daily

  Patients with cyclic or idiopathic neutropenia: recommended starting dose is 5 mcg/kg via SC injection once daily

  Patients acutely exposed to myelosuppressive doses of radiation (i.e., Hematopoietic Syndrome of Acute Radiation Syndrome [HSARS]): recommended dose is 10 mcg/kg via SC injec-tion once daily for patients exposed to myelosuppressive doses of radiation; administer as soon as possible after suspected or confirmed exposure to radiation doses greater than 2 gray (Gy); estimate a patient's absorbed radiation dose (i.e., level of radiation exposure) based on information from public health authorities, biodosimetry if available, or clinical findings such as time to onset of vomiting or lymphocyte depletion kinetics; obtain a baseline CBC and then serial CBCs approximately every 3rd day until the ANC remains >1,000/mm³ for 3 consecutive CBCs; do not delay administration of *filgrastim* if a CBC is not readily available; continue administration until the ANC remains >1,000/mm³ for 3 consecutive CBCs or exceeds 10,000/mm³ after a radiation-induced nadir

Neupogen *Vial:* 300 mcg/ml (1 ml), 480 mcg/1.6 ml (1.6 ml) single-dose (preservative-free); *Prefilled syringe:* 300 mcg/0.5 ml (0.5 ml), 480 mcg/0.8 ml (0.8 ml) single-dose (preservative-free)

▷ *filgrastim-aafi see* **filgastrim (Neupogen)** above for dosing information

Nivestym *Vial:* 300 mcg/ml (1 ml), 480 mcg/1.6 ml (1.6 ml) single-dose (preservative-free); *Prefilled syringe:* 300 mcg/0.5 ml (0.5 ml), 480 mcg/0.8 ml (0.8 ml) single-dose (preservative-free)

▷ *filgrastim-cbqv* (C) *see* **filgrastim (Neupogen)** above for dosing information

Udenyca *Prefilled syringe:* 6 mg/0.6 ml (0.6 ml) single-dose; the needle cap on the prefilled syringe is not made with natural rubber latex (preservative-free)

▷ *filgrastim-sndz* (C) see *filgrastim* **(Neupogen)** above for dosing information

Zarxio *Vial:* 300 mcg/ml (1 ml), 480 mcg/1.6 ml (1.6 ml) single-dose (preservative-free); Prefilled syringe: 300 mcg/0.5 ml (0.5 ml), 480 mcg/0.8 ml (0.8 ml) single-dose (preservative-free)

▷ *tbo-filgrastim* recommended dose: 5 mcg/kg per day via SC injection; administer the first dose no earlier than 24 hours following myelosuppressive chemotherapy; do not administer within 24 hours prior to chemotherapy

Granix *Prefilled syringe:* 300 mcg/0.5 ml (0.5 ml), 480 mcg/0.8 ml (0.8 ml) single-dose (preservative-free)

Comment: **Granix** *(tbo-filgrastim)* is a leukocyte growth factor indicated for reduction in the duration of severe neutropenia in patients with non-myeloid malignancies receiving myelosuppressive anti-cancer drugs associated with a clinically significant incidence of febrile neutropenia. **Granix** should be used during pregnancy only if the potential benefit justifies the potential risk to the fetus. It is not known if *tbo-filgrastim* is excreted in human milk or effects on the breastfed infant.

NON-24 SLEEP-WAKE DISORDER

Comment: For other drug options (stimulants, sedative hypnotics), *see* **Insomnia** *page* 273 or **Sleepiness: Excessive, Shift Work Sleep Disorder** *page* 464

MELATONIN RECEPTOR AGONIST

▷ *tasimelteon* (C) take 1 gelcap before bedtime at the same time every night; do not take with food

Pediatric: <12 years: not established; ≥12 years: same as adult

Hetlioz *Gel cap:* 20 mg

OREXIN RECEPTOR ANTAGONIST

▷ *suvorexant* (C)(IV) use lowest effective dose; take 30 minutes before bedtime; do not take if unable to sleep for ≥7 hours; max 20 mg

Pediatric: <12 years: not recommended; ≥12 years: same as adult

Belsomra *Tab:* 5, 10, 15, 20 mg (30/blister pck)

OBESITY

Comment: Target BMI is 25-30 (≤27 preferred). Approximately 17% of children and adolescents in the US aged 2 to 19 years are obese. Almost 32% of children and adolescents are either overweight or obese, and the proportion of children with severe obesity continues to rise. Obesity in childhood increases the risk of having obesity as an adult and children with obesity are about 5 times more likely to have obesity as adults than children without obesity. The immediate consequences of childhood obesity include increased incidence of psychological issues, asthma, obstructive sleep apnea, orthopedic problems, high blood pressure, elevated lipid levels, and insulin resistance. The US Preventive Services Task Force (USPSTF) recommends that clinicians screen for obesity in children and adolescents 6 years and older and offer or refer them to comprehensive, intensive behavioral interventions (at least 26 hours of contact) to promote improvements in weight status.

REFERENCE
U.S. Preventive Services Task Force. (2017). Screening for obesity in children and adolescents: US Preventive Services Task Force recommendation statement. *Journal of the American Medical Association*, 317(23), 2417–2426. doi:10.1001/jama.2017.6803

STIMULANTS

▷ *amphetamine sulfate* (C)(II)
  Pediatric: <12 years: not recommended; ≥12 years: same as adult
    Evekeo initially 5 mg 30-60 minutes before meals; usually up to 30 mg/day
      Tab: 5, 10 mg

LIPASE INHIBITOR

▷ *orlistat* (X)(G) 1 cap tid 1 hour before or during each main meal containing fat
  Pediatric: <12 years: not recommended; ≥12 years: same as adult
    Alli (OTC) *Cap:* 60 mg
    Xenical *Cap:* 120 mg
  Comment: For use when BMI >30 kg/m^2 or BMI >27 kg/m^2 in the presence of other risk factors (i.e., HTN, DM, dyslipidemia).

ANOREXIGENICS
Sympathomimetics

Comment: ASEs of sympathomimetics include hypertension, tachycardia, restlessness, insomnia, and dry mouth.

▷ *benzphetamine* (X)(III) initially 25-50 mg daily in the mid-morning or mid-afternoon; may increase to bid-tid as needed
  Pediatric: <12 years: not recommended; ≥12 years: same as adult
    Didrex *Tab:* 50*mg
▷ *naltrexone+bupropion* (X)(G) swallow whole; avoid high-fat meals; initially 10 mg bid; evaluate weight loss after 12 weeks; discontinue if less than 5% weight loss
  Pediatric: <18 years: not recommended; ≥18 years: same as adult
    Contrave *Tab:* nal 8 mg+bup 900 mg ext-rel
▷ *methamphetamine* (C)(II) 10-15 mg q AM
  Pediatric: <12 years: not recommended; ≥12 years: same as adult
    Desoxyn *Tab:* 5, 10, 15 mg sust-rel
▷ *phendimetrazine* (C)(III)
  Pediatric: <12 years: not recommended; ≥12 years: same as adult
    Bontril PDM 35 mg bid-tid 1 hour ac; may reduce to 17.5 mg (1/2 tab)/dose; max 210 mg/day in 3 divided doses
      Tab: 35*mg
    Bontril Slow-Release 105 mg in the AM 30-60 minutes before breakfast
      Cap: 105 mg slow-rel
▷ *phentermine* (X)(IV)(G)
  Pediatric: <16 years: not recommended; ≥16 years: same as adult
    Adipex-P 1 cap or tab before breakfast or 1/2 tab bid ac
      Cap: 37.5 mg; *Tab:* 37.5*mg
    Fastin 1 cap before breakfast
      Cap: 30 mg
    Ionamin 1 cap before breakfast or 10-14 hours prior to HS
      Cap: 15, 30 mg
    Suprenza ODT (X)(IV) dissolve 1 tab on top of tongue once daily in the morning, with or without food; use lowest effective dose
      Tab: 15, 30, 37.5 mg orally-disint
  Comment: Contraindicated with history of cardiovascular disease (e.g., coronary artery disease, stroke, arrhythmias, congestive heart failure, uncontrolled hypertension, during or within 14 days following the administration of an MAOI, hyperthyroidism, glaucoma, agitated states, history of drug abuse, pregnancy, nursing).

Sympathomimetic+Antiepileptic Combination

▶ *phentermine+topiramate ext-rel* (X)(IV)(G) initially 3.75/23 daily in the AM x 14 days; then increase to 7.5/46 and evaluate weight loss on this dose after 12 weeks; if ≤3% weight loss from baseline, discontinue or increase dose to 11.25/69 x 14 days; then increase to 15/92 and evaluate weight loss on this dose after 12 weeks; if ≤5% weight loss from baseline, discontinue by taking a dose every other day for at least one week prior to stopping; max 7.5/46 for moderate to severe renal impairment or moderate hepatic impairment.
Pediatric: <16 years: not established; ≥16 years: same as adult
   Qsymia
      Cap: **Qsymia 3.75/23** phen 3.75 mg+topir 23 mg ext-rel
         Qsymia 7.5/46 phen 7.5 mg+topir 46 mg ext-rel
         Qsymia 11.25/69 phen 11.25 mg+topir 69 mg ext-rel
         Qsymia 15/92 phen 15 mg+topir 92 mg ext-rel
      Comment: Side effects include hypertension, tachycardia, restlessness, insomnia, and dry mouth. Contraindicated with glaucoma, hyperthyroidism, and within 14 days of taking an MAOI. **Qsymia 3.75/23** and **Qsymia 11.25/69** are for titration purposes only.

Serotonin 2C Receptor Agonist

▶ *lorcaserin* (X)(G) 10 mg bid; discontinue if 5% weight loss is not achieved by week 12
Pediatric: <18 years: not recommended; ≥18 years: same as adult
   Belviq *Tab:* 10 mg film-coat
   Comment: **Belviq** is indicated as an adjunct to a reduced-calorie diet and increased physical activity for chronic weight management in adults with an initial body mass index (BMI) of 30 kg/m^2 or greater (obese) or 27 kg/m^2 or greater (over weight) in the presence of at least one weight-related comorbid condition (e.g., hypertension, dyslipidemia, type 2 diabetes). Serotonin 2C receptor agonists interact with serotonergic drugs (selective serotonin reuptake inhibitors (SSRIs), serotonin-norepinephrine reuptake inhibitors (SNRIs), monoamine oxidase inhibitors (MAOIs), triptans, **bupropion**, **dextromethorphan**, **St. John's wort**); therefore, use with extreme caution due to the risk of serotonin syndrome.

GLUCAGON-LIKE PEPTIDE-1 (GLP-1) RECEPTOR AGONIST

▶ *liraglutide* (C) administer SC in the upper arm, abdomen, or thigh once daily; escalate dose gradually over 5 weeks to 3 mg SC daily; *Week 1:* 0.6 mg SC daily; *Week 2:* 1.2 mg SC daily; *Week 3:* 1.8 mg SC daily; *Week 4:* 2.4 mg SC daily; *Week 5:* 3 mg SC daily;
Pediatric: <18 years: not recommended
   Saxenda Soln for SC inj: 6 mg/ml multi-dose prefilled pen (3 ml; 3, 5 pens/carton)
   Comment: **Saxenda** is indicated as an adjunct to a reduced-calorie diet and increased physical activity for chronic weight management in adults with an initial body mass index (BMI) of 30 kg/m^2 or greater (obese) or 27 kg/m^2 or greater over weight) in the presence of at least one weight-related comorbid condition (e.g., hypertension, dyslipidemia, type 2 diabetes). Not indicated for treatment of T2DM. Do not use with **Victoza**, other GLP-1 receptor agonists, or insulin. Contraindicated with personal or family history of medullary thyroid carcinoma (MTC) and multiple endocrine neoplasia syndrome (MENS) type 2. Monitor for signs/symptoms pancreatitis. Discontinue if gastroparesis, renal, or hepatic impairment.

◯ OBSESSIVE-COMPULSIVE DISORDER (OCD)

SELECTIVE SEROTONIN REUPTAKE INHIBITORS (SSRIs)

Comment: Co-administration of SSRIs with TCAs requires extreme caution. Concomitant use of MAOIs and SSRIs is absolutely contraindicated. Avoid other serotonergic drugs. A potentially fatal adverse event is *Serotonin Syndrome*, caused by serotonin excess. Milder symptoms require HCP intervention to avert severe symptoms which can be rapidly fatal without urgent/emergent medical care. Symptoms include restlessness, agitation, confusion, hallucinations, tachycardia, hypertension, dilated pupils, muscle twitching, muscle rigidity, loss of muscle coordination, diaphoresis, diarrhea, headache, shivering, piloerection, hyperpyrexia, cardiac arrhythmias, seizures, loss of consciousness, coma, death. Abrupt withdrawal or interruption of treatment with an antidepressant medication is sometimes associated with an *Antidepressant Discontinuation Syndrome* which may be mediated by gradually tapering the drug over a period of two weeks or longer, depending on the dose strength and length of treatment. Common symptoms of the *Serotonin Discontinuation Syndrome* include flu-like symptoms (nausea, vomiting, diarrhea, headaches, sweating), sleep disturbances (insomnia, nightmares, constant sleepiness), mood disturbances (dysphoria, anxiety, agitation), cognitive disturbances (mental confusion, hyperarousal), sensory and movement disturbances (imbalance, tremors, vertigo, dizziness, electric-shock-like sensations in the brain, often described by sufferers as "brain zaps."

► *fluoxetine* (C)(G)

> **Prozac** initially 20 mg daily; may increase after 1 week; doses >20 mg/day may be divided into AM and noon doses; max 80 mg/day
> *Pediatric:* <8 years: not recommended; 8-17 years: initially 10 mg/day; may increase after 2 weeks to 20 mg/day; range 20-60 mg/day; range for lower weight children 20-30 mg/day; >17: same as adult
> > *Cap:* 10, 20, 40 mg; *Tab:* 30*, 60*mg; *Oral soln:* 20 mg/5 ml (4 oz) (mint)
>
> **Prozac Weekly** following daily *fluoxetine* therapy at 20 mg/day for 13 weeks, may initiate **Prozac Weekly** 7 days after the last 20 mg *fluoxetine* dose
> *Pediatric:* <12 years: not recommended; ≥12 years: same as adult
> > *Cap:* 90 mg ent-coat del-rel pellets

► *fluvoxamine* (C)(G)

> **Luvox** initially 50 mg q HS; adjust in 50 mg increments at 4-7 day intervals; range 100-300 mg/day; over 100 mg/day, divide into 2 doses giving the larger dose at HS
> *Pediatric:* <8 years: not recommended; 8-17 years: initially 25 mg q HS; a just in 25 mg increments q 4-7 days; usual range 50-200 mg/day; over 50 mg/day, divide into 2 doses giving the larger dose at HS
> > *Tab:* 25, 50*, 100*mg
>
> **Luvox CR** initially 100 mg once daily at HS; may increase by 50 mg increments at 1 week intervals; max 300 mg/day; swallow whole; do not crush or chew
> *Pediatric:* <18 years: not recommended; ≥18 years: same as adult
> > *Cap:* 100, 150 mg ext-rel

► *paroxetine maleate* (D)(G)

> *Pediatric:* <12 years: not recommended; ≥12 years: same as adult
> **Paxil** initially 20 mg daily in AM; may increase by 10 mg/day at weekly intervals as needed; max 60 mg/day
> > *Tab:* 10*, 20*, 30, 40 mg
>
> **Paxil CR** initially 25 mg daily in AM; may increase by 12.5 mg at weekly intervals as needed; max 62.5 mg/day
> > *Tab:* 12.5, 25, 37.5 mg cont-rel ent-coat
>
> **Paxil Suspension** initially 20 mg daily in AM; may increase by 10 mg/day at weekly intervals as needed; max 60 mg/day
> > *Oral susp:* 10 mg/5 ml (250 ml) (orange)

► *paroxetine mesylate* (D)(G) initially 7.5 mg daily in AM; may increase by 10 mg/day at weekly intervals as needed; max 60 mg/day

> *Pediatric:* <12 years: not recommended; ≥12 years: same as adult
> **Brisdelle** *Cap:* 7.5 mg

► *sertraline* (C) initially 50 mg daily; increase at 1 week intervals if needed; max 200 mg daily

> *Pediatric:* <6 years: not recommended; 6-12 years: initially 25 mg daily; max 200 mg/day; 13-17 years: initially 50 mg daily; max 200 mg/day; >17 years: same as adult
> > **Zoloft** *Tab:* 15*, 50*, 100*mg; *Oral conc:* 20 mg per ml (60 ml [dilute just before administering in 4 oz water, ginger ale, lemon-lime soda, lemonade, or orange juice]) (alcohol 12%)

TRICYCLIC ANTIDEPRESSANTS (TCAs)

► *clomipramine* (C)(G) initially 25 mg daily in divided doses; gradually increase to 100 mg during first 2 weeks; max 250 mg/day; total maintenance dose may be given at HS

> *Pediatric:* <10 years: not recommended; ≥10 years: initially 25 mg daily in divided doses; gradually increase; max 3 mg/kg or 100 mg, whichever is smaller
> **Anafranil** *Cap:* 25, 50, 75 mg

► *imipramine* (C)(G)

> **Tofranil** initially 75 mg/day; max 200 mg/day
> *Pediatric:* adolescents initially 30-40 mg/day; max 100 mg/day
> > *Tab:* 10, 25, 50 mg

Tofranil PM initially 75 mg/day; max 200 mg/day
Pediatric: <12 years: not recommended; ≥12 years: same as adult
Cap: 75, 100, 125, 150 mg

 ONYCHOMYCOSIS (FUNGAL NAIL)

ORAL AGENTS

▷ *griseofulvin, microsize* (C)(G) 1 gm daily for at least 4 months for fingernails and at least 6 months for toenails
Pediatric: 5 mg/lb/day; *see page* 628 *for dose by weight*
Grifulvin V *Tab:* 250, 500 mg; *Oral susp:* 125 mg/5 ml (120 ml; alcohol 0.02%)
▷ *griseofulvin, ultramicrosize* (C) 750 mg in a single or divided doses for at least 4 months for fingernails and at least 6 months for toenails
Pediatric: <2 years: not recommended; ≥2 years: 3.3 mg/lb in a single or divided doses
Gris-PEG *Tab:* 125, 250 mg
▷ *itraconazole* (C)(G) 200 mg daily x 12 consecutive weeks for toenails; 200 mg bid x 1 week, off 3 weeks, then 200 mg bid x 1 additional week for fingernails
Pediatric: <12 years: not recommended; ≥12 years: same as adult
Sporanox *Cap:* 100 mg; *Soln:* 10 mg/ml (150 ml) (cherry-caramel)
Pulse Pack: 100 mg caps (7/pck)
▷ *terbinafine* (B)(G) 250 mg daily x 6 weeks for fingernails; 250 mg daily x 12 weeks for toenails
Pediatric: <12 years: not recommended; ≥12 years: same as adult
Lamisil *Tab:* 250 mg

TOPICAL AGENTS

Comment: File and trim nail while nail is free from drug. Remove unattached infected nail as frequently as monthly. For use with mild to moderate onychomycosis of the fingernails and toenails, without lunula involvement due to *Trichophyton rubrum* immunocompetent patients as part of a comprehensive treatment program. For use on nails and adjacent skin only. Apply evenly to entire onycholytic nail and surrounding 5 mm of skin daily, preferably at HS or 8 hours before washing; apply to nail bed, hyponychium, and under surface of nail plate when it is free of the nail bed; apply over previous coats, then remove with alcohol once per week; treat for up to 48 weeks.
▷ *ciclopirox* (B)
Pediatric: <12 years: not established; ≥12 years: same as adult
Penlac Nail Lacquer *Topical soln (lacquer):* 8% (6.6 ml w. applicator)
▷ *efinaconazole* (C)
Pediatric: <12 years: not established; ≥12 years: same as adult
Jublia *Topical soln:* 5% (10 ml w. brush applicator)
▷ *tavaborole* (C)
Pediatric: <12 years: not established; ≥12 years: same as adult
Kerydin *Topical soln:* 10% (10 ml w. dropper)

 OPHTHALMIA NEONATORUM: CHLAMYDIAL

PROPHYLAXIS

▷ *erythromycin* ophthalmic ointment 0.5-1 cm ribbon into lower conjunctival sac of each eye x 1 application
Ilotycin Ophthalmic Ointment *Ophth oint:* 5 mg/gm (1/8 oz)
Comment: The following treatment regimens are published in the **2015 CDC Sexually Transmitted Diseases Treatment Guidelines**. Treatment regimens are presented by generic drug name first, followed by information about brands and dose forms.

RECOMMENDED TREATMENT REGIMENS
Regimen 1
▷ *erythromycin base* 50 mg/kg/day in 4 doses x 14 days

Regimen 2

 erythromycin ethylsuccinate 50 mg/kg/day in 4 doses x 14 days; *see page 626 for dose by weight*

DRUG BRANDS AND DOSE FORMS

 erythromycin base (B)(G)
> Ery-Tab *Tab:* 250, 333, 500 mg ent-coat
> PCE *Tab:* 333, 500 mg

Comment: *erythromycin* may increase INR with concomitant *warfarin*, as well as increase serum level of *digoxin,* benzodiazepines, and statins.

 erythromycin ethylsuccinate (B)(G)
> EryPed *Oral susp:* 200 mg/5 ml (100, 200 ml) (fruit); 400 mg/5 ml (60, 100, 200 ml)
> (banana); *Oral drops:* 200, 400 mg/5 ml (50 ml) (fruit); *Chew tab:* 200 mg wafer (fruit)
> E.E.S. *Oral susp:* 200, 400 mg/5 ml (100 ml) (fruit)
> E.E.S. Granules *Oral susp:* 200 mg/5 ml (100, 200 ml) (cherry)

Comment: *erythromycin* may increase INR with concomitant *warfarin*, as well as increase serum level of *digoxin,* benzodiazepines, and statins.

OPHTHALMIA NEONATORUM: GONOCOCCAL

Comment: The following prophylaxis and treatment regimens for gonococcal conjunctivitis is published in the **2015 CDC Sexually Transmitted Diseases Treatment Guidelines.**

PROPHYLAXIS

 erythromycin 0.5% ophthalmic ointment 0.5-1 cm ribbon into lower conjunctival sac of each eye x 1 application
> Ilotycin Ophthalmic Ointment *Ophth oint:* 5 mg/gm (1/8 oz)

TREATMENT

 ceftriaxone (B)(G) 25-50 mg/kg IV or IM in a single dose, not to exceed 125 mg
> Rocephin *Vial:* 250, 500 mg; 1, 2 gm

OPIOID DEPENDENCE, OPIOID USE DISORDER (OUD), OPIOID WITHDRAWAL SYNDROME

Comment: Safety labeling for all immediate-release (IR) opioids has been issued by the FDA. The Black Boxed Warning (BBW) includes serious risks of misuse, abuse, addiction, overdose, and death. The dosing section offers clear steps regarding administration and patient monitoring including initial dose, dose changes, and the abrupt cessation of treatment in physical dependence. Chronic maternal use of opioids during pregnancy can lead to potentially life-threatening neonatal opioid withdrawal. The American Pain Society (APS) has released new evidence-based clinical practice guidelines that include 32 recommendations related to post-op pain management in adults and children. The Transmucosal Immediate Release Fentanyl (TIRF) Risk Evaluation and Mitigation Strategy (REMS) program is an FDA-required program designed to ensure informed risk-benefit decisions before initiating treatment, and while patients are treated to ensure appropriate use of TIRF medicines. The purpose of the TIRF REMS Access program is to mitigate the risk of misuse, abuse, addiction, overdose and serious complications due to medication errors with the use of TIRF medicines. You must enroll in the TIRF REMS Access program to prescribe, dispense, or distribute TIRF medicines. To register, call the TIRF REMS Access program at 1-866-822-1483 or register online at https://www.tirfremsaccess.com/TirfUI/rems/home.action.

SELECTIVE ALPHA 2-ADRENERGIC RECEPTOR AGONIST

Comment: **Lucemyra** *(lofexidine)* is the first FDA-approved non-opioid treatment for the management of opioid withdrawal symptoms, for the mitigation of withdrawal symptoms to facilitate abrupt discontinuation of opioids in adults. While **Lucemyra** may lessen the severity of withdrawal symptoms, it may not completely prevent them. This oral selective alpha 2-adrenergic receptor agonist reduces the release of norepinephrine. The actions of norepinephrine in the autonomic nervous system are believed to play a role in many of the symptoms of opioid withdrawal and is only approved for treatment for up to 14 days.

▶ *lofexidine* (C) 0.18 mg x 3 tabs taken orally 4 x/day at 5-to 6-hour intervals; max 14 days with dosing guided by symptoms; discontinue with a gradual dose reduction over 2 to 4 days

    Pediatric: <17 years: not established; ≥17 years: same as adult

      Lucemyra *Tab:* 0.18 mg

      Comment: **Lucemyra** is not a treatment for Opioid Use Disorder (OUD), per se, but can be used as part of a broader, long-term treatment plan for managing OUD. The most common side effects from treatment with **Lucemyra** include hypotension, bradycardia, somnolence, sedation, and dizziness. **Lucemyra** has also been associated with a few cases of syncope. *methadone* and **Lucymra** both prolong the QT interval. Therefore, ECG monitoring is recommended when used concomitantly. Concomitant use of oral *naltrexone* with **Lucemyra** may reduce efficacy of oral naltrexone. Concomitant use of *paroxetine* has resulted in increased plasma levels of **Lucemyra**. Monitor for symptoms of orthostasis and bradycardia with concomitant use of CYP2D6 inhibitors. The safety of **Lucymra** in pregnant women has not been established. There is no information regarding the presence of **Lucemyra** or its metabolites in human milk or effects on the breastfed infant.

OPIOID AGONISTS

Methadone Detoxification and Methadone Maintenance

Comment: *methadone* is not indicated as an as-needed (prn) analgesic. For use in chronic moderately severe-to-severe pain management (e.g., hospice care).

▶ *methadone* (C)(II)(G) A single dose of 20 to 30 mg may be sufficient to suppress with-drawal syndrome; *Narcotic Detoxification:* 15-40 mg daily in decreasing doses not to exceed 21 days; *Narcotic Maintenance:* >21 days; see mfr pkg insert; clinical stability is most commonly achieved at doses between 80 to 120 mg/day; monitor patients with periodic ECGs (e.g., risk of lethal QT interval prolongation, *torsades de pointes*)

    Pediatric: <12: not recommended; ≥12 years: same as adult

      Dolophine *Tab:* 5, 10 mg; *Dispersible tab:* 40 mg (dissolve in 120 ml orange juice or other citrus drink); *Oral soln:* 5, 10 mg/ml; *Oral conc:* 10 mg/ml; *Syr:* 10 mg/30 ml; *Vial:* 10 mg/ml (200 mg/20 ml multi-dose) for injection

      Comment: *methadone* administration is allowed only by approved providers with strict state and federal regulations (as stipulated in 42 CFR 8.12). Black Box Warning (BBW): *Dolophine* exposes users to risks of addiction, abuse, and misuse, which can lead to overdose and death. Assess each patient's risk and monitor regularly for development of these behaviors and conditions. Serious, life-threatening, or fatal respiratory depression may occur. The peak respiratory depressant effect of *methadone* occurs later, and persists longer than the peak analgesic effect. Accidental ingestion, especially by children, can result in fatal overdose. QT interval prolongation and serious arrhythmia (*torsades de pointes*) have occurred during treatment with *methadone*. Closely monitor patients with risk factors for development of prolonged QT interval, a history of cardiac conduction abnormalities, and those taking medications affecting cardiac conduction. Neonatal Opioid Withdrawal Syndrome (NOWS) is an expected and treatable outcome of use of methadone use during pregnancy. NOWS may be life-threatening if not recognized and treated in the neonate. The balance between the risks of NOWS and the benefits of maternal *methadone* use should be considered and the patient advised of the risk of NOWS so that appropriate planning for management of the neonate can occur. *methadone* has been detected in human milk. Concomitant use with CYP3A4, 2B6, 2C19, 2C9 or 2D6 inhibitors or discontinuation of concomitantly used CYP3A4 2B6, 2C19, or 2C9 inducers can result in a fatal overdose of methadone. Concomitant use of opioids with benzodiazepines or other central nervous system (CNS) depressants, including alcohol, may result in profound sedation, respiratory depression, coma, and death.

OPIOID ANTAGONIST

▶ *naltrexone* (C)

    Pediatric: <12 years: not established; ≥12 years: same as adult

      ReVia 50 mg daily

        Tab: 50 mg

      Vivitrol 380 mg IM once monthly; alternate buttocks

        Vial: 380 mg

OPIOID PARTIAL AGONIST-ANTAGONIST

Comment: **Belbuca, Butrans, Probuphine, Sublocade, and Subutex** maintenance are allowed only by approved providers with strict state and federal regulations. These drugs are potentiated by CYP3A4 inhibitors (e.g., azole antifungals, macrolides, HIV protease inhibitors) and antagonized by CYP3A4 inducers (monitor for opioid withdrawal). Concomitant NNRTIs (e.g., *efavirenz, nevirapine, etravirine, delavirdine*) or PIs (e.g., *atazanavir* with or without *ritonavir*): monitor. Risk of respiratory or CNS depression with concomitant opioid analgesics, general anesthetics, benzodiazepines, phenothiazines, other tranquilizers, sedative/hypnotics, alcohol, or other CNS depressants. Risk of serotonin syndrome with concomitant SSRIs, SNRIs, TCAs, 5-HT3 receptor antagonists, *mirtazapine, trazodone, tramadol,* MAO inhibitors.

▷ **buprenorphine (C)(III)**

Belbuca apply buccal film to inside of cheek; do not chew or swallow; *Opioid naïve:* initially 75 mcg once daily-q 12 hours x at least 4 days; then, increase to 150 mcg q 12 hours; may increase in increments of 150 mcg q 12 hours no sooner than every 4 days; max 900 mcg q 12 hours; see mfr pkg insert for conversion from other opioids; *Severe hepatic impairment or oral mucositis:* reduce initial and titration doses by half
Pediatric: <12 years: not established; ≥12 years: same as adult
 Buccal film: 75, 150, 300, 450, 600, 750, 900 mcg (60/pck) (peppermint)
Butrans Transdermal System apply one patch to clean, dry, hairless, intact skin on the upper outer arm, upper chest, upper back, or side of chest every 7 days; rotate sites and do not re-use a site for at least 21 days; *Opioid naïve or oral morphine <30 mg/day or equivalent:* one 5 mcg/hour patch; *Converting from oral morphine equivalents 30-80 mg/day:* taper current opioids for up to 7 days to ≤30 mg/day oral morphine equivalents before starting; then initiate with 10 mcg/hour patch; may use a short-acting analgesic until efficacy is attained; increase dose only after exposure to previous dose x at least 72 hours; max one 20 mcg/hour patch/week; *Conversion from higher opioid doses:* not recommended
Pediatric: <12 years: not established; ≥12 years: same as adult
 Transdermal patch: 5, 7.5, 10, 15, 20 mcg/hour (4/pck)
Probuphine initiate when stable on *buprenorphine* ≤8 mg/day; insertion site is the inner side of the upper arm; 4 implants are intended to be in place for 6 months; remove the implants by the end of the 6th month and insert four new implants on the same day in the contralateral arm; if a new implant is not inserted on the same day as removal of a previous implant, maintain the patient on the previous dose of transmucosal *buprenorphine* (i.e., the dose from which the patient was transferred to **Probuphine** treatment).
Pediatric: <16 years: not established; ≥16 years: same as adult
 Subdermal implant: 74.2 mg of *buprenorphine* (equivalent to 80 mg of *buprenorphine hydrochloride*)
Comment: Healthcare providers who prescribe, perform insertions and/or perform removals of **Probuphine** must successfully complete a live training program, and demonstrate procedural competency prior to inserting or removing the implants. Further information: visit www.ProbuphineREMS.com or call 1-844-859-6341
Subutex (G) 8 mg in a single dose on day 1; then 16 mg in a single dose on day 2; target dose is 16 mg/day in a single dose; dissolve under tongue; do not chew or swallow whole
Pediatric: <12 years: not established; ≥12 years: same as adult
 SL tab (lemon-lime) or SL film (lime): 2, 8 mg (30/pck)
Sublocade verify that patient is clinically stable on transmucosal *buprenorphine* before initiating *Sublocade*; doses must be prepared by an authorized healthcare provider and administered once monthly only by SC injection in the abdominal region; initially, 300 mg SC once monthly x the first 2 months, followed by 100 mg SC once monthly maintenance dose; increasing the maintenance dose to 300 mg once monthly may be considered for patients in which the benefits outweigh the risks
Pediatric: <12 years: not established; ≥12 years: same as adult
 Prefilled syringe: 100 mg/0.5 ml, 300 mg/1.5 ml sust-rel single-dose w. 19 gauge 5/8-inch needle
Comment: Serious harm or death could result if **Sublocade** is administered intravenously. Neonatal opioid withdrawal syndrome (NOWS) is an expected and treatable outcome of prolonged use of opioids during pregnancy. (Not recommended

with moderate-to-severe hepatic impairment. Monitor liver function tests prior to and during treatment. If diagnosed with adrenal insufficiency, treat with physiologic replacement of corticosteroids, and wean patient off of the opioid. **Sublocade** is only available through the restricted SUBLOCADE REMS Program. Healthcare settings and pharmacies that order and dispense **Sublocade** must be certified in this program. To report suspected adverse reactions, contact Indivior Inc. at 1877-782-6966 or FDA at 1-800-FDA-1088 or www.fda.gov/medwatch.

OPIOID PARTIAL AGONIST-ANTAGONIST+OPIOID ANTAGONIST

Comment: **Bunabail, Cassipa, Suboxone, Sucartonone, Troxyca ER,** and **Zubsolv** maintenance may be prescribed only by Drug Addiction Treatment Act (DATA) Certified Providers with strict state and federal regulations. These drugs are potentiated by CYP3A4 inhibitors (e.g., azole antifungals, macrolides, HIV protease inhibitors) and antagonized by CYP3A4 inducers (monitor for opioid withdrawal). Concomitant NNRTIs (e.g., *efavirenz, nevirapine, etravirine, delavirdine*) or PIs (e.g., *atazanavir* with or without *ritonavir*): monitor. Risk of respiratory or CNS depression with concomitant opioid analgesics, general anesthetics, benzodiazepines phenothiazines, other tranquilizers, sedative/ hypnotics, alcohol, or other CNS depressants. Risk of serotonin syndrome with concomitant SSRIs, SNRIs, TCAs, 5-HT3 receptor antagonists, *mirtazapine, trazodone, tramadol,* MAO inhibitors. *buprenorphine/naloxone* products are not recommended in patients with severe hepatic impairment and may not be appropriate for patients with moderate hepatic impairment. *buprenorphine* passes into human breast milk. Neonatal opioid withdrawal syndrome may occur in newborn infants of mothers who are receiving treatment with *buprenorphine.*

▷ *buprenorphine+naloxone* (C)(III)(G)

Bunavail administer one buccal film once daily at the same time each day; target dose is 8.4/1.4 once daily; place the side of the **Bunavail** film with the text (BN2, BN4, or BN6) against the inside of the cheek; press and hold the film in place for 5 seconds; maintenance is usually 2.1/0.3 to 12.6/2.1 once daily

Pediatric: <16 years: not recommended; ≥16 years: same as adult

SL film:
Bunavail 2.1/0.3 bup 2.1 mg+nal 0.3 mg (30/carton)
Bunavail 4.2/0.7 bup 4.2 mg+nal 0.7 mg (30/carton)
Bunavail 6.3/1 bup 6.3 mg+nal 1 mg (30/carton)

Comment: One **Bunavail** 4.2/0.7 mg buccal film provides equivalent *buprenorphine* exposure to a **Sucartonone** 8/2 mg sublingual tablet. **Cassipa** place one film under the tongue, close to the base on the left or right side, and allow to completely dissolve as a single daily dose; initiate only after induction and stabilization of the patient, and the patient has been titrated to a dose of 16 mg *buprenorphine* using another marketed product; do not cut, chew, or swallow whole

Pediatric: <12 years: not recommended; ≥12 years: adjust in 2-4 mg of *buprenorphine*

SL film:
Cassipa 16/4 bupre 16 mg+nalox 4 mg

Suboxone (G) adjust dose in increments/decrements of 2/0.5 or 4/1 once daily *buprenorphine+naloxone,* based on the patient's daily dose of *buprenorphine,* to a level that suppresses opioid withdrawal signs and symptoms; *Recommended target dosage:* 16/4 as a single daily dose; *Maintenance dose:* generally in the range of 4/1 to 24/6 per day; higher once daily doses have not been demonstrated to provide any clinical advantage

Pediatric: <12 years: not established; ≥12 years: same as adult

Suboxone

SL tab, SL film: **Suboxone 2/0.5** bup 2 mg+nal 0.5 mg (30/bottle) (lime)
Suboxone 4/1 bup 4 mg+nal 1 mg (30/bottle) (lime)
Suboxone 8/2 bup 8 mg+nal 2 mg (30/bottle) (lime)
Suboxone 12/3 bup 12 mg+nal 3 mg (30/bottle) (lime)

Sucartonone adjust in 2-4 mg of *buprenorphine*/day in a single dose; usual range is 4-24 mg/day in a single dose; target dose is 6 mg/day in a single dose; dissolve under tongue; do not chew or swallow whole

Pediatric: <16 years: not recommended; ≥16 years: same as adult

Sucartonone

SL film: **Sucartonone 2/0.5** bup 2 mg+nal 0.5 mg (30/pck) (lime)
Sucartonone 4/1 bup 4 mg+nal 1 mg (30/pck) (lime)
Sucartonone 8/2 bup 8 mg+nal 2 mg (30/pck) (lime)
Sucartonone 12/3 bup 12 mg+nal 3 mg (30/pck) (lime)

Zubsolv initial induction with buprenorphine sublingual tabs; administer as a single dose once daily; titrate dose in increments of 1.4/0.36 or 2.9/0.72 per day; recommended target dose is 11.4/2.9 per day; usual max 17.2/4.2 per day
Pediatric: <16 years: not recommended; ≥16 years: same as adult
  Zubsolv
  SL tab: **Zubsolv 1.4/0.36** bup 1.4 mg+nal 0.36 mg
  Zubsolv 2.9/0.72 bup 2.9 mg+nal 0.71 mg
  Zubsolv 5.7/1.4 bup 5.7 mg+nal 1.4 mg
  Zubsolv 8.6/2.1 bup 8.6 mg+nal 2.1 mg
  Zubsolv 11.4/2.9 bup 11.4 mg+nal 2.9 mg
  Comment: One **Subutex 5.7/1.4** SL tab is bioequivalent to one **Sucartonone 8/2** SL film.

▷ *oxycodone+naloxone* (C)(II) *Opioid-naïve and opioid non-tolerant:* initially 10/1.2 q 12 hours; *Opioid tolerant:* single doses greater than 40/4.8, or a total daily dose greater than 80/9.6 are only for use in patients for whom tolerance to an opioid of comparable potency has been established; swallow whole, or sprinkle contents on applesauce and swallow immediately without chewing
Pediatric: <18 years: not recommended; ≥18 years: same as adult
  Troxyca ER
  Cap: **Troxyca ER 10/1.2** oxy 10 mg+nalox 1.2 mg ext-rel
  Troxyca ER 20/1.2 oxy 20 mg+nalox 2.4 mg ext-rel
  Troxyca ER 30/1.2 oxy 30 mg+nalox 3.6 mg ext-rel
  Troxyca ER 40/1.2 oxy 40 mg+nalox 4.8 mg ext-rel
  Troxyca ER 60/1.2 oxy 60 mg+nalox 7.2 mg ext-rel
  Troxyca ER 80/1.2 oxy 80 mg+nalox 9.6 mg ext-rel

Comment: Opioid tolerant patients are those taking, for one week or longer, at least 60 mg oral *morphine* per day, 25 mcg transdermal *fentanyl* per hour, 30 mg oral *oxycodone* per day, 8 mg oral *hydromorphone* per day, 25 mg oral *oxymorphone* per day, 60 mg oral *hydrocodone* per day, or an equianalgesic dose of another opioid.

SELECTIVE ALPHA 2-ADRENERGIC RECEPTOR AGONIST

Comment: **Lucemyra** *(lofexidine)* is the first FDA-approved non-opioid treatment for the management of opioid withdrawal symptoms, for the mitigation of withdrawal symptoms to facilitate abrupt discontinuation of opioids in adults. While **Lucemyra** may lessen the severity of withdrawal symptoms, it may not completely prevent them. This oral selective alpha 2-adrenergic receptor agonist reduces the release of norepinephrine. The actions of norepinephrine in the autonomic nervous system are believed to play a role in many of the symptoms of opioid withdrawal and is only approved for treatment for up to 14 days.

▷ *lofexidine* (C) 0.18 mg x 3 tabs taken orally 4 x/day at 5-to 6-hour intervals; max 14 days with dosing guided by symptoms; discontinue with a gradual dose reduction over 2 to 4 days.
Pediatric: <17 years: not recommended; ≥17 years: same as adult
  Lucemyra *Tab:* 0.18 mg
  Comment: **Lucemyra** is not a treatment for Opioid Use Disorder (OUD), per se, but can be used as part of a broader, long-term treatment plan for managing OUD. The most common side effects from treatment with **Lucemyra** include hypotension, bradycardia, somnolence, sedation, and dizziness. **Lucemyra** has also been associated with a few cases of syncope. *methadone* and **Lucymra** both prolong the QT interval. Therefore, ECG monitoring is recommended when used concomitantly. Concomitant use of oral *naltrexone* with **Lucemyra** may reduce efficacy of oral naltrexone. Concomitant use of *paroxetine* has resulted in increased plasma levels of **Lucemyra**. Monitor for symptoms of orthostasis and bradycardia with concomitant use of CYP2D6 inhibitors. The safety of **Lucymra** in pregnant women has not been established. There is no information regarding the presence of **Lucemyra** or its metabolites in human milk or effects on the breastfed infant.

OPIOID-INDUCED CONSTIPATION (OIC)

► *lubiprostone* (C) swallow whole; take with food and water; initially 24 mcg bid; *Moderate hepatic impairment (Child Pugh Class B):* 16 mg bid; *Severe hepatic impairment (Child Pugh Class C):* 8 mg bid

Amitiza *Cap:* 8, 24 mg

Comment: **Amitiza** increases intestinal fluid and intestinal transit time. Suspend dosing and rehydrate if severe diarrhea occurs. **Amitiza** is contraindicated with known or suspected mechanical GI obstruction. Most common adverse reactions in CIC are nausea, diarrhea, headache, abdominal pain, abdominal distension, and flatulence .

► *methylnaltrexone bromide* (C) one oral dose or one weight-based SC dose every other day as needed; max one dose per 24 hours; administer SC inject into the upper arm, abdomen, or thigh; rotate sites

Chronic Non-cancer Pain: 450 mg po once daily in the morning (take with water on an empty stomach at least 30 minutes before the first meal of the day) or 12 mg SC once daily in the morning; *Severe Hepatic Impairment:* <38 kg: 0.075 mg/kg; 38-<62 kg: 4 mg (0.2 ml); 62-114 kg: 6 mg (0.3 ml); >114 kg: 0.075 mg/kg

Advanced Illness, Receiving Palliative Care: <38 kg: 0.15 mg/kg; 38-<62 kg: 8 mg (0.4 ml); 62-114 kg: 12 mg (0.6 ml); >114 kg: 0.15 mg/kg; *Moderate and Severe Renal Impairment (CrCl<60 mL/min):* <38 kg: 0.075 mg/kg; 38-<62 kg: 4 mg (0.2 ml); 62-114 kg: 6 mg (0.3 ml); >114 kg: 0.075 mg/kg

Pediatric: <18 years: not established; ≥18 years: same as adult

Relistor *Tab:* 150 mg film-coat; *Vial:* 12 mg single-dose (0.6 ml, 7/carton)

Relistor Injection: *Prefilled syringe:* 8 mg (0.4 ml), 12 mg (0.6 ml) (7/carton)

Comment: **Relistor** injection is indicated for patients with advanced illness or pain caused by active cancer who require opioid dosage escalation for palliative care. Relistor is an opioid antagonist indicated for the treatment of opioid-induced constipation (OIC) in adult patients with chronic non-cancer pain, including patients with chronic pain related to prior cancer or its treatment who do not require frequent (e.g., weekly) opioid dosage escalation. *methylnaltrexone* is a selective antagonist of opioid binding at the mu-opioid receptor in the gut. As a quaternary amine, the ability of *methylnaltrexone* to cross the blood-brain barrier is restricted. This allows *methylnaltrexone* to function as a peripherally-acting mu-opioid receptor antagonist in tissues such as the gastrointestinal tract, thereby decreasing the constipating effects of opioids without impacting opioid-mediated analgesic effects on the central nervous system. The pre-filled syringe is only for patients who require a **Relistor** injection dose of 8 mg or 12 mg. Use the vial for patients who require other doses. **Relistor** is contraindicated with known or suspected GI obstruction and patients at increased risk of recurrent obstruction, due to the potential for gastrointestinal perforation. Be within close proximity to toilet facilities once **Relistor** is administered. Discontinue all maintenance laxative therapy prior to initiation. Laxative(s) can be used as needed if there is a suboptimal response after three days. Discontinue if treatment with the opioid pain medication is also discontinued. Safety and effectiveness of **Relistor** have not been established in pediatric patients. Avoid concomitant use with other opioid antagonists because of the potential for additive effects of opioid receptor antagonism and increased risk of opioid withdrawal symptoms (sweating, chills, diarrhea, abdominal pain, anxiety, and yawning). Advise females of reproductive potential, who become pregnant or are planning to become pregnant, that the use of **Relistor** during pregnancy may precipitate opioid withdrawal in a fetus due to the undeveloped blood-brain barrier. Breastfeeding is not recommended during treatment.

► *naldemedine* (C) <12 years: not established; ≥12 years: take one tab once daily; take with or without food; discontinue if opioid pain therapy discontinued

Pediatric: <12 years: not established; ≥12 years: same as adult

Symproic *Tab:* 0.2 mg

Comment: **Symproic** is contraindicated with known or suspected GI obstruction and patients at increased risk for recurrent obstruction. Avoid with severe hepatic impairment (Child-Pugh Class C). Not recommended in pregnancy and breastfeeding (during and 3 days after final dose). There is risk of perforation in persons with conditions associated with reduction in structural integrity the GI tract wall (e.g., peptic ulcer disease [PUD], Ogilvie's syndrome, diverticulitis disease, infiltrative GI tract malignancies, or peritoneal metastases).

► *naloxegol* (C) swallow whole; take on an empty stomach; initially 25 mg once daily in the AM; discontinue other laxatives; *CrCl <60 mL/min:* 12.5 mg

Pediatric: <12 years: not established; ≥12 years: same as adult

>   **Movantik** *Tab:* 12.5, 25 mg

>   Comment: **Movantik** is an opioid antagonist indicated for the treatment of opioid-induced constipation (OIC) in adult patients with chronic non-cancer pain, including patients with chronic pain related to prior cancer or treatment who do not require frequent (e.g., weekly) opioid dosage escalation. Alteration in analgesic dosing regimen prior to starting **Movantik** is not required. Patients receiving opioids for less than 4 weeks may be less responsive to **Movantik**. Take on an empty stomach at least 1 hour prior to the first meal of the day or 2 hours after the meal. For patients who are unable to swallow the **Movantik** tablet whole, the tablet can be crushed and given orally or administered via nasogastric tube (see full prescribing information). Avoid consumption of grapefruit or grapefruit juice. Discontinue if treatment with the opioid pain medication is also discontinued.

OPIOID-INDUCED NAUSEA/VOMITING (OINV)

Comment: Opioid analgesics bind to μ (mu), κ (kappa), or δ (delta) opioid receptors in the brain, spinal cord, and digestive tract. However, opioids cause adverse effects that may interfere with their therapeutic use. Opioid-induced nausea/vomiting (OINV) treatment options include serotonin receptor antagonists, dopamine receptor antagonists, and neurokinin-1 receptor antagonists.

SEROTONIN RECEPTOR ANTAGONISTS

▷ *dolasetron* **(B)** administer 100 mg IV over 30 seconds; max 100 mg/dose
Pediatric: <2 years: not recommended; 2-16 years: 1.8 mg/kg; >16 years: same as adult
>   **Anzemet** *Tab:* 50, 100 mg; *Amp:* 12.5 mg/0.625 ml; *Prefilled carpuject syringe:* 12.5 mg (0.625 ml); *Vial:* 100 mg/5 ml (single-use); *Vial:* 500 mg/25 ml (multi-dose)

▷ *granisetron*
>   **Kytril (B)** administer IV over 30 seconds, 30 min; max 1 dose/week
>   *Pediatric:* <2 years: not recommended; ≥2 years: 10 mcg/kg
>   > *Tab:* 1 mg; *Oral soln:* 2 mg/10 ml (30 ml; orange); *Vial:* 1 mg/ml (1 ml single-dose) (preservative-free); 1 mg/ml (4 ml multi-dose) (benzyl alcohol)
>   **Sancuso (B)** apply 1 patch 24-48 hours before chemo; remove 24 hours (minimum) to 7 days (maximum) after completion of treatment
>   *Pediatric:* <12 years: not recommended; ≥12 years: same as adult
>   > *Transdermal patch:* 3.1 mg/day

▷ *ondansetron* **(C)(G)** 8 mg q 8 hours x 2 doses; then 8 mg q 12 hours
Pediatric: <4 years: not recommended; 4-11 years: 4 mg q 4 hours x 3 doses; then 4 mg q 8 hours
>   **Zofran** *Tab:* 4, 8, 24 mg
>   **Zofran ODT** *ODT:* 4, 8 mg (strawberry) (phenylalanine)
>   **Zofran Oral Solution** *Oral soln:* 4 mg/5 ml (50 ml) (strawberry) (phenylalanine); *Parenteral form:* see mfr pkg insert
>   **Zofran Injection** *Vial:* 2 mg/ml (2 ml single-dose); 2 mg/ml (20 ml multi-dose); 32 mg/50 ml (50 ml multi-dose); *Prefilled syringe:* 4 mg/2 ml, single-use (24/carton)
>   **Zuplenz Oral Soluble Film:** 4, 8 mg oral-dis (10/carton) (peppermint)

>   Comment: The FDA has issued an updated warning against *ondansetron)* use in pregnancy *ondansetron* is a 5-HT3 receptor antagonist approved by the FDA for preventing nausea and vomiting related to cancer chemotherapy and surgery. However, it has been used "off label" to treat the nausea and vomiting of pregnancy. The FDA has cautioned against the use of *onzansetron* in pregnancy in light of studies of *ondansetron* in early pregnancy and associated with congenital cardiac malformations and oral clefts (i.e., cleft lip and cleft palate). Further, there are potential maternal risks in pregnancy with electrolyte imbalance caused by severe nausea and vomiting (as with hyperemesis gravidarum). These risks include serotonin syndrome (a triad of cognitive and behavioral changes including confusion, agitation, autonomic instability, and neuromuscular changes). Therefore, *ondansetron* should not be taken during pregnancy.

▷ *palonosetron* **(B)(G)** administer 0.25 mg IV over 30 seconds; max 1 dose/week
Pediatric: <1 month: not recommended; 1 month to 17 years: 20 mcg/kg; max 1.5 mg/single dose; infuse over 15 minutes
>   **Aloxi** *Vial (single-use):* 0.075 mg/1.5 ml; 0.25 mg/5 ml (mannitol)

DOPAMINE RECEPTOR ANTAGONISTS

▷ *prochlorperazine* (C)(G)

Compazine 5-10 mg tid-qid prn; usual max 40 mg/day
Pediatric: <2 years or <20 lb: not recommended; 20-29 lb: 2.5 mg daily bid prn; max 7.5 mg/day; 30-39 lb: 2.5 mg bid-tid prn; max 10 mg/day; 40-85 lb: 2.5 mg tid or 5 mg bid prn; max 15 mg/day
  Tab: 5, 10 mg; *Syr:* 5 mg/5 ml (4 oz) (fruit)
Compazine Suppository 25 mg rectally bid prn; usual max 50 mg/day
Pediatric: <2 years or <20 lb: not recommended; 20-29 lb: 2.5 mg daily-bid prn; max 7.5; mg/day; 30-39 lb: 2.5 mg bid-tid prn; max 10 mg/day; 40-85 lb: 2.5 mg tid or 5 mg bid prn; max 15 mg/day
  Rectal supp: 2.5, 5, 25 mg
Compazine Injectable 5-10 mg tid or qid prn
Pediatric: <2 years or <20 lb: not recommended; ≥2 years or ≥20 lb: 0.06 mg/kg x 1 dose
  Vial: 5 mg/ml (2, 10 ml)
Compazine Spansule 15 mg q AM prn or 10 mg q 12 hours prn usual max 40 mg/day
Pediatric: <12 years: not recommended; ≥12 years: same as adult
  Spansule: 10, 15 mg sust-rel

NEUROKININ-1 RECEPTOR ANTAGONISTS

▷ *aprepitant* (B)(G) administer with 5HT-3 receptor antagonist; *Day 1:* 125 mg; *Day 2 & 3:* 80 mg in the morning
Pediatric: <6 months: years: not recommended; ≥6 months: use oral suspension (see mfr pkg insert for dose by weight
  Emend *Cap:* 40, 80, 125 mg (2 x 80 mg bi-fold pck; 1 x 25 mg/2 x 80 mg tri-fold pck); *Oral susp:* 125 mg pwdr for oral suspension, single-dose pouch w. dispenser; *Vial:* 150 mg pwdr for reconstitution and IV infusion

 OPIOID OVERDOSE

OPIOID ANTAGONISTS

▷ *nalmefene* (B) initially 0.25 mcg/kg IV, IM, or SC, then incremental doses of 0.25 mcg/kg at 2-5 minute intervals; cumulative max 1 mcg/kg; if opioid dependency suspected use 0.1 mg/70 kg initially and then proceed as usual if no response in 2 minutes
Pediatric: not recommended
  Revex *Amp:* 100 mcg/ml (1 ml); 1 mg/ml (2 ml)
▷ *naloxone* (B)(G) 0.4-2 mg; repeat in 2-3 minutes if no response
Pediatric: 0.01 mg/kg initially, repeat in 2-3 minutes at 0.1 mg/kg if response inadequate
  Evzio *Prefilled autoinjector:* 0.4 mg/0.4, 2 mg/0.4 ml IM/SC only
  Comment: **Evzio** 2 mg/0.4 ml comes with 2 autoinjectors and one trainer. This strength is indicated for the emergency treatment of known or suspected opioid overdose manifested by CNS depression.
  If the electronic voice instruction system does not operate properly, **Evzio** will still deliver the intended dose of *naloxone* when used according to the printed instructions on the flat surface of the autoinjector label. **Evzio** cannot be administered IV. Due to the short duration of action of naloxone, as compared to opioids which are longer acting, monitoring of the patient is critical as the opioid reversal effects of naloxone may wear off before the effects of the opioid.
  Narcan *Vial/Amp:* 0.4 mg/ml (1 ml), 1 mg/ml (2 ml); *Prefilled syringe:* 0.4 mg/ml (1 ml), 1 mg/ml (2 ml) IV, IM, or SC (parabens-free)
  Narcan Nasal Spray position supine with head tilted back; 1 spray in one nostril; if an additional dose is needed, spray into the opposite nostril
    Nasal spray: 4 mg/0.1 ml, single-dose (2 blister pcks, each w a single nasal spray/carton)

ORGAN TRANSPLANT REJECTION PROPHYLAXIS (OTRP)

SELECTIVE IMMUNOMODULATORY AGENTS

Comment: Selective immunosuppressive agents are drugs that suppress the immune system due to a selective point of action. They are used to reduce the risk of rejection in organ transplants, in autoimmune diseases, and can be used as cancer chemotherapy. As immunosuppressive agents lower the immunity, there is increased risk of infection.

CHIMERIC (MURINE/HUMAN) MONOCLONAL ANTIBODY

▶ *basiliximab* (B) recommended regimen is two doses of 20 mg each; the first 20-mg dose should be administered within 2 hours prior to transplantation surgery; the second dose should be administered 4 days after transplantation; the second dose should be withheld if complications such as severe hypersensitivity reactions to **Simulect** or graft loss occurs
Pediatric: <35 kg: two doses of 10 mg each; *≥35 kg:* two doses of 20 mg each; the first dose should be administered within 2 hours prior to transplantation surgery; the second dose should be administered 4 days after transplantation; the second dose should be withheld if complications such as severe hypersensitivity reactions to **Simulect** or graft loss occurs
  Simulect *Vial:* 10, 20 mg (6 ml) for reconstitution and IV infusion (presservative-free 10 mg vial: contains 10 mg *basiliximab*, 3.61 mg monobasic potassium phosphate, 0.50 mg disodium hydrogen phosphate (anhydrous), 0.80 mg sodium chloride, 10 mg sucrose, 40 mg mannitol, 20 mg glycine, to be reconstituted in 2.5 ml of sterile water for injection, USP 20 mg *vial; contains* 20 mg *basiliximab*, 7.21 mg monobasic potassium phosphate, 0.99 mg disodium hydrogen phosphate (anhydrous), 1.61 mg sodium chloride, 20 mg sucrose, 80 mg mannitol and 40 mg glycine, to be reconstituted in 5 ml of sterile water for injection

INOSINE MONOPHOSPHATE DEHYDROGENASE (IMPDH) INHIBITOR)

▶ *mycophenolate mofetil (MMF)* (D) <3 years: not recommended: 3 months-18 years: recommended dose of **CellCept** oral suspension is 600 mg/m2 administered bid (up to total max 2 gm daily); patients with BSA 1.25 m2 to 1.5 m2 may be dosed with **CellCept** capsules at 750 mg bid (total 1.5 gm daily); patients with BSA >1.5 m2 may be dosed with **CellCept** capsules or tablets at 1 gm bid (total 2 gm daily); >18 years: 1.5 gm bid orally (total 3 gm daily) or via IV infusion (infuse over no less than 2 hours; do not administer by bolus or rapid infusion)
  CellCept *Cap:* 250 mg; *Cap:* 500 mg; *Oral susp:* 200 mg/ml (225 ml) after reconstitution w bottle adapter and 2 oral dispensers; *Vial:* 500 mg MMF hcl for IV infusion after reconstitution and dilution in D5W
  Comment: **CellCept** (*mycophenolate mofetil, MMF*)) is the 2-morpholinoethyl ester of mycophenolic acid (MPA), an inosine monophosphate dehydrogenase (IMPDH) inhibitor. MMF has been demonstrated in experimental animal models to prolong the survival of allogeneic transplants (kidney, heart, liver, intestine, limb, small bowel, pancreatic islets, and bone marrow). MMF has demonstrated teratogenic effects in humans; however, there are no adequate and well-controlled studies in pregnancy. Females of reproductive potential must be made aware of the increased risk of first trimester pregnancy loss and congenital malformations and must be counseled regarding pregnancy prevention and planning. To prevent unplanned exposure during pregnancy, females of reproductive potential should have a serum or urine pregnancy test with a sensitivity of at least 25 mIU/ml immediately before starting **CellCept**, repeated testing 8 to 10 days later and during routine follow-up visits. In the event of a positive pregnancy test, females should be counseled with regard to maternal-fetal risk/benefit. Animal studies have shown mycophenolic acid to be excreted in milk. It is not known whether MMF is excreted in human milk. Because of the potential for serious adverse reactions in breastfed infants from MMF exposure, risk/benefit of breastfeeding should be discussed with the patient.

Mammalian Target of Rapamycin (mTOR) Inhibitors (mTORi)

Comment: The most frequently occurring adverse events associated with mTOR inhibitors (≥30%) include aphthous stomatitis, rash, anemia, fatigue, hyperglycemia, hypertriglyceridemia, hypercholesterolemia, decreased appetite, nausea, diarrhea, abdominal pain, headache, peripheral edema, hypertension, increased serum creatinine, fever, urinary tract infection, arthralgia, pain, thrombocytopenia, and interstitial lung disease. There are no adequate and well-controlled studies in pregnant females. Effective contraception must be initiated before mTORi therapy, continued during therapy, and for 12 weeks after therapy has been stopped. It is not known whether *serolimus*-based drugs are excreted in human milk. The pharmacokinetic and safety profiles in breastfed infants are not known; therefore, a decision should be made whether to discontinue nursing or to discontinue the drug, taking into account the importance of the drug to the mother.

▶ *everolimus* (C)(G) administer consistently with or without food at the same time as *cyclosporine* or *tacrolimus*; monitor *everolimus* concentrations: adjust just maintenance dose to achieve trough concentrations within the 3-8 ng/mL target range (using LC/MS/MS assay method); *Mild hepatic impairment:* reduce initial daily dose by one-third; *Moderate or severe hepatic impairment:* reduce initial daily dose by one-half *Kidney Transplant:* indicated for patients at low-moderate immunologic risk; use in combination with *basiliximab*, *cyclosporine* (reduced doses), and *corticosteroids;* starting dose is 0.75 mg bid; initiate as soon as possible after transplantation *Liver Transplant:* use in combination with *tacrolimus* (reduced doses) and *corticosteroids*; starting dose is 1.0 mg bid; initiate 30 days after transplantation

  Pediatric: <18 years: not established/not recommended; ≥18 years: same as adult
     Zortress *Tab:* 0.25, 0.5, 0.75 mg

  Comment: To report suspected adverse reactions, contact Novartis Pharmaceuticals Corporation at 1-888-669-6682 or FDA at 1-800-FDA1088 or www.fda.gov/medwatch.

▶ *serolimus* (C)
  Generic: (for prescribing information, *see* **Rapamune**)
     Tab: 1, 2 mg

     Rapamune administer consistently with or without food at the same time as *cyclosporine (CsA) Low to moderate-immunologic risk: Day 1:* 6 mg as a single loading dose; *Day 2:* initiate 2 mg once daily maintenance; use initially with *cyclosporine* (CsA) and *corticosteroids*; initiate CsA withdrawal over 4-8 weeks beginning 2-4 months post-transplantation *High-immunologic risk: Day 1:* up to 15 mg as a single loading dose; *Day 2:* initiate 5 mg once daily maintenance; use with CsA for the first 12 months post-transplantation

  Pediatric: <13 years: not established/not recommended; ≥13 years: same as
     Tab: 0.5, 1, 2, mg; *Oral soln:* 60 mg/60 ml in amber glass bottle, one oral syringe adapter for fitting into the neck of the bottle, sufficient disposable amber oral syringes and caps for daily dosing, and a carrying case; bottles should be stored protected from light and refrigerated at 2°C to 8°C (36°F to 46°F); once the bottle is opened, the contents should be used within one month; If necessary, bottles may be stored the bottles at room temperatures up to 25°C (77°F) for a short period of time (not more than 15 days)

  Comment: To report suspected adverse reactions, contact Pfizer at 1-800-438-1985 or FDA at 1-800-FDA-1088 or www.fda.gov/medwatch.

CALCINEURIN-INHIBITOR IMMUNOSUPPRESSANTS

Comment: *tacrolimus* products are available in immediate-release (capsule, granules, parenteral form for IV administration) and extended-release tablet form, The forms are not interchangeable. Consider dose reduction or discontinuation in the event of myocardial hypertrophy and discontinue in the event of pure red cell aplasia. Avoid live vaccines during treatment with *tacrolimus*. Monitor for new onset diabetes after transplant. Monitor for acute and/or chronic nephrotoxicity and consider dosage reduction with concomitant nephrotoxic drugs and/or neurotoxic drugs. The most common adverse reactions (incidence 10-15%) have included diarrhea, constipation, anemia, UTI, hypertension, tremor, peripheral edema, hyperkalemia, diabetes mellitus, and headache. Monitor for hypertension, hyperkalemia, other abnormal electrolytes, and QT prolongation. Data from post-marketing surveillance and the TPRI suggest that infants exposed to *tacrolimus in utero* are at risk for prematurity, birth defects/congenital anomalies, low birthweight, and fetal distress. Risk/benefit to mother and infant should be considered. Adult organ recipients and parents of pediatric organ recipients should be encouraged to enroll in The Transplant Pregnancy Registry International (TPRI) by calling 1-877-955-6877 or visiting www.transplantpregnancyregistry.org. Controlled lactation studies have not been conducted in humans; however, *tacrolimus* has been reported in human breast milk and effects on the breastfed infant are unknown. Risk/benefit of maternal health and infant health should be discussed. To report suspected adverse reactions, contact Astellas Pharma US at 1-800-727-7003 or FDA at 1-800-FDA-1088 or visit www.fda.gov/medwatch.

▶ *tacrolimus* see mfr pkg insert for dosing table; dosing is based on: patient age (<18 years or ≥18 years), organ transplanted, whether concomitant with *azathioprine* or MMF/IL-2 receptor antagonist, dosage formulation, whole blood trough concentration range in ng/mL, and specific months in the treatment schedule; see the mfr pkg insert also for dosage adjustments for African-American patients, hepatic and patients with hepatic and/or renal impairment

Envarsus XR take once daily on an empty stomach at the same time of day, preferably in the morning

	Initial Oral Dose	Whole Blood Trough Concentration Range
De novo kidney transplantation with antibody induction	0.14 mg/kg/day	Month 1: 6-11 ng/mL >Month 1: 4-11 ng/mL
Conversion from *tacrolimus* immediate-release formulation	80% of the preconversion dose of *tacrolimus* immediate-release	Titrate to 4-11 ng/mL

Tab: 0.75, 1, 4 mg ext-rel

Comment: **Envarsus XR** (*tacrolimus* extended-release) is indicated to prevent organ rejection in *de novo* kidney transplant patients in combination with other immunosuppressants. **Envarsus XR** was initially approved for the prophylaxis of organ rejection in kidney transplant patients converted from *tacrolimus* **immediate-release** formulations. **Envarsus XR** is not interchangeable with other tacrolimus products.

Prograf *Cap:* 0.5, 1, 5 mg; *Granules:* 0.2, 1 mg unit-dose pkts for oral suspension (50 pkts/caton); *Amp:* 5 mg/ml solution for dilution and IV Infusion (1 ml, 10/box)

Comment: **Prograf** *(tacrolimus)* is indicated for the prophylaxis of organ rejection in patients receiving an allogenic liver, kidney, or heart transplant with other immunosuppressants. Frequent monitoring of trough concentration is recommended. Capsules and suspension should be consistently administered either with or without food. IV administration is intended for patients who are unable to swallow capsules or tablets. **Prograf** is not interchangeable with other extended-release *tacrolimus* products. Monitor for, and implement appropriate management for new onset diabetes, nephrotoxicity, neurotoxicity, hyperkalemia, hypertension, and anaphylaxis. **Prograf** is not recommended with concomitant use of *sirolimus* with liver and heart transplantation due to increased risk of adverse reactions.

OSGOOD-SCHLATTER DISEASE

Acetaminophen for IV Infusion *see Pain page* 352
NSAIDs *see page* 571
Opioid Analgesics *see Pain page* 354
Topical & Transdermal Analgesics *see Pain page* 352
Parenteral Corticosteroids *see page* 577
Oral Corticosteroids *see page* 577
Topical Analgesic and Anesthetic Agents *see page* 569

OSTEOARTHRITIS, ANKYLOSING SPONDYLITIS

Acetaminophen for IV Infusion *see Pain page* 352
NSAIDs *see page* 571
Opioid Analgesics *see Pain page* 354
Topical & Transdermal Analgesics *see Pain page* 352
Parenteral Corticosteroids *see page* 577
Oral Corticosteroids *see page* 577
Topical Analgesic and Anesthetic Agents *see page* 569

TOPICAL & TRANSDERMAL ANALGESICS

 capsaicin (B)(G) apply tid to qid prn to intact skin
Pediatric: <2 years: not recommended; ≥2 years: same as adult
Axsain *Crm:* 0.075% (1, 2 oz)
Capsin *Lotn:* 0.025, 0.075% (59 ml)
Capsaicin-HP (OTC) *Crm:* 0.075% (1.5 oz), 0.025% (45, 90 gm); *Lotn:* 0.075% (2 oz); 0.025% (45, 90 gm)

Capzasin-P (OTC) *Crm:* 0.025% (1.5 oz); *Lotn:* 0.025% (2 oz)
Dolorac *Crm:* 0.025% (28 gm)
Double Cap (OTC) *Crm:* 0.05% (2 oz)
R-Gel *Gel:* 0.025% (15, 30 gm)
Zostrix (OTC) *Crm:* 0.025% (0.7, 1.5, 3 oz)
Zostrix HP (OTC) *Emol crm:* 0.075% (1, 2 oz)

➤ *capsaicin* 8% patch (B) apply up to 4 patches for one 60-minute application to clean dry skin; may prep area with topical anesthetic; wear non-latex gloves; patches may be cut to size/shape; treatment may be repeated every 3 months
   Pediatric: <18 years: not recommended; ≥18 years: same as adult
   Qutenza *Patch:* 8% 1640 mcg/cm (179 mg) (1 or 2 patches w. 1-50 gm tube cleansing gel/carton)

➤ *diclofenac sodium* (C; D ≥30 wks)(G) apply qid prn to intact skin
   Pediatric: <12 years: not established; ≥12 years: same as adult
   Pennsaid 1.5% in 10 drop increments, dispense and rub into front, side, and back of knee: usually; 40 drops (40 mg) qid
      Topical soln: 1.5% (150 ml)
   Pennsaid 2% apply 2 pump actuations (40 mg) and rub into front, side, and back of knee bid
      Topical soln: 2% (20 mg/pump actuation, 112 gm)
   Solaraze Gel massage in to clean skin bid prn
      Gel: 3% (50 gm) (benzyl alcohol)
   Voltaren Gel (G) apply qid prn to intact skin
      Gel: 1% (100 gm)

Comment: *diclofenac* is contraindicated with *aspirin* allergy. As with other NSAIDs, should be avoided in late pregnancy (≥30 weeks) because it may cause premature closure of the ductus arteriosus.

➤ *doxepin* (B) cream apply to affected area qid at intervals of at least 3-4 hours; max 8 days
   Pediatric: <12 years: not recommended; >12 years: same as adult
   Prudoxin *Crm:* 5% (45 gm)
   Zonalon *Crm:* 5% (30, 45 gm)

➤ *pimecrolimus* 1% cream (C)(G) <2 years: not recommended; ≥2 years: apply to affected area bid; do not apply an occlusive dressing
   Elidel *Crm:* 1% (30, 60, 100 gm)

Comment: *pimecrolimus* is indicated for short-term and intermittent long-term use. Discontinue use when resolution occurs. Contraindicated if the patient is immunosuppressed. Change to the 0.1% preparation or if secondary bacterial infection is present.

➤ *trolamine salicylate* apply tid-qid
   Pediatric: <2 years: not recommended; ≥2 years: same as adult
   Mobisyl Creme *Crm:* 10% (100 gm)

ORAL SALICYLATE

➤ *indomethacin* (C) initially 25 mg bid to tid, increase as needed at weekly intervals by 25-50 mg/day; max 200 mg/day
   Pediatric: <14 years: usually not recommended; >2 years, if risk warranted: 1-2 mg/kg/day in divided doses; max 3-4 mg/kg/day (or 150-200 mg/day, whichever is less); <14 years: ER cap not recommended
      Cap: 25, 50 mg; *Susp:* 25 mg/5 ml (pineapple-coconut, mint) (alcohol 1%); *Supp:* 50 mg; *ER Cap:* 75 mg ext-rel

Comment: *indomethacin* is indicated only for acute painful flares. Administer with food and/or antacids. Use lowest effective dose for shortest duration.

ORAL NSAIDs

See more Oral NSAIDs page 571

➤ *diclofenac* (C) take on empty stomach; 35 mg tid; Hepatic impairment: use lowest dose
   Pediatric: <18 years: not recommended; ≥18 years: same as adult
   Zorvolex *Gelcap:* 18, 35 mg

➤ *diclofenac sodium* (C)
   Pediatric: <18 years: not recommended; ≥18 years: same as adult

Voltaren 50 mg bid to qid <u>or</u> 75 mg bid <u>or</u> 25 mg qid with an additional 25 mg at HS if necessary
  Tab: 25, 50, 75 mg ent-coat
Voltaren XR 100 mg once daily; rarely, 100 mg bid may be used
  Tab: 100 mg ext-rel

ORAL NSAIDs+PPI

▷ *esomeprazole+naproxen* (C)(G) 1 tab bid; use lowest effective dose for the shortest duration swallow whole; take at least 30 minutes before a meal
  Pediatric: <18 years: not recommended; ≥18 years: same as adult
    Vimovo *Tab:* nap 375 mg+eso 20 mg ext-rel; nap 500 mg+eso 20 mg ext-rel
    Comment: **Vimovo** is indicated to improve signs/symptoms, and risk of gastric ulcer in patients at risk of developing NSAID-associated gastric ulcer.

COX-2 INHIBITORS

Comment: Cox-2 inhibitors are contraindicated with history of asthma, urticaria, and allergic-type reactions to *aspirin*, other NSAIDs, and sulfonamides, 3rd trimester of pregnancy, and coronary artery bypass graft (CABG) surgery.
▷ *celecoxib* (C)(G) 100-400 mg daily bid; max 800 mg/day
  Pediatric: <18 years: not recommended; ≥18 years: same as adult
    Celebrex *Cap:* 50, 100, 200, 400 mg
▷ *meloxicam* (C)(G)
    Mobic <2 years, <60 kg: not recommended; ≥2, >60 kg: 0.125 mg/kg; max 7.5 mg once daily; ≥18 years: initially 7.5 mg once daily; max 15 mg once daily; *Hemodialysis:* max 7.5 mg/day
      Tab: 7.5, 15 mg; *Oral susp:* 7.5 mg/5 ml (100 ml) (raspberry)
    Vivlodex <18 years: not established; ≥18 years: initially 5 mg qd; may increase to max 10 mg/day; *Hemodialysis:* max 5 mg/day
      Cap: 5, 10 mg

INTRA-ARTICULAR STEROID INJECTIONS

▷ *triamcinolone acetonide* ext-rel injectable synthetic corticosteroid indicated as an intra-articular injection for the management of osteoarthritis pain of the knee
    Zilretta *Vial:* 32 mg single-dose microsphere pwdr for injection + 5 ml diluent and vial adapter/single-use kit
    Comment: **Zilretta** is <u>not</u> intended for repeat administration. **Zilretta** is <u>not</u> interchangeable with other formulations of injectable *triamcinolone acetonide.*

INTRA-ARTICULAR SODIUM HYALURONATE INJECTIONS

Comment: *sodium hyaluronate* intra-articular injection is indicated for the treatment of pain in osteoarthritis (OA) of the knee in patients who have failed to respond adequately to conservative non-pharmacologic therapy and simple analgesics (e.g., acetaminophen), alternative practices and procedures include nonsteroidal anti-inflammatory drugs (NSAIDs), intra-articular injection of corticosteroid, unmodified hyaluronan injections, avoidance of activities that cause joint pain, exercise, weight loss, physical therapy, and removal of excess fluid from the knee. For those patients who have failed the above treatments, surgical interventions such as arthroscopic surgery and total knee replacement surgery are also alternative treatments. Do not inject this product in the knees of patients with infections <u>or</u> skin diseases in the area of the injection site. Potential adverse effects occur in association with intraarticular injections: arthralgia, joint stiffness, joint effusion, joint swelling, joint warmth, injection site pain, arthritis, allergic reaction, and bleeding at the injection site. *sodium hyaluronate* has not been formally assigned to a pregnancy category by the FDA. Animal studies have failed to reveal evidence of fertility impairment <u>or</u> teratogenicity. There are no controlled data in human pregnancy.
▷ *sodium hyaluronate* (B) using strict aseptic technique, administer by intra-articular injection (into the synovial space of the affected knee(s) for the prescribed number of weeks (see mfr pkg insert); after preparing the injection site and attaining local analgesia, remove joint synovial fluid <u>or</u> effusion prior to injection; do not inject intra-vascularly, extra-articularly, <u>or</u> in the synovial tissues <u>or</u> capsule; for at least 48 hours following an injection, avoid

jogging, strenuous activity, or high-impact sports such as soccer or tennis, weight-bearing activity, or standing for longer than 1 hour at a time

Pediatric: <12 years: not recommended; ≥12 years: same as adult

Durolane administer a single intra-articular knee injection
Pediatric: <21 years: not recommended
Prefilled syringe: 60 mg (20 mg/ml, 3 ml) single-use

Euflexxa administer 3 to 5 intra-articular knee injections one week apart
Pediatric: <21 years: not recommended
Prefilled syringe: 20 mg (10 mg/ml, 2.0 ml) single-use

Gel-One administer a single intra-articular knee injection
Pediatric: <21 years: not recommended
Prefilled syringe: 30 mg (10 mg/ml, 3 ml) single-use

GelSyn-3 administer 3 to 5 intra-articular injections one week apart
Pediatric: <21 years: not recommended
Prefilled syringe: 16.5 mg (8.4 mg/ml, 2 ml) single-use

GenVisc 850 administer 3-5 intra-articular knee injections one week apart
Pediatric: <21 years: not recommended
Prefilled syringe: 25 mg (10 mg/ml, 2.5 ml) single-use

Hyalgan administer 3 to 5 intra-articular injections one week apart
Pediatric: <21 years: not recommended
Prefilled syringe: 10 mg/ml (20 mg, 2 ml) single-use

Monovisc administer a single intra-articular knee injection
Pediatric: <21 years: not recommended
Prefilled syringe: 88 mg (22 mg/ml, 4 ml) single-use

Orthovisc administer 3 to 4 intra-articular knee injections one week apart
Pediatric: <21 years: not recommended
Prefilled syringe: 30 mg (15 mg/ml, 2 ml) single-use

Spartz, Supartz FX administer 3- to 5 intra-articular knee injections one week apart
Pediatric: <21 years: not recommended
Prefilled syringe: 25 mg (10 mg/ml, 2.5 ml) single-use

Synvisc administer 3 intra-articular knee injections one week apart
Pediatric: <21 years: not recommended
Prefilled syringe: 16 mg (8 mg/ml, 2 ml) single-use

Synvisc-One administer a single intra-articular knee injection
Pediatric: <21 years: not recommended
Prefilled syringe: 48 mg (8 mg/ml, 6 ml) single-use

Visco-3 administer 3 intra-articular knee injections one week apart
Pediatric: <21 years: not recommended
Prefilled syringe: 25 mg (10 mg/ml, 2.5 ml) single-use

TUMOR NECROSIS FACTOR (TNF) ALPHA BLOCKERS FOR ANKYLOSING SPONDYLITIS

▷ *adalimumab-adaz* (B) 40 mg SC every other week; some patients with RA not receiving **methotrexate** may benefit from increasing the frequency to 40 mg SC every week
Pediatric: <18 years: not recommended; ≥18 years: same as adult

Hyrimox *Prefilled syringe:* 40 mg/0.8 ml single-dose (preservative-free)
Comment: **Hyrimox** is biosimilar to **Humira** *(adalimumab).*

▷ *adalimumab-adbm* (B) initially 80 SC; then, 40 mg SC every other week starting one week after initial dose; inject into thigh or abdomen; rotate sites
Pediatric: <18 years: not recommended; ≥18 years: same as adult

Cyltezo *Prefilled syringe:* 40 mg/0.8 ml single-dose (preservative-free)
Comment: **Cyltezo** is biosimilar to **Humira** *(adalimumab).*

▷ *infliximab (tumor necrosis factor-alpha blocker)* must be refrigerated at 2°C to 8°C (36°F to 46°F); administer dose intravenously over a period of not less than 2 hours; do not use beyond the expiration date as this product contains no preservative; 5 mg/kg at 0, 2 and 6 weeks, then every 8 weeks.
Pediatric: <6 years: not studied; ≥6-17 years: mg/kg at 0, 2 and 6 weeks, then every 8 weeks; ≥18 years: same as adult

Remicade *Vial:* 100 mg for reconstitution to 10 ml administration volume, single-dose (preservative-free)
Comment: **Remicade** is indicated to reduce signs and symptoms, and induce and maintain clinical remission, in adults and children ≥6 years-of-age with moderately to

severely active disease who have had an inadequate response to conventional therapy and reduce the number of draining enterocutaneous and rectovaginal fistulas, and maintain fistula closure, in adults with fistulizing disease. Common adverse effects associated with **Remicade** included abdominal pain, headache, pharyngitis, sinusitis, and upper respiratory infections. In addition, **Remicade** might increase the risk for serious infections, including tuberculosis, bacterial sepsis, and invasive fungal infections. Available data from published literature on the use of *infliximab* products during pregnancy have not reported a clear association with *infliximab* products and adverse pregnancy outcomes. *infliximab* products cross the placenta and infants exposed *in utero* should not be administered live vaccines for at least 6 months after birth. Otherwise, the infant may be at increased risk of infection, including disseminated infection which can become fatal. Available information is insufficient to inform the amount of *infliximab* products present in human milk or effects on the breastfed infant. To report suspected adverse reactions, contact Merck Sharp & Dohme Corp., a subsidiary of Merck & Co. at 1-877-888-4231 or FDA at 1-800-FDA1088 or www.fda.gov/medwatch.

▷ *infliximab-abda (tumor necrosis factor-alpha blocker)* (B)
　　Renflexis: see *infliximab* (**Remicade**) above for full prescribing information
　　Comment: **Renflexis** is a biosimilar to **Remicade** for the treatment of immune-disorders including Crohn's disease, ulcerative colitis, rheumatoid arthritis, ankylosing spondylitis, psoriatic arthritis and plaque psoriasis. **Renflexis** was approved under the FDA category for biosimilars and demonstrated no clinically meaningful differences for use, dosing regimens, strengths, dosage forms, and routes of administration from the FDA-approved biological product **Remicade**.

▷ *infliximab-dyyb (tumor necrosis factor-alpha blocker)* (B)
　　Inflectra: see *infliximab* (**Remicade**) above for full prescribing information
　　Comment: **Inflectra** is a biosimilar to **Remicade** for the treatment of immune-disorders including Crohn's disease, ulcerative colitis, rheumatoid arthritis, ankylosing spondylitis, psoriatic arthritis and plaque psoriasis. **Inflectra** was approved under the FDA category for biosimilars and demonstrated no clinically meaningful differences for use, dosing regimens, strengths, dosage forms, and routes of administration from the FDA-approved biological product **Remicade**.

▷ *infliximab-qbtx (tumor necrosis factor-alpha blocker)* (B)
　　Ifixi: see *infliximab* (**Remicade**) above for full prescribing information
　　Comment: **Ifixi** is a biosimilar to **Remicade** for the treatment of immune disorders including Crohn's disease, ulcerative colitis, rheumatoid arthritis, ankylosing spondylitis, psoriatic arthritis and plaque psoriasis. **Ifixi** was approved under the FDA category for biosimilars and demonstrated no clinically meaningful differences for use, dosing regimens, strengths, dosage forms, and routes of administration from the FDA-approved biological product **Remicade**.

OSTEOPOROSIS

Comment: Indications for bone density screening include: Postmenopausal women not receiving HRT, maternal history of hip fracture, personal history of fragility fracture, presence of high serum markers of bone resorption, smoker, height >67 inches, weight <125 lb, taking a steroid, GnRH agonist, or antiseizure drug, immobilization, hyperthyroidism, posttransplantation, malabsorption syndrome, hyperparathyroidism, prolactinemia. The mnemonic **ABONE** [**A**ge >65, **B**ulk (weight <140 lbs at menopause), and **N**ever **E**strogens (for more than 6 months)], represents other indications for bone density screening. Foods high in calcium include almonds, broccoli, baked beans, salmon, sardines, buttermilk, turnip greens, collard greens, spinach, pumpkin, rhubarb, and bran. Recommended Daily Calcium Intake: 1-3 years: 700 mg; 4-8 years: 1000 mg; 9-18 years: 1300 mg; 19-50 years: 1000 mg; 51-70 years (males): 1000 mg; ≥51 years (females): 1200 mg; pregnancy or nursing: 1000-1300 mg Recommended Daily Vitamin D Intake: >1 year: 600 IU; 50+ years: 800-1000 IU. Prior to initiating, or concomitant prescribing, corticosteroids in patients at risk for, or diagnosed with, osteoporosis, referral to the following ACR guidelines is recommended: ACR Guidelines on Prevention & Treatment of Glucocorticoid-induced Osteoporosis [press release, June 7, 2017]. Atlanta, GA. American College of Rheumatology www.rheumatology.org/About-Us/Newsroom/Press-

Releases/ID/812/ACR-Releases-Guideline-on-Prevention-Treatment-of-Glucocorticoid-Induced-Osteoporosis

ESTROGEN REPLACEMENT THERAPY

Comment: *estrogen* plus progesterone is indicated for postmenopausal women with an intact uterus. *estrogen* monotherapy is indicated in women without a uterus. The following list is not inclusive; for more estrogen replacement therapies *see **Menopause** page* 301)

▷ *estradiol* (X)
    Alora initially 0.05 mg/day apply patch twice weekly to lower abdomen, upper quadrant of buttocks or outer aspect of hip
      Transdermal patch: 0.025, 0.05, 0.075, 0.1 mg/day (8, 24/pck)
    Climara initially 0.025 mg/day patch once/week to trunk
      Transdermal patch: 0.025, 0.0375, 0.05, 0.075, 0.1 mg/day (4, 8, 24/pck)
    Estrace 1-2 mg daily cyclically (3 weeks on and 1 week off)
      Tab: 0.5, 1, 2*mg (tartrazine)
    Estraderm initially apply one 0.05 mg/day patch twice weekly to trunk
      Transdermal patch: 0.05, 0.1 mg/day (8, 24/pck)
    Menostar apply one patch weekly to lower abdomen, below the waist; avoid the breasts; alternate sites; *Transdermal patch:* 14 mcg/day (4/pck)
    Minivelle initially one 0.0375 mg/day patch twice weekly to trunk area; adjust after one month of therapy
      Transdermal patch: 0.025, 0.0375, 0.05, 0.075, 0.1 mg/day (8/pck)
    Vivelle initially one 0.0375 mg/day patch twice weekly to trunk area; use with an oral progestin to prevent endometrial hyperplasia
      Transdermal patch: 0.025, 0.0375, 0.05, 0.075, 0.1 mg/day (8, 48/pck)
    Vivelle-Dot initially one 0.05 mg/day patch twice weekly to lower abdomen, below the waist; use with an oral progestin to prevent endometrial hyperplasia
      Transdermal patch: 0.025, 0.0375, 0.05, 0.075, 0.1 mg/day (8, 24/pck)
▷ *estradiol+levonorgestrel* (X) apply 1 patch weekly to lower abdomen; avoid waistline; alternate sites
    Climara Pro *Transdermal patch:* estra 0.045 mg+levo 0.015 mg per day (4/pck)
▷ *estradiol+norethindrone* (X) 1 tab daily
    Activella (G) *Tab:* estra 1 mg+noreth 0.5 mg
    FemHRT 1/5 *Tab:* estra 5 mcg+noreth 1 mg
▷ *estradiol+norgestimate* (X) one x 1 mg *estradiol* tab daily x 3 days, then 1 x *estradiol* 1 mg+**norgestimate** 0.09 mg tab once daily x 3 days; repeat this pattern continuously
    Ortho-Prefest *Tab:* estra 1 mg+norgest 0.09 mg (30/blister pck)
▷ *estrogen, conjugated (equine)* (X)
    Premarin 1 tab daily
      Tab: 0.3, 0.45, 0.625, 0.9, 1.25, 2.5 mg
▷ *estropipate, piperazine estrone sulfate* (X)(G)
    Ogen 0.625-1.25 mg daily cyclically (3 weeks on and 1 week off)
      Tab: 0.625, 1.25, 2.5 mg
    Ortho-Est 0.75-6 mg daily cyclically (3 weeks on and 1 week off)
      Tab: 0.625, 1.25 mg

ESTROGENS, CONJUGATED+ESTROGEN AGONIST-ANTAGONIST COMBINATION

▷ *estrogen, conjugated+bazedoxifene* (X)
    Duavee 1 tab daily
      Tab: estra, conj 0.45 mg+baze 20 mg

CALCIUM SUPPLEMENTS

Comment: Take *calcium* supplements after meals to avoid gastric upset. Dosages of calcium over 2000 mg/day have not been shown to have any additional benefit. *calcium* decreases *tetracycline* absorption. *calcium* absorption is decreased by corticosteroids.

▷ *calcitonin-salmon* (C)
    Fortical 200 IU intranasally daily; alternate nostrils each day
      Nasal spray: 200 IU/actuation (30 doses, 3.7 ml)
    Miacalcin Nasal spray 200 IU spray in one nostril once daily; alternate nostrils each day
      Nasal spray: 200 IU/actuation (30 doses, 3.7 ml)

Miacalcin Injection 100 units SC or IM every other day
Vial: 200 units/ml (2 ml)

Comment: Supplement diet with calcium (1 gm/day) and vitamin D (400 IU/day).

▷ calcium carbonate (C)(OTC)(G)
Rolaids chew 2 tabs bid; max 14 tabs/day
Chew tab: 550 mg
Rolaids Extra Strength chew 2 tabs bid; max 8 tabs/day
Chew tab: 1000 mg
Tums chew 2 tabs bid; max 16 tabs/day
Chew tab: 500 mg
Tums Extra Strength chew 2 tabs bid; max 10 tabs/day
Chew tab: 750 mg
Tum Sultra chew 2 tabs bid; max 8 tabs/day
Chew tab: 1000 mg
Os-Cal 500 (OTC) 1-2 tab bid to tid
Chew tab: elemental calcium carbonate 500 mg

▷ calcium carbonate+vitamin D (C)(G)
Os-Cal 250+D (OTC) 1-2 tab tid
Tab: calc carb 250 mg+vit d 125 IU
Os-Cal 500+D (OTC) 1-2 tab bid-tid
Tab: calc carb 500 mg+vit d 125 IU
Viactiv (OTC) 1 tab tid
Chew tab: calc carb 500 mg+vit d 100 IU+vit k 40 mcg

▷ calcium citrate (C)(G)
Citracal (OTC) 1-2 tabs bid
Tab: calc cit 200 mg

▷ calcium citrate+vitamin D (C)(G)
Citracal+D (OTC) 1-2 cplts bid
Cplt: calc cit 315 mg+vit d 200 IU
Citracal 250+D (OTC) 1-2 tabs bid
Tab: calc cit 250 mg+vit d 62.3 IU

VITAMIN D ANALOGS

Comment: Concurrent *vitamin D* supplementation is contraindicated for patients taking *calcitriol* or *doxercalciferol* due to the risk of *vitamin D* toxicity.

▷ calcitriol (C) Predialysis: initially 0.25 mcg daily; may increase to 0.5 mcg daily; Dialysis: initially 0.25 mcg daily; may increase by 0.25 mcg/day at 4-8 week intervals; usual mainte-nance 0.5-1 mcg/day; Hypoparathyroidism: initially 0.25 mcg q AM; may increase by 0.25 mcg/day at 4- to 8-week intervals; usual maintenance 0.5-2 mcg/day
Pediatric: Predialysis: <3 years: 10-15 ng/kg/day; ≥3 years: initially 0.25 mcg daily; may in-crease to 0.5 mcg/day; Dialysis: not recommended; Hypoparathyroidism: initially 0.25 mcg daily; may increase by 0.25 mcg/day at 2-4 week intervals; usual maintenance (1-5 years) 0.25-0.75 mcg/day, (≥6 years) 0.5-2 mcg/day
Rocaltrol Cap: 0.25, 0.5 mcg
Rocaltrol Solution Soln: 1 mcg/ml (15 ml, single-use dispensers)

▷ doxercalciferol (C) initially 0.25 mcg q AM; may increase by 0.25 mcg/day at 4-8 week intervals; usual maintenance 0.5-2 mcg/day
Pediatric: initially 0.25 mcg daily; may increase by 0.25 mcg; 0.25 mcg/day at 2-4 week inter-vals; usual maintenance (1-5 years) 0.25-0.75 mcg/day, (≥6 years) 0.5-2 mcg/day
Hectorol Cap: 0.25, 0.5 mcg

BISPHOSPHONATES (CALCIUM MODIFIERS)

Comment: Bisphosphonates should be swallowed whole in the AM with 6-8 oz of plain water 30 minutes before first meal, beverage, or other medications of the day. Monitor serum alkaline phosphatase. Contraindications include abnormalities of the esophagus which delay esophageal emptying such as stricture or achalasia, inability to stand or sit upright for at least 30 minutes post-dose, patients at risk of aspiration, and hypocalcemia. Co-administration of bisphosphonates and *calcium*, antacids, or oral medications containing multivalent cations will interfere with absorption of the bisphosphonate. Therefore, instruct patients to wait at least half hour after taking the bisphosphonate before taking any other oral medications.

▷ *alendronate (as sodium)* (C)(G) take once weekly, in the AM, 30 minutes before the first food, beverage, <u>or</u> medication of the day; do not lie down (remain upright) for at least 30 minutes and after the first food of the day; *CrCl <35 mL/min:* not recommended
Pediatric: <12 years: not recommended; ≥12 years: same as adult

Binosto dissolve the effervescent tab in 4 oz (120 ml) of plain, room temperature, water (not mineral <u>or</u> flavored); wait 5 minutes after the effervescence has subsided, then stir for 10 seconds, then drink
Tab: 70 mg effervescent for buffered solution (4, 12/carton) (strawberry)
Fosamax (G) swallow tab whole; dosing regimens are the same for men and postmenopausal women; *Prevention:* 5 mg once daily <u>or</u> 35 mg once weekly; *Treatment:* 10 mg once daily <u>or</u> 70 mg once weekly
Tab: 5, 10, 35, 40, 70 mg

▷ *alendronate+cholecalciferol (vit d3)* (C)(G) take 1 tab once weekly, in the AM, with plain water (not mineral) 30 minutes before the first food, beverage, <u>or</u> medication of the day; do not lie down (remain upright) for at least 30 minutes and after the first food of the day
Pediatric: <12 years: not recommended; ≥12 years: same as adult

Fosamax Plus D
Tab: **Fosamax Plus D 70/2800** alen 70 mg+chole 2800 IU
Fosamax Plus D 70/5600 alen 70 mg+chole 5600 IU

▷ *ibandronate (as monosodium monohydrate)* (C)(G)
Pediatric: <12 years: not recommended; ≥12 years: same as adult

Boniva take 2.5 mg once daily <u>or</u> 150 mg once monthly on the same day; take in the AM, with plain water (not mineral) 60 minutes before the first food, beverage, <u>or</u> medication of the day; do not lie down (remain upright) for at least 30 minutes and after the first food of the day
Tab: 2.5, 150 mg
Boniva Injection administer 3 mg every 3 months by IV bolus over 15-30 seconds; if dose is missed, administer as soon as possible; then every 3 months from the date of the last dose
Prefilled syringe: 3 mg/3 ml (5 ml)
Comment: Boniva Injection must be administered by a health care professional.

▷ *risedronate (as sodium)* (C)(G) take in the AM; swallow whole with a full glass of plain water (not mineral); do not lie down (remain upright) for 30 minutes afterward
Pediatric: <12 years: not recommended; ≥12 years: same as adult

Actonel take at least 30 minutes before any food <u>or</u> drink; *Women:* 5 mg once daily <u>or</u> 35 mg once weekly <u>or</u> 75 mg on two consecutive days monthly <u>or</u> 150 mg once monthly; *Men:* 35 mg once weekly
Tab: 5, 30, 35, 75, 150 mg
Atelvia 35 mg once weekly immediately after breakfast
Tab: 35 mg del-rel

▷ *risedronate+calcium* (C) 1 x 5 mg *risedronate* tab weekly <u>plus</u> 1 x 500 mg *calcium* tab on days 2-7 weekly

Actonel with Calcium *Tab: risedronate* 5 mg <u>and</u> *Tab: calcium* 500 mg (4 *risedronate* tabs + 30 *calcium* tabs/pck)

▷ *zoledronic acid* (D)(G)
Pediatric: <12 years: not recommended; ≥12 years: same as adult

Reclast administer 5 mg via IV infusion over at least 15 minutes mg once a year (for osteoporosis) <u>or</u> once every 2 years (for osteopenia <u>or</u> prophylaxis)
Bottle: 5 mg/100 ml (single-dose)
Comment: Reclast is indicated for the treatment of postmenopausal osteoporosis in women who are at high risk for fracture and to increase bone mass in men with primary <u>or</u> hypogonadal osteoporosis who are at high risk for fracture. Administered by a health care professional. Contraindicated in hypocalcemia.
Zometa *Bottle:* 4 mg/5 ml administer 4 mg via IV infusion over at least 15 minutes every 3-4 weeks; optimal duration of treatment not known
Vial: 4 mg/5 ml (single-dose)
Comment: Zometa is indicated for the treatment of hypercalcemia of malignancy. The safety and efficacy of **Zometa** in the treatment of hypercalcemia associated with hyperparathyroidism <u>or</u> with other nontumor-related conditions has not been established.

SELECTIVE ESTROGEN RECEPTOR MODULATOR (SERMs)

▷ *raloxifene* (X)(G) 60 mg once daily
   Evista *Tab:* 60 mg

   Comment: Contraindicated in women who have history of, or current, venous thrombotic event.

HUMAN PARATHYROID HORMONE

▷ *teriparatide* (C) 20 mcg SC daily in the thigh or abdomen; may treat for up to 2 years
   Pediatric: <12 years: not recommended; ≥12 years: same as adult
   Forteo Multidose Pen *Multi-dose pen:* 250 mcg/ml (3 ml)

   Comment: Forteo is indicated for the treatment of postmenopausal osteoporosis in women who are at high risk for fracture and to increase bone mass in men with primary or hypogonadal osteoporosis who are at high risk for fracture.

HUMAN PARATHYROID HORMONE RELATED PEPTIDE (PTHrP[1-34]) ANALOG

▷ *abaloparatide* 80 mcg (40 mcl) SC once daily
   Tymlos *Pen:* 80 mcg/40 mcl (1.56 ml, 2,000 mcg/ml) (30 doses) preassembled, sin-gle-patient use, disposable w. glass cartridge

   Comment: Tymlos is a bone building agent for the treatment of postmenopausal women with osteoporosis at high risk for fracture. Tymlos is not indicated for use in females of reproductive potential. There are no human data with use in pregnant women to inform any drug associated risks and animal reproduction studies with *abaloparatide* have not been conducted. There is no information on the presence of *abaloparatide* in human milk, the effects on the breastfed infant, or the effects on milk production; however, breastfeeding is not recommended while using Tymlos. Tymlos is not recommended for use in pediatric patients with open epiphyses or hereditary disorders predisposing to osteosarcoma because of an increased baseline risk of osteosarcoma. Tymlos may cause hypercalciuria. It is unknown whether Tymlos may exacerbate urolithiasis in patients with active or a history of urolithiasis. If active urolithiasis or pre-existing hypercalciuria is suspected, measurement of urinary calcium excretion should be considered. No dosage adjustment is required for patients any degree of renal impairment. Currently, there are no specific drug-drug interaction studies.

BIOENGINEERED REPLICA OF HUMAN PARATHYROID HORMONE

▷ *bioengineered replica of human parathyroid hormone* (C) initially inject mg IM into the thigh once daily; when initiating, decrease dose of active *vitamin D* by 50% if serum *calcium* is above 7.5 mg/dL; monitor serum *calcium* levels every 3 to 7 days after starting or adjusting dose and when adjusting either active *vitamin D* or *calcium* supplements dose
   Pediatric: <18 years: not recommended; ≥18 years: same as adult
   Natpara *Soln for inj:* 25, 50, 75, 100 mcg (2/pkg) multi-dose, dual-chamber glass car-tridge containing a sterile powder and diluent

   Comment: Natpara is indicated as adjunct to *calcium* and *vitamin D* in patients with parathyroidism.

OSTEOCLAST INHIBITOR (RANK LIGAND [RANKL] INHIBITOR)

▷ *denosumab* (X)
   Pediatric: <18 years: not established; treatment with Prolia may impair bone growth in children with open growth plates and may inhibit eruption of dentition. ≥18 years: same as adult
   Prolia for SC route only; should not be administered intravenously, intramuscularly, or intradermally; 60 mcg SC once every 6 months in the upper arm, abdomen, or upper thigh
   Vial/Pen: 60 mg/ml (1 ml) single-dose

   Comment: Prolia is indicated for the treatment of postmenopausal osteoporosis in females who are at high risk for fracture defined as a history of osteoporotic fracture or multiple risk factors for fracture or patients who have failed or are intolerant to other therapy and treatment to increase bone mass in women at high risk for fracture receiving adjuvant aromatase inhibitor therapy for breast cancer.

Prolia is also indicated for treatment to increase bone mass in men at high risk for fracture receiving androgen deprivation therapy for non-metastatic prostate cancer. **Prolia** must be administered by a health care professional. *denosumab* contraindicated with hypocalcemia. Instruct patients to take *calcium* 1,000 mg daily and at least 400 IU *vitamin D* daily. There is no information regarding the presence of *denosumab* in human milk or effects on the breastfed invent. To report suspected adverse reactions, contact Amgen Inc. at 1-800-77-AMGEN (1-800-772-6436) or FDA at 1-800-FDA-1088 or www.fda.gov/medwatch.

Xgeva *Multiple Myeloma and Bone Metastasis from Solid Tumors: admin*ister 120 mg administer SC in the upper arm, abdomen, or upper thigh; SC every 4 weeks; *Giant Cell Tumor of Bone:* administer 120 mg SC 4 every weeks with additional 120 mg doses on Days 8 and 15 of the first month of therapy and administer calcium and vitamin D as necessary to treat or prevent hypocalcemia; *Hypercalcemia of Malignancy:* administer 120 mg every 4 weeks with additional 120 mg doses Days 8 and 15 of the first month of therapy

Pediatric: recommended only for treatment of skeletally mature adolescents with giant cell tumor of bone; treatment with **Xgeva** may impair bone growth in children with open growth plates and may inhibit eruption of dentition

Vial: 120 mg/1.7 ml (70 mg/ml) solution in a single-dose

Comment: Xgeva is indicated for prevention of skeletal-related events in patients with multiple myeloma and in patients with bone metastases from solid tumors, treatment of adults and skeletally mature adolescents with giant cell tumor of bone that is un-resectable or where surgical resection is likely to result in severe morbidity, and treatment of hypercalcemia of malignancy refractory to bisphosphonate therapy. CrCl < 30 mL/min or receiving dialysis are at risk for hypocalcemia. Adequately supplement with calcium and vitamin D. There is no information regarding the presence of *denosumab* in human milk or effects on the breastfed invent. To report suspected adverse reactions, contact Amgen Inc at 1-800-77-AMGEN (1-800-772-6436) or FDA at 1-800-FDA-1088 or www.fda.gov/medwatch.

OTITIS EXTERNA

OTIC ANALGESIC

▶ *antipyrine+benzocaine+zinc acetate dihydrate* (C) fill ear canal with solution; then insert a cotton plug into meatus; may repeat every 1-2 hours prn
Pediatric: same as adult
Otozin *Otic soln:* antipyr 5.4%+benz 1%+zinc1% per ml (10 ml w. dropper)

OTIC ANTI-INFECTIVE

▶ *chloroxylenol+pramoxine* (C) 4-5 drops tid x 5-10 days
Pediatric: <1 year: not recommended; 1-12 years: 5 drops bid x 10 days; ≥12 years: same as adult
PramOtic *Otic drops:* chlorox+pramox (5 ml w. dropper)
▶ *finafloxacin* (C) otic 4-5 drops tid x 5-10 days
Pediatric: <1 year: not recommended; ≥1 year: same as adult
Xtoro *Otic soln:* 0.3% (5, 8 ml)
▶ *ofloxacin* (C)(G) 10 drops bid x 10 days
Pediatric: <1 year: not recommended; 1-12 years: 5 drops bid x 10 days; ≥12 years: same as adult
Floxin Otic *Otic soln:* 0.3% (5, 10 ml w. dropper; 0.25 ml, 5 drop singles, 20/carton)
Comment: Floxin Otic is indicated for adult patients with perforated tympanic membranes and pediatric patients with PE tubes.

OTIC ANTI-INFECTIVE+CORTICOSTEROID COMBINATIONS

▶ *chloroxylenol+pramoxine+hydrocortisone* (C) drops 4 drops tid-qid x 5-10 days
Pediatric: 3 drops tid-qid x 5-10 days

Cortane B, Cortane B Aqueous *Otic soln:* chlo 1 mg+pram 10 mg+hydro 10 mg per ml (10 ml w. dropper)

Comment: **Cortane B Aqueous** may be used to saturate a cotton wick.

▷ *ciprofloxacin+hydrocortisone* (C) susp 3 drops bid x 7 days
  Pediatric: <1 year: not recommended; ≥1 year: same as adult
      Cipro HC Otic *Otic susp:* cipro 0.2%+hydro 1% (10 ml w. dropper)

▷ *ciprofloxacin+dexamethasone* (C) 4 drops bid x 7 days
  Pediatric: <6 months: not recommended; ≥6 months: same as adult
      Ciprodex *Otic susp:* cipro 0.3%+dexa 1% (7.5 ml)

  Comment: **Ciprodex** is indicated for the treatment of otitis media in pediatric patients with tympanostomy tubes.

▷ *colistin+neomycin+hydrocortisone+thonzonium* (C) 5 drops tid or qid x 5-10 days
  Pediatric: 4 drops tid-qid x 5-10 days
      Coly-Mycin S *Otic susp:* 5, 10 ml
      Cortisporin-TC Otic *Otic susp:* colis 3 mg+neo 3.3 mg+hydro 10 mg+thon 0.5 mg per ml (10 ml w. dropper) (thimerosal)

▷ *polymyxin b+neomycin+hydrocortisone* (C) 4 drops tid-qid; max 10 days
  Pediatric: 3 drops tid-qid; max 10 days
      Cortisporin Otic Suspension *Otic susp:* poly b 10,000 u+neo 3.5 mg+hydro 10 mg per 5 ml (10 ml w. dropper)
      Cortisporin Otic Solution *Otic soln:* poly b 10000 u+neo 3.5 mg+hydro 10 mg per 5 ml (10 ml w. dropper)

OTIC ASTRINGENTS

▷ *acetic acid 2% in aluminum sulfate* (C) 4-6 drops q 2-3 hours
  Pediatric: same as adult
      Domeboro Otic *Otic soln:* 60 ml w. dropper

▷ *acetic acid+propylene glycol+benzethonium chloride+sodium acetate* (C) 3-5 drops q 4-6 hours
  Pediatric: same as adult
      VoSol *Otic soln:* acet 2% (15, 30 ml)

▷ *acetic acid+propylene glycol+hydrocortisone+benzethonium chloride+sodium acetate* (C) 3-5 drops q 4-6 hours
  Pediatric: same as adult
      VoSol HC *Otic soln:* acet 2%+hydro 1% (10 ml)

OTIC ANESTHETIC+ANALGESIC COMBINATIONS

▷ *antipyrine+benzocaine+glycerine* (C) fill ear canal and insert cotton plug; may repeat q 1-2 hours as needed
  Pediatric: same as adult
      A/B Otic *Otic soln:* 15 ml w. dropper

▷ *benzocaine* (C) 4-5 drops q 1-2 hours
  Pediatric: <1 year: not recommended; ≥1 year: same as adult
      Americaine Otic *Otic soln:* 20% (15 ml w. dropper)
      Benzotic *Otic soln:* 20% (15 ml w. dropper)

SYSTEMIC ANTI-INFECTIVES

Comment: Used for severe disease or with culture.

▷ *amoxicillin+clavulanate* (B)(G)
      Augmentin 500 mg tid or 875 mg bid x 7-10 days
      Pediatric: 40-45 mg/kg/day divided tid x 10 days or 90 mg/kg/day divided bid x 10 days *see pages 618 for dose by weight*
          Tab: 250, 500, 875 mg; *Chew tab:* 125, 250 mg (lemon-lime); 200, 400 mg (cherry-banana) (phenylalanine); *Oral susp:* 125 mg/5 ml (banana), 250 mg/5 ml (75, 100, 150 ml) (orange); 200, 400 mg/5 ml (50, 75, 100 ml) (orange) (phenylalanine)
      Augmentin ES-600 not recommended for adults
      Pediatric: <3 months: not recommended; ≥3 months, <40 kg: 90 mg/kg/day in 2 divided doses x 7-10 days; ≥40 kg: not recommended
          Oral susp: 42.9 mg/5 ml (50, 75, 100, 125, 150, 200 ml) (strawberry cream) (phenylalanine)
      Augmentin XR 2 tabs q 12 hours x 7-10 days

Pediatric: <16 years: use other forms; ≥16 years: same as adult
    Tab: 1000*mg ext-rel

 cefaclor (B)(G) 250-500 mg q 8 hours x 7-10 days
Pediatric: <1 month: not recommended; 20-40 mg/kg bid <u>or</u> q 12 hours x 10 days; max 1 gm/day; *see page 620 for dose by weight*
    Tab: 500 mg; *Cap:* 250, 500 mg; *Susp:* 125 mg/5 ml (75, 150 ml) (strawberry); 187 mg/5 ml (50, 100 ml) (strawberry); 250 mg/5 ml (75, 150 ml) (strawberry); 375 mg/5 ml (50, 100 ml) (strawberry)
    Cefaclor Extended Release
      Pediatric: <16 years: ext-rel not recommended; ≥16 years: same as adult
      Tab: 375, 500 mg ext-rel

 dicloxacillin (B) 500 mg qid x 7-10 days
Pediatric: 12.5-25 mg/kg/day in 4 divided doses x 7-10 days; *see page 624 for dose by weight*
    Dynapen *Cap:* 125, 250, 500 mg; *Oral susp:* 62.5 mg/5 ml (80, 100, 200 ml)

 trimethoprim+sulfamethoxazole (TMP-SMX) (C)(G)
Pediatric: <2 months: not recommended; ≥2 months: 40 mg/kg/day of *sulfamethoxazole* in 2 doses bid x 10 days; *see page 630 for dose by weight*
    Bactrim, Septra 2 tabs bid x 10 days
      Tab: trim 80 mg+sulfa 400 mg*
    Bactrim DS, Septra DS 1 tab bid x 10 days
      Tab: trim 160 mg+sulfa 800 mg*
    Bactrim Pediatric Suspension, Septra Pediatric Suspension
      Oral susp: trim 40 mg+sulfa 200 mg per 5 ml (100 ml) (cherry) (alcohol 0.3%)
Comment: Sulfonamides are contraindicated in the first trimester of pregnancy, the final month of pregnancy, and infants <8 weeks-of-age. *CrCl 15-30 mL/min:* reduce dose by 1/2; *CrCl <15 mL/min:* not recommended. Contraindicated with G6PD deficiency. A high fluid intake is indicated during sulfonamide therapy to avoid crystallization in the kidneys.

OTITIS MEDIA: ACUTE

OTIC ANALGESIC

 antipyrine+benzocaine+zinc acetate dihydrate otic (C) fill ear canal with solution; then insert cotton plug into meatus; may repeat every 1-2 hours prn
Pediatric: same as adult
    Otozin *Otic soln:* antipyr 5.4%+benz 1%+zinc1% per ml (10 ml w. dropper)

SYSTEMIC ANTI-INFECTIVES

 amoxicillin (B)(G) 500-875 mg bid <u>or</u> 250-500 mg tid x 10 days
Pediatric: <40 kg (88 lb): 20-40 mg/kg/day in 3 divided doses x 10 days <u>or</u> 25-45 mg/kg/day in 2 divided doses x 10 days; *see page 617 for dose by weight*
    Amoxil *Cap:* 250, 500 mg; *Tab:* 875*mg; *Chew tab:* 125, 200, 250, 400 mg (cherry-banana-peppermint) (phenylalanine); *Oral susp:* 125, 250 mg/5 ml (80, 100, 150 ml) (strawberry); 200, 400 mg/5 ml (50, 75, 100 ml) (bubble gum); *Oral drops:* 50 mg/ml (30 ml) (bubble gum)
    Moxatag *Tab:* 775 mg ext-rel
    Trimox *Tab:* 125, 250 mg; *Cap:* 250, 500 mg; *Oral susp:* 125, 250 mg/5 ml (80, 100, 150 ml) (raspberry-strawberry)
Comment: Consider 80-90 mg/kg/day in 3 divided doses for resistant for cases

 amoxicillin+clavulanate (B)(G)
    Augmentin 500 mg tid <u>or</u> 875 mg bid x 7-10 days
    Pediatric: 40-45 mg/kg/day divided tid x 10 days <u>or</u> 90 mg/kg/day divided bid x 10 days *see pages 618 for dose by weight*
    Tab: 250, 500, 875 mg; *Chew tab:* 125, 250 mg (lemon-lime); 200, 400 mg (cherry-banana) (phenylalanine); *Oral susp:* 125 mg/5 ml (banana), 250 mg/5 ml (75, 100, 150 ml) (orange); 200, 400 mg/5 ml (50, 75, 100 ml) (orange) (phenyl-alanine)
    Augmentin ES-600 not recommended for adults
    Pediatric: <3 months: not recommended; ≥3 months, <40 kg: 90 mg/kg/day in 2 divided doses x 7-10 days; ≥40 kg: not recommended

    Oral susp: 42.9 mg/5 ml (50, 75, 100, 125, 150, 200 ml) (strawberry cream) (phenyl-
alanine)

Augmentin XR 2 tabs q 12 hours x 7-10 days
Pediatric: <16 years: use other forms; ≥16 years: same as adult
    Tab: 1000*mg ext-rel

▷ *ampicillin* (B) 250-500 mg qid x 10 days
Pediatric: 50-100 mg/kg/day in 4 divided doses x 10 days; *see page 619 for dose by weight*
    Omnipen, Principen *Cap:* 250, 500 mg; *Oral susp:* 125, 250 mg/5 ml (100, 150, 200 ml)
    (fruit)

▷ *azithromycin* (B)(G) 500 mg x 1 dose on day 1, then 250 mg daily on days 2-5 or 500 mg
daily x 3 days or **Zmax** 2 gm in a single dose
Pediatric: 12 mg/kg/day x 5 days; max 500 mg/day; *see page 619 for dose by weight*
    Zithromax *Tab:* 250, 500, 600 mg; *Oral susp:* 100 mg/5 ml (15 ml); 200 mg/5 ml (15,
    22.5, 30 ml) (cherry); *Pkt:* 1 gm for reconstitution (cherry-banana)
    Zithromax Tri-pak *Tab:* 3 x 500 mg tabs/pck
    Zithromax Z-pak *Tab:* 6 x 250 mg tabs/pck
    Zmax *Oral susp:* 2 gm ext-rel for reconstitution (cherry-banana) (148 mg Na$^+$)

▷ *cefaclor* (B)(G) 250-500 mg q 8 hours x 7-10 days
Pediatric: <1 month: not recommended; 20-40 mg/kg bid or q 12 hours x 10 days; max 1
gm/day; *see page 620 for dose by weight*
    Tab: 500 mg; *Cap:* 250, 500 mg; *Susp:* 125 mg/5 ml (75, 150 ml) (strawberry); 187
    mg/5 ml (50, 100 ml) (strawberry); 250 mg/5 ml (75, 150 ml) (strawberry); 375
    mg/5 ml (50, 100 ml) (strawberry)
    Cefaclor Extended Release
Pediatric: <16 years: ext-rel not recommended
    Tab: 375, 500 mg ext-rel

▷ *cefdinir* (B) 300 mg bid or 600 mg daily x 5-10 days
Pediatric: <6 months: not recommended; 6 months-12 years: 14 mg/kg/day in 1-2 divided
doses x 10 days; *>12 years: same as adult; see page 621 for dose by weight*
    Omnicef *Cap:* 300 mg; *Oral susp:* 125 mg/5 ml (60, 100 ml) (strawberry)

▷ *cefixime* (B)(G)
Pediatric: <6 months: not recommended; 6 months-12 years, <50 kg: 8 mg/kg/day in 1-2
divided doses x 10 days; >12 years, ≥50 kg: same as adult; *see page 621 for dose by weight*
    Suprax *Tab:* 400 mg; *Cap:* 400 mg; *Oral susp:* 100, 200, 500 mg/5 ml (50, 75, 100 ml)
    (strawberry)

▷ *cefpodoxime proxetil* (B) 100 mg bid x 5 days
Pediatric: <2 months: not recommended; 2 months-12 years: 10 mg/kg/day (max 400 mg/
dose) or 5 mg/kg/day bid (max 200 mg/dose) x 5 days; >12 years: same as adult; *see page
622 for dose by weight*
    Vantin *Tab:* 100, 200 mg; *Oral susp:* 50, 100 mg/5 ml (50, 75, 100 ml) (lemon creme)

▷ *cefprozil* (B) 250-500 mg bid or 500 mg daily x 10 days
Pediatric: <2 years: same as adult; 2-12 years: 7.5 mg/kg bid x 10 days; *see page 622 for dose
by weight;* >12 years: same as adult
    Cefzil *Tab:* 250, 500 mg; *Oral susp:* 125, 250 mg/5 ml (50, 75, 100 ml) (bubble gum)
    (phenylalanine)

▷ *ceftibuten* (B) 400 mg daily x 10 days
Pediatric: 9 mg/kg daily x 10 days; max 400 mg/day; *see page 623 for dose by weight*
    Cedax *Cap:* 400 mg; *Oral susp:* 90 mg/5 ml (30, 60, 90, 120 ml); 180 mg/5 ml (30, 60,
    120 ml) (cherry)

▷ *ceftriaxone* (B)(G) 1-2 gm IM x 1 dose; max 4 gm
Pediatric: 50 mg/kg IM x 1 dose
    Rocephin *Vial:* 250, 500 mg; 1, 2 gm

▷ *cephalexin* (B)(G) 250 mg qid x 10 days
Pediatric: 25-50 mg/kg/day in 4 doses x 10 days; *see page 623 for dose by weight*
    Keflex *Cap:* 250, 333, 500, 750 mg; *Oral susp:* 125, 250 mg/5 ml (100, 200 ml) (straw-
berry)

▷ *clarithromycin* (C)(G) 500 mg bid or 500 mg ext-rel once daily x 10 days
Pediatric: <6 months: not recommended; ≥6 months: 7.5 mg/kg divided bid x 7 days; *see
page 624 for dose by weight*
    Biaxin *Tab:* 250, 500 mg
    Biaxin Oral Suspension *Oral susp:* 125, 250 mg/5 ml (50, 100 ml) (fruit-punch)
    Biaxin XL *Tab:* 500 mg ext-rel

Comment: The FDA is advising caution before prescribing *clarithromycin* to patients with heart disease because of a potential increased risk of heart problems <u>or</u> death that can occur years later. This recommendation is based on a review of the results of a 10-year follow-up study of patients with coronary heart disease from a large clinical trial that first observed this safety issue. Consider risk benefit and the use of other antibiotics in such patients.

➤ *erythromycin+sulfisoxazole* (C)(G)
Pediatric: <2 months: not recommended; ≥2 months: 50 mg/kg/day in 3 divided doses x 10 days; *see page 627 for dose by weight*
    Eryzole *Oral susp:* eryth 200 mg+sulfa 600 mg per 5 ml (100, 150, 200, 250 ml)
    Pediazole *Oral susp:* eryth 200 mg+sulfa 600 mg per 5 ml (100, 150, 200 ml) (strawberry-banana)
Comment: *erythromycin* may increase INR with concomitant *warfarin*, as well as increase serum level of *digoxin,* benzodiazepines, and statins. *sulfamethoxazole* is not recommended in pregnancy or lactation. *CrCl 15-30 mL/min:* reduce dose by 1/2; *CrCl <15 mL/min:* not recommended.

➤ *loracarbef* (B) 400 mg bid x 10 days
Pediatric: 30 mg/kg/day in divided bid x 7 days; *see page 628 for dose by weight*
    Lorabid *Pulvule:* 200, 400 mg; *Oral susp:* 100 mg/5 ml (50, 100 ml); 200 mg/5 ml (50, 75, 100 ml) (strawberry bubble gum)

➤ *trimethoprim+sulfamethoxazole (TMP-SMX])* (C)(G)
Pediatric: <2 months: not recommended; >2 months: 40 mg/kg/day of *sulfamethoxazole* in divided doses bid x 10 days; *see page 630 for dose by weight*
    Bactrim, Septra 2 tabs bid x 10 days
      Tab: trim 80 mg+sulfa 400 mg*
    Bactrim DS, Septra DS 1 tab bid x 10 days
      Tab: trim 160 mg+sulfa 800 mg*
    Bactrim Pediatric Suspension, Septra Pediatric Suspension
      Oral susp: trim 40 mg+sulfa 200 mg per 5 ml (100 ml) (cherry) (alcohol 0.3%)
Comment: Sulfonamides are contraindicated in the first trimester of pregnancy, the final month of pregnancy, and infants <8 weeks-of-age. *CrCl 15-30 mL/min:* reduce dose by 1/2; *CrCl <15 mL/min:* not recommended. Contraindicated with G6PD deficiency. A high fluid intake is indicated during sulfonamide therapy to avoid crystallization in the kidneys.

OTIC ANTI-INFECTIVE

➤ *ofloxacin* (C)(G) 10 drops bid x 14 days
    Pediatric: <6 months: not recommended; 6 months-12 years: 5 drops bid x 14 days; >12 years: same as adult
    Floxin Otic *Otic soln:* 0.3% (5, 10 ml w. dropper)

OTIC ANTI-INFECTIVE+CORTICOSTEROID COMBINATIONS

Comment: *neomycin* may cause ototoxicity. Do not use with known <u>or</u> suspected tympanic membrane rupture.

➤ *chloroxylenol+pramoxine+hydrocortisone* (C) 4 drops tid-qid x 5-10 days
Pediatric: 3 drops tid-qid x 5-10 days
    Cortane Ear Drops, *Otic drops:* 10 ml

➤ *ciprofloxacin+hydrocortisone* (C) otic susp 3 drops bid x 7 days
Pediatric: <1 year: not recommended; ≥1 year: same as adult
    Cipro HC *Otic susp:* cipro 0.3%+dexa 0.1% (10 ml)

➤ *ciprofloxacin+dexamethasone* (C) otic susp 4 drops bid x 7 days
Pediatric: <6 months: not recommended; ≥6 months: same as adult
    Ciprodex *Otic susp:* cipro 0.3%+dexa 1% (7.5 ml)
    Comment: Ciprodex is indicated for the treatment of otitis media in pediatric patients with tympanostomy tubes (PE tubes).

➤ *colistin+neomycin+hydrocortisone+thonzonium* (C) 5 drops tid-qid x 5-10 days
Pediatric: 4 drops tid-qid x 5-10 days
    Coly-Mycin S *Otic susp:* 5, 10 ml

➤ *polymyxin b+neomycin+hydrocortisone* (C)(G) 4 drops tid-qid; max 10 days
Pediatric: 3 drops tid-qid; max 10 days
    Cortisporin *Otic susp:* 10 ml w. dropper; *Otic soln:* 10 ml w. dropper
    PediOtic *Otic susp:* 7.5 ml w. dropper

▷ *polymyxin b+neomycin+hydrocortisone+surfactant* (C) 4 drops tid-qid
  Pediatric: 3 drops tid-qid; max 10 days
    Cortisporin-TC *Otic susp:* 10 ml w. dropper

OTIC ANESTHETIC+ANALGESIC COMBINATIONS

▷ *antipyrine+benzocaine+glycerine* (C) fill ear canal and insert cotton plug; may repeat q 1-2 hours as needed
  Pediatric: same as adult
    A/B Otic *Otic soln:* antipy 5.4%+benzo 1.4% 15 ml w. dropper
▷ *benzocaine* (C)(OTC) 4-5 drops q 1-2 hours
  Pediatric: <1 year: not recommended; ≥1 year: same as adult
    Otic drops: 20% (15 ml dropper-top bottle)
    Americaine Otic *Otic soln:* 15 ml w. dropper
    Benzotic *Otic soln:* 20% (15 ml w. dropper)

 OTITIS MEDIA: SEROUS (SOM), OTITIS MEDIA WITH EFFUSION

Anti-infectives *see* **Otitis Media: Acute** *page 347*
Antihistamines & Decongestants *see* **Drugs for the Management of Allergy, Cough, and Cold Symptoms** *page 603*
Oral Corticosteroids *see page 577*

INTRA-TYMPANIC AGENT

▷ *ciprofloxacin otic suspension* <6 months: not recommended; ≥6 months: instill 0.1 ml in each ear, via intra-tympanic administration only by a qualified healthcare professional, following suctioning of the middle ear effusion
    Otiprio *Vial:* 6% otic suspension (6 mg/ml, 1 ml) single-patient use with two 0.1 ml doses in each vial (preservative-free)
    Comment: Otiprio is *ciprofloxacin,* a synthetic fluoroquinolone antibacterial, indicated for the treatment of acute otitis media (AOM) due to *Pseudomonas aeruginosa* and *Staphylococcus aureus* and for intra-tympanic administration in pediatric patients ≥6 months-of-age with bilateral AOM with effusion undergoing tympanostomy tube placement. The bactericidal action of *ciprofloxacin* results from interference with the enzyme DNA gyrase, which is needed for the synthesis of bacterial DNA. *ciprofloxacin* has been shown to be active against most isolates of the following bacteria: Gram-positive Bacteria (i.e., *Staphylococcus aureus, Streptococcus pneumoniae*) and Gram-negative Bacteria (*Haemophilus influenza, Moraxella catarrhalis, Pseudomonas aeruginosa*). **Otiprio** is for intra-tympanic administration only. The most frequently occurring adverse reactions (incidence > 3 %) were nasopharyngitis and irritability. Because of the negligible systemic exposure associated with clinical administration of **Otiprio**, this product is expected to be of minimal risk for maternal and fetal toxicity during pregnancy and nursing infants of mothers receiving **Otiprio** should not be affected. To report suspected adverse reactions, contact Otonomy at 1-800-826-6411 or FDA at 1-800-FDA-1088 or www.fda.gov/medwatch.

 PAGET'S DISEASE: BONE

Comment: Calcium decreases *tetracycline* absorption. *calcium* absorption is decreased by corticosteroids. *calcium* absorption is decreased by foods such as rhubarb, spinach, and bran.

BISPHOSPHONATES (CALCIUM MODIFIERS)

Comment: Bisphosphonates should be swallowed whole in the AM with 6-8 oz of plain water 30 minutes before first meal, beverage, or other medications of the day. Monitor serum alkaline phosphatase. Contraindications include abnormalities of the esophagus which delay esophageal emptying such as stricture or achalasia, inability to stand or sit upright for at least 30 minutes post-dose, patients at risk of aspiration, and hypocalcemia. Co-administration of bisphosphonates and calcium, antacids, or oral medications containing multivalent cations will interfere with absorption of the bisphosphonate. Therefore, instruct patients to wait at least half hour after taking the bisphosphonate before taking any other oral medications.

▷ *alendronate (as sodium)* (C)(G) take once weekly, in the AM, 30 minutes before the first food, beverage, or medication of the day; do not lie down (remain upright) for at least 30 minutes and after the first food of the day; not recommended with *CrCl <35 mL/min*.
Pediatric: <12 years: not recommended; ≥12 years: same as adult
  Binosto dissolve the effervescent tab in 4 oz (120 ml) of plain, room temperature, water (not mineral or flavored); wait 5 minutes after the effervescence has subsided, then stir for 10 seconds, then drink
    Tab: 70 mg effervescent for buffered solution (4, 12/carton) (strawberry)
  Fosamax (G) swallow tab whole; dosing regimens are the same for men and post-menopausal women; *Prevention:* 5 mg once daily or 35 mg once weekly; *Treatment:* 10 mg once daily or 70 mg once weekly
    Tab: 5, 10, 35, 40, 70 mg
▷ *alendronate+cholecalciferol (vit d3)* (C)(G) take 1 tab once weekly, in the AM, with plain water (not mineral) 30 minutes before the first food, beverage, or medication of the day; do not lie down (remain upright) for at least 30 minutes and after the first food of the day
Pediatric: <12 years: not recommended; ≥12 years: same as adult
  Fosamax Plus D
    Tab: **Fosamax Plus D 70/2800** alen 70 mg+chole 2800 IU
  Fosamax Plus D 70/5600 alen 70 mg+chole 5600 IU
▷ *ibandronate (as monosodium monohydrate)* (C)(G)
Pediatric: <12 years: not recommended; ≥12 years: same as adult
  Boniva take 2.5 mg once daily or 150 mg once monthly on the same day; take in the AM, with plain water (not mineral) 60 minutes before the first food, beverage, or medication of the day; do not lie down (remain upright) for at least 30 minutes and after the first food of the day
    Tab: 2.5, 150 mg
  Boniva Injection administer 3 mg every 3 months by IV bolus over 15-30 seconds; if dose is missed, administer as soon as possible, then every 3 months from the date of the last dose
    Prefilled syringe: 3 mg/3 ml (5 ml)
  Comment: **Boniva Injection** must be administered by a qualified health care professional.
▷ *risedronate (as sodium)* (C)(G) take in the AM; swallow whole with a full glass of plain water (not mineral) do not lie down (remain upright) for 30 minutes afterward
Pediatric: <12 years: not recommended; ≥12 years: same as adult
  Actonel take at least 30 minutes before any food or drink; *Women:* 5 mg once daily or 35 mg once weekly or 75 mg on two consecutive days monthly or 150 mg once monthly; *Men:* 35 mg once weekly
    Tab: 5, 30, 35, 75, 150 mg
  Atelvia 35 mg once weekly immediately after breakfast
    Tab: 35 mg del-rel
▷ *risedronate+calcium* (C) 1 x 5 mg *risedronate* tab weekly and 1 x 500 mg *calcium* tab on days 2-7 weekly
  Actonel with Calcium *Tab: risedronate* 5 mg and *Tab: calcium* 500 mg (4 *risedronate* tabs + 30 *calcium* tabs/pck)
▷ *zoledronic acid* (D)(G)
Pediatric: <12 years: not recommended; ≥12 years: same as adult
  Reclast administer 5 mg via IV infusion over at least 15 minutes mg once a year (for osteoporosis) or once every 2 years (for osteopenia or prophylaxis)
    Bottle: 5 mg/100 ml (single-dose)
  Comment: **Reclast** is indicated for the treatment of postmenopausal osteoporosis in women who are at high risk for fracture and to increase bone mass in men with primary or hypogonadal osteoporosis who are at high risk for fracture. Administered by a qualified health care professional. Contraindicated in hypocalcemia.
  Zometa administer 4 mg via IV infusion over at least 15 minutes every 3-4 weeks; optimal duration of treatment not known
    Bottle: 4 mg/5 ml; *Vial:* 4 mg/5 ml (single-dose)
  Comment: **Zometa** is indicated for the treatment of hypercalcemia of malignancy. The safety and efficacy of **Zometa** in the treatment of hypercalcemia associated with hyperparathyroidism or with other non-tumor-related conditions has not been established.

PAIN

Antidepressants *see Depression page* 117
Skeletal Muscle Relaxants *see Muscle Strain page* 311

ACETAMINOPHEN FOR IV INFUSION

▷ *acetaminophen* injectable (B) administer by IV infusion over 15 minutes; 1,000 mg q 6 hours prn or 650 mg q 4 hours prn; max 4,000 mg/day
Pediatric: <2 years: not recommended; 2-13 years <50 kg: 15 mg/kg q 6 hours prn or 2.5 mg/kg q 4 hours prn; max 750 mg/single dose; max 75 mg/kg per day; >13 years: same as adult
  Ofirmev *Vial:* 10 mg/ml (100 ml) (preservative-free)
  Comment: The Ofirmev vial is intended for single-use. If any portion is withdrawn from the vial, use within 6 hours. Discard the unused portion. For pediatric patients, withdraw the intended dose and administer via syringe pump. Do not admix Ofirmev with any other drugs. Ofirmev is physically incompatible with *diazepam* and *chlorpromazine hydrochloride.*

IBUPROFEN FOR IV INFUSION

▷ *ibuprofen* (B) dilute dose in 0.9% NS, D5W, or Lactated Ringers (LR) solution; administer by IV infusion over at least 10 minutes; do not administer via IV bolus or IM; 400-800 mg q 6 hours prn; maximum 3,200 mg/day
Pediatric: <6 months; not recommended; 6 months-<12 years: 10 mg/kg q 4-6 hours prn; max 400 mg/dose; max 40 mg/kg or 2,400 mg/24 hours, whichever is less; 12-17 years: 400 mg q 4-6 hours prn; max 2,400 mg/24 hours
  Caldolor *Vial:* 800 mg/8 ml single-dose
  Comment: Prepare Caldolor solution for IV administration as follows: 100 mg dose: dilute 1 ml of Caldolor in at least 100 ml of diluent (IVF); 200 mg dose: dilute 2 ml of Caldolor in at least 100 ml of diluent; 400 mg dose: dilute 4 ml of Caldolor in at least 100 ml of diluent; 800 mg dose: dilute 8 ml of Caldolor in at least 200 ml of diluent. Caldolor is also indicated for management of fever. For adults with fever, 400 mg via IV infusion, followed by 400 mg q 4-6 hours or 100-200 mg q 4 hours prn.

OCULAR PAIN

▷ *dexamethasone ophthalmic insert* post-surgical insertion in the lower lacrimal punctum and into the canaliculus by a qualified health care provider; insert is resorbable (does not require removal); saline irrigation or manual expression can be performed if removal is necessary; a single insert provides sustained delivery of dexamethasone up to 30 days.
Pediatric: not established
  Dextenza 0.4 mg single dose in a foam carrier within a foil laminate pouch (preservative-free)
  Comment: Dextenza is the first FDA-approved intra-canalicular insert delivering dexamethasone to treat post-surgical ocular pain for up to 30 days with a single administration.
▷ *difluprednate* (C) apply 1 drop to affected eye qid; for postop ocular pain, begin treatment 24 hours postop and continue x 2 weeks; then bid daily x 1 week; then taper
Pediatric: <12 years: not recommended; ≥12 years: same as adult
  Durezol *Ophth emul:* 0.05% (5 ml)
  Comment: Durezol is an ophthalmic steroid.
▷ *nepafenac* (C) apply 1 drop to affected eye tid; for postop ocular pain, begin treatment 24 hours before surgery and continue day of surgery and for two weeks post-op
Pediatric: <10 years: not recommended; ≥10 years: same as adult
  Nevanac *Ophth susp:* 0.1% (3 ml) (benzalkonium chloride)
  Comment: Nevanac is an ophthalmic NSAID.

TOPICAL & TRANSDERMAL ANALGESICS

▷ *capsaicin* (B)(G) apply tid-qid prn to intact skin
Pediatric: <2 years: not recommended; ≥2 years: apply sparingly tid-qid prn

Axsain *Crm:* 0.075% (1, 2 oz)
Capsin (OTC) *Lotn:* 0.025, 0.075% (59 ml)
Capzasin-HP (OTC) *Crm:* 0.075% (1.5 oz), 0.025% (45, 90 gm); *Lotn:* 0.075% (2 oz); 0.025% (45, 90 gm)
Capzasin-P (OTC) *Crm:* 0.025% (1.5 oz); *Lotn:* 0.025% (2 oz)
Dolorac *Crm:* 0.025% (28 gm)
Double Cap (OTC) *Crm:* 0.05% (2 oz)
R-Gel *Gel:* 0.025% (15, 30 gm)
Zostrix (OTC) *Crm:* 0.025% (0.7, 1.5, 3 oz)
Zostrix HP (OTC) *Emol crm:* 0.075% (1, 2 oz)

▷ *capsaicin* 8% patch **(B)** apply up to 4 patches for one 60-minute application to clean dry skin; may prep area with topical anesthetic; wear non-latex gloves; patches may be cut to size/shape; treatment may be repeated every 3 months
Pediatric: <18 years: not recommended; ≥8 years: same as adult
Qutenza *Patch:* 8% 1640 mcg/cm (179 mg) (1 or 2 patches w. 1-50 gm tube cleansing gel/carton)

▷ *diclofenac sodium* **(C; D ≥30 wks)(G)** apply qid prn to intact skin
Pediatric: <12 years: not established; ≥12 years: same as adult
Pennsaid 1.5% in 10 drop increments, dispense and rub into front, side, and back of knee: usually; 40 drops (40 mg) qid
Topical soln: 1.5% (150 ml)
Pennsaid 2% apply 2 pump actuations (40 mg) and rub into front, side, and back of knee bid
Topical soln: 2% (20 mg/pump actuation, 112 gm)
Solaraze Gel massage in to clean skin bid prn
Gel: 3% (50 gm) (benzyl alcohol)
Voltaren Gel (G) apply qid prn to intact skin
Gel: 1% (100 gm)

Comment: *diclofenac* is contraindicated with *aspirin* allergy. As with other NSAIDs, should be avoided in late pregnancy (≥30 weeks) because it may cause premature closure of the ductus arteriosus.

▷ *doxepin* **(B)** cream apply to affected area qid at intervals of at least 3-4 hours; max 8 days
Pediatric: <12 years: not recommended; >12 years: same as adult
Prudoxin *Crm:* 5% (45 gm)
Zonalon *Crm:* 5% (30, 45 gm)

▷ *pimecrolimus* 1% cream **(C)(G)** <2 years: not recommended; ≥2 years: apply to affected area bid; do not apply an occlusive dressing
Elidel *Crm:* 1% (30, 60, 100 gm)

Comment: *pimecrolimus* is indicated for short-term and intermittent long-term use. Discontinue use when resolution occurs. Contraindicated if the patient is immunosuppressed. Change to the 0.1% preparation or if secondary bacterial infection is present.

▷ *trolamine salicylate* apply tid-qid
Pediatric: <2 years: not recommended; ≥2 years: same as adult
Mobisyl Creme *Crm:* 10% (100 gm)

TOPICAL AND TRANSDERMAL ANESTHETICS

Comment: *lidocaine* should not be applied to non-intact skin.

▷ *lidocaine* cream **(B)** apply to affected area bid prn
Pediatric: <12 years: not recommended; ≥12 years: same as adult
LidaMantle *Crm:* 3% (1, 2 oz)
Lidoderm *Crm:* 3% (85 gm)
ZTlido *lidocaine* topical system 1% (30/carton)
Comment: Compared to **Lidoderm** (*lidocaine* patch 5%) which contains 700 mg/patch, **ZTlido** only requires 35 mg per topical system to achieve the same therapeutic dose.

▷ *lidocaine* lotion **(B)** apply to affected area bid prn
Pediatric: <12 years: not recommended; ≥12 years: same as adult
LidaMantle *Lotn:* 3% (177 ml)

▷ *lidocaine* 5% patch **(B)(G)** apply up to 3 patches at one time for up to 12 hours/24-hour period (12 hours on/12 hours off); patches may be cut into smaller sizes before removal of the release liner; do <u>not</u> re-use
Pediatric: <12 years: not recommended; ≥12 years: same as adult
    Lidoderm *Patch:* 5% (10x14 cm; 30/carton)

▷ *lidocaine+dexamethasone* **(B)**
Pediatric: <12 years: not recommended; ≥12 years: same as adult
    Decadron Phosphate with Xylocaine *Lotn:* dexa 4 mg+lido 10 mg per ml (5 ml)

▷ *lidocaine+hydrocortisone* **(B)(G)** apply to affected area bid prn
Pediatric: <12 years: not recommended; ≥12 years: same as adult
    LidaMantle HC *Crm:* lido 3%+hydro 0.5% (1, 3 oz); *Lotn:* (177 ml)

▷ *lidocaine* 2.5%+*prilocaine* 2.5% apply sparingly to the burn bid-tid prn
Pediatric: <12 years: not recommended; ≥12 years: same as adult
    Emla Cream (B) 5, 30 gm/tube

OPIOID ANALGESICS

Comment: According to the American Society of Interventional Pain Physicians (ASIPP), presumptive urine drug testing (UDT) should be performed when opioid therapy for chronic pain is initiated, along with subsequent use as adherence monitoring, using in-office point of service testing, to identify patients who are non-compliant or abusing prescription drugs or illicit drugs.

REFERENCE
Manchikanti, L., Kaye, A. M., Knezevic, N. N., McAnally, H., Slavin, K., Trescot, A.M., . . . Hirsch, J. A. (2017). Responsible, safe, and effective prescription of opioids for chronic non-cancer pain: American Society of Interventional Pain Physicians (ASIPP) guidelines. *Pain Physician, 20*(2S), S3-S92. Retrieved from https://www.painphysicianjournal.com/current/pdf?article=NDIwMg%3D%3D&journal=103

Opiate agonists may produce significant central nervous system and respiratory depression of varying duration, particularly when given in high dosages and/or by rapid intravenous administration. Apnea may result from decreased respiratory drive as well as increased airway resistance, and rigidity of respiratory muscles may occur during rapid IV administration or when these agents are used in the induction of anesthesia. At therapeutic analgesic dosages, the respiratory effects are usually not clinically important except in patients with pre-existing pulmonary impairment. Therapy with opiate agonists should be avoided or administered with extreme caution and initiated at reduced dosages in patients with severe CNS depression (e.g., sleep apnea, hypoxia, anoxia, or hypercapnia, upper airway obstruction, chronic pulmonary insufficiency, limited ventilatory reserve, other respiratory disorders). In the presence of excessive respiratory secretions, the use of opiate agonists may also be problematic because they decrease ciliary activity and reduce the cough reflex. Caution is also advised in patients who may be at increased risk for respiratory depression, such as comatose patients or those with head injury, intracranial lesions, or intracranial hypertension. Clinical monitoring of pulmonary function is recommended, and equipment for resuscitation should be immediately available if parenteral or neuraxial routes are used. *naloxone* may be administered to reverse clinically significant respiratory depression, which may be prolonged depending on the opioid agent, cumulative dose, and route of administration.

▷ *benzhydrocodone+acetaminophen* **(II)** <18 years: not recommended; ≥18 years: initiate treatment with at 1-2 tabs every 4 to 6 hours prn; max 12 tabs/24 hours; max 14 days
    Apadaz *Tab:* benz 6.12 mg+acet 325 mg
Comment: *benzhydrocodone* 6.12 mg is equivalent to 4.54 mg *hydrocodone* or 7.5 mg *hydrocodone bitartrate*. If switching from immediate-release *hydrocodone bitartrate+acetaminophen*, substitute **Apadaz** 6.12 mg/325 mg for 7.5 mg/325 mg *hydrocodone bitartrate+acetaminophen*. Dosage of **Apadaz** should be adjusted according to the severity of the pain and the response of the patient. Do not stop **Apadaz** abruptly in the physically-dependent patient.

▷ *butalbital+acetaminophen* **(C)(G)** 1 tab q 4 hours prn; max 6 tabs/day
Pediatric: <12 years: not recommended; ≥12 years: same as adult
    Tab: but 50 mg+acet 325 mg
    Phrenilin 1-2 tabs q 4 hours prn; max 6 tabs/day
    Tab: but 50 mg+acet 325 mg

Phrenilin Forte 1 tab or cap q 4 hours prn; max 6 caps/day
Cap: but 50 mg+acet 325 mg; *Tab:* but 50 mg+acet 325 mg

▶ *butalbital+acetaminophen+caffeine* (C)(G)
Pediatric: <12: not recommended; ≥12 years: same as adult
Fioricet 1-2 tabs q 4 hours prn; max 6/day
Tab: but 50 mg+acet 325 mg+caf 40 mg
Zebutal q 4 hours prn; max 5/day
Cap: but 50 mg+acet 325 mg+caf 40 mg

▶ *butalbital+aspirin+caffeine* (C)(III)(G)
Pediatric: <12 years: not recommended; ≥12 year: same as adult
Fiorinal 1-2 tabs or caps q 4 hours prn; max 6 caps/day
Tab/Cap: but 50 mg+asp 325 mg+caf 40 mg

Comment: *aspirin*-containing medications are contraindicated with history of allergic-type reaction to *aspirin*, children and adolescents with *Varicella* or other viral illness, and 3rd trimester of pregnancy.

▶ *butalbital+aspirin+codeine+caffeine* (C)(III)(G)
Pediatric: <18 years: not recommended; ≥18 year: same as adult
Fiorinal with Codeine 1-2 caps q 4 hours prn; max 6 caps/day
Cap: but 50 mg+asp 325 mg+cod 30 mg+caf 40 mg

Comment: *Codeine* is known to be excreted in breast milk. <12 years: not recommended; 12-<18: use extreme caution; not recommended for children and adolescents with asthma or other chronic breathing problem. The FDA and the European Medicines Agency (EMA) are investigating the safety of using *codeine* containing medications to treat pain, cough and colds, in children 12-<18 years because of the potential for serious side effects, including slowed or difficult breathing. *aspirin*-containing medications are contraindicated with history of allergic-type reaction to *aspirin*, children and adolescents with *Varicella* or other viral illness, and 3rd trimester of pregnancy.

▶ *codeine sulfate* (C)(III)(G) 15-60 q 4-6 hours prn; max 60 mg/day
Pediatric: <18 years: not recommended; ≥18 year: same as adult
Tab: 15, 30, 60 mg

Comment: *codeine* is known to be excreted in breast milk. <12 years: not recommended; 12-<18: use extreme caution; not recommended for children and adolescents with asthma or other chronic breathing problem. The FDA and the European Medicines Agency (EMA) are investigating the safety of using *codeine* containing medications to treat pain, cough and colds, in children 12-<18 years because of the potential for serious side effects, including slowed or difficult breathing.

▶ *codeine+acetaminophen* (C)(III)(G) 15-60 mg of *codeine* q 4 hours prn; max 360 mg of *codeine*/day
Pediatric: <18 years: not recommended; ≥18 year: same as adult
Tab: **Tylenol #1** cod 7.5 mg+acet 300 mg (sulfites)
Tylenol #2 cod 15 mg+acet 300 mg (sulfites)
Tylenol #3 cod 30 mg+acet 300 mg (sulfites)
Tylenol #4 cod 60 mg+acet 300 mg (sulfites)
Tylenol with Codeine Elixir (C)(III)
Elix: cod 12 mg+acet 120 mg per 5 ml (cherry) (alcohol)

Comment: *codeine* is known to be excreted in breast milk. <12 years: not recommended; 12-<18: use extreme caution; not recommended for children and adolescents with asthma or other chronic breathing problem. The FDA and the European Medicines Agency (EMA) are investigating the safety of using *codeine* containing medications to treat pain, cough and colds, in children 12-<18 years because of the potential for serious side effects, including slowed or difficult breathing.

▶ *dihydrocodeine+acetaminophen+caffeine* (C)(III)(G)
Pediatric: <18 years: not recommended; ≥18 years: same as adult
Panlor DC 1-2 caps q 4-6 hours prn; max 10 caps/day
Cap: dihydro 16 mg+acet 325 mg+caf 30 mg
Panlor SS 1 tab q 4 hours prn; max 5 tabs/day
Tab: dihydro 32 mg+acet 325 mg+caf 60*mg

Comment: *Codeine* is known to be excreted in breast milk. <12 years: not recommended; 12-<18: use extreme caution; not recommended for children and adolescents with asthma or other chronic breathing problem. The FDA and the European Medicines Agency (EMA) are investigating the safety of using *codeine* containing medications to treat pain, cough and colds, in children 12-<18 years because of the potential for serious side effects, including slowed or difficult breathing.

▷ *dihydrocodeine+aspirin+caffeine* (D)(III)(G) 1-2 caps q 4 hours prn
Pediatric: <18 years: not recommended; ≥18 years: same as adult
  Synalgos-DC
    Cap: dihydro 16 mg+asp 356.4 mg+caf 30 mg

Comment: *Codeine* is known to be excreted in breast milk. <12 years: not recommended; 12-<18: use extreme caution; not recommended for children and adolescents with asthma or other chronic breathing problem. The FDA and the European Medicines Agency (EMA) are investigating the safety of using *codeine* containing medications to treat pain, cough and colds, in children 12-<18 years because of the potential for serious side effects, including slowed or difficult breathing. *aspirin*-containing medications are contraindicated with history of allergic-type reaction to *aspirin*, children and adolescents with *Varicella* or other viral illness, and 3rd trimester of pregnancy.

▷ *hydrocodone bitartrate* (C)(II)
Pediatric: <18 years: not recommended; ≥18 years: same as adult
  Hysingla ER swallow whole; 1 tab once daily at the same time each day
    Tab: 20, 30, 40, 60, 80, 100, 120 mg ext-rel
  Vantrela ER swallow whole; 1 tab once daily at the same time each day
    Tab: 15, 30, 45, 60, 90 mg ext-rel
  Zohydro ER swallow whole; *Opioid naïve:* 10 mg q 12 hours; may increase by 10 mg q 12 hours every 3-7 days; when discontinuing, titrate downward every 2-4 days
    Cap: 10, 15, 20, 30, 40, 50 mg ext-rel

▷ *hydrocodone bitartrate+acetaminophen* (C)(II)(G)
Pediatric: <18: not recommended; ≥18 years: same as adult
  Hycet 5/325 1-2 tabs q 4-6 hours prn; max 8 tabs/day
    Tab: hydro 5 mg+acet 325 mg*
  Hycet 7.5/325 1 tab q 4-6 hours prn; max 6 tabs/day
    Tab: hydro 7.5 mg+acet 325 mg*
  Hycet 10/325 1 tab q 4-6 hours prn; max 6 tab/day
    Tab: hydro 10 mg+acet 325 mg*
  Hycet Oral Solution 2.5/325 3 tsp (15 ml) q 4-6 hours prn; max 24 tsp (90 ml)/day (alcohol 7%)
    Liq: hydro 2.5 mg+acet 108 mg per 15 ml (alcohol 7%)
  Hycet Oral Solution 7.5/325 1 tsp (5 ml) q 4-6 hours prn; max 8 tsp (90 ml)/day (alcohol 7%)
    Liq: hydro 7.5 mg+acet 325 mg per 15 ml (alcohol 7%)
  Lorcet 1-2 tabs q 4-6 hours prn; max 8 caps/day*
    Tab: hydro 5 mg+acet 325 mg
  Lorcet Plus 1 tab q 4-6 hours prn; max 6 tabs/day*
    Tab: hydro 7.5 mg+acet 325 mg
  Lorcet-HD 1 cap q 4-6 hours prn; max 6 tabs/day*
    Tab: hydro 10 mg+acet 325 mg
  Lortab 5/325 1-2 tabs q 4-6 hours prn; max 8 tabs/day
    Tab: hydro 5 mg+acet 325 mg*
  Lortab 7.5/325 1 tab q 4-6 hours prn; max 6 tabs/day
    Tab: hydro 7.5 mg+acet 325 mg*
  Lortab 10/500 1 tab q 4-6 hours prn; max 6 tabs/day
    Tab: hydro 10 mg+acet 325 mg*
  Maxidone 1 tab q 4-6 hours prn; max 5 tabs/day
    Tab: hydro 10 mg+acet 750 mg*
  Norco 5/325 1-2 tabs q 4-6 hours prn; max 8 tabs/day
    Tab: hydro 5 mg+acet 325 mg*
  Norco 7.5/325 1 tab q 4-6 hours prn; max 6 tabs/day
    Tab: hydro 7.5 mg+acet 325 mg*
  Norco 10/325 1 tab q 4-6 hours prn; max 6 tabs/day
    Tab: hydro 10 mg+acet 325 mg*
  Vicodin 1-2 tabs q 4-6 hours prn; max 8 tabs/day
    Tab: hydro 5 mg+acet 300 mg*
  Vicodin ES 1 tab q 4-6 hours prn; max 6 tabs/day
    Tab: hydro 7.5 mg+acet 300 mg*

Vicodin HP 1 tab q 4-6 hours prn; max 6 tabs/day
  Tab: hydro 10 mg+acet 300 mg*
Xodol 5/300 1-2 tabs q 4-6 hours prn; max 8 tabs/day
  Tab: hydro 5 mg+acet 300 mg*
Xodol 7.5/300 1 tab q 4-6 hours prn; max 6 tabs/day
  Tab: hydro 7.5 mg+acet 300 mg*
Xodol 10/300 1 tab q 4-6 hours prn; max 6 tabs/day
  Tab: hydro 10 mg+acet 300 mg*
Zamicet Oral Solution 5/163 3 tsp (15 ml) q 4-6 hours prn; max 24 tsp (90 ml)/day
(alcohol 7.7%)
  Liq: hydro 5 mg+acet 325 mg per 163 ml (alcohol 7%)
Zamicet Oral Solution 10/325 3 tsp (15 ml) q 4-6 hours prn; max 24 tsp (90 ml)/day
(alcohol 7.7%)
  Liq: hydro 10 mg+acet 325 mg per 15 ml (alcohol 7%)
Zydone 5/400 1-2 tabs q 4-6 hours prn; max 8 tabs/day
  Tab: hydro 5 mg+acet 400 mg
Zydone 7.5/400 1 tab q 4-6 hours prn; max 6 tabs/day
  Tab: hydro 7.5 mg+acet 400 mg
Zydone 10/400 1 tab q 4-6 hours prn; max 6 tabs/day
  Tab: hydro 10 mg+acet 400 mg

➤ *hydrocodone+ibuprofen* **(C; not for use in 3rd)(II)(G)**
Pediatric: <18: not recommended; ≥18 years: same as adult
    Ibudone 5/200 1 tab q 4-6 hours prn; max 5 tabs/day
      Tab: hydro 5 mg+ibup 200 mg
    Ibudone 10/200 1 tab q 4-6 hours prn; max 5 tabs/day
      Tab: hydro 10 mg+ibup 200 mg
    Reprexain 1 tab q 4-6 hours prn; max 5 tabs/day
      Tab: hydro 5 mg+ibup 200 mg
    Vicoprofen 1 tab q 4-6 hours prn; max 5 tabs/day
      Tab: hydro 7.5 mg+ibup 200 mg

➤ *hydromorphone* **(C)(II)(G)**
Pediatric: <18: not recommended; ≥18 years: same as adult
    Dilaudid initially 2-4 mg q 4-6 hours prn
      Tab: 2, 4, 8 mg (sulfites)
    Dilaudid Oral Liquid 2.5-10 mg q 3-6 hours prn
      Liq: 5 mg/5 ml (sulfites)
    Dilaudid Rectal Suppository 2.5-10 mg q 6-8 hours prn
      Rectal supp: 3 mg
    Dilaudid Injection initially 1-2 mg SC or IM q 4-6 hours prn
      Amp: 1, 2, 4 mg/ml (1 ml)
    Dilaudid-HP Injection initially 1-2 mg SC or IM q 4-6 hours prn
      Amp: 10 mg/ml (1 ml)
    Exalgo initially 8-64 mg once daily
      Tab: 8, 12, 16, 32 mg ext-rel (sulfites)

➤ *meperidine* **(C; D in 2nd, 3rd)(II)(G)** 50-150 mg q 3-4 hours prn
Pediatric: 0.5-0.8 mg/lb q 3-4 hours prn; max adult dose
    Demerol *Tab:* 50, 100 mg; *Syr:* 50 mg/5 ml (banana) (alcohol-free)

➤ *meperidine+promethazine* **(C; D in 2nd, 3rd)(II)(G)**
Pediatric: <18: not recommended; ≥18 years: same as adult
    Mepergan 1-2 tsp q 3-4 hours prn
      Syr: mep 25 mg+prom 25 mg per ml
    Mepergan Fortis 1-2 tsp q 4-6 hours prn
      Tab: mep 50 mg+prom 25 mg

➤ *methadone* **(C)(II)(G)** 2.5-10 mg PO, SC, or IM q 3-4 hours; for use only in chronic moderately severe-to-severe pain management (e.g., hospice care). For opioid naïve patients, initiate **Dolophine** tablets with 2.5 mg every 8 to 12 hours; unlike other opioid analgesics, *methadone* is not indicated as an as-needed (prn) analgesic, per se; titrate slowly with dose increases no more frequent than every 3 to 5 days; to convert to **Dolophine** tablets from another opioid, use available conversion factors to obtain estimated dose (see mfr pkg insert); do not abruptly discontinue **Dolophine** in a physically dependent patient
Pediatric: <18: not recommended; ≥18 years: same as adult

Dolophine *Tab:* 5, 10 mg; *Dispersible tab:* 40 mg (dissolve in 120 ml orange juice or other citrus drink); *Oral soln:* 5, 10 mg/ml; *Oral conc:* 10 mg/ml; *Syr:* 10 mg/30 ml; *Vial:* 10 mg/ml (200 mg/20 ml multi-dose) for injection

Comment: *methadone* administration is allowed only by approved providers with strict state and federal regulations (as stipulated in 42 CFR 8.12). Black Box Warning (BBW): *Dolophine* exposes users to risks of addiction, abuse, and misuse, which can lead to overdose and death. Assess each patient's risk and monitor regularly for development of these behaviors and conditions. Serious, life-threatening, or fatal respiratory depression may occur. The peak respiratory depressant effect of *methadone* occurs later, and persists longer than the peak analgesic effect. Accidental ingestion, especially by children, can result in fatal overdose. QT interval prolongation and serious arrhythmias (*torsades de pointes*) have occurred during treatment with *methadone*. Closely monitor patients with risk factors for development of prolonged QT interval, a history of cardiac conduction abnormalities, and those taking medications affecting cardiac conduction. Neonatal Opioid Withdrawal Syndrome (NOWS) is an expected and treatable outcome of use of methadone use during pregnancy. NOWS may be life-threatening if not recognized and treated in the neonate. The balance between the risks of NOWS and the benefits of maternal *methadone* use should be considered and the patient advised of the risk of NOWS so that appropriate planning for management of the neonate can occur. *methadone* has been detected in human milk. Concomitant use with CYP3A4, 2B6, 2C19, 2C9 or 2D6 inhibitors or discontinuation of concomitantly used CYP3A4 2B6, 2C19, or 2C9 inducers can result in a fatal overdose of *methadone*. Concomitant use of opioids with benzodiazepines or other central nervous system (CNS) depressants, including alcohol, may result in profound sedation, respiratory depression, coma, and death.

▶ *morphine sulfate (immed-release)* (C)(II)(G) usually 15-30 mg q 4 hours prn; solution, usually 10-20 mg q 4 hours prn
Pediatric: <18: not recommended; ≥18 years: same as adult
 Tab: 15*, 30*mg; *Oral soln:* 10 mg/5 ml, 20 mg/5 ml (100, 500 ml), 100 mg/5 ml (30, 120 ml)

▶ *morphine sulfate (immed- and sust-rel)* (C)(II)
Comment: Dosage dependent upon previous opioid dosage; see mfr pkg insert for conversion guidelines; not for prn use; swallow whole or sprinkle contents of caps on applesauce (do not crush, chew, or dissolve). Generic *morphine sulfate* is available in the following forms: *Tab:* 15*, 30*mg; *Oral soln:* 10, 20 mg/5 ml (100 ml); 100 mg/5 ml (30, 120 ml w. oral syringe)
Pediatric: <18 years: not recommended; ≥18 years: same as adult
 Arymo ER swallow whole; 1 tab once daily at the same time each day
  Tab: 15, 30, 60 mg ext-rel
 Duramorph administer per anesthesia
  IV/Intrathecal/Epidural: 0.5, 1 mg/ml
 Infumorph administer per anesthesia
  Intrathecal/Epidural: 10, 20 mg/ml
 Kadian (G) 1 cap every 12-24 hours
  Cap: 10, 20, 30, 50, 60, 80, 100, 200 mg sust-rel
 MS Contin (G) 1 tab every 24 hours
  Tab: 15, 30, 60, 100, 200 mg sust-rel
 MSIR 5-30 mg q 4 hours prn
  Tab: 15*, 30*mg; *Cap:* 15, 30 mg
 MSIR Oral Solution 5-30 mg q 4 hours prn
  Oral soln: 10, 20 mg/5 ml (120 ml)
 MSIR Oral Solution Concentrate 5-30 mg q 4 hours prn
  Oral conc: 20 mg/ml (30, 120 ml w. dropper)
 Oramorph SR 1 cap every 12-24 hours
  Tab: 15, 30, 60, 100 mg sust-rel
 Roxanol Oral Solution 10-30 mg q 4 hours prn
  Oral soln: 20 mg/ml (1, 4, 8 oz)
 Roxanol Rescudose
  Oral soln: 10 mg/2.5 ml (25 single-dose)

▶ *morphine sulfate (ext-rel)* (C)(II)
Pediatric: <18 years: not recommended; ≥18 years: same as adult
 MorphaBond ER *Tab:* 15, 30, 60, 100 mg ext-rel

Comment: **MorphaBond** may be prescribed only by a qualified Healthcare providers knowledgeable in use of potent opioids for management of chronic pain. Do not abruptly discontinue in a physically dependent patient. Instruct patients to swallow **MorphaBond ER** tablets intact and not to cut, break, crush, chew, or dissolve **MorphaBond ER** to avoid the risk of release and absorption of potentially fatal dose of morphine. **MorphaBond ER** 100 mg tablets, a single dose greater than 60 mg, or a total daily dose >120 mg, are only for use in patients in whom tolerance to an opioid of comparable potency has been established. Patients considered opioid-tolerant are those taking, for one week or longer, at least 60 mg oral *morphine* per day, 25 mcg transdermal *fentanyl* per hour, 30 mg oral *oxycodone* per day, 8 mg oral *hydromorphone* per day, 25 mg oral *oxymorphone* per day, 60 mg oral *hydrocodone* per day, or an equianalgesic dose of another opioid. Use the lowest effective dosage for the shortest duration consistent with individual patient treatment goals. Individualize dosing based on the severity of pain, patient response, prior analgesic experience, and risk factors for addiction, abuse, and misuse

➤ *morphine sulfate+naltrexone* (C)(II)
Pediatric: <18 years: not recommended; ≥18 years: same as adult
Embeda 1 cap q 12-24 hours
   Cap: Embeda 20/0.8 morph 20 mg+nal 0.8 mg ext-rel
Embeda 30/1.2 morph 30 mg+nal 1.2 mg ext-rel
Embeda 50/2 morph 50 mg+nal 2 mg ext-rel
Embeda 60/2.4 morph 60 mg+nal 2.4 mg ext-rel
Embeda 80/3.2 morph 80 mg+nal 3.2 mg ext-rel
Embeda 100/4 morph 100 mg+nal 4 mg ext-rel

Comment: **Embeda** is not for prn use; for use in opioid-tolerant patients only; swallow whole or sprinkle contents of caps on applesauce (do not crush, chew, or dissolve); do not administer via NG or gastric tube (PEG tube).

➤ *oxycodone* (B)(II) 5-15 mg q 4-6 hours prn
Comment: Concomitant use of CYP3A4 inhibitors may increase opioid effects and CYP3A4 inducers may decrease effects or possibly cause development of an abstinence syndrome (withdrawal symptoms) in patients who are physically *oxycodone* dependent/addicted.
Pediatric: <18 years: not recommended; ≥18 years: same as adult
Oxaydo *Tab:* 5, 7.5 mg
Comment: **Oxaydo** is the first and only immediate-release oral *oxycodone* that discourages intranasal abuse. **Oxaydo** is formulated with sodium lauryl sulfate, an inactive ingredient that may cause nasal burning and throat irritation when snorted and, thus potentially reducing abuse liability. There is no generic equivalent.
Oxecta *Tab:* 5, 7.5 mg
Oxycodone Oral Solution (G) *Oral soln:* 5 mg/5 ml (15, 30 ml)
OxyIR (G) *Cap:* 5 mg
RoxyBond *Tab:* 5, 15, 30 mg
Comment: The FDA recently approved **RoxyBond** immediate-release tablets for the management of severe pain that does not respond to alternative treatment and requires an opioid analgesic. **RoxyBond** is the first immediate-release opioid analgesic to received FDA approval with a label describing its abuse-deterrent properties under the FDA 2015 Guidance for Industry: Abuse-Deterrent Opioids Evaluation and Labeling. The drug is formulated with inactive ingredients making it more difficult to misuse and abuse. When compared with another approved immediate-release tablet, **RoxyBond** was shown to be more resistant to cutting, crushing, grinding, or breaking, and more resistant to extraction. Adverse events associated with **RoxyBond** include nausea, constipation, vomiting, headache, pruritus, insomnia, dizziness, asthenia, somnolence, and addiction.
Roxycodone *Tab:* 5, 15*, 30*mg; *Oral soln:* 5 mg/ml
Roxycodone Intensol *Oral soln:* 20 mg/ml

➤ *oxycodone cont-rel* (B)(II)(G) dosage dependent upon previous opioid dosages; see mfr pkg insert: <11 years: not recommended; 11-16 years: the child's pain must be severe enough to require around-the-clock, long-term treatment not managed well by other treatments; must already be taking and tolerating minimum opium dose equal to *oxycodone* 20 mg/day x 5 consecutive days; >16 year: same as adult; no previous treatment with *oxycodone* required

OxyContin dose q 12 hours
   Tab: 10, 15, 20, 30, 40, 60, 80 mg cont-rel
OxyFast dose q 6 hours
   Oral conc: 20 mg/ml (30 ml w. dropper)
Xtampza ER dose q 12 hours
   Cap: 10, 15, 20, 30, 40 mg ext-rel
Comment: May open the **Xtampza ER** capsule and sprinkle in water <u>or</u> on soft food.

▷ *oxycodone+acetaminophen* (C)(II)(G)

Comment: Maximum 4 gm acetaminophen per day.
Pediatric: not recommended
   Magnacet 2.5/400 1 tab q 6 hours prn; max 10 tabs/day
     Tab: oxy 2.5 mg+acet 325 mg
   Magnacet 5/400 1 tab q 6 hours prn; max 10 tabs/day
     Tab: oxy 5 mg+acet 325 mg
   Magnacet 7.5/400 1 tab q 6 hours prn; max 8 tabs/day
     Tab: oxy 7.5 mg+acet 325 mg
   Magnacet 10/400 1 tab q 6 hours prn; max 6 tabs/day
     Tab: oxy 10 mg+acet 325 mg
   Percocet 2.5/325 1 tab q 6 hours prn; max 4 gm acet/day
     Tab: oxy 2.5 mg+acet 325 mg
   Percocet 5/325 1 tab q 6 hours prn; max 4 gm acet/day
     Tab: oxy 5 mg+acet 325*mg
   Percocet 7.5/325 1 tab q 6 hours prn; max 4 gm acet/day
     Tab: oxy 7.5 mg+acet 325 mg
   Percocet 7.5/500 1 tabs q 6 hours prn; max 4 gm acet/day
     Tab: oxy 7.5 mg+acet 325 mg
   Percocet 10/325 1 tabs q 6 hours prn; max 4 gm acet/day
     Tab: oxy 10 mg+acet 325 mg
   Percocet 10/650 1 tab q 6 hours prn; max 4 gm acet/day
     Tab: oxy 10 mg+acet 325 mg
   Roxicet 5/325 1 tab/tsp q 6 hours prn
     Tab: oxy 5 mg+acet 325 mg; *Oral soln:* oxy 5 mg+acet 325 mg per 5 ml
   Roxicet 5/500 1 caplet q 6 hours prn
     Cplt: oxy 5 mg+acet 325 mg
   Roxicet Oral Solution 1 tsp q 6 hours prn
     Oral soln: oxy 5 mg+acet 325 mg per 5 ml (alcohol 0.4%)
   Tylox 1 cap q 6 hours prn
     Cap: oxy 5 mg+acet 325 mg
   Xartemis XR 2 tabs q 12 hours prn
     Tab: oxy 7.5 mg+acet 325 mg

▷ *oxycodone+aspirin* (D)(II)(G)
   Percodan 1 tab q 6 hours prn
     Pediatric: not recommended
     Tab: oxy 4.8355 mg+asp 325*mg
   Percodan-Demi 1-2 tabs q 6 hours prn
     Pediatric: 6-12 years: 1/4 tab q 6 hours prn; >12-18 years: 1/2 tab q 6 hours prn
     Tab: oxy 2.25 mg+asp 325 mg

Comment: *aspirin*-containing medications are contraindicated with history of allergic-type reaction to *aspirin*, children and adolescents with *Varicella* or other viral illness, and 3rd trimester of pregnancy.

▷ *oxycodone+ibuprofen* (C)(II)(G)
Pediatric: <14 years: not recommended; ≥14 years: same as adult
   Combunox 1 tab q 6 hours prn
     Tab: oxy 5 mg+ibu 400*mg

▷ *oxycodone+naloxone* (C)(II) 1 tab q 3-4 hours prn
Pediatric: <12 years: not recommended; ≥12 years: same as adult
   Targiniq
     Tab: **Targiniq 10/5** oxy 10 mg+nal 5 mg
       Targiniq 20/10 oxy 20 mg+nal 10 mg
       Targiniq 40/20 oxy 40 mg+nal 20 mg

▷ *oxymorphone* (C)(II)(G)
  Pediatric: <18 years: not recommended; ≥18 years: same as adult
    Numorphan 1 supp q 4-6 hours prn
      Rectal supp: 5 mg; *Vial:* 1 mg/ml (1 ml), *Amp:* 1.5 mg/ml (10 ml);
    Comment: Store in refrigerator in original package. 1 mg of **Numorphan** is
    approximately equivalent in analgesic activity to 10 mg of *morphine sulfate*.
    Opana 1-1 tab q 4-6 hours prn
      Tab: 5, 10 mg
    Opana ER 1 tab q 12 hours prn
      Tab: 5, 7.5, 10, 15, 20, 30, 40 mg ext-rel crush-resist
    Opana Injection initially 0.5 mg IV or IM; 1 x 1 mg IM or IV q 4-6 hours prn
      Amp: 1 mg/ml (1 ml) (paraben/sodium dithionite-free)
▷ *pentazocine+aspirin* (D)(IV) 2 cplts tid or qid prn
  Pediatric: <12 years: not recommended; ≥12 years: same as adult
    Talwin Compound *Cplt:* pent 12.5 mg+asp 325 mg
  Comment: *aspirin*-containing medications are contraindicated with history of allergic-type
  reaction to *aspirin*, children and adolescents with *Varicella* or other viral illness, and 3rd
  trimester of pregnancy.
▷ *pentazocine+naloxone* (C)(IV) 1 tab q 3-4 hours prn
  Pediatric: <12 years: not recommended; ≥12 years: same as adult
    Talwin NX *Tab:* pent 50 mg+nal 0.5*mg
▷ *pentazocine lactate* (C)(IV) 30 mg IM, SC, or IV q 3-4 hours; max 360 mg/day
  Pediatric: <1 year: not recommended; ≥1 year: 0.5 mg/kg IM
    Talwin Injectable *Amp:* pent 30 mg/ml (1, 1.5, 2 ml)
▷ *propoxyphene napsylate+acetaminophen* (C)(IV)(G)
  Comment: Max 4 gm acetaminophen per day.
  Pediatric: <12 years: not recommended; ≥12 years: same as adult
    Balacet 325 1 tab q 4 hours prn; max 6 tabs/day
      Tab: prop 100 mg+acet 325 mg
▷ *tramadol* (C)(IV)(G)
  Comment: *tramadol* is known to be excreted in breast milk. The FDA and the European
  Medicines Agency (EMA) are investigating the safety of using *tramadol*-containing
  medications to treat pain in children 12-18 years because of the potential for serious side
  effects, including slowed or difficult breathing.
    Rybix ODT initially 100 mg once daily; may increase by 100 mg every 5 days; max 300
    mg/day; *CrCl <30 mL/min or severe hepatic impairment:* not recommended; *Cirrhosis:*
    max 50 mg q 12 hours
  Pediatric: <12 years: contraindicated; 12-<18: use extreme caution; not recommended for
  children and adolescents with obesity, asthma, obstructive sleep apnea, or other chronic
  breathing problem, or for post-tonsillectomy/adenoidectomy pain; ≥18 years: same as adult
      ODT: 50 mg (mint) (phenylalanine)
    Ryzolt initially 100 mg once daily; may increase by 100 mg every 5 days; max 300 mg/
    day; *CrCl <30 mL/min or severe hepatic impairment:* not recommended
  Pediatric: <12 years: contraindicated; 12-<18: use extreme caution; not recommended for
  children and adolescents with obesity, asthma, obstructive sleep apnea, or other chronic
  breathing problem, or for post-tonsillectomy/adenoidectomy pain; ≥18 years: same as adult
      Tab: 100, 200, 300 mg ext-rel
    Ultram 50-100 mg q 4-6 hours prn; max 400 mg/day; *CrCl <30 mL/min:* max 100 mg q
    12 hours; *Cirrhosis:* max 50 mg q 12 hours
  Pediatric: <12 years: contraindicated; 12-<18: use extreme caution; not recommended for
  children and adolescents with obesity, asthma, obstructive sleep apnea, or other chronic
  breathing problem, or for post-tonsillectomy/adenoidectomy pain; ≥18 years: same as adult
      Tab: 50*mg
    Ultram ER initially 100 mg once daily; may increase by 100 mg every 5 days; max 300 mg/
    day; *CrCl <30 mL/min or severe hepatic impairment:* not recommended
  Pediatric: <12 years: contraindicated; 12-<18: use extreme caution; not recommended
  for children and adolescents with obesity, asthma, obstructive sleep apnea, or other
  chronic breathing problem, or for post-tonsillectomy/adenoidectomy pain; ≥18 years:
  same as adult
      Tab: 100, 200, 300 mg ext-rel

▷ *tramadol+acetaminophen* (C)(IV)(G) 2 tabs q 4-6 hours; max 8 tabs/day; 5 days; *CrCl <30 mL/min:* max 2 tabs q 12 hours; max 4 tabs/day x 5 days
Pediatric: <12 years: contraindicated; 12-<18: use extreme caution; not recommended for children and adolescents with obesity, asthma, obstructive sleep apnea, or other chronic breathing problem, or for post-tonsillectomy/adenoidectomy pain; ≥18 years: same as adult
    Ultracet *Tab:* tram 37.5+acet 325 mg
  Comment: *tramadol* is known to be excreted in breast milk. The FDA and the European Medicines Agency (EMA) are investigating the safety of using *tramadol*-containing medications to treat pain in children 12-18 years because of the potential for serious side effects, including slowed or difficult breathing.

▷ *buprenorphine* (C)(III) change patch every 7 days; do not increase the dose until previous dose has been worn for at least 72 hours; after removal, do not re-use the site for at least 3 weeks; do not expose the patch to heat
Pediatric: <16 years: not recommended; ≥16 years: same as adult
    Butrans Transdermal System
      Transdermal patch: 5, 10, 20 mcg/hour (4/pck)

▷ *fentanyl* transdermal system (C)(II) apply to clean, dry, non-irritated, intact, skin; hold in place for 30 seconds; start at lowest dose and titrate upward; *Opioid-naïve:* change patch every 3 days (72 hours)
Pediatric: <18 years or <110 lb: not recommended; ≥18 years or ≥110 lb: same as adult
    Duragesic *Transdermal patch:* 12, 25, 37.5, 50, 62.5, 75, 87.5, 100 mcg/hour (5/pck)

▷ *fentanyl iontophoretic transdermal system*
    Ionsys is a transdermal patient-controlled device that sticks to the arm or chest; it is activated when the patient pushes the button
  Comment: **Ionsys** is for in-hospital use only and should be discontinued prior to hospital discharge. It is indicated for post-op pain relief.

TRANSMUCOSAL (SUB-LINGUAL, BUCCAL) OPIOIDS

Comment: For chronic severe pain. For management of breakthrough pain in patients with cancer who are already receiving and who are tolerant to opioid therapy. Opioid-tolerant patients are those taking oral *morphine* ≥60 mg/day, transdermal *fentanyl* ≥25 mcg/hour, *oxycodone* ≥30 mg/day, oral *hydromorphone* ≥8 mg/day, or an equianalgesic dose of another opioid, for ≥1 week

ORAL OPIOID PARTIAL AGONIST-ANTAGONIST

▷ *buprenorphine* (C)
Pediatric: <16 years: not recommended; ≥16 year: same as adult
    Subutex 8 mg in a single dose on day 1; then 16 mg in a single dose on day 2; target dose is 16 mg/day in a single dose; dissolve under tongue; do not chew or swallow whole
      SL tab (lemon-lime) or *SL film (lime):* 2, 8 mg (30/pck)

▷ *fentanyl* buccal soluble film (C)(II) dissolve 1 film on moistened area inside cheek; initially 200 mcg; no more than 4 doses/day at least 2 hours apart; max 1200 mcg/dose; do not cut film
Pediatric: <18 years: not recommended; ≥18 years: same as adult
    Onsolis *Buccal film:* 200, 400, 600, 800, 1200 mcg (30 films/pck)

▷ *fentanyl citrate* transmucosal unit (C)(II)(G) initially one 200 mcg unit placed between cheek and lower gum; move from side to side; suck (not chew); use 6 units before titrating; titrate dose as needed; max 4 units/day
Pediatric: <18 years: not recommended; ≥18 years: same as adult
    Actiq *Unit:* 200, 400, 600, 800, 1200, 1600 mcg (24 units/pck)
    Fentora *Unit:* 100, 200, 400, 600, 800 mcg (24 units/pck)

▷ *fentanyl* sublingual tab (C)(II) initially one 100 mcg dose; if inadequate after 30 minutes, may repeat; titrate in increments of 100 mcg; max 2 doses per episode, up to 4 episodes per day; wait at least 2 hours before treating another episode; *Maintenance:* use only one tablet of appropriate strength; do not chew, suck, or swallow tablets; do not convert from other *fentanyl* products on a mcg-per-mcg basis or interchange with other *fentanyl* products
Pediatric: <18 years: not recommended; ≥18 years: same as adult
    Abstral *SL tab:* 100, 200, 300, 400, 600, 800 mcg (32 tabs/pck)

▷ *fentanyl sublingual spray* (C)(II)
Pediatric: <18 years: not recommended; ≥18 years: same as adult
    Subsys 100, 200, 400, 600, 800 mcg/S L spray

Comment: Subsys is not bioequivalent with other *fentanyl* products. Do not convert patients from other *fentanyl* products to Subsys on a mcg-per-mcg basis. There are no conversion directions available for patients on any other *fentanyl* products other than Actiq. (Note: This includes oral, transdermal, or parenteral formulations of *fentanyl*.)

▷ *sufentanil* 30 mcg sublingually prn; minimum 1 hour between doses; max 12 tablets/24 hours; max 72 hours
Pediatric: <18 years: not established; ≥18 years: same as adult
Dsuvia *SL tab:* 30 mcg in a single use applicator (SDA)
Comment: Dsuvia *(sufentanil)* is a synthetic opioid analgesic formulation for the management of acute severe pain that is severe enough to require an opioid analgesic, and for which alternative treatments are inadequate. Dsuvia is indicated for use only in adults in a certified medically supervised healthcare settings, such as hospitals, surgical centers, and emergency departments. Dsuvia is only available through the Dsuvia REMS Program; Dsuvia is not for home use or for use in children; discontinue treatment with Dsuvia before patients leave the certified medically supervised healthcare setting; Do not discontinue Dsuvia abruptly in the physically-dependent patient. Concomitant use with CYP3A4 inhibitors (or discontinuation of CYP3A4 inducers) can result in a fatal overdose of *sufentanil*. The most commonly reported adverse reactions (incidence ≥ 2%) have been nausea, headache, vomiting, dizziness and hypotension.

PARENTERAL OPIOID AGONIST-ANTAGONISTS

▷ *nalbuphine* (B)(G) 10 mg/70 kg IM, SC, or IV q 3-6 hours prn
Pediatric: <18 years: not recommended; ≥18 years: same as adult
Nubain *Amp:* 10, 20 mg/ml (1 ml) (sulfite-free, parabens-free)
▷ *pentazocine+naloxone* (C)(IV) 1-2 tabs q 3-4 hours prn; max 12 tabs/day
Pediatric: <12 years: not recommended; ≥12 year: same as adult
Talwin-NX *Tab:* pent 50 mg+nal 0.5*mg

TRANSMUCOSAL (INTRA-NASAL) OPIOIDS

▷ *butorphanol tartrate* nasal spray (C)(IV) initially 1 spray (1 mg) in one nostril and may repeat after 60-90 minutes (*Elderly* 90-120 minutes) in opposite nostril if needed or 1 spray in each nostril and may repeat q 3-4 hours prn
Pediatric: <18 years: not recommended; ≥18 years: same as adult
Butorphanol Nasal Spray *Nasal spray:* 1 mg/actuation (10 mg/ml, 2.5 ml)
Stadol Nasal Spray *Nasal spray:* 1 mg/actuation (10 mg/ml, 2.5 ml)
▷ *fentanyl* nasal spray (C)(II) initially 1 spray (100 mcg) in one nostril and may repeat after 2 hours; when adequate analgesia is achieved, use that dose for subsequent breakthrough episodes
Titration steps: 100 mcg using 1 x 100 mcg spray; 200 mcg using 2 x 100 mcg spray (1 in each nostril); 400 mcg using 1 x 400 mcg spray; 800 mcg using 2 x 400 mcg (1 in each nostril); max 800 mcg; limit to ≤4 doses per day
Pediatric: <18 years: not recommended; ≥18 years: same as adult
Lazanda Nasal Spray *Nasal spray:* 100, 400 mcg/100 mcl (8 sprays/bottle)
Comment: Lazanda Nasal Spray is available by restricted distribution program. To enroll, call 855-841-4234 or visit https://www.fda.gov/downloads/drugs/drugsafety/postmarketdrugsafetyinformationforpatientsandproviders/ucm261983.pdf. Lazanda Nasal Spray is indicated for the management of breakthrough pain in cancer patients who are already receiving and who are tolerant to opioid therapy for their underlying persistent cancer pain. Patients considered opioid tolerant are those who are taking at least 60 mg of oral morphine/day, 25 mcg of transdermal *fentanyl*/hour, 30 mg oral *oxycodone*/day, 8 mg oral *hydromorphone*/day, 25 mg oral *oxymorphone*/day, or an equianalgesic dose of another opioid for a week or longer. Patients must remain on around-the-clock opioids when using Lazanda Nasal Spray. As such, it is contraindicated in the management of acute or post-op pain, including headache/migraine, or dental pain.

INTRATHECAL OPIOID

▷ *ziconotide* intrathecal (IT) infusion (C) initially no more than 2.4 mcg/day (0.1 mcg/hour) and titrate to upward by up to 2.4 mcg/day (0.1 mcg/day at intervals of no more than 2-3 times per week, up to a recommended maximum of 19.2 mcg/day (0.8 mcg/hour) by Day

21; dose increases in increments of less than 2.4 mcg/day (0.1 mcg/hour) and increases in dose less frequently than 2-3 times per week may be used.

Pediatric: <12 years: not recommended; ≥12 years: same as adult

Prialt *Vial:* 25 mcg/ml (20 ml), 100 mcg/ml (1, 2, 5 ml)

Comment: Patients with a pre-existing history of psychosis should not be treated with **ziconotide**. Contraindications to the use of IT analgesia include conditions such as the presence of infection at the microinfusion injection site, uncontrolled bleeding diathesis, and spinal canal obstruction that impairs circulation of CSF.

 PANCREATIC ENZYME INSUFFICIENCY

Comment: Seen in chronic pancreatitis, post-pancreatectomy, cystic fibrosis, steatorrhea, post-GI tract bypass surgery, and ductal obstruction from neoplasia. May sprinkle cap; however, do not crush or chew cap or tab. May mix with applesauce or other acidic food; follow with water or juice. Do not let any drug remain in mouth. Take dose just prior to each meal or snack. Base dose on lipase units; adjust per diet and clinical response (i.e., steatorrhea). Pancrelipase products are interchangeable. Contraindicated with pork protein hypersensitivity.

PANCRELIPASE PRODUCTS

▷ *pancreatic enzymes* (C)

Creon 500 units/kg per meal; max 2,500 units/kg per meal or <10,000 units/kg per day or <4,000 units/gm fat ingested per day

Pediatric: <12 months: 2,000-4,000 units per 120 ml formula or per breast-feeding (do not mix directly into formula or breast milk; 12 months to 4 years: 1,000 units/kg per meal; max 2,500 units/kg per meal <10,000 units/kg per day; >4 years: same as adult

    Cap: **Creon 3000** lip 3,000 units+pro 9,500 units+amyl 15,000 units del-rel
        Creon 6000 lip 6,000 units+pro 19,000 units+amyl 30,000 units del-rel
        Creon 12000 lip 12,000 units+pro 38,000 units+amyl 60,000 units del-rel
        Creon 24000 lip 24,000 units+pro 76,000 units+amyl 120,000 units del-rel
        Creon 36000 lip 36,000 units+pro 114,000 units+amyl 180,000 units del-rel

Cotazym 1-3 tabs just prior to each meal or snack

Pediatric: <12 years: not recommended; ≥12 years: same as adult

    Tab: **Cotazym** lip 1,000 units+pro 12,500 units+amyl 12,500 units del-rel
        Cotazym-S lip 5,000 units+pro 20,000 units+amyl 20,000 units del-rel

Donnazyme 1-3 caps just prior to each meal or snack

Pediatric: <12 years: not recommended; ≥12 years: same as adult

    Cap: **Donnazyme** lip 5,000 units+pro 20,000 units+amyl 20,000 units del-rel

Ku-Zyme 1-2 caps just prior to each meal or snack

Pediatric: <12 years: not recommended; ≥12 years: same as adult

    Cap: **Ku-Zyme:** lip 12,000 units+pro 15,000 units+amyl 15,000 units del-rel

Kutrase 1-2 caps just prior to each meal or snack

Pediatric: <12 years: not recommended; ≥12 years: same as adult

    Cap: **Kutrase:** lip 12,000 units+pro 30,000 units+amyl 30,000 units del-rel

Pancreaze 2,500 lipase units/kg per meal or <10,000 lipase units/kg per day or <4,000 lipase units/gm fat ingested per day

Pediatric: <12 months: 2,000-4,000 lipase units per 120 ml formula or per breast-feeding; >12 months to <4 years 1,000 lipase units/kg per meal; >4 years: 500 lipase units/kg per meal; max: adult dose

    Cap: **Pancreaze 4200** lip 4,200 units+pro 10,000 units+amyl 17,500 units ec-microtabs
        Pancreaze 10500 lip 10,500 units+pro 25,000 units+amyl 43,750 units ec-microtabs
        Pancreaze 16800 lip 16,800 units+pro 40,000 units+amyl 70,000 units ec-microtabs
        Pancreaze 21000 lip 21,000 units+pro 37,000 units+amyl 61,000 units ec-microtabs

Pertyze *12 months to 4 years and ≥8 kg:* initially 1,000 lipase units/kg per meal; *≥4 years and ≥16 kg:* initially 500 lipase units/kg per meal; *Both:* 2,500 lipase units/kg per meal or <10,000 units/kg per day or <4,000 lipase units/gm fat ingested per day

    Cap: **Pertyze 8000** lip 8,000 units+pro 28,750 units+amyl 30,250 units del-rel

Pertyze 16000 lip 16,000 units+pro 57,500 units+amyl 65,000 units del-rel
Ultrase 1-3 tabs just prior to each meal or snack
  Pediatric: same as adult
  Cap: **Ultrase** lip 4,500 units+pro 20,000 units+amyl 25,000 units del-rel
      Ultrase MT lip 12,000 units+pro 39,000 units+amyl 39,000 units del-rel
        Ultrase MT 18 lip 18,000 units+pro 58,500 units+amyl 58,500 units del-rel
        Ultrase MT 20 lip 20,000 units+pro 65,000 units+amyl 65,000 units del-rel
Viokace initially 500 lip units/kg per meal; max 2,500 lipase units/kg per meal, or
<10,000 lipase units/kg per meal, or <4,000 units/gm fat ingested per day
  Pediatric: same as adult
  Tab: **Viokace 8** lip 8,000 units+pro 30,000 units+amyl 30,000 units
      Viokace 16 lip 16,000 units+pro 60,000 units+amyl 60,000 units
Viokace 0440 lip 10,440 units+pro 39,150 units amyl 39,150 units
Viokace 20880 lip 20,880 units+pro 78,300 units amyl 78,300 units
Comment: **Viokace 10440** and **Viokase 20880** should be taken with a daily proton
pump inhibitor (PPI).
Viokace Powder 1/4 tsp (0.7 gm) with meals
Viokace Powder lip 16,800 units+pro 70,000 units+amyl 70,000 units per 1/4 tsp (8 oz)
Zenpep initially 500 lipase units/kg per meal; max 2,500 lipase units/kg per meal or
<10,000 units/kg per day or <4,000 units/gm fat ingested per day
  Pediatric: Infant-12 months: infants may be given 3,000 lipase units (one capsule) per
    120 ml of formula or per breast-feeding; do not mix capsule contents directly into
    formula or breast milk prior to administration; *Children >12 months to <4 Years:*
    enzyme dosing should begin with 1,000 lipase units/kg of body weight per meal to a
    maximum of 2,500 lipase units/kg of body weight per meal (or ≤10,000 lipase units/
    kg/day), or <4,000 lipase units/gm fat ingested per day; *Children ≥4 Years:* same as
    adult
  Cap: **Zenpep 3000** lip 3,000 units+pro 10,000 units+amyl 14,000 units del-rel
    Zenpep 5000 lip 5,000 units+pro 17,000 units+amyl 24,000 units
    Zenpep 10000 lip 10,000 units+pro 32,000 units+amyl 42,000 units del-rel
    Zenpep 15000 lip 15,000 units+pro 47,000 units+amyl 63,000 units del-rel
    Zenpep 20000 lip 20,000 units+pro 63,000 units+amyl 84,000 units del-rel
    Zenpep 25000 lip 25,000 units+pro 79,000 units+amyl 105,000 units del-rel
    Zenpep 40000 lip 40,000 units+pro 126,000 units+amyl 168,000 units del-rel
Comment: **Zenpep** is not interchangeable with any other pancrelipase product. Dosing
should not exceed the recommended maximum dosage set forth by the Cystic Fibrosis
Foundation Consensus Conferences Guidelines. **Zenpep** should be swallowed whole.
For infants or patients unable to swallow intact capsules, the contents may be sprinkled
on soft acidic food, e.g., applesauce.
Zymase 1-3 caps just prior to each meal or snack
  Pediatric: <12 years: not recommended; ≥12 years: same as adult
  Cap: **Zymase** lip 12,000 units+prot 24,000 units+amyl 24,000 units del-rel

PANIC DISORDER

Comment: If possible when considering a benzodiazepine to treat anxiety, a short-acting
benzodiazepines should be used only prn to avert intense anxiety and panic for the least
time necessary while a different non-addictive anti-anxiety regimen (e.g., SSRI, SNRI,
TCA, *buspirone*, beta-blocker) is established and effective treatment goals achieved. Co-
administration of SSRIs with TCAs requires extreme caution. Concomitant use of MAOIs
and SSRIs is absolutely contraindicated. Avoid other serotonergic drugs. A potentially fatal
adverse event is **serotonin syndrome,** caused by serotonin excess. Milder symptoms require
HCP intervention to avert severe symptoms which can be rapidly fatal without urgent/
emergent medical care. Symptoms include restlessness, agitation, confusion, hallucinations,
tachycardia, hypertension, dilated pupils, muscle twitching, muscle rigidity, loss of muscle
coordination, diaphoresis, diarrhea, headache, shivering, piloerection, hyperpyrexia, cardiac
arrhythmias, seizures, loss of consciousness, coma, death. Abrupt withdrawal or interruption of
treatment with an antidepressant medication is sometimes associated with an **antidepressant
discontinuation syndrome** which may be mediated by gradually tapering the drug over
a period of two weeks or longer, depending on the dose strength and length of treatment.

Common symptoms of the *serotonin discontinuation syndrome* include flu-like symptoms (nausea, vomiting, diarrhea, headaches, sweating), sleep disturbances (insomnia, nightmares, constant sleepiness), mood disturbances (dysphoria, anxiety, agitation), cognitive disturbances (mental confusion, hyperarousal), sensory and movement disturbances (imbalance, tremors, vertigo, dizziness, electric-shock-like sensations in the brain, often described by sufferers as "brain zaps."

SELECTIVE SEROTONIN REUPTAKE INHIBITORS (SSRIs)

▷ *escitalopram* (C)(G) initially 10 mg daily; may increase to 20 mg daily after 1 week; *Elderly* or *hepatic impairment*: 10 mg once daily
  Pediatric: <12 years: <12 years: not recommended; ≥12 years: same as adult; 12-17 years: initially 10 mg once daily; may increase to 20 mg once daily after 3 weeks
    Lexapro *Tab:* 5, 10*, 20*mg
    Lexapro Oral Solution *Oral soln:* 1 mg/ml (240 ml) (peppermint) (parabens)

▷ *fluoxetine* (C)(G)
    Prozac initially 20 mg daily; may increase after 1 week; doses >20 mg/day should be divided into AM and noon doses; max 80 mg/day
    Pediatric: <8 years: not recommended; 8-17 years: initially 10 mg/day; may increase after 2 weeks to 20 mg/day; range 20-60 mg/day; range for lower weight children 20-30 mg/day; >17 years: same as adult
      Cap: 10, 20, 40 mg; *Tab:* 30*, 60*mg; *Oral soln:* 20 mg/5 ml (4 oz) (mint)
    Prozac Weekly following daily *fluoxetine* therapy at 20 mg/day for 13 weeks, may initiate **Prozac Weekly** 7 days after the last 20 mg *fluoxetine* dose
    Pediatric: <12 years: not recommended; ≥12 years: same as adult
      Cap: 90 mg ent-coat del-rel pellets

▷ *paroxetine maleate* (D)(G)
  Pediatric: <12 years: not recommended; ≥12 years: same as adult
    Paxil initially 20 mg daily in AM; may increase by 10 mg/day at weekly intervals as needed; max 60 mg/day
      Tab: 10*, 20*, 30, 40 mg
    Paxil CR initially 25 mg daily in AM; may increase by 12.5 mg at weekly intervals as needed; max 62.5 mg/day
      Tab: 12.5, 25, 37.5 mg cont-rel ent-coat
    Paxil Suspension initially 20 mg daily in AM; may increase by 10 mg/day at weekly intervals as needed; max 60 mg/day
      Oral susp: 10 mg/5 ml (250 ml) (orange)

▷ *paroxetine mesylate* (D)(G) initially 7.5 mg daily in AM; may increase by 10 mg/day at weekly intervals as needed; max 60 mg/day
  Pediatric: <12 years: not recommended; ≥12 years: same as adult
    Brisdelle *Cap:* 7.5 mg

▷ *sertraline* (C) initially 50 mg daily; increase at 1 week intervals if needed; max 200 mg daily
  Pediatric: <6 years: not recommended; 6-12 years: initially 25 mg daily; max 200 mg/day; 13-17 years: initially 50 mg daily; max 200 mg/day; ≥17 years: same as adult
    Zoloft *Tab:* 15*, 50*, 100*mg; *Oral conc:* 20 mg per ml (60 ml, dilute just before administering in 4 oz water, ginger ale, lemon-lime soda, lemonade, or orange juice) (alcohol 12%)

SEROTONIN-NOREPINEPHRINE REUPTAKE INHIBITORS (SNRIs)

▷ *desvenlafaxine* (C)(G) swallow whole; initially 50 mg once daily; max 120 mg/day
  Pediatric: <12 years: not recommended; ≥12 years: same as adult
    Pristiq *Tab:* 50, 100 mg ext-rel

▷ *venlafaxine* (C)(G)
    Effexor initially 75 mg/day in 2-3 doses; may increase at 4 day intervals in 75 mg increments to 150 mg/day; max 375 mg/day
    Pediatric: <18 years: not recommended; ≥18 years: same as adult
      Tab: 25, 37.5, 50, 75, 100 mg
    Effexor XR initially 75 mg q AM; may start at 37.5 mg daily x 4-7 days, then increase by increments of up to 75 mg/day at intervals of at least 4 days; usual max 375 mg/day
    Pediatric: <18 years: not recommended; ≥18 years: same as adult
      Cap: 37.5, 75, 150 mg ext-rel

TRICYCLIC ANTIDEPRESSANTS (TCAs)

▷ *doxepin* (C)(G)
  Pediatric: <12 years: not recommended; ≥12 years: same as adult
    Cap: 10, 25, 50, 75, 100, 150 mg; *Oral conc:* 10 mg/ml (4 oz w. dropper)
▷ *imipramine* (C)(G)
  Pediatric: <12 years: not recommended; ≥12 years: same as adult
    Tofranil initially 75 mg daily (max 200 mg); *Adolescents:* initially 30-40 mg daily (max 100 mg/day); if maintenance dose exceeds 75 mg daily, may switch to **Tofranil PM** for divided or bedtime dose
      Tab: 10, 25, 50 mg
    Tofranil PM initially 75 mg daily 1 hour before HS; max 200 mg
      Cap: 75, 100, 125, 150
    Tofranil Injection 50 mg IM; lower dose for adolescents; switch to oral form as soon as possible
      Amp: 25 mg/2 ml (2 ml)

FIRST GENERATION ANTIHISTAMINE

▷ *hydroxyzine* (C)(G) 50-100 mg qid; max 600 mg/day
  Pediatric: <6 years: 50 mg/day divided qid; ≥6 years: 50-100 mg/day divided qid
    Atarax *Tab:* 10, 25, 50, 100 mg; *Syr:* 10 mg/5 ml (alcohol 0.5%)
    Vistaril *Cap:* 25, 50, 100 mg; *Oral susp:* 25 mg/5 ml (4 oz) (lemon)
  Comment: *hydroxyzine* is contraindicated in early pregnancy and in patients with a prolonged QT interval. It is not known whether this drug is excreted in human milk; therefore, *hydroxyzine* should not be given to nursing mothers.

AZAPIRONES

▷ *buspirone* (B) initially 7.5 mg bid; may increase by 5 mg/day q 2-3 days; max 60 mg/day
  Pediatric: <6 years: not recommended; 6-17 years: same as adult
    BuSpar *Tab:* 5, 10, 15*, 30*mg

BENZODIAZEPINES

Short Acting

▷ *alprazolam* (D)(IV)(G)
  Pediatric: <18 years: not recommended; ≥18 years: same as adult
    Niravam initially 0.25-0.5 mg tid; may titrate every 3-4 days; max 4 mg/day
      Tab: 0.25*, 0.5*, 1*, 2*mg orally-disint
    Xanax initially 0.25-0.5 mg tid; may titrate every 3-4 days; max 4 mg/day
      Tab: 0.25*, 0.5*, 1*, 2*mg
    Xanax XR initially 0.5-1 mg once daily, preferably in the AM; increase at intervals of at least 3-4 days by up to 1 mg/day. Taper no faster than 0.5 mg every 3 days; max 10 mg/day. When switching from immediate-release *alprazolam*, give total daily dose of immediate-release once daily.
      Tab: 0.5, 1, 2, 3 mg ext-rel
▷ *oxazepam* (C)(IV)(G) 10-15 mg tid-qid for moderate symptoms; 15-30 mg tid-qid for severe symptoms
  Pediatric: <12 years: not recommended; ≥12 years: same as adult
    Tab: 15 mg; Cap: 10, 15, 30 mg

Intermediate-Acting

▷ *lorazepam* (D)(IV)(G) 1-10 mg/day in 2-3 divided doses
  Pediatric: <12 years: not recommended; ≥12 years: same as adult
    Ativan *Tab:* 0.5, 1*, 2*mg
    Lorazepam Intensol *Oral conc:* 2 mg/ml (30 ml w. graduated dropper)

Long-Acting

▷ *chlordiazepoxide* (D)(IV)(G)
  Pediatric: <6 years: not recommended; ≥6 years: 5 mg bid-qid; increase to 10 mg bid-tid
    Librium 5-10 mg tid-qid for moderate symptoms; 20-25 mg tid-qid for severe symptoms
      Cap: 5, 10, 25 mg
    Librium Injectable 50-100 mg IM or IV; then 25-50 mg IM tid-qid prn; max 300 mg/day
      Inj: 100 mg

▷ *chlordiazepoxide+clidinium* (D)(IV) 1-2 caps tid-qid: max 8 caps/day
    Pediatric: <12 years: not recommended; ≥12 years: same as adult
        Librax *Cap:* chlor 5 mg+clid 2.5 mg
▷ *clonazepam* (D)(IV)(G) initially 0.25 mg bid; increase to 1 mg/day after 3 days
    Pediatric: <18 years: not recommended; ≥18 years: same as adult
        Klonopin *Tab:* 0.5*, 1, 2 mg
        Klonopin Wafers dissolve in mouth with <u>or</u> without water
           Wafer: 0.125, 0.25, 0.5, 1, 2 mg orally-disint
▷ *clorazepate* (D)(IV)(G) 30 mg/day in divided doses; max 60 mg/day
    Pediatric: <9 years: not recommended; ≥9 years: same as adult
        Tranxene *Tab:* 3.75, 7.5, 15 mg
        Tranxene SD do not use for initial therapy
           Tab: 22.5 mg ext-rel
        Tranxene SD Half Strength do not use for initial therapy
           Tab: 11.25 mg ext-rel
        Tranxene T-Tab *Tab:* 3.75*, 7.5*, 15*mg
▷ *diazepam* (D)(IV)(G) 2-10 mg bid to qid
    Pediatric: <12 years: not recommended; ≥12 years: same as adult
        Diastat *Rectal gel delivery system:* 2.5 mg
        Diastat AcuDial *Rectal gel delivery system:* 10, 20 mg
        Valium *Tab:* 2*, 5*, 10*mg
        Valium Injectable *Vial:* 5 mg/ml (10 ml); *Amp:* 5 mg/ml (2 ml); *Prefilled syringe:* 5 mg/ml (5 ml)
        Valium Intensol Oral Solution *Conc oral soln:* 5 mg/ml (30 ml w. dropper) (alcohol 19%)
        Valium Oral Solution *Oral soln:* 5 mg/5 ml (500 ml) (wintergreen spice)

PHENOTHIAZINES

▷ *prochlorperazine* (C)(G)
    Pediatric: <12 years: not recommended; ≥12 years: same as adult
        Compazine 5 mg tid-qid
           Tab: 5 mg; *Syr:* 5 mg/5 ml (4 oz) (fruit); *Rectal supp:* 2.5, 5, 25 mg
        Compazine Spansule 15 mg q AM or 10 mg q 12 hours
           Spansule: 10, 15 mg sust-rel
▷ *trifluoperazine* (C)(G) 1-2 mg bid; max 6 mg/day; max 12 weeks
    Pediatric: <12 years: not recommended; ≥12 years: same as adult
        Stelazine *Tab:* 1, 2, 5, 10 mg

 PARKINSON'S DISEASE (PD)

Parkinson's Disease-associated Dementia, *see Dementia page* 115
Comment: When administering *carbidopa* and *levodopa* separately, administer each at the same time. Titrate daily dose ratio of 1:10 *carbidopa* to *levodopa*. Max daily *carbidopa* 200 mg. Most patients will require *levodopa* 400 to 1600 mg/day in divided doses every 4 to 8 hours. After titrating both drugs to the desired effects without intolerable side effects, switch to a *carbidopa+levodopa* combination form.

DOPAMINE PRECURSOR (LEVODOPA)

▷ *levodopa* (C)(G)
    Tab: 125, 150, 200 mg

DECARBOXYLASE INHIBITOR (CARBIDOPA)

▷ *carbidopa* (C)(G)
    Lodosyn *Tab:* 25 mg

TREATMENT OF DOPAMINE OFF EPISODES

▷ *levodopa inhalation powder* for oral inhalation <u>only</u>; do <u>not</u> swallow capsules; administer capsules <u>only</u> with the **Inhibra** inhaler; max 1 dose (2 capsules) for any OFF period; max 5 doses (10 capsules , 420 mg)/day
    Inbrija *Inhal cap:* 42 mg inhal pwdr (60 caps—4 caps/foil blister card, 15 cards/carton) w. **Inbrija** inhaler

Comment: **Inbrija** is an aromatic amino acid oral inhalation powder for the intermittent (on-demand) treatment of OFF episodes in people with Parkinson's disease treated with *carbidopa/levodopa*. OFF episodes, also known as OFF periods, are defined as the return of Parkinson's symptoms that result from low levels of dopamine between doses of oral carbidopa/levodopa, the standard oral baseline Parkinson's treatment. **Inbrija** is not recommended for patients with asthma, COPD, or other chronic underlying lung disease. **Inbrija** is contraindicated within 14 days before and 7 days after taking a non-selective monoamine oxidase inhibitor (MOAI). Monitor patients on MAO-B inhibitors for orthostatic hypotension. Concomitant dopamine D2 antagonists, respiratory tract infection, and discolored sputum.

DOPAMINE RECEPTOR AGONISTS

▷ *amantadine* (C)

Comment: *amantadine* is a chrono-synchronous amantadine therapy for the treatment of levodopa-induced dyskinesia (LID) in patients with Parkinson's disease.

Gocovri take once daily at bedtime; initially 137 mg; after 1 week, increase to the recommended daily dosage of 274 mg; swallow whole; may sprinkle contents on soft food; take with or without food; avoid use with alcohol; a lower dosage is recommended for patients with moderate or severe renal impairment; Contraindicated in patients with end-stage renal disease

    Cap: 68.5, 137 mg ext-rel

Osmolex ER initial dose 129 mg orally once daily in the morning; may be increase dose in weekly intervals; max daily dose 322 mg in the morning; dose frequency reduction and monitoring required for renal impairment; swallow whole; do not chew, crush, or divide

    Tab: 129, 193, 258 mg ext-rel

Comment: **Osmolex ER** is not interchangeable with other *amantadine* immediate- or extended-release products. Most common adverse reactions (incidence ≥ 5%) are nausea, dizziness/ lightheadedness, and insomnia. **Osmolex ER** is contraindicated in patients with end-stage renal disease (ESRD). Advise patients prior to treatment about potential for falling asleep during activities of daily living (ADLs) and somnolence and discontinue **Osmolex ER** if occurs. Monitor patients for depressed mood, depression, and suicidal ideation or behavior. Patients with major psychotic disorder should ordinarily not be treated with **Osmolex ER**; observe patients throughout treatment for the occurrence of hallucinations, especially at initiation and after dose increases. Monitor patients for dizziness and orthostatic hypotension, especially after starting **Osmolex ER** or increasing the dose. Avoid sudden withdrawal/discontinuation due to risk of Withdrawal-Emergent Hyperpyrexia and confusion: Monitor patient for development of impulse control/ compulsive behaviors. Ask patients about increased gambling urges, sexual urges, uncontrolled spending or other urges and consider dose reduction or discontinuation if any occur. Increased risk of anticholinergic effects may require reduction of **Osmolex ER** or dose of the anticholinergic drug(s). Excretion of *amantadine* increases with acidic urine resulting in possible accumulation with urine change towards alkaline. Live Attenuated Influenza Vaccines (LAVs) are not recommended during treatment with **Osmolex ER**. Concomitant use of alcohol is not recommended due to increased potential for CNS effects. There are no adequate data on the developmental risk associated with use of *amantadine* in pregnant women. Animal studies suggest a potential risk for fetal harm with *amantadine*. *Amantadine* is excreted in human milk, but amounts have not been quantified. There is no information on the risk to the breastfed infant. To report suspected reactions, contact Vertical Pharmaceuticals, LLC at 1-877-482-3788 or FDA at 1-800-FDA-1088 or www.fda.gov/medwatch.

Symadine (G) initially 100 mg bid; may increase after 1-2 weeks by 100 mg/day; max 400 mg/day in divided doses; for extrapyramidal effects, 100 mg bid; max 300 mg/day in divided doses

    Cap: 100 mg

Symmetrel (G) initially 100 mg bid; may increase after 1-2 weeks by 100 mg/day; max 400 mg/day in divided doses; for extrapyramidal effects, 100 mg bid; max 300 mg/day in divided doses

    Cap: 100 mg; *Syr:* 50 mg/5 ml (16 oz) (raspberry)

▷ *bromocriptine* (B)(G) initially 1.25 mg bid to 2.5 mg tid with meals; increase as needed every 2-4 weeks by 2.5 mg/day; max 100 mg/day

Parlodel *Tab:* 2.5*mg; *Cap:* 5 mg

▷ *pramipexole* (C)(G) initially 0.125 mg tid; increase at intervals q 5-7 days; max 1.5 mg tid

Mirapex *Tab:* 0.125, 0.25*, 0.5*, 1*, 1.5*mg

▷ *ropinirole* (C) initially 0.25 mg tid for first week; then 0.5 mg tid for second week; then 0.75 mg tid for third week; then 1 mg tid for fourth week; may increase by 1.5 mg/day at 1 week intervals to 9 mg/day; then increase up to 3 mg/day at 1 week intervals; max 24 mg/day

Requip *Tab:* 0.25, 0.5, 1, 2, 4, 5 mg

▷ *rotigotine* transdermal patch (C) apply to clean, dry, intact skin on abdomen, thigh, hip, flank, shoulder, or upper arm; rotate sites and allow 14 days before reusing site; if hairy, shave site at least 3 days before application to site; avoid abrupt cessation; taper by 2 mg/24 hr every other day; *Early stage:* initially 2 mg/24 hr patch once daily; may increase weekly by 2 mg/24 hr if needed; max 6 mg/24 hr once daily; *Advanced stage:* initially 4 mg/24 hr patch once daily; may increase weekly by 2 mg/24 hr if needed; max 8 mg/24 hr once daily

Neupro *Trans patch:* 1 mg/24 hr, 2 mg/24 hr, 3 mg/24 hr, 4 mg/24 hr, 6 mg/24 hr, 8 mg/24 hr (30/carton) (sulfites)

DOPA-DECARBOXYLASE INHIBITORS

Comment: Contraindicated in narrow-angle glaucoma. Use with caution with sympathomimetics and antihypertensive agents.

▷ *carbidopa+levodopa* (C)(G) usually 400-1600 mg *levodopa*/day

Duopa *Ent susp:* carb 4.63 mg+levo 20 mg single-use cassettes for use w. CADD Legacy 1400 Pump

Sinemet 10/100 initially 1 tab tid-qid; increase if needed daily or every other day up to qid

Tab: carb 10 mg+levo 100 mg*

Sinemet 25/100 initially 1 tab bid-tid; increase if needed daily or every other day up to qid

Tab: carb 25 mg+levo 100 mg*

Sinemet 25/250 1 tab tid-qid

Tab: carb 25 mg+levo 250 mg*

Sinemet CR 25/100 initially one 25/100 tab bid; allow 3 days between dosage adjustments

Tab: carb 25 mg+levo 100 mg cont-rel

Sinemet CR 50/200 initially one 50/200 tab bid; allow 3 days between dosage adjustments

Tab: carb 50 mg+levo 200 mg cont-rel*

DOPA-DECARBOXYLASE INHIBITOR+DOPAMINE PRECURSOR+COMT INHIBITOR COMBINATION

▷ *carbidopa+levodopa+entacapone* (C) titrate individually with separate components; then switch to corresponding strength *levodopa* and *carbidopa*; max 8 tabs/day

Tab: **Stalevo 50** carb 12.5 mg+levo 50 mg+enta 200 mg

Stalevo 75 carb 12.5 mg+levo 75 mg+enta 200 mg

Stalevo 100 carb 12.5 mg+levo 100 mg+enta 200 mg

Stalevo 125 carb 12.5 mg+levo 125 mg+enta 200 mg

Stalevo 150 carb 12.5 mg+levo 150 mg+enta 200 mg

Stalevo 200 carb 12.5 mg+levo 200 mg+enta 200 mg

MONOAMINE OXIDASE INHIBITORS (MAOIs)

▷ *rasagiline* (C)(G) usual maintenance: 0.5-1 mg/day; max: 1 mg/day; initial dose for patients on concomitant *levodopa*: 0.5 mg daily; initial dose for patients not on concomitant *levodopa*: 1 mg daily

Azelect *Tab:* 0.5, 1 mg

Comment: Azelect is indicated as monotherapy or as adjunct to *levodopa*. With mild hepatic dysfunction (Child-Pugh Class 5-6), limit Azelect dose to 0.5 mg daily. With moderate to severe hepatic dysfunction (Child-Pugh Class 7-15), Azelect is not recommended. Contraindications include co-administration with *meperidine, methadone, mirtazapine, propoxyphene, tramadol, dextromethorphan*, St. John's wort, *cyclobenzaprine, methylphenidate, dexmethylphenidate*, or other MAOIs.

▷ *selegiline* (C)(G) 5 mg at breakfast and at lunch; max 10 mg/day
> *Tab/Cap:* 5 mg

▷ *selegiline* (C)(G) 1.25 mg daily; max 2.5 mg/day
> Zelapar *ODT:* 1.25 mg orally-disint (phenylalanine)

MONOAMINE OXIDASE TYPE B (MOA-B) INHIBITOR

▷ *safinamide* (C) initially 50 mg once daily at the same time each day; after 2 weeks, dose may be increased to 100 mg once daily based on individual need and tolerability; *Moderate Hepatic Impairment:* do not exceed 50 mg once daily; *Severe Hepatic Impairment:* contraindicated
> Xadago *Tab:* 50, 100 mg
>
> Comment: Xadago *(safinamide)* has not been shown to be effective as monotherapy; it is adjunctive treatment to *levodopa/carbodopa* in patients experiencing OFF episodes. Xadago drug interactions: SSRIs (monitor for serotonin syndrome); sympathomimetics (monitor for hypertension); tyramine: (monitor for severe hypertension); substrates of breast cancer resistance protein [BCRP]): potential for increase plasma concentration of BRCP substrate. Xadago is contraindicated with concomitant use of other MAOIs or other drugs that are potent inhibitors of monoamine oxidase (e.g., *linezolid; isoniazid* has some monoamine oxidase inhibiting activity), opioids and their derivatives, SNRIs, tri- or tetra-cyclic or triazolopyridine antidepressants, *cyclobenzaprine, methylphenidate*, and *amphetamine* and their derivatives, *dextromethorphan*, St. John's Wort, and severe hepatic impairment (Child-Pugh Class C). The most common adverse effects (incidence ≥2%) are dyskinesia, fall, nausea, and insomnia. Other adverse side effects include falling asleep during activities of daily living (ADLs), hallucinations, psychotic behavior, compulsive and impulsive behaviors, and withdrawal-emergent hyperpyrexia and confusion. Dopaminergic antagonists (e.g., antipsychotics, *metoclopramide*) may decrease the effectiveness of Xadago and exacerbate symptoms of Parkinson's disease. Dopaminergic antagonists (e.g., antipsychotics, *metoclopramide*) may decrease the effectiveness of Xadago and exacerbate symptoms of Parkinson's disease. There are no adequate and well-controlled human studies of Xadago use in pregnancy. Based on animal studies, Xadago may cause fetal harm. It is not known whether Xadago is present in human milk or effects on the breastfed infant. Mothers should be advised regarding the risk/benefit to mother and infant, and decide whether or not to discontinue the Xadago or breastfeeding. To report suspected adverse reactions, contact US WorldMeds at 1-888-492-3246 or FDA at 1-800-FDA-1088 or visit www.fda.gov/medwatch.

COMT INHIBITORS

▷ *entacapone* (C) 1 tab with each dose of *levodopa* or *carbidopa*; max 8 tabs/day
> Comtan *Tab:* 200 mg
>
> Comment: Comtan is an adjunct to *levodopa+carbidopa* in patients with end-of-dose wearing off.

▷ *tolcapone* (C)(G) 100-200 mg tid; max 600 mg/day
> Tasmar *Tab:* 100, 200 mg
>
> Comment: Monitor LFTs every 2 weeks. Withdraw Tasmar if no substantial improvement in the first 3 weeks of treatment.

CENTRALLY-ACTING ANTICHOLINERGICS

▷ *benztropine mesylate* (C) initially 0.5-1 mg q HS, increase if needed; for extrapyramidal disorders 1-4 mg once daily-bid; max 6 mg/day
> Cogentin *Tab:* 0.5*, 1*, 2*mg

▷ *biperiden hydrochloride* (C) initially 1 tab tid or qid, then increase as needed; max 8 tabs/day
> Akineton *Tab:* 2 mg

▷ *procyclidine* (C) initially 2.5 mg tid; may increase as needed to 5 mg tid-qid every 3-5 days; max 15 mg/day
> Kemadrin *Tab:* 5 mg

▷ *trihexyphenidyl* (C)(G) initially 1 mg; increase as needed by 2 mg every 3-5 days; max 15 mg/day
> Artane *Tab:* 2*, 5*mg

PSEUDOBULBAR AFFECT (PBA)

Comment: Pseudobulbar affect (PBA), emotional lability, labile affect, or emotional incontinence refers by to a neurologic disorder characterized by involuntary crying or uncontrollable episodes of crying and/or laughing, or other emotional outbursts. PBA occurs secondary to a neurologic disease or brain injury such as traumatic brain injury (TBI), stroke, Parkinson's disease, multiple sclerosis, and amyotrophic lateral sclerosis (ALS, or Lou Gehrig's disease).

▷ *dextromethorphan+quinidine* (C)(G) 1 cap once daily x 7 days; then starting on day 8, 1 cap bid
Pediatric: <12 years: not recommended; ≥12 years: same as adult
  Nuedexta *Cap:* dextro 20 mg+quini 10 mg
  Comment: *dextromethorphan hydrobromide* is an uncompetitive NMDA receptor antagonist and sigma-1 agonist. *quinidine sulfate* is a CYP450 2D6 inhibitor. Nuedexta is contraindicated with an MAOI or within 14 days of stopping an MAOI, with prolonged QT interval, congenital long QT syndrome, history suggestive of torsades de pointes, or heart failure, complete atrioventricular (AV) block without implanted pacemaker or patients at high risk of complete AV block, and concomitant drugs that both prolong QT interval and are metabolized by CYP2D6 (e.g., *thioridazine* or *pimozide*). Discontinue Nuedexta if the following occurs: hepatitis or thrombocytopenia or any other hypersensitivity reaction. Monitor ECG in patients with left ventricular hypertrophy (LVH) or left ventricular dysfunction (LVD). *desipramine* exposure increases Nuedexta 8-fold; reduce *desipramine* dose and adjust based on clinical response. Use of Nuedexta with selective serotonin reuptake inhibitors (SSRIs) or tricyclic antidepressants (TCAs) increases the risk of serotonin syndrome. *paroxetine* exposure increases Nuedexta 2-fold; therefore, reduce paroxetine dose and adjust based on clinical response *digoxin* exposure may increase *digoxin* substrate plasma concentration. Nuedexta is not recommended in pregnancy or breastfeeding. Safety and effectiveness of Nuedexta in children have not been established. To report suspected adverse reactions, contact Avanir Pharmaceuticals at 1-866-388-5041 or FDA at 1-800-FDA-1088 or www.fda.gov/medwatch.

PARKINSON'S PSYCHOSIS
Atypical Anti-Psychotic

▷ *pimavanserin* take 34 mg once daily with or without food; no titration is needed
  Nuplazid *Tab:* 10, (2 x 17 mg tabs); *Cap:* 34 mg
  Comment: Nuplazid (*pimavanserin*) is an atypical antipsychotic indicated for the treatment of hallucinations and delusions associated with Parkinson's disease psychosis. Nuplazid is not indicated for dementia-related psychosis unrelated to Parkinson's disease as elderly patients with dementia-related psychosis treated with antipsychotic drugs are at increased risk of death. There is risk of QT interval prolongation with Nuplazid; therefore, avoid use in patients with risk factors for prolonged QT interval and concomitant use of other drugs that also increase the QT interval. Nuplazid does not affect motor function. Reduce Nuplazid dose by one-half with strong CYP3A4 inhibitors (e.g., *ketoconazole*). Strong CYP3A4 inducers may reduce efficacy of Nuplazid; increase in Nuplazid dosage may be needed. No Nuplazid dose adjustment is needed in patients with mild-to-moderate renal impairment. Nuplazid is not recommended for use in patients with severe renal impairment or hepatic impairment. There are no data on Nuplazid use in pregnancy that would allow assessment of the drug-associated risk of major congenital malformations or miscarriage, presence of *pimavanserin* in human milk, or effects on the breastfed infant. The most common adverse reactions (incidence ≥5%) are peripheral edema and confusional state. To report suspected adverse reactions, contact Acadia Pharmaceuticals at 1-844-422-2342 or FDA at 1-800-FDA-1088 or visit www.fda.gov/medwatch.

PARONYCHIA (PERIUNGUAL ABSCESS)

▷ *cephalexin* (B)(G) 500 mg bid x 10 days
  Pediatric: 25-50 mg/day in 2 divided doses x 10 days
  Keflex *Cap:* 250, 333, 500, 750 mg; *Oral susp:* 125, 250 mg/5 ml (100, 200 ml) (strawberry)

➤ *clindamycin* (B)(G) 150-300 mg q 6 hours x 10 days
Pediatric: 8-16 mg/kg/day in 3-4 divided doses x 10 days
   Cleocin *Cap:* 75 (tartrazine), 150 (tartrazine), 300 mg
   Cleocin Pediatric Granules *Oral susp:* 75 mg/5 ml (100 ml) (cherry)
➤ *dicloxacillin* (B)(G) 500 mg q 6 hours x 10 days
Pediatric: 12.5-25 mg/kg/day in 4 divided doses x 10 days; *see page 624 for dose by weight*
   Dynapen *Cap:* 125, 250, 500 mg; *Oral susp:* 62.5 mg/5 ml (80, 100, 200 ml)
➤ *erythromycin base* (B)(G) 500 mg q 6 hours x 10 days
Pediatric: <45 kg: 30-50 mg in 2-4 doses x 10 days; ≥45 kg: same as adult
   Ery-Tab *Tab:* 250, 333, 500 mg ent-coat
   PCE *Tab:* 333, 500 mg
Comment: *erythromycin* may increase INR with concomitant **warfarin**, as well as increase serum level of **digoxin**, benzodiazepines, and statins.
➤ *erythromycin ethylsuccinate* (B)(G) 400 mg q 6 hours x 10 days
Pediatric: 30-50 mg/kg/day in 4 divided doses q 6 hours x 10 days; may double dose with severe infection; max 100 mg/kg/day; *see page 626 for dose by weight*
   EryPed *Oral susp:* 200 mg/5 ml (100, 200 ml) (fruit); 400 mg/5 ml (60, 100, 200 ml) (banana); *Oral drops:* 200, 400 mg/5 ml (50 ml) (fruit); *Chew tab:* 200 mg wafer (fruit)
   E.E.S. *Oral susp:* 200, 400 mg/5 ml (100 ml) (fruit)
   E.E.S. Granules *Oral susp:* 200 mg/5 ml (100, 200 ml) (cherry)
   E.E.S. 400 Tablets *Tab:* 400 mg
Comment: *erythromycin* may increase INR with concomitant **warfarin**, as well as increase serum level of **digoxin**, benzodiazepines, and statins.

PAROXYSMAL NOCTURNAL HEMOGLOBINURIA (PNH)

COMPLEMENT INHIBITOR

➤ *eculizumab* (C) dilute to a final admixture concentration of 5 mg/ml using the following steps: (1) withdraw the required amount of **Soliris** from the vial into a sterile syringe; (2) transfer the dose to an infusion bag; (3) add IV fluid equal to the drug volume (0.9% NaCl or 0.45% NaCl or D5W or Ringer's Lactate); the final admixed **Soliris** 5 mg/ml infusion volume is: 300 mg dose (60 ml), 600 mg dose (120 ml), 900 mg dose (180 ml), 1200 mg dose (240 ml)
Pediatric: <18 years: safety and effectiveness not established
   Soliris *Vial:* 300 mg (10 mg/ml, 30 ml), single-use, concentrated solution for intravenous infusion (preservative-free)
   Comment: **Soliris** *(eculizumab)* is a complement inhibitor indicated for the treatment of patients with paroxysmal nocturnal hemoglobinuria (PNH) to reduce hemolysis, patients with atypical hemolytic uremia syndrome (aHUS) to inhibit complement-mediated thrombotic microangiopathy (TMA), and adult patients with generalized myasthenia gravis (gMG) who are anti-acetylcholine receptor (AchR) antibody positive. **Soliris** *(eculizumab)* should be administered at the above recommended dosage regimen time points or within 2 days of each time point. Supplemental dosing of **Soliris** is required in the setting of concomitant support with plasmapheresis (PI) or plasma exchange (PE) or fresh frozen plasma (FFP) infusion. See mfr pkg insert for supplemental dosing. **Soliris** is not indicated for the treatment of patients with Shiga toxin *E. coli*-related hemolytic uremic syndrome (STEC-HUS). **Soliris** is contraindicated in patients with unresolved *Neisseria meningitides* infection and patients who are not currently vaccinated against *Neisseria meningitides,* unless the risks of delaying **Soliris** treatment outweigh the risks of developing meningococcal infection. Prescribers must enroll in the **Soliris** REMS Program (1-888-SOLIRIS, 1-888-765-4747), counsel patients about the risk of meningococcal infection, provide patients with **Soliris** REMS educational materials, and ensure that patients are vaccinated with a meningococcal vaccine. The most frequently reported adverse reactions in the PNH randomized trial (incidence ≥10%) are headache, nasopharyngitis, back pain, and nausea. The most frequently reported adverse reactions in aHUS single-arm prospective trials (incidence ≥15%) are hypertension, URI, diarrhea, headache, anemia, vomiting,

nausea, UTI, and leukopenia. There are no adequate and well-controlled human studies of **Soliris** in pregnancy or effects on the breastfed infant. Based on animal studies, **Soliris** may cause fetal harm. It is not known whether Soliris is excreted in human milk. IgG is excreted in human milk, so it is expected that **Soliris** will be present in human milk. However, published data suggest that antibodies in human milk do not enter the neonatal and infant circulation in substantial amounts. Caution should be exercised when **Soliris** is administered to the breastfeeding patient. To report suspected adverse reactions, contact Alexion Pharmaceuticals at 1-888-SOLIRIS (1-888-765-4747 or FDA at 1-800-FDA-1088 or visit www.fda.gov/medwatch.

➢ *ravulizumab-cwvz* withdraw the calculated volume of **Ultomiris** from the appropriate number of vials (according to the weight-based reference table) and dilute in an infusion bag using 0.9%NS to a final concentration of 5 mg/ml; administer all doses via IV infusion only; starting 2 weeks after administration of the loading dose, begin maintenance doses at once every 8-week intervals; the dosing schedule is allowed to occasionally vary within 7 days of the scheduled infusion day (except for the first maintenance dose of **Ultomiris**) but the subsequent dose should be administered according to the original schedule; for patients switching from *eculizumab* (**Soliris**) to **Ultomiris**, administer the loading dose of **Ultomiris** 2 weeks after the last *eculizumab* (**Soliris**) infusion, and then administer maintenance doses once every 8 weeks, starting 2 weeks after loading dose administration; dilute the appropriate number of vials to a final concentration of 5 mg/ml prior to administration

Weight-Based Dosing Regimen

	Loading	Maintenance
≥40-<60 mg/kg:	2,400 mg	3,000 mg
≥60-<100 mg/kg:	2,700 mg	3,300 mg
≥100 mg/kg:	3,000 mg	3,600 mg

Pediatric: <18 years: not recommended; ≥18 years: same as adult

Ultomiris *Vial:* 300 mg/30 ml (10 mg/ml) in a single-dose

Comment: Ultomiris (*ravulizumab-cwvz*) is a long-acting C5 complement inhibitor for the treatment of paroxysmal nocturnal hemoglobinuria (PNH). Vaccinate patients for meningococcal disease according to current ACIP guidelines to reduce the risk of serious infection. Provide 2 weeks of antibacterial drug prophylaxis to patients if **Ultomoris** must be initiated immediately and vaccines are administered less than 2 weeks before starting **Ultomiris** therapy. There are no available data on **Ultomiris** use in pregnant women to inform a drug-associated risk of major birth defects, miscarriage, or adverse maternal or fetal outcomes (PNH in pregnancy is associated with adverse maternal outcomes, including worsening cytopenias, thrombotic events, infections, bleeding, miscarriages, and increased maternal mortality, and adverse fetal outcomes, including fetal death and premature delivery). There are no data on the presence of *ravulizumab-cwvz* in human milk or effect on the breastfed infant. However, breastfeeding should be discontinued during treatment and for 8 months after the final dose. Healthcare professionals who prescribe **Ultomiris** must enroll in the **Ultomiris** REMS program by telephone at 1-888-765-4747 or by visiting www.ultomirisrems.com.

**PEDICULOSIS HUMANUS CAPITIS (HEAD LICE),
PEDICULOSIS PHTHIRUS (PUBIC LICE)**

➢ *ivermectin* (C) thoroughly wet hair; leave on for 10 minutes; then rinse off with water; do not re-treat
Pediatric: <6 months, <33 lbs: not recommended; ≥6 months, ≥33 lbs: same as adult
   Sklice *Lotn:* 0.5% (4 oz, 117 gm, laminate tube)
➢ *lindane* (C)(G) apply, leave on for 4 minutes, then thoroughly wash off
Pediatric: <2 years: not recommended; ≥2 years: same as adult
   Kwell Shampoo *Shampoo:* 1% (60 ml)
➢ *malathion* (B)(G) thoroughly wet hair; allow to dry naturally; shampoo and rinse after 8-12 hours; use a fine tooth comb to remove lice and nits; if lice persist after 7-9 days, may repeat treatment
Pediatric: same as adult
   Ovide (OTC) *Lotn:* 59% (2 oz)

▶ *permethrin* (B)(G) apply to washed and towel-dried hair; allow to remain on for 10 minutes, then rinse off; repeat after 7 days if needed
Pediatric: <2 months: not recommended; ≥2 months: same as adult
    Nix (OTC) *Crm rinse:* 1% (2 oz w. comb)
▶ *pyrethrins with piperonyl butoxide* (C)(G) apply and leave on for 10 minutes, then wash off
    A-200 *Shampoo:* pyr 0.33%+pip but 3%
    Rid Mousse *Shampoo:* pyr 0.33%+pip but 4%
    Rid Shampoo *Shampoo:* pyr 0.33%+pip but 3%
Comment: To remove nits, soak hair in equal parts white vinegar and water for 15-20 minutes.

PELVIC INFLAMMATORY DISEASE (PID)

Comment: The following treatment regimens are published in the **2015 CDC Sexually Transmitted Diseases Treatment Guidelines.** Treatment regimens are presented by generic drug name first, followed by information about brands and dose forms. Treat all sexual partners. Because of the high risk for maternal morbidity and preterm delivery, pregnant women who have suspected PID should be hospitalized and treated with parenteral antibiotics. HIV-infected women with PID respond equally well to standard parenteral and antibiotic regimens as HIV-negative women.

OUTPATIENT REGIMENS

Regimen 1

▶ *ceftriaxone* 250 mg IM in a single dose plus *doxycycline*
▶ *doxycycline* 100 mg bid x 14 days with or without *metronidazole*
▶ *metronidazole* 500 mg PO bid x 14 days

Regimen 2

▶ *cefoxitin* 2 gm IM in a single dose plus *probebecid*
▶ *probenecid* 1 gm PO in a single dose administered concurrently plus *doxycycline* 100 mg bid x 14 days with or without *metronidazole*
▶ *metronidazole* 500 mg PO bid x 14 days

Regimen 3

▶ Other parenteral third-generation cephalosporin (e.g., *ceftizoxime* or *cefotaxime*) in a single dose) plus *doxycycline*
▶ *doxycycline* 100 mg bid x 14 days with or without *metronidazole*
▶ *metronidazole* 500 mg PO bid x 14 days

DRUG BRANDS AND DOSE FORMS

▶ *cefoxitin* (B)(G)
    Mefoxin *Vial:* 1, 2 g
▶ *ceftriaxone* (B)(G)
    Rocephin Vials 250, 500 mg; 1, 2 gm
▶ *doxycycline* (D)(G)
    Acticlate *Tab:* 75, 150**mg
    Adoxa *Tab:* 50, 75, 100, 150 mg ent-coat
    Doryx *Tab:* 50, 75, 100, 150, 200 mg del-rel
    Doxteric *Tab:* 50 mg del-rel
    Monodox *Cap:* 50, 75, 100 mg
    Oracea *Cap:* 40 mg del-rel
    Vibramycin *Tab:* 100 mg; *Cap:* 50, 100 mg; *Syr:* 50 mg/5 ml (raspberry-apple) (sulfites); *Oral susp:* 25 mg/5 ml (raspberry)
    Vibra-Tab *Tab:* 100 mg film-coat
Comment: *doxycycline* is contraindicated <8 years-of-age, in pregnancy, and lactation (discolors developing tooth enamel). A side effect may be photosensitivity (photophobia). Do not take with antacids, calcium supplements, milk or other dairy, or within 2 hours of taking another drug.

> *metronidazole* (not for use in 1st; B in 2nd, 3rd)
> > **Flagyl** *Tab:* 250*, 500*mg
> > **Flagyl 375** *Cap:* 375 mg
> > **Flagyl ER** *Tab:* 750 mg ext-rel
>
> Comment: Alcohol is contraindicated during treatment with oral *metronidazole* and for 72 hours after therapy due to a possible *disulfiram*-like reaction (nausea, vomiting, flushing, headache).

> *probenecid* (B)(G)
> > **Benemid** *Tab:* 500*mg; *Cap:* 500 mg

PEMPHIGUS VULGARIS (PV), PEMPHIGUS FOLIACEUS (PF)

Comment: Pemphigus is a rare bullous autoimmune disorder that has no cure and is fatal if left untreated. It is characterized by auto-antibody-mediated blistering of the skin (primarily affecting the chest and back; usually sparing the palms and soles of the feet) and oral mucosa. There are two histologic subtypes. Pemphigus vulgaris (PV), accounting for 70% of pemphigus cases, affects the mid-to-deep layers of the epidermis. The hallmark of PV is involvement of the oral mucosa. Pemphigus foliaceus (PF) affects the superficial skin layers and does not affect the oral mucosa. Systemic administration of corticosteroids is the standard first-line treatment to suppress the immune response. Adjuvant nonsteroidal immunosuppressants may be used (e.g., *azathioprine*, *cyclophosphamide*, *mycophenolate mofetil* [MMF], *dapsone*).

GLUCOCORTICOSTEROID

> *prednisone* 1.0-1.5 mg/kg (oral or parenteral) daily with slow tapering and discontinuation after lesions have resolved

MYCOPHENOLIC ACID

> *azathioprine* (D) 1 mg/kg/day in a single or divided doses; may increase by 0.5 mg/kg/day q 4 weeks; max 2.5 mg/kg/day; minimum trial to ascertain effectiveness is 12 weeks; administer IV doses over no less than 2 hours
> *Pediatric:* <12 years: not recommended; >12 years: same as adult
> > **Azasan** *Tab* 75*, 100*mg
> > **Imuran** *Tab* 50*mg

> *cyclophosphamide* (D)(G) *Oral:* Usually 1 mg per kg per day to 5 mg per kg per day for both initial and maintenance dosing; *Intravenous:* initial course for patients with no hematologic deficiency: 40 mg/kg to 50 mg/kg in divided doses over 2 to 5 days; *Other regimens include:* 10 mg/kg to 15 mg/kg every 7 to 10 days or 3 mg/kg to 5 mg/kg twice weekly
> > *Tab:* 25, 50 mg; *Vial:* 500 mg; 1, 2 gm pwdr for reconstitution and IV infusion

SULFONE

> *dapsone* topical (C)(G) apply to affected area bid
> *Pediatric:* <12 years: not recommended; ≥12 years: same as adult
> > **Aczone** *Gel:* 5, 7.5% (30, 60, 90 gm pump)

CD20-DIRECTED CYTOLYTIC MONOCLONAL ANTIBODY

> *rituximab* initially (Month 0) 1000 mg x 2 IV infusions separated by 2 weeks in combination with a tapering course of glucocorticoids; then a 500 mg IV infusion at Month 12 and every 6 months thereafter or based on clinical evaluation; *Relapse:* 1000 mg IV infusion with considerations to resume or increase the glucocorticoid dose based on clinical evaluation; subsequent infusions may be no sooner than 16 weeks after the previous infusion; methylprednisolone 100 mg IV or equivalent glucocorticoid recommended 30 minutes prior to each infusion
> *Pediatric:* <6 years: not recommended; ≥6 years: same as adult
> > **Rituxan** *Vial:* 100 mg/10 ml (10 ml), 50 mg/50 ml (50 ml) single-use
> > Comment: **Rituxan** *(rituximab)* is a CD20-targeting cytolytic monoclonal antibody that received FDA Breakthrough Therapy Designation for treatment of PV in 2017.

Safety and efficacy in recalcitrant PV has been demonstrated in approximately 500 patients across several small trials and case studies, with clinical remission occurring within six weeks in up to 95% of cases. In a recent phase 2 trial comparing *rituximab* plus *prednisone* with *prednisone* alone in patients with newly diagnosed PV, a 55% increase in 2-year remission rate (89% vs 34%) was observed in those receiving *rituximab* plus *prednisone*. Consider intravenous immunoglobulin (e.g., IVIG).

INTERLEUKIN-6 (IL-6) RECEPTOR ANTAGONIST

▷ *tocilizumab* (B) *<100 kg:* 162 mg SC every other week on the same day followed by an increase according to clinical response; *≥100 kg:* 162 mg SC once weekly on the same day; SC injections may be self-administered after being trained and supervised by a qualified health care provider

    Actemra *Vial:* 80 mg/4 ml, 200 mg/10 ml, 400 mg/20 ml, single-use, for IV infusion after dilution; *Prefilled syringe:* 162 mg (0.9 ml, single-dose)

    Comment: Actemra *(tocilizumab)* has received FDA Orphan Drug Designation in PV and is currently being investigated in a phase 2 trial. It is indicated for active recalcitrant pemphigus vulgaris has that has failed 2 lines of prior treatment comprising *prednisone, mycophenolate mofetil MMF)*, and IV immunoglobulin.

B-LYMPHOCYTE STIMULATOR (BLyS)-SPECIFIC INHIBITOR

▷ *belimumab SC administration:* 200 mg SC once weekly; may be self- administered by the patient in the home setting; *IV infusion:* 10 mg/kg at 2-week inter- by a qualified healthcare provider

Pediatric: <18 years: not established; ≥18 years: same as adult

    Benlysta *Prefilled syringe:* 200 mg/ml (1 ml) single-dose (4/carton); *Auto injector:* 200 mg (1 ml) single-dose (4/carton); *Vial:* 120 mg/5 ml, 400 mg/20 ml, single-dose, pwdr for reconstitution and IV infusion (4/carton)

    Comment: Benlysta *(belimumab)* is an IgG1-lambda monoclonal antibody that prevents the survival of B lymphocytes by blocking the binding of soluble human B lymphocyte stimulator protein (BLyS) to receptors on B lymphocytes. This reduces the activity of B-cell mediated immunity and the autoimmune response. Benlysta was initially approved as an intravenous formulation administered in a hospital or clinic setting as a weight-dosed IV infusion every four weeks. Patients can now self-administer Benlysta as a once weekly SC injection after being trained and supervised by a qualified health care provider.

 PEPTIC ULCER DISEASE (PUD)

Helicobacter pylori **Eradication Regimens** *see page* 203
Antacids *see* GERD *page* 170

H2 ANTAGONISTS

▷ *cimetidine* (B)(G)

    Pediatric: <16 years: not recommended; ≥16 years: same as adult

    Tagamet 800 mg bid <u>or</u> 400 mg qid; max 2.4 gm/day
      Tab: 300, 400*, 800*mg

    Tagamet HB (OTC) *Prophylaxis:* 1 tab ac; *Treatment:* 1 tab bid
      Tab: 200 mg

    Tagamet HB Oral Suspension (OTC) *Prophylaxis:* 1 tsp ac; *Treatment:* 1 tsp bid
      Oral susp: 200 mg/20 ml (12 oz)

    Tagamet Liquid *Liq:* 300 mg/5 ml (mint-peach) (alcohol 2.8%)

▷ *famotidine* (B)(G) 20 mg bid <u>or</u> 40 mg q HS; *max* 6 weeks

    Pediatric: 0.5 mg/kg/day q HS <u>or</u> in 2 divided doses; max 40 mg/day

    Pepcid *Tab:* 20, 40 mg; *Oral susp:* 40 mg/5 ml (50 ml)

    Pepcid AC (OTC) 1 tab ac; max 2 doses/day
      Tab/Rapid dissolv tab: 10 mg

    Pepcid Complete (OTC) 1 tab ac; max 2 doses/day
      Tab: fam 10 mg+$CaCO_2$ 800 mg+mag hydrox 165 mg

Pepcid RPD
Tab: 20, 40 mg rapid-dissolv
▷ *nizatidine* (B)(G) 150 mg bid; max 12 weeks
Pediatric: <12 years: not recommended; ≥12 years: same as adult
Axid *Cap:* 150, 300 mg
Axid AR (OTC) 1 tab ac; max 150 mg/day
Tab: 75 mg
▷ *ranitidine* (B)(G)
Pediatric: <1 month: not recommended; 1 month-16 years: 2-4 mg/kg/day in 2 divided doses; max 300 mg/day; *Duodenal/Gastric Ulcer:* 2-4 mg/kg/day divided bid; max 300 mg/day; *Erosive Esophagitis:* 5-10 mg/kg/day divided bid; max 300 mg/day; >16 years: same as adult
Zantac 150 mg bid or 300 mg q HS
Tab: 150, 300 mg
Zantac 75 (OTC) 1 tab ac
Tab: 75 mg
Zantac EFFERdose dissolve 25 mg tab in 5 ml water; dissolve 150 mg tab in 6-8 oz water
Efferdose: 25, 150 mg effervescent (phenylalanine)
Zantac Syrup *Syr:* 15 mg/ml (peppermint) (alcohol 7.5%)
▷ *ranitidine bismuth citrate* (C) 400 mg bid
Pediatric: <12 years: not recommended; ≥12 years: same as adult
Tritec *Tab:* 400 mg

PROTON PUMP INHIBITORS (PPIs)

Comment: If hepatic impairment, or if patient is Asian, consider reducing the PPI dosage. Research has demonstrated associations between PPI use and fractures of the hip, wrist, and spine, hypomagnesemia, kidney injuries and chronic kidney disease, possible cardiovascular drug interactions, and infections (e.g., *Clostridium difficile* and pneumonia). Reducing the acidity of the stomach allows bacteria to thrive and spread to other organs like the lungs and intestines. This risk is increased with high dose and chronic use and greatest in the elderly. The most recent class-wide FDA warning cites reports of cutaneous and systemic lupus erythematosis (CLS/SLE) associates with PPIs in patients with both new onset and exacerbation of existing autoimmune disease. PPI treatment should be discontinued and the patient should be referred to a specialist (http://www.fda.gov/Drugs/DrugSafety/InformationbyDrugClass/ucm213259.htm).

▷ *dexlansoprazole* (B)(G) 30-60 mg daily for up to 4 weeks
Pediatric: <18 years: not recommended; ≥18 years: same as adult
Dexilant *Cap:* 30, 60 mg ent-coat del-rel granules; may open and sprinkle on applesauce; do not crush or chew granules
Dexilant SoluTab *Tab:* 30 mg del-rel orally-disint
▷ *esomeprazole* (B)(OTC)(G) 20-40 mg daily; max 8 weeks; take 1 hour before food; swallow whole or mix granules with food or juice and take immediately; do not crush or chew granules
Pediatric: <1 year: not recommended; 1-11 years: <20 kg: 10 mg; ≥20 kg: 10-20 mg once daily; 12-17 years: 20-40 mg once daily; max 8 weeks; >17 years: same as adult
Nexium *Cap:* 20, 40 mg ent-coat del-rel pellets
Nexium for Oral Suspension *Oral susp:* 10, 20, 40 mg ent-coat del-rel granules/pkt (30 pkt/carton); mix in 2 tbsp water and drink
▷ *lansoprazole* (B)(OTC)(G) 15-30 mg daily for up to 8 weeks; may repeat course; take before eating
Pediatric: <1 year: not recommended; 1-11, <30 kg: 15 mg once daily; ≥12 years: same as adult
Prevacid *Cap:* 15, 30 mg ent-coat del-rel granules; swallow whole or mix granules with food or juice and take immediately; do not crush or chew granules; follow with water
Prevacid for Oral Suspension *Oral susp:* 15, 30 mg ent-coat del-rel granules/pkt (30 pkt/carton); mix in 2 tbsp water and drink immediately; (strawberry)
Prevacid SoluTab *ODT:* 15, 30 mg (strawberry) (phenylalanine)
Prevacid 24HR 15 mg ent-coat del-rel granules; swallow whole or mix granules with food or juice and take immediately; do not crush or chew granules; follow with water
▷ *omeprazole* (C)(OTC)(G) 20-40 mg daily; take before eating; swallow whole or mix granules with applesauce and take immediately; do not crush or chew; follow with water

Pediatric: <1 year: not recommended; 5-<10 kg: 5 mg daily; 10-<20 kg: 10 mg daily; ≥20 kg: same as adult
> **Prilosec** *Cap:* 10, 20, 40 mg ent-coat del-rel granules
> **Prilosec OTC** *Tab:* 20 mg del-rel (regular, wild berry)

▷ *pantoprazole* (B)(G) initially 40 mg bid
Pediatric: <12 years: not recommended; ≥12 years: same as adult
> **Protonix** *Tab:* 40 mg ent-coat del-rel
> **Protonix for Oral Suspension** *Oral susp:* 40 mg ent-coat del-rel granules/pkt; mix in 1 tsp apple juice for 5 seconds <u>or</u> sprinkle on 1 tsp apple sauce, and swallow immediately; do not mix in water <u>or</u> any other liquid <u>or</u> food; take approximately 30 minutes prior to a meal; 30 pkt/carton

▷ *rabeprazole* (B)(OTC)(G) initially 20 mg daily; then titrate; may take 100 mg daily in divided doses <u>or</u> 60 mg bid
Pediatric: <12 years: not recommended; ≥12 years: 20 mg once daily; max 8 weeks
> **AcipHex** *Tab:* 20 mg ent-coat del-rel
> **AcipHex Sprinkle** *Cap:* 5, 10 mg del-rel

OTHER AGENTS

▷ *glycopyrrolate* (B)(G) initially 1-2 mg bid-tid; *Maintenance:* 1 mg bid; max 8 mg/day
Pediatric: <12 years: not recommended; ≥12 years: same as adult
> **Robinul** *Tab:* 1 mg (dye-free)
> **Robinul Forte** *Tab:* 2 mg (dye-free)

Comment: *glycopyrrolate* is an anticholinergic adjunct to PUD treatment.

▷ *mepenzolate* (B)(G) 25-50 mg divided qid, with meals and at HS
> **Cantil** *Tab:* 25 mg

▷ *sucralfate* (B)(G) **Active ulcer:** 1 gm qid; *Maintenance:* 1 gm bid
> **Carafate** *Tab:* 1*g; *Oral susp:* 1 gm/10 ml (14 oz)

PROPHYLAXIS

▷ *misoprostol* (X) 200 mg qid with food for prevention of NSAID-induced gastric ulcers
> **Cytotec** *Tab:* 100, 200 mg

Comment: *misoprostol* is a prostaglandin E1 analog indicated for the prevention of NSAID-induced gastric ulcers. Females of childbearing potential should have a negative serum pregnancy test within 2 weeks before starting and first dose on the 2nd <u>or</u> 3rd day of next the menstrual period. A contraceptive method should be maintained during therapy. Risks to pregnant females include: spontaneous abortion, premature birth, fetal anomalies, and uterine rupture.

PERIPHERAL NEURITIS, DIABETIC NEUROPATHIC PAIN, PERIPHERAL NEUROPATHIC PAIN

▷ **Acetaminophen for IV Infusion** *see Pain page 352*
▷ **Ibuprophen for IV Infusion** *see Pain page 352*
▷ *acetaminophen* (B)(G) *see Fever page 163*

▷ *aspirin* (D)(G) *see Fever page 164*
Comment: *aspirin*-containing medications are contraindicated with history of allergic-type reaction to *aspirin*, children and adolescents with *Varicella* or other viral illness, and 3rd trimester of pregnancy.

ALPHA-2 DELTA LIGAND

▷ *pregabalin (GABA analog)* (C)(V) initially 150 mg daily divided bid-tid; may titrate within one week; max 600 mg divided bid-tid; discontinue over one week
Pediatric: <18 years: not recommended; ≥18 years: same as adult
> **Lyrica** *Cap:* 25, 50, 75, 100, 150, 200, 225, 300 mg; *Oral soln:* 20 mg/ml

SEROTONIN-NOREPINEPHRINE REUPTAKE INHIBITOR (SNRI)

▷ *duloxetine* (C) swallow whole; 30-60 mg once daily; may increase by 30 mg at 1 week intervals; usual target 60 mg daily; max 120 mg/day
Pediatric: <12 years: not recommended; ≥12 years: same as adult

Cymbalta *Cap:* 20, 30, 60 mg ent-coat pellets

Comment: **Cymbalta** is indicated for chronic pain syndromes (e.g., arthritis, fibromyalgia, lowback pain).

TOPICAL & TRANSDERMAL ANALGESICS

▶ *capsaicin* (B)(G) apply tid-qid prn to intact skin
  Pediatric: <2 years: not recommended; ≥2 years: apply sparingly tid-qid prn
    Axsain *Crm:* 0.075% (1, 2 oz)
    Capsin *Lotn:* 0.025, 0.075% (59 ml)
    Capzasin-HP (OTC) *Crm:* 0.075% (1.5 oz), 0.025 (45, 90 gm); *Lotn:* 0.075% (2 oz);
    0.025% (45, 90 gm)
    Capzasin-P (OTC) *Crm:* 0.025% (1.5 oz); *Lotn:* 0.025% (2 oz)
    Dolorac *Crm:* 0.025% (28 gm)
    Double Cap (OTC) *Crm:* 0.05% (2 oz)
    R-Gel *Gel:* 0.025% (15, 30 gm)
    Zostrix (OTC) *Crm:* 0.025% (0.7, 1.5, 3 oz)
    Zostrix HP (OTC) *Emol crm:* 0.075% (1, 2 oz)
▶ *capsaicin* 8% patch (B) apply up to 4 patches for one 60-minute application to clean dry
  skin; may prep area with topical anesthetic; wear non-latex gloves; patches may be cut to
  size/shape; treatment may be repeated every 3 months
  Pediatric: <18 years: not recommended; ≥18 years: same as adult
    Qutenza *Patch:* 8% 1640 mcg/cm (179 mg) (1 or 2 patches w. 1-50 gm tube cleansing
    gel/carton)
▶ *diclofenac sodium* (C; D ≥30 wks)(G) apply qid prn to intact skin
  Pediatric: <12 years: not established; ≥12 years: same as adult
    Pennsaid 1.5% in 10 drop increments, dispense and rub into front, side, and back of
    knee: usually; 40 drops (40 mg) qid
      Topical soln: 1.5% (150 ml)
    Pennsaid 2% apply 2 pump actuations (40 mg) and rub into front, side, and back of
    knee bid
      Topical soln: 2% (20 mg/pump actuation, 112 gm)
    Solaraze Gel massage in to clean skin bid prn
      Gel: 3% (50 gm) (benzyl alcohol)
    Voltaren Gel (G) apply qid prn to intact skin
      Gel: 1% (100 gm)

Comment: *diclofenac* is contraindicated with *aspirin* allergy. As with other NSAIDs, should
be avoided in late pregnancy (≥30 weeks) because it may cause premature closure of the
ductus arteriosus.

▶ *doxepin* (B) cream apply to affected area qid at intervals of at least 3-4 hours; max 8 days
  Pediatric: <12 years: not recommended; >12 years: same as adult
    Prudoxin *Crm:* 5% (45 gm)
    Zonalon *Crm:* 5% (30, 45 gm)
▶ *pimecrolimus* 1% cream (C)(G) <2 years: not recommended; ≥2 years: apply to affected area
  bid; do not apply an occlusive dressing
    Elidel *Crm:* 1% (30, 60, 100 gm)

Comment: *pimecrolimus* is indicated for short-term and intermittent long-term use.
Discontinue use when resolution occurs. Contraindicated if the patient is immunosuppressed. Change to the 0.1% preparation or if secondary bacterial infection is present.

▶ *trolamine salicylate* apply tid-qid
  Pediatric: <2 years: not recommended; ≥2 years: same as adult
    Mobisyl Creme *Crm:* 10% (100 gm)

TOPICAL AND TRANSDERMAL ANESTHETICS

Comment: *lidocaine* should not be applied to non-intact skin.

▶ *lidocaine* cream (B) apply to affected area bid prn
  Pediatric: <12 years: not recommended; ≥12 years: same as adult
    LidaMantle *Crm:* 3% (1, 2 oz)
    Lidoderm *Crm:* 3% (85 gm)
    ZTlido *lidocaine* topical system 1% (30/carton)

Comment: Compared to **Lidoderm** (*lidocaine* patch 5%) which contains 700 mg/patch, **ZTlido** only requires 35 mg per topical system to achieve the same therapeutic dose.

▷ *lidocaine* lotion (B) apply to affected area bid prn
   Pediatric: <12 years: not recommended; ≥12 years: same as adult
     LidaMantle *Lotn:* 3% (177 ml)

▷ *lidocaine* 5% patch (B)(G) apply up to 3 patches at one time for up to 12 hours/24-hour period (12 hours on/12 hours off); patches may be cut into smaller sizes before removal of the release liner; do not re-use
   Pediatric: <12 years: not recommended; ≥12 years: same as adult
     Lidoderm *Patch:* 5% (10x14 cm; 30/carton)

▷ *lidocaine+dexamethasone* (B)
   Pediatric: <12 years: not recommended; ≥12 years: same as adult
     Decadron Phosphate with Xylocaine *Lotn:* dexa 4 mg+lido 10 mg per ml (5 ml)

▷ *lidocaine+hydrocortisone* (B)(G) apply to affected area bid prn
   Pediatric: <12 years: not recommended; ≥12 years: same as adult
     LidaMantle HC *Crm:* lido 3%+hydro 0.5% (1, 3 oz); *Lotn:* (177 ml)

▷ *lidocaine 2.5%+prilocaine 2.5%* apply sparingly to the burn bid-tid prn
   Pediatric: <12 years: not recommended; ≥12 years: same as adult
     Emla Cream (B) 5, 30 gm/tube

ORAL ANALGESICS

▷ *tramadol* (C)(IV)(G)
   Comment: *tramadol* is known to be excreted in breast milk. The FDA and the European Medicines Agency (EMA) are investigating the safety of using *tramadol*-containing medications to treat pain in children 12-18 years because of the potential for serious side effects, including slowed or difficult breathing.
     Rybix ODT initially 100 mg once daily; may increase by 100 mg every 5 days; max 300 mg/day; *CrCl <30 mL/min or severe hepatic impairment:* not recommended; *Cirrhosis:* max 50 mg q 12 hours
   Pediatric: <12 years: contraindicated; 12-<18: use extreme caution; not recommended for children and adolescents with obesity, asthma, obstructive sleep apnea, or other chronic breathing problem, or for post-tonsillectomy/adenoidectomy pain; ≥18 years: same as adult
     ODT: 50 mg (mint) (phenylalanine)
     Ryzolt initially 100 mg once daily; may increase by 100 mg every; 5 days; max 300 mg/day; *CrCl <30 mL/min or severe hepatic impairment:* not recommended
   Pediatric: <18 years: not recommended; ≥18 years: same as adult
     Tab: 100, 200, 300 mg ext-rel
     Ultram 50-100 mg q 4-6 hours prn; max 400 mg/day; *CrCl <30 mL/min:* max 100 mg q 12 hours; *Cirrhosis:* max 50 mg q 12 hours
   Pediatric: <18 years: not recommended; ≥18 years: same as adult
     Tab: 50 mg
     Ultram ER initially 100 mg once daily; may increase by 100 mg every 5 days; max 300 mg/day; *CrCl <30 mL/min or severe hepatic impairment:* not recommended
   Pediatric: <18 years: not recommended; ≥18 years: same as adult
     Tab: 100, 200, 300 mg ext-rel

▷ *tramadol+acetaminophen* (C)(IV)(G) 2 tabs q 4-6 hours; max 8 tabs/day; 5 days; *CrCl <30 mL/min:* max 2 tabs q 12 hours; max 4 tabs/day x 5 days
   Pediatric: <18 years: not recommended; ≥18 years: same as adult
     Ultracet *Tab:* tram 37.5+acet 325 mg
   Comment: *tramadol* is known to be excreted in breast milk. The FDA and the European Medicines Agency (EMA) are investigating the safety of using *tramadol*-containing medications to treat pain in children 12-18 years because of the potential for serious side effects, including slowed or difficult breathing.

MU-OPIOID AGONIST+NOREPINEPHRINE REUPTAKE INHIBITOR COMBINATION

▷ *tapentadol* (C)
   Pediatric: <18 years: not recommended; ≥18 years: same as adult

Nucynta 50-100 mg q 4-6 hours prn; max 700 mg/day on the first day; 600 mg/day on subsequent days
  Tab: 50, 75, 100 mg
Nucynta ER *Opioid-naïve:* initially 50 mg q 12 hours, then titrate to optimal dose within therapeutic range; usual therapeutic range 100-250 mg q 12 hours; doses >500 mg not recommended; *Converting from Nucynta:* divide total **Nucynta** daily dose into 2 **Nucynta ER** doses and administer q 12 hours; converting from *oxycodone CR* and other opioids, see mfr recommendations
  Tab: 50, 100, 150, 200, 250 mg ext-rel

PERIPHERAL VASCULAR DISEASE (PVD, ARTERIAL INSUFFICIENCY, INTERMITTENT CLAUDICATION)

ANTIPLATELET THERAPY

▷ *aspirin* (D)(OTC) usually 81 mg once daily; range 75-325 mg once daily
  Ecotrin *Tab/Cap:* 81, 325, 500 mg ent-coat
  Comment: *aspirin*-containing medications are contraindicated with history of allergic-type reaction to *aspirin*, children and adolescents with *Varicella* or other viral illness, and 3rd trimester of pregnancy.
▷ *cilostazol* (C) 100 mg bid 1/2 hour before or 2 hours after breakfast or dinner; may reduce to 50 mg bid if used with CYP 3A4 (e.g., azole antifungals, macrolides, *diltiazem, fluvoxamine, fluoxetine, nefazodone, sertraline*) or CYP 2C19 (e.g., *omeprazole*) inhibitors
  Tab: 50, 100 mg
  Comment: *cilostazol* may be used with *aspirin*. Cautious use with other antiplatelet agents and anticoagulants.
▷ *clopidogrel* (B) 75 mg daily
  Plavix *Tab:* 75 mg
▷ *dipyridamole* (B)(G) 25-100 mg tid-qid
  Persantine *Tab:* 25, 50, 75 mg
  Comment: *dipyridamole* does not potentiate *warfarin* and may be taken concomitantly. Do not administer *dipyridamole* concomitantly with *aspirin*.
▷ *pentoxifylline* (C) 400 mg tid with food
  PentoPak *Tab:* 400 mg ext-rel
  Trental *Tab:* 400 mg sust-rel
▷ *ticlopidine* (B) 250 mg bid with food
  Ticlid *Tab:* 250 mg
  Comment: Monitor for neutropenia; resolves after discontinuation.
▷ *warfarin* (X) adjust dose to maintain INR in recommended range; *see Anticoagulation Therapy* page 596
  Coumadin *Tab:* 1*, 2*, 2.5*, 5*, 7.5*, 10*mg
  Coumadin for Injection *Vial:* 2 mg/ml (5 mg) pwdr for reconstitution
  Comment: Treatment for over-anticoagulation with *warfarin* is *vitamin K*.

PERLECHE (ANGULAR STOMATITIS)

Comment: Perleche is a form of intertrigo. This localized tissue inflammation and maceration is characterized by constant exposure to saliva, which normally contains bacteria, yeast, and other organisms, in the natural anatomical furrow at the corners of the mouth. Perleche is often misdiagnosed as yeast infection, but almost never responds to anti-yeast agents. Patients with severe vitamin deficiencies (e.g., chronic alcoholism, malnutrition) are often at increased risk. Sensitivities or allergies to toothpaste may be contributing irritants.

Treatment: apply a small amount of a combination of 2.5% *hydrocortisone* cream and *miconazole* cream (which kills yeast, fungi, and many bacteria) to the affected area twice a day. Once the area is clear, recurrence can be prevented with local application of petroleum jelly.

PERTUSSIS (WHOOPING COUGH)

Prophylaxis *see Childhood Immunizations page 558*

POST-EXPOSURE PROPHYLAXIS & TREATMENT

Comment: Antibiotics do not alter the course of illness, but they do prevent transmission. Infected persons should be isolated until after the fifth day of antibiotic treatment.

➤ *azithromycin* (B)(G) 500 mg x 1 dose on day 1, then 250 mg daily on days 2-5 or 500 mg daily x 3 days
    Pediatric: 12 mg/kg/day x 5 days; max 500 mg/day; *see page 619 for dose by weight*
        Zithromax *Tab:* 250, 500, 600 mg; *Oral susp:* 100 mg/5 ml (15 ml); 200 mg/5 ml (15, 22.5, 30 ml) (cherry); *Pkt:* 1 gm for reconstitution (cherry-banana)
        Zithromax Tri-pak *Tab:* 3 x 500 mg tabs/pck
        Zithromax Z-pak *Tab:* 6 x 250 mg tabs/pck
        Zmax *Oral susp:* 2 gm ext-rel for reconstitution (cherry-banana) (148 mg Na⁺)
    Comment: *azithromycin* is the drug of choice for infants <1 month-of-age.

➤ *clarithromycin* (C)(G) 250 mg bid or 500 mg ext-rel once daily x 10 days
    Pediatric: <6 months: not recommended; ≥6 months: 7.5 mg/kg divided bid x 10 days; *see page 624 for dose by weight*
        Biaxin *Tab:* 250, 500 mg
        Biaxin Oral Suspension *Oral susp:* 125, 250 mg/5 ml (50, 100 ml) (fruit-punch)
        Biaxin XL *Tab:* 500 mg ext-rel
    Comment: The FDA is advising caution before prescribing *clarithromycin* to patients with heart disease because of a potential increased risk of heart problems or death that can occur years later. This recommendation is based on a review of the results of a 10-year follow-up study of patients with coronary heart disease from a large clinical trial that first observed this safety issue. Consider risk benefit and the use of other antibiotics in such patients.

➤ *erythromycin base* (B)(G) 1 gm/day divided qid x 14 days
    Pediatric: 40 mg/kg/day in divided doses x 14 days
        Ery-Tab *Tab:* 250, 333, 500 mg ent-coat
        PCE *Tab:* 333, 500 mg
    Comment: *erythromycin* may increase INR with concomitant *warfarin*, as well as increase serum level of *digoxin*, benzodiazepines, and statins.

➤ *erythromycin ethylsuccinate* (B)(G) 1 gm/day in 4 divided doses x 14 days
    Pediatric: 40-50 mg/kg/day in 4 divided doses x 7 days; may double dose with severe infection; max 100 mg/kg/day; *see page 626 for dose by weight*
        EryPed *Oral susp:* 200 mg/5 ml (100, 200 ml) (fruit); 400 mg/5 ml (60, 100, 200 ml) (banana); *Oral drops:* 200, 400 mg/5 ml (50 ml) (fruit); *Chew tab:* 200 mg wafer (fruit)
        E.E.S. *Oral susp:* 200, 400 mg/5 ml (100 ml) (fruit)
        E.E.S. Granules *Oral susp:* 200 mg/5 ml (100, 200 ml) (cherry)
        E.E.S. 400 Tablets *Tab:* 400 mg
    Comment: *erythromycin* may increase INR with concomitant *warfarin*, as well as increase serum level of *digoxin,* benzodiazepines, and statins.

➤ *trimethoprim+sulfamethoxazole (TMP-SMX)* (C)(G)
    Pediatric: <2 months: not recommended; ≥2 months: 40 mg/kg/day of *sulfamethoxazole* in 2 doses bid x 10 days; *see page 630 for dose by weight*
        Bactrim, Septra 2 tabs bid x 10 days
            Tab: trim 80 mg+sulfa 400 mg*
        Bactrim DS, Septra DS 1 tab bid x 10 days
            Tab: trim 160 mg+sulfa 800 mg
        Bactrim Pediatric Suspension, Septra Pediatric Suspension
            Oral susp: trim 40 mg+sulfa 200 mg per 5 ml (100 ml) (cherry) (alcohol 0.3%)
    Comment: Sulfonamides are contraindicated in the first trimester of pregnancy, the final month of pregnancy, and infants <8 weeks-of-age. *CrCl 15-30 mL/min:* reduce dose by 1/2; *CrCl <15 mL/min:* not recommended. Contraindicated with G6PD deficiency. A high fluid intake is indicated during sulfonamide therapy to avoid crystallization in the kidneys.

 PHARYNGITIS: GONOCOCCAL

Comment: Treat all sexual contacts. Empiric therapy requires concomitant treatment for *Chlamydia*. Post-treatment culture recommended with PMHx history rheumatic fever.

PRIMARY THERAPY

▷ **azithromycin** (B)(G) 1 gm x 1 dose

Pediatric: 12 mg/kg/day x 5 days; max 500 mg/day; *see page 619 for dose by weight*

 Zithromax *Tab:* 250, 500, 600 mg; *Oral susp:* 100 mg/5 ml (15 ml); 200 mg/5 ml (15, 22.5, 30 ml) (cherry); *Pkt:* 1 gm for reconstitution (cherry-banana)

 Zithromax Tri-pak *Tab:* 3 x 500 mg tabs/pck

 Zithromax Z-pak *Tab:* 6 x 250 mg tabs/pck

 Zmax *Oral susp:* 2 gm ext-rel for reconstitution (cherry-banana) (148 mg Na⁺)

Comment: Per the CDC 2015 STD Treatment Guidelines, *azithromycin* should be used with *ceftriaxone* 250 mg.

▷ **ceftriaxone** (B)(G) 250 mg IM x 1 dose

Pediatric: <45 kg: 125 mg IM x 1 dose; ≥45 kg: same as adult

 Rocephin *Vial:* 250, 500 mg; 1, 2 gm

PHARYNGITIS: STREPTOCOCCAL (STREP THROAT)

Comment: Acute rheumatic fever is a rare but serious autoimmune disease that may occur following a group A *streptococcal* throat infection. It causes inflammatory lesions in connective tissue, especially that of the heart, kidneys, joints, blood vessels, and subcutaneous tissue. Prior to the broad availability of penicillin, rheumatic fever was a leading cause of death in children and one of the leading causes of acquired heart disease in adults. Strep throat is highly responsive to the penicillins and cephalosporins.

▷ **amoxicillin** (B)(G) 500-875 mg bid or 250-500 mg tid x 10 days

Pediatric: <40 kg (88 lb): 20-40 mg/kg/day in 3 divided doses x 10 days or 25-45 mg/kg/day in 2 divided doses x 10 days; ≥40 kg: same as adult; *see page 617 for dose by weight*

 Amoxil *Cap:* 250, 500 mg; *Tab:* 875*mg; *Chew tab:* 125, 200, 250, 400 mg (cherry-banana-peppermint) (phenylalanine); *Oral susp:* 125, 250 mg/5 ml (80, 100, 150 ml) (strawberry); 200, 400 mg/5 ml (50, 75, 100 ml) (bubble gum); *Oral drops:* 50 mg/ml (30 ml) (bubble gum)

 Moxatag *Tab:* 775 mg ext-rel

 Trimox *Tab:* 125, 250 mg; *Cap:* 250, 500 mg; *Oral susp:* 125, 250 mg/5 ml (80, 100, 150 ml) (raspberry-strawberry)

▷ **amoxicillin+clavulanate** (B)(G)

 Augmentin 500 mg tid or 875 mg bid x 7-10 days

Pediatric: 40-45 mg/kg/day divided tid x 10 days or 90 mg/kg/day divided bid x 10 days *see pages 618 for dose by weight*

  Tab: 250, 500, 875 mg; *Chew tab:* 125, 250 mg (lemon-lime); 200, 400 mg (cherry-banana) (phenylalanine); *Oral susp:* 125 mg/5 ml (banana), 250 mg/5 ml (75, 100, 150 ml) (orange); 200, 400 mg/5 ml (50, 75, 100 ml) (orange) (phenylalanine)

 Augmentin ES-600 not recommended for adults

Pediatric: <3 months: not recommended; ≥3 months, <40 kg: 90 mg/kg/day in 2 divided doses x 7-10 days; ≥40 kg: not recommended

  Oral susp: 42.9 mg/5 ml (50, 75, 100, 125, 150, 200 ml) (strawberry cream) (phenyl-alanine)

 Augmentin XR 2 tabs q 12 hours x 7-10 days

Pediatric: <16 years: use other forms; ≥16 years: same as adult

  Tab: 1000*mg ext-rel

▷ **azithromycin** (B)(G) 500 mg x 1 dose on day 1, then 250 mg daily on days 2-5 or 500 mg daily x 3 days

Pediatric: 12 mg/kg/day x 5 days; max 500 mg/day; *see page 619 for dose by weight*

 Zithromax *Tab:* 250, 500, 600 mg; *Oral susp:* 100 mg/5 ml (15 ml); 200 mg/5 ml (15, 22.5, 30 ml) (cherry); *Pkt:* 1 gm for reconstitution (cherry-banana)

 Zithromax Tri-pak *Tab:* 3 x 500 mg tabs/pck

 Zithromax Z-pak *Tab:* 6 x 250 mg tabs/pck

 Zmax *Oral susp:* 2 gm ext-rel for reconstitution (cherry-banana) (148 mg Na⁺)

▷ **cefaclor** (B)(G) 250 mg tid or 375 mg bid x 5 days

Pediatric: <1 month: not recommended; 20-40 mg/kg bid or q 12 hours x 10 days; max 1 gm/day; *see page 620 for dose by weight*

 Tab: 500 mg; *Cap:* 250, 500 mg; *Susp:* 125 mg/5 ml (75, 150 ml) (strawberry); 187 mg/5 ml (50, 100 ml) (strawberry); 250 mg/5 ml (75, 150 ml) (strawberry); 375 mg/5 ml (50, 100 ml) (strawberry)

Cefaclor Extended Release
Pediatric: <16 years: ext-rel not recommended; ≥16 years: same as adult
Tab: 375, 500 mg ext-rel

➤ *cefadroxil* (B) 1 gm in 1-2 doses x 10 days
Pediatric: 30 mg/kg/day in 2 divided doses x 10 days; *see page 620 for dose by weight*
Duricef *Cap:* 500 mg; *Tab:* 1 gm; *Oral susp:* 250 mg/5 ml (100 ml); 500 mg/5 ml (75, 100 ml) (orange-pineapple)

➤ *cefdinir* (B) 300 mg bid x 10 days
Pediatric: <6 months: not recommended; 6 months-12 years: 14 mg/kg/day in 1-2 doses x 10 days; *see page 621 for dose by weight;* >12 years: same as adult
Omnicef *Cap:* 300 mg; *Oral susp:* 125 mg/5 ml (60, 100 ml) (strawberry)

➤ *cefditoren pivoxil* (B) 200 mg bid x 10 days
Pediatric: <12 years: not recommended; ≥12 years: same as adult
Spectracef *Tab:* 200 mg
Comment: **Spectracef** is contraindicated with milk protein allergy or carnitine deficiency.

➤ *cefixime* (B)(G) 400 mg daily x 5 days
Pediatric: <6 months: not recommended; 6 months-12 years, <50 kg: 8 mg/kg/day in 1-2 divided doses x 10 days; *see page 621 for dose by weight;* >12 years, ≥50 kg: same as adult
Suprax *Tab:* 400 mg; *Cap:* 400 mg; *Oral susp:* 100, 200, 500 mg/5 ml (50, 75, 100 ml) (strawberry)

➤ *cefpodoxime proxetil* (B) 100 mg bid x 5-7 days
Pediatric: <2 months: not recommended; 2 months-12 years: 10 mg/kg/day in 2 divided doses x 5-7 days; *see page 622 for dose by weight;* >12 years: same as adult
Vantin *Tab:* 100, 200 mg; *Oral susp:* 50, 100 mg/5 ml (50, 75, 100 ml) (lemon creme)

➤ *cefprozil* (B) 500 mg daily x 10 days
Pediatric: <2 years: not recommended; 2-12 years: 7.5 mg/kg divided bid x 10 days; *see page 622 for dose by weight;* >12 years: same as adult
Cefzil *Tab:* 250, 500 mg; *Oral susp:* 125, 250 mg/5 ml (50, 75, 100 ml) (bubble gum) (phenylalanine)

➤ *ceftibuten* (B) 400 mg daily x 5 days
Pediatric: 9 mg/kg daily x 5 days; *see page 623 for dose by weight*
Cedax *Cap:* 400 mg; *Oral susp:* 90 mg/5 ml (30, 60, 90, 120 ml); 180 mg/5 ml (30, 60, 120 ml) (cherry)

➤ *cephalexin* (B)(G) 500 mg bid x 10 days
Pediatric: 25-50 mg/kg/day in 2 divided doses x 10 days; *see page 623 for dose by weight*
Keflex *Cap:* 250, 333, 500, 750 mg; *Oral susp:* 125, 250 mg/5 ml (100, 200 ml) (strawberry)

➤ *clarithromycin* (C)(G) 250 mg bid or 500 mg ext-rel once daily x 10 days
Pediatric: <6 months: not recommended; ≥6 months: 7.5 mg/kg divided bid x 10 days; *see page 624 for dose by weight*
Biaxin *Tab:* 250, 500 mg
Biaxin Oral Suspension *Oral susp:* 125, 250 mg/5 ml (50, 100 ml) (fruit-punch)
Biaxin XL *Tab:* 500 mg ext-rel
Comment: The FDA is advising caution before prescribing *clarithromycin* to patients with heart disease because of a potential increased risk of heart problems or death that can occur years later. This recommendation is based on a review of the results of a 10-year follow-up study of patients with coronary heart disease from a large clinical trial that first observed this safety issue. Consider risk benefit and the use of other antibiotics in such patients.

➤ *dirithromycin* (C)(G) 500 mg daily x 10 days
Pediatric: <12 years: not recommended; ≥12 years: same as adult
Dynabac *Tab:* 250 mg

➤ *erythromycin base* (B)(G) 500 mg qid x 10 days
Pediatric: <45 kg: 30-50 mg divided bid-qid x 10 days; ≥45 kg: same as adult
Ery-Tab *Tab:* 250, 333, 500 mg ent-coat
PCE *Tab:* 333, 500 mg
Comment: *erythromycin* may increase INR with concomitant *warfarin*, as well as increase serum level of *digoxin*, benzodiazepines, and statins.

➤ *erythromycin estolate* (B)(G) 250-500 mg qid x 10 days
Pediatric: 20-50 mg/kg divided q 6 hours x 10 days; *see page 625 for dose by weight*
Ilosone *Pulvule:* 250 mg; *Tab:* 500 mg; *Liq:* 125, 250 mg/5 ml (100 ml)

Comment: *erythromycin* may increase INR with concomitant *warfarin*, as well as increase serum level of *digoxin,* benzodiazepines, and statins.

▷ *erythromycin ethylsuccinate* (B)(G) 400 mg qid or 800 mg bid x 10 days
Pediatric: 30-50 mg/kg/day in 4 divided doses x 7 days; may double dose with severe infection; max 100 mg/kg/day; *see page 626 for dose by weight*
> **EryPed** *Oral susp:* 200 mg/5 ml (100, 200 ml) (fruit); 400 mg/5 ml (60, 100, 200 ml) (banana); *Oral drops:* 200, 400 mg/5 ml (50 ml) (fruit); *Chew tab:* 200 mg wafer (fruit)
> **E.E.S.** *Oral susp:* 200, 400 mg/5 ml (100 ml) (fruit)
> **E.E.S. Granules** *Oral susp:* 200 mg/5 ml (100, 200 ml) (cherry)
> **E.E.S. 400 Tablets** *Tab:* 400 mg

Comment: *erythromycin* may increase INR with concomitant *warfarin,* as well as increase serum level of *digoxin,* benzodiazepines, and statins.

▷ *loracarbef* (B) 200 mg bid x 5 days
Pediatric: 15 mg/kg/day in 2 divided doses x 5 days; *see page 628 for dose by weight*
> **Lorabid** *Pulvule:* 200, 400 mg; *Oral susp:* 100 mg/5 ml (50, 100 ml); 200 mg/5 ml (50, 75, 100 ml) (strawberry bubble gum)

▷ *penicillin g (benzathine)* (B)(G) 1.2 million units IM x 1 dose
Pediatric: <60 lb: 300,000-600,000 units IM x 1 dose; ≥60 lb: 900,000 units x 1 dose
> **Bicillin L-A** *Cartridge-needle unit:* 600,000 units (1 ml); 1.2 million units (2 ml)

▷ *penicillin g (benzathine and procaine)* (B)(G) 2.4 million units IM x 1 dose
Pediatric: <30 lb: 600,000 units IM x 1 dose; 30-60 lb: 900,000 units-1.2 million units IM x 1 dose; >60 lb: same as adult
> **Bicillin C-R** *Cartridge-needle unit:* 600,000 units (1 ml); 1.2 million units; (2 ml); 2.4 million units (4 ml)

▷ *penicillin v potassium* (B)(G) 500 mg bid or 250 mg qid x 10 days
Pediatric: <12 years: 25-50 mg/kg day in 4 divided doses x 10 days; *see page 629 for dose by weight;* >12 years: same as adult
> **Pen-Vee K** *Tab:* 250, 500 mg; *Oral soln:* 125 mg/5 ml (100, 200 ml); 250 mg/5 ml (100, 150, 200 ml)
> **Veetids** *Tab:* 250, 500 mg; *Oral soln:* 125, 250 mg/5 ml (100, 200 ml)

PHENYLKETONURIA (PKU)

PHENYLALANINE-METABOLIZING ENZYME

Comment: **Palynziq** (*pegvaliase epbx*) is a phenylalanine-metabolizing enzyme indicated to reduce blood phenylalanine (PHa) concentrations in adult patients with phenylketonuria who have uncontrolled blood phenylalanine concentrations >600 micromol/L on existing management. **Palynziq** is to be used in conjunction with a Pha-restricted diet.

▷ *pegvaliase epbx* recommended initial dosage is 2.5 mg SC once weekly x 4 weeks; titrate dosage in a step-wise manner over at least 5 weeks based on tolerability to achieve a dosage of 20 mg SC once daily; see mfr pkg insert for titration regimen; consider increasing the dosage to max 40 mg SC once daily in patients who have been on 20 mg once daily continuously for at least 24 weeks and who have not achieved either a 20% reduction in blood phenylalanine concentration from pre-treatment baseline or a blood phenylalanine concentration ≤600 micromol/L; discontinue **Palynziq** in patients who have not achieved at least a 20% reduction in blood phenylalanine concentration from pre-treatment baseline or a blood phenylalanine concentration ≤ 600 micromol/L after 16 weeks of continuous treatment with the maximum dosage of 40 mg once daily; reduce the dosage and/or modify dietary protein and phenylalanine intake, as needed, to maintain blood phenylalanine concentrations within a clinically acceptable range and >30 micromol/L *ALWAYS co-prescribe auto-injectable epinephrine.*
Pediatric: <18 years: not recommended; ≥18 years: same as adult
> **Palynziq** *Prefilled syringe:* 2.5, 10 mg/0.5 ml; 20 mg/ml, single-dose (preservative-free)

Comment: Obtain blood phenylalanine concentrations every 4 weeks until a maintenance dosage is established. After a maintenance dosage is established, periodically monitor blood phenylalanine concentrations. Counsel patients to monitor dietary protein and phenylalanine intake, and adjust as directed by their healthcare provider. Anaphylaxis has been reported after administration of **Palynziq** and may occur at any time during treatment. Administer the initial dose under the supervision of a healthcare provider equipped to manage anaphylaxis, and closely observe patients for at least 60 min following injection. Prior to self-injection, confirm patient competency with self-administration, and the patient's and observer's (if applicable) ability to recognize signs and symptoms of anaphylaxis and to administer auto-injectable epinephrine, if needed. *Prescribe auto-injectable epinephrine.* Prior to first dose, instruct the patient and observer (if applicable) on its appropriate use. Instruct the patient to seek immediate medical care upon its use. Instruct patients to carry auto-injectable epinephrine with them at all times during **Palynziq** treatment. **Palynziq** is available only through the restricted Palynziq REMS program. **Palynziq** may cause fetal harm when administered to a pregnant woman. Limited available data with *pegvaliase-pqpz* use in pregnant women are insufficient to inform a drug-associated risk of adverse developmental outcomes. There are risks to the fetus associated with poorly controlled phenylalanine concentrations in women with PKU during pregnancy including increased risk for miscarriage, major birth defects (including microcephaly, major cardiac malformations), intrauterine fetal growth retardation, and future intellectual disability with low IQ; therefore, phenylalanine concentrations should be closely monitored in women with PKU during pregnancy. There are no data on the presence of *pegvaliase-pqpz* in human milk or the effects on the breastfed infant.

PENYLALANINE HYDROXYLASE ACTIVATOR (PHA)

Comment: Kuvan (sapropterin) is a phenylalanine hydroxylase activator (PHA) indicated to reduce blood phenylalanine (Phe) levels in patients with hyperphenylalaninemia (HPA) due to tetrahydrobiopterin- (BH4-) responsive Phenylketonuria (PKU). Kuvan is to be used in conjunction with a Phe-restricted diet

▷ **sapropterin** recommended starting dose is 10 mg/kg/day taken once daily; doses may be adjusted in the range of 5 to 20 mg/kg taken once daily. Blood Phe must be monitored regularly; take with food to increase absorption; tabs may be swallowed whole or dissolved in 4 to 8 oz (120-240 ml) of water or apple juice; once dissolved, dose should be taken within 15 minutes; pwdr for oral soln should be dissolved in 4 to 8 oz (120-240 m) of water or apple juice and consumed within 30 minutes of preparation
Pediatric: <18 years: not recommended; ≥18 years: same as adult
   Kuvan *Tab:* 100 mg; *Pwdr for Oral Soln:* 100 mg/unit dose pkt

 PHEOCHROMOCYTOMA

ALPHA-BLOCKER

▷ **phenoxybenzamine** (C) initially 10 mg bid; increase every other day as needed; usually 20-40 mg bid-tid
Pediatric: <18 years: not established; ≥18 years: same as adult
   Dibenzyline *Cap:* 10 mg
   Comment: Dibenzyline *(phenoxybenzamine hydrochloride)* is a long-acting, adrenergic, alpha-receptor blocking agent, which can produce and maintain "chemical sympathectomy" by oral administration. It increases blood flow to the skin, mucosa and abdominal viscera, and lowers both supine and erect blood pressures. It has no effect on the parasympathetic system. **Dibenzyline** is indicated in the treatment of pheochromocytoma, to control episodes of hypertension and sweating. If tachycardia is excessive, it may be necessary to use a *beta*-blocking agent concomitantly. **Dibenzyline**-induced *alpha*-adrenergic blockade leaves *beta*-adrenergic receptors unopposed. Compounds that stimulate both types of receptors may, therefore, produce an exaggerated hypotensive response and tachycardia.

 PHEOCHROMOCYTOMA: UNRESECTABLE, LOCALLY ADVANCED, OR METASTATIC

ALPHA-BLOCKER

▷ **phenoxybenzamine** (C) initially 10 mg bid; increase every other day as needed; usually 20-40 mg bid-tid
Pediatric: <18 years: not established; ≥18 years: same as adult
   Dibenzyline *Cap:* 10 mg
   (see **PHEOCHROMOCYTOMA** for comment)

ANTINEOPLASIA AGENT

 iobenguane I 131 to be administered <u>only</u> by a qualified health care professional; verify pregnancy status in females of reproductive potential prior to administration; initiate thyroid-blocking medication prior to **Azedra** administration and continue after each dose. do <u>not</u> administer if platelet count <80,000/mcL <u>or</u> absolute neutrophil count <1,200/mcL; administer intravenously as a dosimetric dose followed by two therapeutic doses administered 90 days apart

> *Recommended **Dosimetric** Dose:*
>   *>50 kg:* 185 to 222 MBq (5 to 6 mCi)
>   *≤50 kg:* 3.7 MBq/kg (0.1 mCi/kg)
> *Recommended Therapeutic Dose for each of the 2 doses:*
>   *> 62.5 kg:* 18,500 MBq (500 mCi)
>   *≤62.5 kg:* 296 MBq/kg (8 mCi/kg)
> Adjust therapeutic doses based on radiation dose estimates results from dosimetry, if needed
> *Pediatric:* <12 years: not established; ≥12 years: same as adult
>   **Azedra** *Vial:* 555 MBq/ml (15 mCi/ml) single-dose for IV infusion

> Comment: **Azedra** *(iobenguane I 131)* is a radioactive therapeutic agent indicated for the treatment of patients with iobenguane scan-positive, unresectable, locally advanced, <u>or</u> metastatic pheochromocytoma <u>or</u> paraganglioma who require systemic anti-cancer therapy. Monitor for hypothyroidism and thyroid-stimulating hormone (TSH) before starting **Azedra** and annually thereafter. Monitor blood pressure frequently during the first 24 hours after each dose. **Azedra** can cause fetal harm; advise females <u>and</u> males of reproductive potential of the potential risk to a fetus and to use effective contraception. **Azendra** may cause infertility. Advise women <u>not</u> to breastfeed.

PINWORM (*ENTEROBIUS VERMICULARIS*)

Comment: Treatment of all family members is recommended.

ANTHELMINTICS

Comment: Oral bioavailability of anthelmintics is enhanced when administered with a fatty meal (estimated fat content 40 gm). Treatment of all family members is recommended. Some clinicians recommend all household contacts of infected patients receive treatment, especially when multiple <u>or</u> repeated symptomatic infections occur, since such contacts commonly also are infected; retreatment after 14 to 21 days may be needed.

▶ *albendazole* (C) 400 mg x 1 dose; may repeat in 2-3 weeks if needed; take with a meal
  Pediatric: <20 kg: 200 mg as a single dose; ≥20 kg: same as adult
    Albenza *Tab:* 200 mg

▶ *mebendazole* (C) chew, swallow, <u>or</u> mix with food; 100 mg x 1 dose; may repeat in 3 weeks if needed; take with a meal
  Pediatric: <2 years: not recommended; ≥2 years: same as adult
    Emverm *Chew tab:* 100 mg
    Vermox (G) *Chew tab:* 100 mg

▶ *pyrantel pamoate* (C) 11 mg/kg x 1 dose; max 1 gm/dose; may repeat in 2-3 weeks if needed; take with a meal
  Pediatric: 25-37 lb: 1/2 tsp x 1 dose; 38-62 lb: 1 tsp x 1 dose; 63-87 lb: 1 tsp x 1 dose; 88-112 lb: 2 tsp x 1 dose; 113-137 lb: 2 tsp x 1 dose; 138-162 lb: 3 tsp x 1 dose; 163-187 lb: 3 tsp x 1 dose; >187 lb: 4 tsp x 1 dose
    Pin-X (OTC); *Cap:* 180 mg; *Liq:* 50 mg/ml (30 ml); 144 mg/ml (30 ml); *Oral susp:* 50 mg/ml (30 ml)

▶ *thiabendazole* (C) 50 mg/kg x 1 dose after a meal; max 3 gm; may repeat in 2-3 weeks if needed; take with a meal
  Pediatric: same as adult
    Mintezol *Chew tab:* 500*mg (orange); *Oral susp:* 500 mg/5 ml (120 ml) (orange)

Comment: *thiabendazole* is not for prophylaxis and should not be used as first-line therapy for pinworms. May impair mental alertness. May not be available in the US.

PITYRIASIS ALBA

Topical Corticosteroids see page 574

Comment: Pityriasis alba is a chronic skin disorder seen in children with a genetic predisposition to atopic disease. Treatment is directed toward controlling roughness and pruritus. There is no known treatment for the associated skin pigment changes. Pityriasis alba resolves spontaneously and permanently in the 2nd or 3rd decade of life.

COAL TAR PREPARATIONS

▶ *coal tar* (C)
Pediatric: same as adult
    Scytera (OTC) apply qd-qid; use lowest effective dose
      Foam: 2%
    T/Gel Shampoo Extra Strength (OTC) use every other day; max 4 x/week; massage into affected area for 5 minutes; rinse; repeat
      Shampoo: 1%
    T/Gel Shampoo Original Formula (OTC) use every other day; max 7 x/week; massage into affected area for 5 minutes; rinse; repeat
      Shampoo: 0.5%
    T/Gel Shampoo Stubborn Itch Control (OTC) use every other day; max 7 x/week; massage into affected area for 5 minutes; rinse; repeat
      Shampoo: 0.5%

EMOLLIENTS AND OTHER MOISTURIZING AGENTS

see **Dermatitis: Atopic** *page* 121

PITYRIASIS ROSEA

Topical Corticosteroids *see page* 574
Antihistamines *see* **Drugs for the Management of Allergy, Cough, and Cold Symptoms** *see page* 603

PLAGUE (*YERSINIA PESTIS*)

Comment: *Yersinia pestis* is transmitted via the bite of a flea from an infected rodent or the bite, lick, or scratch of an infected cat. Untreated bubonic plague may progress to secondary pneumonic plague, which may be transmitted via contaminated respiratory droplet spread.
▶ *streptomycin* (C)(G) 15 mg/kg IM bid x 10 days
Pediatric: same as adult
Amp: 1 gm/2.5 ml or 400 mg/ml (2.5 ml)
Comment: For patients with renal impairment, reduce dose of *streptomycin* to 20 mg/kg/day if mild and 8 mg/kg/day q 3 days if advanced). For patients who are pregnant or who have hearing impairment, shorten the course of treatment to 3 days after fever has resolved.
▶ *moxifloxacin* (C)(G) 400 mg daily x 10 days
Pediatric: <18 years: not recommended; ≥18 years: same as adult
Avelox *Tab:* 400 mg; IV soln: 400 mg/250 mg (latex-free, preservative-free)
▶ *tetracycline* (D)(G) 500 mg qid or 25-50 mg/kg/day divided q 6 hours x 10 days
Pediatric: <8 years: not recommended; ≥8 years: same as adult
Comment: *tetracycline* is contraindicated <8 years-of-age, in pregnancy, and lactation (discolors developing tooth enamel). A side effect may be photosensitivity (photophobia). Do not take with antacids, calcium supplements, milk or other dairy, or within two hours of taking another drug.

PNEUMONIA: BACTERIAL, HOSPITAL-ACQUIRED (HABP)

PARENTERAL CEPHALOSPORIN ANTIBACTERIAL+BETA-LACTIMASE INHIBITOR

▶ *ceftazidime+avibactam* (B) infuse dose over 2 hours; recommended duration of treatment: 5 to 4 days; *CrCl 31-50 mL/min:* 1.25 gm every 8 hours; *CrCl 16-30 mL/min:* 0.94 gm every 12 hours; *CrCl 6-15 mL/min:* 0.94 gm every 24 hours; *CrCl ≤5 mL/min:* 0.94 gm every 48 hours; both *ceftazidime* and *avibactam* are hemodialyzable; thus, administer **Avycaz** after hemodialysis on hemodialysis days
Pediatric: <18 years: not recommended; ≥18 years: same as adult

Avycaz *Vial:* 2.5 gm, single-dose, pwdr for reconstitution and IV infusion

Comment: Avycaz 2.5 gm contains *ceftazidime* (a cephalosporin) 2 grams (equivalent to 2.635 grams of *ceftazidime pentahydrate/sodium carbonate powder*) and *avibactam* (a beta lactam inhibitor) 0.5 grams (equivalent to 0.551 grams of *avibactam sodium*). As only limited clinical safety and efficacy data for **Avycaz** are currently available, reserve **Avycaz** for use in patients who have limited or no alternative treatment options. To reduce the development of drug-resistant bacteria and maintain the effectiveness of **Avycaz** and other antibacterial drugs, **Avycaz** should be used only to treat infections that are proven or strongly suspected to be caused by susceptible bacteria. Seizures and other neurologic events may occur, especially in patients with renal impairment. Adjust dose in patients with renal impairment. Decreased efficacy in patients with baseline CrCl 30--≤50 mL/min. Monitor CrCl at least daily in patients with changing renal function and adjust the dose of **Avycaz** accordingly. Monitor for hypersensitivity reactions, including anaphylaxis and serious skin reactions. Cross-hypersensitivity may occur in patients with a history of penicillin allergy. If an allergic reaction occurs, discontinue **Avycaz**. *Clostridium difficile*-associated diarrhea CDAD) has been reported with nearly all systemic antibacterial agents, including **Avycaz**. There are no adequate and well-controlled studies of **Avycaz**, *ceftazidime*, <u>or</u> *avibactam* in pregnant females. *ceftazidime* is excreted in human milk in low concentrations. It is not known whether *avibactam* is excreted into human milk. There are no studies to inform effects on the breastfed infant.

PNEUMONIA: BACTERIAL, VENTILATOR-ASSOCIATED (VABP)

PARENTERAL CEPHALOSPORIN ANTIBACTERIAL+BETA-LACTIMASE INHIBITOR

▷ *ceftazidime+avibactam* (B) infuse dose over 2 hours; recommended duration of treatment: 5 to 4 days; *CrCl 31-50 mL/min:* 1.25 gm every 8 hours; *CrCl 16-30 mL/min:* 0.94 gm every 12 hours; *CrCl 6-15 mL/min:* 0.94 gm every 24 hours; *CrCl ≤5 mL/min:* 0.94 gm every 48 hours; both *ceftazidime* and *avibactam* are hemodialyzable; thus, administer **Avycaz** after hemodialysis on hemodialysis days

Pediatric: <18 years: not recommended; ≥18 years: same as adult

Avycaz *Vial:* 2.5 gm, single-dose, pwdr for reconstitution and IV infusion

Comment: Avycaz 2.5 gm contains *ceftazidime* (a cephalosporin) 2 grams (equivalent to 2.635 grams of *ceftazidime pentahydrate/sodium carbonate powder*) and *avibactam* (a beta lactam inhibitor) 0.5 grams (equivalent to 0.551 grams of *avibactam sodium*). As only limited clinical safety and efficacy data for **Avycaz** are currently available, reserve **Avycaz** for use in patients who have limited or no alternative treatment options. To reduce the development of drug-resistant bacteria and maintain the effectiveness of **Avycaz** and other antibacterial drugs, **Avycaz** should be used only to treat infections that are proven or strongly suspected to be caused by susceptible bacteria. Seizures and other neurologic events may occur, especially in patients with renal impairment. Adjust dose in patients with renal impairment. Decreased efficacy in patients with baseline CrCl 30--≤50 mL/min. Monitor CrCl at least daily in patients with changing renal function and adjust the dose of **Avycaz** accordingly. Monitor for hypersensitivity reactions, including anaphylaxis and serious skin reactions. Cross-hypersensitivity may occur in patients with a history of penicillin allergy. If an allergic reaction occurs, discontinue **Avycaz**. *Clostridium difficile*-associated diarrhea CDAD) has been reported with nearly all systemic antibacterial agents, including **Avycaz**. There are no adequate and well-controlled studies of **Avycaz**, *ceftazidime*, <u>or</u> *avibactam* in pregnant females. *ceftazidime* is excreted in human milk in low concentrations. It is not known whether *avibactam* is excreted into human milk. There are no studies to inform effects on the breastfed infant.

PNEUMONIA: CHLAMYDIAL

RECOMMENDED REGIMEN

▷ *erythromycin base* (B)(G) 500 mg qid hours x 10-14 days

Pediatric: <45 kg: 50 mg in 4 divided doses x 10-14 days; ≥45 kg: same as adult

Ery-Tab *Tab:* 250, 333, 500 mg ent-coat

PCE *Tab:* 333, 500 mg

Comment: *erythromycin* may increase INR with concomitant *warfarin*, as well as increase serum level of *digoxin,* benzodiazepines, and statins.

➤ *erythromycin ethylsuccinate* (B)(G) 400 mg qid x 10-14 days
Pediatric: <45 kg: 50 mg/kg/day in 4 divided doses x 10-14 days; ≥45 kg: same as adult; *see page 626 for dose by weight*
　　EryPed *Oral susp:* 200 mg/5 ml (100, 200 ml) (fruit); 400 mg/5 ml (60, 100, 200 ml) (banana); *Oral drops:* 200, 400 mg/5 ml (50 ml) (fruit); *Chew tab:* 200 mg wafer (fruit)
　　E.E.S. *Oral susp:* 200, 400 mg/5 ml (100 ml) (fruit)
　　E.E.S. Granules *Oral susp:* 200 mg/5 ml (100, 200 ml) (cherry)
　　E.E.S. 400 Tablets *Tab:* 400 mg
Comment: *erythromycin* may increase INR with concomitant *warfarin*, as well as increase serum level of *digoxin*, benzodiazepines, and statins.

ALTERNATE REGIMENS

➤ *azithromycin* (B)(G) 500 mg once daily x 10 days
Pediatric: 20 mg/kg per dose once daily x 3 days; max 500 mg/day; *see page 619 for dose by weight*
　　Zithromax *Tab:* 250, 500, 600 mg; *Oral susp:* 100 mg/5 ml (15 ml); 200 mg/5 ml (15, 22.5, 30 ml) (cherry); Pkt: 1 gm for reconstitution (cherry-banana)
　　Zithromax Tri-pak *Tab:* 3 x 500 mg tabs/pck
　　Zithromax Z-pak *Tab:* 6 x 250 mg tabs/pck
　　Zmax *Oral susp:* 2 gm ext-rel for reconstitution (cherry-banana) (148 mg Na+)
➤ *levofloxacin* (C) *Uncomplicated:* 500 mg daily x 7 days; *Complicated:* 750 mg daily x 7 days
Pediatric: <18 years: not recommended; ≥18 years: same as adult
　　Levaquin *Tab:* 250, 500, 750 mg; *Oral soln:* 25 mg/ml (480 ml) (benzyl alcohol); *Inj conc:* 25 mg/ml for IV infusion after dilution (20, 30 ml single-use vial) (preservative-free); *Premix soln:* 5 mg/ml for IV infusion (50, 100, 150 ml) (preservative-free)
Comment: *levofloxacin* is contraindicated <18 years-of-age, and during pregnancy and lactation. Risk of tendonitis or tendon rupture.

PNEUMONIA: COMMUNITY ACQUIRED (CAP) AND COMMUNITY ACQUIRED BACTERIAL PNEUMONIA (CABP)

Comment: Over 70% of patients with uncomplicated community-acquired pneumonia (CAP) received prescriptions for antibiotics that exceeded national duration recommendations, according to a retrospective study that included 22,128 patients from 18 to 64 years-of-age with private insurance and 130,746 patients aged >65 years with Medicare, who were hospitalized with uncomplicated CAP. Length of antibiotic therapy (LOT) during hospital stay was estimated using the MarketScan Hospital Drug Database and outpatient LOT was determined using prescriptions filled at discharge. The researchers defined excessive duration as a LOT of more than 3 days.

REFERENCE

Yi, S. H., Hatfield, K. M., Baggs, J., Hicks, L. A., Srinivasan, A., Reddy, S., & Jernigan, J. A. (2017). Duration of antibiotic use among adults with uncomplicated community-acquired pneumonia requiring hospitalization in the United States. *Clinical Infectious Diseases, 66*(9), 1333–1341. doi:10.1093/cid/cix986

ANTI-INFFECTIVES

➤ *amoxicillin* (B)(G) 500-875 mg bid or 250-500 mg tid x 3-10 days
Pediatric: <40 kg (88 lb): 20-40 mg/kg/day in 3 divided doses x 3-10 days or 25-45 mg/kg/day in 2 divided doses x 3-10 days; ≥40 kg: same as adult
　　Amoxil *Cap:* 250, 500 mg; *Tab:* 875 mg; *Chew tab:* 125, 200, 250, 400 mg (cherry-banana-peppermint) (phenylalanine); *Oral susp:* 125, 250 mg/5 ml (80, 100, 150 ml) (strawberry); 200, 400 mg/5 ml (50, 75, 100 ml) (bubble gum); *Oral drops:* 50 mg/ml (30 ml) (bubble gum)
　　Moxatag *Tab:* 775 mg ext-rel
　　Trimox *Tab:* 125, 250 mg; *Cap:* 250, 500 mg; *Oral susp:* 125, 250 mg/5 ml (80, 100, 150 ml) (raspberry-strawberry)
➤ *amoxicillin+clavulanate* (B)(G) 500 mg tid or 875 mg bid x 3-10 days
　　Augmentin 500 mg tid or 875 mg bid x 3-10 days
　　Pediatric: 40-45 mg/kg/day divided tid x 10 days or 90 mg/kg/day divided bid x 10 days
　　see pages 618 for dose by weight

Tab: 250, 500, 875 mg; *Chew tab:* 125, 250 mg (lemon-lime); 200, 400 mg (cherry-banana) (phenylalanine); *Oral susp:* 125 mg/5 ml (banana), 250 mg/5 ml (75, 100, 150 ml) (orange); 200, 400 mg/5 ml (50, 75, 100 ml) (orange) (phenylalanine)

Augmentin ES-600 not recommended for adults

Pediatric: <3 months: not recommended; ≥3 months, <40 kg: 90 mg/kg/day in 2 divided doses x 3-10 days; ≥40 kg: not recommended

Oral susp: 42.9 mg/5 ml (50, 75, 100, 125, 150, 200 ml) (strawberry cream) (phenylalanine)

Augmentin XR 2 tabs q 12 hours x 3-10 days

Pediatric: <16 years: use other forms; ≥16 years: same as adult

Tab: 1000*mg ext-rel

➤ *azithromycin* (B)(G) *Day 1,* 500 mg as a single dose and *Days 2-5,* 250 mg once daily or 500 mg once daily x 3 days

Pediatric: <6 months: not recommended; ≥6 months: 10 mg/kg x 1 dose on day 1; then 5 mg/kg/day on days 2-5; max 500 mg/day; *see page 619 for dose by weight*

Zithromax *Tab:* 250, 500, 600 mg; *Oral susp:* 100 mg/5 ml (15 ml); 200 mg/5 ml (15, 22.5, 30 ml) (cherry); *Pkt:* 1 gm for reconstitution (cherry-banana)

Zithromax Tri-pak *Tab:* 3 x 500 mg tabs/pck

Zithromax Z-pak *Tab:* 6 x 250 mg tabs/pck

Zmax *Oral susp:* 2 gm ext-rel for reconstitution (cherry-banana) (148 mg Na⁺)

➤ *cefaclor* (B)(G) 250 mg tid or 375 mg bid 3-10 days

Pediatric: <1 month: not recommended; 1 month-12 years: 20-40 mg/kg divided bid or q 12 hours x 3-10 days; max 1 gm/day; *see page 620 for dose by weight;* >12 years: same as adult

Tab: 500 mg; *Cap:* 250, 500 mg; *Susp:* 125 mg/5 ml (75, 150 ml) (strawberry); 187 mg/5 ml (50, 100 ml) (strawberry); 250 mg/5 ml (75, 150 ml) (strawberry); 375 mg/5 ml (50, 100 ml) (strawberry)

Cefaclor Extended Release 375-500 mg bid x 3-10 days

Pediatric: <16 years: ext-rel not recommended; ≥16 years: same as adult

Tab: 375, 500 mg ext-rel

➤ *cefdinir* (B) 300 mg bid or 600 mg daily x 3-10 days

Pediatric: <6 months: not recommended; 6 months-12 years: 14 mg/kg/day in a single or 2 divided doses x 3-10 days; *see page 621 for dose by weight;* >12 years: same as adult

Omnicef *Cap:* 300 mg; *Oral susp:* 125 mg/5 ml (60, 100 ml) (strawberry)

➤ *cefpodoxime proxetil* (B) 200 mg bid x 3-10 days

Pediatric: 2 months-12 years: 10 mg/kg/day in 2 divided doses x 3-5 days; *see page 622 for dose by weight;* >12 years: same as adult

Vantin *Tab:* 100, 200 mg; *Oral susp:* 50, 100 mg/5 ml (50, 75, 100 ml) (lemon creme)

➤ *ceftaroline fosamil* (B) administer by IV infusion after reconstitution every 12 hours x 3-10 days; *CrCl ≥50 mL/min:* 600 mg; *CrCl >30-<50 mL/min:* 400 mg; *CrCl: >15-<30 mL/min:* 300 mg; ES RD: 200 mg

Pediatric: <18 years: not recommended; ≥18 years: same as adult

Teflaro *Vial:* 400, 600 mg

➤ *ceftriaxone* (B)(G) 1-2 gm IM daily; x 1-3 days

Pediatric: 50-75 mg/kg IM in 2 divided doses; max 2 gm/day x 1-3 days

Rocephin *Vial:* 250, 500 mg; 1, 2 gm

➤ *clarithromycin* (C)(G) 500 mg bid or 500 mg ext-rel once daily x 3-10 days

Pediatric: <6 months: not recommended; ≥6 months: 7.5 mg/kg bid x 3-10 days

Biaxin *Tab:* 250, 500 mg

Biaxin Oral Suspension *Oral susp:* 125, 250 mg/5 ml (50, 100 ml) (fruit-punch)

Biaxin XL *Tab:* 500 mg ext-rel

Comment: The FDA is advising caution before prescribing *clarithromycin* to patients with heart disease because of a potential increased risk of heart problems or death that can occur years later. This recommendation is based on a review of the results of a 10-year follow-up study of patients with coronary heart disease from a large clinical trial that first observed this safety issue. Consider risk benefit and the use of other antibiotics in such patients.

➤ *dirithromycin* (C)(G) 500 mg daily x 3-10 days

Pediatric: <12 years: not recommended; ≥12 years: same as adult

Dynabac *Tab:* 250 mg

➤ *doxycycline* (D)(G) 100 mg bid x 3-10 days

Pediatric: <8 years: not recommended; ≥8 years, ≤100 lb: 2 mg/lb on first day in 2 divided doses, followed by 1 mg/lb/day in 1-2 divided doses; ≥8 years, >100 lb: same as adult; *see page 625 for dose by weight*

Acticlate *Tab:* 75, 150**mg
Adoxa *Tab:* 50, 75, 100, 150 mg ent-coat
Doryx *Tab:* 50, 75, 100, 150, 200 mg del-rel
Doxteric *Tab:* 50 mg del-rel
Monodox *Cap:* 50, 75, 100 mg
Oracea *Cap:* 40 mg del-rel
Vibramycin *Tab:* **100 mg;** *Cap:* 50, 100 mg; *Syr:* 50 mg/5 ml (raspberry-apple) (sulfites); *Oral susp:* 25 mg/5 ml (raspberry)
Vibra-Tab *Tab:* 100 mg film-coat

Comment: *doxycycline* is contraindicated <8 years-of-age, in pregnancy, and lactation (discolors developing tooth enamel). A side effect may be photosensitivity (photophobia). Do not take with antacids, calcium supplements, milk or other dairy, or within 2 hours of taking another drug.

▷ *ertapenem* (B)(G) 1 gm daily; *CrCl <30 mL/min:* 500 mg daily x 3-10 days; may switch to an oral antibiotic after 3 days if warranted; *IV infusion:* administer over 30 minutes; *IM injection:* reconstitute with *lidocaine* only
Invanz *Vial:* 1 gm pwdr for reconstitution

▷ *erythromycin base* (B)(G) 500 mg q 6 hours x 14-21 days; <45 kg: 30-50 mg in 2-4 doses x 3-10 days; ≥45 kg: same as adult
Ery-Tab *Tab:* 250, 333, 500 mg ent-coat
PCE *Tab:* 333, 500 mg

Comment: **erythromycin** may increase INR with concomitant *warfarin*, as well as increase serum level of *digoxin*, benzodiazepines, and statins.

▷ *erythromycin estolate* (B) 500 mg q 6 hours x 3-10 days
Ilosone *Pulvule:* 250 mg; *Tab:* 500 mg; *Liq:* 125, 250 mg/5 ml (100 ml)

Comment: **erythromycin** may increase INR with concomitant *warfarin*, as well as increase serum level of *digoxin*, benzodiazepines, and statins.

▷ *gemifloxacin* (C)(G) 320 mg daily x 3-10 days
Pediatric: <18 years: not recommended; ≥18 years: same as adult
Factive *Tab:* 320*mg

▷ *levofloxacin* (C) 250 mg once daily x 3-10 days
Pediatric: <18 years: not recommended; ≥18 years: same as adult
Levaquin *Tab:* 250, 500, 750 mg; *Oral soln:* 25 mg/ml (480 ml) (benzyl alcohol); *Inj conc:* 25 mg/ml for IV infusion after dilution (20, 30 ml single-use vial) (preservative-free); *Premix soln:* 5 mg/ml for IV infusion (50, 100, 150 ml) (preservative-free)

▷ *linezolid* (C)(G) 400-600 mg q 12 hours x 10-14 days
Pediatric: <5 years: 10 mg/kg q 8 hours x 10-14 days; 5-11 years: 10 mg/kg q 12 hours x 10-14 days; >11 years: same as adult
Zyvox *Tab:* 400, 600 mg; *Oral susp:* 100 mg/5 ml (150 ml) (orange) (phenylalanine)

Comment: *linezolid* is indicated to treat susceptible vancomycin-resistant *E. faecium* infections.

▷ *loracarbef* (B) 400 mg bid x 3-10 days
Pediatric: <12 years: 15 mg/kg/day in 2 divided doses x 7 days; *see page 628 for dose by weight table;* ≥12 years: 200 mg bid x 7 days
Lorabid *Pulvule:* 200, 400 mg; *Oral susp:* 100 mg/5 ml (50, 100 ml); 200 mg/5 ml (50, 75, 100 ml) (strawberry bubble gum)

▷ *moxifloxacin* (C)(G) 400 mg daily x 3-10 days
Pediatric: <18 years: not recommended; ≥18 years: same as adult
Avelox *Tab:* 400 mg; IV soln: 400 mg/250 mg (latex-free, preservative-free)

▷ *ofloxacin* (C)(G) 400 mg bid x 3-10 days
Pediatric: <18 years: not recommended; ≥18 years: same as adult
Floxin *Tab:* 200, 300, 400 mg

▷ *penicillin v potassium* (B) 250-500 mg q 6 hours x 3-10 days
Pediatric: <12 years: 25-75 mg/kg day divided q 6-8 hours x 5-7 days; *see page 629 for dose by weight table;* ≥12 years: same as adult
Pen-VK *Tab:* 250, 500 mg; *Oral soln:* 125 mg/5 ml (100, 200 ml); 250 mg/5 ml (100, 150, 200 ml)

▷ *tedizolid phosphate* (B) administer 200 mg once daily x 6 days, via PO or IV infusion over 1 hour
Sivextro *Tab:* 200 mg (6/blister pck)

Comment: **Sivextro** is indicated for the treatment of community acquired bacterial pneumonia (CABP)

▷ *telithromycin* (C) 2 x 400 mg tabs in a single dose once daily x 3-5 days
  Pediatric: <8 years: not recommended; ≥8 years: same as adult
    Ketek *Tab:* 300, 400 mg
  Comment: *telithromycin* is contraindicated with PMHx hepatitis or jaundice associated with macrolide use.

▷ *tigecycline* (D)(G) 100 mg once; then 50 mg q 12 hours x 3-5 days; *Severe hepatic impairment (Child-Pugh Class C):* 100 mg once; then 25 mg q 12 hours x 3-5 days
  Pediatric: <18 years: not recommended; ≥18 years: same as adult
    Tygacil *Vial:* 50 mg pwdr for reconstitution and IV infusion (preservative-free)
    Comment: **Tygacil** is indicated only for the treatment of adults (≥18 years-of-age) with community acquired bacterial pneumonia (CABP). *tigecycline* is contraindicated in pregnancy, and lactation (discolors developing tooth enamel). A side effect may be photo-sensitivity (photophobia). Do not give with antacids, calcium supplements, milk or other dairy, or within two hours of taking another drug.

▷ *trimethoprim+sulfamethoxazole* (TMP-SMX) (C)(G)
  Pediatric: <2 months: not recommended; ≥2 months: 40 mg/kg/day of *sulfamethoxazole* in 2 doses bid x 3-10 days; *see page 630 for dose by weight*
    Bactrim, Septra 2 tabs bid x 3-10 days
      Tab: trim 80 mg+sulfa 400 mg*
    Bactrim DS, Septra DS 1 tab bid x 3-10 days
      Tab: trim 160 mg+sulfa 800 mg*
    Bactrim Pediatric Suspension, Septra Pediatric Suspension 160/800 bid x 3-10 days
      Oral susp: trim 40 mg+sulfa 200 mg per 5 ml (100 ml) (cherry) (alcohol 0.3%)
  Comment: Sulfonamides are contraindicated in the first trimester of pregnancy, the final month of pregnancy, and infants <8 weeks-of-age. *CrCl 15-30 mL/min:* reduce dose by 1/2; *CrCl <15 mL/min:* not recommended. Contraindicated with G6PD deficiency. A high fluid intake is indicated during sulfonamide therapy to avoid crystallization in the kidneys.

AMINOMETHYLCYCLINE TETRACYCLINE

▷ *omadacycline Loading Dose, Day 1:* 200 mg via IV infusion over 60 minutes or 100 mg via IV infusion over 30 minutes twice; *Maintenance:* 100 mg via IV infusion over 30 minutes once daily or 300 mg orally once daily; total treatment duration 7-14 days; before oral dosing, fast x at least 4 hours and then take tablets with water; after oral dosing, no food or drink (except water) x 2 hours and no dairy products, antacids, or multivitamins x 4 hours
  Pediatric: <18 years: not recommended; ≥18 years: same as adult
    Nuzyra *Tab:* 150 mg; *Vial:* 100 mg single dose for reconstitution, dilution, and IV infusion
    Comment: **Nuzyra** *(omadacycline)* is an aminomethylcycline tetracycline antibiotic for the treatment of community-acquired bacterial pneumonia (CABP) and acute bacterial skin and skin structure infection (ABSSSI). The most common adverse reactions (incidence ≥2%) are nausea, vomiting, infusion site reactions, alanine aminotransferase (ALT) increased, aspartate aminotransferase (AST) increased, gamma-glutamyl transferase (GGT) increased, hypertension, headache, diarrhea, insomnia, and constipation. Like other tetracycline-class antibacterial drugs, **Nuzyra** may cause discoloration of deciduous teeth and reversible inhibition of bone growth when administered during the second and third trimester of pregnancy. The limited available data of **Nuzyra** use in pregnancy is insufficient to inform drug-associated risk of major birth defects and miscarriages. There is no information on the presence of *omadacycline* in human milk or effects on the breastfed infant.

 PNEUMONIA: LEGIONELLA

ANTI-INFECTIVES

▷ *ciprofloxacin* (C) 500 mg bid x 14-21 days
  Pediatric: <18 years: not recommended; ≥18 years: same as adult
    Cipro (G) *Tab:* 250, 500, 750 mg; *Oral susp:* 250, 500 mg/5 ml (100 ml) (strawberry)
    Cipro XR *Tab:* 500, 1000 mg ext-rel
    ProQuin XR *Tab:* 500 mg ext-rel

➤ *clarithromycin* (C)(G) 500 mg bid or 500 mg ext-rel once daily x 14-21 days
   Biaxin *Tab:* 250, 500 mg
   Biaxin Oral Suspension *Oral susp:* 125, 250 mg/5 ml (50, 100 ml) (fruit-punch)
   Biaxin XL *Tab:* 500 mg ext-rel

Comment: The FDA is advising caution before prescribing *clarithromycin* to patients with heart disease because of a potential increased risk of heart problems or death that can occur years later. This recommendation is based on a review of the results of a 10-year follow-up study of patients with coronary heart disease from a large clinical trial that first observed this safety issue. Consider risk benefit and the use of other antibiotics in such patients.

➤ *dirithromycin* (C)(G) 500 mg once daily x 14-21 days
   Dynabac *Tab:* 250 mg

➤ *erythromycin base* (B)(G) 500 mg qid x 14-21 days
   Pediatric: <45 kg: 30-50 mg in 2-4 divided doses x 14-21 days; ≥45 kg: same as adult
   Ery-Tab *Tab:* 250, 333, 500 mg ent-coat
   PCE *Tab:* 333, 500 mg

Comment: *erythromycin* may increase INR with concomitant *warfarin*, as well as increase serum level of *digoxin*, benzodiazepines, and statins.

➤ *erythromycin estolate* (B)(G) 1-2 gm daily in divided doses x 14-21 days
   Pediatric: 30-50 mg/kg/day in divided doses x 14-21 days; *see page 625 for dose by weight*
   Ilosone *Pulvule:* 250 mg; *Tab:* 500 mg; *Liq:* 125, 250 mg/5 ml (100 ml)

Comment: *erythromycin* may increase INR with concomitant *warfarin*, as well as increase serum level of *digoxin*, benzodiazepines, and statins.

➤ *trimethoprim+sulfamethoxazole (TMP-SMX)* (C)(G)
   Pediatric: <2 months: not recommended; ≥2 months: 40 mg/kg/day of *sulfamethoxazole* in 2 doses bid x 10 days
   Bactrim, Septra 2 tabs bid x 10 days
      Tab: trim 80 mg+sulfa 400 mg*
   Bactrim DS, Septra DS 1 tab bid x 10 days
      Tab: trim 160 mg+sulfa 800 mg*
   Bactrim Pediatric Suspension, Septra Pediatric Suspension
      Oral susp: trim 40 mg+sulfa 200 mg per 5 ml (100 ml) (cherry) (alcohol 0.3%)

Comment: Sulfonamides are contraindicated in the first trimester of pregnancy, the final month of pregnancy, and infants <8 weeks-of-age. *CrCl 15-30 mL/min:* reduce dose by 1/2; *CrCl <15 mL/min:* not recommended. Contraindicated with G6PD deficiency. A high fluid intake is indicated during sulfonamide therapy to avoid crystallization in the kidneys.

PNEUMONIA: MYCOPLASMA

ANTI-INFECTIVES

➤ *azithromycin* (B)(G) 500 mg x 1 dose on day 1, then 250 mg daily on days 2-5 or 500 mg daily x 3 days or **Zmax** 2 gm in a single dose
   Pediatric: 12 mg/kg/day x 5 days; max 500 mg/day; *see page 619 for dose by weight*
   Zithromax *Tab:* 250, 500, 600 mg; *Oral susp:* 100 mg/5 ml (15 ml); 200 mg/5 ml (15, 22.5, 30 ml) (cherry); *Pkt:* 1 gm for reconstitution (cherry-banana)
   Zithromax Tri-pak *Tab:* 3 x 500 mg tabs/pck
   Zithromax Z-pak *Tab:* 6 x 250 mg tabs/pck
   Zmax *Oral susp:* 2 gm ext-rel for reconstitution (cherry-banana) (148 mg Na⁺)

➤ *clarithromycin* (C)(G) 500 mg bid or 500 mg ext-rel once daily x 14-21 days
   Pediatric: <6 months: not recommended; ≥6 months: 7.5 mg/kg bid x 7 days; *see page 624 for dose by weight*
   Biaxin *Tab:* 250, 500 mg
   Biaxin Oral Suspension *Oral susp:* 125, 250 mg/5 ml (50, 100 ml) (fruit-punch)
   Biaxin XL *Tab:* 500 mg ext-rel

Comment: The FDA is advising caution before prescribing *clarithromycin* to patients with heart disease because of a potential increased risk of heart problems or death that can occur years later. This recommendation is based on a review of the results of a 10-year follow-up study of patients with coronary heart disease from a large clinical trial that first observed this safety issue. Consider risk benefit and the use of other antibiotics in such patients.

➤ *erythromycin base* (B)(G) 500 mg q 6 hours x 14-21 days
   Pediatric: <45 kg: 30-50 mg in 2-4 doses x 14-21 days; ≥45 kg: same as adult

Ery-Tab *Tab:* 250, 333, 500 mg ent-coat
PCE *Tab:* 333, 500 mg

Comment: *erythromycin* may increase INR with concomitant *warfarin*, as well as increase serum level of *digoxin,* benzodiazepines, and statins.

▶ *erythromycin ethylsuccinate* (B)(G) 400 mg qid x 14-21 days
Pediatric: 30-50 mg/kg/day in 4 divided doses x 14-21 days; may double dose with severe infection; max 100 mg/kg/day; *see page 626 for dose by weight*
EryPed *Oral susp:* 200 mg/5 ml (100, 200 ml) (fruit); 400 mg/5 ml (60, 100, 200 ml) (banana); *Oral drops:* 200, 400 mg/5 ml (50 ml) (fruit); *Chew tab:* 200 mg wafer (fruit)
E.E.S. *Oral susp:* 200, 400 mg/5 ml (100 ml) (fruit)
E.E.S. Granules *Oral susp:* 200 mg/5 ml (100, 200 ml) (cherry)
E.E.S. 400 Tablets *Tab:* 400 mg

Comment: *erythromycin* may increase INR with concomitant *warfarin*, as well as increase serum level of *digoxin,* benzodiazepines, and statins.

▶ *tetracycline* (D)(G) 500 mg qid
Pediatric: <8 years: not recommended; ≥8 years, <100 lb: 25-50 mg/kg/day in 2-4 divided doses; ≥8 years, ≥100 lb: same as adult; *see page 630 for dose by weight*
Achromycin V *Cap:* 250, 500 mg
Sumycin *Tab:* 250, 500 mg; *Cap:* 250, 500 mg; *Oral susp:* 125 mg/5 ml (100, 200 ml) (fruit) (sulfites)

Comment: *tetracycline* is contraindicated <8 years-of-age, in pregnancy, and lactation (discolors developing tooth enamel). A side effect may be photo-sensitivity (photophobia). Do not take with antacids, calcium supplements, milk or other dairy, or within two hours of taking another drug.

PNEUMONIA: PNEUMOCOCCAL

TREATMENT
see CAP/CABP *page* 391

PROPHYLAXIS
▶ *pneumococcal* vaccine (C) 0.5 ml IM or SC in deltoid x 1 dose
Pneumovax
Pediatric: <2 years: not recommended; ≥2 years: same as adult
Vial: 25 mcg/0.5 ml (single-dose, 10/pck; multi-dose, 2.5 ml, 10/pck)
Pnu-Imune 23
Pediatric: <2 years: not recommended; ≥2 years: same as adult
Vial: 25 mcg/0.5 ml (0.5 ml single-dose, 5/pck; 2.5 ml)
Prevnar 13 for adults ≥50 years of age
Pediatric: total 4 doses: 2, 4, 6, and 12-15 months-of-age; may start at 6 weeks of age; administer first 3 doses 4-8 weeks apart and the 4th dose at least 2 months after the 3rd dose
Vial: 25 mcg/0.5 ml (single-dose, 10/pck); *Prefilled syringe:* (single-dose, 10/pck; 2.5 ml, multi-dose)

Comment: Pneumococcal vaccine contains 23 polysaccharide isolates representing approximately 85-90% of common U.S. isolates. Administer the pneumococcal vaccine in the anterolateral aspect of the thigh for infants and the deltoid for toddlers, children, and adults.

PNEUMONIA (*PNEUMOCYSTIS JIROVECI*)

QUINONE ANTIMICROBIAL
▶ *atovaquone* (C)(G) take as a single dose with food or a milky drink at the same time each day; repeat dose if vomited within 1 hour; *Prophylaxis:* 1,500 mg once daily; *Treatment:* 750 mg bid x 21 days
Pediatric: <12 years: not recommended; ≥12 years: same as adult
Mepron *Susp:* 750 mg/5 ml (210 ml; 5 ml pouches) (citrus)

Comment: **Mepron** *(atovaquone)* suspension is a quinone antimicrobial drug indicated for the prevention of *Pneumocystis jiroveci* pneumonia (PCP), and treatment of mild-to-moderate PCP, in adults and adolescents ≥13 years-of-age who cannot tolerate *trimethoprim+sulfamethoxazole* (TMP-SMX). Treatment of severe PCP (alveolar arterial oxygen diffusion gradient [(A-a)DO$_2$] >45 mm Hg) with **Mepron**, and the efficacy of **Mepron** in subjects who are failing therapy with TMPSMX, have not been studied. Elevated liver chemistry tests and cases of hepatitis and fatal liver failure have been reported. Failure to administer **Mepron** suspension with food may result in lower plasma *atovaquone* concentrations and may limit response to therapy. Patients with gastrointestinal disorders may have limited absorption resulting in suboptimal *atovaquone* concentrations. Concomitant administration of the following drugs reduce *atovaquone* concentrations: *rifampin* and *rifabutin*, *tetracyclines*, *metoclopramide*. Concomitant administration of *indinavir* reduces *indinavir* trough concentrations. The most frequent adverse reactions (≥25% that required discontinuation) attributed to **Mepron** taken for prophylaxis have been diarrhea, rash, headache, nausea, and fever. The most frequent adverse reactions (≥14% that required discontinuation) attributed to **Mepron** taken for prophylaxis have been rash (including maculopapular), nausea, diarrhea, headache, vomiting, and fever. There are no adequate and well-controlled studies of **Mepron** use in pregnancy. *atovaquone* was not teratogenic and did not cause reproductive toxicity in animal studies at plasma concentrations up to 2 to 3 times the estimated human exposure (dose of 1,000 mg/kg/day). However, **Mepron** should be used during pregnancy only if the potential benefit justifies the potential risk to the fetus. It is not known whether *atovaquone* is excreted into human milk or effects on the breastfed infant. In an animal study (with doses of 10 and 250 mg/kg), *atovaquone* concentrations in milk were 30% of the concurrent *atovaquone* concentrations in maternal plasma at both doses; therefore, caution should be exercised when **Mepron** is administered to patients who are breastfeeding. To report suspected adverse reactions, contact GlaxoSmithKline at 1-888-825-5249 or FDA at 1-800-FDA-1088 or visit www.fda.gov/medwatch

▷ *trimethoprim+sulfamethoxazole (TMP-SMX)* (C)(G) Prophylaxis: 1 tab 3 x/week; Treatment: 1 tab daily x 3 weeks; *Septra* can be given if intolerable to *Bactrim*
Pediatric: <2 months: not recommended; ≥2 months: 40 mg/kg/day of *sulfamethoxazole* in 2 doses bid x 10 days

    Bactrim, Septra 2 tabs bid x 10 days
      Tab: trim 80 mg+sulfa 400 mg*
    Bactrim DS, Septra DS 1 tab bid x 10 days
      Tab: trim 160 mg+sulfa 800 mg*
    Bactrim Pediatric Suspension, Septra Pediatric Suspension
      Oral susp: trim 40 mg+sulfa 200 mg per 5 ml (100 ml) (cherry) (alcohol 0.3%)

Comment: Sulfonamides are contraindicated in the first trimester of pregnancy, the final month of pregnancy, and infants <8 weeks-of-age. *CrCl 15-30 mL/min:* reduce dose by 1/2; *CrCl <15 mL/min:* not recommended. Contraindicated with G6PD deficiency. A high fluid intake is indicated during sulfonamide therapy to avoid crystallization in the kidneys.

POLIOMYELITIS

PROPHYLAXIS

▷ *trivalent poliovirus vaccine, inactivated (type 1, 2, and 3)* (C)
Pediatric: <6 weeks: not recommended; ≥6 weeks: one dose at 2, 4, 6-18 months and 4-6 years of age
    Ipol 0.5 ml SC or IM in deltoid area

POLYCYSTIC KIDNEY DISEASE, AUTOSOMAL DOMINANT (ADPKD)

SELECTIVE VASOPRESSIN V2 RECEPTOR ANTAGONIST

▷ *tolvaptan* usual starting dose is 15 mg once daily with or without food; may titrate the dose once daily after at least 24 hours to 30 mg; then may titrate once daily dose to 60 mg as needed to achieve the desired level of serum sodium; do not administer for more than 30 days to minimize the risk of liver injury; initiation and re-initiation of therapy to should occur in a hospital environment to evaluate the therapeutic response and because too rapid correction of hyponatremia can cause osmotic demyelination resulting in dysarthria, mutism, dysphagia, lethargy, affective changes, spastic quadriparesis, seizures, coma and death; avoid fluid restriction during the first 24 hours of therapy. Patients receiving *tolvaptan* should be advised that they can continue ingestion of fluid in response to thirst; following discontinuation from *tolvaptan*, patients should be advised to resume fluid restriction and should be monitored for changes in serum sodium and volume status

Pediatric: <18 years: not established; ≥18 years: same as adult

    Jynarque *Tab:* 15, 30, 45, 60, 90 mg (7, 28/pck)

    Samsca *Tab:* 15, 30 mg

Comment: *tolvaptan* is indicated to slow kidney function decline patients at risk of rapidly progressing autosomal dominant polycystic kidney disease (ADPKD). Further, *tolvaptan* is indicated for the treatment of clinically significant hypervolemic and euvolemic hyponatremia [serum sodium <125 mEq/L or less marked hyponatremia that is symptomatic and has resisted correction with fluid restriction], including patients with heart failure and Syndrome of Inappropriate Antidiuretic Hormone (SIAD). Contraindications to *tolvaptan* include use in in patients with autosomal dominant polycystic kidney disease (ADPKD) outside of FDA approved REMS, patients requiring intervention to raise serum sodium urgently to prevent or to treat serious neurological symptoms , patients unable to respond appropriately to thirst, hypovolemic hyponatremia, concomitant use of strong CYP 3A inhibitors, anuria, and hypersensitivity to the drug. Avoid use in patients with underlying liver disease; if hepatic injury is suspected, discontinue. Avoid use with CYP 3A inducers and moderate CYP 3A inhibitors. Dehydration and hypovolemia may require intervention. Avoid use with hypertonic saline. Consider dose reduction if co-administered with P-gp inhibitors. Monitor serum K$^+$ in patients with potassium >5 mEq/L or on drugs known to increase potassium. Based on animal data, *tolvaptan* may cause fetal harm. Discontinue *tolvaptan* or breastfeeding taking into consideration importance of the drug to mother.

POLYCYSTIC OVARIAN SYNDROME (PCOS, STEIN-LEVENTHAL DISEASE)

See **Contraceptives** *page 559*
See **Type 2 Diabetes Mellitus** *page 501*

POLYMYALGIA RHEUMATICA

Oral Corticosteroids *see page 577*
Calcium and Vitamin D Supplementation see **Hypocalcemia** *page 256*

Comment: Initial treatment is low-dose prednisone at 12-25 mg/day. May attempt a very slow tapering regimen after 2-4 weeks. If relapse occurs, increase the daily dose of corticosteroid to the previous effective dose. Most people with polymyalgia rheumatica need to continue corticosteroid treatment for at least a year. Approximately 30-60% of people will have at least one relapse during corticosteroid tapering. Joint guidelines from the American Academy of Rheumatology (AAR) and the European League Against Rheumatism (ELAR) suggest using concomitant *methotrexate* (MTX) along with corticosteroids in some patients. It may be useful early in the course of treatment or later, if the patient relapses or does not respond to corticosteroids. The American Academy of Rheumatology (AAR) recommends the following daily doses for anyone on a chronic oral corticosteroid regimen: Calcium 1,200-1,500 mg/day and vitamin D 800-1,000 IU/day.

▶ *methotrexate* (X) 7.5 mg x 1 dose per week or 2.5 mg x 3 at 12 hour intervals once a week; max 20 mg/week; therapeutic response begins in 3-6 weeks; administer methotrexate injection SC only into the abdomen or thigh

    Pediatric: <2 years: not recommended; ≥2 years: 10 mg/m^2 once weekly; max 20 mg/m^2

    Rasuvo *Autoinjector:* 7.5 mg/0.15 ml, 10 mg/0.20 ml, 12.5 mg/0.25 ml, 15 mg/0.30 ml, 17.5 mg/0.35 ml, 20 mg/0.40 ml, 22.5 mg/0.45 ml, 25 mg/0.50 ml, 27.5 mg/0.55 ml, 30 mg/0.60 ml (solution concentration for SC injection is 50 mg/ml)

Rheumatrex *Tab:* 2.5*mg (5, 7.5, 10, 12.5, 15 mg/week, 4/card unit dose pack)
TrexallR *Tab:* 5*, 7.5*, 10*, 15*mg (5, 7.5, 10, 12.5, 15 mg/week, 4/card unit dose pack)
Comment: *methotrexate* (MTX) is contraindicated with immunodeficiency, blood dyscrasias, alcoholism, and chronic liver disease.

POLYNEUROPATHY, CHRONIC INFLAMMATORY DEMYELINATING (CIDP)

IMMUNE GLOBULIN, HUMAN

➤ *immune globulin subcutaneous [human] 20% liquid* <18 years: not recommended; ≥18 years: administer once weekly via SC infusion only; *Infusion sites:* abdomen, thigh, upper arm, *and/or* lateral hip; may use up to 8 injection sites simultaneously, with at least 2 inches between sites; *Infusion volume:* for the first infusion, up to 15 ml per injection site; may increase to 20 ml per site after the fourth infusion; max 25 ml per site as tolerated; *Infusion rate:* first infusion, up to 15 ml/hr per site; may increase, to max 25 ml/hr per site as tolerated; however, maximum flow rate is not to exceed a total of 50 ml/hr for all sites combined; before switching to **Hizentra**, obtain the patient's serum IgG trough level to guide subsequent dose adjustments; adjust the dose: based on clinical response and serum IgG trough levels; initiate therapy 1 week after the last IGIV infusion; recommended subcutaneous dose is 0.2 g/kg (1 ml/kg) per week; in the clinical study after transitioning from IGIV to **Hizentra**, a dose of 0.4 g/kg (2 ml/kg) per week was also safe and effective to prevent CIDP relapse; If CIDP symptoms worsen, consider re-initiating treatment with an IGIV approved for the treatment of CIDP, while discontinuing **Hizentra**; if improvement and stabilization are observed during IGIV treatment, consider reinitiating **Hizentra** at 0.4 g/kg per week, while discontinuing IGIV; if CIDP symptoms worsen on 0.4 g/kg per week, consider reinitiating **Hizentra** therapy with IGIV, while discontinuing **Hizentra**; monitor patient's clinical response and adjust duration of therapy based on patient need

Hizentra *Vial:* 0.2 mg/ml (20%; 5, 10, 20, 50 ml)

Comment: IgA-deficient patients with anti-IgA antibodies are at greater risk of severe hypersensitivity and anaphylactic reactions. Thrombosis may occur following treatment with immune globulin products, including **Hizentra**. Aseptic meningitis syndrome has been reported with IGIV and IGSC, including **Hizentra**. Monitor renal function in patients at risk of acute renal failure (ARF). Monitor for clinical signs and symptoms of hemolysis. Monitor for pulmonary adverse reactions (transfusion-related acute lung injury [TRALI]). **Hizentra** is made from human blood and may contain infectious agents (e.g., viruses, the variant Creutzfeldt-Jakob disease (vCJD) agent and, theoretically, the Creutzfeldt-Jakob disease (CJD) agent). Monitor for clinical signs and symptoms of hemolysis. The most common adverse reactions observed in ≥5% of study subjects were local infusion site reactions, headache, diarrhea, fatigue, back pain, nausea, pain in extremity, cough, upper respiratory tract infection, rash, pruritus, vomiting, abdominal pain (upper), migraine, arthralgia, pain, fall and nasopharyngitis. No human or animal reproduction studies have not been conducted with **Hizentra**. It is not known whether **Hizentra** can cause fetal harm when administered during pregnancy. No human data are available to inform maternal use of **Hizentra** on the breastfed infant. Safety and effectiveness of weekly **Hizentra** administration have not been established in children <2 years of age. To report suspected adverse reactions, contact CSL Behring Pharmacovigilance at 1-866-915-6958 or FDA at 1-800-FDA-1088 or www.fda.gov/medwatch.

POLYPS: NASAL

LONG-ACTING CORTICOSTEROID SINUS IMPLANT

➤ *mometasone furoate* the Sinuva Sinus Implant must be inserted by a physician trained in otolaryngology; the implant is loaded into a sterile delivery system supplied with the implant and placed in the ethmoid sinus under endoscopic visualization; the implant is left in the sinus to gradually release the corticosteroid over 90 days; the implant is removed at Day 90 or earlier at the physician's discretion using standard surgical instruments; repeat administration has not been studied.
Pediatric: <18 years: not established: ≥18 years: same as adult
Sinuva Sinus Implant *Sinus implant:* 1350 mcg w. sterile delivery system

Comment: **Sinuva** is a corticosteroid-eluting sinus implant indicated for the treatment of recurrent nasal polyp disease in patients who have ethmoid sinus surgery. Monitor nasal mucosa adjacent to the **Sinuva Sinus Implant** for any signs of bleeding (epistaxis), irritation, infection, or perforation. Avoid use in patients with nasal ulcers or trauma. Monitor patients with a change in vision or with a history of increased intraocular pressure, glaucoma, and/or cataracts closely. Potential worsening of existing tuberculosis; fungal, bacterial, viral, parasitic infection, or ocular herpes simplex. More serious or even fatal course of chickenpox or measles in susceptible patients. If corticosteroid effects such as hypercorticism and adrenal suppression appear in patients, consider sinus implant removal. To report suspected adverse reactions, contact Intersect ENT at 1-866 531-6004 or FDA at 1-800-FDA-1088 or www.fda.gov/medwatch.

NASAL SPRAY CORTICOSTEROIDS

▶ *beclomethasone dipropionate* (C)

Beconase 1 spray in each nostril bid-qid
Pediatric: <6 years: not recommended; 6-12 years: 1 spray in each nostril tid; >12 years: same as adult
   Nasal spray: 42 mcg/actuation (6.7 gm, 80 sprays; 16.8 gm, 200 sprays)

Beconase AQ 1-2 sprays in each nostril bid
Pediatric: <6: not recommended; ≥6 years: same as adult
   Nasal spray: 42 mcg/actuation (25 gm, 180 sprays)

Beconase Inhalation Aerosol 1-2 sprays in each nostril bid to qid
Pediatric: <6: not recommended; 6-12 years: 1 spray in each nostril tid; >12 years: same as adult
   Nasal spray: 42 mcg/actuation (6.7 gm, 80 sprays; 16.8 gm, 200 sprays)

Vancenase AQ 1-2 sprays in each nostril bid
Pediatric: <6 years: not recommended; ≥6 years: same as adult
   Nasal spray: 84 mcg/actuation (25 gm, 200 sprays)

Vancenase AQ DS 1-2 sprays in each nostril once daily
Pediatric: <6 years: not recommended; ≥6 years: same as adult
   Nasal spray: 84, 168 mcg/actuation (19 gm, 120 sprays)

Vancenase Pockethaler 1 spray in each nostril bid or qid
Pediatric: <6: not recommended; ≥6 years: 1 spray in each nostril tid
   Pockethaler: 42 mcg/actuation (7 gm, 200 sprays)

QNASL Nasal Aerosol 2 sprays, 80 mcg/spray, in each nostril once daily
Pediatric: <12 years: 2 sprays, 40 mcg/spray, in each nostril once daily; ≥12 years: same as adult
   Nasal spray: 40 mcg/actuation (4.9 gm, 60 sprays); 80 mcg/actuation (8.7 gm, 120 sprays)

▶ *budesonide* (C)

Rhinocort initially 2 sprays in each nostril bid in the AM and PM, or 4 sprays in each nostril in the AM; max 4 sprays each nostril/day; use lowest effective dose
Pediatric: <6 years: not recommended; ≥6 years: same as adult
   Nasal spray: 32 mcg/actuation (7 gm, 200 sprays)

Rhinocort Aqua Nasal Spray initially 1 spray in each nostril once daily; max 4 sprays in each nostril once daily
Pediatric: <6 years: not recommended; ≥6-12 years: initially 1 spray in each nostril once daily; max 2 sprays in each nostril once daily
   Nasal spray: 32 mcg/actuation (10 ml, 60 sprays)

▶ *ciclesonide* (C)
Pediatric: <6 years: not recommended; ≥6 years: same as adult

Omnaris 2 sprays in each nostril once daily
   Nasal spray: 50 mcg/actuation (12.5 gm, 120 sprays)

Zetonna 1-2 sprays in each nostril once daily
   Nasal spray: 37 mcg/actuation (6.1 gm, 60 sprays) (HFA)

▶ *dexamethasone* (C) 2 sprays in each nostril bid-tid; max 12 sprays/day; maintain at lowest effective dose
Pediatric: <6 years: not recommended; ≥6-12 years: 1-2 sprays in each nostril bid; max 8 sprays/day; maintain at lowest effective dose; >12 years: same as adult
   Dexacort Turbinaire *Nasal spray:* 84 mcg/actuation (12.6 gm, 170 sprays)

▶ *flunisolide* (C) 2 sprays in each nostril bid; may increase to 2 sprays in each nostril tid; max 8 sprays/nostril/day

Pediatric: <6 years: not recommended; 6-14 years: initially 1 spray in each nostril tid or 2 sprays in each nostril bid; max 4 sprays/nostril/day; >14 years: same as adult

    Nasalide *Nasal spray:* 25 mcg/actuation (25 ml, 200 sprays)
    Nasarel *Nasal spray:* 25 mcg/actuation (25 ml, 200 sprays)

▶ *fluticasone furoate* (C) 2 sprays in each nostril once daily; may reduce to 1 spray each nostril once daily

Pediatric: <2 years: not recommended; ≥2-11 years: 1 spray in each nostril once daily; ≥12 years: same as adult

    Veramyst *Nasal spray:* 27.5 mcg/actuation (10 gm, 120 sprays) (alcohol-free)

▶ *fluticasone propionate* (C)

    Flonase (OTC)(G) initially 2 sprays in each nostril once daily or 1 spray bid; maintenance 1 spray once daily

Pediatric: <4 years: not recommended; ≥4 years: initially 1 spray in each nostril once daily; may increase to 2 sprays in each nostril once daily; maintenance 1 spray in each nostril once daily; max 2 sprays in each nostril/day

    Nasal spray: 50 mcg/actuation (16 gm, 120 sprays)

    Xhance 1 spray per nostril bid (total daily dose 372 mcg); 2 sprays per nostril bid may also be effective in some patients (total daily dose 744 mcg)

Pediatric: <12 years: not established; ≥12 years: same as adult

    Nasal spray: 93 mcg/actuation (16 ml, 120 metered sprays)

Comment: Available data from published literature on the use of inhaled or intranasal *fluticasone propionate* in pregnant women have not reported a clear association with adverse developmental outcomes. There are no available data on the presence of *fluticasone propionate* in human milk or effects on the breastfed child. The safety and efficacy of **Xhance** in pediatric patients have not been established.

▶ *mometasone furoate* (C)(G) 2 sprays in each nostril once daily

Pediatric: <2 years: not recommended; 2-11 years: 1 spray in each nostril once daily; max 2 sprays in each nostril once daily; >11 years: same as adult

    Nasonex *Nasal spray:* 50 mcg/actuation (17 gm, 120 sprays)

▶ *olopatadine* (C) 2 sprays in each nostril bid

Pediatric: <6 years: not recommended; 6-11 years: 1 spray each nostril bid; >11 years: same as adult

    Patanase *Nasal spray:* 0.6%; 665 mcg/actuation (30.5 gm, 240 sprays) (benzalkonium chloride)

▶ *triamcinolone acetonide* (C)(G) initially 2 sprays in each nostril once daily; max 4 sprays in each nostril once daily or 2 sprays in each nostril bid or 1 spray in each nostril qid; maintain at lowest effective dose

Pediatric: <6 years: not recommended; ≥6 years: 1 spray in each nostril once daily; max 2 sprays in each nostril once daily

    Nasacort Allergy 24HR (OTC) *Nasal spray:* 55 mcg/actuation (10 gm, 120 sprays)
    Tri-Nasal *Nasal spray:* 50 mcg/actuation (15 ml, 120 sprays)

POLYURIA: NOCTURNAL

VASOPRESSIN ANALOG

▶ **desmopressin acetate** administer a single sublingual dose 1 hour prior to bedtime *Females:* 27.7 mcg; *Males:* 55.3 mcg

    Nocdurna *SL tab:* 27.7, 55.3 mcg

    Comment: **Nocdurna** (*desmopressin acetate*) a vasopressin analog and the first sublingual tab indicated for the treatment of nocturia due to nocturnal polyuria in adults. **Nocdurna** is indicated for patients ≥18 years-of-age with nocturnal polyuria who awaken at least 2 x/night to void. **Nocdurna** is available in two strengths: 27.7 mcg of *desmopressin acetate* (equivalent to 25 mcg of *desmopressin*) and 55.3 mcg of *desmopressin acetate* and dose is gender-based. **Nocdurna** is contraindicated with the following conditions: hyponatremia or a history of hyponatremia, polydipsia, concomitant use with loop diuretics or systemic or inhaled glucocorticoids, EGFR <50 mL/min/1.73 m², syndrome of inappropriate antidiuretic hormone secretion (SIADH), during illnesses that can cause fluid or electrolyte imbalance, heart failure (HF), uncontrolled hypertension. **Nocdurna** can cause hyponatremia, which may be life-threatening if severe. Ensure serum sodium concentration is normal before starting or resuming **Nocdurna**. Measure serum sodium within one week and approximately 1 month after initiating therapy and periodically during treatment. Monitor serum sodium more frequently in patients ≥65 years-of-age and in patients at increased risk of hyponatremia. Monitor serum sodium more frequently when **Nocdurna** is concomitantly used with drugs that may increase the risk of hyponatremia (e.g., tricyclic antidepressants (TCAs), selective serotonin re-uptake inhibitors (SSRIs), *chlorpromazine*, opiate analgesics, thiazide diuretics, NSAIDs, *lamotrigine*, *chlorpropamide* and, *carbamazepine*). **Nocdurna** is not recommended in patients at risk of increased intracranial pressure or history of urinary retention. Limit fluid intake to a minimum from 1 hour before until 8 hours after administration; treatment without concomitant reduction of fluid intake may lead to fluid retention and hyponatremia. If hyponatremia occurs, **Nocdurna** may need to be temporarily or permanently discontinued. Use of **Nocdurna** is not recommended and **Nocdurna** is not recommended for the treatment of nocturia in pregnancy (nocturia is usually related to normal, physiologic changes during pregnancy that do not require treatment). There are no data with **Nocdurna** use in pregnancy to inform any drug-associated risks. *desmopressin* is present in small amounts in human milk; however, there is no information on the effects of desmopressin on the breastfed infant. To report suspected adverse reactions, contact Ferring at 1-888-337-7464 or FDA at 1-800-FDA-1088 or visit www.fda.gov/medwatch.

POST-HERPETIC NEURALGIA (PHN)

Acetaminophen for IV Infusion *see Pain page 352*
Oral Analgesics *see Pain page 352*

GAMMA AMINOBUTYRIC ACID ANALOG

 gabapentin (C) CrCl 30-60 mL/min: 600-1800 mg; CrCl <30 mL/min or on hemodialysis: not recommended; avoid abrupt cessation of *gabapentin* and *gabapentin enacarbil*; to discontinue, withdraw gradually over 1 week or longer.
> **Gralise** initially 300 mg on Day 1; then 600 mg on Day 2; then 900 mg on Days 3-6; then 1200 mg on Days 7-10; then 1500 mg on Days 11-14; titrate up to 1800 mg on Day 15; take entire dose once daily with the evening meal; do not crush, split, or chew
> *Pediatric:* <18 years: not recommended; ≥18 years: same as adult
> *Tab:* 300, 600 mg
> **Neurontin** (G) 300 mg daily x 1 day, then 300 mg bid x 1 day, then 300 mg tid continuously; max 1,800 mg/day in 3 divided doses; taper over 7 days
> *Pediatric:* <3 years: not recommended; 3-12 years: initially 10-15 mg/kg/day in 3 divided doses; max 12 hours between doses; titrate over 3 days; 3-4 years: titrate to 40 mg/kg/day; 5-12 years: titrate to 25-35 mg/kg/day; max 50 mg/kg/day
>> *Tab:* 600*, 800*mg; *Cap:* 100, 300, 400 mg; *Oral soln:* 250 mg/5 ml (480 ml) (strawberry-anise)

▷ *gabapentin enacarbil* (C) 600 mg once daily at about 5:00 PM; if dose not taken at recommended time, next dose should be taken the following day; swallow whole; take with food; CrCl 30-59 mL/min: 600 mg on Day 1, Day 3, and every day thereafter; avoid abrupt cessation of *gabapentin enacarbil;* to discontinue, withdraw gradually over 1 week or longer; CrCl <30 mL/min: or on hemodialysis: not recommended
Pediatric: <18 years: not recommended; ≥18 years: same as adult
> **Horizant** *Tab:* 600 ext-rel

Tricyclic Antidepressants (TCAs)

Comment: Co-administration of SSRIs and TCAs requires extreme caution.

▷ *amitriptyline* (C)(G) initially 75 mg/day in divided doses of 50-100 mg/day q HS; max 300 mg/day
Pediatric: <12 years: not recommended; ≥12 years: same as adult
> *Tab:* 10, 25, 50, 75, 100, 150 mg
▷ *amoxapine* (C) initially 50 mg bid-tid; after 1 week may increase to 100 mg bid-tid; usual effective dose 200-300 mg/day; if total dose exceeds 300 mg/day, give in divided doses (max 400 mg/day); may give as a single bedtime dose (max 300 mg q HS)
Pediatric: <12 years: not recommended; ≥12 years: same as adult
> *Tab:* 25, 50, 100, 150 mg

▷ *desipramine* (C)(G) 100-200 mg/day in single or divided doses; max 300 mg/day
　　Pediatric: <12 years: not recommended; ≥12 years: same as adult
　　　　Norpramin *Tab:* 10, 25, 50, 75, 100, 150 mg
▷ *doxepin* (C)(G) 75 mg/day; max 150 mg/day
　　Pediatric: <12 years: not recommended; ≥12 years: same as adult
　　　　Cap: 10, 25, 50, 75, 100, 150 mg; Oral conc: 10 mg/ml (4 oz w. dropper)
▷ *imipramine* (C)(G)
　　Pediatric: <12 years: not recommended; ≥12 years: same as adult
　　　　Tofranil initially 75 mg daily (max 200 mg); adolescents initially 30-40 mg daily (max 100 mg/day); if maintenance dose exceeds 75 mg daily, may switch to **Tofranil PM** for divided or bedtime dose
　　　　　　Tab: 10, 25, 50 mg
　　　　Tofranil PM initially 75 mg daily 1 hour before HS; max 200 mg
　　　　　　Cap: 75, 100, 125, 150 mg
　　　　Tofranil Injection 50 mg IM; lower dose for adolescents; switch to oral form as soon as possible
　　　　　　Amp: 25 mg/2 ml (2 ml)
▷ *nortriptyline* (D)(G) initially 25 mg tid-qid; max 150 mg/day
　　Pediatric: <12 years: not recommended; ≥12 years: same as adult
　　　　Pamelor *Cap:* 10, 25, 50, 75 mg; *Oral soln:* 10 mg/5 ml (16 oz)
▷ *protriptyline* (C) initially 5 mg tid; usual dose 15-40 mg/day in 3-4 divided doses; max 60 mg/day
　　Pediatric: <12 years: not recommended; ≥12 years: same as adult
　　　　Vivactil *Tab:* 5, 10 mg
▷ *trimipramine* (C) initially 75 mg/day in divided doses; max 200 mg/day
　　Pediatric: <12 years: not recommended; ≥12 years: same as adult
　　　　Surmontil *Cap:* 25, 50, 100 mg

ALPHA-2 DELTA LIGAND

▷ *pregabalin (GABA analog)* (C)(V) initially 150 mg daily divided bid-tid and may titrate within one week; max 600 mg divided bid-tid; discontinue over one week
　　Pediatric: <18 years: not recommended; ≥18 years: same as adult
　　　　Lyrica *Cap:* 25, 50, 75, 100, 150, 200, 225, 300 mg; *Oral soln:* 20 mg/ml

TOPICAL AND TRANSDERMAL ANALGESICS

▷ *capsaicin* 8% patch (B) apply up to 4 patches for one 60-minute application to clean dry skin; may prep area with topical anesthetic; wear non-latex gloves; patches may be cut to size/shape; treatment may be repeated every 3 months
　　Pediatric: <18 years: not recommended; ≥18 years: same as adult
　　　　Qutenza *Patch:* 8% 1640 mcg/cm (179 mg) (1 or 2 patches w. 1-50 gm tube cleansing gel/carton)
▷ *diclofenac sodium* (C; D ≥30 wks)(G) apply qid prn to intact skin
　　Pediatric: <12 years: not established; ≥12 years: same as adult
　　　　Pennsaid 1.5% in 10 drop increments, dispense and rub into front, side, and back of knee: usually; 40 drops (40 mg) qid
　　　　　　Topical soln: 1.5% (150 ml)
　　　　Pennsaid 2% apply 2 pump actuations (40 mg) and rub into front, side, and back of knee bid
　　　　　　Topical soln: 2% (20 mg/pump actuation, 112 gm)
　　　　Solaraze Gel massage in to clean skin bid prn
　　　　　　Gel: 3% (50 gm) (benzyl alcohol)
　　　　Voltaren Gel (G) apply qid prn to intact skin
　　　　　　Gel: 1% (100 gm)
　　Comment: *diclofenac* is ontraindicated with *aspirin* allergy. As with other NSAIDs, should be avoided in late pregnancy (≥30 weeks) because it may cause premature closure of the ductus arteriosus.
▷ *doxepin* (B) cream apply to affected area qid at intervals of at least 3-4 hours; max 8 days
　　Pediatric: <12 years: not recommended; >12 years: same as adult
　　　　Prudoxin *Crm:* 5% (45 gm)
　　　　Zonalon *Crm:* 5% (30, 45 gm)

404 ■ Post-Herpetic Neuralgia (PHN)

▶ *pimecrolimus* 1% cream (C)(G) <2 years: not recommended; ≥2 years: apply to affected area bid; do not apply an occlusive dressing
    Elidel *Crm:* 1% (30, 60, 100 gm)
Comment: *pimecrolimus* is indicated for short-term and intermittent long-term use. Discontinue use when resolution occurs. Contraindicated if the patient is immunosuppressed. Change to the 0.1% preparation or if secondary bacterial infection is present.
▶ *trolamine salicylate* apply tid-qid
Pediatric: <2 years: not recommended; ≥2 years: same as adult
    Mobisyl Creme *Crm:* 10% (100 gm)

TOPICAL & TRANSDERMAL ANESTHETICS

Comment: *lidocaine* should not be applied to non-intact skin.
▶ *lidocaine* cream (B) apply to affected area bid prn
Pediatric: <12 years: not recommended; ≥12 years: same as adult
    LidaMantle *Crm:* 3% (1, 2 oz)
    Lidoderm *Crm:* 3% (85 gm)
    ZTlido *lidocaine* topical system 1% (30/carton)
    Comment: Compared to **Lidoderm** (*lidocaine* patch 5%) which contains 700 mg/patch, ZTlido only requires 35 mg per topical system to achieve the same therapeutic dose.
▶ *lidocaine* lotion (B) apply to affected area bid prn
Pediatric: <12 years: not recommended; ≥12 years: same as adult
    LidaMantle *Lotn:* 3% (177 ml)
▶ *lidocaine* 5% patch (B)(G) apply up to 3 patches at one time for up to 12 hours/24-hour period (12 hours on/12 hours off); patches may be cut into smaller sizes before removal of the release liner; do not re-use
Pediatric: <12 years: not recommended; ≥12 years: same as adult
    Lidoderm *Patch:* 5% (10x14 cm; 30/carton)
lidocaine+dexamethasone (B)
Pediatric: <12 years: not recommended; ≥12 years: same as adult
    Decadron Phosphate with Xylocaine *Lotn:* dexa 4 mg+lido 10 mg per ml (5 ml)
▶ *lidocaine+hydrocortisone* (B)(G) apply to affected area bid prn
Pediatric: <12 years: not recommended; ≥12 years: same as adult
    LidaMantle HC *Crm:* lido 3%+hydro 0.5% (1, 3 oz); *Lotn:* (177 ml)
▶ *lidocaine* 2.5%+*prilocaine* 2.5% apply sparingly to the burn bid-tid prn
Pediatric: <12 years: not recommended; ≥12 years: same as adult
    Emla Cream (B) 5, 30 gm/tube

ORAL ANALGESICS

▶ *acetaminophen* (B)(G) *see Fever page 163*
▶ *aspirin* (D)(G) *see Fever page 164*
Comment: *aspirin*-containing medications are contraindicated with history of allergic-type reaction to *aspirin*, children and adolescents with *Varicella* or other viral illness, and 3rd trimester of pregnancy.
▶ *tramadol* (C)(IV)(G)
Comment: *tramadol* is known to be excreted in breast milk. The FDA and the European Medicines Agency (EMA) are investigating the safety of using *tramadol*-containing medications to treat pain in children 12-18 years because of the potential for serious side effects, including slowed or difficult breathing.
    Rybix ODT initially 100 mg once daily; may increase by 100 mg every 5 days; max 300 mg/day; *CrCl <30 mL/min or severe hepatic impairment:* not recommended; *Cirrhosis:* max 50 mg q 12 hours
Pediatric: <18 years: not recommended; ≥18 years: same as adult
    ODT: 50 mg (mint) (phenylalanine)
    Ryzolt initially 100 mg once daily; may increase by 100 mg every 5 days; max 300 mg/day; *CrCl <30 mL/min or severe hepatic impairment:* not recommended
Pediatric: <18 years: not recommended; ≥18 years: same as adult
    Tab: 100, 200, 300 mg ext-rel
    Ultram 50-100 mg q 4-6 hours prn; max 400 mg/day; *CrCl <30 mL/min:* max 100 mg q 12 hours; *Cirrhosis:* max 50 mg q 12 hours
Pediatric: <18 years: not recommended; ≥18 years: same as adult
    Tab: 50*mg

Ultram ER initially 100 mg once daily; may increase by 100 mg every 5 days; max 300 mg/day; *CrCl <30 mL/min: or severe hepatic impairment:* not recommended
Pediatric: <18 years: not recommended; ≥18 years: same as adult
Tab: 100, 200, 300 mg ext-rel

➤ *tramadol+acetaminophen* (C)(IV)(G) 2 tabs q 4-6 hours; max 8 tabs/day; 5 days; *CrCl <30 mL/min:* max 2 tabs q 12 hours; max 4 tabs/day x 5 days
Pediatric: <18 years: not recommended; ≥18 years: same as adult
Ultracet *Tab:* tram 37.5+acet 325 mg

Comment: *tramadol* is known to be excreted in breast milk. The FDA and the European Medicines Agency (EMA) are investigating the safety of using *tramadol*-containing medications to treat pain in children 12-18 years because of the potential for serious side effects, including slowed or difficult breathing.

TRICYCLIC ANTIDEPRESSANTS (TCAs)

Comment: Co-administration of TCAs with SSRIs requires extreme caution.
➤ *amitriptyline* (C)(G) titrate to achieve pain relief; max 300 mg/day
Pediatric: <12 years: not recommended; ≥12 years: same as adult
Tab: 10, 25, 50, 75, 100, 150 mg
➤ *amoxapine* (C) titrate to achieve pain relief; if total dose exceeds 300 mg/day, give in divided doses; max 400 mg/day
Pediatric: <12 years: not recommended; ≥12 years: same as adult
Tab: 25, 50, 100, 150 mg
➤ *desipramine* (C)(G) titrate to achieve pain relief; max 300 mg/day
Pediatric: <12 years: not recommended; ≥12 years: same as adult
Norpramin *Tab:* 10, 25, 50, 75, 100, 150 mg
➤ *doxepin* (C)(G) titrate to achieve pain relief; max 150 mg/day
Pediatric: <12 years: not recommended; ≥12 years: same as adult
Cap: 10, 25, 50, 75, 100, 150 mg; *Oral conc:* 10 mg/ml (4 oz w. dropper)
➤ *imipramine* (C)(G)
Pediatric: <12 years: not recommended; ≥12 years: same as adult
Tofranil titrate to achieve pain relief; max 200 mg/day; adolescents max 100 mg/day; if maintenance dose exceeds 75 mg/day, may switch to Tofranil PM at bedtime
Tab: 10, 25, 50 mg
Tofranil PM titrate to achieve pain relief; initially 75 mg at HS; max 200 mg at HS
Cap: 75, 100, 125, 150 mg
Tofranil Injection 50 mg IM; lower dose for adolescents; switch to oral form as soon as possible
Amp: 25 mg/2 ml (2 ml)
➤ *nortriptyline* (D)(G) titrate to achieve pain relief; initially 10-25 mg tid-qid; max 150 mg/day; lower doses for elderly and adolescents
Pediatric: <12 years: not recommended; ≥12 years: same as adult
Pamelor titrate to achieve pain relief; max 150 mg/day
Cap: 10, 25, 50, 75 mg; *Oral soln:* 10 mg/5 ml (16 oz)
➤ *protriptyline* (C) titrate to achieve pain relief; initially 5 mg tid; max 60 mg/day
Pediatric: <12 years: not recommended; ≥12 years: same as adult
Vivactil *Tab:* 5, 10 mg
➤ *trimipramine* (C) titrate to achieve pain relief; max 200 mg/day
Pediatric: <12 years: not recommended; ≥12 years: same as adult
Surmontil *Cap:* 25, 50, 100 mg

POST-TRAUMATIC STRESS DISORDER (PTSD)

Comment: No one pharmacological agent has emerged as the best treatment for PTSD. A combination of pharmacological agents (e.g., antidepressants, non-adrenergic agents, antipsychosis drugs) may comprise an individualized treatment plan to successfully manage core symptoms of PTSD as well as associated anxiety, depression, sleep disturbances, and co-occurring psychiatric disorders.

SELECTIVE SEROTONIN REUPTAKE INHIBITORS (SSRIs)

Comment: The FDA has approved two SSRIs for the treatment of PTSD: *paroxetine* and *sertraline*. However, the safety and efficacy of other SSRIs (*fluoxetine, citalopram, escitalopram, fluvoxamine*) have been tested in clinical practice. Co-administration of SSRIs with TCAs requires extreme caution. Concomitant use of MAOIs and SSRIs is absolutely contraindicated. Avoid St. John's wort and other serotonergic agents. A potentially fatal adverse event is *serotonin syndrome*, caused by serotonin excess. Milder symptoms require HCP intervention to avert severe symptoms which can be rapidly fatal without urgent/ emergent medical care. Symptoms include restlessness, agitation, confusion, hallucinations, tachycardia, hypertension, dilated pupils, muscle twitching, muscle rigidity, loss of muscle coordination, diaphoresis, diarrhea, headache, shivering, piloerection, hyperpyrexia, cardiac arrhythmias, seizures, loss of consciousness, coma, death. Abrupt withdrawal or interruption of treatment with an antidepressant medication is sometimes associated with an *Antidepressant Discontinuation Syndrome* which may be mediated by gradually tapering the drug over a period of two weeks or longer, depending on the dose strength and length of treatment. Common symptoms of the *serotonin discontinuation Syndrome* include flu-like symptoms (nausea, vomiting, diarrhea, headaches, sweating), sleep disturbances (insomnia, nightmares, constant sleepiness), mood disturbances (dysphoria, anxiety, agitation), cognitive disturbances (mental confusion, hyperarousal), sensory and movement disturbances (imbalance, tremors, vertigo, dizziness, electric-shock-like sensations in the brain, often described by sufferers as "brain zaps."

▷ *paroxetine maleate* (D)(G)
    Pediatric: <12 years: not recommended; ≥12 years: same as adult
        Paxil initially 20 mg daily in AM; may increase by 10 mg/day at weekly intervals as needed; max 60 mg/day
          Tab: 10*, 20*, 30, 40 mg
        Paxil CR initially 25 mg daily in AM; may increase by 12.5 mg at weekly intervals as needed; max 62.5 mg/day
          Tab: 12.5, 25, 37.5 mg cont-rel ent-coat
        Paxil Suspension initially 20 mg daily in AM; may increase by 10 mg/day at weekly intervals as needed; max 60 mg/day
          Oral susp: 10 mg/5 ml (250 ml; orange)
▷ *paroxetine mesylate* (D)(G) initially 7.5 mg daily in AM; may increase by 10 mg/day at weekly intervals as needed; max 60 mg/day
    Pediatric: <12 years: not recommended; ≥12 years: same as adult
        Brisdelle *Cap:* 7.5 mg
▷ *sertraline* (C) initially 50 mg daily; increase at 1 week intervals if needed; max 200 mg daily
    Pediatric: <6 years: not recommended; 6-12 years: initially 25 mg daily; max 200 mg/day; 13-17 years: initially 50 mg daily; max 200 mg/day; ≥17 years: same as adult
        Zoloft *Tab:* 15*, 50*, 100*mg; *Oral conc:* 20 mg per ml (60 ml [dilute just before administering in 4 oz water, ginger ale, lemon-lime soda, lemonade, or orange juice]) (alcohol 12%)

ATYPICAL ANTIPSYCHOSIS DRUGS

▷ *olanzapine* (C)(G) initially 2.5-5 mg once daily at HS; increase by 5 mg every week to 20 mg at HS; usual maintenance 10-20 mg/day
        Zyprexa *Tab:* 2.5, 5, 7.5, 10, 15, 20 mg
        Zyprexa Zydis *ODT:* 5, 10, 15, 20 mg (phenylalanine)
▷ *quetiapine* (C)(G) initially 25 mg bid; increase total daily dose by 50 mg, as needed and tolerated, to max 300-600 mg/day
        Seroquel *Tab:* 25, 100, 200, 300 mg
        Seroquel XR *Tab:* 50, 150, 200, 300, 400 mg ext-rel
▷ *risperidone* (C)(G) initially 0.5-1 mg bid; titrate to 3 mg bid by the end of the first week; usual maintenance 4-6 mg/day
        Risperdal *Tab:* 0.25, 0.5, 1, 2, 3, 4 mg; *Soln:* 1 mg/ml (30 ml w. pipette); *Consta (Inj):* 25, 37.5, 50 mg
        Risperdal M-Tabs *M-tab:* 0.5, 1, 2, 3, 4 mg orally-disint (phenylalanine)

NON-ADRENERGIC AGENTS

ALPHA-1 ANTAGONISTS

Comment: *prazosin* is useful in reducing combat-trauma nightmares, normalizing dreams for combat veterans, and mediating other sleep disturbances.
▷ *prazosin* (C)(G) first dose at HS, 1 mg bid-tid; increase dose slowly; usual range 6-15 mg/ day in divided doses; max 20-40 mg/day

Pediatric: <12 years: not recommended; ≥12 years: same as adult
    Minipress *Cap:* 1, 2, 5 mg

CENTRAL ALPHA-2 AGONISTS

Comment: *clonidine* is useful to reduce nightmares, hypervigilance, startle reactions, and outbursts of rage.
▷ *clonidine* (C)
    Pediatric: <12 years: not recommended; ≥12 years: same as adult
        Catapres initially 0.1 mg bid; usual range 0.2-0.6 mg/day in divided doses; max 2.4 mg/day *Tab:* 0.1*, 0.2*, 0.3*mg
        Catapres-TTS initially 0.1 mg patch weekly; increase after 1-2 weeks if needed; max 0.6 mg/day
          Patch: 0.1, 0.2 mg/day (12/carton); 0.3 mg/day (4/carton)
        Kapvay (G) initially 0.1 mg bid; usual range 0.2-0.6 mg/day in divided doses; max 2.4 mg/day *Tab:* 0.1, 0.2 mg
        Nexiclon XR initially 0.18 mg (2 ml) suspension <u>or</u> 0.17 mg tab once daily; usual max 0.52 mg (6 ml suspension) once daily
          Tab: 0.17, 0.26 mg ext-rel; *Oral susp:* 0.09 mg/ml ext-rel (4 oz)

BETA-ADRENERGIC BLOCKER (NON-CARDIOSELECTIVE)

Comment: *propranolol* is useful to mediate hyperarousal. For other non-cardioselective beta-adrenergic blockers, *see* **Hypertension**, *page 241*
▷ *propranolol* (C)(G) 40-240 mg daily
    Pediatric: <12 years: not recommended; ≥12 years: same as adult
        Inderal *Tab:* 10*, 20*, 40*, 60*, 80*mg
        Inderal LA initially 80 mg daily in a single dose; increase q 3-7 days; usual range 120-160 mg/day; max 320 mg/day in a single dose

SEROTONIN-NOREPINEPHRINE REUPTAKE INHIBITORS (SNRIs)

▷ *desvenlafaxine* (C)(G) swallow whole; initially 50 mg once daily; max 120 mg/day
    Pediatric: <12 years: not recommended; ≥12 years: same as adult
        Pristiq *Tab:* 50, 100 mg ext-rel
▷ *duloxetine* (C)(G) swallow whole; initially 30 mg once daily x 1 week; then increase to 60 mg once daily; max 120 mg/day
    Pediatric: <12 years: not recommended; ≥12 years: same as adult
        Cymbalta *Cap:* 20, 30, 40, 60 mg del-rel
▷ *venlafaxine* (C)(G)
        Effexor initially 75 mg/day in 2-3 divided doses; may increase at 4-day intervals in 75 mg increments to 150 mg/day; max 225 mg/day
    Pediatric: <18 years: not recommended; ≥18 years: same as adult
          Tab: 37.5, 75, 150, 225 mg
        Effexor XR initially 75 mg q AM; may start at 37.5 mg daily x 4-7 days, then increase by increments of up to 75 mg/day at intervals of at least 4 days; usual max 375 mg/day
    Pediatric: <18 years: not recommended; ≥18 years: same as adult
          Tab/Cap: 37.5, 75, 150 mg ext-rel

5HT2/3 RECEPTOR BLOCKERS

▷ *mirtazapine* (C) initially 15 mg q HS; increase at intervals of 1-2 weeks; 1-2 weeks; usual range 15-60 mg/day; max 60 mg/day
    Pediatric: <12 years: not recommended; ≥12 years: same as adult
        Remeron *Tab:* 15*, 30*, 45*mg
        Remeron SolTab *ODT:* 15, 30, 45 mg (orange) (phenylalanine)

SERTONIN+ACETYLCHOLINE+NOREPINEPHRINE+DOPAMINE BLOCKER

▷ *trazodone* (C)(G) initially 150 mg/day in divided doses with food; increase by 50 mg/day q 3-4 days; max 400 mg/day in divided doses <u>or</u> 50-400 mg at HS
    Pediatric: <18 years: not recommended; ≥18 years: same as adult
        Oleptro *Tab:* 50, 100*, 150*, 200, 250, 300 mg

TRICYCLIC ANTIDEPRESSANTS (TCAs)

▷ *amitriptyline* (C)(G) 10-20 mg at HS
Pediatric: <12 years: not recommended; ≥12 years: same as adult
Tab: 10, 25, 50, 75, 100, 150 mg
▷ *doxepin* (C)(G) 10-200 mg at HS
Pediatric: <12 years: not recommended; ≥12 years: same as adult
Cap: 10, 25, 50, 75, 100, 150 mg; *Oral conc:* 10 mg/ml (4 oz w. dropper)
▷ *imipramine* (C)(G) 10-200 mg q HS
Tofranil 100-300 mg at HS or divided bid or tid
Pediatric: <6 years: not recommended; 6-12 years: initially 25 mg; >12 years: 50 mg max
2.5 mg/kg/day
Tab: 10, 25, 50 mg
Tofranil PM initially 75 mg daily 1 hour before HS; max 200 mg
Pediatric: <12 years: not recommended; ≥12 years: same as adult
Cap: 75, 100, 125, 150 mg
Tofranil Injection 50 mg IM; lower dose for adolescents; switch to oral form as soon as
possible
Amp: 25 mg/2 ml (2 ml)
▷ *nortriptyline* (D)(G) 10-150 mg q HS
Pediatric: <12 years: not recommended; ≥12 years: same as adult
Pamelor *Cap:* 10, 25, 50, 75 mg; *Oral soln:* 10 mg/5 ml

MONOAMINE OXIDASE INHIBITORS (MAOIs)

Comment: Many drug and food interactions with this class of drugs, use cautiously. MAOIs
should be reserved for refractory depression that has not responded to other classes of
antidepressants. Concomitant use of MAOIs and SSRIs is contraindicated. See mfr pkg insert
for drug and food interactions. MAOIs have been used to reduce recurrent recollections of the
trauma, nightmares, flashbacks, numbing, sleep disturbances, and social withdrawal in PTSD.
▷ *phenelzine* (C)(G) initially 15 mg tid; max 90 mg/day
Pediatric: <16 years: not recommended; ≥16 years: same as adult
Nardil *Tab:* 15 mg
▷ *selegiline* (C) initially 10 mg tid; max 60 mg/day
Pediatric: <12 years: not recommended; ≥12 years: same as adult
Emsam *Transdermal patch:* 6 mg/24 hrs, 9 mg/24 hrs, 12 mg/24 hrs
Comment: At the **Emsam** transdermal patch 6 mg/24 hrs dose, the dietary restrictions
commonly required when using nonselective MAOIs are not necessary.

 PRECOCIOUS PUBERTY, CENTRAL (CPP)

Comment: GnRH-dependent CPP is defined by pubertal development occurring before
the age of 8 years in girls and 9 years in boys. It is characterized by early pubertal changes
such as breast development and start of menses in girls and increased testicular and penile
growth in boys, appearance of pubic hair, as well as acceleration of growth velocity and bone
maturation and tall stature during childhood, which often results in reduced adult height due
to premature fusion of the growth plates.

GONADOTROPIN RELEASING HORMONE (GnRH) AGONIST

▷ *triptorelin* (X)
Pediatric: <2 years: not recommended; ≥2 years: administer as a single 22.5 mg IM injection once every 24 weeks; must be administered under the supervision of a physician;
monitor response with LH levels after a GnRH or GnRH agonist stimulation test, basal LH,
or serum concentration of sex steroid levels beginning 1 to 2 months following initiation
of therapy, during therapy as necessary to confirm maintenance of efficacy, and with each
subsequent dose; measure height every 3-6 months and monitor bone age periodically; see
mfr pkg insert for reconstitution and administration instructions
Triptodur Single-use kit: 1 single-dose vial of **triptorelin** 22.5 mg w. Flip-Off seal containing sterile lyophilized white to slightly yellow powder cake, 1 sterile, glass syringe prefilled
with 2 ml of sterile water for injection, 2 sterile 21 gauge, 1½" needles (thin-wall) with
safety cover

Comment: **Triptodur** is contraindicated in females who are pregnant since expected hormonal changes that occur with *triptorelin* treatment increase the risk for pregnancy loss. Available data with *triptorelin* use in pregnant females are insufficient to determine a drug-associated risk of adverse developmental outcomes. Based on mechanism of action in humans and findings of increased pregnancy loss in animal studies, *triptorelin* may cause fetal harm when administered to pregnant females. Advise pregnant females of the potential risk to a fetus. The estimated background risk of major birth defects and miscarriage is unknown. There are no data on the presence of *triptorelin* in human milk or the effects of the drug on the breastfed infant. The developmental and health benefits of breastfeeding should be considered along with the mother's clinical need for *triptorelin* and any potential adverse effects on the breastfed child from *triptorelin* or from the underlying maternal condition. During the early phase of therapy, gonadotropins and sex steroids rise above baseline because of the initial stimulatory effect of the drug. Therefore, a transient increase in clinical signs and symptoms of puberty, including vaginal bleeding, may be observed during the first weeks of therapy. Post-marketing reports with this class of drugs include symptoms of emotional lability, such as crying, irritability, impatience, anger, and aggression. Monitor for development or worsening of psychiatric symptoms during treatment with **Triptodur.** Post-marketing reports of convulsions have been observed in patients receiving GnRH agonists, including *triptorelin.* These included patients with a history of seizures, epilepsy, cerebrovascular disorders, central nervous system anomalies or tumors, and patients on concomitant medications that have been associated with convulsions such as bupropion and SSRIs. Convulsions have also been reported in patients in the absence of any of the conditions mentioned above.

 PREGNANCY

See **Prescription Prenatal Vitamins** *page 600*
Comment: Prenatal vitamins should have at least 400 mcg of folic acid content. Take one dose once daily. It is recommended that prenatal vitamins be started at least 3 months prior to conception to improve preconception nutritional status, and continued throughout pregnancy and the postnatal period, in lactating and nonlactating women, and throughout the childbearing years.

NAUSEA/VOMITING

➤ *doxyalamine succinate+pyridoxine* (A)(G) do not crush or chew; take on an empty stomach with water; initially 2 tabs at HS on day 1; may increase to 1 tab AM and 2 tabs at HS day 2; may increase to 1 tab AM, 1 tab mid-afternoon, 2 tabs at HS; max 4 tabs/day
   Diclegis *Tab:* doxyl 10 mg+pyri 10 mg del-rel
   Comment: **Diclegis** is the only FDA-approved drug for the treatment of morning sickness. It has not been studied in women with hyperemesis gravidarum.
➤ *promethazine* (C)(G) 12.5-50 mg PO/IM/rectally q 4-6 hours prn
   Phenergan *Tab:* 12.5*, 25*, 50 mg; *Plain syr:* 6.25 mg/5 ml; *Fortis syr:* 25 mg/5 ml; *Rectal supp:* 12.5, 25, 50 mg; *Amp:* 25, 50 mg/ml (1 ml)
Comment: *promethazine* is contraindicated in children with uncomplicated nausea, dehydration, Reye's syndrome, history of sleep apnea, asthma, and lower respiratory disorders in children. *promethazine* lowers the seizure threshold in children, may cause cholestatic jaundice, anticholinergic effects, extrapyramidal effects, and potentially fatal respiratory depression.

 PREMENSTRUAL DYSPHORIC DISORDER (PMDD)

NSAIDs *see page 571*
Opioid Analgesics *see* **Pain** *page 354*
Oral Contraceptives *see page 559*

ORAL ESTROGEN+PROGESTERONE COMBINATIONS

Comment: **Rajani** (a generic form of **Beyaz**) and **Yaz**; also available in generic Forms (**Gianvi, Ocella, Syeda, Vestura, Yasmin, Zarah**) have an FDA indication for treatment of PMDD in females who choose to use an OCP. Contraindicated with renal and adrenal insufficiency.

Monitor K⁺ level during the first cycle if the patient is at risk for hyperkalemia for any reason. If the patient is taking a drug that increase serum potassium (e.g., ACEIs, ARBS, NSAIDs, K⁺ sparing diuretics), the patient is at risk for hyperkalemia.

▷ *ethinyl estradiol+drospirenone* (X)(G) Pre-menarchal: not indicated; Post-menarchal: 1 tab once daily x 28 days; repeat cycle; start on first Sunday after menses begins or on first day of next menses

  Yaz *Tab*: ethin estra 20 mcg+drospir 3 mg

▷ *ethinyl+estradiol+drospirenone+levomefolate calcium* (X)(G) Pre-menarchal: not indicated; Post-menarchal: 1 tab once daily x 28 days; repeat cycle; start on first Sunday after menses begins or on first day of next menses preceded by a negative pregnancy test

  Beyaz *Tab*: ethin estra 20 mcg+drospir 3 mg+levo 0.451 mg
  Rajani *Tab*: ethin estra 20 mcg+drospir 3 mg+levo 0.451 mg

DIURETICS

▷ *spironolactone* (D)(G) initially 50-100 mg once daily or in divided doses; titrate at 2-week intervals
Pediatric: <12 years: not recommended; ≥12 years: same as adult

  Aldactone *Tab*: 25, 50*, 100*mg

ANTIDEPRESSANTS

▷ *fluoxetine* (C)(G)

  Prozac initially 20 mg daily; may increase after 1 week; doses >20 mg/day should be divided into AM and noon doses; max 80 mg/day
  Pediatric: <8 years: not recommended; 8-17 years: initially 10 or 20 mg/day; start lower weight children at 10 mg/day; if starting at 10 mg/day, may increase after 1 week to 20 mg/day; ≥17 years: same as adult

    Tab: 10*mg; *Cap*: 10, 20, 40 mg; *Oral soln*: 20 mg/5 ml (4 oz) (mint)

  Prozac Weekly following daily *fluoxetine* therapy at 20 mg/day for 13 weeks, may initiate Prozac Weekly 7 days after the last 20 mg *fluoxetine* dose
  Pediatric: <12 years: not recommended; ≥12 years: same as adult

    Cap: 90 mg ent-coat del-rel pellets

  Sarafem administer daily or 14 days before expected menses and through first full day of menses; initially 20 mg/day; max 80 mg/day
  Pediatric: <8 years: not recommended; 8-17 years: initially 10 or 20 mg/day; start lower weight children at 10 mg/day; if starting at 10 mg/day, may increase after 1 week to 20 mg/day

    Tab: 10, 15, 20 mg; *Cap*: 20 mg

▷ *paroxetine maleate* (D)(G)
Pediatric: <12 years: not recommended; ≥12 years: same as adult

  Paxil initially 20 mg daily in AM; may increase by 10 mg/day at weekly intervals as needed; max 60 mg/day

    Tab: 10*, 20*, 30, 40 mg

  Paxil CR initially 25 mg daily in AM; may increase by 12.5 mg at weekly intervals as needed; max 62.5 mg/day; may start 14 days before and continue through day one of menses

    Tab: 12.5, 25, 37.5 mg cont-rel ent-coat

  Paxil Suspension initially 20 mg daily in AM; may increase by 10 mg/day at weekly intervals as needed; max 60 mg/day

    Oral susp: 10 mg/5 ml (250 ml) (orange)

▷ *paroxetine mesylate* (D)(G) initially 7.5 mg daily in AM; may increase by 10 mg/day at weekly intervals as needed; max 60 mg/day
Pediatric: <12 years: not recommended; ≥12 years: same as adult

  Brisdelle *Cap*: 7.5 mg

▷ *sertraline* (C)

  For 2 weeks prior to onset of menses: initially 50 mg daily x 3; then increase to 100 mg daily for remainder of the cycle; *For full cycle*: initially 50 mg daily; then may increase by 50 mg/day each cycle to max 150 mg/day
  Pediatric: <12 years: not recommended; ≥12 years: same as adult

    Zoloft *Tab*: 25*, 50*, 100*mg; *Oral conc*: 20 mg per ml (60 ml) (alcohol 12%); dilute just before administering in 4 oz water, ginger ale, lemon-lime soda, lemonade, or orange juice

➤ *nortriptyline* (D)(G) initially 25 mg tid-qid; max 150 mg/day
   Pediatric: <12 years: not recommended; ≥12 years: same as adult
      Pamelor *Cap:* 10, 25, 50, 75 mg; *Oral soln:* 10 mg/5 ml

CALCIUM SUPPLEMENTS

➤ *calcium* (C) 1200 mg/day
see Osteoporosis page 340

 PROCTITIS: ACUTE (PROCTOCOLITIS, ENTERITIS)

Comment: The following regimen for the treatment of proctitis, proctocolitis, and enteritis is published in the **2015 CDC Sexually Transmitted Diseases Treatment Guidelines**.

RECOMMENDED REGIMEN

➤ *ceftriaxone* (B)(G) 250 mg IM in a single dose
   Rocephin *Vial:* 250, 500 mg; 1, 2 gm
     plus
➤ *doxycycline* 100 mg bid x 7 days
   Acticlate *Tab:* 75, 150**mg
   Adoxa *Tab:* 50, 75, 100, 150 mg ent-coat
   Doryx *Tab:* 50, 75, 100, 150, 200 mg del-rel
   Doxteric *Tab:* 50 mg del-rel
   Monodox *Cap:* 50, 75, 100 mg
   Oracea *Cap:* 40 mg del-rel
   Vibramycin *Tab:* 100 mg; *Cap:* 50, 100 mg; *Syr:* 50 mg/5 ml (raspberry-apple) (sulfites); *Oral susp:* 25 mg/5 ml (raspberry)
   Vibra-Tab *Tab:* 100 mg film-coat

 PROSTATE CANCER: METASTATIC, CASTRATION-RESISTANT (CRPC), METASTATIC HIGH-RISK CASTRATION-SENSITIVE PROSTATE CANCER (CSPC)

CYP17 INHIBITOR

➤ *abiraterone acetate*
   Comment: Patients receiving treatment with *abiraterone acetate* should also receive a gonadotropin-releasing hormone (GnRH) analog concurrently or should have had a bilateral orchiectomy. Avoid concomitant strong CYP3A4 inducers; if a strong CYP3A4 must be co-administered, increase the *abiraterone acetate* dosing frequency. Avoid co-administration of *abiraterone acetate* with CYP2D6 substrates that have a narrow therapeutic index; if an alternative treatment cannot be used, exercise caution and consider a dose reduction of the CYP2D6 substrate. Hepatotoxicity can be severe and fatal. Do not initiate *abiraterone acetate* in patients with baseline severe hepatic impairment Child-Pugh C). *abiraterone acetate* should be discontinued if patients develop severe hepatotoxicity. Monitor liver function and modify, interrupt, or discontinue *abiraterone acetate* dosing as recommended. Advise males with female partners of reproductive potential to use effective contraception during treatment and for 3 weeks after the last dose. Based on animal studies, *abiraterone acetate* may impair reproductive function and fertility in males of reproductive potential.
   Yonsa recommended dose: 500 mg (4 x 125 mg tabs) administered once daily (in combination with *methylprednisolone* 4 mg administered orally twice daily); take with or without food; swallow whole with water; do not crush or chew
    Tab: 125 mg
   Comment: Yonsa is an ultramicrosize formulation of the oral CYP17 inhibitor *abiraterone acetate* (FDA-approved as **Zytiga**) used in combination with *methylprednisolone* for the treatment of metastatic castration-resistant prostate cancer (CRPC). The most common adverse side effects (incidence ≥10%) are fatigue, joint swelling or discomfort, edema, hot flush, diarrhea, vomiting, cough, hypertension, dyspnea, UTI, and confusion. The most common laboratory abnormalities (incidence >20%) are anemia, elevated alkaline phosphatase, hypertriglyceridemia, lymphopenia, hypercholesterolemia, hyperglycemia, elevated AST and ALT, hyperkalemia, and hypophosphatemia. Monitor for signs and symptoms of mineralocorticoid excess

and adrenocortical insufficiency and treat as appropriate. To report suspected adverse reactions, contact Sun Pharmaceutical Industries at 1-800-818-4555 or FDA at 1-800-FDA-1088 or visit www.fda.gov/medwatch.

Zytiga recommended dose: *CRPC:* 1000 mg (4 x 250 mg or 2 x 500 mg tabs) administered once daily (in combination with *prednisone* 5 mg administered orally twice daily); *CSPC:* 1000 mg (4 x 250 mg or 2 x 500 mg tabs) administered once daily (in combination with *prednisone* 5 mg administered orally once daily); take on an empty stomach, at least 1 hour before or 2 hours after a meal; swallow whole with water; do not crush or chew

  Tab: 250, 500 mg

Comment: **Zytiga** (*abiraterone acetate*) is an oral CYP17 inhibitor used in combination with *prednisone* for the treatment of metastatic castration-resistant prostate cancer (CRPC) and metastatic high-risk castration-sensitive prostate cancer (CSPC). The most common adverse reactions (incidence ≥10%) are fatigue, arthralgia, hypertension, nausea, edema, hypokalemia, hot flush, diarrhea, vomiting, upper respiratory infection, cough, and headache. The most common laboratory abnormalities (incidence ≥20%) are anemia, elevated alkaline phosphatase, hypertriglyceridemia, lymphopenia, hypercholesterolemia, hyperglycemia, and hypokalemia. Monitor for signs and symptoms of mineralocorticoid excess and adrenocortical insufficiency and treat as appropriate. To report suspected adverse reactions, contact Janssen Biotech at 1-800-526-7736 (1-800-JANSSEN) or FDA at 1-800-FDA1088 or visit www.fda.gov/medwatch.

ANDROGEN RECEPTOR INHIBITOR

▷ *apalutamide* administer 240 mg (4 x 60 mg tablets) once daily; swallow tablets whole, do not crush or chew; take with or without food.

  Erleada *Tab:* 60 mg

  Comment: **Erleada** (*apalutamide*) is the first FDA-approved treatment for non-metastatic, castration-resistant prostate cancer. Patients should also receive a gonadotropin-releasing hormone (GnRH) analog concurrently or should have had bilateral orchiectomy. Concomitant use of **Erleada** with medications that are sensitive substrates of CYP3A4, CYP2C19, CYP2C9, UGT, P-gp, BCRP, or OATP1B1 may result in loss of activity of these medications. The most common adverse reactions (incidence ≥10%) have been fatigue, hypertension, rash, diarrhea, nausea, weight decreased, arthralgia, fall, hot flush, decreased appetite, fracture, and peripheral edema. Falls (16%) and fractures (12%) have occurred in patients receiving **Erleada**. Evaluate patients for fall and fracture risk, and treat patients with bone-targeted agents according to established guidelines. Seizure has occurred in 0.2% of patients receiving **Erleada**. Permanently discontinue **Erleada** in patients who develop a seizure during treatment. Advise males with female partners of reproductive potential to use effective contraception.

◯ PROSTATITIS: ACUTE

ANTI-INFECTIVES

▷ *ciprofloxacin* (C) 500 mg bid x 4-6 weeks
  Pediatric: <18 years: not recommended; ≥18 years: same as adult
    Cipro (G) *Tab:* 250, 500, 750 mg; *Oral susp:* 250, 500 mg/5 ml (100 ml) (strawberry)
    Cipro XR *Tab:* 500, 1000 mg ext-rel
    ProQuin XR *Tab:* 500 mg ext-rel
  Comment: *ciprofloxacin* is contraindicated <18 years-of-age, and during pregnancy and lactation. Risk of tendonitis or tendon rupture.

▷ *norfloxacin* (C) 400 mg bid x 28 days
  Pediatric: <18 years: not recommended; ≥18 years: same as adult
    Noroxin *Tab:* 400 mg
  Comment: *norfloxacin* is contraindicated <18 years-of-age, and during pregnancy and lactation. Risk of tendonitis or tendon rupture.

▷ *ofloxacin* (C)(G) 300 mg x bid x 6 weeks
  Pediatric: <18 years: not recommended; ≥18 years: same as adult
    Floxin *Tab:* 200, 300, 400 mg
  Comment: *ofloxacin* is contraindicated <18 years-of-age, and during pregnancy and lactation. Risk of tendonitis or tendon rupture.

▷ *trimethoprim+sulfamethoxazole (TMP-SMX)* (C)(G)
 Pediatric: <12 years: not recommended; ≥12 years: same as adult
 Bactrim, Septra 2 tabs bid x 10 days
  Tab: trim 80 mg+sulfa 400 mg*
 Bactrim DS, Septra DS 1 tab bid x 10 days
  Tab: trim 160 mg+sulfa 800 mg*
 Bactrim Pediatric Suspension, Septra Pediatric Suspension
  Oral susp: trim 40 mg+sulfa 200 mg per 5 ml (100 ml) (cherry) (alcohol 0.3%)
Comment: Sulfonamides are contraindicated in the first trimester of pregnancy, the final month of pregnancy, and infants <8 weeks-of-age. *CrCl 15-30 mL/min:* reduce dose by 1/2; *CrCl <15 mL/min:* not recommended. Contraindicated with G6PD deficiency. A high fluid intake is indicated during sulfonamide therapy to avoid crystallization in the kidneys.

PROSTATITIS: CHRONIC

ANTI-INFECTIVES

▷ *carbenicillin* (B) 2 tabs qid x 4-12 weeks
 Geocillin *Tab:* 382 mg
▷ *ciprofloxacin* (C) 500 mg bid x 3 or more months
 Pediatric: <18 years: not recommended; ≥18 years: same as adult
 Cipro (G) *Tab:* 250, 500, 750 mg; *Oral susp:* 250, 500 mg/5 ml (100 ml) (strawberry)
 Cipro XR *Tab:* 500, 1000 mg ext-rel
 ProQuin XR *Tab:* 500 mg ext-rel
Comment: *ciprofloxacin* is contraindicated <18 years-of-age, and during pregnancy and lactation. Risk of tendonitis or tendon rupture.
▷ *norfloxacin* (C) 400 mg bid x 4-12 weeks
 Pediatric: <18 years: not recommended; ≥18 years: same as adult
 Noroxin *Tab:* 400 mg
Comment: *norfloxacin* contraindicated <18 years-of-age, and during pregnancy and lactation. Risk of tendonitis or tendon rupture.
▷ *ofloxacin* (C)(G) 300 mg bid x 4-12 weeks
 Pediatric: <18 years: not recommended; ≥18 years: same as adult
 Floxin *Tab:* 200, 300, 400 mg
Comment: *ofloxacin* is contraindicated <18 years-of-age, and during pregnancy and lactation. Risk of tendonitis or tendon rupture.
▷ *trimethoprim+sulfamethoxazole* (C)(G)
 Pediatric: <18 years: See Appendix ___ for dose by weight; ≥18 years: same as adult
 Bactrim, Septra 2 tabs bid x 10 days
  Tab: trim 80 mg+sulfa 400 mg*
 Bactrim DS, Septra DS 1 tab bid x 10 days
  Tab: trim 160 mg+sulfa 800 mg
 Bactrim Pediatric Suspension, Septra Pediatric Suspension 20 ml bid x 10 days
  Oral susp: trim 40 mg+sulfa 200 mg per 5 ml (100 ml) (cherry) (alcohol 0.3%)
Comment: Sulfonamides are contraindicated in the first trimester of pregnancy, the final month of pregnancy, and infants <8 weeks-of-age. *CrCl 15-30 mL/min:* reduce dose by 1/2; *CrCl <15 mL/min:* not recommended. Contraindicated with G6PD deficiency. A high fluid intake is indicated during sulfonamide therapy to avoid crystallization in the kidneys.

SUPPRESSION THERAPY

▷ *trimethoprim+sulfamethoxazole (TMP-SMX)* (C)(G)
 Pediatric: <18 years: not recommended; ≥18 years: same as adult
 Bactrim, Septra 2 tabs bid x 10 days
  Tab: trim 80 mg+sulfa 400 mg*
 Bactrim DS, Septra DS 1 tab bid x 10 days
  Tab: trim 160 mg+sulfa 800 mg*
 Bactrim Pediatric Suspension, Septra Pediatric Suspension 20 ml bid x 10 days
  Oral susp: trim 40 mg+sulfa 200 mg per 5 ml (100 ml) (cherry) (alcohol 0.3%)
Comment: Sulfonamides are contraindicated in the first trimester of pregnancy, the final month of pregnancy, and infants <8 weeks-of-age. *CrCl 15-30 mL/min:* reduce dose by 1/2; *CrCl <15 mL/min:* not recommended. Contraindicated with G6PD deficiency. A high fluid intake is indicated during sulfonamide therapy to avoid crystallization in the kidneys.

PRURITUS

Antihistamines *See* Drugs for the Management of Allergy, Cough, and Cold Symptoms *page* 603
Topical Corticosteroids *see page* 574
Parenteral Corticosteroids *see page* 577
Oral Corticosteroids *see page* 577
OTC Antihistamines
OTC Eucerin Products
OTC Lac-Hydrin Products
OTC Lubriderm Products
OTC Aveeno Products

TOPICAL OIL

▷ *fluocinolone acetonide* 0.01% topical oil (C)
   Pediatric: <6 years: not recommended; ≥6 years: apply sparingly bid for up to 4 weeks
      Derma-Smoothe/FS Topical Oil apply sparingly tid
         Topical oil: 0.01% (4 oz) (peanut oil)

TOPICAL AND TRANSDERMAL ANALGESICS

▷ *capsaicin* (B)(G) apply tid-qid prn to intact skin
   Pediatric: <2 years: not recommended; ≥2 years: same as adult
      Axsain *Crm:* 0.075% (1, 2 oz)
      Capsin (OTC) *Lotn:* 0.025, 0, 075% (59 ml)
      Capzasin-HP (OTC) *Crm:* 0.075% (1.5 oz); Lotn: 0.075% (2 oz) 0.025% (45, 90 gm)
      Capzasin-P (OTC) *Crm:* 0.025% (1.5 oz); Lotn: 0.025% (2 oz)
      Dolorac *Crm:* 0.025% (28 gm)
      Double Cap (OTC) *Crm:* 0.05% (2 oz)
      R-Gel *Gel:* 0.025% (15, 30 gm)
      Zostrix (OTC) *Crm:* 0.025% (0.7, 1.5, 3 oz) **Zostrix HP (OTC)** *Emol crm:* 0.075% (1, 2 oz)
▷ *capsaicin* 8% patch (B) apply up to 4 patches for one 60-minute application to clean dry skin; may prep area with topical anesthetic; wear non-latex gloves; patches may be cut to size/shape; treatment may be repeated every 3 months
   Pediatric: <18 years: not recommended; ≥18 years: same as adult
      Qutenza *Patch:* 8% 1640 mcg/cm (179 mg) (1 or 2 patches w. 1-50 gm tube cleansing gel/carton)
▷ *diclofenac sodium* (C; D ≥30 wks)(G) apply qid prn to intact skin
   Pediatric: <12 years: not established; ≥12 years: same as adult
      Pennsaid 1.5% in 10 drop increments, dispense and rub into front, side, and back of knee: usually; 40 drops (40 mg) qid
         Topical soln: 1.5% (150 ml)
      Pennsaid 2% apply 2 pump actuations (40 mg) and rub into front, side, and back of knee bid
         Topical soln: 2% (20 mg/pump actuation, 112 gm)
      Solaraze Gel massage in to clean skin bid prn
         Gel: 3% (50 gm) (benzyl alcohol)
      Voltaren Gel (G) apply qid prn to intact skin
         Gel: 1% (100 gm)
   Comment: *diclofenac* is contraindicated with *aspirin* allergy. As with other NSAIDs, should be avoided in late pregnancy (≥30 weeks) because it may cause premature closure of the ductus arteriosus.
▷ *doxepin* (B) cream apply to affected area qid at intervals of at least 3-4 hours; max 8 days
   Pediatric: <12 years: not recommended; >12 years: same as adult
      Prudoxin *Crm:* 5% (45 gm)
      Zonalon *Crm:* 5% (30, 45 gm)
▷ *pimecrolimus* 1% cream (C)(G) <2 years: not recommended; ≥2 years: apply to affected area bid; do not apply an occlusive dressing
      Elidel *Crm:* 1% (30, 60, 100 gm)
   Comment: *pimecrolimus* is indicated for short-term and intermittent long-term use. Discontinue use when resolution occurs. Contraindicated if the patient is

immunosuppressed. Change to the 0.1% preparation or if secondary bacterial infection is present.

▶ *trolamine salicylate* apply tid-qid
  Pediatric: <2 years: not recommended; ≥2 years: same as adult
    Mobisyl Creme *Crm:* 10% (100 gm)

PSEUDOBULBAR AFFECT (PBA) DISORDER

Comment: Pseudobulbar affect (PBA), emotional lability, labile affect, or emotional incontinence refers by to a neurologic disorder characterized by involuntary crying or uncontrollable episodes of crying and/or laughing, or other emotional outbursts. PBA occurs secondary to a neurologic disease or brain injury such as traumatic brain injury (TBI), stroke, Parkinson's disease, multiple sclerosis, amyotrophic lateral sclerosis (ALS, Lou Gehrig's disease).

▶ *dextromethorphan+quinidine* (C)(G) 1 cap once daily x 7 days; then starting on day 8, 1 cap bid
  Pediatric: <12 years: not recommended; ≥12 years: same as adult
    Nuedexta *Cap:* dextro 20 mg+quini 10 mg

Comment: *dextromethorphan hydrobromide* is an uncompetitive NMDA receptor antagonist and sigma-1 agonist. *quinidine sulfate* is a CYP450 2D6 inhibitor. **Nuedexta** is contraindicated with an MAOI or within 14 days of stopping an MAOI, with prolonged QT interval, congenital long QT syndrome, history suggestive of torsades de pointes, or heart failure, complete atrioventricular (AV) block without implanted pacemaker or patients at high risk of complete AV block, and concomitant drugs that both prolong QT interval and are metabolized by CYP2D6 (e.g., *thioridazine* or *pimozide*). Discontinue **Nuedexta** if the following occurs: hepatitis or thrombocytopenia or any other hypersensitivity reaction. Monitor ECG in patients with left ventricular hypertrophy (LVH) or left ventricular dysfunction (LVD). *desipramine* exposure increases **Nuedexta** 8-fold; reduce *desipramine* dose and adjust based on clinical response. Use of **Nuedexta** with selective serotonin reuptake inhibitors (SSRIs) or tricyclic antidepressants (TCAs) increases the risk of serotonin syndrome. *paroxetine* exposure increases **Nuedexta** 2-fold; therefore, reduce **paroxetine** dose and adjust based on clinical response (*digoxin* exposure may increase *digoxin* substrate plasma concentration. **Nuedexta** is not recommended in pregnancy or breastfeeding. Safety and effectiveness of **Nuedexta** in children have not been established. To report suspected adverse reactions, contact Avanir Pharmaceuticals at 1-866-388-5041 or FDA at 1-800-FDA-1088 or www.fda.gov/medwatch.

PSEUDOGOUT

Injectable Acetaminophen *see Pain page* 352
NSAIDs *see page* 571
Opioid Analgesics *see Pain page* 354
Topical and Transdermal Analgesics *see Pain page* 352
Parenteral Corticosteroids *see page* 577
Oral Corticosteroids *see page* 577
Topical Analgesic and Anesthetic Agents *see page* 569

PSEUDOMEMBRANOUS COLITIS

Comment: Staphylococcal enterocolitis and antibiotic-associated pseudomembranous colitis caused by *C. difficile*.

ANTI-INFECTIVES

▶ *metronidazole* (not for use in 1st; B in 2nd, 3rd)(G) 500 mg tid x 14 days
    Flagyl *Tab:* 250*, 500*mg
    Flagyl 375 *Cap:* 375 mg
    Flagyl ER *Tab:* 750 mg ext-rel

Comment: Alcohol is contraindicated during treatment with oral *metronidazole* and for 72 hours after therapy due to a possible *disulfiram*-like reaction (nausea, vomiting, flushing, headache).

▶ *vancomycin hcl capsule* (B)(G) 500 mg to 2 gm in 3-4 doses x 7-10 days; max 2 gm/day
  Pediatric: 40 mg/kg/day in 3-4 doses x 7-10 days; max 2 gm/day; use caps or oral solution
  as appropriate
      Vancocin *Cap:* 125, 250 mg

GLYCOPEPTIDE ANTIBACTERIAL AGENT

Comment: Firvanq *(vancomycin hcl oral solution)* is a glycopeptide antibacterial agent
FDA approved to treat *C. difficile*-associated diarrhea (CDAD) and enterolitis caused by
Staphylococcus aureus, including methicillin-resistant strains (MRSA). **Firvanq** should be
used only to treat or prevent infections that are proven or strongly suspected to be caused
by susceptible bacteria. Orally administered *vancomycin hcl* is not effective for treatment
of other types of infections. Prescribing **Firvanq** in the absence of a proven or strongly
suspected bacterial infection is unlikely to provide benefit to the patient and increases the
risk of the development of drug-resistant bacteria.

▶ *vancomycin hcl oral solution* see mfr pkg insert for preparation and important administration information; *CDAD* 125 mg orally 4 x/day x 10 days; *Staphylococcal enterocolitis:*
  500 mg to 2 gm orally in 3 or 4 divided doses x 7-10 days
  Pediatric: <18 years: *CDAD and Staphylococcal enterocolitis:* 40 mg/kg orally in 3 or 4
  divided doses x 7-10 days; total daily dosage max 2 gm; ≥18 years: same as adult
      Firvanq *Kit w. pwdr for oral soln:* 25, 50 mg/ml (150, 300 ml) equivalent to 3.75, 7.5,
      10.5, or 15 gm *vancomycin hcl*, and grape-flavored diluent
  Comment: Nephrotoxicity has occurred following oral *vancomycin hcl* therapy and
  can occur either during or after completion of therapy. The risk is increased in geriatric
  patients. Monitor renal function. Ototoxicity has occurred in patients receiving *vancomycin hcl*. Assessment of auditory function may be appropriate in some instances. The most
  common adverse reactions (≥10%) have been nausea (17%), abdominal pain (15%) and
  hypokalemia (13%). There are no available data on **Firvanq** use in pregnant women to
  inform a drug associated risk of major birth defects or miscarriage. Available published
  data on *vancomycin hcl* use in pregnancy during the second and third trimesters have not
  shown an association with adverse pregnancy related outcomes. There are insufficient data
  to inform the levels of *vancomycin hcl* in human milk. However, systemic absorption of
  vancomycin hcl following oral administration is expected to be minimal. There are no data
  on the effects of **Firvanq** on the breastfed infant.

PSITTACOSIS

ANTI-INFECTIVES

▶ *tetracycline* (D)(G) 250 mg qid or 500 mg tid x 7-14 days
  Pediatric: <8 years: not recommended; ≥8 years, <100 lb: 25-50 mg/kg/day in 4 doses x
  7-14 days; ≥8 years, ≥100 lb: same as adult
      Achromycin V *Cap:* 250, 500 mg
      Sumycin *Tab:* 250, 500 mg; *Cap:* 250, 500 mg; *Oral susp:* 125 mg/5 ml (100, 200 ml) (fruit)
      (sulfites)
  Comment: *tetracycline* is contraindicated <8 years-of-age, in pregnancy, and lactation
  (discolors developing tooth enamel). A side effect may be photo-sensitivity (photophobia).
  Do not take with antacids, calcium supplements, milk or other dairy, or within two hours of
  taking another drug.

PSORIASIS, PLAQUE PSORIASIS

Emollients *see Dermatitis: Atopic page* 121
Topical Corticosteroids *see page* 574

TOPICAL HIGH POTENCY CORTICOSTEROID

▶ *clobetasol propionate* (C)(G) apply a thin layer to the affected skin areas bid; rub in gently
  and completely; wash hands after each application; discontinue when control is achieved;
  max 50 gm/week; max 2 consecutive weeks per treatment course; do not use if atrophy is
  present at the treatment site; do not bandage, cover, or wrap the treated skin area; avoid use
  on the face, scalp, axilla, groin, or other intertriginous areas; topical use only; not for oral,
  ophthalmic, or intravaginal use

Pediatric: <18 years: not recommended; ≥18 years: same as adult
Impoyz *Crm:* 0.025% (60, 112 gm)
Comment: **Impoyz** (*clobetasol propionate 0.025%*) cream is a high potency corticosteroid indicated for the treatment of moderate-to-severe plaque psoriasis.

VITAMIN D-3 DERIVATIVES

➤ *calcipotriene* (C)
Pediatric: <12 years: not recommended; ≥12 years: same as adult
Dovonex apply bid to lesions and gently rub in completely
Crm: 0.005% (30, 120 gm)

VITAMIN D-3 DERIVATIVE+CORTICOSTEROID COMBINATIONS

➤ *calcipotriene+betamethasone dipropionate* (C)(G)
Pediatric: <18 years: not recommended; ≥18 years: same as adult
Enstilar apply to affected area and gently rub in once daily x up to 4 weeks; limit treatment area to 30% of body surface area; do not occlude; do not use on face, axillae, groin, or atrophic skin; max 100 gm/week
Foam: calci 0.005%+beta 0.064% (60 gm spray can)
Taclonex apply to affected area and gently rub in once daily as needed, up to 4 weeks
Taclonex Ointment apply bid to lesions and gently rub in completely; limit treatment area to 30% of body surface area; do not occlude; do not use on face, axillae, groin, or atrophic skin; max 100 gm/week
Oint: calci 0.005%+beta 0.064% (60, 100 gm)
Taclonex Scalp Topical Suspension apply to affected area and gently rub in once daily x 2 weeks or until cleared; max 8 weeks; limit treatment area to 30% of body surface area; do not occlude; do not use on face, axillae, groin, or atrophic skin; max 100 gm/week
Bottle: (30, 60 gm; 120 gm [2 x 60 gm])
➤ *calcitriol* (C) apply bid to lesions and gently rub in completely; max weekly dose should not exceed 200 gm
Pediatric: <18 years: not recommended; ≥18 years: same as adult
Vectical *Oint:* 3 mcg/gm (100 gm)

HIGH-POTENCY TOPICAL STEROID

For other high-potency Topical Corticosteroids *see page* 574

➤ *clobetasol propionate* apply a thin layer to the affected skin areas bid; rub in gently and completely; wash hands after each application; discontinue when control is achieved; max 50 gm/week; max 2 consecutive weeks per treatment course; do not use if atrophy is present at the treatment site; do not bandage, cover, or wrap the treated skin area; avoid use on the face, scalp, axilla, groin, or other intertriginous areas; topical use only; not for oral, ophthalmic, or intravaginal use
Pediatric: <18 years: not recommended; ≥18 years: same as adult
Impoyz *Crm:* 0.025% (60, 112 gm)
Comment: **Impoyz** (*clobetasol propionate 0.025%*) cream is a high potency corticosteroid specifically indicated for the treatment of moderate-to-severe plaque psoriasis.
➤ *halobetasol propionate* apply a thin layer to the affected skin areas bid; rub in gently and completely; wash hands after each application; discontinue when control is achieved; max 50 gm/week; max 2 consecutive weeks per treatment course; do not use if atrophy is present at the treatment site; do not bandage, cover, or wrap the treated skin area; avoid use on the face, scalp, axilla, groin, or other intertriginous areas; topical use only; not for oral, ophthalmic, or intravaginal use
Pediatric: <18 years: not recommended; ≥18 years: same as adult
Bryhali *Lotn:* 0.01% (60, 112 gm)
Comment: **Bryhali** (*halobetasol propionate 0.01%*) cream is a high potency corticosteroid specifically indicated for the treatment of moderate-to-severe plaque psoriasis.

IMMUNOSUPPRESSANTS

➤ *alefacept* (B) 7.5 mg IV bolus or 15 mg IM once weekly x 12 weeks; may re-treat x 12 weeks
Pediatric: <12 years: not recommended; ≥12 years: same as adult

Amevive *IV dose pack:* 7.5 mg single-use (w. 10 ml sterile water diluents [use 0.6 ml]; 1, 4/pck); *IM dose pack:* 15 mg single-use (w. 10 ml sterile water diluent [use 0.6 ml]; 1, 4/pck

Comment: CD4+ and T-lymphocyte count should be checked prior to initiating treatment with *alefacept* and then monitored. Treatment should be withheld if CD4+ T-lymphocyte counts are below 250 cells/mcl.

▷ *cyclosporine* (C) 1.25 mg/kg bid; may increase after 4 weeks by 0.5 mg/kg/day; then adjust at 2-week intervals; max 4 mg/kg/day; administer with meals
    Pediatric: <18 years: not recommended; ≥18 years: same as adult
        Neoral *Cap:* 25, 100 mg (alcohol)
        Neoral Oral Solution *Oral soln:* 100 mg/ml (50 ml) may dilute in room temperature apple juice or orange juice (alcohol)

ANTIMITOTICS

▷ *anthralin* (C) apply once daily
    Pediatric: <12 years: not recommended; ≥12 years: same as adult
        Zithranol-RR *Crm:* 1.2% (15, 45 gm)

RETINOIDS

▷ *acitretin* (X)(G) 25-50 mg once daily with main meal
    Pediatric: <12 years: not recommended; ≥12 years: same as adult
        Soriatane *Cap:* 10, 25 mg
▷ *tazarotene* (X)(G) apply once daily at HS
    Pediatric: <12 years: not recommended; ≥12 years: same as adult
        Avage Cream *Crm:* 0.1% (30 gm)
        Tazorac Cream *Crm:* 0.05, 0.1% (15, 30, 60 gm)
        Tazorac Gel *Gel:* 0.05, 0.1% (30, 100 gm)

COAL TAR PREPARATIONS

▷ *coal tar* (C)(G)
    Pediatric: same as adult
        Scytera (OTC) apply qd-qid; use lowest effective dose
          Foam: 2%
        T/Gel Shampoo Extra Strength (OTC) use every other day; max 4 x/week; massage into affected areas for 5 minutes; rinse; repeat *Shampoo:* 1%
        T/Gel Shampoo Original Formula (OTC) use every other day; max 7 x/week; massage into affected areas for 5 minutes; rinse; repeat *Shampoo:* 0.5%
        T/Gel Shampoo Stubborn Itch Control (OTC) use every other day; max 7 x/week; massage into affected areas for 5 minutes; rinse; repeat *Shampoo:* 0.5%

HUMANIZED INTERLEUKIN-17A ANTAGONIST

▷ *brodalumab* (B) inject SC into the upper arm, abdomen, or thigh; rotate sites; administer 210 mg SC (as two separate 150 mg SC injections) at weeks 0, 1, and 2; then 210 mg every 2 weeks
    Pediatric: <18 years: not recommended; ≥18 years: same as adult
        Siliq *Prefilled pen:* 210 mg/1.5 ml solution, single-use (2/carton) (preservative-free)
        Comment: **Siliq** is currently indicated for plaque psoriasis only. **Siliq** is contraindicated with Crohn's disease. *Black Box Warning (BBW):* Suicidal ideation and behavior, including completed suicides, have occurred in patients treated with **Siliq**. Prior to prescribing, weigh potential risks and benefits in patients with a history of depression and/or suicidal ideation or behavior. Patients with new or worsening suicidal thoughts and behavior should be referred to a mental health professional, as appropriate. Advise patients and caregivers to seek medical attention for manifestations of suicidal ideation or behavior, new onset or worsening depression, anxiety, or other mood changes. Avoid using live vaccines concurrently with **Siliq** therapy. There are no human data on **Siliq** use in pregnant women to inform a drug associated risk. Human IgG antibodies are known to cross the placental barrier; therefore, **Siliq** may be transmitted from the mother to the developing fetus. There are no data on the presence of *brodalumab* in human milk or effects on the breastfed infant. **Siliq** is available only through the restricted **Siliq** REMS Program.

▷ *ixekizumab* <18 years: not recommended; ≥18 years: recommended dose is 160 mg (2 x 80 mg injections) SC at Week 0, followed by 80 mg at weeks 2, 4, 6, 8, 10, and 12, then 80 mg SC every 4 weeks

Pediatric: <18 years: not recommended; ≥18 years: same as adult

Taltz *Prefilled pen/Prefilled autoinjector:* 80 mg/ml (1 ml) single-dose

Comment: Taltz injection the first and only treatment approved by the FDA for moderate-to-severe plaque psoriasis involving the genital area. This indication is based upon positive results from a randomized, double-blind, placebo-controlled study in moderate-to-severe psoriasis involving the genital area which involved 149 patients with plaque psoriasis who were candidates for phototherapy or systemic therapy but failed to respond to or were intolerant to at least 1 topical therapy. There are no available data on Taltz use in pregnancy to inform any drug associated risks. Human IgG is known to cross the placental barrier; therefore, Taltz may be transmitted from the mother to the developing fetus. There are no data on the presence of *ixekizumab* in human milk or effects on the breastfed infant.

▷ *secukinumab* (B) inject SC into the upper arm, abdomen, or thigh; rotate sites; administer 300 mg SC (as two separate 150 mg SC injections) at weeks 0, 1, 2, 3, and 4; then 300 mg every 4 weeks; for some patients, 150 mg/dose may be sufficient

Pediatric: <18 years: not recommended; ≥18 years: same as adult

Cosentyx *Vial:* 150 mg/ml pwdr for SC inj after reconstitution single-use (preservative-free)

Comment: Cosentyx may be used as monotherapy or in combination with *methotrexate* (MTX). Avoid using live vaccines concurrently with Siliq therapy. For professional preparation and administration only.

INTERLEUKIN-23 ANTAGONIST

▷ *guselkumab injection* administer 100 mg SC at Week 0, Week 4 and every 8 weeks thereafter

Tremfya *Prefilled syringe:* 100 mg/ml (1 ml) single-dose

Comment: Tremfya is an interleukin-23 blocker indicated for the treatment of patients >18 years-of-age with moderate-to-severe plaque psoriasis who are candidates for systemic therapy or phototherapy. Evaluate for TB prior to initiating treatment with Tremfya. Tremfya may increase the risk of infection. Instruct patients to seek medical advice if signs or symptoms of clinically important chronic or acute infection occur. If a serious infection develops, discontinue Tremfya until the infection resolves. Avoid use of live vaccines in patients treated with Tremfya. The most common (≥1%) adverse reactions associated with Tremfya include upper respiratory infections, headache, injection site reactions, arthralgia, diarrhea, gastroenteritis, tinea infections, and herpes simplex infections. The safety and efficacy of Tremfya in pediatric patients (<18 years-of-age) have not been established. There are no available data on Tremfya use in pregnancy to inform a drug-associated risk of adverse developmental outcomes, presence of *guselkumab* in human milk, or effects on the breastfed infant. To report suspected adverse reactions, contact Janssen Biotech at 1-800-JANSSEN (1-800-526-7736) or FDA at 1-800-FDA1088 or visit www.fda.gov/medwatch.

▷ *tildrakizumab-asmn* inject SC; rotate sites; recommended dose is 100 mg at Weeks 0, 4, and every 12 weeks thereafter.

Pediatric: <18 years: not recommended; ≥18 years: same as adult

Ilumya *Prefilled syringe:* 100 mg/ml (1 ml) single-use (preservative-free)

Comment: Ilumya is an interleukin-23 (IL-23) antagonist indicated for the treatment of adults with moderate-to-severe plaque psoriasis who are candidates for systemic therapy or phototherapy. Ilumya acts by selectively binding to the p19 subunit of IL-23 and inhibiting its interaction with the Il-23 receptor, blocking the release of pro-inflammatory cytokines and chemokines. Most common adverse reactions associated with Ilumya treatment are upper respiratory infections, injection site reactions, and diarrhea. Avoid use of live vaccines in patients treated with Ilumya. If a serious allergic reaction occurs, discontinue Ilumya immediately and initiate appropriate therapy. Ilumya may increase the risk of infection. Evaluate for TB prior to initiating treatment. Instruct patients to seek medical advice if signs or symptoms of clinically important chronic or acute infection occur. If a serious infection develops, consider discontinuing Ilumya until the infection resolves. Limited available data with Ilumya use in pregnant women are insufficient to inform a drug associated risk of adverse developmental outcomes. Human IgG is known to cross the placental barrier; therefore, **Ilumya** may be transferred from the mother to the fetus. There are no data on the presence of *tildrakizumab- asmn* in human milk or effects on the breastfed infant. To report suspected adverse reactions, contact Merck Sharp & Dohme, a subsidiary of Merck, at 1-877-888-4231 or FDA at 1-800-FDA-1088 or www.fda.gov/medwatch.

INTERLEUKIN-12+INTERLEUKIN-23 ANTAGONIST

▷ *ustekinumab* (B) inject SC; rotate sites; <100 kg: 45 mg once; then 4 weeks later; then every 12 weeks; ≥100 kg: 90 mg once; then 4 weeks later; then every 12 weeks
   Pediatric: <18 years: not recommended; ≥18 years: same as adult
      Stelara *Vial:* 45 mg/0.5 ml single-use (preservative-free)
      Comment: **Stelara** may be used as monotherapy or in combination with *methotrexate* (MTX).

TUMOR NECROSIS FACTOR (TNF) BLOCKERS

▷ *adalimumab* (B) initially 80 mg SC once followed by 40 mg once every other week starting one week after initial dose; inject into thigh or abdomen; rotate sites
   Pediatric: <18 years: not recommended; ≥18 years: same as adult
      Humira *Prefilled syringe:* 20 mg/0.4 ml; 40 mg/0.8 ml single-dose (2/pck; 2, 6/starter pck) (preservative-free)
▷ *adalimumab-adaz* (B) initially 80 SC; then, 40 mg SC every other week starting one week after initial dose; inject into thigh or abdomen; rotate sites
   Pediatric: <18 years: not recommended; ≥18 years: same as adult
      Hyrimoz *Prefilled syringe/Prefilled pen:* 40 mg/0.8 ml, single-dose (preservative-free)
      Comment: **Hymirox** is biosimilar to **Humira** *(adalimumab)*.
▷ *adalimumab-adbm* (B) initially 80 SC; then, 40 mg SC every other week starting one week after initial dose; inject into thigh or abdomen; rotate sites
   Pediatric: <18 years: not recommended; ≥18 years: same as adult
      Cyltezo *Prefilled syringe:* 40 mg/0.8 ml single-dose (preservative-free)
      Comment: **Cyltezo** is biosimilar to **Humira** *(adalimumab)*.
▷ *etanercept* (B) inject SC into thigh, abdomen, or upper arm; rotate sites; initially 50 mg twice weekly (3-4 days apart) for 3 months; then 50 mg/week maintenance or 25 mg or 50 mg per week for 3 months; then 50 mg/week maintenance
   Pediatric: <4 years: not recommended; 4-17 years: Chronic moderate-to-severe plaque psoriasis; >17 years: same as adult
      Enbrel *Vial:* 25 mg pwdr for SC injection after reconstitution (4/carton w. supplies) (preservative-free, diluent contains benzyl alcohol); *Prefilled syringe:* 25, 50 mg/ml (preservative-free); *SureClick autoinjector:* 50 mg/ml (preservative-free)
▷ *golimumab* (B) administer SC or IV infusion (in combination with *methotrexate [MTX]*)
   Pediatric: <18 years: not recommended; ≥18 years: same as adult
      Simponi 50 mg SC once monthly; rotate sites
         Prefilled syringe, SmartJect autoinjector: 50 mg/0.5 ml, single-use (preservative-free)
      Simponi Aria 2 mg/kg IV infusion week 0 and week 4; then every 8 weeks thereafter
         Vial: 50 mg/4 ml, single-use, soln for IV infusion after dilution (latex-free, preservative-free)
▷ *infliximab* (*tumor necrosis factor-alpha blocker*) must be refrigerated at 2ºC to 8ºC (36ºF to 46ºF); administer dose intravenously over a period of not less than 2 hours; do not use beyond the expiration date as this product contains no preservative; administer in conjunction with *methotrexate*, infuse 3 mg/kg at 0, 2 and 6 weeks; then every 8 weeks; some patients may benefit from increasing the dose up to 10 mg/kg or treatment as often as every 4 weeks
   Pediatric: <6 years: not studied; ≥6-17 years: 3 mg/kg at 0, 2 and 6 weeks, then every 8 weeks; ≥18 years: same as adult
      Remicade *Vial:* 100 mg for reconstitution to 10 ml administration volume, single-dose (preservative-free)
      Comment: **Remicade** is indicated to reduce signs and symptoms, and induce and maintain clinical remission, in adults and children ≥6 years-of-age with moderately to severely active disease who have had an inadequate response to conventional therapy and reduce the number of draining enterocutaneous and rectovaginal fistulas, and maintain fistula closure, in adults with fistulizing disease. Common adverse effects associated with **Remicade** included abdominal pain, headache, pharyngitis, sinusitis,

and upper respiratory infections. In addition, **Remicade** might increase the risk for serious infections, including tuberculosis, bacterial sepsis, and invasive fungal infections. Available data from published literature on the use of *infliximab* products during pregnancy have not reported a clear association with *infliximab* products and adverse pregnancy outcomes. *infliximab* products cross the placenta and infants exposed *in utero* should not be administered live vaccines for at least 6 months after birth. Otherwise, the infant may be at increased risk of infection, including disseminated infection which can become fatal. Available information is insufficient to inform the amount of *infliximab* products present in human milk or effects on the breastfed infant. To report suspected adverse reactions, contact Merck Sharp & Dohme Corp., a subsidiary of Merck & Co. at 1-877-888-4231 or FDA at 1-800-FDA1088 or www.fda.gov/medwatch.

▶ *infliximab-abda (tumor necrosis factor-alpha blocker)* **(B)**
  Renflexis: see *infliximab* (**Remicade**) above for full prescribing information
  Comment: **Renflexis** is a biosimilar to **Remicade** for the treatment of immune-disorders including Crohn's disease, ulcerative colitis, rheumatoid arthritis, ankylosing spondylitis, psoriatic arthritis and plaque psoriasis. **Renflexis** was approved under the FDA category for biosimilars and demonstrated no clinically meaningful differences for use, dosing regimens, strengths, dosage forms, and routes of administration from the FDA-approved biological product **Remicade**.

▶ *infliximab-dyyb (tumor necrosis factor-alpha blocker)* **(B)**
  Inflectra: see *infliximab* (**Remicade**) above for full prescribing information
  Comment: **Inflectra** is a biosimilar to **Remicade** for the treatment of immune-disorders including Crohn's disease, ulcerative colitis, rheumatoid arthritis, ankylosing spondylitis, psoriatic arthritis and plaque psoriasis. **Inflectra** was approved under the FDA category for biosimilars and demonstrated no clinically meaningful differences for use, dosing regimens, strengths, dosage forms, and routes of administration from the FDA-approved biological product **Remicade**.
  Renflexis *see infliximab* (**Remicade**) above for full prescribing information
  Comment: **Inflectra** is a biosimilar to **Remicade** for the treatment of immune-disorders including Crohn's disease, ulcerative colitis, rheumatoid arthritis, ankylosing spondylitis, psoriatic arthritis and plaque psoriasis. **Inflectra** was approved under the FDA category for biosimilars and demonstrated no clinically meaningful differences for use, dosing regimens, strengths, dosage forms, and routes of administration from the FDA-approved biological product **Remicade**.

▶ *infliximab-qbtx (tumor necrosis factor-alpha blocker)* **(B)**
  Ifixi: see *infliximab* (**Remicade**) above for full prescribing information
  Comment: **Ifixi** is a biosimilar to **Remicade** for the treatment of immune disorders including Crohn's disease, ulcerative colitis, rheumatoid arthritis, ankylosing spondylitis, psoriatic arthritis and plaque psoriasis. **Ifixi** was approved under the FDA category for biosimilars and demonstrated no clinically meaningful differences for use, dosing regimens, strengths, dosage forms, and routes of administration from the FDA-approved biological product **Remicade**.

MOISTURIZING AGENTS

Aquaphor Healing Ointment (OTC) *Oint:* (1.75, 3.5, 14 oz) (alcohol)
Eucerin Daily Sun Defense (OTC) *Lotn:* 6 oz (fragrance-free)
Comment: **Eucerin Daily Sun Defense** is a moisturizer with SPF 15.
Eucerin Facial Lotion (OTC) *Lotn:* 4 oz
Eucerin Light Lotion (OTC) *Lotn:* 8 oz
Eucerin Lotion (OTC) *Lotn:* 8, 16 oz
Eucerin Original Creme (OTC) *Crm:* 2, 4, 16 oz (alcohol)
Eucerin Plus Creme *Crm:* 4 oz
Eucerin Plus Lotion (OTC) *Lotn:* 6, 12 oz
Eucerin Protective Lotion (OTC) *Lotn:* 4 oz (alcohol)
Comment: **Eucerin Protective Lotion** is a moisturizer with SPF 25.
Lac-Hydrin Cream (OTC) *Crm:* 280, 385 gm
Lac-Hydrin Lotion (OTC) *Lotn:* 225, 400 gm
Lubriderm Dry Skin Scented (OTC) *Lotn:* 6, 10, 16, 32 oz
Lubriderm Dry Skin Unscented (OTC) *Lotn:* 3.3, 6, 10, 16 oz (fragrance-free)
Lubriderm Sensitive Skin Lotion (OTC) *Lotn:* 3.3, 6, 10, 16 oz (lanolin-free)

Lubriderm Dry Skin (OTC) *Lotn (scented):* 2.5, 6, 10, 16 oz;
Lotn (fragrance-free): 1, 2.5, 6, 10, 16 oz
Lubriderm Bath 1-2 capfuls in bath or rub onto wet skin as needed; then rinse (8 oz)

PSORIATIC ARTHRITIS

Injectable Acetaminophen *see Pain page 352*
NSAIDs *see page 571*
Opioid Analgesics *see Pain page 354*
Topical & Transdermal Analgesics *see Pain page 352*
Parenteral Corticosteroids *see page 577*
Oral Corticosteroids *see page 577*
Topical Analgesic and Anesthetic Agents *see page 569*

TOPICAL AND TRANSDERMAL ANALGESICS

▷ *capsaicin* (B)(G) apply tid-qid prn to intact skin
  Pediatric: <2 years: not recommended; ≥2 years: same as adult
      Axsain *Crm:* 0.075% (1, 2 oz)
      Capsin *Lotn:* 0.025, 0.075% (59 ml)
      Capzasin-HP (OTC) *Crm:* 0.075% (1.5 oz), 0.025% (45, 90 gm); *Lotn:* 0.075% (2 oz);
      0.025% (45, 90 gm)
      Capzasin-P (OTC) *Crm:* 0.025% (1.5 oz); *Lotn:* 0.025% (2 oz)
      Dolorac *Crm:* 0.025% (28 gm)
      Double Cap (OTC) *Crm:* 0.05% (2 oz)
      R-Gel *Gel:* 0.025% (15, 30 gm)
      Zostrix (OTC) *Crm:* 0.025% (0.7, 1.5, 3 oz)
      Zostrix HP (OTC) *Emol crm:* 0.075% (1, 2 oz)
▷ *capsaicin* 8% patch (B) apply up to 4 patches for one 60-minute application to clean dry
  skin; may prep area with topical anesthetic; wear non-latex gloves; patches may be cut to
  size/shape; treatment may be repeated every 3 months
  Pediatric: <18 years: not recommended; ≥18 years: same as adult
      Qutenza *Patch:* 8% 1640 mcg/cm (179 mg) (1 or 2 patches w. 1-50 gm tube cleansing
      gel/carton)
▷ *diclofenac sodium* (C; D ≥30 wks)(G) apply qid prn to intact skin
  Pediatric: <12 years: not established; ≥12 years: same as adult
      Pennsaid 1.5% in 10 drop increments, dispense and rub into front, side, and back of
      knee: usually; 40 drops (40 mg) qid
          Topical soln: 1.5% (150 ml)
      Pennsaid 2% apply 2 pump actuations (40 mg) and rub into front, side, and back of
      knee bid
          Topical soln: 2% (20 mg/pump actuation, 112 gm)
      Solaraze Gel massage in to clean skin bid prn
          Gel: 3% (50 gm) (benzyl alcohol)
      Voltaren Gel (G) apply qid prn to intact skin
          Gel: 1% (100 gm)
  Comment: *diclofenac* is contraindicated with *aspirin* allergy. As with other NSAIDs, should
  be avoided in late pregnancy (≥30 weeks) because it may cause premature closure of the
  ductus arteriosus.
▷ *doxepin* (B) cream apply to affected area qid at intervals of at least 3-4 hours; max 8 days
  Pediatric: <12 years: not recommended; >12 years: same as adult
      Prudoxin *Crm:* 5% (45 gm)
      Zonalon *Crm:* 5% (30, 45 gm)
▷ *pimecrolimus* 1% cream (C)(G) <2 years: not recommended; ≥2 years: apply to affected
  area bid; do not apply an occlusive dressing
      Elidel *Crm:* 1% (30, 60, 100 gm)
  Comment: *pimecrolimus* is indicated for short-term and intermittent long-term use.
  Discontinue use when resolution occurs. Contraindicated if the patient is immunosuppressed. Change to the 0.1% preparation or if secondary bacterial infection is present.
▷ *trolamine salicylate* apply tid-qid
  Pediatric: <2 years: not recommended; ≥2 years: same as adult
      Mobisyl Creme *Crm:* 10% (100 gm)

ORAL SALICYLATE

▷ *indomethacin* (C) initially 25 mg bid-tid, increase as needed at weekly intervals by 25-50 mg/day; max 200 mg/day
Pediatric: <14 years: usually not recommended; >2 years, if risk warranted: 1-2 mg/kg/day in divided doses; max 3-4 mg/kg/day or 150-200 mg/day, whichever is less; <14 years: ER cap not recommended
    Cap: 25, 50 mg; *Susp:* 25 mg/5 ml (pineapple-coconut, mint) (alcohol 1%); *Supp:* 50 mg; *ER Cap:* 75 mg ext-rel
Comment: *indomethacin* is indicated only for acute painful flares. Administer with food and/or antacids. Use lowest effective dose for shortest duration.

ORAL NSAIDs

See more **Oral NSAIDs** page 571

▷ *diclofenac sodium* (C)
    Voltaren 50 mg bid-qid or 75 mg bid or 25 mg qid with an additional 25 mg at HS if necessary
    Tab: 25, 50, 75 mg ent-coat
    Voltaren XR 100 mg once daily; rarely, 100 mg bid may be used
    Tab: 100 mg ext-rel

NSAID+PPI

▷ *esomeprazole+naproxen* (C)(G) 1 tab bid; use lowest effective dose for the shortest duration swallow whole; take at least 30 minutes before a meal
Pediatric: <18 years: not recommended; ≥18 years: same as adult
    Vimovo *Tab:* nap 375 mg+eso 20 mg ext-rel; nap 500 mg+eso 20 mg ext-rel
    Comment: **Vimovo** is indicated to improve signs/symptoms, and risk of gastric ulcer in patients at risk of developing NSAID-associated gastric ulcer.

COX-2 INHIBITORS

Comment: Cox-2 inhibitors are contraindicated with history of asthma, urticaria, and allergic-type reactions to **aspirin**, other NSAIDs, and sulfonamides, 3rd trimester of pregnancy, and coronary artery bypass graft (CABG) surgery.
▷ *celecoxib* (C)(G) 50-400 mg once daily-bid; max 800 mg/day
Pediatric: <18 years: not recommended; ≥18 years: same as adult
    Celebrex *Cap:* 50, 100, 200, 400 mg
▷ *meloxicam* (C)(G)
Pediatric: <18 years: not recommended; ≥18 years: same as adult
    Mobic <2 years, <60 kg: not recommended; ≥2, ≥60 kg: 0.125 mg/kg; max 7.5 mg once daily; ≥18 years: initially 7.5 mg once daily; max 15 mg once daily; *Hemodialysis:* max 7.5 mg/day
    Tab: 7.5, 15 mg; *Oral susp:* 7.5 mg/5 ml (100 ml) (raspberry)
    Vivlodex <18 years: not established; ≥18 years: initially 5 mg qd; may increase to max 10 mg/day; *Hemodialysis:* max 5 mg/day
    Cap: 5, 10 mg

PHOSPHODIESTERASE 4 (PDE4) INHIBITOR

▷ *apremilast* (C) swallow whole; initial titration over 5 days; maintenance 30 mg bid; *Day 1:* 10 mg in AM; *Day 2:* 10 mg AM and 10 mg PM; *Day 3:* 10 mg AM and 20 mg PM; *Day 4:* 20 mg AM and 20 mg PM; *Day 5:* 20 mg AM and 30 mg PM; *Day 6 and ongoing:* 30 mg AM and 30 mg PM
Pediatric: <12 years: not recommended; ≥12 years: same as adult
    Otezla *Tab:* 10, 20, 30 mg; *2-Week Starter Pack*
    Comment: Register pregnant patients exposed to by calling 877-311-8972.

INTERLEUKIN-12 & INTERLEUKIN-23 ANTAGONIST

▷ *ustekinumab* (B) inject SC; rotate sites; <100 kg: 45 mg once; then 4 weeks later; then every 12 weeks; ≥100 kg: 90 mg once; then 4 weeks later; then every 12 weeks
Pediatric: <18 years: not recommended; ≥18 years: same as adult
    Stelara *Vial:* 45 mg/0.5 ml single-use (preservative-free)
    Comment: **Stelara** may be used as monotherapy or in combination with **methotrexate** (MTX).

TUMOR NECROSIS FACTOR (TNF) BLOCKERS

▷ **adalimumab (B)** 40 mg SC once every other week; may increase to once weekly without **methotrexate** (MTX); administer in abdomen or thigh; rotate sites; 2-17 years, supervise first dose
Pediatric: <2 years, <10 kg: not recommended; 10-<15 kg: 10 mg every other week; 15-<30 kg: 20 mg every other week; 30 kg: 40 mg every other week
  Humira *Prefilled syringe:* 20 mg/0.4 ml; 40 mg/0.8 ml single-dose (2/pck; 2, 6/starter pck) (preservative-free)
  Comment: Humira may use with **methotrexate** (MTX), DMARDS, corticoids, salicylates, NSAIDs, or analgesics.

▷ **adalimumab-adaz (B)** 40 mg SC every other week; some patients with RA not receiving **methotrexate** may benefit from increasing the frequency to 40 mg SC every week
Pediatric: <18 years: not recommended; ≥18 years: same as adult
  Hyrimox *Prefilled syringe/Prefilled pen:* 40 mg/0.8 ml single-dose (preservative-free)
  Comment: Hyrimox is biosimilar to **Humira** *(adalimumab).*

▷ **adalimumab-adbm (B)** initially 80 SC; then, 40 mg SC every other week starting one week after initial dose; inject into thigh or abdomen; rotate sites
Pediatric: <18 years: not recommended; ≥18 years: same as adult
  Cyltezo *Prefilled syringe:* 40 mg/0.8 ml single-dose (preservative-free)
  Comment: Cyltezo is biosimilar to **Humira** *(adalimumab).*

▷ **etanercept (B)** 25 mg SC twice weekly (72-96 hours apart) or 50 mg SC weekly; rotate sites
Pediatric: <4 years: not recommended; 4-17 years: 0.4 mg/kg SC twice weekly, 72-96 hours apart (max 25 mg/dose) or 0.8 mg/kg SC weekly (max 50 mg/dose); >17 years: same as adult
  Enbrel *Vial:* 25 mg pwdr for SC injection after reconstitution (4/carton w. supplies) (preservative-free; diluent contains benzyl alcohol); *Prefilled syringe:* 25, 50 mg/ml (preservative-free); *SureClick Autoinjector:* 50 mg/ml (preservative-free)
  Comment: *etanercept* reduces pain, morning stiffness, and swelling. May be administered in combination with **methotrexate.** Live vaccines should not be administered concurrently. Do not administer with active infection.

▷ **golimumab (B)** administer SC or IV infusion (in combination with **methotrexate [MTX]**)
Pediatric: <18 years: not recommended; ≥18 years: same as adult
  Simponi 50 mg SC once monthly; rotate sites
    Prefilled syringe, SmartJect autoinjector: 50 mg/0.5 ml, single-use (preservative-free)
  Simponi Aria 2 mg/kg IV infusion week 0 and week 4; then every 8 weeks thereafter
    Vial: 50 mg/4 ml, single-use, soln for IV infusion after dilution (latex-free, preservative-free)
  Comment: Corticosteroids, non-biologic DMARDs, and/or NSAIDs may be continued during treatment with **golimumab.**

▷ **infliximab (tumor necrosis factor-alpha blocker)** must be refrigerated at 2°C to 8°C (36°F to 46°F); administer dose intravenously over a period of not less than 2 hours; do not use beyond the expiration date as this product contains no preservative; 5 mg/kg at 0, 2 and 6 weeks, then every 8 weeks; some adult patients who initially respond to treatment may benefit from increasing the dose to 10 mg/kg if response is lost later
Pediatric: <6 years: not studied; ≥6-17 years: mg/kg at 0, 2 and 6 weeks, then every 8 weeks; ≥18 years: same as adult
  Remicade *Vial:* 100 mg for reconstitution to 10 ml administration volume, single-dose (preservative-free)
  Comment: Remicade is indicated to reduce signs and symptoms, and induce and maintain clinical remission, in adults and children ≥6 years-of-age with moderately to severely active disease who have had an inadequate response to conventional therapy and reduce the number of draining enterocutaneous and rectovaginal fistulas, and maintain fistula closure, in adults with fistulizing disease. Common adverse effects associated with **Remicade** included abdominal pain, headache, pharyngitis, sinusitis, and upper respiratory infections. In addition, **Remicade** might increase the risk for serious infections, including tuberculosis, bacterial sepsis, and invasive fungal infections. Available data from published literature on the use of **infliximab** products during pregnancy have not reported a clear association with **infliximab** products and adverse pregnancy outcomes. **infliximab** products cross the placenta and infants exposed *in utero* should not be administered live vaccines for at least 6 months after birth. Otherwise, the infant may be at increased risk of infection, including disseminated

infection which can become fatal. Available information is insufficient to inform the amount of *infliximab* products present in human milk or effects on the breastfed infant. To report suspected adverse reactions, contact Merck Sharp & Dohme Corp., a subsidiary of Merck & Co. at 1-877-888-4231 or FDA at 1-800-FDA1088 or www.fda. gov/medwatch.

➤ *infliximab-abda (tumor necrosis factor-alpha blocker)* (B)
 Renflexis: see *infliximab* (Remicade) above for full prescribing information
 Comment: **Renflexis** is a biosimilar to **Remicade** for the treatment of immune-disorders including Crohn's disease, ulcerative colitis, rheumatoid arthritis, ankylosing spondylitis, psoriatic arthritis and plaque psoriasis. **Renflexis** was approved under the FDA category for biosimilars and demonstrated no clinically meaningful differences for use, dosing regimens, strengths, dosage forms, and routes of administration from the FDA-approved biological product **Remicade**.

➤ *infliximab-dyyb (tumor necrosis factor-alpha blocker)* (B)
 Inflectra: see *infliximab* (Remicade) above for full prescribing information
 Comment: **Inflectra** is a biosimilar to **Remicade** for the treatment of immune-disorders including Crohn's disease, ulcerative colitis, rheumatoid arthritis, ankylosing spondylitis, psoriatic arthritis and plaque psoriasis. **Inflectra** was approved under the FDA category for biosimilars and demonstrated no clinically meaningful differences for use, dosing regimens, strengths, dosage forms, and routes of administration from the FDA-approved biological product **Remicade**.

➤ *infliximab-qbtx (tumor necrosis factor-alpha blocker)* (B)
 Ifixi: see *infliximab* (Remicade) above for full prescribing information
 Comment: **Ifixi** is a biosimilar to **Remicade** for the treatment of immune disorders including Crohn's disease, ulcerative colitis, rheumatoid arthritis, ankylosing spondylitis, psoriatic arthritis and plaque psoriasis. **Ifixi** was approved under the FDA category for biosimilars and demonstrated no clinically meaningful differences for use, dosing regimens, strengths, dosage forms, and routes of administration from the FDA-approved biological product **Remicade**.

Selective Costimulation Modulator

➤ *abatacept* (C) administer as an IV infusion over 30 minutes at weeks 0, 2, and 4; then every 4 weeks thereafter; <60 kg, administer 500 mg/dose; 60-100 kg, administer 750 mg/dose; >100 kg, administer 1 gm/dose
 Pediatric: <6 years: not recommended; 6-17 years: administer as an IV infusion over 30 minutes at weeks 0, 2, and 4; then every 4 weeks thereafter; <75 kg, administer 10 mg/kg; same as adult (max 1 gm); >17 years: same as adult
  Orencia *Vial:* 250 mg pwdr for IV infusion after reconstitution (silicone-free) (pre-servative-free); *Prefilled syringe:* 125 mg/ml soln for SC injection (preservative-free); *ClickJect Autoinjector:* 125 mg/ml soln for SC injection

CD20-DIRECTED CYTOLYTIC MONOCLONAL ANTIBODY

➤ *rituximab* (C) administer corticosteroid 30 minutes prior to each infusion; concomitant *methotrexate* therapy, administer a 1,000 mg IV infusion at 0 and 2 weeks; then every 24 weeks or based on response, but not sooner than every 16 weeks.
 Pediatric: <6 years: not recommended; ≥6 years: same as adult
  Rituxan *Vial:* 10 mg/ml (10, 50 ml) (preservative-free)
 Comment: *rituximab* is a B-cell targeting chimeric monoclonal antibody that acts against CD20 and reduces antibody titers. B-cell depletion by *rituximab* may also set the stage for production of interleukin 10–secreting B cells that do not interact with T cells, which further reduces production of antidesmoglein antibodies. *rituximab* carries a black box warning regarding fatal infusion reactions, severe mucocutaneous reactions, hepatitis B virus reactivation, and progressive multifocal leukoencephalopathy. However, serious adverse events are rare. There was no evidence of increased mortality with longer exposure to *rituximab* or to multiple courses of therapy.

PULMONARY ARTERIAL HYPERTENSION (PAH) (WHO GROUP I)

ENDOTHELIAL RECEPTOR ANTAGONIST (ERA)

➤ *bosentan* (G) initiate at 62.5 mg orally twice daily; for patients weighing greater than 40 kg, increase to 125 mg orally twice daily after 4 weeks

Pediatric: <3 years: not established; 3-12: initiate at 62.5 mg orally twice daily; for patients weighing > 40 kg, increase to 125 mg orally twice daily after 4 weeks; >12 years: same as adult

Tracleer *Tab:* 62.5, 125 mg film-coat; *Tab for oral suspension:* 32 mg

Comment: *bosentan* is an endothelin receptor antagonist (ERA) indicated for the treatment of pulmonary arterial hypertension (PAH) (WHO Group 1). **Tracleer** is the first ERA indicated for the treatment of PAH in patients aged 3 years and older with idiopathic or congenital PAH to improve pulmonary vascular resistance (PVR), which is expected to result in an improvement in exercise ability. The most common adverse events associated with **Tracleer** in clinical trials include respiratory tract infections, headache, edema, chest pain, syncope, flushing, hypotension, sinusitis, arthralgia, abnormal serum aminotransferases, palpitations, and anemia. Monitor hemoglobin levels after 1 and 3 months of treatment, then every 3 months thereafter. If signs of pulmonary edema occur, consider the diagnosis of associated pulmonary veno-occlusive disease (PVOD) and consider discontinuing **Tracleer**. Measure liver aminotransferases prior to initiation of treatment and then monthly. Reduce the dose and closely monitor patients developing aminotransferase elevations >3 x ULN. Co-administration of **Tracleer** with drugs metabolized by CYP2C9 and CYP3A can increase exposure to **Tracleer** and/or the co-administered drug. **Tracleer** use decreases contraceptive exposure and reduces effectiveness. There are no data on the presence of *bosentan* in human milk or the effects on the breastfed infant. However, because of the potential for serious adverse reactions, such as fluid retention and hepatotoxicity in breastfed infants, advise women not to breastfeed during treatment with **Tracleer** and pregnancy is contraindicated while taking **Tracleer**. To prevent pregnancy, females of reproductive potential must use two reliable forms of contraception during treatment and for one month after stopping **Tracleer** Due to the risks of hepatotoxicity and birth defects, **Tracleer** includes a boxed warning and is only available through the restricted **Tracleer** Risk Evaluation and Mitigation Strategy REMS Program, a restricted distribution program. Patients, prescribers, and pharmacies must enroll in the program to receive and administer **Tracleer**: www.tracleerrems.com/prescribers.aspx. To report adverse side effects, pregnancy, or other complications contact Actelion at 1-866-228-3546 or call 1-800-FDA-1088 or visit www.fda.gov/medwatch.

PROSTACYCLIN RECEPTOR AGONIST

▷ *selexipag* (X) initially 200 mcg bid; increase by 200 mcg bid to highest tolerated dose up to 1600 mcg bid; *Moderate hepatic impairment (Child-Pugh Class B):* initially 200 mcg once daily; increase by 200 mcg once daily at weekly intervals as tolerated; swallow whole; may take with food to improve tolerability
Pediatric: <12 years: not recommended; ≥12 years: same as adult

Uptravi
Tab: 200, 400, 600, 800, 1000, 1200, 1400, 1600 mcg; *Titration pck:* 140 x 200 mcg + 60 x 800 mcg)

Comment: Discontinue **Uptravi** if pulmonary veno-occlusive disease is confirmed or severe hepatic impairment (Child-Pugh Class C). May be potentiated by concomitant strong CYP2C8 inhibitors (e.g., gemfibrozil); *Nursing mothers:* not recommended. Discontinue breastfeeding or discontinue the drug.

ENDOTHELIN RECEPTOR ANTAGONIST, SELECTIVE FOR THE ENDOTHELIN TYPE-A (ETA) RECEPTOR

▷ *ambrisentan* (X)(G) initiate treatment at 5 mg once daily, with or without *tadalafil* 20 mg once daily; at 4-week intervals, either the dose of **Letairis** or *tadalafil* can be increased, as needed and tolerated, to **Letairis** 10 mg or *tadalafil* 40 mg; do not split, crush, or chew
Pediatric: <12 years: not recommended; ≥12 years: same as adult

Letairis *Tab:* 5, 10 mg film-coat

Comment: In patients with PAH, plasma ET-1 concentrations are increased as much as 10-fold and correlate with increased mean right atrial pressure and disease severity. ET-1 and ET-1 mRNA concentrations are increased as much as 9-fold in the lung tissue of patients with PAH, primarily in the endothelium of pulmonary arteries. These findings suggest that ET-1 may play a critical role in the pathogenesis and progression of PAH. When taken with *tadalafil*, **Letairis** is indicated to reduce the risk of disease progression and hospitalization, to reduce the risk of hospitalization due to worsening PAH, and to improve exercise tolerance. **Letairis** is contraindicated in idiopathic pulmonary fibrosis (IPF).

Exclude pregnancy before the initiation of treatment with **Letairis**. Females of reproductive potential must use acceptable methods of contraception during treatment with **Letairis** and for one month after treatment. Obtain monthly pregnancy tests during treatment and 1 month after discontinuation of treatment. Females can only receive **Letairis** through the **Letairis** Risk Evaluation and Mitigation Strategy (REMS) Program, a restricted distribution program, because of the risk of embryo-fetal toxicity: www.Letairisrems.com or 1-866-664-5327.

Guanylate Cyclase Stimulator

▶ *riociguat* **(X)** initially 0.5-1 mg tid; titrate every 2 weeks as tolerated (SBP ≥95 and absence of hypotensive symptoms) to highest tolerated dose; max 2.5 mg tid
  Pediatric: <12 years: not recommended; ≥12 years: same as adult
  Adempas *Tab:* 0.5, 1, 1.5, 2, 2.5 mg
  Comment: If **Adempas** is interrupted for ≥3 days, re-titrate. Consider titrating to dosage higher than 2.5 mg tid, if tolerated, in patients who smoke. Consider a starting dose of 0.5 mg tid when initiating **Adempas** in patients receiving strong cytochrome P450 (CYP) and P-glycoprotein/breast cancer resistance protein (P-gp/BCRP) inhibitors such as azole antimycotics (e.g., *ketoconazole, itraconazole*) or HIV protease inhibitors (e.g., *ritonavir*). Monitor for signs and symptoms of hypotension with strong CYP and P-gp/BCRP inhibitors. Obtain pregnancy tests prior to initiation and monthly during treatment. **Adempas** has consistently shown to have teratogenic effects when administered to animals. Females can only receive **Adempas** through the Adempas Risk Evaluation and Mitigation Strategy (REMS) Program, a restricted distribution program: **www.AdempasREMS.com** or 855-4 ADEMPAS. It is not known if **Adempas** is present in human milk; however, *riociguat* or its metabolites were present in the milk of rats. Because of the potential for serious adverse reactions in nursing infants from *riociguat*, discontinue nursing or **Adempas**. In placebo-controlled clinical trials, serious bleeding has occurred (including hemoptysis, hematemesis, vaginal hemorrhage, catheter site hemorrhage, subdural hematoma, and intra-abdominal hemorrhage. Safety and efficacy have not been demonstrated in patients with creatinine clearance <15 mL/min or on dialysis or severe hepatic impairment (Child-Pugh Class C).

PHOSPHODIESTERASE TYPE 5 (PDE5) INHIBITORS, CGMP-SPECIFIC DRUGS

▶ *sildenafil citrate* **(B)(G)** *Orally:* initially 5 or 20 mg tid, 4-6 hours apart; max 20 mg tid; *IV bolus:* 2.5 mg or 10 mg bolus injection tid, 4-6 hours apart; max 10 mg tid; the dose does not need to be adjusted for body weight
  Pediatric: <12 years: not recommended; ≥12 years: same as adult
  Revatio *Tab:* 20 mg film-coat; *Oral susp:* 10 mg/ml pwdr for reconstitution (1.12 gm, 112 ml) (grape) (sorbitol); *Vial:* 10 mg/12.5 ml (0.8 mg/ml)
  Comment: A 10 mg IV dose is predicted to provide pharmacological effect equivalent to the 20 mg oral dose. **Revatio** is contraindicated with concomitant nitrate drugs including *nitroglycerin, isosorbide dinitrate*, isosorbide mononitrate, and some recreational drugs such as "poppers." Taking **Revatio** with a nitrate can cause a sudden and serious decrease in blood pressure. **Revatio** is contraindicated with concomitant guanylate cyclase stimulator drugs such as *riociguat* (**Adempas**). Avoid the use of grapefruit products while taking **Revatio**. Stop **Revatio** and get emergency medical help if sudden vision loss. **Revatio** is contraindicated with other phosphodiesterase type 5 (PDE5) Inhibitors, cGMP-specific drugs such as *avanafil* (Stendra), *tadalafil* (Cialis) or *vardenafil* (Levitra). Caution with history of recent MI, stroke, life-threatening arrhythmia, hypotension, hypertension, cardiac failure, unstable angina, retinitis pigmentosa, CYP3A4 inhibitors (e.g., *cimetidine*, the azoles, *erythromycin*, protease inhibitors (e.g., *ritonavir*), CYP3A4 inducers (e.g., *rifampin, carbamazepine, phenytoin, phenobarbital*), alcohol, antihypertensive agents. Side effects include headache, flushing, nasal congestion, rhinitis, dyspepsia, and diarrhea. Use **Revatio** with caution in patients with anatomical deformation of the penis (e.g., angulation, cavernosal fibrosis, or Peyronie's disease) or in patients who have conditions, which may predispose them to priapism (e.g., sickle cell anemia, multiple myeloma, or leukemia). In the event of an erection that persists longer than 4 hours, the patient should seek immediate medical assistance. If priapism (painful erection greater than 6 hours in duration) is not treated immediately, penile tissue damage and permanent loss of potency could result.

▷ *tadalafil* (B)(G) 40 mg once daily; *CrCl 31–80 mL/min:* initially 20 mg once daily; increase to 40 mg once daily if tolerated; *CrCl <30 mL/min:* not recommended; *Mild or moderate hepatic cirrhosis (Child-Pugh Class A or B):* initially 20 mg once daily. *Severe hepatic cirrhosis (Child-Pugh Class C):* not recommended; *use with ritonavir; Receiving ritonavir for at least 1 week:* initiate *tadalafil* at 20 mg once daily; may increase to 40 mg once daily if tolerated; *Already on tadalafil:* stop *tadalafil* at least 24 hours prior to initiating *ritonavir;* resume *tadalafil* at 20 mg once daily after at least 1 week; may increase to 40 mg once daily if tolerated
Pediatric: <12 years: not recommended; ≥12 years: same as adult
    Adcirca *Tab:* 20 mg
  Comment: Contraindicated with concomitant organic nitrates and guanylate cyclase stimulators (e.g., *riociguat*).

▷ *treprostinil* (B) swallow whole; take with food
    Orenitram *Tab:* 0.125, 0.25, 1, 2.5 mg ext-rel
    Comment: **Orenitram** is indicated to improve exercise capacity. It is contraindicated with severe hepatic impairment (Child-Pugh Class C). **Orenitram** inhibits platelet aggregation and increases the risk of bleeding. Concomitant administration of **Orenitram** with diuretics, antihypertensive agents or other vasodilators increases the risk of symptomatic hypotension.

PULMONARY FIBROSIS, IDIOPATHIC (IPF)

Parenteral Corticosteroids *see page* 577
Oral Corticosteroids *see page* 577

Comment: Idiopathic pulmonary fibrosis (IPF) is a chronic, progressive, interstitial lung disease of unknown etiology. There are few effective therapies and the mortality rate is high. New treatments for IPF are urgently needed. Antiinflammatory therapy with corticosteroids or immunosuppressants fails to significantly improve the survival time of patients with IPF. Other pharmacological interventions, which *nintedanib* (Ofev), *etanercept* (Enbrel), *warfarin*, *imatinib mesylate* (Gleevec), and *bosentan* (Tracleer) remain controversial. *pirfenidone* was approved by the European Medicines Agency in 2011. In a 2016 study, *N-Acetylcysteine* was found to have a significant effect only on decreases in percentage of predicted vital capacity and 6 minutes walking test distance. *N-acetylcysteine* showed no beneficial effect on changes in forced vital capacity, changes in predicted carbon monoxide diffusing capacity, rates of adverse events, or death rates.

REFERENCES
Canestaro, W. J., Forrester, S. H., Raghu, G., Ho, L., & Devine, B. E. (2016). Drug treatment of idiopathic pulmonary fibrosis: Systematic review and network meta-analysis. *Chest, 149*(3), 756–766. doi:10.1016/j.chest.2015.11.013
Sun, T., Liu, J., & Zhao, D. W. (2016). Efficacy of *N*-Acetylcysteine in idiopathic pulmonary fibrosis: A systematic review and meta-analysis. *Medicine, 95*(19), e3629. doi:10.1097/md.0000000000003629

▷ *azathioprine* (D) 1 mg/kg/day in a single or divided doses; may increase by 0.5 mg/kg/day q 4 weeks; max 2.5 mg/kg/day; minimum trial to ascertain effectiveness is 12 weeks
Pediatric: <12 years: not recommended; ≥12 years: same as adult
    Azasan *Tab* 75*, 100*mg
    Imuran *Tab* 50*mg

▷ *nintedanib* (D) recommended dose is 150 mg bid, approximately 12 hours apart, with food; *Mild Hepatic Impairment (Child-Pugh A):* 100 mg bid, approximately 12 hours apart, with food; *Moderate or Severe Hepatic Impairment (Child-Pugh B or C):* not recommended; consider temporary dose reduction to 100 mg, treatment interruption, or discontinuation for management of adverse reactions; prior to initiation of treatment, perform a pregnancy test; Monitor LFTs and bilirubin before and during treatment
Pediatric: <12 years: not established; ≥12 years: same as adult
    Ofev *Cap:* 100, 150 mg
    Comment: Monitor liver enzymes. If elevated LFTs (3 < AST/ALT <5 XULN) without severe liver damage, interrupt therapy or reduce dose to 100 mg bid. When liver enzymes return to baseline, restart at 100 mg bid and titrate up. Diarrhea, nausea, and vomiting have occurred with **Ofev**. Treat patients at first signs with adequate hydration and antidiarrheal medicine (e.g., *loperamide*) or anti-emetics. Discontinue **Ofev** if severe diarrhea, nausea, or vomiting persists despite symptomatic treatment.

Gastrointestinal perforation has been reported. Use **Ofev** with caution when treating patients with recent abdominal surgery. Discontinue **Ofev** in patients who develop gastrointestinal perforation. Only use **Ofev** in patients with known risk of gastrointestinal perforation if the anticipated benefit outweighs the potential risk. Arterial thromboembolic events have been reported. Use caution when treating patients at higher cardiovascular risk including known coronary artery disease (CAD). Bleeding events have been reported. Use **Ofev** in patients with known bleeding risk only if anticipated benefit outweighs the potential risk. There are no human data to inform safety on the use of **Ofev** in pregnancy; however; based on animal studies and the mechanism of action, the use of **Ofev** in pregnancy can cause fetal harm (structural damage during organogenesis and embryo-fetal death). Advise patients of the potential risks to the developing fetus vs patient need/benefit and advise females of reproductive potential to use effective contraception. There is no information on the presence of ***nintedanib*** in human milk or effects on the breastfed infant; breastfeeding is not recommended. Safety and efficacy of **Ofev** have not been studied in patients with severe renal impairment and end-stage renal disease (ESRD). Decreased exposure has been noted in smokers which may alter the efficacy profile of **Ofev**. The most common adverse reactions (≥5%) are: diarrhea, nausea, abdominal pain, vomiting, liver enzyme elevation, decreased appetite, headache, weight decreased, and hypertension. To report suspected adverse reactions, contact Boehringer Ingelheim Pharmaceuticals at (800) 542-6257 or (800) 459-9906 TTY or FDA at 1-800-FDA-1088 or visit www.fda.gov/medwatch.

➤ ***pirfenidone*** (C) take with food at the same time each day; *Days 1-7:* 1 cap tid; *Days 8-14:* 2 caps tid; *Days 15 and ongoing:* 3 caps tid; max 9 caps/day
   Pediatric: <12 years: not established; ≥12 years: same as adult
   Esbriet *Gelcap:* 267 mg

 PYELONEPHRITIS: ACUTE

URINARY TRACT ANALGESIA

➤ ***phenazopyridine*** (B)(G) 95-200 mg q 6 hours prn; max 2 days
   Pediatric: <12 years: not recommended; ≥12 years: same as adult
   AZO Standard, Prodium, Uristat (OTC) *Tab:* 95 mg
   AZO Standard Maximum Strength (OTC) *Tab:* 97.5 mg
   Pyridium, Urogesic *Tab:* 100, 200 mg
   Urogesic *Tab:* 100, 200 mg

OUTPATIENT ANTI-INFECTIVE TREATMENT

Comment: Acute pyelonephritis can be treated with a single IM antibiotic administration followed by a PO antibiotic regimen and close follow up. Example: **Rocephin** 1 gm IM followed by **Bactrim DS**, *cephalexin, ciprofloxacin, levofloxacin,* or *loracarbef.*

➤ ***cephalexin*** (B)(G) 1-4 gm/day in 4 divided doses x 10-14 days
   Pediatric: 25-50 mg/kg/day in 4 divided doses x 10-14 days; *see page 623 for dose by weight*
   Keflex *Cap:* 250, 333, 500, 750 mg; *Oral susp:* 125, 250 mg/5 ml (100, 200 ml) (strawberry)
➤ ***ciprofloxacin*** (C) 500 mg bid or 1000 mg XR once daily x 3-14 days
   Pediatric: <18 years: not recommended; ≥18 years: same as adult
   Cipro (G) *Tab:* 250, 500, 750 mg; *Oral susp:* 250, 500 mg/5 ml (100 ml) (strawberry)
   Cipro XR *Tab:* 500, 1000 mg ext-rel
   ProQuin XR *Tab:* 500 mg ext-rel
➤ ***levofloxacin*** (C) *Uncomplicated:* 500 mg once daily x 10 days; *Complicated:* 750 mg once daily x 10 days
   Pediatric: <18 years: not recommended; ≥18 years: same as adult
   Levaquin *Tab:* 250, 500, 750 mg; *Oral soln:* 25 mg/ml (480 ml) (benzyl alcohol);
   Inj conc: 25 mg/ml for IV infusion after dilution for IV infusion (50, 100, 150 ml) (preservative-free)
➤ ***loracarbef*** (B) 400 mg bid x 14 days
   Pediatric: 15 mg/kg/day in 2 divided doses x 14 days; *see page 628 for dose by weight*
   Lorabid *Pulvule:* 200, 400 mg; *Oral susp:* 100 mg/5 ml (50, 100 ml); 200 mg/5 ml (50, 75, 100 ml) (strawberry bubble gum)

▷ *trimethoprim+sulfamethoxazole (TMP-SMX)* (D)(G) bid x 10 days
  Pediatric: <2 months: not recommended; ≥2 months: 40 mg/kg/day of *sulfamethoxazole* in
  2 divided doses x 10 days; *see page 630 for dose by weight*
    Bactrim, Septra 2 tabs bid x 10 days
      Tab: trim 80 mg+sulfa 400 mg*
    Bactrim DS, Septra DS 1 tab bid x 10 days
      Tab: trim 160 mg+sulfa 800 mg*
    Bactrim Pediatric Suspension, Septra Pediatric Suspension
      Oral susp: trim 40 mg+sulfa 200 mg per 5 ml (100 ml) (cherry) (alcohol 0.3%)
  Comment: Sulfonamides are contraindicated in the first trimester of pregnancy, the final
  month of pregnancy, and infants <8 weeks-of-age. *CrCl 15-30 mL/min:* reduce dose by 1/2;
  CrCl <15 mL/min: not recommended. Contraindicated with G6PD deficiency. A high fluid
  intake is indicated during sulfonamide therapy to avoid crystallization in the kidneys.

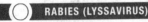

RABIES (LYSSAVIRUS)

PRE-EXPOSURE PROPHYLAXIS (PrEP) AND POST-EXPOSURE PROPHYLAXIS (PEP)

Comment: Have *epinephrine* 1:1000 readily available. Every exposure to possible rabies
infection must be individually evaluated. Rabies vaccine and **Rabies Immune Globulin
(Human) (HRIG)** should be given to all persons suspected of exposure to rabies with one
exception: persons who have been previously immunized with rabies vaccine and have a
confirmed adequate rabies antibody titer should receive only vaccine. Recommendations
for use of passive and active immunization after exposure to an animal suspected of
having rabies have been detailed by the Health Canada National Advisory Committee on
Immunization19 and the U.S. Public Health Service Immunization Practices Advisory
Committee (ACIP). HRIG should be used in conjunction with rabies vaccine and can be
administered through the seventh day after the first dose of vaccine is administered. Beyond
the seventh day, HRIG is not indicated since an antibody response to cell culture vaccine is
presumed to have occurred. If the patient has previously received HRIG, and has a confirmed
adequate rabies antibody titer, administer only the vaccine. HRIG should be administered
as promptly as possible after exposure, but can be administered up to the eighth day after
the first dose of vaccine is administered. Repeated doses of rabies immune globulin should
not be administered once vaccine treatment has been initiated as this could prevent the full
expression of active immunity expected from the rabies vaccine. Administer HRIG via IM
injection only. Do not give intravenously. The recommended HRIG dose 20 IU/kg (0.133
mL/kg) of body weight administered at the time of the first vaccine dose. It may also be given
through the seventh day after the first dose of vaccine is given. If anatomically feasible, up to
one-half the HRIG dose should be thoroughly infiltrated in the area around the wound and
the rest should be administered intramuscularly in the gluteal area or lateral thigh muscle
using a separate syringe and needle. Because of risk of injury to the sciatic nerve, only the
upper, outer quadrant should be used. **HRIG** should never be administered in the same
syringe or needle or in the same anatomical site as vaccine. Because of interference with
active antibody production, the recommended dose should not be exceeded. It is not known
whether rabies immune globulin can cause fetal harm when administered to a pregnant
female or can affect reproduction capacity. It should be administered in pregnancy only if
clearly needed. Safety and effectiveness in the pediatric population have not been established.

PRE-EXPOSURE PROPHYLAXIS (PrEP)

Comment: Postpone pre-exposure prophylaxis during acute febrile illness or infection. Have
epinephrine 1:1000 readily available.

▷ *rabies vaccine, human diploid cell [HDVC]* (C) *Infants and Young Children:* administer IM
  in the vastus lateralis; *All others:* administer IM in the deltoid; do not inject the vaccine into
  the gluteal area as administration in this area may result in lower neutralizing antibody
  titers; *Not previously immunized: Day 0,* administer 1 ml IM as soon as possible after exposure; then repeat on days 7, and 21 or 28; administer 1st dose with rabies immune globulin,
  human (HRIG); *Previously immunized:* only 2 doses are administered; Day 0, Administer 1
  ml IM immediately after exposure and again 3 days later; no HRIG is needed
    Imovax, RabAvert *Vial:* 2.5 IU/ml (1 ml) (2.5 IU of freeze-dried vaccine w. diluent) for
    IM injection after reconstitution (preservative-free)

Comment: Administer vaccine immediately after reconstitution. If not used, discard. It is also not known whether rabies vaccine can cause fetal harm when administered to a pregnant female or can affect reproductive capacity. Rabies vaccine 10 should be given to a pregnant woman only if potential benefits outweigh potential risks. All serious systemic neuroparalytic or anaphylactic reactions to a rabies vaccine should be immediately reported to VAERS at 1-800-822-7967 (http://vaers.hhs.gov) or Sanofi Pasteur at 1-800-VACCINE (1-800-822-2463).

POST-EXPOSURE PROPHYLAXIS (PEP)

Rabies Immune Globulin, Human (HRIG)

▷ *rabies immune globulin, human (HRIG)* (C) administer 20 IU/kg infiltrated into wound area as much as feasible, then remaining dose administered IM at site remote from vaccine administration

    BayRab, KamRAB, Imogam Rabies HT *Vial:* 150 IU/ml (2, 10 ml)

    Comment: Administer *rabies immune globulin, human (HRIG)* concurrently with a full course of rabies vaccine if the patient have not previously received the rabies vaccine and has confirmed adequate antibodies, administer only the vaccine.

    HyperRAB S/D *Vial:* 300 IU/2 ml (2 ml); 1500 IU/10 ml (10 ml), single-dose

    Comment: **HyperRAB S/D** is a high-potency rabies immunoglobulin.

Comment: If the patient has previously received rabies vaccine, and has a confirmed adequate rabies antibody titer, administer only the vaccine. Repeated dosing of *immune globulin, human (HRIG)* after administration of rabies vaccine may suppress the immune response to the vaccine. If the patient has not previously received rabies vaccine, administer **HRIG** concurrently with a full course of rabies vaccine. Defer live vaccine (measles, mumps, rubella) administration for 4 months. There are no data with **HRIG** use in pregnant women to inform a drug-associated risk. There is no information regarding the presence of HRIG in human milk or effect on the breastfed infant.

TETANUS PROPHYLAXIS VACCINE

See Tetanus page 478 for patients not vaccinated within the past 5 years.

RESPIRATORY SYNCYTIAL VIRUS (RSV)

PROPHYLAXIS

▷ *palivizumab* 15 mg/kg IM administered monthly throughout the RSV season
    Synagis *Vial:* 100 mg/ml

TREATMENT

See Bronchiolitis page 60

RESTLESS LEGS SYNDROME (RLS)

GAMMA AMINOBUTYRIC ACID ANALOGS

▷ *gabapentin* (C)(G) 100 mg once daily x 1 day; then 100 mg bid x 1 day; then 100 mg tid thereafter; max 900 mg tid

    Gralise (C) initially 300 mg on Day 1; then 600 mg on Day 2; then 900 mg on Days 3-6; then 1200 mg on Days 7-10; then 1500 mg on Days 11-14; titrate up to 1800 mg on Day 15; take entire dose once daily with the evening meal; do not crush, split, or chew
    Pediatric: <12 years: not recommended; ≥12 years: same as adult
        Tab: 300, 600 mg

    Neurontin (G) 100 mg daily x 1 day, then 100 mg bid x 1 day, then 100 mg tid continuously; max 900 mg tid
    Pediatric: <3 years: not recommended; 3-12 years: initially 10-15 mg/kg/day in 3 divided doses; max 12 hours between doses; titrate over 3 days; 3-4 years: titrate to 40 mg/kg/day; 5-12 years: titrate to 25-35 mg/kg/day; max 50 mg/kg/day;

▷ *gabapentin enacarbil* (C) 600 mg once daily at about 5:00 PM; if dose not taken at recommended time, next dose should be taken the following day; swallow whole; take with food; *CrCl 30-59 mL/min:* 600 mg on Day 1, Day 3, and every day thereafter; *CrCl <30 mL/min* or on hemodialysis: not recommended

Pediatric: <12 years: not recommended; ≥12 years: same as adult

   Horizant *Tab:* 600 ext-rel

Comment: Avoid abrupt cessation of *gabapentin* and *gabapentin enacarbil*. To discontinue, withdraw gradually over 1 week or longer.

DOPAMINE RECEPTOR AGONISTS

▷ *pramipexole dihydrochloride* (C)(G) initially 0.125 mg once daily 2-3 hours before bedtime; may double dose every 4-7 days; max 0.75 mg/day
   Pediatric: <12 years: not recommended; ≥12 years: same as adult
   Mirapex *Tab:* 0.125, 0.25*, 0.5*, 0.75*, 1*, 1.5*mg

▷ *ropinirole* (C) take once daily 1-3 hours prior to bedtime; initially 0.25 mg on days 1 and 2; then 0.5 mg on days 3-7; increase by 0.5 mg/day at 1 week intervals to 3 mg; max 4 mg/day
   Pediatric: <12 years: not recommended; ≥12 years: same as adult
   Requip *Tab:* 0.25, 0.5, 1, 2, 3, 4, 5 mg

▷ *rotigotine* transdermal patch (C) apply to clean, dry, intact skin on abdomen, thigh, hip, flank, shoulder, or upper arm; initially 1 mg/24 Hrs patch once daily; may increase weekly by 1 mg/24 Hrs if needed; max 3 mg/24 Hrs once daily; rotate sites and allow 14 days before reusing site; if hairy, shave site at least 3 days before application to site; avoid abrupt cessation; reduce by 1 mg/24 Hrs every other day
   Pediatric: <12 years: not recommended; ≥12 years: same as adult
   Neupro *Trans patch:* 1 mg/24 Hrs, 2 mg/24 Hrs, 3 mg/24 Hrs, 4 mg/24 Hrs, 6 mg/24 Hrs, 8 mg/24 Hrs (30/carton) (sulfites)

◯ RETINITIS: CYTOMEGALOVIRUS (CMV)

Comment: *cidofovir* and *valganciclovir* are nucleoside analogs and prodrugs of *ganciclovir* indicated for the treatment of AIDS-related *cytomegalovirus* (CMV) retinitis and prevention of CMV disease in adult kidney, heart, and kidney-pancreas transplant patients at high risk, and for prevention of CMV disease in pediatric kidney and heart transplant patients at high risk. *letermovir* is a CMV DNA terminase complex inhibitor indicated for prophylaxis of CMV infection and disease in adult CMV-seropositive recipients [R+] of an allogeneic hemato-poietic stem cell transplant (HSCT).

▷ *cidofovir* (C) administer via IV infusion over 1 hour; pre-treat with oral *probenecid* (2 gm, 3 hours prior to starting the *cidofovir* infusion and 1 gm, 2 and 8 hours after the infusion is ended) and 1 liter of IV NaCl should be infused immediately before each dose of *cidofovir* (a 2nd liter of NaCl should also be infused either during or after each dose of *cidofovir* if a fluid load is tolerable); *Induction:* 5 mg/kg once weekly for 2 consecutive weeks; *Maintenance:* 5 mg/kg once every 2 weeks; reduce to 3 mg/kg if serum creatinine (sCr) increases 0.3-0.4 mg/dL above baseline; discontinue if sCr increases to >0.5 mg/dL above baseline or if >3+ proteinuria develops
   Pediatric: <12 years: not recommended; ≥12 years: same as adult
   Vistide *Vial:* 75 mg/ml (5 ml) (preservative-free)
   Comment: *cidofovir* is a nucleoside analog indicated for treatment of AIDS-related *cytomegalovirus* (CMV) retinitis.

▷ *valganciclovir* (C)(G) take with food; *Induction:* 900 mg bid x 21 days; *Maintenance:* 900 mg daily; CrCl <60 mL/min: reduce dose (see mfr pkg insert; hemodialysis or CrCl <10 mL/min not recommended (use *ganciclovir*)
   Pediatric: <4 months: not recommended; 4 months-16 years: see mfr pkg insert for dosing calculation equation
   Valcyte *Tab:* 450 mg (preservative-free); *Oral pwdr for reconstitution:* 50 mg/ml (tutti-frutti)

CMV DNA TERMINASE VOMPLRX INHIBITOR

Comment: *letermovir* is a CMV DNA terminase complex inhibitor indicated for prophylaxis of CMV infection and disease in adult CMV-seropositive recipients [R+] of an allogeneic hemato-poietic stem cell transplant (HSCT).

▷ *cidofovir* (C) administer via IV infusion over 1 hour; pre-treat with oral probenecid (2 gm, 3 hours prior to starting the cidofovir infusion and 1 gm, 2 and 8 hours after the infusion is ended) and 1 liter of IV NaCl should be infused immediately before each dose of cidofovir (a 2nd liter of NaCl should also be infused either during or after each dose of cidofovir if a fluid load is tolerable); Induction: 5 mg/kg once weekly for 2 consecutive weeks; Maintenance: 5 mg/kg once every 2 weeks; reduce to 3 mg/kg if serum creatinine (sCr) increases 0.3-0.4 mg/dL above baseline; discontinue if sCr increases to >0.5 mg/dL above baseline or if >3+ proteinuria develops

Pediatric: <12 years: not recommended; >12 years: same as adult

    Vistide *Vial:* 75 mg/ml (5 ml) (preservative-free)

Comment: cidofovir is a nucleoside analog indicated for treatment of AIDS-related cytomegalovirus (CMV) retinitis.

➤ *letermovir* administer dose orally or as an IV infusion over 1 hour; dose is 480 mg once daily through 100 days post-transplant; if co-administered with *cyclosporine*, decrease the *letermovir* dose to 240 mg once daily

Pediatric: <18 years: not recommended; ≥18 years: same as adult

    Prevymis *Tab:* 240, 450 mg; *Vial:* 240 mg/12 ml (20 mg/ml), 480 mg/24 ml (20 mg/ml), single-dose

Comment: Closely monitor serum creatinine levels in patients with CrCL <50 mL/min using **Prevymis** injection for IV infusion. **Prevymis** is not recommended for patients with severe (Child-Pugh C) hepatic impairment. **Prevymis** is contraindicated with *pimozide*, ergot alkaloids, and *pitavastatin* and *simvastatin* when co-administered with *cyclosporine*. Most common adverse events (10%) have been nausea, diarrhea, vomiting, peripheral edema, cough, head ache, fatigue, and abdominal pain. No adequate human data are available to inform whether **Prevymis** poses a risk to pregnancy outcomes. It is not known whether *letermovir* is present in human breast milk or effects the breastfed infant. To report suspected adverse reactions, contact Merck Sharp & Dohme, a subsidiary of Merck, at 1-877888-4231 or FDA at 1-800-FDA-1088 or visit www.fda.gov/medwatch.

➤ *valganciclovir* (C)(G) take with food; Induction: 900 mg bid x 21 days; Maintenance: 900 mg daily; CrCl <60 mL/min: reduce dose (see mfr pkg insert; hemodialysis or CrCl <10 mL/min not recommended (use ganciclovir)

Pediatric: <4 months: not recommended; 4 months-16 years: see mfr pkg insert for dosing calculation equation

    Valcyte *Tab:* 450 mg (preservative-free); Oral pwdr for reconstitution: 50 mg/ml (tutti-frutti)

RHEUMATOID ARTHRITIS (RA)

Injectable Acetaminophen *see Pain page 352*
NSAIDs *see page 571*
Opioid Analgesics *see Pain page 354*
Topical & Transdermal Analgesics *see Pain page 352*
Parenteral Corticosteroids *see page 577*
Oral Corticosteroids *see page 577*
Topical Analgesic and Anesthetic Agents *see page 569*

TOPICAL AND TRANSDERMAL ANALGESICS

➤ *capsaicin* cream (B)(G) apply tid-qid prn to intact skin

Pediatric: <2 years: not recommended; ≥2 years: same as adult

    Axsain *Crm:* 0.075% (1, 2 oz)
    Capsin *Lotn:* 0.025, 0.075% (59 ml)
    Capzasin-HP (OTC) *Crm:* 0.075% (1.5 oz), 0.025% (45, 90 gm); *Lotn:* 0.075% (2 oz); 0.025% (45, 90 gm)
    Capzasin-P (OTC) *Crm:* 0.025% (1.5 oz); *Lotn:* 0.025% (2 oz)
    Dolorac *Crm:* 0.025% (28 gm)
    Double Cap (OTC) *Crm:* 0.05% (2 oz)
    R-Gel *Gel:* 0.025% (15, 30 gm)
    Zostrix (OTC) *Crm:* 0.025% (0.7, 1.5, 3 oz)
    Zostrix HP (OTC) *Emol crm:* 0.075% (1, 2 oz)

➤ *capsaicin* 8% patch (B) apply up to 4 patches for one 60-minute application to clean dry skin; may prep area with topical anesthetic; wear non-latex gloves; patches may be cut to size/shape; treatment may be repeated every 3 months

Pediatric: <18 years: not recommended; ≥18 years: same as adult

Qutenza *Patch:* 8% 1640 mcg/cm (179 mg) (1 or 2 patches w. 1-50 gm tube cleansing gel/carton)

▷ *diclofenac sodium* (C; D ≥30 wks)(G) apply qid prn to intact skin
Pediatric: <12 years: not established; ≥12 years: same as adult

Pennsaid 1.5% in 10 drop increments, dispense and rub into front, side, and back of knee: usually; 40 drops (40 mg) qid
Topical soln: 1.5% (150 ml)

Pennsaid 2% apply 2 pump actuations (40 mg) and rub into front, side, and back of knee bid
Topical soln: 2% (20 mg/pump actuation, 112 gm)

Solaraze Gel massage in to clean skin bid prn
Gel: 3% (50 gm) (benzyl alcohol)

Voltaren Gel (G) apply qid prn to intact skin
Gel: 1% (100 gm)

Comment: *diclofenac* is contraindicated with *aspirin* allergy. As with other NSAIDs, should be avoided in late pregnancy (≥30 weeks) because it may cause premature closure of the ductus arteriosus.

▷ *doxepin* (B) cream apply to affected area qid at intervals of at least 3-4 hours; max 8 days
Pediatric: <12 years: not recommended; >12 years: same as adult

Prudoxin *Crm:* 5% (45 gm)
Zonalon *Crm:* 5% (30, 45 gm)

▷ *pimecrolimus* 1% cream (C)(G) <2 years: not recommended; ≥2 years: apply to affected area bid; do not apply an occlusive dressing
Elidel *Crm:* 1% (30, 60, 100 gm)

Comment: *pimecrolimus* is indicated for short-term and intermittent long-term use. Discontinue use when resolution occurs. Contraindicated if the patient is immunosuppressed. Change to the 0.1% preparation or if secondary bacterial infection is present.

▷ *trolamine salicylate* apply tid-qid
Pediatric: <2 years: not recommended; ≥2 years: same as adult
Mobisyl Creme *Crm:* 10% (100 gm)

ORAL SALICYLATE

▷ *indomethacin* (C) initially 25 mg bid-tid, increase as needed at weekly intervals by 25-50 mg/day; max 200 mg/day
Pediatric: <14 years: usually not recommended; >2 years, if risk warranted: 1-2 mg/kg/day in divided doses; max 3-4 mg/kg/day (or 150-200 mg/day, whichever is less; <14 years: ER cap not recommended
Cap: 25, 50 mg; *Susp;* 25 mg/5 ml (pineapple-coconut, mint) (alcohol 1%); *Supp:* 50 mg; *ER Cap:* 75 mg ext-rel

Comment: *indomethacin* is indicated only for acute painful flares. Administer with food and/or antacids. Use lowest effective dose for shortest duration.

ORAL NSAID

See more **Oral NSAIDs** *page 571*

▷ *diclofenac sodium* (C)(G)
Voltaren 50 mg bid-qid or 75 mg bid or 25 mg qid with an additional 25 mg at HS if necessary
Pediatric: <12 not recommended; ≥12 years: same as adult
Tab: 25, 50, 75 mg ent-coat
Voltaren XR 100 mg once daily; rarely, 100 mg bid may be used
Pediatric: <18 not recommended; ≥18 years: same as adult
Tab: 100 mg ext-rel

ORAL NSAID+PPI

▷ *esomeprazole+naproxen* (C)(G) 1 tab bid; use lowest effective dose for the shortest duration swallow whole; take at least 30 minutes before a meal
Pediatric: <18 not recommended; ≥18 years: same as adult
Vimovo *Tab:* nap 375 mg+eso 20 mg ext-rel; nap 500 mg+eso 20 mg ext-rel
Comment: **Vimovo** is indicated to improve signs/symptoms, and risk of gastric ulcer in patients at risk of developing NSAID-associated gastric ulcer.

COX-2 INHIBITORS

Comment: Cox-2 inhibitors are contraindicated with history of asthma, urticaria, and allergic-type reactions to *aspirin*, other NSAIDs, and sulfonamides, 3rd trimester of pregnancy, and coronary artery bypass graft (CABG) surgery.

▶ *celecoxib* (C)(G) 50-400 mg once daily-bid; max 800 mg/day
   Pediatric: <18 years: not recommended; ≥18 years: same as adult
      Celebrex *Cap:* 50, 100, 200, 400 mg

▶ *meloxicam* (C)(G)
      Mobic <2 years, <60 kg: not recommended; ≥2, ≥60 kg: 0.125 mg/kg; max 7.5 mg once daily; ≥18 years: initially 7.5 mg once daily; max 15 mg once daily; *Hemodialysis:* max 7.5 mg/day
         Tab: 7.5, 15 mg; *Oral susp:* 7.5 mg/5 ml (100 ml) (raspberry)
      Vivlodex <18 years: not established; ≥18 years: initially 5 mg qd; may increase to max 10 mg/day; Hemodialysis: max 5 mg/day
         Cap: 5, 10 mg

JANUS KINASE (JAK) INHIBITOR (JAKI)

▶ *baricitinib* recommended dose is 2 mg once daily; avoid initiation or interrupt **Olumiant** in patients with Hgb <8 gm/dL and/or absolute lymphocyte count (ALC) <500 cells/mm³, and/or absolute neutropenia count (ANC)
      Olumiant *Tab:* 2 mg <1000 cells/mm³.

   Comment: **Olumiant** *(baricitinib)* is indicated for the treatment pf patients ≥18 years-of-age with moderate-to-severe active RA who have had an inadequate response to one or more TNF antagonist therapies. **Olumiant** may be used as monotherapy or in combination with *methotrexate* (MTX) or other DMARDs; **Olumiant** is not recommended in combination with other JAK inhibitors, biologic DMARDs, potent immunosuppressants (e.g., *azathioprine, cyclosporine*), or strong organic anion transporter 3 (OAT3) inhibitors (e.g., probenecid). **Olumiant** is not recommended with moderate-to-severe renal impairment or severe hepatic impairment. Adverse reactions (incidence ≥1%) include nausea, upper respiratory infections (URIs), herpes simplex, and herpes zoster. Laboratory assessments are recommended due to potential for changes in lymphocytes, neutrophils, hemoglobin, liver enzymes, and lipids. Avoid use of **Olumiant** with active serious infection including localized infection or tuberculosis (TB). If infection occurs, halt the **Olumiant** until the infection is controlled or resolved. Avoid use of **Olumiant** with live vaccines. Use caution in patients who might be at risk for thrombosis or gastrointestinal perforation. Limited human data on use of **Olumiant** in pregnancy are not sufficient to inform drug-associated risk for major birth defects or miscarriage. No information is available on the presence of **Olumiant** in human milk or effects on the breastfed infant. To report suspected adverse reactions contact Eli Lilly and Company at 1-800-LillyRx (1-800-545-5979) or FDA at 1-800-FDA-1088 or visit www.fda.gov/medwatch.

▶ *tofacitinib* (C) 5 mg twice daily or 11 mg once daily; discontinue after 16 weeks if adequate therapeutic benefit is not achieved; use the lowest effective dose to maintain response; see mfr pkg insert for dosage adjustments for patients receiving CYP2C19 and/or CYP3A4 inhibitors; in patients with moderate or severe renal impairment or moderate hepatic impairment, and patients with lymphopenia, neutropenia, or anemia; use of **Xeljanz/Xeljanz XR** in patients with severe hepatic impairment is not recommended in any patient population

   Comment: FDA has issued a MedWatch Alert to the public that a recent safety clinical trial found an increased risk of blood clots in the lungs and death when a 10 mg twice daily dose of *tofacitinib* (Xeljanz, Xeljanz XR) was administered to patients with rheumatoid arthritis (RA). FDA has not approved the 10 mg twice daily dosing regimen for RA; this dosing regimen is only approved for patients with ulcerative colitis (UC).
   Pediatric: <18 years: not recommended; ≥18 years: same as adult
      Xeljanz *Tab:* 5 mg
      Xeljanz XR *Tab:* 11 mg ext-rel

   Comment: **Xeljanz** is indicated for moderate-to-severe RA as monotherapy in patients who have inadequate response or intolerance to *methotrexate* (MTX) and/or in combination with other non-biologic DMARDs. Use **Xeljanz** with caution in patients that may be at increased risk for gastrointestinal perforation. The most common adverse events associated with **Xeljanz** treatment are diarrhea, elevated cholesterol level, headache, herpes zoster (shingles), increased blood creatine phosphokinase, nasopharyngitis, rash, and upper respiratory tract infection (URI). Avoid use of **Xeljanz/Xeljanz XR** during an active serious infection, including localized infection. Patients treated with **Xeljanz** are at increased risk for developing serious infections that may lead to hospitalization or death. **Xeljanz** has a BBW for serious infections (e.g., opportunistic infections), and malignancy (e.g., lymphoma). Use of **Xeljanz** in combination with biological therapies or with potent immunosuppressants, such as *azathioprine* and *cyclosporine*, is not recommended. Avoid live vaccine administration during treatment with **Xeljanz**. Prior to starting **Xeljanz**, perform a test for latent tuberculosis; if it is positive, start treatment for tuberculosis latent tuberculosis test is negative. Recommend lab monitoring due to potential for changes in lymphocytes, neutrophils, hemoglobin, liver enzymes, and lipids. Do not initiate **Xeljanz** if absolute lymphocyte count <500 cells/mm^3, an absolute neutrophil count (ANC) <1000 cells/mm3 or Hgb <9 gm/dL. The safety and effectiveness of **Xeljanz/Xeljanz XR** in pediatric patients have not been established. Available data with **Xeljanz** use in pregnancy are insufficient to establish a drug associated risk of major birth defects, miscarriage, or adverse maternal or fetal outcomes. In animal reproduction studies, fetocidal, and teratogenic effects were noted. There is a pregnancy exposure registry that monitors pregnancy outcomes in females exposed to **Xeljanz/Xeljanz XR** during pregnancy. Consider pregnancy planning and prevention for females of reproductive potential. Patients should be encouraged to enroll in the **Xeljanz/Xeljanz XR** pregnancy registry if they become pregnant. To enroll or obtain information from the registry, patients can call the toll free number 1-877-311-8972. There are no data on the presence of *tofacitinib* in human milk or the effects on a breastfed infant; however, patients should be advised not to breastfeed. To report suspected adverse reactions, contact Pfizer at 1-800-438-1985 or FDA at 1-800-FDA-1088 or visit www.fda.gov/medwatch.

DISEASE MODIFYING ANTI-RHEUMATIC DRUGS (DMARDs)

Comment: DMARDs are first-line treatment options for RA. DMARDs include penicillamine, gold salts (*auranofin*, *aurothio-glucose*), immunosuppressants, and *hydroxychloroquine*. The DMARDs reduce ESR, reduce RF, and favorably affect the outcome of RA. Immunosuppressants may require 6 weeks to affect benefits and 6 months for full improvement.

▶ *auranofin (gold salt)* (C) 3 mg bid or 6 mg once daily; if inadequate response after 6 months, increase to 3 mg tid
Pediatric: <12 years: not recommended; ≥12 years: same as adult
Ridaura *Vial:* 100 mg/20 ml

▶ *azathioprine* (D) 1 mg/kg/day in a single or divided doses; may increase by 0.5 mg/kg/day q 4 weeks; max 2.5 mg/kg/day; minimum trial to ascertain effectiveness is 12 weeks
Pediatric: <12 years: not recommended; ≥12 years: same as adult
Azasan *Tab* 75*, 100*mg
Imuran *Tab* 50*mg

▶ *cyclosporine (immunosuppressant)* (C) 1.25 mg/kg bid; may increase after 4 weeks by 0.5 mg/kg/day; then adjust at 2 week intervals; max 4 mg/kg/day; administer with meals
Pediatric: <12 years: not recommended; ≥12 years: same as adult
Neoral *Cap:* 25, 100 mg (alcohol)
Neoral Oral Solution *Oral soln:* 100 mg/ml (50 ml) may dilute in room temperature apple juice or orange juice (alcohol)
Comment: **Neoral** is indicated for RA unresponsive to *methotrexate (MTX)*.

▶ *hydroxychloroquine* (C) 400-600 mg/day
Pediatric: <12 years: not recommended; ≥12 years: same as adult
Plaquenil *Tab:* 200 mg
Comment: May require several weeks to achieve beneficial effects. If no improvement in 6 months, discontinue.

▶ *leflunomide* (X)(G) initially 100 mg once daily x 3 days; maintenance dose 20 mg once daily; max 20 mg daily
Pediatric: <18 years: not recommended; ≥18 years: same as adult
Arava *Tab:* 10, 20, 100 mg
Comment: **Arava** is contraindicated with breastfeeding.

▷ **methotrexate (MTX) (X)** 7.5 mg x 1 dose per week <u>or</u> 2.5 mg x 3 at 12 hour intervals once a week; max 20 mg/week; therapeutic response begins in 3-6 weeks; administer **methotrexate** injection SC only into the abdomen <u>or</u> thigh

Pediatric: <2 years: not recommended; ≥2 years: 10 mg/m² once weekly; max 20 mg/m²

   Rasuvo *Autoinjector:* 7.5 mg/0.15 ml, 10 mg/0.20 ml, 12.5 mg/0.25 ml, 15 mg/0.30 ml, 17.5 mg/0.35 ml, 20 mg/0.40 ml, 22.5 mg/0.45 ml, 25 mg/0.50 ml, 27.5 mg/0.55 ml, 30 mg/0.60 ml (solution concentration for SC injection is 50 mg/ml)

   Rheumatrex *Tab:* 2.5*mg (5, 7.5, 10, 12.5, 15 mg/week, 4/card unit-of-use dose pack)

   Trexall *Tab:* 5*, 7.5*, 10*, 15*mg (5, 7.5, 10, 12.5, 15 mg/week, 4/card unit-of-use dose pack)

Comment: **methotrexate (MTX)** is contraindicated with immunodeficiency, blood dyscrasias, alcoholism, and chronic liver disease.

▷ **penicillamine** administer on an empty stomach, at least one hour before meals <u>or</u> two hours after meals, <u>and</u> at least one hour apart from any other drug, food, milk, antacid, zinc or iron-containing preparation ; maintenance dosage must be individualized, and may require adjustment during the course of treatment. *initially*, a single daily dose of 125-250 mg; then, increase at 1-3 month intervals by 125-250 mg/day, as patient response and tolerance indicate; if a satisfactory remission of symptoms is achieved, the dose associated with the remission should be continued as the patient's maintenance therapy; if there is <u>no</u> improvement, and there are <u>no</u> signs of potentially serious toxicity after 2-3 months of treatment with doses of 500-750 mg/day, increase by 250 mg/day at 2-3 month intervals until a satisfactory remission occurs <u>or</u> signs of toxicity develop; if there is <u>no</u> discernible improvement after 3-4 months of treatment with 1000-1500 mg/day, discontinue **Cuprimine**. Changes in maintenance dosage levels may <u>not</u> be reflected clinically <u>or</u> in the erythrocyte sedimentation rate (ESR) for 2-3 months after each dosage adjustment.

   Cuprimine *Cap:* 125, 250 mg

   Depen: 250 mg

Comment: The use of **penicillamine** has been associated with fatalities due to certain diseases such as aplastic anemia, agranulocytosis, thrombocytopenia, Goodpasture's syndrome, and myasthenia gravis. Because of the potential for serious hematological and renal adverse reactions to occur at any time, routine urinalysis, white and differential blood cell count, hemoglobin, and direct platelet count must be checked twice weekly, together with monitoring of the patient's skin, lymph nodes and body temperature, during the first month of therapy, every two weeks for the next five months, and monthly thereafter. Patients should be instructed to report promptly the development of signs and symptoms of granulocytopenia and/or thrombocytopenia such as fever, sore throat, chills, bruising or bleeding; the above laboratory studies should then be promptly repeated.

▷ **sulfasalazine (C; D in 2nd, 3rd)(G)** initially 0.5 gm once daily bid; gradually increase every 4 days; usual maintenance 2-3 gm/day in equally divided doses at regular intervals; max 4 gm/day

Pediatric: <6 years: not recommended; 6-16 years: initially 1/4 to 1/3 of maintenance dose; increase weekly; maintenance 30-50 mg/kg/day in 2 divided doses at regular intervals; max 2 gm/day; >16 years: same as adult

   Azulfidine *Tab:* 500 mg

   Azulfidine EN *Tab:* 500 mg ent-coat

TUMOR NECROSIS FACTOR (TNF) BLOCKERS

▷ **adalimumab (B)** 40 mg SC once every other week; may increase to once weekly without **methotrexate** (MTX); administer in abdomen <u>or</u> thigh; rotate sites; 2-17 years, supervise first dose

Pediatric: <2 years, <10 kg: not recommended; 10-<15 kg: 10 mg every other week; 15-<30 kg: 20 mg every other week; ≥30 kg: 40 mg every other week

   Humira *Prefilled syringe:* 20 mg/0.4 ml; 40 mg/0.8 ml single-dose (2/pck; 2, 6/starter pck) (preservative-free)

Comment: **Humira** may use with **methotrexate** (MTX), DMARDs, corticosteroids, salicylates, NSAIDs, <u>or</u> analgesics.

▷ **adalimumab-adbm (B)** initially 80 SC; then, 40 mg SC every other week starting one week after initial dose; inject into thigh or abdomen; rotate sites

Pediatric: <18 years: not recommended; ≥18 years: same as adult

   Cyltezo *Prefilled syringe:* 40 mg/0.8 ml single-dose (preservative-free)

Comment: **Cyltezo** is biosimilar to **Humira** (*adalimumab*).

▶ *certolizumab pegol* (B) 400 mg SC on day 1, at week 2, and at week 4; then 200 mg every other week; rotate sites
Pediatric: <12 years: not recommended; ≥12 years: same as adult
    Cimzia *Vial:* 200 mg single-dose w. supplies (2/pck, 2, 6/starter pck); *Prefilled syringe:* 200 mg single-dose w. supplies (2/pck, 2, 6/starter pck) (preservative-free)

▶ *etanercept* (B) 25 mg SC twice weekly, 72-96 hours apart or 50 mg SC weekly; rotate sites
Pediatric: <4 years: not recommended; 4-17 years: 0.4 mg/kg SC twice weekly, 72-96 hours apart (max 25 mg/dose) or 0.8 mg/kg SC weekly (max 50 mg/dose)
    Enbrel *Vial:* 25 mg pwdr for SC injection after reconstitution (4/carton w. supplies) (preservative-free; diluent contains benzyl alcohol); *Prefilled syringe:* 50 mg/ml (preservative-free); *SureClick autoinjector:* 50 mg/ml (preservative-free)

Comment: *etanercept* reduces pain, morning stiffness, and swelling. May be administered in combination with *methotrexate*. Live vaccines should not be administered concurrently. Do not administer with active infection.

▶ *golimumab* (B) administer SC or IV infusion (in combination with *methotrexate* [MTX])
Pediatric: <12 years: not recommended; ≥12 years: same as adult
    Simponi 50 mg SC once monthly; rotate sites
      Prefilled syringe, SmartJect autoinjector: 50 mg/0.5 ml, single-use (preservative-free)
    Simponi Aria 2 mg/kg IV infusion week 0 and week 4; then every 8 weeks thereafter
      Vial: 50 mg/4 ml, single-use, soln for IV infusion after dilution (latex-free, preservative-free)

Comment: corticosteroids, non-biologic DMARDs, and/or NSAIDs may be continued during treatment with *golimumab*.

▶ *infliximab (tumor necrosis factor-alpha blocker)* must be refrigerated at 2°C to 8°C (36°F to 46°F); administer dose intravenously over a period of not less than 2 hours; do not use beyond the expiration date as this product contains no preservative; 5 mg/kg at 0, 2 and 6 weeks, then every 8 weeks.
Pediatric: <6 years: not studied; ≥6-17 years: mg/kg at 0, 2 and 6 weeks, then every 8 weeks; ≥18 years: same as adult
    Remicade *Vial:* 100 mg for reconstitution to 10 ml administration volume, single-dose (preservative-free)

Comment: Use *infliximab* concomitantly with *methotrexate* when there has been insufficient response to *methotrexate* alone. Remicade is indicated to reduce signs and symptoms, and induce and maintain clinical remission, in adults and children ≥6 years-of-age with moderately to severely active disease who have had an inadequate response to conventional therapy and reduce the number of draining enterocutaneous and rectovaginal fistulas, and maintain fistula closure, in adults with fistulizing disease. Common adverse effects associated with Remicade included abdominal pain, headache, pharyngitis, sinusitis, and upper respiratory infections. In addition, Remicade might increase the risk for serious infections, including tuberculosis, bacterial sepsis, and invasive fungal infections. Available data from published literature on the use of *infliximab* products during pregnancy have not reported a clear association with *infliximab* products and adverse pregnancy outcomes. *infliximab* products cross the placenta and infants exposed *in utero* should not be administered live vaccines for at least 6 months after birth. Otherwise, the infant may be at increased risk of infection, including disseminated infection which can become fatal. Available information is insufficient to inform the amount of *infliximab* products present in human milk or effects on the breastfed infant. To report suspected adverse reactions, contact Merck Sharp & Dohme Corp., a subsidiary of Merck & Co. at 1-877-888-4231 or FDA at 1-800-FDA1088 or www.fda.gov/medwatch.

▶ *infliximab-abda (tumor necrosis factor-alpha blocker)* (B)
    Renflexis: see *infliximab* (Remicade) above for full prescribing information
    Comment: Renflexis is a biosimilar to Remicade for the treatment of immune-disorders including Crohn's disease, ulcerative colitis, rheumatoid arthritis, ankylosing spondylitis, psoriatic arthritis and plaque psoriasis. Renflexis was approved under the FDA category for biosimilars and demonstrated no clinically meaningful differences for use, dosing regimens, strengths, dosage forms, and routes of administration from the FDA-approved biological product Remicade.

▶ *infliximab-dyyb (tumor necrosis factor-alpha blocker)* (B)
    Inflectra: see *infliximab* (Remicade) above for full prescribing information
    Comment: Inflectra is a biosimilar to Remicade for the treatment of immune-disorders including Crohn's disease, ulcerative colitis, rheumatoid arthritis, ankylosing

spondylitis, psoriatic arthritis and plaque psoriasis. **Inflectra** was approved under the FDA category for biosimilars and demonstrated no clinically meaningful differences for use, dosing regimens, strengths, dosage forms, and routes of administration from the FDA-approved biological product **Remicade**.

▷ *infliximab-qbtx (tumor necrosis factor-alpha blocker)* **(B)**
Ifixi: see *infliximab* **(Remicade)** above for full prescribing information
Comment: **Ifixi** is a biosimilar to **Remicade** for the treatment of immune disorders including Crohn's disease, ulcerative colitis, rheumatoid arthritis, ankylosing spondylitis, psoriatic arthritis and plaque psoriasis. **Ifixi** was approved under the FDA category for biosimilars and demonstrated no clinically meaningful differences for use, dosing regimens, strengths, dosage forms, and routes of administration from the FDA-approved biological product **Remicade**.

Interleukin-1 Receptor Antagonist

▷ *anakinra (interleukin-1 receptor antagonist)* **(B)** 100 mg SC once daily; discard any unused portion
Pediatric: <12 years: not recommended; ≥12 years: same as adult
  Kineret *Prefilled syringe:* 100 mg/single-dose syringe (7, 28/pck) (preservative-free)

Interleukin-6 Receptor Antagonists

▷ *sarilumab* 200 mg SC every 2 weeks on the same day; if necessary, the dosage can be reduced 150 mg every 2 weeks to manage potential laboratory abnormalities, such as neutropenia, thrombocytopenia, and liver enzyme elevations; SC injections may be self-administered
Pediatric: <18 years: not recommended; ≥18 years: same as adult
  Kevzara *Prefilled syringe:* 150, 200 mg (1.4 ml, single-use)
Comment: *sarilumab* is a human monoclonal antibody that binds to the interleukin-6 receptor (IL-6R), and has been shown to inhibit IL-6R mediated signaling. IL-6 is a cytokine in the body that, in excess and over time, can contribute to the inflammation associated with RA. **Kevzara** received FDA approval in May, 2017 for use in patients with active moderate-to-severe rheumatoid arthritis (RA) in adults who have had an inadequate response or intolerance to one or more disease modifying antirheumatic drugs (DMARDs). **Kevzara** may be used as monotherapy or in combination with *methotrexate* or other conventional DMARDs. Monitor patient for dose related laboratory changes including elevated LFTs, neutropenia, and thrombocytopenia. **Kevzara** should not be initiated in patients with an absolute neutrophil count (ANC) <2000/mm³, platelet count <150,000/mm³, or liver transaminases above 1.5 times the upper limit of normal (ULN). Registration in the Pregnancy Exposure Registry (1-877-311-8972) is encouraged for monitoring pregnancy outcomes in women exposed to **Kevzara** during pregnancy. Negative side effects of **Kevzara** should be reported to the FDA at www.fda.gov/medwatch or call 1-800-FDA-1088 or call Sanofi-Aventis at 1-800-633-1610. The limited available data with **Kevzara** in pregnant women are not sufficient to determine whether there is a drug-associated risk for major birth defects and miscarriage. Monoclonal antibodies, such as *sarilumab*, are actively transported across the placenta during the third trimester of pregnancy and may affect immune response in the infant exposed *in utero*. It is not known whether *sarilumab* passes into breast milk; therefore, breastfeeding is not recommended while using **Kevzara**.

▷ *tocilizumab* **(B)** *IV Infusion:* administer over 1 hour; do not administer as bolus or IV push; *Adults, PJIA, and SJIA, ≥30 kg:* dilute to 100 mL in 0.9% or 0.45% NaCl. *PJIA and SJIA, <30 kg:* dilute to 50 mL in 0.9% or 0.45% NaCl.
Adults: IV Infusion: Whether used in combination with DMARDs or as monotherapy, the recommended IV infusion starting dose is 4 mg/kg IV every 4 weeks followed by an increase to 8 mg/kg IV every 4 weeks based on clinical response; Max 800 mg per infusion in RA patients; *SC Administration:* ≥100 kg: 162 mg SC once weekly on the same day; <100 kg: 162 mg SC every other week on the same day followed by an increase according to clinical response; SC injections may be self-administered
Pediatric: <2 years: not recommended; ≥2 years: weight-based dosing according to diagnosis: *PJIA:* ≥30 kg: 8 mg/kg SC every 4 weeks; <30 kg: 10 mg/kg SC every 4 weeks; *SJIA:* ≥30 kg: 8 mg/kg SC every 2 weeks; <30 kg: 12 mg/kg SC every 2 weeks
  Actemra *Vial:* 80 mg/4 ml, 200 mg/10 ml, 400 mg/20 ml, single-use, for IV infusion after dilution; *Prefilled syringe:* 162 mg (0.9 ml, single-dose)

Comment: *tocilizumab* is an interleukin-6 receptor-α inhibitor indicated for use in moderate-to-severe rheumatoid arthritis (RA) that has not responded to conventional therapy, and also for some subtypes of juvenile idiopathic arthritis (JIA). **Actemra** may be used alone or in combination with *methotrexate* and in RA, other DMARDs may be used. Monitor patient for dose related laboratory changes including elevated LFTs, neutropenia, and thrombocytopenia. **Actemra** should not be initiated in patients with an absolute neutrophil count (ANC) below 2000 per mm³, platelet count below 100,000 per mm³, or who have ALT or AST above 1.5 times the upper limit of normal (ULN). Registration in the Pregnancy Exposure Registry (1-877-311-8972) is encouraged for monitoring pregnancy outcomes in women exposed to **Actemra** during pregnancy. The limited available data with **Actemra** in pregnant women are not sufficient to determine whether there is a drug-associated risk for major birth defects and miscarriage. Monoclonal antibodies, such as *tocilizumab*, are actively transported across the placenta during the third trimester of pregnancy and may affect immune response in the infant exposed *in utero*. It is not known whether *tocilizumab* passes into breast milk; therefore, breastfeeding is not recommended while using **Actemra**.

Selective Co-stimulation Modulator

▷ *abatacept* (C) administer as an IV infusion over 30 minutes at weeks 0, 2, and 4; then every 4 weeks thereafter; <60 kg, administer 500 mg/dose; 60-100 kg, administer 750 mg/dose; >100 kg, administer 1 gm/dose
Pediatric: <6 years: not recommended; 6-17 years: administer as an IV infusion over 30 minutes at weeks 0, 2, and 4; then every 4 weeks thereafter; <75 kg, administer 10 mg/kg; same as adult (max 1 gm)
   Orencia *Vial:* 250 mg pwdr for IV infusion after reconstitution (silicone-free) (preservative-free); *Prefilled syringe:* 125 mg/ml soln for SC injection (preservative-free); *ClickJect Autoinjector:* 125 mg/ml soln for SC injection

CD20 ANTIBODY

▷ *rituximab* (C) administer corticosteroid 30 minutes prior to each infusion; concomitant *methotrexate* therapy, administer a 1000 mg IV infusion at 0 and 2 weeks; then every 24 weeks or based on response, but not sooner than every 16 weeks.
Pediatric: <6 years: not recommended; ≥6 years: same as adult
   Rituxan *Vial:* 10 mg/ml (10, 50 ml) (preservative-free)

INTRA-ARTICULAR INJECTION

▷ *sodium hyaluronate* 20 mg as intra-articular injection weekly x 5 weeks
Pediatric: <12 years: not recommended; ≥12 years: same as adult
   Hyalgan *Prefilled syringe:* 20 mg/2 ml
   Comment: Remove joint effusion and inject with *lidocaine* if possible before injecting **Hyalgan**.

 RHINITIS/SINUSITIS: ALLERGIC

Drugs for the Management of Allergy, Cough, and Cold Symptoms *see page* 603
Parenteral Corticosteroids *see page* 577
Oral Corticosteroids *see page* 577

Comment: The Joint Task Force on Practice Parameters, which comprises representatives of the American Academy of Allergy, Asthma and Immunology (AAAAI) and the American College of Allergy, Asthma and Immunology (ACAAI), has provided guidance to healthcare providers on the initial pharmacologic treatment of seasonal allergic rhinitis in patients aged ≥12 years. For initial treatment of seasonal allergic rhinitis in persons aged ≥12 years: routinely prescribe monotherapy with an intranasal corticosteroid rather than an intranasal corticosteroid in combination with an oral antihistamine. For initial treatment of seasonal allergic rhinitis in persons aged ≥15 years: recommend an intranasal corticosteroid over a leukotriene. For initial treatment of seasonal allergic rhinitis in persons aged ≥15 years: recommend an intranasal corticosteroid over a leukotriene receptor antagonist. For initial treatment of moderate to severe seasonal allergic rhinitis in persons aged ≥12 years: recommend a combination of an intranasal corticosteroid and an intranasal antihistamine.

REFERENCE

Wallace, D. V., Dykewicz, M. S., Oppenheimer, J., Portnoy, J. M., & Lang, D. M. (2017). Pharmacologic treatment of seasonal allergic rhinitis: Synopsis of guidance from the 2017 Joint Task Force on Practice Parameters. *Annals of Internal Medicine, 167*(12), 876–881. doi:10.7326/m17-2203

SECOND GENERATION ANTIHISTAMINES

Comment: The following drugs are second generation antihistamines. As such they minimally sedating, much less so than the first generation antihistamines. All antihistamines are excreted into breast milk.

▶ *cetirizine* (C)(OTC)(G) initially 5-10 mg once daily; 5 mg once daily; ≥65 years: use with caution
Pediatric: <6 years: not recommended; ≥6 years: same as adult
  cetirizine Cap: 10 mg
  Children's Zyrtec Chewable *Chew tab:* 5, 10 mg (grape)
  Children's Zyrtec Allergy Syrup *Syr:* 1 mg/ml (4 oz) (grape, bubble gum) (sugar-free, dye-free)
  Zyrtec *Tab:* 10 mg
  Zyrtec Hives Relief *Tab:* 10 mg
  Zyrtec Liquid Gels *Liq gel:* 10 mg

▶ *desloratadine* (C)
  Clarinex 1/2-1 tab once daily
  Pediatric: <6 years: not recommended; ≥6 years: same as adult
    Tab: 5 mg
  Clarinex RediTabs 5 mg once daily
  Pediatric: <6 years: not recommended; 6-12 years: 2.5 mg once daily; ≥12 years: same as adult
    ODT: 2.5, 5 mg (tutti-frutti) (phenylalanine)
  Clarinex Syrup 5 mg (10 ml) once daily
  Pediatric: <6 months: not recommended; 6-11 months: 1 mg (2 ml) once daily; 1-5 years: 1.25 mg (2.5 ml) once daily; 6-11 years: 2.5 mg (5 ml) once daily; ≥12 years: same as adult
    Syr: 0.5 mg per ml (4 oz) (tutti-frutti) (phenylalanine)
  Desloratadine ODT 1 tab once daily
  Pediatric: <6 years: not recommended; 6-11 years: 1/2 tab once daily; ≥12 years: same as adult
    ODT: 5 mg

▶ *fexofenadine* (C)(OTC)(G) 60 mg once daily-bid or 180 mg once daily; *CrCl <90 mL/min:* 60 mg once daily
Pediatric: <6 months: not recommended; 6 months-2 years: 15 mg bid; *CrCl ≤90 mL/min:* 15 mg once daily; 2-11 years: 30 mg bid; *CrCl ≤90 mL/min:* 30 mg once daily; ≥12 years: same as adult
  Allegra *Tab:* 30, 60, 180 mg film-coat
  Allegra Allergy *Tab:* 60, 180 mg film-coat
  Allegra ODT *ODT:* 30 mg (phenylalanine)
  Allegra Oral Suspension *Oral susp:* 30 mg/5 ml (6 mg/ml) (4 oz)

▶ *levocetirizine* (B)(OTC)(G) administer dose in the PM; *Seasonal Allergic Rhinitis:* <2 years: not recommended; may start at ≥2 years; *Chronic Idiopathic Urticaria (CIU), Perennial Allergic Rhinitis:* <6 months: not recommended; may start at ≥ 6 months; *Dosing by Age:* 6 months-5 years: max 1.25 mg once daily; 6-11 years: max 2.5 mg once daily; ≥12 years: 2.5-5 mg once daily; *Renal Dysfunction <12 years:* contraindicated; *Renal Dysfunction ≥12 years:* CrCl 50-80 ml/min: 2.5 mg once daily; CrCl 30-50 mL/min: 2.5 mg every other day; CrCl: 10-30 mL/min: 2.5 mg twice weekly (every 3-4 days); CrCl <10 mL/min, ESRD or hemodialysis: contraindicated
  Children's Xyzal Allergy 24HR *Oral Soln:* 0.5 mg/ml (150 ml)
  Xyzal Allergy 24HR *Tab:* 5*mg

▶ *loratadine* (C)(OTC)(G) 5 mg bid or 10 mg once daily; *Hepatic or Renal Insufficiency:* see mfr pkg insert
Pediatric: <2 years: not recommended; 2-5 years: 5 mg once daily; ≥6 years: same as adult
  Children's Claritin Chewables *Chew tab:* 5 mg (grape) (phenylalanine)
  Children's Claritin Syrup 1 mg/ml (4 oz) (fruit) (sugar-free, alcohol-free, dye-free; sodium 6 mg/5 ml)
  Claritin *Tab:* 10 mg

Claritin Hives Relief *Tab:* 10 mg
Claritin Liqui-Gels *Liq gel:* 10 mg
Claritin RediTabs 12 Hours *ODT:* 5 mg (mint)
Claritin RediTabs 24 Hours *ODT:* 10 mg (mint)

FIRST GENERATION ANTIHISTAMINES

▷ *diphenhydramine* (B)(G) 25-50 mg q 6-8 hours; max 100 mg/day
Pediatric: <2 years: not recommended; 2-6 years: 6.25 mg q 4-6 hours; max 37.5 mg/day;
>6-12 years: 12.5-25 mg q 4-6 hours; max 150 mg/day; >12 years: same as adult
Benadryl (OTC) *Chew tab:* 12.5 mg (grape) (phenylalanine); *Liq:* 12.5 mg/5 ml (4, 8 oz); *Cap:* 25 mg; *Tab:* 25 mg; *Dye-free soft gel:* 25 mg; *Dye-free liq:* 12.5 mg/5 ml (4, 8 oz)
▷ *diphenhydramine injectable* (B)(G) 25-50 mg IM immediately; then q 6 hours prn
Pediatric: <12 years: *See mfr pkg insert:* 1.25 mg/kg up to 25 mg IM x 1 dose; then q 6 hours
prn; ≥12 years: same as adult
Benadryl Injectable *Vial:* 50 mg/ml (1 ml single-use); 50 mg/ml (10 ml multidose);
Amp: 10 mg/ml (1 ml); *Prefilled syringe:* 50 mg/ml (1 ml)
▷ *hydroxyzine* (C)(G) 50-100 mg/day divided qid prn
Pediatric: <6 years: 50 mg/day divided qid prn; ≥6 years-12 years: 50 mg/day divided qid
prn; >12 years: same as adult
Atarax *Tab:* 10, 25, 50, 100 mg; *Syr:* 10 mg/5 ml (alcohol 0.5%)
Vistaril *Cap:* 25, 50, 100 mg; *Oral susp:* 25 mg/5 ml (4 oz) (lemon)
Comment: *hydroxyzine* is contraindicated in early pregnancy and in patients with a
prolonged QT interval. It is not known whether this drug is excreted in human milk;
therefore, *hydroxyzine* should not be given to nursing mothers.

ALLERGEN EXTRACTS

Comment: Allergen extracts (**Grastek, Oralair, Ragwitek**) are not for immediate relief of
allergic symptoms. Contraindicated with severe, unstable, and uncontrolled asthma, history
of eosinophilic esophagitis, and severe local or systemic reaction. First dose under supervision
HCP and observe ≥30 minutes. Subsequent doses may be taken at home.
▷ *short ragweed pollen allergen extract* (C) one SL tab once daily
Pediatric: <18 years: not established; ≥18 years: same as adult
Ragwitek *SL tab: Ambrosia artemisiifolia 12 amb a 1-unit* (30, 90/blister pck)
Comment: Initiate **Ragwitek** at least 12 weeks before onset of ragweed pollen season
and continue throughout season.
▷ *sweet vernal, orchard, perennial rye, timothy, Kentucky blue grass mixed pollen allergen
extract* (C) 300 IR once daily
Pediatric: <10 years: not established; 10-17 years: Day 1: 100 IR; Day 2: 200 IR; Day 3 and
thereafter: 300 IR once daily
Oralair *SL tab:* 100, 300 IR (index of reactivity) (30/blister pck)
Comment: **Oralair** is indicated for grass pollen-induced allergic rhinitis with or without
conjunctivitis confirmed by positive skin test. Initiate **Oralair** at least 4 months before
onset of grass pollen season and continue throughout season.
▷ *Timothy grass pollen allergen extract* (C) one SL tab once daily
Pediatric: <5 years: not established; ≥5 years: same as adult
Grastek *SL tab:* 2800 bioequivalent allergy units (BAUS) (30/blister pck)
Comment: **Grastek** is indicated for grass pollen-induced allergic rhinitis with or without
conjunctivitis confirmed by positive skin test. Initiate **Grastek** at least 12 weeks before
onset of grass pollen season and continue throughout season.

NASAL DECONGESTANT

▷ *tetrahydrozoline* (C)
Tyzine 2-4 drops or 3-4 sprays in each nostril q 3-8 hours prn
Pediatric: <6 years: not recommended; ≥6 years: same as adult
Nasal spray: 0.1% (15 ml); *Nasal drops:* 0.1% (30 ml)
Tyzine Pediatric Nasal Drops 2-3 sprays or drops in each nostril q 3-6 hours prn
Nasal drops: 0.05% (15 ml)

LEUKOTRIENE RECEPTOR ANTAGONISTS (LRAs)

Comment: For prophylaxis and chronic treatment only. Not for primary (rescue) treatment of
acute asthma attack.

▷ *montelukast* (B)(G) 10 mg once daily in the PM; for EIB, take at least 2 hours before exercise; max 1 dose/day
  Pediatric: <12 months: not recommended; 12-23 months: one 4 mg granule pkt daily; 2-5 years: one 4 mg chew tab or granule pkt daily; 6-14 years: one 5 mg chew tab daily; ≥15 years: same as adult
    Singulair *Tab:* 10 mg
    Singulair Chewable *Chew tab:* 4, 5 mg (cherry, phenylalanine)
    Singulair Oral Granules: 4 mg/pkt; take within 15 minutes of opening pkt; may mix with applesauce, carrots, rice, or ice cream
▷ *zafirlukast* (B)(G) 20 mg bid, 1 hour ac or 2 hours pc
  Pediatric: <7 years: not recommended; 7-11 years: 10 mg bid 1 hour ac or 2 hours pc; >11 years: same as adult
    Accolate *Tab:* 10, 20 mg
▷ *zileuton* (C)(G)
  Pediatric: <12 years: not recommended; ≥12 years: same as adult
    Zyflo 1 tab qid (total 2400 mg/day)
      Tab: 600 mg
    Zyflo CR 2 tab bid (total 2400 mg/day)
      Tab: 600 mg ext-rel

NASAL CORTICOSTEROIDS

▷ *beclomethasone dipropionate* (C)
    Beconase 1 spray in each nostril bid-qid
      Pediatric: <6 years: not recommended; 6-12 years: 1 spray in each nostril tid; >12 years: same as adult
      Nasal spray: 42 mcg/actuation (6.7 gm, 80 sprays; 16.8 gm, 200 sprays)
    Beconase AQ 1-2 sprays in each nostril bid
      Pediatric: <6: not recommended; ≥6 years: same as adult
      Nasal spray: 42 mcg/actuation (25 gm, 180 sprays)
    Beconase Inhalation Aerosol 1-2 sprays in each nostril bid to qid
      Pediatric: <6: not recommended; 6-12 years: 1 spray in each nostril tid; >12 years: same as adult
      Nasal spray: 42 mcg/actuation (6.7 gm, 80 sprays; 16.8 gm, 200 sprays)
    Vancenase AQ 1-2 sprays in each nostril bid
      Pediatric: <6 years: not recommended; ≥6 years: same as adult
      Nasal spray: 84 mcg/actuation (25 gm, 200 sprays)
    Vancenase AQ DS 1-2 sprays in each nostril once daily
      Pediatric: <6 years: not recommended; ≥6 years: same as adult
      Nasal spray: 84, 168 mcg/actuation (19 gm, 120 sprays)
    Vancenase Pockethaler 1 spray in each nostril bid or qid
      Pediatric: <6: not recommended; ≥6 years: 1 spray in each nostril tid
      Pockethaler: 42 mcg/actuation (7 gm, 200 sprays)
    QNASL Nasal Aerosol 2 sprays, 80 mcg/spray, in each nostril once daily
      Pediatric: <12 years: 2 sprays, 40 mcg/spray, in each nostril once daily; ≥12 years: same as adult
      Nasal spray: 40 mcg/actuation (4.9 gm, 60 sprays); 80 mcg/actuation (8.7 gm, 120 sprays)
▷ *budesonide* (C)
    Rhinocort initially 2 sprays in each nostril bid in the AM and PM, or 4 sprays in each nostril in the AM; max 4 sprays each nostril/day; use lowest effective dose
      Pediatric: <6 years: not recommended; ≥6 years: same as adult
      Nasal spray: 32 mcg/actuation (7 gm, 200 sprays)
    Rhinocort Aqua Nasal Spray initially 1 spray in each nostril once daily; max 4 sprays in each nostril once daily
      Pediatric: <6 years: not recommended; ≥6-12 years: initially 1 spray in each nostril once daily; max 2 sprays in each nostril once daily
      Nasal spray: 32 mcg/actuation (10 ml, 60 sprays)
▷ *ciclesonide* (C)
  Pediatric: <6 years: not recommended; ≥6 years: same as adult
    Omnaris 2 sprays in each nostril once daily
      Nasal spray: 50 mcg/actuation (12.5 gm, 120 sprays)

>> **Zetonna** 1-2 sprays in each nostril once daily
>> *Nasal spray:* 37 mcg/actuation (6.1 gm, 60 sprays) (HFA)

▷ *dexamethasone* (C) 2 sprays in each nostril bid-tid; max 12 sprays/day; maintain at lowest effective dose
Pediatric: <6 years: not recommended; ≥6-12 years: 1-2 sprays in each nostril bid; max 8 sprays/day; maintain at lowest effective dose; >12 years: same as adult
>> **Dexacort Turbinaire** *Nasal spray:* 84 mcg/actuation (12.6 gm, 170 sprays)

▷ *fluticasone furoate* (C) 2 sprays in each nostril once daily; may reduce to 1 spray each nostril once daily
Pediatric: <2 years: not recommended; ≥2-11 years: 1 spray in each nostril once daily; ≥12 years: same as adult
>> **Veramyst** *Nasal spray:* 27.5 mcg/actuation (10 gm, 120 sprays) (alcohol-free)

▷ *fluticasone propionate* (C)(OTC)(G) initially 2 sprays in each nostril once daily or 1 spray bid; maintenance 1 spray once daily
Pediatric: <4 years: not recommended; ≥4 years: initially 1 spray in each nostril once daily; may increase to 2 sprays in each nostril once daily; maintenance 1 spray in each nostril once daily; max 2 sprays in each nostril/day
>> **Flonase** *Nasal spray:* 50 mcg/actuation (16 gm, 120 sprays)

▷ *flunisolide* (C) 2 sprays in each nostril bid; may increase to 2 sprays in each nostril tid; max 8 sprays/nostril/day
Pediatric: <6 years: not recommended; 6-14 years: initially 1 spray in each nostril tid or 2 sprays in each nostril bid; max 4 sprays/nostril/day; >14 years: same as adult
>> **Nasalide** *Nasal spray:* 25 mcg/actuation (25 ml, 200 sprays)
>> **Nasarel** *Nasal spray:* 25 mcg/actuation (25 ml, 200 sprays)

▷ *mometasone furoate* (C)(G) 2 sprays in each nostril once daily
Pediatric: <2 years: not recommended; 2-11 years: 1 spray in each nostril once daily; max 2 sprays in each nostril once daily; >11 years: same as adult
>> **Nasonex** *Nasal spray:* 50 mcg/actuation (17 gm, 120 sprays)

▷ *olopatadine* (C) 2 sprays in each nostril bid
Pediatric: <6 years: not recommended; 6-11 years: 1 spray each nostril bid; >11 years: same as adult
>> **Patanase** *Nasal spray:* 0.6%; 665 mcg/actuation (30.5 gm, 240 sprays) (benzalkonium chloride)

▷ *triamcinolone acetonide* (C)(G) initially 2 sprays in each nostril once daily; max 4 sprays in each nostril once daily or 2 sprays in each nostril bid or 1 spray in each nostril qid; maintain at lowest effective dose
Pediatric: <6 years: not recommended; ≥6 years: 1 spray in each nostril once daily; max 2 sprays in each nostril once daily
>> **Nasacort Allergy 24HR (OTC)** *Nasal spray:* 55 mcg/actuation (10 gm, 120 sprays)
>> **Tri-Nasal** *Nasal spray:* 50 mcg/actuation (15 ml, 120 sprays)

NASAL MAST CELL STABILIZERS

▷ *cromolyn sodium* (B)(OTC) 1 spray in each nostril tid-qid; max 6 sprays in each nostril/day
Pediatric: <2 years: not recommended; ≥2 years: same as adult
>> **Children's NasalCrom, NasalCrom** *Nasal spray:* 5.2 mg/spray (13 ml, 100 sprays; 26 ml, 200 sprays)

Comment: Begin 1-2 weeks before exposure to known allergen. May take 2-4 weeks to achieve maximum effect.

NASAL ANTIHISTAMINES

▷ *azelastine* (C)
>> **Astelin Ready Spray** 2 sprays in each nostril bid
>> *Pediatric:* <5 years: not recommended; ≥5-12 years: 1 spray in each nostril once daily bid; >12 years: same as adult
>>> *Nasal spray:* 137 mcg/actuation (30 ml, 200 sprays) (benzalkonium chloride)
>> **Astepro 0.15% Nasal Spray** 1 or 2 sprays each nostril once daily bid
>> *Pediatric:* <12 years: not recommended; ≥12 years: same as adult
>>> *Nasal spray:* 205.5 mcg/actuation (17 ml, 106 sprays; 30 ml, 200 sprays) (benzalkonium chloride)

NASAL ANTIHISTAMINE+CORTICOSTEROID COMBINATION

➤ *azelastine/fluticasone* (C)(G) 1 spray in each nostril bid
    Pediatric: <6 years: not recommended; ≥6 years: same as adult
        Dymista *Nasal spray:* azel 137 mcg/*flutic* 50 mcg per actuation (23 gm, 120 sprays)
        (benzalkonium chloride)

NASAL ANTICHOLINERGICS

➤ *ipratropium bromide* (B)(G)
        Atrovent Nasal Spray 0.03% 2 sprays in each nostril bid-tid
        Pediatric: <6 years: not recommended; ≥6 years: same as adult
          Nasal spray: 21 mcg/actuation (30 ml, 345 sprays)
        Atrovent Nasal Spray 0.06% 2 sprays in each nostril tid-qid; max 5-7 days
        Pediatric: <5 years: not recommended; ≥5-11 years: 2 sprays in each nostril tid; >11
    years: same as adult
          Nasal spray: 42 mcg/actuation (15 ml, 165 sprays)
  Comment: Avoid use with narrow-angle glaucoma, prostate hyperplasia, and bladder neck
obstruction.

RHINITIS MEDICAMENTOSA

Comment: The nasal/oral regimen selected should be instituted with concurrent weaning
from the nasal decongestant.

Nasal Corticosteroids *see Rhinitis, Sinusitis: Allergic page* 443
Oral Corticosteroids *see page* 577
Parenteral Corticosteroids *see page* 577
OTC **Decongestants**
OTC **Antihistamine+Decongestant Combinations**

NASAL ANTICHOLINERGICS

➤ *ipratropium bromide* (B)(G)
        Atrovent Nasal Spray 0.03% stop nasal decongestant; 2 sprays in each nostril bid-tid
        with progressive weaning as tolerated
        Pediatric: <6 years: not recommended; ≥6 years: same as adult
          Nasal spray: 21 mcg/actuation (30 ml, 345 sprays)
        Atrovent Nasal Spray 0.06% stop nasal decongestant; 2 sprays in each nostril tid-qid
        with progressive weaning as tolerated
        Pediatric: <5 years: not recommended; ≥5-11 years: 2 sprays in each nostril tid; ≥11
    years: same as adult
          Nasal spray: 42 mcg/actuation (15 ml, 165 sprays)
  Comment: Avoid use with narrow-angle glaucoma, prostate hyperplasia, and bladder neck
obstruction

NASAL ANTIHISTAMINE

➤ *azelastine* (C) 2 sprays in each nostril bid
    Pediatric: <5 years: not recommended; ≥5-12 years: 1 spray in each nostril bid
        Astelin Ready Spray *Nasal spray:* 137 mcg/actuation (30 ml, 200 sprays)

FIRST GENERATION ANTIHISTAMINES

➤ *diphenhydramine* (B)(G) 25-50 mg q 6-8 hours; max 100 mg/day
    Pediatric: <2 years: not recommended; 2-6 years: 6.25 mg q 4-6 hours; max 37.5 mg/day;
    >6-12 years: 12.5-25 mg q 4-6 hours; max 150 mg/day; >12 years: same as adult
        Benadryl (OTC) *Chew tab:* 12.5 mg (grape) (phenylalanine); *Liq:* 12.5 mg/5 ml
        (4, 8 oz); *Cap:* 25 mg; *Tab:* 25 mg; *Dye-free soft gel:* 25 mg; *Dye-free liq:* 12.5 mg/5 ml
        (4, 8 oz)
➤ *diphenhydramine* injectable (B)(G) 25-50 mg IM immediately; then q 6 hours prn
    Pediatric: <12 years: See mfr pkg insert: 1.25 mg/kg up to 25 mg IM x 1 dose; then q 6 hours
    prn; ≥12 years:

    Benadryl Injectable *Vial:* 50 mg/ml (1 ml single-use); 50 mg/ml (10 ml multi-dose);
    Amp: 10 mg/ml (1 ml); *Prefilled syringe:* 50 mg/ml (1 ml)

▷ *hydroxyzine* (C)(G) 25 mg tid prn; max 600 mg/day
    Pediatric: <6 years: 50 mg/day divided qid prn; ≥6 years: 50-100 mg/day divided qid prn;
max 600 mg/day
    Atarax *Tab:* 10, 25, 50, 100 mg; *Syr:* 10 mg/5 ml (alcohol 0.5%)
    Vistaril *Cap:* 25, 50, 100 mg; *Oral susp:* 25 mg/5 ml (4 oz) (lemon)

SECOND GENERATION ANTIHISTAMINES

Comment: Second generation antihistamines are sedating, but much less so than the first
generation antihistamines. All antihistamines are excreted into breast milk.

▷ *cetirizine* (C)(OTC)(G) <6 years: not recommended; ≥6-<65 years: initially 5-10 mg once
daily; ≥65 years: 5 mg once daily
    cetirizine Cap: 10 mg
    Children's Zyrtec Chewable *Chew tab:* 5, 10 mg (grape)
    Children's Zyrtec Allergy Syrup *Syr:* 1 mg/ml (4 oz) (grape, bubble gum) (sugar-free,
    dye-free)
    Zyrtec *Tab:* 10 mg
    Zyrtec Hives Relief *Tab:* 10 mg
    Zyrtec Liquid Gels *Liq gel:* 10 mg

▷ *desloratadine* (C)
    Clarinex <6 years: not recommended; ≥6 years: 1/2-1 tab once daily
      Tab: 5 mg
    Clarinex RediTabs <6 years: not recommended; 6-12 years: 2.5 mg once daily; ≥12
    years: 5 mg once daily
      ODT: 2.5, 5 mg (tutti-frutti) (phenylalanine)
    Clarinex Syrup <6 months: not recommended; 6-11 months: 1 mg (2 ml) once daily;
    1-5 years: 1.25 mg (2.5 ml) once daily; 6-11 years: 2.5 mg (5 ml) once daily; ≥12 years: 5
    mg (10 ml) once daily
      Tab: 0.5 mg per ml (4 oz) (tutti-frutti) (phenylalanine)
    Desloratadine ODT

▷ *fexofenadine* (C)(OTC)(G) 6 months-2 years: 15 mg bid; *CrCl ≤90 mL/min:* 15 mg once
daily; 2-11 years: 30 mg bid; *CrCl ≤90 mL/min:* 30 mg once daily ≥12 years and older: ≥12
years: 60 mg once daily-bid or 180 mg once daily; *CrCl <90 mL/min:* 60 mg once daily
Allegra *Tab:* 30, 60, 180 mg film-coat
    Allegra Allergy *Tab:* 60, 180 mg film-coat
    Allegra ODT *ODT:* 30 mg (phenylalanine)
    Allegra Oral Suspension *Oral susp:* 30 mg/5 ml (6 mg/ml) (4 oz)

▷ *levocetirizine* (B)(OTC)(G) administer dose in the PM; *Seasonal Allergic Rhinitis:* <2 years:
not recommended; may start at ≥2 years; *Chronic Idiopathic Urticaria (CIU), Perennial
Allergic Rhinitis:* <6 months: not recommended; may start at ≥ 6 months; *Dosing by Age:*
6 months-5 years: max 1.25 mg once daily; 6-11 years: max 2.5 mg once daily; ≥12 years:
2.5-5 mg once daily; *Renal Dysfunction <12 years:* contraindicated; *Renal Dysfunction ≥12
years:* CrCl 50-80 ml/min: 2.5 mg once daily; CrCl 30-50 mL/min: 2.5 mg every other day;
CrCl: 10-30 mL/min: 2.5 mg twice weekly (every 3-4 days); CrCl <10 mL/min, ESRD or
hemodialysis: contraindicated
    Children's Xyzal Allergy 24HR *Oral Soln:* 0.5 mg/ml (150 ml)
    Xyzal Allergy 24HR *Tab:* 5*mg

▷ *loratadine* (C)(OTC)(G) 5 mg bid or 10 mg once daily; *Hepatic or Renal Insufficiency:* see
mfr pkg insert
    Pediatric: <2 years: not recommended; 2-5 years: 5 mg once daily; ≥6 years: same as
adult
    Children's Claritin Chewables *Chew tab:* 5 mg (grape) (phenylalanine)
    Children's Claritin Syrup 1 mg/ml (4 oz) (fruit) (sugar-free, alcohol-free, dye-free,
    sodium 6 mg/5 ml)
    Claritin *Tab:* 10 mg
    Claritin Hives Relief *Tab:* 10 mg
    Claritin Liqui-Gels *Liq gel:* 10 mg
    Claritin RediTabs 12 Hours *ODT:* 5 mg (mint)
    Claritin RediTabs 24 Hours *ODT:* 10 mg (mint)

RHINITIS: VASOMOTOR

NASAL ANTICHOLINERGICS

Comment: Avoid use with narrow-angle glaucoma, prostate hyperplasia, and bladder neck obstruction

▷ *ipratropium bromide* (B)(G)
> **Atrovent Nasal Spray 0.03%** stop nasal decongestant; 2 sprays in each nostril bid-tid with progressive weaning as tolerated
> *Pediatric:* <6 years: not recommended; ≥6 years: same as adult
>> *Nasal spray:* 21 mcg/actuation (30 ml, 345 sprays)
> **Atrovent Nasal Spray 0.06%** stop nasal decongestant; 2 sprays in each nostril tid-qid with progressive weaning as tolerated
> *Pediatric:* <5 years: not recommended; ≥5-11 years: 2 sprays in each nostril tid; >11 years: same as adult
>> *Nasal spray:* 42 mcg/actuation (15 ml, 165 sprays)

RIVER BLINDNESS (ONCHOCERCIASIS)

ANTHELMINTIC

▷ *moxidectin* (G) take 8 mg (4 x 2 mg tablets) as a single dose, with or without food
> *Pediatric:* <12 years: not recommended; ≥12 years: same as adult
>> *Tab:* 2 mg

Comment: *moxidectin* is a macrocyclic lactone anthelmintic medicine indicated for the treatment of river blindness (onchocerciasis) due to *Onchocerca volvulus* in patients ≥12 years-of-age. *moxidectin* does not kill adult *O. volvulus* parasites. Follow-up is advised. The safety and efficacy of repeat administration of *moxidectin* tablets in patients with *O. volvulus* has not been studied. Cutaneous, ophthalmological and/or systemic adverse reactions of varying severity (Mazzotti Reaction) have occurred in patients with onchocerciasis following treatment. Episodes of symptomatic orthostatic hypotension, including inability to stand without support, may occur in patients following treatment. Serious or even fatal encephalopathy following treatment may occur in patients co-infected with *Loa loa* (assess patients for loiasis in *Loa loa* endemic areas prior to treatment. Patients with hyper-reactive onchodermatitis (sowda) may be more likely than others to experience severe edema and aggravation of onchodermatitis. Limited available data on the use of *moxidectin* in pregnant patients are insufficient to establish whether there is a *moxidectin*-associated risk for major birth defects and miscarriage. *moxidectin* has been detected in human milk following a single 8 mg dose. There are no data on the effects of *moxidectin* on breastfed infants. Risk/benefit of the developmental and health benefits of breastfeeding should be considered along with the mother's clinical need for *moxidectin*. The most common adverse reactions (incidence > 10%) have been eosinophilia, pruritus, musculoskeletal pain, headache, lymphopenia, tachycardia, rash, abdominal pain, hypotension, pyrexia, leukocytosis, influenza-like illness, neutropenia, cough, lymph node pain, dizziness, diarrhea, hyponatremia, and peripheral swelling. To report suspected adverse reactions, contact Medicines Development for Global Health at 1-800-MDGH-456 or FDA at 1-800-FDA-1088 or visit www.fda.gov/medwatch.

ROCKY MOUNTAIN SPOTTED FEVER (RMSF, *RICKETTSIA RICKETTSII*)

ANTI-INFECTIVES

▷ *doxycycline* (D)(G) 200 mg on first day; then 100 mg bid x 7-10 days
> *Pediatric:* <8 years: not recommended; ≥8 years, <100 lb: 2-2.5 mg/kg q 12 hours x 7-10 days; ≥8 years, ≥100 lb: same as adult
>> **Acticlate** *Tab:* 75, 150**mg
>> **Adoxa** *Tab:* 50, 75, 100, 150 mg ent-coat
>> **Doryx** *Tab:* 50, 75, 100, 150, 200 mg del-rel
>> **Doxteric** *Tab:* 50 mg del-rel
>> **Monodox** *Cap:* 50, 75, 100 mg
>> **Oracea** *Cap:* 40 mg del-rel

Vibramycin *Tab:* 100 mg; *Cap:* 50, 100 mg; *Syr:* 50 mg/5 ml (raspberry-apple) (sulfites); *Oral susp:* 25 mg/5 ml (raspberry)
Vibra-Tab *Tab:* 100 mg film-coat

Comment: *doxycycline* contraindicated <8 years-of-age, in pregnancy, and lactation (discolors developing tooth enamel). A side effect may be photosensitivity (photophobia). Do <u>not</u> take with antacids, calcium supplements, milk or other dairy, or within 2 hours of taking another drug.

 tetracycline **(D)(G)** 500 mg q 6 hours x 7-10 days
Pediatric: <8 years: not recommended; ≥8 years, <100 lb: 10 mg/kg/day q 6 hours x 7-10 days; ≥8 years, ≥100 lb: same as adult
Achromycin V *Cap:* 250, 500 mg
Sumycin *Tab:* 250, 500 mg; *Cap:* 250, 500 mg; *Oral susp:* 125 mg/5 ml (100, 200 ml) (fruit) (sulfites)

Comment: *tetracycline* is contraindicated <8 years-of-age, in pregnancy, and lactation (discolors developing tooth enamel). A side effect may be photosensitivity (photophobia). Do <u>not</u> take with antacids, calcium supplements, milk or other dairy, or within two hours of taking another drug.

ROSEOLA INFANTUM (EXANTHEM SUBITUM)

Antipyretics *see Fever page* 163

Comment: Roseola infantum (also known as exanthem subitum, sixth disease, pseudorubella, exanthem criticum, and three-day fever) is a generally mild clinical syndrome, commonly occurring in children <3 years-of-age, characterized by sudden onset of high fever (may exceed 40°C [104°F]) that lasts 3 days and resolves abruptly, and is followed by development of a rash lasting ≤3 days. Roseola usually is caused by human herpesvirus 6 (HHV-6). Treatment is antipyretics (aspirin is contraindicated) and adequate hydration. Monitor for febrile seizures. As with the common cold, roseola spreads from person to person through contact with an infected person's respiratory secretions or saliva. The disease can occur at any time of year.

ROTAVIRUS GASTROENTERITIS

PROPHYLAXIS

Comment: **RotaTeq** targets the most common strains of rotavirus (G1, G2, G3, G4), which are responsible for more than 90% of rotavirus disease in the United States.

 rotavirus vaccine, live not recommended for adults
Pediatric: <6 weeks <u>or</u> >32 weeks: not recommended; >6 weeks and <32 weeks: administer 1st dose at 6-12 weeks of age; administer 2nd and 3rd doses at 4-10-week intervals for a total of 3 doses; if an incomplete dose is administered, do not administer a replacement dose, but continue with the remaining doses in the recommended series
RotaTeq *Oral susp:* 2 ml single-use tube (fetal bovine serum [trace], preservative-free, thimerosal-free)

ROUNDWORM (*ASCARIASIS*)

ANTHELMINTICS

Comment: Oral bioavailability of anthelmintics is enhanced when administered with a fatty meal (estimated fat content 40 gm).

 albendazole **(C)** take with a meal; swallow, chew, crush, or mix with food; 400 mg once daily x 7 days
Pediatric: <2 years: 200 mg once daily x 3 days; may repeat in 3 weeks if needed; 2-12 years: 400 mg once daily x 3 days; may repeat in 3 weeks if needed; >12 years: same as adult
Albenza *Tab:* 200 mg

 mebendazole **(C)** take with a meal; swallow, chew, crush, or mix with food; 100 mg bid x 3 days; may repeat in 3 weeks if needed
Pediatric: <2 years: not recommended; ≥2 years: same as adult
Emverm *Chew tab:* 100 mg
Vermox (G) *Chew tab:* 100 mg

► *pyrantel pamoate* (C) take with a meal; may open capsule and sprinkle or mix with food; treat x 3 days; may repeat in 2-3 weeks if needed; 11 mg/kg once daily x 3 days; max 1 gm/dose

Pediatric: 25-37 lb: 1/2 tsp x 1 dose; 38-62 lb: 1 tsp x 1 dose; 63-87 lb: 1 tsp x 1 dose; 88-112 lb: 2 tsp x 1 dose; 113-137 lb: 2 tsp x 1 dose; 138-162 lb: 3 tsp x 1 dose; 163-187 lb: 3 tsp x 1 dose; >187 lb: 4 tsp x 1 dose

  Antiminth (OTC) *Cap:* 180 mg; *Liq:* 50 mg/ml (30 ml); 144 mg/ml (30 ml); *Oral susp:* 50 mg/ml (60 ml)

  Pin-X (OTC) *Cap:* 180 mg; *Liq:* 50 mg/ml (30 ml); 144 mg/ml (30 ml); *Oral susp:* 50 mg/ml (30 ml)

► *thiabendazole* (C) 25 mg/kg bid x 7 days; max 1.5 gm/dose; max 3000 mg/day; take with a meal

Pediatric: same as adult

  Mintezol *Chew tab:* 500*mg (orange); *Oral susp:* 500 mg/5 ml (120 ml) (orange)

  Comment: *thiabendazole* is not for prophylaxis. May impair mental alertness. May not be available in the US.

RUBELLA (GERMAN MEASLES)

Antipyretics *see* **Fever** *page* 163
See **Childhood Immunizations** *page* 558

Comment: Rubella is highly contagious and highly teratogenic. Quarantine is mandatory to prevent a community outbreak. Herd immunity is the best prevention.

PROPHYLAXIS VACCINE

Comment: <12 months: not recommended; ≥12 months: 25 mcg SC; if vaccinated <12 months, re-vaccinate at 12 months; administer in the upper posterior arm.

► *rubella virus, live, attenuated+neomycin* vaccine (C)
Pediatric: <12 months: not recommended (if vaccinated <12 months, revaccinate at 12 months); ≥12 months: 25 mcg SC

  Meruvax II 25 mcg SC

► *measles, mumps, rubella, live, attenuated, neomycin vaccine* (C)
  MMR II 25 mcg SC (preservative-free)

  Comment: Contraindications: hypersensitivity to *neomycin* or eggs, primary or acquired immune deficiency, immunosuppressant therapy, bone marrow or lymphatic malignancy, and pregnancy (within 3 months following vaccination).

  see **Childhood Immunizations** *page* 558

PRE- AND POST-EXPOSURE PROPHYLAXIS
Immune Globulin

► *immune globulin (human)* administer via intramuscular injection only (never intravenously); ensure adequate hydration prior to administration

Household and Institutional Rubella Case Contacts: promptly administer 0.55 ml/kg IM as a single dose

Planned Travel to Rubella Endemic Area: administer 0.55 ml/kg as a single dose at least 6 days prior to travel

Pediatric: 0.25 ml/kg IM (0.5 mg/kg in immunocompromised children)

  GamaSTAN S/D *Vial:* 2, 10 ml single-dose

  Comment: **GamaSTAN S/D** is the only *gammaglobulin* product FDA-approved for measles and HAV post-exposure prophylaxis (PEP). **GamaSTAN S/D** is also FDA-approved for varicella post-exposure prophylaxis (PEP). Other **GamaSTAN S/D** indications: to prevent or modify measles in a susceptible person exposed fewer than 6 days previously; to modify varicella; to modify rubella in exposed women who will not consider a therapeutic abortion. **GamaSTAN S/D** is not indicated for routine prophylaxis or treatment of viral hepatitis B, rubella, poliomyelitis, mumps or varicella. Contraindications to **GamaSTAN S/D** include persons with cancer, chronic liver disease, and persons allergic to *gammaglobulin*, the HAV vaccine, or a component of the HAV vaccine. Dosage is higher for HAV PEP than for measles and varicella PEP based on recently observed decreasing concentrations of HAV antibodies in **GamaSTAN S/D**, attributed to the decreasing prevalence of previous HAV infection among plasma donors.

RUBEOLA (RED MEASLES)

Antipyretics *see* **Fever** *page 163*
See **Childhood Immunizations** *page 558*

PROPHYLAXIS VACCINE

▷ *measles, mumps, rubella, live, attenuated, neomycin vaccine* (C)
    MMR II 25 mcg SC (preservative-free)
    Comment: Contraindications: hypersensitivity to *neomycin* or eggs, primary or acquired immune deficiency, immunosuppressant therapy, bone marrow or lymphatic malignancy, and pregnancy (within 3 months following vaccination).

PRE- AND POST-EXPOSURE PROPHYLAXIS
Immune Globulin (Human)

▷ *immune globulin (human)* administer via intramuscular injection <u>only</u> (<u>never</u> intravenously); ensure adequate hydration prior to administration
    Household and Institutional Measles Case Contacts: promptly administer 0.025 ml/kg IM as a single dose
    Planned Travel to Measles Endemic Area: administer 0.025 ml/kg IM as a single dose at least 6 days prior to travel
    Pediatric: 0.25 ml/kg IM (0.5 mg/kg in immunocompromised children)
        GamaSTAN S/D *Vial:* 2, 10 ml single-dose
        Comment: **GamaSTAN S/D** is the only *gammaglobulin* product FDA-approved for measles and HAV post-exposure prophylaxis (PEP). **GamaSTAN S/D** is also FDA-approved for varicella post-exposure prophylaxis (PEP). Other **GamaSTAN S/D** indications: to prevent or modify measles in a susceptible person exposed fewer than 6 days previously; to modify varicella; to modify rubella in exposed women who will <u>not</u> consider a therapeutic abortion. **GamaSTAN S/D** is <u>not</u> indicated for routine prophylaxis or treatment of viral hepatitis B, rubella, poliomyelitis, mumps or varicella. Contraindications to **GamaSTAN S/D** include persons with cancer, chronic liver disease, and persons allergic to *gammaglobulin*, the HAV vaccine, or a component of the HAV vaccine. Dosage is higher for HAV PEP than for measles and varicella PEP based on recently observed decreasing concentrations of HAV antibodies in **GamaSTAN S/D**, attributed to the decreasing prevalence of previous HAV infection among plasma donors.

SALMONELLOSIS

ANTI-INFECTIVES

▷ *ciprofloxacin* (C) 500 mg bid x 3-5 days
    Pediatric: <18 years: not recommended; ≥18 years: same as adult
        Cipro (G) *Tab:* 250, 500, 750 mg; *Oral susp:* 250, 500 mg/5 ml (100 ml) (strawberry)
        Cipro XR *Tab:* 500, 1000 mg ext-rel
        ProQuin XR *Tab:* 500 mg ext-rel
    Comment: *ciprofloxacin* is contraindicated <18 years-of-age, and during pregnancy and lactation. Risk of tendonitis or tendon rupture.
▷ *trimethoprim+sulfamethoxazole* (TMP-SMX) (D)(G)
    Pediatric: <2 months: not recommended; ≥2 months: 40 mg/kg/day of *sulfamethoxazole* in 2 divided doses bid x 10 days; *see page 630 for dose by weight*
        Bactrim, Septra 2 tabs bid x 10 days
            Tab: trim 80 mg+sulfa 400 mg*
        Bactrim DS, Septra DS 1 tab bid x 10 days
            Tab: trim 160 mg+sulfa 800 mg*
        Bactrim Pediatric Suspension, Septra Pediatric Suspension
            Oral susp: trim 40 mg+sulfa 200 mg per 5 ml (100 ml) (cherry) (alcohol 0.3%)

Comment: Sulfonamides are contraindicated in the first trimester of pregnancy, the final month of pregnancy, and infants <8 weeks-of-age. *CrCl 15-30 mL/min:* reduce dose by 1/2; *CrCl <15 mL/min:* not recommended. Contraindicated with G6PD deficiency. A high fluid intake is indicated during sulfonamide therapy to avoid crystallization in the kidneys.

SCABIES (*SARCOPTES SCABIEI*)

Comment: This section presents treatment regimens for scabies infestation published in the 2015 CDC Sexually Transmitted Diseases Treatment Guidelines, as well as other available treatments.

RECOMMENDED REGIMEN

▷ *permethrin* (B)(G) massage into skin from head to soles of feet; leave on x 8-14 hours, then rinse off
   Pediatric: <2 months: not recommended; ≥2 months: same as adult
      Acticin, Elimite *Crm:* 5% (60 gm)

ALTERNATIVE REGIMEN

▷ *lindane* (B)(G) 1 oz of lotion or 30 gm of cream apply to all skin surfaces from neck down to the soles of the feet; leave on x 8 hours, then wash off thoroughly; may repeat if needed in 14 days
   Pediatric: <2 months: not recommended; ≥2 months: same as adult
      Kwell *Lotn:* 1% (60, 473 ml); *Crm:* 1% (60 gm); *Shampoo:* 1% (60, 473 ml)

OTHER TOPICAL TREATMENTS

▷ *crotamiton* (C) massage into skin from chin down; repeat in 24 hours
   Pediatric: <12 years: not recommended; ≥12 years: same as adult
      Eurax *Lotn:* 10% (60 gm); *Crm:* 10% (60 gm)

SCARLET FEVER (SCARLATINA)

Comment: Microorganism responsible for scarlet fever is Group A beta-hemolytic *Streptococcus* (GABHS). Strep cultures and screens will be positive.
▷ *azithromycin* (B)(G) 500 mg x 1 dose on day 1, then 250 mg once daily on days 2-5 or 500 mg once daily x 3 days
   Pediatric: 12 mg/kg/day x 5 days; max 500 mg/day; *see page 619 for dose by weight*
      Zithromax *Tab:* 250, 500, 600 mg; *Oral susp:* 100 mg/5 ml (15 ml); 200 mg/5 ml (15, 22.5, 30 ml) (cherry); *Pkt:* 1 gm for reconstitution (cherry-banana)
      Zithromax Tri-pak *Tab:* 3 x 500 mg tabs/pck
      Zithromax Z-pak *Tab:* 6 x 250 mg tabs/pck
      Zmax *Oral susp:* 2 gm ext-rel for reconstitution (cherry-banana) (148 mg Na⁺)
▷ *cefadroxil* (B)
   Pediatric: 15-30 mg/kg/day in 2 divided doses x 10 days; *see page 620 for dose by weight*
      Duricef *Cap:* 500 mg; *Tab:* 1 gm; *Oral susp:* 250 mg/5 ml (100 ml); 500 mg/5 ml (75, 100 ml) (orange-pineapple)
▷ *cephalexin* (B)(G)
   Pediatric: 25-50 mg/kg/day in 2 divided doses x 10 days; *see page 623 for dose by weight*
      Keflex *Cap:* 250, 333, 500, 750 mg; *Oral susp:* 125, 250 mg/5 ml (100, 200 ml) (strawberry)
▷ *clarithromycin* (C)(G) 250 mg bid or 500 mg ext-rel once daily x 10 days
   Pediatric: <6 months: not recommended; ≥6 months: 7.5 mg/kg bid x 10 days; *see page 624 for dose by weight*
      Biaxin *Tab:* 250, 500 mg
      Biaxin Oral Suspension *Oral susp:* 125, 250 mg/5 ml (50, 100 ml) (fruit punch)
      Biaxin XL *Tab:* 500 mg ext-rel
   Comment: The FDA is advising caution before prescribing *clarithromycin* to patients with heart disease because of a potential increased risk of heart problems or death that can occur years later. This recommendation is based on a review of the results of a 10-year follow-up

study of patients with coronary heart disease from a large clinical trial that first observed this safety issue. Consider risk benefit and the use of other antibiotics in such patients.

➤ *clindamycin* (B)(G) 150-300 mg q 6 hours x 10 days
Pediatric: 8-16 mg/kg/day in 3-4 divided doses x 10 days
   Cleocin *Cap:* 75 (tartrazine), 150 (tartrazine), 300 mg
   Cleocin Pediatric Granules *Oral susp:* 75 mg/5 ml (100 ml) (cherry)

➤ *erythromycin estolate* (B)(G) 250 mg q 6 hours x 10 days
Pediatric: 20-50 mg/kg q 6 hours x 10 days; *see page 625 for dose by weight*
   Ilosone *Pulvule:* 250 mg; *Tab:* 500 mg; *Liq:* 125, 250 mg/5 ml (100 ml)
Comment: *erythromycin* may increase INR with concomitant *warfarin*, as well as increase serum level of *digoxin,* benzodiazepines, and statins.

➤ *erythromycin ethylsuccinate* (B)(G) 400 mg qid or 800 mg bid x 10 days
Pediatric: 30-50 mg/kg/day in 4 divided doses x 10 days; may double dose with severe infection; max 100 mg/kg/day; *see page 626 for dose by weight*
   EryPed *Oral susp:* 200 mg/5 ml (100, 200 ml) (fruit); 400 mg/5 ml (60, 100, 200 ml) (banana); *Oral drops:* 200, 400 mg/5 ml (50 ml) (fruit); *Chew tab:* 200 mg wafer (fruit)
   E.E.S. *Oral susp:* 200, 400 mg/5 ml (100 ml) (fruit)
   E.E.S. Granules *Oral susp:* 200 mg/5 ml (100, 200 ml) (cherry)
   E.E.S. 400 Tablets *Tab:* 400 mg
Comment: *erythromycin* may increase INR with concomitant *warfarin*, as well as increase serum level of *digoxin,* benzodiazepines, and statins.

➤ *penicillin g (benzathine and procaine)* (B)(G) 2.4 million units IM x 1 dose
Pediatric: <30 lb: 600,000 units IM x 1 dose; 30-60 lb: 900,000-1.2 million units IM x 1 dose
   Bicillin C-R Cartridge-needle unit: 600,000 units (1 ml); 1.2 million units; (2 ml); 2.4 million units (4 ml)

➤ *penicillin v potassium* (B) 250 mg tid x 10 days
Pediatric: 25-50 mg/kg day in 4 divided doses x 10 days; ≥12 years: same as adult; *see page 629 for dose by weight*
   Pen-Vee K *Tab:* 250, 500 mg; *Oral soln:* 125 mg/5 ml (100, 200 ml); 250 mg/5 ml (100, 150, 200 ml)

SCHISTOSOMIASIS

TREMATODICIDE

Comment: *praziquantel* is a trematodicide indicated for the treatment of infections due to all species of genus *Schistosoma* (e.g., *Schistosoma mekongi, Schistosoma japonicum, Schistosoma mansoni,* and *Schistosoma hematobium)* and infections due to liver flukes (i.e., *Clonorchis sinensis, Opisthorchis viverrini). praziquantel* induces a rapid contraction of schistosomes by a specific effect on the permeability of the cell membrane. The drug further causes vacuolization and disintegration of the schistosome tegument.

➤ *praziquantel* (B) 20 mg/kg tid as a one-day treatment; take the 3 doses at intervals of not less than 4 hours and not more than 6 hours; swallow whole with water during meals; holding the tablets in the mouth leaves a bitter taste which can trigger gagging or vomiting.
Pediatric: <4 years: not established; ≥4 years: same as adult
   Biltricide *Tab:* 600 mg film-coat
Comment: Concomitant administration with strong Cytochrome P450 (P450) inducers, such as *rifampin,* is contraindicated since therapeutically effective blood levels of *praziquantel* may not be achieved. In patients receiving *rifampin* who need immediate treatment for schistosomiasis, alternative agents for schistosomiasis should be considered. However, if treatment with *praziquantel* is necessary, *rifampin* should be discontinued 4 weeks before administration of *praziquantel*. Treatment with *rifampin* can then be restarted one day after completion of *praziquantel* treatment.
Concomitant administration of other P450 inducers (e.g., antiepileptic drugs such as *phenytoin, phenobarbital, carbamazepine)* and *dexamethasone*, may also reduce plasma levels of *praziquantel*. Concomitant administration of P450 inhibitors (e.g., *cimetidine, ketoconazole, itraconazole, erythromycin)* may increase plasma levels of *praziquantel*. Patients should be warned not to drive a car or operate machinery on the day of **Biltricide** treatment and the following day. There are no adequate or well-controlled studies in pregnant women. This drug should be used during pregnancy only if clearly needed. *praziquantel*

appears in the milk of nursing women at a concentration of about 1/4 that of maternal serum. It is not known whether a pharmacological effect is likely to occur in children. Women should not nurse on the day of **Biltricide** treatment and during the subsequent 72 hours.

SCHIZOPHRENIA, SCHIZOPHRENIA WITH CO-MORBID PERSONALITY DISORDER

Other Antipsychosis Drugs *see* **Antipsychosis Drugs** *pages* 589
Tardive Dyskinesia *see page* 473

Comment: A team of researchers examined the effects of antipsychotics on mortality risk in schizophrenia patients. They studied data on 29,823 patients with schizophrenia in Sweden, aged 16 to 64 years and found mortality among patients with schizophrenia was 40% lower when they used antipsychotics as compared to when they did not. Long-acting injection (LAI) use was associated with an approximately 33% lower risk of death compared with the oral use of the same medication. The lowest mortality was observed with use of once-monthly *paliperidone* LAI, oral aripiprazole, and risperidone LAI.

REFERENCE
Taipale, H., Mittendorfer-Rutz, E., Alexanderson, K., Majak, M., Mehtälä, J., Hoti, F., . . . Tiihonen, J. (2018). Antipsychotics and mortality in a nationwide cohort of 29,823 patients with schizophrenia. *Schizophrenia Research, 197*, 274–280. doi:10.1016/j.schres.2017.12.010

ATYPICAL ANTIPSYTICS

▶ *aripiprazole* (C)(G) initially 15 mg once daily; may increase to max 30 mg/day
Pediatric: <10 years: not recommended; ≥10-17 years: initially 2 mg/day in a single dose for 2 days; then increase to 5 mg/day in a single dose for 2 days; then increase to target dose of 10 mg/day in a single dose; may increase by 5 mg/day at weekly intervals as needed to max 30 mg/day

> **Abilify** *Tab:* 2, 5, 10, 15, 20, 30 mg
> **Abilify Discmelt** *Tab:* 15 mg orally-disint (vanilla) (phenylalanine)
> **Abilify Maintena** *Vial:* 300, 400 mg ext-rel pwdr for IM injection after reconstitution; 300, 400 mg single-dose prefilled dual-chamber syringes w. supplies

▶ *aripiprazole lauroxil* (C)
ALERT: aripiprazole lauroxil is available in two parenteral delivery forms, **Aristada** and **Aristada Initio**, with differing doses and frequently of administration. Therefore, **Aristada Initio** is not interchangeable with **Aristada**. **Aristada Initio** is a smaller particle-size version of extended-release injectable *aripiprazole*). It is the first and only long-acting atypical antipsychotic that can be initiated on day one. Combining **Aristada Initio** with a single 30 mg dose of oral *aripiprazole* provides an alternative regimen to initiate patients onto any dose of **Aristada** on day one. Previously, the initiation process for the older *aripiprazole* product was to give the first dose and to then give oral *aripiprazole* for 21 consecutive days. **Aristada Initio** releases relevant levels of *aripiprazole* within 4 days of initiation. **Aristada Initio** carries a warning that it is not approved for use by older patients with dementia-related psychosis, as this patient population is at risk for increased mortality when treated with antipsychotics. For patients naïve to *aripiprazole*, establish tolerability with oral *aripiprazole* prior to initiating treatment with **Aristada Initio**.
Pediatric: <18 years: not recommended; ≥18 years: same as adult

> **Aristada** administer by IM injection in the deltoid (441 mg dose only) or gluteal (441 mg, 662 mg, 882 mg or 1064 mg) muscle by a qualified healthcare professional; initiate at a dose of 441 mg, 662 mg or 882 mg administered monthly, or 882 mg every 6 weeks, or 1064 mg every 2 months
> *Prefilled syringe:* 441, 662, 882, 1064 mg single-use, ext-rel susp
> **Aristada Initio** administer a single 675 mg **Aristada Initio** injection (plus a single 30 mg dose of oral *aripiprazole* in conjunction with the first **Aristada Initio** injection); administer the IM injection into the deltoid or gluteal muscle; must be administered only by a qualified healthcare professional; **Aristada Initio** is only to be used as a single dose and is not for repeated dosing
> *Prefilled pen:* 675 mg/2.4 ml ext-rel single-dose

Comment: Aristada and **Aristada Initio** are atypical antipsychotics. **Aristada** is available in 4 doses with 3 dosing duration options for flexible dosing. **Aristada initio** is a single-dose *longer-acting* form of *aripiprazole lauroxil* For patients naïve to *aripiprazole*, establish tolerability with oral *aripiprazole* prior to initiating treatment with **Aristada**. **Aristada** can be initiated at any of the 4 doses at the appropriate dosing duration option. In conjunction with the first injection, administer treatment with oral *aripiprazole* for 21 consecutive days for all 4 dose sizes. The most common adverse event associated with **Aristada/Aristada Initio** is akathisia. Patients are also at increased risk for developing neuroleptic malignant syndrome, tardive dyskinesia, pathological gambling or other compulsive behaviors, orthostatic hypotension, hyperglycemic, dyslipidemia, and weight gain. Hypersensitive reactions can occur and range from pruritus or urticaria to anaphylaxis. Stroke, transient ischemic attacks, and falls have been reported in elderly patients with dementia-related psychosis who were treated with *apriprazole*. **Aristada/Aristada Initio** are *not* for treatment of people who have lost touch with reality (psychosis) *due to* confusion and memory loss dementia). Avoid use in known CYP2D6 poor metabolizers. Avoid use with strong CYP2D6 or CYP 3A4 inhibitors and strong CYP3A4 inducers. *aripiprazole* may cause extrapyramidal and/or withdrawal symptoms in neonates exposed in utero in the third trimester of pregnancy. *aripiprazole* is present in human breast milk; however, there are insufficient data to assess the amount in human milk or the effects on the breastfed infant. The development and health benefits of breastfeeding should be considered along with the mother's clinical need for *aripiprazole* and any potential adverse effects on the breastfed infant from **Aristada/Aristada Initio** or from the underlying maternal condition. For more information or to report suspected ASEs, contact the National Pregnancy Registry for Atypical Antipsychotics at 1-866-961-2388 or visit http://womensmentalhealth.org/clinical-and-research programs/ pregnancy registry. Limited published data on *aripiprazole* use in pregnant women are *not* sufficient to inform any drug-associated risks for birth defects or miscarriage. To report suspected adverse reactions, contact Alkermes at 1-866-274-7823 or FDA at 1-800-FDA-1088 or www.fda.gov/medwatch.

▷ *lurasidone* (B)(G) initially 40 mg once daily; usual range 40 to max 160 mg/day; take with food; *CrCl <50 mL/min, moderate hepatic impairment (Child-Pugh 7-9)*: max 80 mg/day; *Child-Pugh 10-15)*: max 40 mg/day
Pediatric: <13 years: not established; 13-17 years: initially 40 mg once daily; may titrate up to max 80 mg/day

    Latuda *Tab*: 20, 40, 60, 80, 120 mg

    Comment: **Latuda** is contraindicated with concomitant strong CYP3A4 inhibitors (e.g., *ketoconazole, voriconazole, clarithromycin, ritonavir*) and inducers (e.g., *phenytoin, carbamazepine, rifampin, St. John's wort*); see mfr pkg insert if patient taking moderate CYP3A4 inhibitors (e.g., *diltiazem, atazanavir, erythromycin, fluconazole, verapamil*).

SEIZURE DISORDER

Status Epilepticus see *Status Epilepticus* page 466
Anticonvulsant Drugs see page 591

SEXUAL ASSAULT (STD/STI/VD EXPOSURE)

Comment: The following treatment regimens for victims of sexual assault are published in the 2015 CDC Sexually Transmitted Diseases Treatment Guidelines.

RECOMMENDED PROPHYLAXIS REGIMEN

▷ *ceftriaxone* 250 mg IM in a single dose plus *metronidazole* 2 gm in a single dose plus *azithromycin* 1 gm in a single dose

ALTERNATE PROPHYLAXIS REGIMENS

Regimen 1

▷ *ceftriaxone* 250 mg IM in a single dose plus *metronidazole* 2 gm in a single dose plus *doxycycline* 100 mg bid x 7 days

Regimen 2

▷ *cefixime* 400 mg in a single dose plus *metronidazole* 2 gm in a single dose plus *azithromycin* 1 gm in a single dose

Regimen 3

▷ *cefixime* 400 mg in a single dose plus *metronidazole* 2 gm in a single dose plus *doxycycline* 100 mg bid x 7 days

Regimen 4

▷ *azithromycin* (B) 1 gm as a single dose plus *metronidazole* 2 gm in a single dose

DRUG BRANDS AND DOSE FORMS

▷ *azithromycin* (B)(G)

   Zithromax *Tab:* 250, 500, 600 mg; *Oral susp:* 100 mg/5 ml (15 ml); 200 mg/5 ml (15, 22.5, 30 ml) (cherry); *Pkt:* 1 gm for reconstitution (cherry-banana)
   Zithromax Tri-pak *Tab:* 3 x 500 mg tabs/pck
   Zithromax Z-pak *Tab:* 6 x 250 mg tabs/pck
   Zmax *Oral susp:* 2 gm ext-rel for reconstitution (cherry-banana) (148 mg Na⁺)

▷ *cefixime* (B)(G)

   Suprax *Tab:* 400 mg; *Cap:* 400 mg; *Oral susp:* 100, 200, 500 mg/5 ml (50, 75, 100 ml) (strawberry)

▷ *ceftriaxone* (B)(G)

   Rocephin *Vial:* 250, 500 mg; 1, 2 gm

▷ *doxycycline* (D)(G)

   Acticlate *Tab:* 75, 150**mg
   Adoxa *Tab:* 50, 75, 100, 150 mg ent-coat
   Doryx *Tab:* 50, 75, 100, 150, 200 mg del-rel
   Doxteric *Tab:* 50 mg del-rel
   Monodox *Cap:* 50, 75, 100 mg
   Oracea *Cap:* 40 mg del-rel
   Vibramycin *Tab:* 100 mg; *Cap:* 50, 100 mg; *Syr:* 50 mg/5 ml (raspberry-apple) (sulfites); *Oral susp:* 25 mg/5 ml (raspberry)
   Vibra-Tab *Tab:* 100 mg film-coat

Comment: *doxycycline* is contraindicated <8 years-of-age, in pregnancy, and lactation (discolors developing tooth enamel). A side effect may be photosensitivity (photophobia). Do not take with antacids, calcium supplements, milk or other dairy, or within 2 hours of taking another drug.

▷ *metronidazole* (not for use in 1st; B in 2nd, 3rd)(G)

   Flagyl *Tab:* 250*, 500*mg
   Flagyl 375 *Cap:* 375 mg
   Flagyl ER *Tab:* 750 mg ext-rel

Comment: Alcohol is contraindicated during treatment with oral *metronidazole* and for 72 hours after therapy due to a possible *disulfiram*-like reaction (nausea, vomiting, flushing, headache).

⬤ SHIGELLOSIS (GENUS *SHIGELLA*)

ANTI-INFECTIVES

▷ *azithromycin* (B)(G) 500 mg x 1 dose on day 1, then 250 mg once daily on days 2-5 or 500 mg once daily x 3 days or **Zmax** 2 gm in a single dose
   Pediatric: <6 months: not recommended; ≥6 months: 10 mg/kg x 1 dose on day 1; then 5 mg/kg/day on days 2-5; max 500 mg/day; *see page 619* for dose by weight
   Zithromax *Tab:* 250, 500, 600 mg; *Oral susp:* 100 mg/5 ml (15 ml); 200 mg/5 ml (15, 22.5, 30 ml) (cherry); *Pkt:* 1 gm for reconstitution (cherry-banana)
   Zithromax Tri-pak *Tab:* 3 x 500 mg tabs/pck
   Zithromax Z-pak *Tab:* 6 x 250 mg tabs/pck
   Zmax *Oral susp:* 2 gm ext-rel for reconstitution (cherry-banana) (148 mg Na⁺)

▷ *ciprofloxacin* (C) 500 mg bid x 3 days
   Pediatric: <18 years: not recommended; ≥18 years: same as adult
   Cipro (G) *Tab:* 250, 500, 750 mg; *Oral susp:* 250, 500 mg/5 ml (100 ml) (strawberry)
   Cipro XR *Tab:* 500, 1000 mg ext-rel
   ProQuin XR *Tab:* 500 mg ext-rel

▷ *ofloxacin* (C)(G) 400 mg bid x 3 days
   Pediatric: <18 years: not recommended; ≥18 years: same as adult
   Floxin *Tab:* 200, 300, 400 mg

▶ *tetracycline* (D)(G) 250-500 mg qid x 5 days
  Pediatric: <8 years: not recommended; ≥8 years, <100 lb: 25-50 mg/kg/day in 4 divided
  doses x 5 days; ≥8 years, ≥100 lb: same as adult; *see page 630 for dose by weight*
    Achromycin V *Cap:* 250, 500 mg
    Sumycin *Tab:* 250, 500 mg; *Cap:* 250, 500 mg; *Oral susp:* 125 mg/5 ml (100, 200 ml)
    (fruit) (sulfites)
  Comment: *tetracycline* is contraindicated <8 years-of-age, in pregnancy, and lactation
  (discolors developing tooth enamel). A side effect may be photosensitivity (photophobia).
  Do <u>not</u> take with antacids, calcium supplements, milk or other dairy, or within two hours of
  taking another drug.
▶ *trimethoprim+sulfamethoxazole* (TMP-SMX) (D)(G)
    Bactrim, Septra 2 tabs bid x 10 days
      Tab: trim 80 mg+sulfa 400 mg*
    Bactrim DS, Septra DS 1 tab bid x 10 days
      Tab: trim 160 mg+sulfa 800 mg*
    Bactrim Pediatric Suspension, Septra Pediatric Suspension 20 ml bid x 10 days
      Oral susp: trim 40 mg+sulfa 200 mg per 5 ml (100 ml) (cherry) (alcohol 0.3%)
  Comment: Sulfonamides are contraindicated in the first trimester of pregnancy, the final
  month of pregnancy, and infants <8 weeks-of-age. *CrCl 15-30 mL/min:* reduce dose by 1/2;
  CrCl <15 mL/min: not recommended. Contraindicated with G6PD deficiency. A high fluid
  intake is indicated during sulfonamide therapy to avoid crystallization in the kidneys.

SHOCK: SEPTIC, DISTRIBUTIVE

Comment: Septic shock is the most common form of distributive shock and is characterized
by considerable mortality (treated, around 30%; untreated, probably >80%). In the United
States, septic shock is the leading cause of non-cardiac death in intensive care units. **Giapreza**
(angiotensin II) *received accelerated review and FDA approval December 2017* to increase
blood pressure, when added to conventional interventions used to raise blood pressure, to
prevent/treat dangerously low hypotension resulting from septic and other distributive shock
states. There is a potential for venous and arterial thrombotic and thromboembolic events in
patients who receive **Giapreza**. Therefore, use concurrent venous thromboembolism (VTE)
prophylaxis. **Giapreza** became available March 2018.

ANGIOTENSIN II

▶ *angiotensin II* dilute in 0.9% NaCl; must be administered as an IV infusion; initial infusion rate
20 ng/kg/min; titrate as frequently as every 5 minutes by increments of up to 15 ng/kg/min
as needed; during the first 3 hours, max 80 ng/kg/min; max maintenance dose 40 ng/kg/min;
diluted solution may be stored at room temperature or refrigerated; discard after 24 hours.
Dilution/Concentration:
  Giapreza 1 ml (2.5 mg/ml) in 500 ml 0.9%NaCl = 5,000 ng/ml
        1 ml (2.5.mg/ml in 250 ml 0.9%NaCl = 10,000 ng/ml
        2 ml (5 mg/ml) in 500 ml 0.9%NaCl = 10,000 ng/ml
    Giapreza *Vial:* 2.5 mg in ml, 5 mg/2 ml (2.5 mg/ml)
  Comment: The safety and efficacy of **Giapreza** in pediatric patients have not been established.
  It is not known whether **Giapreza** is present in human milk and no data are available on
  the effects of angiotensin II on the breastfed child. The published data on angiotensin II
  use in pregnant women are not sufficient to determine a drug-associated risk of adverse
  developmental outcomes. However, Delaying treatment in pregnant women with hypotension
  associated with septic or other distributive shock is likely to increase the risk of shock-
  associated maternal and fetal morbidity and mortality.

SICKLE CELL DISEASE (SCD)

▶ *hydroxyurea*
  Comment: *hydroxyurea* has an FDA-approved "orphan drug" designation for the treatment
  of sickle cell disease SCD). It is an antimetabolite indicated to reduce the frequency of
  painful crises and to reduce the need for blood transfusions in patients with sickle cell
  anemia SCA) with recurrent moderate to severe painful crises. *Blac Box Warning (BBW):*
  hydroxyurea may cause severe myelosuppression. Do not administer if bone marrow
  function is markedly depressed. Monitor blood counts at baseline and every 2 weeks

throughout treatment. Blood counts within an acceptable range are defined as: *neutrophils* ≥ 2,500 cells/mm3, *platelets* ≥95,000 cells/mm3, *Hgb* ≥5.3 gm/dL, *reticulocytes* ≥95,000 cells/mm3 if the Hgb <9 gm/dL. Discontinue *hydroxyurea* until hematologic recovery if blood counts are considered toxic. Treatment may be resumed after reducing the *hydroxyurea* dose by 2.5 mg/kg/day from the dose associated with hematological toxicity. *CrCl <60 mL/min:* reduce dose by 50%. *hydroxyurea* is carcinogenic. Advise sun protection and monitor patients for malignancies. Avoid live vaccines when using *hydroyurea.* Discontinue *hydroxyurea* if vasculitic toxicity occurs. Risks with concomitant use of antiretroviral drugs: pancreatitis, hepatotoxicity, and neuropathy. Monitor for signs and symptoms in patients with HIV infection using antiretroviral drugs. If patients with HIV infection are treated with *hydroxyurea,* and in particular, in combination with *didanosine* and/or *stavudine,* close monitoring for signs and symptoms of pancreatitis is recommended. Permanently discontinue *hydroxyurea* in patients who develop signs and symptoms of pancreatitis. *hydroxyurea* can cause fetal harm (embryotoxic and teratogenic effects in animal studies). Advise patients regarding potential risk to a fetus and use of effective contraception during and after treatment with **hydroxyurea** for at least 6 months after therapy is ended. Advise females to immediately report pregnancy. *Hydroxyurea* may damage spermatozoa and testicular tissue, resulting in possible genetic abnormalities. Azoospermia or oligospermia, sometimes reversible, has been observed in men. Inform male patients about the possibility of sperm conservation before the initiation of *hydroxyurea* therapy. Males with female sexual partners of reproductive potential should use effective contraception during and after treatment for at least 1 year. *hydroxyurea* is excreted in human milk. Discontinue breastfeeding during treatment. To report suspected adverse reactions, contact Bristol-Myers Squibb at 1-800-721-5072 or FDA at 1-800-FDA-1088 or www.fda.gov/medwatch. *Droxia* use actual or ideal body weight (whichever is less) for dosing; initially 15 mg/kg once daily; if the blood counts are within an acceptable range, increase the dose by 5 mg/kg/day every 12 weeks to the highest dose that does not produce toxic blood counts over 24 consecutive weeks (dosage should not exceed 35 mg/kg/day)
Pediatric: <18 years: not established; ≥18 years: same as adult
  Cap: 200, 300, 400 mg

Hydrea (see **Droxia** for prescribing information)
  Tab: **500 mg**

Siklos use actual or ideal body weight (whichever is less) for dosing. *initially* 20 mg/kg once daily; may be increased by 5 mg/kg/day every 8 weeks, or sooner if a severe painful crisis occurs, until a maximum tolerated dose or 35 mg/kg/day is reached; reduce the dose of Siklos by 50% (10 mg) in patients with CrCl <60 mL/min or with ESRD
Pediatric: <2 years: not recommended; ≥2 years: same as adult
  Tab: 100 mg; 1,000***mg

Comment: Safety and effectiveness of **Siklos** have been established in pediatric patients aged 2-18 years with sickle cell anemia (SSA) with recurrent moderate to severe painful crises and is the only *hydroxyurea* approved for use in children. Use of **Siklos** in these age groups is supported by evidence from a non-interventional cohort study, the European Sickle Cell Disease prospective Cohort study, ESCORT-HU, in which 405 pediatric patients ages 2 to <18 were treated with **Siklos**: n = 274 children (2-11 years) and n = 108 adolescents 12-16 years). Pediatric patients aged 2-16 years had a higher risk of neutropenia than patients >16 years. Continuous follow-up of the growth of treated children is recommended.

AMINO ACID

▷ *L-glutamine powder* take 5-15 gm orally, twice daily, based on body weight; <30 kg, <66 lb (1 pkt bid), 30-65 kg, 66-143 lb (2 pkts bid), >65 kg, >143 lb (3 pkts bid); mix each dose in 8 oz. (240 ml) of cold or room temperature beverage or 4-6 oz of food before ingestion
Pediatric: <5 years: not established; ≥5 years: same as adult
  Endari *Oral Powder:* 5 gm/paper-foil-plastic laminate pkt (60 pkts/carton)
  Comment: **Endari** is an amino acid indicated to reduce the acute complications of sickle cell disease. Common adverse reactions include constipation, nausea, abdominal pain, headache, cough, pain in extremity, back pain, chest pain There are no available data on **Endari** use in pregnancy to inform a drug-associated risk of major birth defects and miscarriage. There are no data on the presence of **Endari** in human milk or effects on the breastfed infant. The developmental and health benefits from breastfeeding should be considered along with the mother's clinical need for **Endari** and any potential adverse effects on the breastfed child from **Endari** or from the underlying maternal

condition. To report suspected adverse reactions, contact Emmaus Medical at 1-877-420-6493 or FDA at 1-800-FDA-1088 or www.fda.gov/medwatch.

CHIMERIC (MURINE/HUMAN) MONOCLONAL ANTIBODY

▷ *basiliximab* (B)
  Pediatric: <6 months: not recommended; 6 months-12 years: 14 mg/kg/day in a single or 2 divided doses x 10 days; 12 years: same as adult
    Simulect *Vial:* 10, 20 mg (6 ml) for reconstitution and IV infusion (preservative-free 10 mg vial: contains 10 mg *basiliximab*, 3.61 mg monobasic potassium phosphate, 0.50 mg disodium hydrogen phosphate (anhydrous), 0.80 mg sodium chloride, 10 mg sucrose, 40 mg mannitol, 20 mg glycine, to be reconstituted in 2.5 mL of Sterile Water for Injection, USP 20 mg *vial; contains* 20 mg *basiliximab*, 7.21 mg monobasic potassium phosphate, 0.99 mg disodium hydrogen phosphate (anhydrous), 1.61 mg sodium chloride, 20 mg sucrose, 80 mg mannitol and 40 mg glycine, to be reconstituted in 5 mL of Sterile Water for Injection, US
    Comment: **Simulect** is indicated for the prophylaxis of acute organ rejection in patients receiving renal transplantation when used as part of an immunosuppressive regimen that includes *cyclosporine* (modified) and corticosteroids. The efficacy of **Simulect** for the prophylaxis of acute rejection in recipients of other solid organ allografts has not been demonstrated. No dose adjustment is necessary when Simulect is added to triple immunosuppression regimens including *cyclosporine*, corticosteroids, and either *azathioprine* or *mycophenolate mofetil*. It is not known whether **Simulect** is excreted in human milk. A decision should be made to discontinue nursing or to discontinue the drug, taking into account the importance of the drug to the mother.

SINUSITIS, RHINOSINUSITIS: ACUTE BACTERIAL (ABRS)

ANTI-INFECTIVES

▷ *amoxicillin* (B)(G) 500-875 mg bid or 250-500 mg tid x 10 days
  Pediatric: <40 kg (88 lb): 20-40 mg/kg/day in 3 divided doses x 10 days or 25-45 mg/kg/day in 2 divided doses x 10 days; *see page 617 for dose by weight*
    Amoxil *Cap:* 250, 500 mg; *Tab:* 875*mg; *Chew tab:* 125, 200, 250, 400 mg (cherry-banana-peppermint) (phenylalanine); *Oral susp:* 125, 250 mg/5 ml (80, 100, 150 ml) (strawberry); 200, 400 mg/5 ml (50, 75, 100 ml) (bubble gum); *Oral drops:* 50 mg/ml (30 ml) (bubble gum)
    Moxatag *Tab:* 775 mg ext-rel
    Trimox *Tab:* 125, 250 mg; *Cap:* 250, 500 mg; *Oral susp:* 125, 250 mg/5 ml (80, 100, 150 ml) (raspberry-strawberry)
▷ *amoxicillin+clavulanate* (B)(G)
    Augmentin 500 mg tid or 875 mg bid x 10 days
    Pediatric: 40-45 mg/kg/day divided tid x 10 days or 90 mg/kg/day divided bid x 10 days
    see pages 618 for dose by weight
      Tab: 250, 500, 875 mg; *Chew tab:* 125, 250 mg (lemon-lime); 200, 400 mg (cherry-banana) (phenylalanine); *Oral susp:* 125 mg/5 ml (banana), 250 mg/5 ml (75, 100, 150 ml) (orange); 200, 400 mg/5 ml (50, 75, 100 ml) (orange) (phenylalanine)
    Augmentin ES-600 not recommended for adults
    Pediatric: <3 months: not recommended; ≥3 months, <40 kg: 90 mg/kg/day in 2 divided doses x 10 days; ≥40 kg: not recommended
      Oral susp: 42.9 mg/5 ml (50, 75, 100, 125, 150, 200 ml) (strawberry cream) (phenylalanine)
    Augmentin XR 2 tabs q 12 hours x 10 days
    Pediatric: <16 years: use other forms; ≥16 years: same as adult
      Tab: 1000*mg ext-rel
▷ *cefaclor* (B)(G) 250-500 mg q 8 hours x 10 days; max 2 gm/day
  Pediatric: <1 month: not recommended; 20-40 mg/kg bid or q 12 hours x 10 days; max 1 gm/day; *see page 620 for dose by weight*
  Tab: 500 mg; *Cap:* 250, 500 mg; *Susp:* 125 mg/5 ml (75, 150 ml) (strawberry); 187 mg/5 ml (50, 100 ml) (strawberry); 250 mg/5 ml (75, 150 ml) (strawberry); 375 mg/5 ml (50, 100 ml) (strawberry)
  Pediatric: <16 years: ext-rel not recommended; ≥16 years: same as adult
    Cefaclor Extended Release *Tab:* 375, 500 mg ext-rel

▷ *cefdinir* (B) 300 mg bid or 600 mg once daily x 10 days
Pediatric: <6 months: not recommended; 6 months-12 years: 14 mg/kg/day in a single or 2 divided doses x 10 days; 12 years: same as adult; *see page 621 for dose by weight*
Omnicef *Cap:* 300 mg; *Oral susp:* 125 mg/5 ml (60, 100 ml) (strawberry)

▷ *cefixime* (B)(G) 400 mg once daily x 10 days
Pediatric: <6 months: not recommended; 6 months-12 years, <50 kg: 8 mg/kg/day in 1-2 divided doses x 10 days; *see page 621 for dose by weight;* >12 years, >50 kg: same as adult
Suprax *Tab:* 400 mg; *Cap:* 400 mg; *Oral susp:* 100, 200, 500 mg/5 ml (50, 75, 100 ml) (strawberry)

▷ *cefpodoxime proxetil* 200 mg bid x 10 days
Pediatric: <2 months: not recommended; 2 months-12 years: 10 mg/kg/day (max 400 mg/dose) or 5 mg/kg/day bid (max 200 mg/dose) x 10 days; *see page 622 for dose by weight*
Vantin *Tab:* 100, 200 mg; *Oral susp:* 50, 100 mg/5 ml (50, 75, 100 mg) (lemon creme)

▷ *cefprozil* (B) 250-500 mg bid x 10 days
Pediatric: <6 months: not recommended; 6 months-12 years: *Mild:* 7.5 mg/kg bid x 10 days; *Moderate/Severe:* 15 mg/kg q 12 hours x 10 days; *see page 622 for dose by weight;* >12 years: same as adult
Cefzil *Tab:* 250, 500 mg; *Oral susp:* 125, 250 mg/5 ml (50, 75, 100 ml) (bubble gum) (phenylalanine)

▷ *ceftibuten* (B) 400 mg once daily x 10 days
Pediatric: <12 years: 9 mg/kg once daily x 10 days; max 400 mg/day; *see page 623 for dose by weight;* ≥12 years: 400 mg once daily x 10 days
Cedax *Cap:* 400 mg; Oral susp: 90 mg/5 ml (30, 60, 90, 120 ml); 180
Cedax *Cap:* 400 mg; *Oral susp:* 90 mg/5 ml (30, 60, 90, 120 ml); 180 mg/5 ml (30, 60, 120 ml) (cherry)

▷ *ciprofloxacin* (C) 500 mg bid x 10 days
Pediatric: <18 years: not recommended; ≥18 years: same as adult
Cipro (G) *Tab:* 250, 500, 750 mg; *Oral susp:* 250, 500 mg/5 ml (100 ml) (strawberry)
Cipro XR *Tab:* 500, 1000 mg ext-rel
ProQuin XR *Tab:* 500 mg ext-rel
Comment: ciprofloxacin is contraindicated <18 years-of-age, and during pregnancy and lactation. Risk of tendonitis or tendon rupture.

▷ *clarithromycin* (C)(G) 500 mg bid or 1000 mg ext-rel once daily x 10 days
Pediatric: <6 months: not recommended; ≥6 months: 7.5 mg/kg bid x 10 days; *see page 624 for dose by weight*
Biaxin *Tab:* 250, 500 mg
Biaxin Oral Suspension *Oral susp:* 125, 250 mg/5 ml (50, 100 ml) (fruit punch)
Biaxin XL *Tab:* 500 mg ext-rel
Comment: The FDA is advising caution before prescribing *clarithromycin* to patients with heart disease because of a potential increased risk of heart problems or death that can occur years later. This recommendation is based on a review of the results of a 10-year follow-up study of patients with coronary heart disease from a large clinical trial that first observed this safety issue. Consider risk benefit and the use of other antibiotics in such patients.

▷ *levofloxacin* (C) *Uncomplicated:* 500 mg once daily x 10-14 days; *Complicated:* 750 mg once daily x 10-14 days
Pediatric: <18 years: not recommended; ≥18 years: same as adult
Levaquin *Tab:* 250, 500, 750 mg; *Oral soln:* 25 mg/ml (480 ml) (benzyl alcohol); *Inj conc:* 25 mg/ml for IV infusion after dilution (20, 30 ml single-use vial) (preservative-free); *Premix soln:* 5 mg/ml for IV infusion (50, 100, 150 ml) (preservative-free)
Comment: *levofloxacin* is contraindicated <18 years-of-age, and during pregnancy and lactation. Risk of tendonitis or tendon rupture.

▷ *loracarbef* (B) 400 mg bid x 10 days
Pediatric: 15 mg/kg/day in 2 divided doses x 10 days; *see page 628 for dose by weight*
Lorabid *Pulvule:* 200, 400 mg; *Oral susp:* 100 mg/5 ml (50, 100 ml); 200 mg/5 ml (50, 75, 100 ml) (strawberry bubble gum)

▷ *moxifloxacin* (C)(G) 400 mg once daily x 10 days
Pediatric: <18 years: not recommended; ≥18 years: same as adult
Avelox *Tab:* 400 mg
Comment: *moxifloxacin* is contraindicated <18 years-of-age, and during pregnancy and lactation. Risk of tendonitis or tendon rupture.

▶ *trimethoprim+sulfamethoxazole (TMP-SMX)* (D)(G)
Pediatric: <2 months: not recommended; ≥2 months: 40 mg/kg/day of *sulfamethoxazole* in
2 divided doses bid x 10 days; *see page 630 for dose by weight*
    Bactrim, Septra 2 tabs bid x 10 days
      Tab: trim 80 mg+sulfa 400 mg*
    Bactrim DS, Septra DS 1 tab bid x 10 days
      Tab: trim 160 mg+sulfa 800 mg*
    Bactrim Pediatric Suspension, Septra Pediatric Suspension
      Oral susp: trim 40 mg+sulfa 200 mg per 5 ml (100 ml) (cherry) (alcohol 0.3%)
Comment: Sulfonamides are contraindicated in the first trimester of pregnancy, the final
month of pregnancy, and infants <8 weeks-of-age. *CrCl 15-30 mL/min:* reduce dose by 1/2;
CrCl <15 mL/min: not recommended. Contraindicated with G6PD deficiency. A high fluid
intake is indicated during sulfonamide therapy to avoid crystallization in the kidneys.

SJÖGREN-LARSSON-SYNDROME (SLS)

Comment: Sjögren-Larsson-Syndrome is a chronic autoimmune disorder that causes the
white blood cells to attack the moisture-producing glands. Sjögren's syndrome can occur
in association with other autoimmune diseases, including systemic lupus erythematosus,
rheumatoid arthritis, scleroderma, systemic sclerosis, cryoglobulinemia, or polyarteritis
nodosa. The disease can affect the eyes, mouth, parotid gland, pancreas, gastrointestinal
system, blood vessels, lungs, kidneys, skin, and nervous system. Erythrocyte sedimentation
rate (ESR) is elevated in 80% of patients. Rheumatoid factor is present in 52% of primary
cases and 98% of secondary-type cases. A mild normochromic normocytic anemia is present
in 50% of patients, and leukopenia occurs in up to 42% of patients. Creatinine clearance
is diminished in up to 50% of patients. Anti-nuclear antibody (ANA) is positive in 70% of
patients. SS-A and SS-B are marker antibodies for Sjögren's syndrome—70% of patients are
positive for SS-A and 40% are positive for SS-B.

CHOLINERGIC (MUSCARINIC) AGONIST COMBINATION

▶ *cevimeline* (C)(G) 30 mg tid
    Evoxac *Cap:* 30 mg
Comment: *cevimeline* is contraindicated in acute iritis, narrow angle glaucoma, and
uncontrolled asthma.
▶ *pilocarpine* (C)(G) 5 mg qid *or* 7.5 mg tid
    Salagen *Tab:* 5, 7.5 mg

ORAL ENZYME RINSE

▶ *xylitol+solazyme+selectobac* swish 5 ml for 30 seconds bid-tid
    Orazyme Dry Mouth Rinse *Oral soln:* 1.5, 16 oz

SKIN: CALLUSED

KERATOLYTICS

▶ *salicylic acid* (C)(OTC) apply lotion, cream *or* gel to affected area once daily-bid; apply
patch to affected area and leave on x 48 hours with max 5 applications/14 days
Pediatric: <12 years: not recommended; ≥12 years: same as adult
▶ *urea* (C)
Pediatric: <12 years: not recommended; ≥12 years: same as adult
    Carmol 40 apply to affected area with applicator stick provided once daily-tid; smooth
over until cream is absorbed; protect surrounding tissue; may cover with adhesive
bandage or gauze secured with adhesive tape
      Crm/Gel: 40% (30 gm)
    Keratol 40 apply to affected area with applicator stick provided once daily-tid; smooth
over until cream is absorbed; protect surrounding tissue; may cover with adhesive
bandage or gauze secured with adhesive tape
      Crm: 40% (1, 3, 7 oz); *Gel:* 40% (15 ml); *Lotn:* 40% (8 oz)
Comment: The moisturizing effect of **Carmol 40** and **Keratol 40** is enhanced by
applying while the skin is still moist (after washing *or* bathing).

SKIN INFECTION: BACTERIAL (CARBUNCLE, FOLLICULITIS, FURUNCLE)

Comment: Abscesses usually require surgical incision and drainage.

ANTIBACTERIAL SKIN CLEANSERS

▸ *hexachlorophene* (C) dispense 5 ml into wet hand, work up into lather; then apply to area to be cleansed; rinse thoroughly
    pHisoHex *Liq clnsr:* 5, 16 oz

TOPICAL ANTI-INFECTIVES

▸ *mupirocin* (B)(G) apply to lesions bid
    Pediatric: same as adult
        Bactroban *Oint:* 2% (22 gm); *Crm:* 2% (15, 30 gm)
        Centany *Oint:* 2% (15, 30 gm)
▸ *polymyxin b+neomycin* (C) oint apply once daily-tid
    Neosporin (OTC) *Oint:* 15 gm

ORAL ANTI-INFECTIVES

▸ *amoxicillin* (B)(G) 500-875 mg bid or 250-500 mg tid x 10 days
    Pediatric: <40 kg (88 lb): 20-40 mg/kg/day in 3 divided doses x 10 days or 25-45 mg/kg/day in 2 divided doses x 10 days; *see page 617 for dose by weight*
        Amoxil *Cap:* 250, 500 mg; *Tab:* 875*mg; *Chew tab:* 125, 200, 250, 400 mg (cherry-banana-peppermint) (phenylalanine); *Oral susp:* 125, 250 mg/5 ml (80, 100, 150 ml) (strawberry); 200, 400 mg/5 ml (50, 75, 100 ml) (bubble gum); *Oral drops:* 50 mg/ml (30 ml) (bubble gum)
        Moxatag *Tab:* 775 mg ext-rel
        Trimox *Tab:* 125, 250 mg; *Cap:* 250, 500 mg; *Oral susp:* 125, 250 mg/5 ml (80, 100, 150 ml) (raspberry-strawberry)
▸ *azithromycin* (B)(G) 500 mg x 1 dose on day 1, then 250 mg once daily on days 2-5 or 500 mg once daily x 3 days or **Zmax** 2 gm in a single dose
    Pediatric: 12 mg/kg/day x 5 days; max 500 mg/day; *see page 619 for dose by weight*
        Zithromax *Tab:* 250, 500, 600 mg; *Oral susp:* 100 mg/5 ml (15 ml); 200 mg/5 ml (15, 22.5, 30 ml) (cherry); *Pkt:* 1 gm for reconstitution (cherry-banana)
        Zithromax Tri-pak *Tab:* 3 x 500 mg tabs/pck
        Zithromax Z-pak *Tab:* 6 x 250 mg tabs/pck
        Zmax *Oral susp:* 2 gm ext-rel for reconstitution (cherry-banana) (148 mg Na$^+$)
▸ *cefaclor* (B)(G) 250-500 mg q 8 hours x 10 days; max 2 gm/day
    Pediatric: <1 month: not recommended; 20-40 mg/kg bid or q 12 hours x 10 days; max 1 gm/day; *see page 620 for dose by weight*
        Tab: 500 mg; *Cap:* 250, 500 mg; *Susp:* 125 mg/5 ml (75, 150 ml) (strawberry); 187 mg/5 ml (50, 100 ml) (strawberry); 250 mg/5 ml (75, 150 ml) (strawberry); 375 mg/5 ml (50, 100 ml) (strawberry)
        Cefaclor Extended Release
            Pediatric: <16 years: ext-rel not recommended; ≥16 years: same as adult
            Tab: 375, 500 mg ext-rel
▸ *cefadroxil* (B) 1-2 gm in a single or 2 divided doses x 10 days
    Pediatric: 15-30 mg/kg/day in 2 divided doses x 10 days; *see page 620 for dose by weight*
        Duricef *Cap:* 500 mg; *Tab:* 1 gm; *Oral susp:* 250 mg/5 ml (100 ml); 500 mg/5 ml (75, 100 ml) (orange-pineapple)
▸ *cefdinir* (B) 300 mg bid x 10 days
    Pediatric: <6 months: not recommended; 6 months-12 years: 14 mg/kg/day in 1-2 divided doses x 10 days; *see page 621 for dose by weight*
        Omnicef *Cap:* 300 mg; *Oral susp:* 125 mg/5 ml (60, 100 ml) (strawberry)
▸ *cefditoren pivoxil* (B) 200 mg bid x 10 days
    Pediatric: <12 years: not recommended; ≥12 years: same as adult
        Spectracef *Tab:* 200 mg
    Comment: Contraindicated with milk protein allergy or carnitine deficiency.

▷ *cefpodoxime proxetil* (B) 400 mg bid x 7-14 days
  Pediatric: <2 months: not recommended; 2 months-12 years: 10 mg/kg/day (max 400 mg/dose) or 5 mg/kg/day bid (max 200 mg/dose) x 7-14 days; *see page 622 for dose by weight*
    Vantin *Tab:* 100, 200 mg; *Oral susp:* 50, 100 mg/5 ml (50, 75, 100 mg) (lemon creme)
▷ *cefprozil* (B) 250-500 mg bid or 500 mg once daily x 10 days
  Pediatric: 2-12 years: 7.5 mg/kg bid x 10 days; >12 years: same as adult; *see page 622 for dose by weight*
    Cefzil *Tab:* 250, 500 mg; *Oral susp:* 125, 250 mg/5 ml (50, 75, 100 ml) (bubble gum) (phenylalanine)
▷ *ceftriaxone* (B)(G) 1-2 gm IM once daily; max 4 gm/day
  Pediatric: 50-75 mg/kg IM in 1-2 divided doses; max 2 gm/day
    Rocephin *Vial:* 250, 500 mg; 1, 2 gm
▷ *cephalexin* (B)(G) 500 mg bid x 10 days
  Pediatric: 25-50 mg/kg/day in 4 divided doses x 10 days; *see page 623 for dose by weight*
    Keflex *Cap:* 250, 333, 500, 750 mg; *Oral susp:* 125, 250 mg/5 ml (100, 200 ml) (strawberry)
▷ *clarithromycin* (C)(G) 250-500 mg bid or 500-1000 mg ext-rel once daily x 7-14 days
  Pediatric: <6 months: not recommended; ≥6 months: 7.5 mg/kg bid x 7-14 days; *see page 624 for dose by weight*
    Biaxin *Tab:* 250, 500 mg
    Biaxin Oral Suspension *Oral susp:* 125, 250 mg/5 ml (50, 100 ml) (fruit punch)
    Biaxin XL *Tab:* 500 mg ext-rel
  Comment: The FDA is advising caution before prescribing *clarithromycin* to patients with heart disease because of a potential increased risk of heart problems or death that can occur years later. This recommendation is based on a review of the results of a 10-year follow-up study of patients with coronary heart disease from a large clinical trial that first observed this safety issue. Consider risk benefit and the use of other antibiotics in such patients.
▷ *dicloxacillin* (B) 500 mg qid x 10 days
  Pediatric: 12.5-25 mg/kg/day in 4 divided doses x 10 days; *see page 624 for dose by weight*
    Dynapen *Cap:* 125, 250, 500 mg; *Oral susp:* 62.5 mg/5 ml (80, 100, 200 ml)
▷ *dirithromycin* (C)(G) 500 mg once daily x 5-7 days
  Pediatric: <12 years: not recommended; ≥12 years: same as adult
    Dynabac *Tab:* 250 mg
▷ *doxycycline* (D)(G) 100 mg bid x 9 days
  Pediatric: <8 years: not recommended; ≥8 years, <100 lb: 1 mg/lb in a single dose once daily x 9 days; *see page 625 for dose by weight*; >8 years, ≥100 lb: same as adult
    Acticlate *Tab:* 75, 150**mg
    Adoxa *Tab:* 50, 75, 100, 150 mg ent-coat
    Doryx *Tab:* 50, 75, 100, 150, 200 mg del-rel
    Doxteric *Tab:* 50 mg del-rel
    Monodox *Cap:* 50, 75, 100 mg
    Oracea *Cap:* 40 mg del-rel
    Vibramycin *Tab:* 100 mg; *Cap:* 50, 100 mg; *Syr:* 50 mg/5 ml (raspberry-apple) (sulfites); *Oral susp:* 25 mg/5 ml (raspberry)
    Vibra-Tab *Tab:* 100 mg film-coat
  Comment: *doxycycline* is contraindicated <8 years-of-age, in pregnancy, and lactation (discolors developing tooth enamel). A side effect may be photosensitivity (photophobia). Do not take with antacids, calcium supplements, milk or other dairy, or within 2 hours of taking another drug.
▷ *erythromycin base* (B)(G) 250-500 mg tid x 10 days
  Pediatric: 30-50 mg/kg/day in 2-4 divided doses x 10 days
    Ery-Tab *Tab:* 250, 333, 500 mg ent-coat
    PCE *Tab:* 333, 500 mg
  Comment: *erythromycin* may increase INR with concomitant *warfarin*, as well as increase serum level of *digoxin*, benzodiazepines, and statins.
▷ *erythromycin estolate* (B)(G) 250-500 mg q 6 hours x 10 days
  Pediatric: 20-50 mg/kg q 6 hours x 10 days; *see page 625 for dose by weight*
    Ilosone *Pulvule:* 250 mg; *Tab:* 500 mg; *Liq:* 125, 250 mg/5 ml (100 ml)
  Comment: *erythromycin* may increase INR with concomitant *warfarin*, as well as increase serum level of *digoxin*, benzodiazepines, and statins.

➤ *erythromycin ethylsuccinate* (B)(G) 400 mg qid x 10 days
Pediatric: 30-50 mg/kg/day in 4 divided doses x 10 days; may double dose with severe
infection; max 100 mg/kg/day; *see page 626 for dose by weight*
   EryPed *Oral susp:* 200 mg/5 ml (100, 200 ml) (fruit); 400 mg/5 ml (60, 100, 200 ml)
   (banana); *Oral drops:* 200, 400 mg/5 ml (50 ml) (fruit); *Chew tab:* 200 mg wafer (fruit)
   E.E.S. *Oral susp:* 200, 400 mg/5 ml (100 ml) (fruit)
   E.E.S. Granules *Oral susp:* 200 mg/5 ml (100, 200 ml) (cherry)
   E.E.S. 400 Tablets *Tab:* 400 mg

Comment: *erythromycin* may increase INR with concomitant *warfarin,* as well as increase
serum level of *digoxin,* benzodiazepines, and statins.

➤ *gemifloxacin* (C)(G) 320 mg once daily x 5-7 days
Pediatric: <18 years: not recommended; ≥18 years: same as adult
   Factive *Tab:* 320*mg

Comment: *gemifloxacin* is contraindicated <18 years-of-age, and during pregnancy and
lactation. Risk of tendonitis or tendon rupture.

➤ *levofloxacin* (C) *Uncomplicated:* 500 mg once daily x 7-10 days; *Complicated:* 750 mg once
daily x 7-10 days
Pediatric: <18 years: not recommended; ≥18 years: same as adult
   Levaquin *Tab:* 250, 500, 750 mg; *Oral soln:* 25 mg/ml (480 ml) (benzyl alcohol);
   Inj conc: 25 mg/ml for IV infusion after dilution (20, 30 ml single-use vial)
   (preservative-free); *Premix soln:* 5 mg/ml for IV infusion (50, 100, 150 ml)
   (preservative-free)

Comment: *levofloxacin* is contraindicated <18 years-of-age, and during pregnancy and
lactation. Risk of tendonitis or tendon rupture.

➤ *linezolid* (C)(G) 400-600 mg q 12 hours x 10-14 days
Pediatric: <5 years: 10 mg/kg q 8 hours x 10-14 days; 5-11 years: 10 mg/kg q 12 hours x 10-
14 days; >11 years: same as adult
   Zyvox *Tab:* 400, 600 mg; *Oral susp:* 100 mg/5 ml (150 ml) (orange) (phenylalanine)

Comment: *linezolid* is indicated to treat susceptible vancomycin-resistant *E. faecium* infections.

➤ *loracarbef* (B) 200 mg bid x 7 days
Pediatric: 15 mg/kg/day in 2 divided doses x 7 days; *see page 628 for dose by weight*
   Lorabid *Pulvule:* 200, 400 mg; *Oral susp:* 100 mg/5 ml (50, 100 ml); 200 mg/5 ml (50,
   75, 100 ml) (strawberry bubble gum)

➤ *minocycline* (D)(G) 200 mg on first day; then 100 mg q 12 hours x 9 more days
Pediatric: <8 years: not recommended; ≥8 years, <100 lb: 2 mg/lb on first day in 2 divided
doses, followed by 1 mg/lb q 12 hours x 9 more days; ≥8 years, ≥100 lb: same as adult
   Dynacin *Cap:* 50, 100 mg
   Minocin *Cap:* 50, 75, 100 mg; *Oral susp:* 50 mg/5 ml (60 ml) (custard) (sulfites, alcohol 5%)

Comment: *minocycline* is contraindicated <8 years-of-age, in pregnancy, and lactation
(discolors developing tooth enamel). A side effect may be photosensitivity (photophobia).
Do not take with antacids, calcium supplements, milk or other dairy, or within two hours of
taking another drug.

➤ *moxifloxacin* (C)(G) 400 mg once daily x 10 days
Pediatric: <18 years: not recommended; ≥18 years: same as adult
   Avelox *Tab:* 400 mg

Comment: *moxifloxacin* is contraindicated <18 years-of-age, and during pregnancy and
lactation. Risk of tendonitis or tendon rupture.

➤ *ofloxacin* (C)(G) 400 mg bid x 10 days
Pediatric: <18 years: not recommended; ≥18 years: same as adult
   Floxin *Tab:* 200, 300, 400 mg

Comment: *ofloxacin* is contraindicated <18 years-of-age, and during pregnancy and
lactation. Risk of tendonitis or tendon rupture.

➤ *tetracycline* (D)(G) 500 mg qid x 10 days
Pediatric: <8 years: not recommended; ≥8 years, <100 lb: 25-50 mg/kg/day in 4 divided
doses x 10 days; ≥8 years, ≥100 lb: same as adult; *see page 630 for dose by weight*
   Achromycin V *Cap:* 250, 500 mg
   Sumycin *Tab:* 250, 500 mg; *Cap:* 250, 500 mg; *Oral susp:* 125 mg/5 ml (100, 200 ml)
   (fruit) (sulfites)

Comment: *tetracycline* is contraindicated <8 years-of-age, in pregnancy, and lactation
(discolors developing tooth enamel). A side effect may be photosensitivity (photophobia).

Do not take with antacids, calcium supplements, milk or other dairy, or within two hours of taking another drug.

SLEEP APNEA: OBSTRUCTIVE (HYPOPNEA SYNDROME)

ANTI-NARCOLEPTIC AGENTS
▷ *armodafinil* (C)(IV)(G) *OSAHS:* 150-250 mg once daily in the AM; *SWSD:* 150 mg 1 hour before starting shift; reduce dose with severe hepatic impairment
  Pediatric: <17 years: not recommended; ≥17 years: same as adult
    Nuvigil *Tab:* 50, 150, 200, 250 mg
▷ *modafinil* (C)(IV) 100-200 mg q AM; max 400 mg/day
  Pediatric: <16 years: not recommended; ≥16 years: same as adult
    Provigil *Tab:* 100, 200*mg
  Comment: *modafinil* promotes wakefulness in patients with excessive sleepiness due to obstructive sleep apnea/hypopnea syndrome.

SLEEPINESS: EXCESSIVE, SHIFT WORK SLEEP DISORDER (SWSD)

ANTI-NARCOLEPTIC AGENT
▷ *armodafinil* (C)(IV)(G) *OSAHS:* 150-250 mg once daily in the AM; *SWSD:* 150 mg 1 hour before starting shift; reduce dose with severe hepatic impairment
  Pediatric: <17 years: not recommended; ≥17 years: same as adult
    Nuvigil *Tab:* 50, 150, 200, 250 mg
▷ *modafinil* (C)(IV) 100-200 mg q AM; max 400 mg/day
  Pediatric: <16 years: not recommended; ≥16 years: same as adult
    Provigil *Tab:* 100, 200*mg
  Comment: **Provigil** promotes wakefulness in patients with narcolepsy, shift work sleep disorder, and excessive sleepiness due to obstructive sleep apnea/hypopnea syndrome.

SMALLPOX (*VARIOLA MAJOR*)

PROPHYLAXIS
▷ *vaccina virus* vaccine *(dried, calf lymph type)* (C)
  Pediatric: <12 months: not recommended; 12 months-18 years, non-emergency: not recommended
    DRYvax
      Kit: vial dried smallpox vaccine (1), 0.25 ml diluent in syringe (1), vented needle (1), 100 individually wrapped bifurcated needles (5 needles/strip, 20 strips) (poly-myxin b sulfate+dihydrostreptomycin+sulfate, chlortetracycline HCL+neomycin sulfate+glycerin+phenol)
  Comment: **DRYvax** is a dried live vaccine with approximately 100 million *Infectious vaccina* viruses (pock-forming units [pfu] per ml). Contact with immunosuppressed individuals should be avoided until the scab has separated from the skin (2 to 3 weeks) and/or a protective occlusive dressing covers the inoculation site. Scarification only. Do not inject IV, IM, or SC. Revaccination is recommended every 10 years.

TREATMENT
Comment: July 11, 2018, the U.S. Food and Drug Administration approved **Tpoxx** *(tecovirimat)*, the first drug with an indication for treatment of smallpox. Though the World Health Organization declared smallpox, a contagious and sometimes fatal infectious disease, eradicated in 1980, there have been longstanding concerns that smallpox could be used as a bioweapon. To address the risk of bioterrorism, Congress has taken steps to enable the development and approval of countermeasures to thwart pathogens that could be employed as weapons. **Tpoxx** is the first product to be awarded a Material Threat Medical Countermeasure priority review voucher.

▷ *tecovirimat* 600 mg bid x 14 days; take within 30 minutes after a full meal of moderate or high fat
  Pediatric: <13 kg: not recommended; 13 kg to < 25 kg: 200 mg bid x 14 days; 25 kg to < 40 kg: 400 mg bid x 14 days; ≥40 kg: 600 mg bid x 14 days

Tpoxx *Cap:* 200 mg

Comment: **Tpoxx** is an inhibitor of the orthopoxvirus VP37 envelope wrapping protein and is indicated for the treatment of human smallpox disease in adults and pediatric patients weighing ≥ 13 kg. The effectiveness of **Tpoxx** for treatment of smallpox disease has not been determined in humans because adequate and well-controlled field trials have not been feasible, and inducing smallpox disease in humans to study the drug's efficacy is not ethical. **Tpoxx** efficacy may be reduced in immunocompromised patients based on studies demonstrating reduced efficacy in immunocompromised animal models. Co-administration of **Tpoxx** with *repaglinide* may cause hypoglycemia. Monitor blood glucose and monitor for hypoglycemic symptoms during co-administration. No adequate and well-controlled studies in pregnancy have been conducted; therefore there are no human data to establish the presence or absence of **Tpoxx** associated risk. In animal reproduction studies, no embryo fetal developmental toxicity has been observed. There are no data to assess the presence of *tecovirimat* in human milk or effects on the breastfed infant; however, *tecovirimat* has been found in animal milk. Developmental and health benefits of breastfeeding should be considered along with the mother's clinical need for **Tpoxx** and any potential adverse effects on the breastfed infant from **Tpoxx** or from the underlying maternal condition. Common adverse reactions in healthy adult subjects (incidence ≥ 2%) were headache, nausea, abdominal pain, and vomiting. To report suspected adverse reactions, contact SIGA Technologies at 1-541-753-2000 or FDA at 1-800-FDA-1088 or www.fda.gov/medwatch.

SPINAL MUSCULAR ATROPHY (SMA)

Comment: Spinal muscular atrophy (SMA) is a group of inherited disorders characterized by motor neuron loss in the spinal cord and lower brainstem, muscle weakness, and atrophy. Survival motor neuron (SMN) protein is essential for the maintenance of motor neurons. Because of a defect in, or loss of, the SMN1 gene, patients with SMA do not produce enough SMN protein. It is the most common genetic cause of death in infants, but can affect people at any age. **Spinraza** (*nusinersen*) is the first FDA-approved drug to treat SMA.

SURVIVAL MOTOR NEURON-2 (SMN2)-DIRECTED ANTISENSE OLIGONUCLEOTIDE

▷ *nusinersen* 12 mg per intrathecal administration; initially four loading doses: the first 3 loading doses administered at 14-day intervals; the 4th loading dose administered 30 days after the 3rd loading dose; the maintenance dose is administered every 4 months after the 4th loading dose; prior to administration, 5 ml cerebral spinal fluid (CSF) should be removed; the intrathecal bolus injection should be administered over 1-3 minutes using a spinal anesthetic needle.
Pediatric: same as adult

Spinraza *Vial:* 12 mg/5 ml (2.4 mg/ml) single-dose, solution for intrathecal administration (preservative-free)

Comment: At baseline and prior to each dose, obtain a platelet count and coagulation laboratory testing (there is increased risk for thrombocytopenia and coagulation abnormalities) and quantitative spot urine protein testing (to monitor for renal toxicity). Store **Spinraza** in a refrigerator between 2°C to 8°C (36°F to 46°F) in the original carton to protect from light. Do not freeze. Prior to administration, unopened vials of **Spinraza** can be removed from and returned to the refrigerator, if necessary. If removed from the original carton, the total combined time out of refrigeration should not exceed 30 hours at a temperature that does not exceed 25°C (77°F). **Spinraza** has no labeled contraindications. **Spinraza** has not been studied in pregnant or lactating females, or in patients with renal or hepatic impairment.

SPRAIN

Comment: RICE: Rest; Ice; Compression; Elevation.

Injectable Acetaminophen *see Pain page* 352
NSAIDs *see page* 571
Opioid Analgesics *see Pain page* 354
Topical and Transdermal Analgesics *see Pain page* 352
Parenteral Corticosteroids *see page* 577
Oral Corticosteroids *see page* 577
Topical Analgesic and Anesthetic Agents *see page* 569

STATUS ASTHMATICUS

Inhaled Beta-2 Agonists (Bronchodilators) *see* Asthma *page* 30
Oral Beta-2 Agonists (Bronchodilators) *see* Asthma *page* 36
Inhaled Anticholinergics *see* Asthma *page* 31
Inhaled Anticholinergic+Beta-2 Agonist Combination *see* Asthma *page* 30
Methylxanthines *see* Asthma *page* 30
Parenteral Corticosteroids *see page* 577
Oral Corticosteroids *see page* 577

EPINEPHRINE

▷ *epinephrine* (C)(G) 0.3-0.5 mg (0.3-0.5 ml of a 1:1000 soln) SC q 20-30 minutes as needed
up to 3 doses
Pediatric: <2 years: 0.05-0.1 ml; 2-6 years: 0.1 ml; 6-12 years: 0.2 ml; All: q 20-30 minutes as
needed up to 3 doses; >12 years: same as adult

ANAPHYLAXIS EMERGENCY TREATMENT KITS

▷ *epinephrine* (C) 0.3 ml IM or SC in thigh; may repeat if needed
Pediatric: 0.01 mg/kg SC or IM in thigh; may repeat if needed; <15 kg: not recommended;
15-30 kg: 0.15 mg; >30 kg: same as adult
   AdrenaClick *Auto-injector:* 0.15, 0.3 mg (1 mg/ml; 2/carton) (sulfites)
   Auvi-Q *Auto-injector:* 0.15, 0.3 mg (1 mg/ml; 2/carton w. 1 non active training device)
   (sulfites)
   EpiPen *Autoinjector* 0.3 mg (epi 1:1000, 0.3 ml (2/carton) (sulfites)
   EpiPen Jr *Autoinjector* 0.15 mg (epi 1:2000, 0.3 ml (2/carton) (sulfites)
   Twinject *Autoinjector:* 0.15, 0.3 mg (epi 1:1000, 2/carton) (sulfites)
▷ *epinephrine+chlorpheniramine* (C) epinephrine 0.3 ml SC or IM plus 4 tabs *chlorpheni-
ramine* by mouth
Pediatric: infants-2 years: 0.05-0.1 ml SC or IM; 2-6 years: 0.15 ml SC or IM plus 1 tab
chlor; 6-12 years: 0.2 ml SC or IM plus 2 tabs chlor; >12 years: same as adult
   Ana-Kit: 0.3 ml syringes of *epi* 1:1000 (2/carton) for self-injection plus chlor 2 mg
   chewable tabs x 4

 STATUS EPILEPTICUS

Anticonvulsant Drugs *see page* 591
▷ *diazepam* injectable (D)(IV) initially 5-10 mg IV in large vein; may repeat q 10-15 minutes; max 30 mg; may repeat in 2-4 hours if needed; do not dilute; may give IM if IV not
accessible
Pediatric: 1 month-5 years: 0.2-0.5 mg IV q 2-5 minutes; max 5 mg; >5 years: 1 mg IV q 2-5
minutes; max 10 mg; may repeat in 2-4 hours if needed
   Diastat *Rectal gel delivery system:* 2.5 mg
   Diastat AcuDial *Rectal gel delivery system:* 10, 20 mg
   Valium Injectable *Vial:* 5 mg/ml (10 ml); *Amp:* 5 mg/ml (2 ml); *Prefilled syringe:* 5 mg/
   ml (5 ml)
   Valium Intensol Oral Solution *Conc oral soln:* 5 mg/ml (30 ml w. dropper) (alcohol
   19%)
   Valium Oral Solution *Oral soln:* 5 mg/5 ml (500 ml) (wintergreen-spice)
▷ *lorazepam* injectable (D)(IV) 4 mg IV over 2 minutes (dilute first); may repeat in 10-15
minutes; may give IM if needed (undiluted)
Pediatric: <18 years: not recommended; ≥18 years: same as adult
   Ativan Injectable *Vial:* 2 mg/ml (1, 10 ml); *Tubex:* 2 mg/ml (0.5 ml); *Cartridge:* 2, 4 mg/
   ml (1 ml)
▷ *phenytoin (injectable)* (D)(G) 10-15 mg/kg IV, not to exceed 50 mg/minute; follow with
100 mg orally or IV q 6-8 hours; do not dilute in IV fluid
Pediatric: 15-20 mg/kg IV, not to exceed 1-2 mg/kg/minute
   Dilantin *Vial:* 50 mg/ml (2, 5 ml); *Amp:* 50 mg/ml (2 ml)
   COMMENT: Monitor *phenytoin* serum levels. Therapeutic serum level: 10-20 gm/ml. Side
   effects include gingival hyperplasia.

STYE (HORDEOLUM)

OPHTHALMIC ANTI-INFECTIVES

➤ *erythromycin* ophthalmic ointment **(B)** 1 cm up to 6 x/day
  Pediatric: same as adult
    Ilotycin Ophthalmic Ointment *Ophth oint:* 5 mg/gm (1/8 oz)
➤ *erythromycin* ophthalmic solution **(B)** initially 1-2 drops q 1-2 hours; may then increase
  dose interval
  Pediatric: same as adult
    Isopto Cetamide Ophthalmic Solution *Ophth soln:* 15% (15 ml)
➤ *gentamicin* ophthalmic ointment **(C)** 1 cm bid-tid
  Pediatric: same as adult
    Garamycin Ophthalmic Ointment *Ophth oint:* 3 mg/gm (3.5 gm)
    Genoptic Ophthalmic Ointment *Ophth oint:* 3 mg/gm (3.5 gm)
    Gentacidin Ophthalmic Ointment *Ophth oint:* 3 mg/gm (3.5 gm)
➤ *polymyxin b+bacitracin* ophthalmic ointment **(C)** apply 1/2 inch q 3-4 hours
  Pediatric: same as adult
    Polysporin *Ophth oint:* poly b 10,000 U+bac 500 units per gm (3.75 gm)
➤ *polymyxin b+bacitracin+neomycin* ophthalmic ointment **(C)(G)** apply 1/2 inch q 3-4
  hours
  Pediatric: same as adult
    Neosporin Ophthalmic Ointment *Ophth oint:* poly b 10,000 U+bac 400 U+neo 3.5 mg/
    gm (3.75 gm)
➤ *polymyxin b+neomycin+gramicidin* ophthalmic solution **(C)** 1-2 drops 2-3 times q 1 hour;
  then 1-2 drops bid-qid x 7-10 days
  Pediatric: same as adult
    Neosporin Ophthalmic Solution
    Ophth soln: poly b 10,000 U+neo 1.75 mg/gm 0.025 mg/ml (10 ml)
➤ *sodium sulfacetamide* ophthalmic solution and ointment **(C)**
    Bleph-10 Ophthalmic Solution 2 drops q 4 hour x 7-14 days
    Pediatric: <2 years: not recommended; ≥2 years: 1-2 drops q 2-3 hours during the day
      Ophth soln: 10% (2.5, 5, 15 ml; benzalkonium chloride)
    Bleph-10 Ophthalmic Ointment apply 1/2 inch qid and HS
    Pediatric: <2 years: not recommended; ≥2 years: apply 1/4-1/3 inch qid and HS
      Ophth oint: 10% (3.5 gm) (phenylmercuric acetate)

SUNBURN

➤ *prednisone* **(C)(G)** 10 mg qid x 4-6 days if severe and extensive
➤ *silver sulfadiazine* **(C)(G)** apply topically to burn once daily-bid
  Pediatric: <12 years: not recommended; ≥12 years: same as adult
    Silvadene *Crm:* 1% (20, 50, 85, 400, 1000 gm jar; 20 gm tube)
Comment: *silver sulfadiazine* is contradicted in sulfa allergy, late pregnancy, within the first
2 months after birth, premature infants.

SYPHILIS (*TREPONEMA PALLIDUM*)

Comment: The following treatment regimens for *T. pallidum* are published in the **2015 CDC
Sexually Transmitted Diseases Treatment Guidelines**. Treat all sexual contacts. Consider testing
for other STDs. *Penicillin g*, administered parenterally, is the preferred drug for treating all stages
of syphilis. The preparation used (i.e., benzathine, aqueous procaine, or aqueous crystalline),
the dosage, and the length of treatment depend on the stage and clinical manifestations of
the disease. Combinations of *benzathine penicillin*, *procaine penicillin*, and oral *penicillin*
preparations are not appropriate (e.g., **Bicillin C-R**). All women should be screened serologically
for syphilis early in pregnancy. There are no proven alternatives to *penicillin* for the treatment of
syphilis during pregnancy. Pregnant patients who are allergic to penicillin should be desensitized
and treated with *penicillin*. Sexual transmission of *T. pallidum* is thought to occur only when
mucocutaneous syphilis at any stage should be evaluated clinically and serologically and treated
with a recommended regimen according to CDC guidelines.

PRIMARY, SECONDARY, AND EARLY LATENT (<1 YEAR) SYPHILIS

Regimen 1

▷ *penicillin g (benzathine)* 2.4 million units IM in a single dose

LATE LATENT, LATENT SYPHILIS OF UNKNOWN DURATION, AND TERTIARY SYPHILIS

Regimen 1

▷ *penicillin g (benzathine)* 7.2 million units total administered in 3 divided doses of 2.4 million units each IM at 1 week intervals

REGIMEN: ADULT, NEUROSYPHILIS

Regimen 1

▷ *aqueous crystalline penicillin g* 18-24 million units per day, administered as 3-4 million units IV every 4 hours or continuous IV infusion, for 10-14 days

ALTERNATIVE REGIMEN: ADULT, NEUROSYPHILIS

Regimen 1

▷ *penicillin g (procaine)* 2.4 million units IM once daily x 10-14 days plus *probenecid* 500 mg qid x 10-14 days

PRIMARY AND SECONDARY SYPHILIS IN HIV-INFECTED PERSONS

Regimen 1

▷ *penicillin g (benzathine)* 2.4 million units IM in a single dose

LATENT SYPHILIS AMONG HIV-INFECTED PERSONS

Comment: Treatment is the same as for HIV-negative persons.

CONGENITAL SYPHILIS

Regimen 1

▷ *aqueous crystalline penicillin g* 100,000-150,000 units/kg/day, administered as 50,000 units IV every 12 hours during the first 7 days of life and every 8 hours thereafter for a total of 10 days

ALTERNATE REGIMEN

Regimen 1

▷ *penicillin g (benzathine)* 50,000 units/kg IM in a single dose

Regimen 2

▷ *penicillin g (procaine)* 50,000 units/kg/dose IM, administered in a single daily dose x 10 days

OLDER INFANTS AND CHILDREN

Regimen 1

▷ *aqueous crystalline penicillin g* 200,000-300,000 units/kg/day, administered as 50,000 units IV every 12 hours during the first 7 days of life and every 4-6 hours thereafter for a total of 10 days

DRUG BRANDS AND DOSE FORMS

▷ *aqueous crystalline penicillin g* (B)(G)
▷ *penicillin g (benzathine)* (B)(G)
   Bicillin L-A *Cartridge-needle unit:* 600,000 million units (1 ml); 1.2 million units (2 ml); 2.4 million units (4 ml)
▷ *penicillin g (procaine)* (B)(G)
   Bicillin C-R Cartridge-needle unit: 600,000 units (1 ml); 1.2 million units; (2 ml); 2.4 million units (4 ml)
▷ *probenecid* (B)(G)
   Benemid *Tab:* 500*mg; *Cap:* 500 mg

SYSTEMIC LUPUS ERYTHEMATOSIS (SLE)

NSAIDs *see page* 571
Oral Corticosteroids *see page* 577

Comment: All SLE patients should routinely be given *hydroxychloroquine* HCQ and supplemental vitamin D as low levels of vitamin D are associated with higher rates of ESRD; supplemental vitamin D reduces urine protein (the best predictor of future renal failure). Vitamin D insufficiency and deficiency are more common in patients with SLE than in the general population. Vitamin D supplementation may decrease disease activity and improve fatigue. In addition, supplementation may improve endothelial function, which may reduce cardiovascular disease. A disease-modifying anti-rheumatic drug (DMARD) should be added when a patient's prednisone dose cannot be tapered and also when hemolysis is present and hemoglobin is abnormally low in the setting of mild-to-moderate hematological involvement. Other DMARDs, such as *methotrexate (MTX)*, *azathioprine*, *mycophenolate mofetil* (MMF), *cyclosporine* (CYC), and other calcineurin-inhibitors should be considered in cases of arthritis, cutaneous disease, serositis, vasculitis, or cytopaenias if HCQ is insufficient. For refractory cases, *belimumab* (Benlysta) or *rituximab* (Rituxan), may be considered. The recommended dose of *rituximab*, if required, is either 750 mg/m^2 (to a maximum of 1 gm per day) at day 1 and day 15, or 375 mg/m^2 once a week for 4 doses. In patients with SLE without major organ manifestations, glucocorticoids and antimalarial agents may be beneficial. NSAIDs may be used for short periods in patients at low risk for complications from these drugs. Consider immunosuppressive agents (e.g., *azathioprine*, MMF, MTX) in refractory cases or when steroid doses cannot be reduced to levels for long-term use.

REFERENCES

Gordon, C., Amissah-Arthur, M.-B., Gayed, M., Brown, S., Bruce, I. N., D'Cruz, D., . . . Isenberg, D. (2018). The British Society for Rheumatology guideline for the management of systemic lupus erythematosus in adults. *Rheumatology, 57*(1), e1–e45. doi:10.1093/rheumatology/kex286

Groot, N., de Graeff, N., Avcin, T., Bader-Meunier, B., Brogan, P., Dolezalova, P., . . . Beresford, M. W. (2017). European evidence-based recommendations for diagnosis and treatment of childhood-onset systemic lupus erythematosus: The SHARE initiative. *Annals of the Rheumatic Diseases, 76*(11), 1788–1796. doi:10.1136/annrheumdis-2016-210960

Leach, M. Z. (2017, November 7). First UK guidelines for adults with lupus. *Rheumatology Network*. Retrieved from http://www.rheumatologynetwork.com/article/first-uk-guidelines-adults-lupus

CD20 ANTIBODY

▷ *rituximab* (C) administer corticosteroid 30 minutes prior to each infusion; concomitant *methotrexate* therapy, administer a 1000 mg IV infusion at 0 and 2 weeks; then every 24 weeks or based on response, but not sooner than every 16 weeks.
  Pediatric: <6 years: not recommended; >6 years: same as adult
    Rituxan *Vial:* 10 mg/ml (10, 50 ml) (preservative-free)

B-LYMPHOCYTE STIMULATOR (BLyS)-SPECIFIC INHIBITOR

▷ *belimumab*
    SC administration: 200 mg SC once weekly. May be self-administered by the patient in the home setting.
  Comment: **Benlysta** was initially approved as an intravenous formulation administered in a hospital or clinic setting as a weight-dosed IV infusion every four weeks. Patients can now self-administer **Benlysta** as a once weekly SC injection after being trained by a health care provider.
    IV infusion: 10 mg/kg at 2-week intervals for the first 3 doses and at 4-week intervals thereafter; reconstitute, dilute, and administer as an intravenous infusion over a period of 1 hour. Consider administering premedication for prophylaxis against infusion reactions and hypersensitivity reactions. Must be administered in a hospital or clinic setting by a qualified healthcare provider
  Pediatric: <18 years: not established; ≥18 years: same as adult
    Benlysta Prefilled syringe: 200 mg/ml (1 ml) single-dose (4/carton); *Autoinjector:* 200 mg (1 ml) single-dose (4/carton); *Vial:* 120 mg/5 ml, 400 mg/ 20 ml, single-dose, pwdr for reconstitution and IV infusion (4/carton)

Comment: **Benlysta** is indicated for the treatment of patients >18 years-of-age with active, autoantibody-positive, systemic lupus erythematosus who are receiving standard therapy. Common adverse reactions include nausea, diarrhea, pyrexia, nasopharyngitis, bronchitis, insomnia, pain in extremity, depression, migraine, and pharyngitis. The efficacy of **Benlysta** has not been evaluated in patients with severe active lupus nephritis or severe active central nervous system lupus. **Benlysta** has not been studied in combination with other biologics or intravenous *cyclophosphamide*. Therefore, use of Benlysta is not recommended in these situations. Limited data on use of **Benlysta** in pregnancy women, from observational studies, published case reports, and post-marketing surveillance, is insufficient to determine whether there is a drug-associated risk for major birth defects or miscarriage. Monoclonal antibodies, such as *belimumab,* are actively transported across the placenta during the third trimester of pregnancy and may affect immune response in the in utero-exposed infant. Monoclonal antibodies are increasingly transported across the placenta as pregnancy progresses, with the largest amount transferred during the third trimester. No information is available on the presence of *belimumab* in human milk or the effects of the drug on the breastfed infant. As there are risks to the mother and fetus associated with SLE, risks and benefits should be considered prior to administering live or live-attenuated vaccines to infants exposed to **Benlasta** in utero. Monitor the infant of a treated mother for B-cell reduction and other immune dysfunction. There is a pregnancy exposure registry that monitors pregnancy outcomes in females exposed to **Benlysta** during pregnancy. Healthcare professionals are encouraged to register patients by calling 1-877-681-6296. To report suspected adverse reactions, contact GlaxoSmithKline at 1-877-423-6597 or FDA at 1-800-FDA-1088 or www.fda.gov/medwatch.

DISEASE MODIFYING ANTI-RHEUMATIC DRUGS (DMARDs)

Comment: DMARDs include *penicillamine*, gold salts (*auranofin, aurothioglucose*), immunosuppressants, and *hydroxychloroquine*. The DMARDs reduce ESR, reduce RF, and favorably affect SLE symptoms. Immunosuppressants may require 6 weeks to affect benefits and 6 months for full improvement.

➤ *auranofin (gold salt)* (C) 3 mg bid or 6 mg once daily; if inadequate response after 6 months, increase to 3 mg tid
  Pediatric: <12 years: not recommended; ≥12 years: same as adult
    Ridaura *Vial:* 100 mg/20 ml

➤ *azathioprine* (D) 1 mg/kg/day in a single or divided doses; may increase by 0.5 mg/kg/day q 4 weeks; max 2.5 mg/kg/day; minimum trial to ascertain effectiveness is 12 weeks
  Pediatric: <12 years: not recommended; ≥12 years: same as adult
    Azasan *Tab* 75*, 100*mg
    Imuran *Tab* 50*mg

➤ *cyclosporine (immunosuppressant)* (C) 1.25 mg/kg bid; may increase after 4 weeks by 0.5 mg/kg/day; then adjust at 2 week intervals; max 4 mg/kg/day; administer with meals
  Pediatric: <12 years: not recommended; ≥12 years: same as adult
    Neoral *Cap:* 25, 100 mg (alcohol)
    Neoral Oral Solution *Oral soln:* 100 mg/ml (50 ml) may dilute in room temperature apple juice or orange juice (alcohol)
    Comment: **Neoral** is indicated for RA unresponsive to *methotrexate* (MTX).

➤ *leflunomide* (X)(G) initially 100 mg once daily x 3 days; maintenance dose 20 mg once daily; max 20 mg daily
  Pediatric: <18 years: not recommended; ≥18 years: same as adult
    Arava *Tab:* 10, 20, 100 mg
    Comment: **Arava** is contraindicated with breastfeeding.

➤ *methotrexate* (X) 7.5 mg x 1 dose per week or 2.5 mg x 3 at 12 hour intervals once a week; max 20 mg/week; therapeutic response begins in 3-6 weeks; administer *methotrexate* injection SC only into the abdomen or thigh
  Pediatric: <2 years: not recommended; ≥2 years: 10 mg/m² once weekly; max 20 mg/m²
    Rasuvo *Autoinjector:* 7.5 mg/0.15 ml, 10 mg/0.20 ml, 12.5 mg/0.25 ml, 15 mg/0.30 ml, 17.5 mg/0.35 ml, 20 mg/0.40 ml, 22.5 mg/0.45 ml, 25 mg/0.50 ml, 27.5 mg/0.55 ml, 30 mg/0.60 ml (solution concentration for SC injection is 50 mg/ml)

Rheumatrex *Tab:* 2.5*mg (5, 7.5, 10, 12.5, 15 mg/week, 4/card unit-of-use dose pack)
Trexall *Tab:* 5*, 7.5*, 10*, 15*mg (5, 7.5, 10, 12.5, 15 mg/week, 4/card unit-of-use dose pack)

Comment: *methotrexate* (MTX) is contraindicated with immunodeficiency, blood dyscrasias, alcoholism, and chronic liver disease.

▶ *penicillamine* administer on an empty stomach, at least one hour before meals <u>or</u> two hours after meals, <u>and</u> at least one hour apart from any other drug, food, milk, antacid, zinc or iron-containing preparation; maintenance dosage must be individualized, and may require adjustment during the course of treatment. *initially*, a single daily dose of 125-250 mg; then, increase at 1-3 month intervals by 125-250 mg/day, as patient response and tolerance indicate; if a satisfactory remission of symptoms is achieved, the dose associated with the remission should be continued as the patient's maintenance therapy; if there is <u>no</u> improvement, and there are <u>no</u> signs of potentially serious toxicity after 2-3 months of treatment with doses of 500-750 mg/day, increase by 250 mg/day at 2-3 month intervals until a satisfactory remission occurs <u>or</u> signs of toxicity develop; if there is <u>no</u> discernible improvement after 3-4 months of treatment with 1000-1500 mg/day, discontinue **Cuprimine**. Changes in maintenance dosage levels may <u>not</u> be reflected clinically <u>or</u> in the erythrocyte sedimentation rate (ESR) for 2-3 months after each dosage adjustment.

Cuprimine *Cap:* 125, 250 mg
Depen: 250 mg

Comment: The use of *penicillamine* has been associated with fatalities due to certain diseases such as aplastic anemia, agranulocytosis, thrombocytopenia, Goodpasture's syndrome, and myasthenia gravis. Because of the potential for serious hematological and renal adverse reactions to occur at any time, routine urinalysis, white and differential blood cell count, hemoglobin, and direct platelet count must be checked twice weekly, together with monitoring of the patient's skin, lymph nodes and body temperature, during the first month of therapy, every two weeks for the next five months, and monthly thereafter. Patients should be instructed to report promptly the development of signs and symptoms of granulocytopenia and/or thrombocytopenia such as fever, sore throat, chills, bruising or bleeding; the above laboratory studies should then be promptly repeated.

▶ *sulfasalazine* (C; D in 2nd, 3rd)(G) initially 0.5 gm once daily bid; gradually increase every 4 days; usual maintenance 2-3 gm/day in equally divided doses at regular intervals; max 4 gm/day
Pediatric: <6 years: not recommended; 6-16 years: initially 1/4 to 1/3 of maintenance dose; increase weekly; maintenance 30-50 mg/kg/day in 2 divided doses at regular intervals; max 2 gm/day

Azulfidine *Tab:* 500 mg
Azulfidine EN *Tab:* 500 mg ent-coat

ANTIMALARIALS

▶ *atovaquone* (C)(G) take as a single dose with food <u>or</u> a milky drink at the same time each day; repeat dose if vomited within 1 hour; *Prophylaxis:* 1,500 mg once daily; *Treatment:* 750 mg bid x 21 days
Pediatric: <13 years: not established; ≥13 years: same as adult
Mepron *Susp:* 750 mg/5 ml

▶ *atovaquone+proguanil* (C)(G) >40 kg: take as a single dose with food <u>or</u> a milky drink at the same time each day; repeat dose if vomited within 1 hour; *Prophylaxis:* 1 tab daily starting 1-2 days before entering endemic area, during stay, and for 7 days after return; *Treatment (acute, uncomplicated):* 4 tabs daily x 3 days
Pediatric: <5 kg: not recommended; 5-40 kg:
Prophylaxis: daily dose starting 1-2 days before entering endemic area, during stay, and for 7 days after return; 5-20 kg: 1 ped tab; 21-30 kg: 2 ped tabs; 31-40 kg: 3 ped tabs; ≥40 kg: same as adult; *Treatment (acute, uncomplicated):* daily dose x 3 days; 5-8 kg: 2 ped tabs; 9-10 kg: 3 ped tabs; 11-20 kg: 1 adult tab; 21-30 kg: 2 adult tabs; 31-40 kg: 3 adult tabs; >40 kg: same as adult

Malarone *Tab:* atov 250 mg+prog 100 mg
Malarone Pediatric *Tab:* atov 62.5 mg+prog 25 mg

Comment: *atovaquone* is antagonized by *tetracycline* and *metoclopramide*. Concomitant *rifampin* is not recommended (may elevate LFTs).

▶ *chloroquine* (C)(G) *Prophylaxis:* 500 mg once weekly (on the same day of each week); start 2 weeks prior to exposure, continue while in the endemic area, and continue 4 weeks after

departure; *Treatment:* initially 1 gm; then 500 mg 6 hours, 24 hours, and 48 hours after initial dose or initially 200-250 mg IM; may repeat in 6 hours; max 1 gm in first 24 hours; continue to 1.875 gm in 3 days
Pediatric: Suppression: 8.35 mg/kg (max 500 mg) weekly (on the same day of each week); *Treatment:* initially 16.7 mg/kg (max 1 gm); then 8.35 mg/kg (max 500 mg) 6 hours, 24 hours, and 48 hours after initial dose, or initially 6.25 mg/kg IM; may repeat in 6 hours; max 12.5 mg/kg/day
Pediatric:
    Aralen *Tab:* 500 mg; *Amp:* 50 mg/ml (5 ml)
Comment: There are no adequate and well-controlled studies evaluating the safety and efficacy of *chloroquine* in pregnant women. Usage of *chloroquine* during pregnancy should be avoided except in the suppression or treatment of malaria when the benefit outweighs the potential risk to the fetus. Because of the potential for serious adverse reactions in nursing infants from chloroquine, a decision should be made whether to discontinue nursing or to discontinue the drug, taking into account the potential clinical benefit of the drug to the mother. Since this drug is known to concentrate in the liver, it should be used with caution in patients with hepatic disease or alcoholism or in conjunction with known hepatotoxic drugs.

▷ *hydroxychloroquine* (C)(G) 400-600 mg/day
Pediatric: <12 years: not recommended; ≥12 years: same as adult
    Plaquenil *Tab:* 200 mg
Comment: May require several weeks to achieve beneficial effects. If no improvement in 6 months, discontinue.

▷ *mefloquine* (C) *Prophylaxis:* 250 mg once weekly (on the same day of each week); start 1 week prior to exposure, continue while in the endemic area, and continue for 4 weeks after departure; *Treatment:* 1,250 mg as a single dose
Pediatric: <6 months: not recommended; *Prophylaxis:* ≥6 months: 3-5 mg/kg (max 250 mg) weekly (on the same day of each week); start 1 week prior to exposure, continue while in the endemic area, and continue for 4 weeks after departure; *Treatment:* ≥6 months: 25-50 mg/kg as a single dose; max 250 mg
    Lariam *Tab:* 250*mg
Comment: *mefloquine* is contraindicated with active or recent history of depression, generalized anxiety disorder, psychosis, schizophrenia or any other psychiatric disorder or history of convulsions.

▷ *quinine sulfate* (C)(G) 1 tab or cap every 8 hours x 7 days
Pediatric: <16 years: not recommended; ≥16 years: same as adult
    Tab: 260 mg; *Cap:* 260, 300, 325 mg
    Qualaquin *Cap:* 324 mg
    Comment: *Qualaquin* is indicated in the treatment of uncomplicated *P. falciparum* malaria (including chloroquine-resistant strains).

TAKAYASU ARTERITIS

Comment: TA is a rare yet well-described large-vessel vasculitis with a predilection for the aorta and its primary branches. Treatment options focus on preventing disease progression. There is no consensus on regimen, but high-dose pulse corticosteroid therapy is favored for induction, and long-term therapy includes immunosuppressants and biologics such as *cyclophosphamide, mycophenolate mofetil, methotrexate, infliximab* or *tocilizumab*, as well as revascularization surgery. Disease recurrence is common, and mortality rates can range from 16% to 40%. Therefore, prompt identification and treatment is imperative to prevent further morbidity and mortality.

REFERENCE

Mihalek, A, Parisky, A, McDermott, A, & Shaham B. (2017, July 3). Takayasu arteritis in a child. *Consultant for Pediatricians.* https://www.consultant360.com/articles/takayasu-arteritis-child

TAPEWORM (CESTODE)

ANTHELMINTICS

Comment: Oral bioavailability of anthelmintics is enhanced when administered with a fatty meal (estimated fat content 40 gm).

▷ *albendazole* (C)(G) take with a meal; may crush and mix with food; 400 mg bid x 7 days; may repeat in 3 weeks if needed
Pediatric: <2 years: 200 mg once daily x 3 days; may repeat in 3 weeks; ≥2-12 years: 400 mg once daily x 3 days; may repeat in 3 weeks; ≥12 years: same as adult
    Albenza *Tab:* 200 mg
    Comment: *albendazole* is a broad-spectrum benzimidazole carbamate anthelmintic.
▷ *nitazoxanide* (B) take with a meal; may crush and mix with food; 500 mg q 12 hours x 3 days
Pediatric: <12 months: not recommended; ≥12 months: treat q 12 hours x 3 days; <11 years: [susp] 12-47 months: 5 ml; 4-11 years: 10 ml; ≥11 years: [tab/susp] 500 mg
    Alinia *Tab:* 500 mg; *Oral susp:* 100 mg/5 ml (60 ml)
▷ *praziquantel* (B)(G) take with a meal; may crush and mix with food; 5-10 mg/kg as a single dose
Pediatric: <4 years: not established; ≥4 years: same as adult
    Biltricide *Tab:* 600 mg film-coat (scored for half or quarter dose)
    Comment: Therapeutically effective levels of **Biltricide** may not be achieved when administered concomitantly with strong P450 inducers, such as *rifampin.* Females should not breastfeed on the day of **Biltricide** treatment and during the subsequent 72 hours. Use caution with hepatosplenic patients who have moderate to severe liver impairment (Child-Pugh Class B and C).

TARDIVE DYSKINESIA

Comment: Tardive dyskinesia is a treatable, albeit irreversible, neurological disorder characterized by repetitive involuntary movements, usually of the jaw, lips and tongue, such as grimacing, sticking out the tongue and smacking the lips. Some affected people also experience involuntary movement of the extremities or difficulty breathing. This condition is most often an adverse side effect associated with the older "typical" antipsychotic drugs. Risk is decreased with the newer "atypical" antipsychotic drugs. The first and only FDA-approved treatment for this disorder is *valbenazine* (**Ingrezza**), a vesicular monoamine transporter 2 (VMAT2) inhibitor.

REFERENCE

Davis, M. C., Miller, B. J., Kalsi, J. K., Birkner, T., & Mathis, M. V. (2017). Efficient trial design—FDA approval of valbenazine for tardive dyskinesia. *New England Journal of Medicine, 376*(26), 2503–2506. doi:10.1056/NEJMp1704898

VESICULAR MONOAMINE TRANSPORTER 2 (VMAT2) INHIBITOR

▷ *valbenazine* initially 40 mg once daily; after one week, increase to the recommended 80 mg once daily; take with or without food; recommended dose for patients with moderate or severe hepatic impairment is 40 mg once daily; consider dose reduction based on tolerability in known CYP2D6 poor metabolizers; concomitant use of strong CYP3A4 inducers is not recommended; avoid concomitant use of MAOIs
Pediatric: <18 years: not established; ≥18 years: same as adult
    Ingrezza *Cap:* 40 mg
    Comment: Safety and effectiveness of **Ingrezza** have not been established in pediatric patients. No dose adjustment is required for elderly patients. The limited available data on **Ingrezza** use in pregnant women are insufficient to inform a drug-associated risk. There is no information regarding the presence of **Ingrezza** or its metabolites in human milk, the effects on the breastfed infant, or the effects on milk production. However, women are advised not to breastfeed during treatment and for 5 days after the final dose. To report suspected adverse reactions, contact Neurocrine Biosciences, Inc. at 877-641-3461 or FDA at 1-800-FDA-1088 or www.fda.gov/medwatch.

TEMPOROMANDIBULAR JOINT (TMJ) DISORDER

Injectable Acetaminophen *see Pain page* 352
NSAIDs *see page* 571
Opioid Analgesics *see Pain page* 354
Topical and Transdermal Analgesics *see Pain page* 352
Parenteral Corticosteroids *see page* 577
Oral Corticosteroids *see page* 577
Topical Analgesic and Anesthetic Agents *see page* 569

SKELETAL MUSCLE RELAXANTS

▷ *baclofen* (C)(G) 5 mg tid; titrate up by 5 mg every 3 days to 20 mg tid; max 80 mg/day
Pediatric: <12 years: not recommended; ≥12 years: same as adult
   Lioresal *Tab:* 10*, 20*mg
Comment: *baclofen* is indicated for muscle spasm pain and chronic spasticity associated with multiple sclerosis and spinal cord injury or disease. Potential for seizures or hallucinations on abrupt withdrawal.

▷ *carisoprodol* (C)(G) 1 tab tid or qid
Pediatric: <12 years: not recommended; ≥12 years: same as adult
   Soma *Tab:* 350 mg

▷ *chlorzoxazone* (G) 1 caplet qid; max 750 mg qid
Pediatric: <12 years: not recommended; ≥12 years: same as adult
   Parafon Forte DSC *Cplt:* 500*mg

▷ *cyclobenzaprine* (B)(G) 10 mg tid; usual range 20-40 mg/day in divided doses; max 60 mg/day x 2-3 weeks or 15 mg ext-rel once daily; max 30 mg ext-rel/day x 2-3 weeks
Pediatric: <15 years: not recommended; ≥15 years: same as adult
   Amrix *Cap:* 15, 30 mg ext-rel
   Fexmid *Tab:* 7.5 mg
   Flexeril *Tab:* 5, 10 mg

▷ *dantrolene* (C) 25md daily x 7 days; then 25 mg tid x 7 days; then 50 mg tid x 7 days; max 100 mg qid
Pediatric: 0.5 mg/kg daily x 7 days; then 0.5 mg/kg tid x 7 days; then 1 mg/kg tid x 7 days; then 2 mg/kg tid; max 100 mg qid
   Dantrium *Tab:* 25, 50, 100 mg
Comment: *dantrolene* is indicated for chronic spasticity associated with multiple sclerosis and spinal cord injury or disease.

▷ *diazepam* (C)(IV) 2-10 mg bid-qid; may increase gradually
Pediatric: <6 months: not recommended; ≥6 months: initially 1-2.5 mg bid-qid; may increase gradually
   Diastat *Rectal gel delivery system:* 2.5 mg
   Diastat AcuDial *Rectal gel delivery system:* 10, 20 mg
   Valium *Tab:* 2, 5, 10 mg
   Valium Intensol Oral Solution *Conc oral soln:* 5 mg/ml (30 ml w. dropper) (alcohol 19%)
   Valium Oral Solution *Oral soln:* 5 mg/5 ml (500 ml) (wintergreen spice)

▷ *metaxalone* (B) 1 tab tid-qid
Pediatric: <12 years: not recommended; ≥12 years: same as adult
   Skelaxin *Tab:* 800*mg

▷ *methocarbamol* (C)(G) initially 1.5 gm qid x 2-3 days; maintenance, 750 mg every 4 hours or 1.5 gm 3 x daily; max 8 gm/day
Pediatric: <16 years: not recommended; ≥16 years: same as adult
   Robaxin *Tab:* 500 mg
   Robaxin 750 *Tab:* 750 mg
   Robaxin Injection 10 ml IM or IV; max 30 ml/day; max 3 days; max 5 ml/ gluteal injection q 8 hours; max IV rate 3 ml/min
      Vial: 100 mg/ml (10 ml)

▷ *nabumetone* (C)
Pediatric: <12 years: not recommended; ≥12 years: same as adult
   Relafen *Tab:* 500, 750 mg
   Relafen 500 *Tab:* 500 mg

▷ *orphenadrine citrate* (C)(G) 1 tab bid
Pediatric: <12 years: not recommended; ≥12 years: same as adult
   Norflex *Tab:* 100 mg sust-rel

▷ *tizanidine* (C) 1-4 mg q 6-8 hours; max 36 mg/day
Pediatric: <12 years: not recommended; ≥12 years: same as adult
   Zanaflex *Tab:* 2*, 4**mg; *Cap:* 2, 4, 6 mg

SKELETAL MUSCLE RELAXANT+NSAID COMBINATIONS

Comment: *aspirin*-containing medications are contraindicated with history of allergic-type reaction to *aspirin*, children and adolescents with *Varicella* or other viral illness, and 3rd trimester of pregnancy.

➤ *carisoprodol+aspirin* (C)(III)(G) 1-2 tabs qid
  Pediatric: <12 years: not recommended; ≥12 years: same as adult
    Soma Compound *Tab:* caris 200 mg+asp 325 mg (sulfites)
➤ *meprobamate+aspirin* (D)(IV) 1-2 tabs tid or qid
  Pediatric: <12 years: not recommended; ≥12 years: same as adult
    Equagesic *Tab:* mepro 200 mg+asp 325*mg

SKELETAL MUSCLE RELAXANT+NSAID+CAFFEINE COMBINATIONS

Comment: *aspirin*-containing medications are contraindicated with history of allergic-type reaction to *aspirin*, children and adolescents with *Varicella* or other viral illness, and 3rd trimester of pregnancy.
➤ *orphenadrine+aspirin+caffeine* (D)(G)
  Pediatric: <12 years: not recommended; ≥12 years: same as adult
    Norgesic 1-2 tabs tid-qid
      Tab: orphen 25 mg+asp 385 mg+caf 30 mg
    Norgesic Forte 1 tab tid or qid; max 4 tabs/day
      Tab: orphen 50 mg+asp 770 mg+caf 60*mg

SKELETAL MUSCLE RELAXANT+NSAID+CODEINE COMBINATIONS

➤ *carisoprodol+aspirin+codeine* (D)(III)(G) 1-2 tabs qid prn
  Pediatric: <18 years: not recommended; ≥18 years: not recommended
    Soma Compound w. Codeine *Tab:* caris 200 mg+asp 325 mg+cod 16 mg (sulfites)
Comment: *Codeine* is known to be excreted in breast milk. <12 years: not recommended; 12-<18: use extreme caution; not recommended for children and adolescents with asthma or other chronic breathing problem. The FDA and the European Medicines Agency (EMA) are investigating the safety of using *codeine* containing medications to treat pain, cough and colds, in children 12-<18 years because of the potential for serious side effects, including slowed or difficult breathing. *aspirin*-containing medications are contraindicated with history of allergic-type reaction to *aspirin*, children and adolescents with *Varicella* or other viral illness, and 3rd trimester of pregnancy.

◯ TESTOSTERONE DEFICIENCY, HYPOTESTOSTERONEMIA, HYPOGONADISM

Comment: *testosterone* is contraindicated in male breast cancer and prostate cancer. *testosterone* replacement therapy is indicated in males with primary hypogonadism (congenital or acquired due to cryptorchidism, bilateral torsion, orchitis, vanishing testis syndrome, or orchidectomy), or hypogonadotropic hypogonadism (congenital or acquired), and delayed puberty not secondary to a pathological disorder (x-ray of the hand and wrist to determine bone age should be obtained every 6 months to assess the effect of treatment on the epiphyseal centers).

ORAL ANDROGENS

➤ *fluoxymesterone* (X)(III) *Hypogonadism:* <12 years: use by specialist only; *Puberty:* 5-20 mg once daily; *Delayed puberty:* use low dose and limit duration to 4-6 months
    Halotestin *Tab:* 2*, 5*, 10*mg (tartrazine)
➤ *methyltestosterone* (X)(III) usually 10-50 mg once daily; for delayed puberty, use low dose and limit duration to 4-6 months
    Android *Cap:* 10 mg
    Methitest *Tab:* 10*mg
    Testred *Cap:* 10 mg
➤ *testosterone* (X)(III) 30 mg q 12 hours to gum region, just above the incisor tooth on either side of the mouth; hold system in place for 30 seconds; rotate sites with each application
    Striant *Buccal tab:* 30 mg (6 blister pks; 10 buccal systems/blister pck)
Comment: Serum total *testosterone* concentrations may be checked 4 to 12 weeks after initiating treatment with **Striant**. To capture the maximum serum concentration, an early morning sample (just prior to applying the AM dose) is recommended.

TOPICAL ANDROGENS

Comment: Wash hands after application. Allow solution to dry before it touches clothing. Do not wash site for at least 2 hours after application. Pregnant and nursing women, and children, must avoid skin contact with application sites on men. If there is contact, wash the area as soon as possible with soap and water.

▷ *testosterone* (X)(III)(G)

> *Pediatric:* <18 years: not recommended; ≥18 years: same as adult
>
> > **AndroGel 1% (G)** initially apply 25 mg once daily in the AM to clean, dry, intact skin of the shoulders, upper arms, and/or abdomen; do not apply to scrotum; may increase to 75 mg/day and then to 100 mg/day if needed
> >
> > > *Gel:* 25 mg/2.5 gm pkt (30 pkts/carton); 50 mg/5 gm pkt (30 pkts/carton)
> >
> > **AndroGel 1.62% (G)** initially apply 25 mg once daily in the AM to clean, dry, skin of the shoulders and upper arms intact skin of the upper arms; do not apply to abdomen or genitals; may adjust dose between 1 and 4 pump actuations based on the pre-dose morning serum testosterone concentration at approximately 14 and 28 days after starting treatment or adjusting dose
> >
> > > *Gel:* 20.25 mg/1.25 gm pkt; 40.5 mg/2.5 gm pkt; *20.25* mg/1.25 gm pump actuation (60 metered dose actuations)
> >
> > **Axiron** apply to clean dry intact skin of the axillae; do not apply to the scrotum, penis, abdomen, shoulders, or upper arms; initially apply 60 mg (30 mg/axilla) once daily in the AM; adjust dose based on serum testosterone concentration 2 to 8 hours after applying and at least 14 days after starting therapy or following dose adjustment; may increase dose in 30 mg increments if serum testosterone <300 ng/dL up to 120 mg; reduce dose to 30 mg if levels >1050 ng/dL; discontinue if serum testosterone remains at >1050 ng/dL; to apply a 120 mg dose, apply 30 mg to each axilla and allow to dry, then repeat
> >
> > > *Soln:* 30 mg/1.5 ml pump actuation (60 metered dose actuations) (alcohol, latex-free)
> >
> > **Fortesta (G)** initially 40 mg of testosterone (4 pump actuations) applied to the thighs once daily in the AM; may adjust between 10 mg minimum and 70 mg maximum
> >
> > > *Gel:* 10 mg/0.5 gm pump actuation (120 metered dose actuations) (ethanol)
> >
> > **Comment:** The **Fortesta** dose should be based on the serum *testosterone* concentration 2 hours after applying **Fortesta** and at approximately 14 days and 35 days after starting treatment or following dose adjustment. Dose adjustment criteria: ≤500 ng/dL, increase daily dose by 10 mg; 500-≤1250 ng/dL, no change; 1250-≤2500 ng/dL, decrease daily dose by 10 mg; ≥2500 ng/dL, decrease daily dose by 20 mg.
> >
> > **Testim (G)** initially apply 5 gm once daily in the AM to clean, dry, intact skin of the shoulders and/or upper arms; do not apply to the genitals or abdomen; may increase to 10 gm after 2 weeks
> >
> > > *Gel:* 1%, clear, hydroalcoholic (5 mg/5 gm pkt, 30 pkts/carton)
> >
> > **Vogelxo Gel (G)** 1% initially apply 5 gm once daily in the AM to clean, dry, intact skin of the shoulders, upper arms, and/or abdomen; do not apply to scrotum; may increase to 7.5 gm/day and then to 10 gm/day if needed
> >
> > > *Gel:* 50 mg/5 gm pkt (30 pkts/carton); 50 mg/5 gm tube (30 tubes/carton); *Pump:* 12.5 mg/1.25 gm pump actuation, 60 metered dose actuations)

INTRANASAL ANDROGENS

▷ *testosterone (nasal gel)* (X)(III) initially one pump actuation each nostril (33 mg) 3 x/day, at least 6-8 hours apart, at the same times each day max: 6 pump actuation/day

> *Pediatric:* <18 years: not established; ≥18 years: same as adult
>
> > **Natesto** *Gel:* 5.5 mg/0.122 gm pump actuation (60 metered dose actuations)

TRANSDERMAL ANDROGEN PATCH

▷ *testosterone* (X)(III)

> > **Androderm** initially apply 4 mg nightly at approximately 10 PM to clean, dry area of the arm, back, or upper buttocks; leave on x 24 hours; may increase to 7.5 mg or decrease to 2.5 mg based on confirmed AM serum testosterone concentrations
> >
> > *Pediatric:* <15 years: not recommended; ≥15 years: same as adult
> >
> > > *Transdermal patch:* 2, 4 mg/24 Hr

PARENTERAL ANDROGENS

Comment: Contraindications include males with carcinoma of the breast or known or suspected carcinoma of the prostate and women who are pregnant (exogenous testosterone may cause fetal harm). *Prior to initiation of treatment:* confirm the diagnosis of hypogonadism by ensuring that serum testosterone has been measured in the morning on at least two separate days and that these concentrations are below the normal range. *Starting dose:* administer 75 mg subcutaneously in the abdominal region once weekly. Avoid intramuscular and intravascular administration. *Dose Adjustment:* Based upon total testosterone trough concentrations (measured 7 days after most recent dose) obtained following 6 weeks of dosing and periodically thereafter. **testosterone enanthate** and **testosterone cypionate** are long-acting testosterone esters suspended in oil to prolong absorption. Peak levels occur about 72 hours after intramuscular injection and are followed by a slow decline during the subsequent 1 to 2 weeks. For complete androgen replacement, the regimen should be between 50 and 100 mg of **testosterone enanthate** administered every 7 to 10 days, which will achieve relatively normal levels of testosterone throughout the time interval between injections. Longer time intervals are more convenient but are associated with greater fluctuations in testosterone levels. Higher doses of testosterone produce longer-term effects but also higher peak levels and wider swings between peak and nadir circulating testosterone levels; the result is fluctuating symptoms in many patients. The use of 100 to 150 mg of testosterone every 2 weeks is a reasonable compromise. Use of 300 mg injections every 3 weeks is associated with wider fluctuations of testosterone levels and is generally inadequate to ensure a consistent clinical response. With use of these longer-interval regimens, many men will have pronounced symptoms during the week preceding the next injection. In such instances, a smaller dose at closer intervals should be tried. When full androgen replacement is not required, patients should receive lower doses of testosterone. One such category includes male patients with pre-pubertal onset of hypogonadism who are going through puberty for the first time during therapy and who often may require psychologic counseling, especially when a spouse is involved as well. In these patients, testosterone therapy should be initiated at 50 mg every 3 to 4 weeks and then gradually increased during subsequent months, as tolerated, up to full replacement within 1 year. Men with appreciable benign prostatic hypertrophy who have hypogonadism and symptoms may be given 50 to 100 mg of testosterone every 2 weeks as an initial regimen and maintained on this dosage with careful monitoring of urinary symptoms and prostate examinations; therapy can be withdrawn if necessary. Attaining full virilization in the patient with hypogonadism may take as long as 3 to 4 years. Follow-up intervals should be between 4 and 6 months to monitor progress, review compliance, and determine whether any complications or psychologic adjustment problems are present. As a guide, testosterone levels should be above the lower limit of normal, in the range of 250 to 300 ng/dL, just before the next injection. Excessive peak levels and side effects should also be monitored and used to adjust the dosing regimens. During exogenous administration of androgens, endogenous testosterone release is inhibited through feedback inhibition of pituitary luteinizing hormone (LH). At large doses of exogenous androgens, spermatogenesis may also be suppressed through feedback inhibition of pituitary follicle stimulating hormone (FSH). Androgen therapy should be used very cautiously in pediatric patients and only by specialists who are aware of the adverse effects on bone maturation. Skeletal maturation must be monitored every six months by an X-ray of the hand and wrist. There is a lack of substantial evidence that androgens are effective in fractures, surgery, convalescence, and functional uterine bleeding.

▷ **testosterone cypionate** (X)(III)

Comment: **testosterone cypionate** is the oil-soluble 17 (beta)-cyclopentyl propionate ester of the androgenic hormone testosterone. The half-life of **testosterone cypionate** when injected intramuscularly is approximately 8 days. **Depot-Testosterone Injection (G)** *Usual Starting Dose:* 75-100 mg deep IM in the gluteal muscle; *Dose/Frequency Adjustment:* dose and frequency based upon morning total testosterone trough concentrations (measured 7 days after most recent dose) periodically thereafter; *Maintenance:* usually 100-400 mg deep IM in the gluteal muscle every 4 weeks; total doses above 400 mg per month are not required because of the prolonged action of the preparation; injections more frequently than every two weeks are rarely indicated

Pediatric: <12 years: not established; ≥12 years: same as adult

Vial: 100, 200 mg/ml (5 ml) (benzyl alcohol)

▷ **testosterone enanthate** (X)(III)

Comment: The half-life of **testosterone enanthate** when injected intramuscularly is approximately 4.5 days.

Delatestryl (G) *Usual Starting Dose:* 75-100 mg deep IM in the gluteal muscle; *Dose/Frequency Adjustment:* dose and frequency based upon morning total testosterone trough concentrations (measured 7 days after most recent dose) periodically thereafter; *Maintenance:* usually 100-400 mg deep IM in the gluteal muscle every 4 weeks; total doses above 400 mg per month are <u>not</u> required because of the prolonged action of the preparation; injections more frequently than every two weeks are rarely indicated

Pediatric: <12 years: not established; ≥12 years: same as adult

    Vial: 100, 200 mg/ml (5 ml) (chlorobutanol [chloral derivative] as preservative)

Xyosted *Initially:* 75 mg SC in the abdominal region once weekly; *Dose Adjustment:* based upon morning total testosterone trough concentrations (measured 7 days after most recent dose) obtained following 6 weeks of dosing and periodically thereafter

Pediatric: <18 years: not established; ≥18 years: same as adult

    Autoinjector: 50, 75, 100 mg/0.5 ml single-dose (4/carton) (preservative-free)

Comment: Use **Xyosted** only for the treatment of hypogonadal conditions associated with structural or genetic etiologies. Safety and efficacy of **Xyosted** in males with "age-related hypogonadism" (also referred to as "late-onset hypogonadism") have <u>not</u> been established.

 TETANUS (*CLOSTRIDIUM TETANI*)

PROPHYLAXIS

see **Childhood Immunizations** *page* 558

POSTEXPOSURE PROPHYLAXIS IN PREVIOUSLY NONIMMUNIZED PERSONS

▷ *tetanus immune globulin, human* (C) 250 mg deep IM in a single dose

    Pediatric: >7 years: same as adult

      BayTET, Hyper-TET

      Vial: 250 units single-dose; *Prefilled syringe:* 250 units

▷ *tetanus toxoid vaccine* (C) 0.5 ml IM x 3 dose series

    Vial: 5 Lf units/0.5 ml (0.5, 5 ml); *Prefilled syringe:* 5 Lf units/0.5 ml (0.5 ml)

Comment: Dose of **BayTET/HyperTET** S/D is calculated as 4 units/kg. However, it may be advisable to administer the entire contents of the syringe of **BayTET/HyperTET** S/D (250 units) regardless of the child's size, since theoretically the same amount of toxin will be produced in the child's body by the infecting tetanus organism as it will in an adult's body. At the same time but in a different extremity and with a different syringe, administer Diphtheria and Tetanus Toxoids and Pertussis Vaccine Adsorbed (DTP) or Diphtheria and Tetanus Toxoids Adsorbed (For Pediatric Use) (DT), if pertussis vaccine is contraindicated, should be administered per mfr pkg insert. Tetanus immune globulin may interact with live viral vaccines such as measles, mumps, rubella, and polio. It is also unknown if **BayTET/HyperTET** can cause fetal harm when administered to a pregnant woman <u>or</u> can affect reproduction capacity. The single injection of tetanus toxoid only initiates the series for producing active immunity in the recipient. Impress upon the patient the need for further toxoid injections in 1 month and 1 year, otherwise the active immunization series is incomplete. If a contraindication to using tetanus toxoid-containing preparations exists for a person who has not completed a primary series of tetanus toxoid immunization, and that person has a wound that is neither clean nor minor, only passive immunization should be given using tetanus immune globulin.

 THREADWORM (*STRONGYLOIDES STERCORALIS*)

ANTHELMINTICS

Comment: Oral bioavailability of anthelmintics is enhanced when administered with a fatty meal (estimated fat content 40 gm).

▷ *albendazole* (C) take with a meal; may crush and mix with food; may repeat in 3 weeks if needed; 400 mg bid x 7 days

Pediatric: <2 years: 200 mg bid x 7 days; 2-12 years: 400 mg once daily x 7 days; >12 years: same as adult

    Albenza *Tab:* 200 mg

Comment: *albendazole* is a broad-spectrum benzimidazole carbamate anthelmintic.

▷ *ivermectin* (C) take with water; chew or crush and mix with food; may repeat in 3 months if needed; 200 mcg/kg as a single dose

Pediatric: <15 kg: not recommended; ≥15 kg: same as adult

    Stromectol *Tab:* 3, 6*mg

▷ *mebendazole* (C)(G) take with a meal; chew or crush and mix with food; may repeat in 3 weeks if needed; 100 mg bid x 3 days

Pediatric: <2 years: not recommended; ≥2 years: same as adult

Emverm *Chew tab*: 100 mg

Vermox *Chew tab*: 100 mg

▶ *praziquantel* (B)(G) take with a meal; may crush and mix with food; 5-10 mg/kg as a single dose

Pediatric: <4 years: not established; ≥4 years: same as adult

Biltricide *Tab*: 600**mg film-coat (cross-scored for half or quarter dose)

Comment: Therapeutically effective levels of **Biltricide** may not be achieved when administered concomitantly with strong P450 inducers, such as rifampin. Females should not breastfeed on the day of **Biltricide** treatment and during the subsequent 72 hours. Use caution with hepatosplenic patients who have moderate to severe liver impairment (Child-Pugh Class B and C).

▶ *pyrantel pamoate* (C) take with a meal; may open capsule and sprinkle or mix with food; treat x 3 days; may repeat in 2-3 weeks if needed; treat x 3 days; 11 mg/kg/dose; max 1 gm/dose; <25 lb: not recommended; 25-37 lb: 1/2 tsp/dose; 38-62 lb: 1 tsp/dose; 63-87 lb: 1 tsp/dose; 88-112 lb: 2 tsp/dose; 113-137 lb: 2 tsp/dose; 138-162 lb: 3 tsp/dose; 163-187 lb: 3 tsp/dose; >187 lb: 4 tsp/dose

Antiminth *Cap*: 180 mg; Liq: 50 mg/ml (30 ml); 144 mg/ml (30 ml); *Oral susp*: 50 mg/ml (60 ml)

Pin-X *Cap*: 180 mg; Liq: 50 mg/ml (30 ml); 144 mg/ml (30 ml); *Oral susp*: 50 mg/ml (30 ml)

▶ *nitazoxanide* (B) take with a meal; may crush and mix with food; <12 months: not recommended; ≥12 months: treat q 12 hours x 3 days; <11 years: [use suspension]; 1-3 years: 5 ml; 4-11 years: 10 ml; >11 years: [use tab or suspension] 500 mg

Alinia *Tab*: 500 mg; *Oral susp*: 100 mg/5 ml (60 ml)

▶ *thiabendazole* (C) take with a meal; may crush and mix with food; treat x 7 days; <30 lb: consult mfr pkg insert; ≥30 lb: 25 mg/kg/dose bid with meals; 30-50 lb: 250 mg bid with meals; >50 lb: 10 mg/lb/dose bid with meals; max 1.5 gm/dose; max 3 gm/day

Mintezol *Chew tab*: 500*mg (orange); *Oral susp*: 500 mg/5 ml (120 ml) (orange)

Comment: *thiabendazole* is not for prophylaxis. May impair mental alertness. May not be available in the US.

THROMBOCYTOPENIA PURPURA, IDIOPATHIC (IMMUNE) (ITP)

THROMBOPOIETIN (TPO) RECEPTOR AGONIST

Comment: **Doptelet** *(avatrombopage)* is the first oral thrombopoietin (TPO) receptor agonist approved by the FDA for the treatment of adults with chronic liver disease who are scheduled to undergo a procedure. **Doptelet** is a second generation, once-daily, orally administered TPO receptor agonist that works by increasing platelet counts to the target level of greater or equal to 50,000 per microliter.

▶ *avatrombopag* <18 years: not recommended; ≥18 years: begin dosing 10 to 13 days prior to a scheduled procedure; the patient should undergo the procedure within 5 to 8 days after the last dose; take with food, as a single dose x 5 consecutive days; PLT count <40 x 10^9/L: 60 mg (3 tabs) once daily x 5 days; PLT count 40-50 x 10^9/L: 40 mg (2 tabs) once daily x 5 days

Doptelet *Tab*: 20 mg film-coat

Comment: TPO receptor agonists have been associated with thrombotic and thromboembolic complications in patients with chronic liver disease. Monitor platelet counts and for thromboembolic events and institute treatment promptly. Potential adverse reactions include pyrexia, abdominal pain, nausea, headache, fatigue, and peripheral edema. Based on animal studies, *avatrombopag* may cause fetal harm when administered to a pregnant female. There are no information regarding the presence of *avatrombopag* in human milk or effects on the breastfed infant. However, breastfeeding is not recommended during treatment with **Doptelet** and for at least 2 weeks after the last dose. Safety and effectiveness in patients (<18 years-of-age) have not been established. To report suspected adverse reactions, contact Dova Pharmaceuticals at 1-844-506-3682 or FDA at 1-800-FDA-1088 or visit www.fda.gov/medwatch.

▶ *lusutrombopag* 3 mg orally once daily with or without food x 7 days; administer first dose 8-14 days prior to the scheduled procedure; the procedure should occur 2-8 days after the last dose

Pediatric: <18 years: not established; ≥18 years: same as adult

Mulpleta *Tab:* 3 mg

Comment: **Mulpleta** *(lusutrombopag)* is a thrombopoietin (TPO) receptor agonist indicated for the treatment of thrombocytopenia in adult patients with chronic liver disease who are scheduled to undergo a procedure. TPO receptor agonists have been associated with thrombotic and thromboembolic complications in patients with chronic liver disease. Monitor platelet counts and for thromboembolic events and institute treatment promptly. The most common adverse reaction (incidence 3%) is headache. There are no available data on **Mulpleta** in pregnant women to inform drug-associated fetal risk. However, in animal reproduction studies, oral administration of *lusutrombopag* during organogenesis and the lactation period resulted in adverse developmental fetal outcomes. Advise pregnant women of the potential risk to a fetus Breastfeeding is not recommended during treatment. To report suspected adverse reactions, contact Shionogi at 1-800-849-9707 or FDA at 1-800-FDA-1088 or www.fda.gov/medwatch.

SPLEEN TYROSINE KINASE (SYK) INHIBITOR

▷ *fostamatinib disodium hexahydrate* <18 years: not recommended; ≥18yrs: Initially 100mg twice daily. Increase to 150mg twice daily if platelet count not at ≥50x10⁹/L after 4 weeks. Discontinue if insufficient increase in platelet count after 12 weeks. Dose modifications: see full labeling.

Tavalisse *Tab:* 100, 150mg

Comment: **Tavalisse** *(fostamatinib)* is an oral spleen tyrosine kinase (SYK) inhibitor for the treatment of patients with chronic idiopathic (immune) thrombocytopenia purpura (ITP). Monitor CBCs, including platelets, monthly until stable count (≥50 x 10⁹/L) achieved, then periodically thereafter. Monitor LFTs monthly. Discontinue if AST/ALT >5XULN for ≥2 wrks or ≥3XULN and total bilirubin >2XULN. Monitor blood pressure every 2 weeks until stable dose established, then monthly thereafter. Interrupt or discontinue dose if hypertensive crisis (>180/120 mm Hg) occurs; discontinue if repeat BP >160/100 mm Hg for >4 weeks. Temporarily interrupt if severe diarrhea (Grade ≥3) occurs; resume at next lower daily dose if improved to Grade 1. Monitor ANC monthly and for infection. Temporarily interrupt if ANC <1 x 10⁹/L occurs and remains low after 72 hours until resolved; resume at next lower daily dose. Use lowest effective dose. Due to potential for embryo-fetal toxicity, use effective contraception during and for ≥1 months after last dose. Confirm negative pregnancy status prior to initiation. Breast-feeding not recommended (during and for ≥1 month after last dose). Concomitant strong CYP3A4 inducers: not recommended. Concomitant strong CYP3A4 inhibitors or substrates; monitor for toxicity. May potentiate concomitant BCRP (e.g., rosuvastatin) or P-gp (e.g., digoxin) substrates: monitor for toxicity. Adverse reactions include diarrhea, hypertension, nausea, respiratory infection, dizziness, ALT/AST increase, rash, abdominal pain, fatigue, chest pain, neutropenia.

THROMBOCYTOPENIA PURPURA, THROMBOTIC, ACQUIRED AUTOIMMUNE (aTTP)

VON WILLEBRAND FACTOR (vWF)-DIRECTED ANTIBODY FRAGMENT

▷ *caplacizumab-yhdp* initial administration should be upon the initiation of plasma exchange therapy, by a qualified health care provider
First day of treatment: 11 mg via IV bolus at least 15 minutes *prior to* plasma exchange; followed by 11 mg SC *after completion* of plasma exchange
Subsequent treatment: during daily plasma exchange: 11 mg SC once daily once daily following plasma exchange
Treatment after the plasma exchange period: 11 mg SC once daily x 30 days beyond the last plasma exchange
After initial treatment course: if signs of persistent underlying disease, such as suppressed ADAMTS13 activity levels, remain present, treatment may be extended for a maximum 28 days
Discontinue treatment with Cablivi: if the patient experiences more than 2 recurrences of aTTP
Pediatric: not established

Cablivi *Vial:* 11 mg powder, a single-dose, for reconstitution and IV or SC administration
Comment: **Cablivi** *(caplacizumab-yhdp)* is indicated for the treatment of adult patients with acquired autoimmune thrombotic thrombocytopenic purpura (aTTP), in combination with plasma exchange and immunosuppressive therapy. The *ADAMTS13* gene provides instructions for making an enzyme that is involved in blood clotting. The most common adverse reactions to **Cablivi** (incidence >15%) are epistaxis, headache, and gingival bleeding. Severe bleeding can occur; risk is increased in patients with underlying coagulopathies and patients taking an anticoagulant. The most common adverse reactions (incidence >15%) are epistaxis, headache, and gingival bleeding. If clinically significant bleeding occurs, interrupt treatment. Withhold **Cablivi** for 7 days prior to elective surgery, dental procedures, or any other invasive intervention. Monitor pregnant patients/fetus and neonates closely for signs of bleeding. There is no information regarding the presence of *caplacizumab-yhdp* in human milk or effects on the breastfed infant. Developmental and health benefits of breastfeeding should be considered along with the mother's clinical need for **Cablivi,** potential adverse effects on the breastfed child, and the underlying maternal condition.

CD20-TARGETING MONOCLONAL ANTIBODY

➤ *rituximab* initially (Month 0) 1000 mg x 2 IV infusions separated by 2 weeks in combination with a tapering course of glucocorticoids; then a 500 mg IV infusion at Month 12 and every 6 months thereafter or based on clinical evaluation; *Relapse:* 1000 mg IV infusion with considerations to resume or increase the glucocorticoid dose based on clinical evaluation; subsequent infusions may be no sooner than 16 weeks after the previous infusion; methylprednisolone 100 mg IV or equivalent glucocorticoid recommended 30 minutes prior to each infusion
Pediatric: <6 years: not recommended; ≥6 years: same as adult
Rituxan *Vial:* 100 mg/10 ml (10 ml), 50 mg/50 ml (50 ml) single-use

Comment: **Rituxan** *(rituximab)* is a CD20-targeting cytolytic monoclonal antibody that received FDA Breakthrough Therapy Designation for treatment of PV in 2017. Safety and efficacy in recalcitrant PV has been demonstrated in approximately 500 patients across several small trials and case studies, with clinical remission occurring within six weeks in up to 95% of cases. In a recent phase 2 trial comparing *rituximab* plus *prednisone* with *prednisone* alone in patients with newly diagnosed PV, a 55% increase in 2-year remission rate (89% vs 34%) was observed in those receiving *rituximab* plus *prednisone.* Consider intravenous immunoglobulin (e.g., IVIG).

 TINEA CAPITIS

Comment: Tinea capitis must be treated with a systemic anti-fungal.

FOR SEVERE KERION PRURITUS

➤ *prednisone* (C) 1 mg/kg/day for 7-14 days
see **Oral Corticosteroids** *page 577*

SYSTEMIC ANTI-FUNGALS

➤ *griseofulvin, microsize* (C)(G) 500 mg once daily x 4-6 weeks or longer; max 1 gm/day
Pediatric: <30 lb: 5 mg/lb/day; 30-50 lb: 125-250 mg/day; >50 lb: 250-500 mg/day; 5 mg/lb/day x 4-6 weeks or longer; *see page 628 for dose by weight*
Grifulvin V *Tab:* 250, 500 mg; *Oral susp:* 125 mg/5 ml (120 ml) (alcohol 0.02%)
➤ *griseofulvin, ultramicrosize* (C)(G) 375 mg/day in a single or divided doses x 4-6 weeks or longer
Pediatric: <2 years: not recommended; ≥2 years: 3.3 mg/lb/day in a single or divided doses x 4-6 weeks or longer
Gris-PEG *Tab:* 125, 250 mg

Comment: *griseofulvin* should be taken with fatty foods (e.g., milk, ice cream). Liver enzymes should be monitored.
➤ *ketoconazole* (C)(G) initially 200 mg once daily; max 400 mg/day x 4 weeks
Pediatric: <2 years: not recommended; ≥2 years: 3.3-6.6 mg/kg once daily x 4 weeks
Nizoral *Tab:* 200 mg

Comment: Caution with *ketoconazole* due to concerns about potential for hepatotoxicity.

TINEA CORPORIS

TOPICAL ANTI-FUNGALS

▷ *butenafine* (C)(G) apply bid x 1 week or once daily x 4 weeks
Pediatric: <12 years: not recommended; ≥12 years: same as adult
    Lotrimin Ultra (OTC) *Crm:* 1% (12, 24 gm)
    Mentax *Crm:* 1% (15, 30 gm)
Comment: *butenafine* is a benzylamine, not an azole. Fungicidal activity continues for at least 5 weeks after last application.
▷ *ciclopirox* (B)
    Loprox Cream apply bid; max 4 weeks
    Pediatric: <10 years: not recommended; ≥10 years: same as adult
      Crm: 0.77% (15, 30, 90 gm)
    Loprox Lotion apply bid; max 4 weeks
    Pediatric: <10 years: not recommended; ≥10 years: same as adult
      Lotn: 0.77% (30, 60 ml)
    Loprox Gel apply bid; max 4 weeks
    Pediatric: <16 years: not recommended; ≥16 years: same as adult
      Gel: 0.77% (30, 45 gm)
▷ *clotrimazole* (B)(G) apply to affected area bid x 7 days
Pediatric: same as adult
    Lotrimin *Crm:* 1% (15, 30, 45 gm)
    Lotrimin AF (OTC) *Crm:* 1% (12 gm); *Lotn:* 1% (10 ml); *Soln:* 1% (10 ml)
▷ *econazole* (C) apply once daily x 14 days
Pediatric: same as adult
    Spectazole *Crm:* 1% (15, 30, 85 gm)
▷ *ketoconazole* (C) apply once daily x 14 days
Pediatric: <12 years: not recommended; ≥12 years: same as adult
    Nizoral Cream *Crm:* 2% (15, 30, 60 gm)
▷ *luliconazole* (C) apply to affected area and 1 inch into the immediate surrounding area(s) once daily
Pediatric: <18 years: not recommended; ≥18 years: same as adult
    Luzu Cream 1% *Crm:* 1% (30, 60 gm)
▷ *miconazole* 2% (C) apply once daily-bid x 2 weeks
Pediatric: same as adult
    Lotrimin AF Spray Liquid (OTC) *Spray liq:* 2% (113 gm) (alcohol 17%)
    Lotrimin AF Spray Powder (OTC) *Spray pwdr:* 2% (90 gm) (alcohol 10%)
    Monistat-Derm *Crm:* 2% (1, 3 oz); *Spray liq:* 2% (3.5 oz); *Spray pwdr:* 2% (3 oz)
▷ *naftifine* (B)(G)
Pediatric: <12 years: not recommended; ≥12 years: same as adult
    Naftin Cream apply once daily x 14 days
      Crm: 1% (15, 30, 60 gm)
    Naftin Gel apply bid x 14 days
      Gel: 1% (20, 40, 60 gm)
▷ *oxiconazole nitrate* (B)(G) apply once daily-bid x 2 weeks
Pediatric: same as adult
    Oxistat *Crm:* 1% (15, 30, 60 gm); *Lotn:* 1% (30 ml)
▷ *sulconazole* (C) apply once daily-bid x 3 weeks
Pediatric: <12 years: not recommended; ≥12 years: same as adult
    Exelderm *Crm:* 1% (15, 30, 60 gm); *Lotn:* 1% (30 mg)
▷ *terbinafine* (B)(G)
Pediatric: <12 years: not recommended; ≥12 years: same as adult
    Lamisil Cream (OTC) apply to affected and surrounding area once daily-bid x 1-4 weeks until significantly improved
      Crm: 1% (15, 30 gm)
    Lamisil AT Cream (OTC) apply to affected and surrounding area once daily-bid x 1-4 weeks until significantly improved
      Crm: 1% (15, 30 gm)
    Lamisil Solution (OTC) apply to affected and surrounding area once daily x 1 week
      Soln: 1% (30 ml spray bottle)

TOPICAL ANTIFUNGAL+STEROID COMBINATION

➤ *clotrimazole+betamethasone* (C)(G) apply bid x 2 weeks; max 4 weeks
Pediatric: <12 years: not recommended; ≥12 years: same as adult
Lotrisone *Crm:* clotrim 1 mg+beta 0.5 mg (15, 45 gm); *Lotn:* clotrim 1 mg+beta 0.5 mg (30 ml)

SYSTEMIC ANTIFUNGALS

➤ *griseofulvin, microsize* (C)(G) 500 mg/day x 2-4 weeks; max 1 gm/day
Pediatric: <30 lb: 5 mg/lb/day; 30-50 lb: 125-250 mg/day; >50 lb: 250-500 mg/day; *see page 628 for dose by weight*
Grifulvin V *Tab:* 250, 500 mg; *Oral susp:* 125 mg/5 ml (120 ml) (alcohol 0.02%)
➤ *griseofulvin, ultramicrosize* (C)(G) 375 mg/day in a single or divided doses x 2-4 weeks
Pediatric: <2 years: not recommended; ≥2 years: 3.3 mg/lb/day in a single or divided doses
Gris-PEG *Tab:* 125, 250
Comment: *griseofulvin* should be taken with fatty foods (e.g., milk, ice cream). Liver enzymes should be monitored.
➤ *ketoconazole* (C) initially 200 mg once daily; max 400 mg/day x 4 weeks
Pediatric: <2 years: not recommended; ≥2 years: 3.3-6.6 mg/kg/day x 4 weeks
Nizoral *Tab:* 200 mg
Comment: Caution with *ketoconazole* due to concerns about potential for hepatotoxicity.

TINEA CRURIS (JOCK ITCH)

TOPICAL ANTIFUNGALS

➤ *butenafine* (B)(G) apply bid x 1 week or once daily x 4 weeks
Pediatric: <12 years: not recommended; ≥12 years: same as adult
Lotrimin Ultra (C)(OTC) *Crm:* 1% (12, 24 gm)
Mentax *Crm:* 1% (15, 30 gm)
Comment: *butenafine* is a benzylamine, not an azole. Fungicidal activity continues for at least 5 weeks after last application.
➤ *ciclopirox* (B)
Loprox Cream apply bid; max 4 weeks
Pediatric: <10 years: not recommended; ≥10 years: same as adult
Crm: 0.77% (15, 30, 90 gm)
Loprox Lotion apply bid; max 4 weeks
Pediatric: <10 years: not recommended; ≥10 years: same as adult
Lotn: 0.77% (30, 60 ml)
Loprox Gel apply bid; max 4 weeks
Pediatric: <16 years: not recommended; ≥16 years: same as adult
Gel: 0.77% (30, 45 gm)
➤ *clotrimazole* (B)(G) apply to affected area bid x 7 days
Pediatric: same as adult
Lotrimin *Crm:* 1% (15, 30, 45 gm)
Lotrimin AF (OTC) *Crm:* 1% (12 gm); *Lotn:* 1% (10 ml); *Soln:* 1% (10 ml)
➤ *econazole* (C) apply once daily x 2 weeks
Pediatric: same as adult
Spectazole *Crm:* 1% (15, 30, 85 gm)
➤ *ketoconazole* (C)(G) apply bid x 4 weeks
Pediatric: <12 years: not recommended; ≥12 years: same as adult
Nizoral Cream *Crm:* 2% (15, 30, 60 gm)
➤ *luliconazole* (C) apply to affected area and 1 inch into the immediate surrounding area(s) once daily
Pediatric: <18 years: not recommended; ≥18 years: same as adult
Luzu Cream 1% *Crm:* 1% (30, 60 gm)
➤ *miconazole 2%* (C)(G) apply once daily-bid x 2 weeks
Pediatric: same as adult
Lotrimin AF Spray Liquid (OTC) *Spray liq:* 2% (113 gm) (alcohol 17%)
Lotrimin AF Spray Powder (OTC) *Spray pwdr:* 2% (90 gm) (alcohol 10%)
Monistat-Derm *Crm:* 2% (1, 3 oz); *Spray liq:* 2% (3.5 oz); *Spray pwdr:* 2% (3 oz)

▷ *naftifine* (B)(G)
  Pediatric: <12 years: not recommended; ≥12 years: same as adult
    Naftin Cream apply once daily x 2 weeks
      Crm: 1% (15, 30, 60 gm)
    Naftin Gel apply bid x 2 weeks
      Gel: 1% (20, 40, 60 gm)
▷ *oxiconazole nitrate* (B)(G) apply once daily-bid x 2 weeks
  Pediatric: same as adult
    Oxistat *Crm:* 1% (15, 30, 60 gm); *Lotn:* 1% (30 ml)
▷ *sulconazole* (C) apply once daily-bid x 3 weeks
  Pediatric: <12 years: not recommended; ≥12 years: same as adult
    Exelderm *Crm:* 1% (15, 30, 60 gm); *Lotn:* 1% (30 mg)
▷ *terbinafine* (B)(G)
  Pediatric: <12 years: not recommended; ≥12 years: same as adult
    Lamisil Cream (OTC) apply bid x 1-4 weeks
      Crm: 1% (15, 30 gm)
    Lamisil AT Cream (OTC) apply to affected and surrounding area once daily-bid x 1-4
    weeks until significantly improved
      Crm: 1% (15, 30 gm)
    Lamisil Solution (OTC) apply to affected and surrounding area once daily x 1 week
      Soln: 1% (30 ml spray bottle)
▷ *tolnaftate* (C)(OTC)(G) apply sparingly bid x 2-4 weeks
  Pediatric: <2 years: not recommended; ≥2 years: same as adult
    Tinactin *Crm:* 1% (15, 30 gm); *Pwdr:* 1% (45, 90 gm); *Soln:* 1% (10 ml); *Aerosol liq:* 1%
    (4 oz); *Aerosol pwdr:* 1% (3.5, 5 oz)
▷ *undecylenic acid* apply bid x 4 weeks
  Pediatric: same as adult
    Desenex (OTC) *Pwdr:* 25% (1.5, 3 oz); *Spray pwdr:* 25% (2.7 oz); *Oint:* 25% (0.5, 1 oz)

TOPICAL ANTIFUNGAL+ANTI-INFLAMMATORY AGENTS

▷ *clotrimazole+betamethasone* (C)(G) apply bid x 4 weeks; max 4 weeks
  Pediatric: <12 years: not recommended; ≥12 years: same as adult
  Crm: clotrim 10 mg+beta 0.5 mg (15, 45 gm); *Lotn:* clotrim 10 mg+beta 0.5 mg (30 ml)

SYSTEMIC ANTIFUNGALS

▷ *griseofulvin, microsize* (C)(G) 1 gm once daily x 2 weeks
  Pediatric: <30 lb: 5 mg/lb/day; 30-50 lb: 125-250 mg/day; >50 lb: 250-500 mg/day; 5 mg/lb/
  day x 4-6 weeks *or* longer; *see page* 628 *for dose by weight*
    Grifulvin V *Tab:* 250, 500 mg; *Oral susp:* 125 mg/5 ml (120 ml) (alcohol 0.02%)
▷ *griseofulvin, ultramicrosize* (C) 375 mg/day in a single *or* divided doses x 2 weeks
  Pediatric: <2 years: not recommended; ≥2 years: 3.3 mg/lb/day in a single *or* divided doses
    Gris-PEG *Tab:* 125, 250 mg
  Comment: *griseofulvin* should be taken with fatty foods (e.g., milk, ice cream). Liver
  enzymes should be monitored.
▷ *ketoconazole* (C) initially 200 mg once daily; max 400 mg once daily x 4 weeks
  Pediatric: <2 years: not recommended; ≥2 years: 3.3-6.6 mg/kg/day
    Nizoral *Tab:* 200 mg
  Comment: Caution with *ketoconazole* due to concerns about potential for hepatotoxicity.

◯ TINEA PEDIS (ATHLETE'S FOOT)

TOPICAL ANTIFUNGALS

▷ *butenafine* (B)(G) apply bid x 1 week *or* once daily x 4 weeks
  Pediatric: <12 years: not recommended; ≥12 years: same as adult
    Lotrimin Ultra (C)(OTC) *Crm:* 1% (12, 24 gm)
    Mentax *Crm:* 1% (15, 30 gm)
  Comment: *butenafine* is a benzylamine, not an azole. Fungicidal activity continues for at
  least 5 weeks after last application.
▷ *Burrows solution* wet dressings
▷ *ciclopirox* (B)
    Loprox Cream apply bid; max 4 weeks

Pediatric: <10 years: not recommended; ≥10 years: same as adult
    Crm: 0.77% (15, 30, 90 gm)
Loprox Lotion apply bid; max 4 weeks
    Pediatric: <10 years: not recommended; ≥10 years: same as adult
    Lotn: 0.77% (30, 60 ml)
Loprox Gel apply bid; max 4 weeks
    Pediatric: <16 years: not recommended; ≥16 years: same as adult
    Gel: 0.77% (30, 45 gm)

➤ *clotrimazole* (C)(G) apply bid to affected area x 4 weeks
  Pediatric: same as adult
    Desenex *Crm:* 1% (0.5 oz)
    Lotrimin *Crm:* 1% (15, 30, 45, 90 gm); *Lotn:* 1% (30 ml); *Soln:* 1% (10, 30 ml)
    Lotrimin AF (OTC) *Crm:* 1% (15, 30, 45, 90 gm); *Lotn:* 1% (20 ml); *Soln:* 1% (20 ml)

➤ *econazole* (C) apply once daily x 4 weeks
  Pediatric: same as adult
    Spectazole *Crm:* 1% (15, 30, 85 gm)

➤ *ketoconazole* (C) apply once daily x 6 weeks
  Pediatric: <12 years: not recommended; ≥12 years: same as adult
    Nizoral Cream *Crm:* 2% (15, 30, 60 gm)

➤ *luliconazole* (C) apply to affected area and 1 inch into the immediate surrounding area(s) once daily
  Pediatric: <18 years: not recommended; ≥18 years: same as adult
    Luzu Cream 1% *Crm:* 1% (30, 60 gm)

➤ *miconazole 2%* (C)(G) apply bid x 4 weeks
  Pediatric: same as adult
    Lotrimin AF Spray Liquid (OTC) *Spray liq:* 2% (113 gm) (alcohol 17%)
    Lotrimin AF Spray Powder (OTC) *Spray pwdr:* 2% (90 gm; alcohol 10%)
    Monistat-Derm *Crm:* 2% (1, 3 oz); *Spray liq:* 2% (3.5 oz); *Spray pwdr:* 2% (3 oz)

➤ *naftifine* (B)(G)
  Pediatric: <12 years: not recommended; ≥12 years: same as adult
    Naftin Cream apply once daily x 4 weeks
      Crm: 1% (15, 30, 60 gm)
    Naftin Gel apply bid x 4 weeks
      Gel: 1% (20, 40, 60 gm)

➤ *oxiconazole nitrate* (B)(G) apply once daily-bid x 4 weeks
  Pediatric: same as adult
    Oxistat *Crm:* 1% (15, 30, 60 gm); *Lotn:* 1% (30 ml)

➤ *sertaconazole* (C) apply once daily-bid x 4 weeks
  Pediatric: <12 years: not recommended; ≥12 years: same as adult
    Ertaczo *Crm:* 2% (15, 30 gm)

➤ *sulconazole* (C) apply once daily-bid x 4 weeks
  Pediatric: <12 years: not recommended; ≥12 years: same as adult
    Exelderm *Crm:* 1% (15, 30, 60 gm); *Lotn:* 1% (30 mg)

➤ *terbinafine* (B)(G)
  Pediatric: <12 years: not recommended; ≥12 years: same as adult
    Lamisil Cream (OTC) apply bid x 1-4 weeks
      Crm: 1% (15, 30 gm)
    Lamisil AT Cream (OTC) apply to affected and surrounding area once daily-bid x 1-4 weeks until significantly improved
      Crm: 1% (15, 30 gm)
    Lamisil Solution (OTC) apply to affected and surrounding area bid x 1 week
      Soln: 1% (30 ml spray bottle)

➤ *tolnaftate* (C)(OTC)(G) apply sparingly bid x 2-4 weeks
  Pediatric: <2 years: not recommended; ≥2 years: same as adult
    Tinactin *Crm:* 1% (15, 30 gm); *Pwdr:* 1% (45, 90 gm); *Soln:* 1% (10 ml); *Aerosol liq:* 1% (4 oz); *Aerosol pwdr:* 1% (3.5, 5 oz)

TOPICAL ANTIFUNGAL+ANTI-INFLAMMATORY COMBINATION

➤ *clotrimazole+betamethasone* (C)(G) apply bid x 4 weeks; max 4 weeks
  Pediatric: <12 years: not recommended; ≥12 years: same as adult
    Lotrisone *Crm:* clotrim 1 mg+beta 0.5 mg (15, 45 gm); *Lotn:* clotrim 1 mg+beta 0.5 mg (30 ml)

SYSTEMIC ANTIFUNGALS

▷ *griseofulvin, microsize* (C)(G) 1 gm once daily x 4-8 weeks
Pediatric: <30 lb: 5 mg/lb/day; 30-50 lb: 125-250 mg/day; >50 lb: 250-500 mg/day; 5 mg/lb/day x 4-6 weeks or longer; *see page* 628 *for dose by weight*
    Grifulvin V *Tab:* 250, 500 mg; *Oral susp:* 125 mg/5 ml (120 ml) (alcohol 0.02%)
▷ *griseofulvin, ultramicrosize* (C) 750 mg/day in a single or divided doses x 4-6 weeks
Pediatric: <2 years: not recommended; ≥2 years: 3.3 mg/lb/day in a single or divided doses
    Gris-PEG *Tab:* 125, 250
Comment: *griseofulvin* should be taken with fatty foods (e.g., milk, ice cream). Liver enzymes should be monitored.
▷ *ketoconazole* (C) initially 200 mg once daily; max 400 mg/day x 4 weeks
Pediatric: <2 years: not recommended; ≥2 years: 3.3-6.6 mg/kg once daily x 4 weeks
    Nizoral *Tab:* 200 mg
Comment: Caution with **ketoconazole** due to concerns about potential for hepatotoxicity.

TINEA VERSICOLOR

Comment: Resolution may take 3-6 months.

TOPICAL ANTIFUNGALS

▷ *butenafine* (G) apply once daily x 2 weeks
Pediatric: <12 years: not recommended; ≥12 years: same as adult
    Lotrimin Ultra (C)(OTC) *Crm:* 1% (12, 24 gm)
    Mentax (B) *Crm:* 1% (15, 30 gm)
Comment: *butenafine* is a benzylamine, not an azole. Fungicidal activity continues for at least 5 weeks after last application.
▷ *ciclopirox* (B)
    Loprox Cream apply bid; max 4 weeks
    Pediatric: <10 years: not recommended; ≥10 years: same as adult
      Crm: 0.77% (15, 30, 90 gm)
    Loprox Lotion apply bid; max 4 weeks
    Pediatric: <10 years: not recommended; ≥10 years: same as adult
      Lotn: 0.77% (30, 60 ml)
    Loprox Gel apply bid; max 4 weeks
    Pediatric: <16 years: not recommended; ≥16 years: same as adult
      Gel: 0.77% (30, 45 gm)
▷ *clotrimazole* (B)(G) apply bid x 7 days
Pediatric: same as adult
    Lotrimin *Crm:* 1% (15, 30, 45 gm)
    Lotrimin AF (OTC) *Crm:* 1% (12 gm); *Lotn:* 1% (10 ml); *Soln:* 1% (10 ml)
▷ *econazole* (C) apply once daily x 2 weeks
Pediatric: same as adult
    Spectazole *Crm:* 1% (15, 30, 85 gm)
▷ *miconazole* 2% (C)(G) apply once daily x 2 weeks
Pediatric: same as adult
    Lotrimin AF Spray Liquid (OTC) *Spray liq:* 2% (113 gm) (alcohol 17%)
    Lotrimin AF Spray Powder (OTC) *Spray pwdr:* 2% (90 gm) alcohol 10%)
    Monistat-Derm *Crm:* 2% (1, 3 oz); *Spray liq:* 2% (3.5 oz); *Spray pwdr:* 2% (3 oz)
▷ *ketoconazole* (C)(G)
Pediatric: <12 years: not recommended; ≥12 years: same as adult
    Nizoral Cream apply once daily x 2 weeks
      Crm: 2% (15, 30, 60 gm)
    Nizoral Shampoo lather into area and leave on 5 minutes x 1 application
      Shampoo: 2% (4 oz)
▷ *oxiconazole nitrate* (B)(G) apply once daily x 2 weeks
Pediatric: same as adult
    Oxistat *Crm:* 1% (15, 30, 60 gm); *Lotn:* 1% (30 ml)

▷ *selenium sulfide* shampoo (C)(G) apply after shower, allow to dry, leave on overnight; then scrub off vigorously in AM; repeat in 1 week and again q 3 months until resolution occurs
Pediatric: same as adult
  Selsun Blue *Shampoo:* 1% (120, 210, 240, 330 ml); 2.5% (120 ml)
▷ *sulconazole* (C) apply once daily-bid x 3 weeks
Pediatric: <12 years: not recommended; ≥12 years: same as adult
  Exelderm *Crm:* 1% (15, 30, 60 gm); *Lotn:* 1% (30 mg)
▷ *terbinafine* (B) apply bid to affected and surrounding area x 1 week
Pediatric: <12 years: not recommended; ≥12 years: same as adult
  Lamisil Solution (OTC) *Soln:* 1% (30 ml spray bottle)

ORAL ANTI-FUNGALS

▷ *ketoconazole* (C) initially 200 mg once daily; max 400 mg/day x 4 weeks
Pediatric: <2 years: not recommended; ≥2 years: 3.3-6.6 mg/kg once daily x 4 weeks
  Nizoral *Tab:* 200 mg

 TOBACCO DEPENDENCE, TOBACCO CESSATION, NICOTINE WITHDRAWAL SYNDROME

Comment: According to findings from the Population Assessment of Tobacco and Health (PATH) Study (respondents = 10, 384, mean age = 14.3), any use of e-cigarettes, hookah, non-cigarette combustible tobacco, or smokeless tobacco was independently associated with traditional cigarette smoking 1 year later and use of more than 1 of these products increases the odds of progressing to traditional cigarette use.

REFERENCE

Watkins, S. L., Glantz, S. A., & Chaffee, B. W. (2018). Association of noncigarette tobacco product use with future cigarette smoking among youth in the Population Assessment of Tobacco and Health (PATH) Study, 2013–2015. *JAMA Pediatrics, 172*(2), 181–187. doi:10.1001/jamapediatrics.2017.4173

NON-NICOTINE PRODUCTS

Alpha4-Beta4 Nicotinic Acetylcholine Receptor Partial Agonist

▷ *varenicline* (C) set target quit date; begin therapy 1 week prior to target quit date; take after eating with a full glass of water; initially 0.5 mg once daily for 3 days; then 0.5 mg bid x 4 days; then 1 mg bid; treat x 12 weeks; may continue treatment for 12 more weeks
Pediatric: <16 years: not studied; ≥16 years: same as adult
  Chantix *Tab:* 0.5, 1 mg; *Starting Month Pak:* 0.5 mg x 11 tabs + 1 mg x 42 tabs; *Continuing Month Pak:* 1 mg x 56 tabs
  Comment: Caution with **Chantix** due to potential risk for anxiety or suicidal ideation.

AMINOKETONES

▷ *bupropion HBr* (C)(G)
Pediatric: Safety and effectiveness in the pediatric population have not been established. When considering the use of **Aplenzin** in a child or adolescent, balance the potential risks with the clinical need
  Aplenzin initially 100 mg bid for at least 3 days; may increase to 375 or 400 mg/day after several weeks; then after at least 3 more days, 450 mg in 4 divided doses; max 450 mg/day, 174 mg/single dose
  Tab: 174, 348, 522 mg
▷ *bupropion HCl* (C)(G)
Pediatric: Safety and effectiveness in the pediatric population have not been established. When considering the use of **Forfivo XL** in a child or adolescent, balance the potential risks with the clinical need
  Forfivo XL do not use for initial treatment; use immediate-release *bupropion* forms for initial titration; switch to **Forfivo XL** 450 mg once daily when total dose/day reaches 450 mg; may switch to **Forfivo XL** when total dose/day reaches 300 mg for 2 weeks and patient needs 450 mg/day to reach therapeutic target; swallow whole, do not crush or chew
  Tab: 450 mg ext-rel

Wellbutrin initially 100 mg bid for at least 3 days; may increase to 375 or 400 mg/day after several weeks; then after at least 3 more days, 450 mg in 4 divided doses; max 450 mg/day, 150 mg/single dose
Tab: 75, 100 mg
Wellbutrin SR initially 150 mg in AM for at least 3 days; may increase to 150 mg bid if well tolerated; usual dose 300 mg/day; max 400 mg/day
Tab: 100, 150 mg sust-rel
Wellbutrin XL initially 150 mg in AM for at least 3 days; increase to 150 mg bid if well tolerated; usual dose 300 mg/day; max 400 mg/day
Tab: 150, 300 mg sust-rel
Zyban 150 mg once daily x 3 days; then 150 mg bid x 7-12 weeks; max 300 mg/day
Tab: 150 mg sust-rel

Comment: Contraindications to *bupropion* include seizure disorder, eating disorder, concurrent MAOI and alcohol use. Smoking should be discontinued after the 7th day of therapy with *bupropion*. Avoid bedtime dose.

TRANSDERMAL NICOTINE SYSTEMS (D)

Habitrol (OTC) initially one 21 mg/24 hr patch/day x 4-6 weeks; then one 14 mg/24 hr patch/day x 2-4 weeks; then one 7 mg/24 hr patch/day x 2-4 weeks; then discontinue
Pediatric: <12 years: not recommended; ≥12 years: same as adult
Transdermal patch: 7, 14, 21 mg/24 hr
Nicoderm CQ (OTC) initially one 21 mg/24 hr patch/day x 6 weeks, then one 14 mg/24 hr patch/day x 2 weeks; then one 7 mg/24 hr patch/day x 2 weeks
Pediatric: <12 years: not recommended; ≥12 years: same as adult
Transdermal patch: 7, 14, 21 mg/24 hr

Comment: Nicoderm CQ is available as a clear patch.
Nicotrol Step-down Patch (OTC) 1 patch/day x 6 weeks
Pediatric: <12 years: not recommended; ≥12 years: same as adult
Transdermal patch: 5, 10, 15 mg/16 hr (7/pck)
Nicotrol Transdermal (OTC) 1 patch/day x 6 weeks
Pediatric: <12 years: not recommended; ≥12 years: same as adult
Transdermal patch: 15 mg/16 hour (7/pck)
Prostep initially one 22 mg/24 hr patch/day x 4-8 weeks; then discontinue or one 11 mg/24 hr patch/day x 2-4 additional weeks
Pediatric: <12 years: not recommended; ≥12 years: same as adult
Transdermal patch: 11, 22 mg/24 hr (7/pck)

NICOTINE GUM

▷ *nicotine polacrilex* (D) chew one piece of gum slowly and intermittently over 30 minutes q 1-2 hours x 6 weeks; then q 2-4 hours x 3 weeks; then q 4-8 hours x 3 weeks; max 24 pieces/day; 2 mg if smoked <25 cigarettes/day; 4 mg if smoked >24 cigarettes/day
Pediatric: <12 years: not recommended; ≥12 years: same as adult
Nicorette (OTC) *Gum squares:* 2, 4 mg (108 piece starter kit and 48 piece refill) (orange, mint, or original, sugar-free)

NICOTINE LOZENGE

▷ *nicotine polacrilex* (X)(OTC)(G) dissolve over 20-30 minutes; minimize swallowing; do not eat or drink for 15 min before and during use; Use 2 mg lozenge if first cigarette smoked >30 minutes after waking; Use 4 mg lozenge if first cigarette smoked within 30 min of waking; 1 lozenge q 1-2 hours (at least 9/day) x 6 weeks; then q 2-4 hours x 3 weeks; then q 4-8 hours x 3 weeks; then stop; max 5 lozenges/6 hours and 20 lozenges/day
Pediatric: <18 years: not recommended; ≥18 years: same as adult
Commit Lozenge *Loz:* 2, 4 mg (72/pck) (phenylalanine)
Nicorette Mini Lozenge (G) *Loz:* 2, 4 mg (72/pck) (mint; phenylalanine)

NICOTINE INHALATION PRODUCTS

▷ *nicotine* 0.5 mg aqueous nasal spray (D)
Pediatric: <12 years: not recommended; ≥12 years: same as adult
Nicotrol NS 1-2 doses/hour nasally; max 5 doses/hour or 40 doses/day; usual max 3 months
Nasal spray: 0.5 mg/spray; 10 mg/ml (10 ml, 200 doses)

➤ *nicotine* 10 mg inhalation system (D)
Pediatric: <12 years: not recommended; ≥12 years: same as adult
    Nicotrol Inhaler individualize therapy; at least 6 cartridges/day x 3-6 weeks; max 16 cartridges/day x first 12 weeks; then reduce gradually over 12 more weeks
      Inhaler: 10 mg/cartridge, 4 mg delivered (42 cartridge/pck) (menthol)
    Comment: **Nicotrol Inhaler** is a smoking replacement; to be used with decreasing frequency. Smoking should be discontinued before starting therapy. Side effects include cough, nausea, mouth, or throat irritation. This system delivers nicotine, but no tars or carcinogens. Each cartridge lasts about 20 minutes with frequent continuous puffing and provides nicotine equivalent to 2 cigarettes.

TONSILLITIS: ACUTE

ANTI-INFECTIVES

➤ *amoxicillin* (B)(G) 500-875 mg bid or 250-500 mg tid x 10 days
Pediatric: <40 kg (88 lb): 20-40 mg/kg/day in 3 divided doses x 10 days or 25-45 mg/kg/day in 2 divided doses x 10 days; *see page 617 for dose by weight*
    Amoxil *Cap:* 250, 500 mg; *Tab:* 875*mg; *Chew tab:* 125, 200, 250, 400 mg (cherry-banana-peppermint) (phenylalanine); *Oral susp:* 125, 250 mg/5 ml (80, 100, 150 ml) (strawberry); 200, 400 mg/5 ml (50, 75, 100 ml) (bubble gum); *Oral drops:* 50 mg/ml (30 ml) (bubble gum)
    Moxatag *Tab:* 775 mg ext-rel
    Trimox *Tab:* 125, 250 mg; *Cap:* 250, 500 mg; *Oral susp:* 125, 250 mg/5 ml (80, 100, 150 ml) (raspberry-strawberry)
➤ *azithromycin* (B)(G) 500 mg x 1 dose on day 1, then 250 mg once daily on days 2-5 or 500 mg once daily x 3 days or **Zmax** 2 gm in a single dose
Pediatric: 12 mg/kg/day x 5 days; max 500 mg/day; *see page 619 for dose by weight*
    Zithromax *Tab:* 250, 500, 600 mg; *Oral susp:* 100 mg/5 ml (15 ml); 200 mg/5 ml (15, 22.5, 30 ml) (cherry); *Pkt:* 1 gm for reconstitution (cherry-banana)
    Zithromax Tri-pak *Tab:* 3 x 500 mg tabs/pck
    Zithromax Z-pak *Tab:* 6 x 250 mg tabs/pck
    Zmax *Oral susp:* 2 gm ext-rel for reconstitution (cherry-banana) (148 mg Na⁺)
➤ *cefaclor* (B)(G) 250-500 mg q 8 hours x 10 days; max 2 gm/day
Pediatric: <1 month: not recommended; 20-40 mg/kg bid or q 12 hours x 10 days; max 1 gm/day; *see page 620 for dose by weight*
Tab: 500 mg; *Cap:* 250, 500 mg; *Susp:* 125 mg/5 ml (75, 150 ml) (strawberry); 187 mg/5 ml (50, 100 ml) (strawberry); 250 mg/5 ml (75, 150 ml) (strawberry); 375 mg/5 ml (50, 100 ml) (strawberry)
    Cefaclor Extended Release *Tab:* 375, 500 mg ext-rel
    Pediatric: <16 years: ext-rel not recommended; ≥16 years; same as adult
➤ *cefadroxil* (B) 1 gm once daily or divided bid x 10 days
Pediatric: 30 mg/kg/day in 2 divided doses x 10 days; *see page 620 for dose by weight*
    Duricef *Cap:* 500 mg; *Tab:* 1 gm; *Oral susp:* 250 mg/5 ml (100 ml); 500 mg/5 ml (75, 100 ml) (orange-pineapple)
➤ *cefdinir* (B) 300 mg bid x 5-10 days or 600 mg once daily x 10 days
Pediatric: <6 months: not recommended; 6 months-12 years: 14 mg/kg/day in a single or 2 divided doses x 10 days; >12 years: same as adult; *see page 621 for dose by weight*
    Omnicef *Cap:* 300 mg; *Oral susp:* 125 mg/5 ml (60, 100 ml) (strawberry)
➤ *cefditoren pivoxil* (B) 200 mg bid x 10 days
Pediatric: <12 years: not recommended; ≥12 years: same as adult
    Spectracef *Tab:* 200 mg
    Comment: Contraindicated with milk protein allergy or carnitine deficiency.
➤ *ceftibuten* (B) 200 mg once daily x 10 days
Pediatric: 9 mg/kg once daily x 10 days; max 400 mg/day; *see page 623 for dose by weight*
    Cedax *Cap:* 400 mg; *Oral susp:* 90 mg/5 ml (30, 60, 90, 120 ml); 180 mg/5 ml (30, 60, 120 ml) (cherry)
➤ *cefixime* (B)(G) 400 mg once daily x 10 days
Pediatric: <6 months: not recommended; 6 months-12 years, <50 kg: 8 mg/kg/day in a single or 2 divided doses x 10 days; *see page 621 for dose by weight*; >12 years, >50 kg: same as adult
    Suprax *Tab:* 400 mg; *Cap:* 400 mg; *Oral susp:* 100, 200, 500 mg/5 ml (50, 75, 100 ml) (strawberry)

▷ *cefpodoxime proxetil* (B) 200 mg bid x 5-7 days
  Pediatric: <2 months: not recommended; 2 months-12 years: 10 mg/kg/day (max 400 mg/dose) or 5 mg/kg/day bid (max 200 mg/dose) x 5-7 days; *see page 622 for dose by weight*
    Vantin *Tab:* 100, 200 mg; *Oral susp:* 50, 100 mg/5 ml (50, 75, 100 mg) (lemon creme)
▷ *cefprozil* (B) 500 mg once daily x 10 days
  Pediatric: 2-12 years: 7.5 mg/kg bid x 10 days; >12 years: same as adult; *see page 622 for dose by weight*
    Cefzil *Tab:* 250, 500 mg; *Oral susp:* 125, 250 mg/5 ml (50, 75, 100 ml) (bubble gum) (phenylalanine)
▷ *cephalexin* (B)(G) 250 mg tid x 10 days
  Pediatric: 25-50 mg/kg/day in 4 divided doses x 10 days; *see page 623 for dose by weight*
    Keflex *Cap:* 250, 333, 500, 750 mg; *Oral susp:* 125, 250 mg/5 ml (100, 200 ml) (strawberry)
▷ *clarithromycin* (C)(G) 250 mg bid or 500 mg ext-rel once daily x 10 days
  Pediatric: <6 months: not recommended; ≥6 months: 7.5 mg/kg bid x 10 days; *see page 624 for dose by weight*
    Biaxin *Tab:* 250, 500 mg
    Biaxin Oral Suspension *Oral susp:* 125, 250 mg/5 ml (50, 100 ml) (fruit punch)
    Biaxin XL *Tab:* 500 mg ext-rel

Comment: The FDA is advising caution before prescribing *clarithromycin* to patients with heart disease because of a potential increased risk of heart problems or death that can occur years later. This recommendation is based on a review of the results of a 10-year follow-up study of patients with coronary heart disease from a large clinical trial that first observed this safety issue. Consider risk benefit and the use of other antibiotics in such patients.

▷ *dirithromycin* (C)(G) 500 mg once daily x 10 days
  Pediatric: <12 years: not recommended; ≥12 years: same as adult
    Dynabac *Tab:* 250 mg
▷ *erythromycin base* (B)(G) 300-400 mg tid x 10 days
  Pediatric: 30-50 mg/kg/day in 2-4 divided doses x 10 days
    Ery-Tab *Tab:* 250, 333, 500 mg ent-coat
    PCE *Tab:* 333, 500 mg

Comment: *erythromycin* may increase INR with concomitant *warfarin*, as well as increase serum level of *digoxin*, benzodiazepines, and statins.

▷ *erythromycin ethylsuccinate* (B)(G) 400 mg qid x 7 days
  Pediatric: 30-50 mg/kg/day in 4 divided doses x 7 days; may double dose with severe infection; max 100 mg/kg/day; *see page 626 for dose by weight*
    EryPed *Oral susp:* 200 mg/5 ml (100, 200 ml) (fruit); 400 mg/5 ml (60, 100, 200 ml) (banana); *Oral drops:* 200, 400 mg/5 ml (50 ml) (fruit); *Chew tab:* 200 mg wafer (fruit)
    E.E.S. *Oral susp:* 200, 400 mg/5 ml (100 ml) (fruit)
    E.E.S. Granules *Oral susp:* 200 mg/5 ml (100, 200 ml) (cherry)
    E.E.S. 400 Tablets *Tab:* 400 mg

Comment: *erythromycin* may increase INR with concomitant *warfarin*, as well as increase serum level of *digoxin*, benzodiazepines, and statins.

▷ *loracarbef* (B) 200 mg bid x 10 days
  Pediatric: 15 mg/kg/day in 2 divided doses x 10 days; *see page 628 for dose by weight*
    Lorabid *Pulvule:* 200, 400 mg; *Oral susp:* 100 mg/5 ml (50, 100 ml); 200 mg/5 ml (50, 75, 100 ml) (strawberry bubble gum)
▷ *penicillin v potassium* (B)(G) 250 mg tid x 10 days
  Pediatric: 25-50 mg/kg day in 4 divided doses x 10 days; ≥12 years: same as adult; *see page 629 for dose by weight*
    Pen-Vee K *Tab:* 250, 500 mg; *Oral soln:* 125 mg/5 ml (100, 200 ml); 250 mg/5 ml (100, 150, 200 ml)

TRICHINOSIS (*TRICHINELLA SPIRALIS*)

Comment: Trichinosis is caused by eating raw or undercooked pork or wild game infected with the larvae of a parasitic worm, *Trichinella spiralis*. The initial symptoms are abdominal discomfort, nausea, vomiting, diarrhea, fatigue, and fever beginning one to two days following ingestion. These parasites then invade other organs (e.g., muscles) causing muscle aches, itching, fever, chills, and joint pains that begins about two to eight weeks after ingestion. The treatment is oral anthelmintics which may cause abdominal pain, diarrhea, and (rarely) hypersensitivity reactions, convulsions, neutropenia, agranulocytosis, and hepatitis.

ANTHELMINTICS

Comment: Oral bioavailability of anthelmintics is enhanced when administered with a fatty meal (estimated fat content 40 gm).

▷ *albendazole* (C) take with a meal; may crush and mix with food; may repeat in 3 weeks if needed; 400 mg as once daily x 7 days
Pediatric: <2 years: 200 mg once daily x 3 days; may repeat in 3 weeks; 2-12 years: 400 mg once daily x 3 days; may repeat in 3 weeks; >12 years: same as adult
   Albenza *Tab:* 200 mg
Comment: *albendazole* is a broad-spectrum benzimidazole carbamate anthelmintic.

▷ *ivermectin* (C) take with water; chew or crush and mix with food; may repeat in 3 months if needed; 200 mcg/kg as a single dose
Pediatric: <15 kg: not recommended; ≥15 kg: same as adult
   Stromectol *Tab:* 3, 6*mg

▷ *mebendazole* (C)(G) take with a meal; chew or crush and mix with food; may repeat in 3 weeks if needed; <2 years: not recommended; ≥2 years: 100 mg bid x 3 days
Pediatric: <2 years: not recommended; ≥2 years: same as adult
   Emverm *Chew tab:* 100 mg
   Vermox (G) *Chew tab:* 100 mg

▷ *pyrantel pamoate* (C) take with a meal; may open capsule and sprinkle or mix with food; treat x 3 days; may repeat in 2-3 weeks if needed; treat x 3 days; 11 mg/kg/dose; max 1 gm/dose; <25 lb: not recommended; 25-37 lb: 1/2 tsp/dose; 38-62 lb: 1 tsp/dose; 63-87 lb: 1 tsp/dose; 88-112 lb: 2 tsp/dose; 113-137 lb: 2 tsp/dose; 138-162 lb: 3 tsp/dose; 163-187 lb: 3 tsp/dose; >187 lb: 4 tsp/dose
   Antiminth *Cap:* 180 mg; *Liq:* 50 mg/ml (30 ml); 144 mg/ml (30 ml); *Oral susp:* 50 mg/ml (60 ml)
   Pin-X (OTC) *Cap:* 180 mg; *Liq:* 50 mg/ml (30 ml); 144 mg/ml (30 ml); *Oral susp:* 50 mg/ml (30 ml)

▷ *thiabendazole* (C) take with a meal; may crush and mix with food; treat x 7 days; 25 mg/kg bid x 7 days; max 1.5 gm/dose; take with a meal
Pediatric: same as adult; <30 lb: consult mfr pkg insert; ≥30 lb: 25 mg/kg in 2 divided doses/day with meals; 30-50 lbs: 250 mg bid with meals; >50 lb: 10 mg/lb/dose bid with meals; max 3 gm/day
   Mintezol *Chew tab:* 500*mg (orange); *Oral susp:* 500 mg/5 ml (120 ml) (orange)
Comment: *thiabendazole* is not for prophylaxis. May impair mental alertness. May not be available in the US.

◯ TRICHOMONIASIS (*TRICHOMONAS VAGINALIS*)

Comment: The following treatment regimens for *Trichomoniasis* are published in the **2015 CDC Sexually Transmitted Diseases Treatment Guidelines**. Treat all sexual contacts. A multi-dose treatment regimen should be considered in HIV-positive women.

RECOMMENDED REGIMENS (NON-PREGNANT)
Regimen 1
▷ *metronidazole* 2 gm once in a single dose

Regimen 2
▷ *tinidazole* 2 gm once in a single dose

RECOMMENDED ALTERNATE REGIMEN
Regimen 1
▷ *metronidazole* 500 mg bid x 7 days

DRUG BRANDS AND DOSE FORMS
▷ *metronidazole* (not for use in 1st; B in 2nd, 3rd)(G)
   Flagyl *Tab:* 250*, 500*mg

Flagyl 375 *Cap*: 375 mg
Flagyl ER *Tab*: 750 mg ext-rel
➤ *tinidazole* (not for use in 1st; B in 2nd, 3rd)
Tindamax *Tab*: 250*, 500*mg

RECOMMENDED REGIMENS: PREGNANCY/LACTATION

Comment: All pregnant women should be considered for treatment. Women can be treated with 2 gm *metronidazole* in a single dose at any stage of pregnancy. Lactating women who are administered *metronidazole* should be instructed to interrupt breastfeeding for 12-24 hours after receiving the 2 gm dose of *metronidazole*.

 TRICHOTILLOMANIA

Comment: Trichotillomania is on the obsessive-compulsive spectrum within the larger DS-5 category, Anxiety Disorders, and depression is frequently a co-morbid disorder. Hence, medications used to treat OCD can be helpful in treating trichotillomania. Recommended psychotropic agents include *clomipramine* (Anafranil) and *fluvoxamine* (Luvox). Other medications that research suggests may have some benefit include the SSRIs *fluoxetine* (Prozac), *sertraline* (Zoloft), *paroxetine* (Paxil), the mood stabilizer **lithium carbonate** (Lithobid, Eskalith), the OTC supplement **N-acetylcysteine**, an amino acid that influences neurotransmitters related to mood, **olanzapine** (Zyprexa), an atypical anti-psychotic, and *valproate* (Depakote), an anticonvulsant.

TRICYCLIC ANTIDEPRESSANT (TCA) COMBINATIONS

➤ *clomipramine* (C)(G) initially 25 mg daily in divided doses; gradually increase to 100 mg during first 2 weeks; max 250 mg/day; total maintenance dose may be given at HS
Pediatric: <10 years: not recommended; ≥10 years: initially 25 mg daily in divided doses; gradually increase; max 3 mg/kg or 100 mg, whichever is smaller
Anafranil *Cap*: 25, 50, 75 mg

SELECTIVE SEROTONIN REUPTAKE INHIBITORS (SSRIs)

➤ *fluoxetine* (C)(G)
Prozac initially 20 mg daily; may increase after 1 week; doses >20 mg/day should be divided into AM and noon doses; max 80 mg/day
Pediatric: <8 years: not recommended; 8-17 years: initially 10 mg/day; may increase after 1 week to 20 mg/day; range 20-60 mg/day; range for lower weight children, 20-30 mg/day
Cap: 10, 20, 40 mg; *Tab*: 30*, 60*mg; *Oral soln*: 20 mg/5 ml (4 oz) (mint)
Prozac Weekly following daily fluoxetine therapy at 20 mg/day for 13 weeks, may initiate Prozac Weekly 7 days after the last 20 mg fluoxetine dose
Pediatric: <12 years: not recommended; ≥12 years: same as adult
Cap: 90 mg ent-coat del-rel pellets
➤ *fluvoxamine* (C)(G)
Comment: fluvoxamine has a specific FDA indication for OCD.
Luvox initially 50 mg q HS; adjust in 50 mg increments at 4-7 day intervals; range 100-300 mg/day; over 100 mg/day, divide into 2 doses giving the larger dose at HS
Pediatric: <8 years: not recommended; 8-17 years: initially 25 mg q HS; adjust in 25 mg increments q 4-7 days; usual range 50-200 mg/day; over 50 mg/day, divide into 2 doses giving the larger dose at HS; >17 years: same as adult
Tab: 25, 50*, 100*mg
Luvox CR initially 100 mg once daily at HS; may increase by 50 mg increments at 1 week intervals; max 300 mg/day; swallow whole
Pediatric: <18 years: not recommended; ≥18 years: same as adult
Cap: 100, 150 mg ext-rel
➤ *paroxetine maleate* (D)(G)
Pediatric: <12 years: not recommended; ≥12 years: same as adult
Paxil initially 20 mg daily in AM; may increase by 10 mg/day at weekly intervals as needed; max 60 mg/day
Tab: 10*, 20*, 30, 40 mg

Paxil CR initially 25 mg daily in AM; may increase by 12.5 mg at weekly intervals as needed; max 62.5 mg/day
Tab: 12.5, 25, 37.5 mg cont-rel ent-coat

Paxil Suspension initially 20 mg daily in AM; may increase by 10 mg/day at weekly intervals as needed; max 60 mg/day
Oral susp: 10 mg/5 ml (250 ml) (orange)

▶ *paroxetine mesylate* (D)(G) <12 years: not recommended; ≥12 years: initially 7.5 mg daily in AM; may increase by 10 mg/day at weekly intervals as needed; max 60 mg/day
Brisdelle *Cap:* 7.5 mg

▶ *sertraline* (C)(G) initially 50 mg daily; increase at 1 week intervals if needed; max 200 mg daily; dilute oral concentrate immediately prior to administration in 4 oz water, ginger ale, lemon-lime soda, lemonade, or orange juice
Pediatric: <6 years: not recommended; 6-12 years: initially 25 mg daily; max 200 mg/day; 13-17 years: initially 50 mg daily; max 200 mg/day; >17 years: same as adult
Zoloft *Tab:* 25*, 50*, 100*mg; *Oral conc:* 20 mg per ml (60 ml) (alcohol 12%)

Lithium Salts Mood Stabilizer

▶ *lithium carbonate* (D)(G) swallow whole; *Usual maintenance:* 900-1200 mg/day in 2-3 divided doses
Pediatric: <12 years: not recommended; ≥12 years: same as adult
Lithobid *Tab:* 300 mg slow-rel

Comment: Signs and symptoms of *lithium* toxicity can occur below 2 mEq/L and include blurred vision, tinnitus, weakness, dizziness, nausea, abdominal pains, vomiting, diarrhea to (severe) hand tremors, ataxia, muscle twitches, nystagmus, seizures, slurred speech, decreased level of consciousness, coma, death.

Valproate Mood Stabilizer

▶ *divalproex sodium* (D)(G) take once daily; swallow ext-rel form whole; initially 25 mg/kg/day in divided doses; max 60 mg/kg/day; *Elderly:* reduce initial dose and titrate slowly
Pediatric: <12 years: not recommended; ≥12 years: same as adult
Depakene *Cap:* 250 mg; *Syr:* 250 mg/5 ml (16 oz)
Depakote *Tab:* 125, 250 mg
Depakote ER *Tab:* 250, 500 mg ext-rel
Depakote Sprinkle *Cap:* 125 mg

ANTIPSYCHOTIC

▶ *olanzapine* (C) initially 2.5-10 mg daily; increase to 10 mg/day within a few days; then by 5 mg/day at weekly intervals; max 20 mg/day
Zyprexa *Tab:* 2.5, 5, 7.5, 10 mg
Zyprexa Zydis *ODT:* 5, 10, 15, 20 mg (phenylalanine)

TRIGEMINAL NEURALGIA (TIC DOULOUREUX)

ANTICONVULSANTS

▶ *baclofen* (C)(G) initially 5-10 mg tid with food; usual dose 10-80 mg/day
Pediatric: <12 years: not recommended; ≥12 years: same as adult
Lioresal *Tab:* 10*, 20*mg

Comment: Potential for seizures or hallucinations on abrupt withdrawal of *baclofen*.

▶ *carbamazepine* (C)
Carbatrol initially 200 mg bid; may increase weekly as needed by 200 mg/day; usual maintenance 800 mg-1.2 gm/day
Pediatric: <12 years: max <35 mg/kg/day; use ext-rel form above 400 mg/day; 12-15 years: max 1 gm/day in 2 divided doses; >15 years: usual maintenance 1.2 gm/day in 2 divided doses
Cap: 200, 300 mg ext-rel

Tegretol (G) initially 100 mg bid or 1/2 tsp susp qid; may increase dose by 100 mg q 12 hours or by 1/2 tsp susp q 6 hours; usual maintenance 400-800 mg/day; max 1200 mg/day
Pediatric: <6 years: initially 10-20 mg/kg/day in 2 divided doses; increase weekly as needed in 3-4 divided doses; max 35 mg/kg/day in 3-4 divided doses; ≥6 years: initially

100 mg bid; increase weekly as needed by 100 mg/day in 3-4 divided doses; max 1 gm/day in 3-4 divided doses

   Tab: 200*mg; *Chew tab:* 100*mg; *Oral susp:* 100 mg/5 ml (450 ml) (citrus-vanilla)

Tegretol XR (G) initially 200 mg bid; may increase weekly by 200 mg/day in 2 divided doses

   Pediatric: <6 years: use other forms; ≥6 years: initially 100 mg bid; may increase weekly by 100 mg/day in 2 divided doses; max 1 gm/day

   Tab: 100, 200, 400 mg ext-rel

▷ *clonazepam* (D)(IV)(G) initially 0.25 mg bid; increase to 1 mg/day after 3 days

   Pediatric: <10 years, <30 kg: initially 0.1-0.3 mg/kg/day; may increase up to 0.05 mg/kg/day bid-tid; usual maintenance 0.1-0.2 mg/kg/day tid

   Klonopin *Tab:* 0.5*, 1, 2 mg

   Klonopin Wafers dissolve in mouth with or without water

      Wafer: 0.125, 0.25, 0.5, 1, 2 mg orally-disint

▷ *divalproex sodium* (D) initially 250 mg bid; gradually increase to max 1000 mg/day if needed

   Pediatric: <10 years: not recommended; ≥10 years: same as adult

   Depakene *Cap:* 250 mg; *Syr:* 250 mg/5 ml

   Depakote *Tab:* 125, 250 mg

   Depakote ER *Tab:* 250, 500 mg ext-rel

   Depakote Sprinkle *Cap:* 125 mg

▷ *phenytoin* (D) 400 mg/day in divided doses

   Dilantin *Cap:* 30, 100 mg; *Oral susp:* 125 mg/5 ml (8 oz); *Infatab:* 50 mg

   Comment: Monitor *phenytoin* serum levels. Therapeutic serum level: 10-20 gm/ml. Side effects include gingival hyperplasia.

▷ *valproic acid* (D) initially 15 mg/kg/day; may increase weekly by 5-10 mg/kg/day; max 60 mg/kg/day or 250 mg/day

   Depakene *Cap:* 250 mg; *Syr:* 250 mg/5 ml

TRICYCLIC ANTIDEPRESSANTS (TCAs)

Comment: Co-administration of TCAs with SSRIs requires extreme caution.

▷ *amitriptyline* (C)(G) titrate to achieve pain relief; max 300 mg/day

   Pediatric: <12 years: not recommended; ≥12 years: same as adult

   Tab: 10, 25, 50, 75, 100, 150 mg

▷ *amoxapine* (C) titrate to achieve pain relief; if total dose exceeds 300 mg/day, give in divided doses; max 400 mg/day

   Pediatric: <12 years: not recommended; ≥12 years: same as adult

   Tab: 25, 50, 100, 150 mg

▷ *desipramine* (C)(G) titrate to achieve pain relief; max 300 mg/day

   Pediatric: <12 years: not recommended; ≥12 years: same as adult

   Norpramin *Tab:* 10, 25, 50, 75, 100, 150 mg

▷ *doxepin* (C)(G) titrate to achieve pain relief; max 150 mg/day

   Pediatric: <12 years: not recommended; ≥12 years: same as adult

   Cap: 10, 25, 50, 75, 100, 150 mg; *Oral conc:* 10 mg/ml (4 oz w. dropper)

▷ *imipramine* (C)(G)

   Pediatric: <12 years: not recommended; ≥12 years: same as adult

   Tofranil titrate to achieve pain relief; max 200 mg/day; adolescents max 100 mg/day; if maintenance dose exceeds 75 mg/day, may switch to **Tofranil PM** at bedtime

      Tab: 10, 25, 50 mg

   Tofranil PM titrate to achieve pain relief; initially 75 mg at HS; max 200 mg at HS

      Cap: 75, 100, 125, 150 mg

   Tofranil Injection 50 mg IM; lower dose for adolescents; switch to oral form as soon as possible

      Amp: 25 mg/2 ml (2 ml)

▷ *nortriptyline* (D)(G) titrate to achieve pain relief; initially 10-25 mg tid-qid; max 150 mg/day; lower doses for elderly and adolescents

   Pediatric: <12 years: not recommended; ≥12 years: same as adult

   Pamelor titrate to achieve pain relief; max 150 mg/day

      Cap: 10, 25, 50, 75 mg; *Oral soln:* 10 mg/5 ml (16 oz)

▷ *protriptyline* (C) titrate to achieve pain relief; initially 5 mg tid; max 60 mg/day

   Pediatric: <12 years: not recommended; ≥12 years: same as adult

   Vivactil *Tab:* 5, 10 mg

▷ *trimipramine* (C) titrate to achieve pain relief; max 200 mg/day
   Pediatric: <12 years: not recommended; ≥12 years: same as adult
     Surmontil *Cap:* 25, 50, 100 mg

TUBERCULOSIS (TB): PULMONARY (*MYCOBACTERIUM TUBERCULOSIS*)

SCREENING

▷ *purified protein derivative (PPD)* (C) 0.1 ml intradermally; examine inoculation site for
  induration at 48 to 72 hours.
   Pediatric: same as adult
     Aplisol, Tubersol *Soln:* 5 US units/0.1 ml (1, 5 ml)

PROPHYLAXIS VACCINE

The only tuberculosis vaccine uses attenuation of the related organism *Mycobacterium bovis*
by culture in bile-containing media to create the *Bacillus Calmette-Guerin* (BCG) vaccination
strain. It was first used experimentally in 1921 by Albert Calmette and Camille Guerin and
is currently in widespread use outside of the United States. It is not available in the US. The
BCG vaccine protects newborns against tuberculosis-related meningitis and other systemic
tuberculosis infections, but it has limited protection against active pulmonary disease. Once
vaccinated, the patient will be PPD positive.

ANTI-TUBERCULAR AGENTS

Comment: Avoid *streptomycin* in pregnancy. *pyridoxine* (*vitamin B6*) 25 mg once daily x
6 months should be administered concomitantly with *INH* for prevention of side effects.
rifapentine produces red-orange discoloration of body tissues and body fluids and may stain
contact lenses.
▷ *bedaquiline* (B)(G)
     Sirturo *Tab:* 100 mg
   Comment: *bedaquiline* is a diarylquinoline antimycobacterial ATP synthase for the
   treatment of pulmonary multi-drug resistant TB (MDR-TB).
▷ *ethambutol (EMB)* (B)(G)
     Myambutol *Tab:* 100, 400*mg
▷ *isoniazid (INH)* (C) *Tab:* 300*mg
▷ *pyrazinamide (PZA)* (C) *Tab:* 500*mg
▷ *rifampin (RIF)* (C)(G)
     Rifadin, Rimactane *Cap:* 150, 300 mg
▷ *rifapentine* (C)
     Priftin *Tab:* 150 mg (24, 32 pck)
   Comment: The 32-count packs of **Priftin** are intended for patients with active
   tuberculosis infection (TB). The 24-count packs are intended for patients with latent
   tuberculosis infection (LTBI) who are at high risk for progression to tuberculosis
   disease. **Priftin** for active TB is indicated for patients ≥12 years-of-age. **Priftin** for LTBI
   is indicated for patients ≥2 years-of-age.
▷ *rilpivirine* (C) *Tab:* 25 mg
     Rifabutin *Cap:* 150 mg
▷ *streptomycin (SM)* (C)(G) *Amp:* 1 gm/2.5 ml <u>or</u> 400 mg/ml (2.5 ml)

COMBINATION AGENTS

▷ *rifampin+isoniazid* (C)
     Rifamate *Cap:* rif 300 mg+iso 150 mg
▷ *rifampin+isoniazid+pyrazinamide* (C)
     Rifater *Tab:* rif 120 mg+iso 50 mg+pyr 300 mgss

PROPHYLAXIS AFTER EXPOSURE TO TUBERCULOSIS, WITH NEGATIVE PPD

▷ *isoniazid* (C) 300 mg once daily in a single dose x at least 6 months
   Pediatric: 10-20 mg/kg/day x 9 months

PROPHYLAXIS AFTER EXPOSURE, WITH NEW PPD CONVERSION

▷ *isoniazid* (C) 300 mg once daily in a single dose x 12 months
   Pediatric: 10-20 mg/kg/day x 9 months
   Tab: 100, 300*mg; *Syr:* 50 mg/5 ml; *Inj:* 100 mg/ml

▷ *rifampin* (C) 600 mg once daily + *isoniazid* (C) 300 mg once daily x 4 months
  Pediatric: rifampin (C) 10-20 mg/kg + *isoniazid* (C) 10-20 mg/kg once daily x 4 months

▷ *rifapentine* (C) 600 mg once weekly + *isoniazid* (C) 300 mg once weekly x 12 weeks
  Pediatric: ≤12 years: Treat x 12 weeks; 10-14 kg: *rifapentine* (C) 300 mg once weekly +
  isoniazid (C) 25 mg/kg (max 900 mg) once weekly; 14.1-25 kg: *rifapentine* (C) 450 mg
  once weekly + *isoniazid* (C) 25 mg/kg (max 900 mg) once weekly; 25.1-32 kg: *rifapentine*
  (C) 600 mg once weekly + *isoniazid* (C) 25 mg/kg (max 900 mg) once weekly; 32.1-50 kg:
  rifapentine (C) 750 mg once weekly + *isoniazid* (C) 25 mg/kg (max 900 mg) once weekly;
  >50 kg: *rifapentine* (C) 900 mg once weekly + *isoniazid* (C) 25 mg/kg (max 900 mg) once
  weekly; >12 years: same as adult

TREATMENT REGIMENS (≥12 YEARS)

Regimen 1

▷ *rifampin* (C) 600 mg + *isoniazid* (C) 300 mg + *pyrazinamide* (C) 2 gm + *ethambutol* (C)
  15-25 mg/kg or *streptomycin* (C) 1 gm once daily x 8 weeks; then *isoniazid* (C) 300 mg +
  rifampin (C) 600 mg once daily x 16 weeks or *isoniazid* 900 mg + *rifampin* (C) 600 mg 2-3
  x/week x 16 weeks

Regimen 2

▷ *rifampin* 600 mg + *isoniazid* 300 mg + *pyrazinamide* 2 gm + *ethambutol* 15-25 mg/kg
  or *streptomycin* 1 gm once daily x 2 weeks; then *rifampin* 600 mg + *isoniazid* 900 mg +
  pyrazinamide 4 gm + *ethambutol* 50 mg/kg or *streptomycin* 1.5 gm 2 x/week x 6 weeks;
  then *isoniazid* 300 mg + *rifampin* 600 mg once daily x 16 weeks or 2 x/week x 16 weeks
  rifampin 600 mg once daily x 16 weeks or 2 x/week x 16 weeks

Regimen 3

▷ *rifampin* 600 mg + *isoniazid* 900 mg + *pyrazinamide* 3 gm + *ethambutol* 25-30 mg/kg
  or *streptomycin* 1.5 gm 3 x/week x 6 months

Regimen 4 (for smear and culture negative for pulmonary TB in adult)

▷ Options 1, 2, or 3 x 8 weeks; then *isoniazid* 300 mg + *rifampin* 600 mg once daily x 16 weeks;
  then *rifampin* 600 mg + *isoniazid* 300 mg + *pyrazinamide* 2 gm + *ethambutol* 15-25 mg/kg
  or *streptomycin* 1 gm once daily x 8 weeks or 2-3 x/week x 8 weeks

Regimen 5 (for smear and culture negative for pulmonary TB in adult)

▷ *rifapentine* 600 mg twice weekly x 2 months (at least 72 hours between doses) + once daily
  isoniazid 300 mg, *ethambutol* 15-25 mg/kg + *pyrazinamide* 2 gm; then *rifapentine* 600 mg
  once weekly x 4 months + once daily *isoniazid* 300 mg + another appropriate anti-tuberculosis agent for susceptible organisms

Regimen 6 (when pyrazinamide is contraindicated)

▷ *rifampin* 600 mg + *isoniazid* 300 mg + *ethambutol* 15-25 mg/kg + *streptomycin* 1 gm once
  daily x 4-8 weeks; then *isoniazid* 300 mg + *rifampin* 600 mg once daily x 24 weeks or 2 x/
  week x 24 weeks

PEDIATRIC TREATMENT REGIMENS (<12 YEARS)

Regimen 1

▷ *rifampin* 10-20 mg/kg + *isoniazid* 10-20 mg/kg + *pyrazinamide* 15-20 mg/kg + *ethambutol*
  15-25 mg/kg or *streptomycin* 20-40 mg/kg once daily x 8 weeks; then *isoniazid* 10-20 mg/
  kg + *rifampin* 10-20 mg/kg once daily x 16 weeks or *isoniazid* 20-40 mg/kg + *rifampin*
  10-20 mg/kg 2-3 x/week x 16 weeks

Regimen 2

▷ *rifampin* 10-20 mg/kg + *isoniazid* 10-20 mg/kg + *pyrazinamide* 15-30 mg/kg + *ethambutol*
  15-25 mg/kg or *streptomycin* 20-40 mg/kg once daily x 2 weeks; then *rifampin* 10-20 mg/kg +
  isoniazid 20-40 mg/kg + *pyrazinamide* 50-70 mg/kg + *ethambutol* 50 mg/kg or *streptomycin*
  25-30 mg/kg 2 x/week x 6 weeks; then *isoniazid* 10-20 mg/kg + *rifampin* 10-20 mg/kg once
  daily x 16 weeks or *rifampin* 10-20 mg/kg + *isoniazid* 20-40 mg/kg 2 x/week x 16 weeks

Regimen 3

▷ *rifampin* 10-20 mg/kg + *isoniazid* 20-40 mg/kg + *pyrazinamide* 50-70 mg/kg + *ethambutol*
  25-30 mg/kg or *streptomycin* 25-30 mg/kg 3 x/week x 6 months

Regimen 4 (when pyrazinamide is contraindicated)

➤ *rifampin* 10-20 mg/kg + *isoniazid* 10-20 mg/kg + *ethambutol* 15-25 mg/kg + *streptomycin* 20-40 mg/kg once daily x 4-8 weeks; then *isoniazid* 10-20 mg/kg + *rifampin* 10-20 mg/kg once daily x 24 weeks or *rifampin* 10-20 mg/kg + *isoniazid* 20-40 mg/kg 2 x/week x 24 weeks

POLYPEPTIDE ANTIBIOTIC ISOLATED FROM STREPTOMYCES CAPREOLUS

Comment: *capreomycin sulfate* is a complex of 4 microbiologically active components which have been characterized in part; however, complete structural determination of all the components has not been established. **Capastat Sulfate**, which is to be used concomitantly with other appropriate anti-tuberculosis agents, is indicated in pulmonary infections caused by *capreomycin*-susceptible strains of *M. tuberculosis* when the primary agents (i.e., *isoniazid, rifampin, ethambutol, aminosalicylic acid*, and *streptomycin*) have been ineffective or cannot be used because of toxicity or the presence of resistant tubercle bacilli.

➤ *capreomycin sulfate* (C)(G) may be administered deep IM in a large muscle mass after reconstitution with 2 ml 0.9%NS or sterile water or via IV infusion over 60 minutes after reconstitution and dilution in 100 ml 0.9%NS; usual dose is 1 gm daily (not to exceed 20 mg/kg/day) via IM or IV infusion for 60 to 120 days; see mfr pkg insert for dosage table based on kg body weight and route of administration
Pediatric: <18 years: not recommended; ≥18 years: same as adult

    Capastat *Vial:* 1 gm pwdr for reconstitution with 2 ml 0.9%NS or sterile water

Comment: Black Box Warning (BBW): The use of *capreomycin sulfate* in patients with renal insufficiency or preexisting auditory impairment must be undertaken with great caution, and the risk of additional cranial nerve VIII impairment or renal injury should be weighed against the benefits to be derived from therapy. Since other parenteral antituberculosis agents (e.g., *streptomycin, viomycin*) also have similar and sometimes irreversible toxic effects, particularly on cranial nerve VIII and renal function, simultaneous administration of these agents with **Capastat Sulfate** is not recommended. Use with non-antituberculosis drugs (e.g., *polymyxin A sulfate, colistin sulfate, amikacin, gentamicin, tobramycin, vancomycin, kanamycin*, and *neomycin*) having ototoxic or nephrotoxic potential should be undertaken only with great caution. Audiometric measurements and assessment of vestibular function should be performed prior to initiation of therapy with **Capastat Sulfate** and at regular intervals during treatment. Renal injury, with tubular necrosis, elevation of the blood urea nitrogen (BUN) or serum creatinine, and abnormal urinary sediment, has been noted. Slight elevation of the BUN and serum creatinine (sCr) has been observed in a significant number of patients receiving prolonged therapy. The appearance of casts, red cells, and white cells in the urine has been noted in a high percentage of these cases. The safety of the use of **Capastat Sulfate** in pregnancy has not been determined. Safety and effectiveness in pediatric patients have not been established. It is not known whether this drug is excreted in human milk.

TYPE 1 DIABETES MELLITUS (T1DM)

Comment: Target glycosylated hemoglobin (HbA1c) is <7%. Addition of daily ACE-I and/or ARB therapy is strongly recommended for renal protection. Insulin may be indicated in the management of Type 2 diabetes with or without concomitant oral anti-diabetic agents.

TREATMENT FOR ACUTE HYPOGLYCEMIA

➤ *glucagon (recombinant)* (B) administer SC, IM, or IV; if patient does not respond in 15 minutes, may administer a single dose or 2 divided doses; <20 kg: 0.5 mg or 20-30 mg/kg; ≥20 kg: 1 mg
Pediatric: same as adult

INHALED INSULIN

Rapid-Acting Inhalation Powder Insulin

➤ *insulin human (inhaled)* (C) one inhaler may be used for up to 15 days, then discard; dose at meal times as follows: *Insulin naïve:* initially 4 units at each meal; adjust according to blood glucose monitoring
Conversion from SC to inhaled mealtime insulin:
SC 1-4 units: inhal 4 units
SC 5-8 units: inhal 8 units

SC 9-12 units: inhal 12 units
SC 13-16 units: inhal 16 units
SC 17-20 units: inhal 20 units
SC 21-24 units: inhal 24 units
Pediatric: <18 years: not established; ≥18 years: same as adult

Afrezza Inhalation Powder administer at the beginning of the meal; *Mealtime insulin naïve:* initially 4 units at each meal; *Using SC prandial insulin:* convert dose to **Afrezza** using a conversion table (see mfr pkg insert); *Using SC pre-mixed:* divide 1/2 of total daily injected pre-mixed insulin equally among 3 meals of the day; administer 1/2 total injected pre-mixed dose as once daily injected basal insulin dose

Inhal: 4, 8, 12 unit single-inhalation color-coded cartridges (30, 60, 90/pkg w. 2 disposable inhalers)

Comment: **Afrezza** is not a substitute for long-acting insulin. **Afrezza** must be used in combination with long-acting insulin in patients with T1DM. **Afrezza** is not recommended for the treatment of diabetic ketoacidosis. **Afrezza** is contraindicated with chronic lung disease because of the risk of acute bronchospasm. The use of **Afrezza** is not recommended in patients who smoke or who have recently stopped smoking. Each card contains 5 blister strips with 3 cartridges each (total 15 cartridges). The doses are color-coded. **Afrezza** is contraindicated with chronic respiratory disease (e.g., asthma, COPD) and patients prone to episodes of hypoglycemia.

INJECTABLE INSULINS

Rapid-Acting Insulins

▷ *insulin aspart (recombinant)* (B) onset <15 minutes; peak 1-3 hours; duration 3-5 hours; administer 5-10 minutes prior to a meal; SC or infusion pump or IV infusion
Pediatric: <3 years: not recommended; ≥3 years: same as adult

NovoLog *Vial:* 100 U/ml (10 ml); *PenFill cartridge:* 100 U/ml (3 ml, 5/pck) (zinc, m-cresol)

▷ *insulin glulisine (rDNA origin)* (C) onset <15 minutes; peak 1 hour; duration 2-4 hours; administer up to 15 minutes before, or within 20 minutes after starting a meal; use with an intermediate or long-acting insulin; SC only; may administer via insulin pump; do not dilute or mix with other insulin in pump
Pediatric: <4 years: not recommended; ≥4 years: same as adult

Apidra *Vial:* 100 U/ml (10 ml); *Cartridge:* 100 U/ml (3 ml, 5/pck; m-cresol)

▷ *insulin lispro (recombinant)* (B) onset <15 minutes; peak 1 hour; duration 3.5-4.5 hours; administer up to 15 minutes before, or immediately after, a meal; SC or IV infusion pump only
Pediatric: <3 years: not recommended; ≥3 years: same as adult

Admelog *Vial:* 100 U/ml (10 ml) (zinc, m-cresol); *Prefilled disposable SoloStar pen (disposable):* 100 U/ml (3 ml) (5/carton) (zinc, m-cresol)

Humalog *Vial:* 100 U/ml (10 ml); *Prefilled disposable KwikPen:* 100 U/ml (3 ml, 5/pck) (zinc, m-cresol); *HumaPen Memoir* and *HumaPen Luxura* HD inj device for *Humulog cartridges* (100 U/ml, 3 ml 5/pck) (zinc, m-cresol)

▷ *insulin regular* (B)

Humulin R U-100 *(human, recombinant)* (OTC) onset 30 minutes; peak 2-4 hours; duration up to 6-8 hours; SC or IV or IM
Vial: 100 U/ml (10 ml)

Humulin R U-500 *(human, recombinant)* onset 30 minutes; peak 1.75-4 hours; duration up to 24 hours; SC only; for in-hospital use only
Vial: 500 U/ml (20 ml); *KwikPen:* 3 ml (2, 5/carton)

Comment: **Humulin R U-500** formulation is 5 times more concentrated than standard U-100 concentration, indicated for adults and children who require ≥200 units of insulin/day, allowing patients to inject 80% less liquid to receive the desired dose. Recommend using U-500 syringe (BD, Eli Lilly). The U-500 syringe (0.5 ml, 6 mm x 31 gauge) is marked in 5 unit increments and allows for dosing up to 250 units.

Iletin II Regular *(pork)* (OTC) onset 30 minutes; peak 2-4 hours; duration 6-8 hours; SC, IV or IM
Vial: 100 U/ml (10 ml)

Novolin R *(human)* (OTC) onset 30 minutes; peak 2.5-5 hours; duration 8 hours; SC, IV, or IM
Vial: 100 U/ml (10 ml); *PenFill cartridge:* 100 U/ml (1.5 ml, 5/pck); *Prefilled syringe:* 100 U/ml (1.5 ml, 5/pck)

▷ *pramlintide (amylin analog/amylinomimetic)* (C) administer immediately before major meals (≥250 kcal or ≥30 gm carbohydrates); initially 15 mcg; titrate in 15 mcg increments for 3 days if no significant nausea occurs; if nausea occurs at 45 or 60 mcg, reduce to 30 mcg; if not tolerated, consider discontinuing therapy; *Maintenance:* 60 mcg (30 mcg *only* if 60 mcg not tolerated)

    Symlin *Vial:* 0.6 mg/ml (5 ml) (m-cresol, mannitol)

    Comment: **Symlin** is indicated as adjunct to mealtime insulin with or without a sulfo-nylurea and/or *metformin* when blood glucose control is suboptimal despite optimal insulin therapy. Do not mix with insulin. When initiating **Symlin**, reduce prepran-dial short/rapid-acting insulin dose by 50% and monitor pre- and post-prandial and bedtime blood glucose. Do not use in patients with poor compliance, HgbA1c is >9%, recurrent hypoglycemia requiring assistance in the previous 6 months, or if taking a prokinetic drug. With Type 2 DM, initial therapy is 60 mcg/dose and max is 120 mcg/dose.

RAPID-ACTING+INTERMEDIATE-ACTING INSULIN

Insulin Aspart Protamine Suspension+Insulin Aspart Combinations

▷ *insulin aspart protamine suspension 70%/insulin aspart 30% (recombinant)* (B)(G) onset 15 min; peak 2.4 hours; duration up to 24 hours; SC only
Pediatric: not recommended

    NovoLog Mix 70/30 (OTC) *Vial:* 100 U/ml (10 ml)

    NovoLog Mix 70/30 FlexPen (OTC) *Prefilled disposable pen:* 100 U/ml (3 ml, 5/pck); *PenFill cartridge:* 100 U/ml (3 ml, 5/pck)

LONG-ACTING INSULINS

▷ *insulin detemir (human)* (B) administer SC once daily with evening meal or at HS as a basal insulin; may administer twice daily (AM/PM); administer in the deltoid, abdomen, or thigh; onset 1-2 hours; peak 6-8 hours; duration 24 hours; switching from another basal insulin, dose should be the same on a unit-to-unit basis; may need more *insulin detemir* when switching from NPH; *Type 1:* starting dose 1/3 of total daily insulin requirements; rapid-acting or short-acting, pre-meal insulin should be used to satisfy the remainder of daily insulin requirements; *Type 2 (inadequately controlled on oral antidiabetic agents):* initially 10 units or 0.1-0.2 units/kg, once daily in the evening or divided twice daily (AM/PM); do not add-mix or dilute *insulin detemir* with other insulins.
Pediatric: <2 years: not recommended; ≥2 years: same as adult

    Levemir *Vial:* 100 U/ml (10 ml); *FlexPen:* 100 U/ml (3 ml, 5/pck; (zinc, m-cresol)

▷ *insulin glargine (recombinant)* (C)

    Basaglar administer SC once daily, at the same time each day, as a basal insulin in the deltoid, abdomen, or thigh; onset 1-1.5 hours, no pronounced peak, duration 20-24 hours; *T1DM (adults and children >6 years-of-age):* initially 1/3 of total daily insulin dose; administer the remainder of the total dose as short- or rapid-acting pre-prandial insulin; *T2DM (adults only):* initially 2 units/kilogram or up to 10 units once daily; *Switching from once daily insulin glargine 300 units/ml (i.e., **Toujeo**) to 100 units/ml:* initially 80% of the insulin glargine 300 units/ml; *Switching from twice daily NPH:* initially 80% of the total daily NPH dose; do not add-mix or dilute *insulin glargine* with other insulins.

    Pediatric: <6 years: not established; ≥6 years: individualize and adjust as needed

        Prefilled KwikPen (disposable), 100 U/ml (3 ml) (5/carton) (m-cresol)

    Lantus administer SC once daily at the same time each day as a basal insulin; onset 1-1.5 hours, no pronounced peak, duration 20-24 hours; initial average starting dose 10 units for insulin-naïve patients; *Switching from once daily NPH or Ultralente insulin:* initial dose of *insulin glargine* should be on a unit-for-unit basis; *Switching from twice daily NPH insulin:* start at 20% lower than the total daily NPH dose

    Pediatric: <6 years: not recommended; ≥6 years: same as adult

        Vial: 100 U/ml (10 ml); *Cartridge:* 100 U/ml (3 ml, for use in the *OptiPen One Insulin Delivery Device)* (5/carton) (m-cresol); *SoloStar pen (disposable):* 100 U/ml (3 ml) (5/carton)

    Toujeo administer SC once daily at the same time each day as a basal insulin; in the upper arm, abdomen, or thigh; onset of action 6 hours; duration 20-24 hours; *T2DM, insulin naïve:* initially 0.2 units/kg; titrate every 3-4 days; *T1DM, insulin naïve:* initially 1/3-1/2 total daily insulin dose; remainder as short-acting insulin divided between each meal; *Switch from once daily long- or intermediate-acting insulin:* on a unit-for-unit basis; *Switching from Lantus:* a higher daily dose is expected; *Switching from twice daily NPH:* reduce initial dose by 20% of total daily NPH dose

Pediatric: <18 years: not established; ≥18 years: same as adult

> *Soln for SC injection:* 450 units/1.5 ml prefilled disposable SoloStar pen (1.5 ml, 3/pck); 300 units/ml prefilled Max SoloStar pen (3 ml, 2/pck)

Comment: The Toujeo Max SoloStar pen contains 900 units of *insulin glargine* for administration of up to 160 units in a single injection and need for fewer prescribed pens and fewer refills.

▷ *insulin isophane suspension (NPH)* (B)

Pediatric: <18 years: not recommended; ≥18 years: same as adult

> **Humulin N** *(human, recombinant)* (OTC) onset 1-2 hours; peak 6-12 hours; duration 18-24 hours; SC only
>
> *Vial:* 100 U/ml (10 ml); *Prefilled disposable pen:* 100 U/ml (3 ml, 5/pck)
>
> **Novolin N** *(recombinant)* (OTC) onset 1.5 hours; peak 4-12 hours; duration 24 hours; SC only
>
> *Vial:* 100 U/ml (10 ml); *PenFill cartridge:* 1.5 ml (5/pck); *KwikPens:* 1.5 ml (5/pck)
>
> **Iletin II NPH** *(pork)* (OTC) onset 1-2 hours; peak 6-12 hours; duration 18-26 hours; SC only
>
> *Vial:* 100 U/ml (10 ml)

▷ *insulin zinc suspension (lente)* (B)

Pediatric: <18 years: not recommended; ≥18 years: same as adult

> **Humulin L** *(human)* (OTC) onset 1-3 hours; peak 6-12 hours; duration 18-24 hours; SC only
>
> *Vial:* 100 U/ml (10 ml)
>
> **Iletin II Lente** *(pork)* (OTC) onset 1-3 hours; peak 6-12 hours; duration 18-26 hours; SC only
>
> *Vial:* 100 U/ml (10 ml)
>
> **Novolin L** *(human)* (OTC) onset 2.5 hours; peak 7-15 hours; duration 22 hours; SC only
>
> *Vial:* 100 U/ml (10 ml)

Ultra Long-Acting Insulin

▷ *insulin degludec (insulin analog)* (C) administer by SC injection once daily at any time of day, with *or* without food, into the upper arm, abdomen, *or* thigh; titrate every 3-4 days; *Insulin naïve with type 1 diabetes:* initially 1/3-1/2 of total daily insulin dose, usually 0.2-0.4 units/kg; administer the remainder of the total dose as short-acting insulin divided between each daily meal; *Insulin naive with type 2 diabetes:* initially 10 units once daily; adjust dose of concomitant oral antidiabetic agent; *Already on insulin (type 1 or type 2):* initiate at same unit dose as total daily long- *or* intermediate-acting insulin unit dose

Pediatric: <1 year: not established; ≥1 year: same as adult

> **Tresiba FlexTouch** *Pen:* 100 U/ml (3 ml, 5 pens/carton), 200 U/ml (3 ml, 3 pens/carton) (zinc, m-cresol)

Comment: Tresiba U-200 FlexTouch is the only long-acting insulin in a 160-unit pen allowing up to 160 units in a single injection. The U-200 dose counter always shows the desired dose (i.e., no conversion from U/100 to U-200 is required)

▷ *insulin extended zinc suspension (Ultralente) (human)* (B) onset 4-6 hours; peak 8-20 hours; duration 24-48 hours; SC only

Pediatric: <18 years: not recommended; ≥18 years: same as adult

> **Humulin U** (OTC) *Vial:* 100 U/ml (10 ml)

Insulin Lispro Protamine+Insulin Lispro Combinations

▷ *insulin lispro protamine 75%+insulin lispro 25%* (B)

Pediatric: <18 years: not recommended; ≥18 years: same as adult

> **Humalog Mix 75/25** *(human)* onset 15 minutes; peak 30 minutes to 1 hour; duration 24 hours; SC only
>
> *Vial:* 100 U/ml (10 ml); *Prefilled disposable KwikPen:* 100 U/ml (3 ml, 5/pck) (zinc, m-cresol); *HumaPen Memoir* and *HumaPen Luxura* HD inj device for *Humalog cartridges* (100 U/ml, 3 ml, 5/pck) (zinc, m-cresol)

▷ *insulin lispro protamine 50%+insulin lispro 50%* (B)

Pediatric: <18 years: not recommended; ≥18 years: same as adult

> **Humalog Mix 50/50** *(recombinant)* (B) onset 15 minutes; peak 2.3 hours; range 1-5 hours; SC only

Vial: 100 U/ml (10 ml); *Prefilled disposable KwikPen:* 100 U/ml (3 ml, 5/pck) (zinc, m-cresol); *HumaPen Memoir* and *HumaPen LUXURA* HD inj device for *Humalog cartridges* (100 U/ml, 3 ml, 5/pck) (zinc, m-cresol)

Insulin Isophane Suspension (NPH)+Insulin Regular Combinations

▷ *NPH* 70%+*regular* 30% **(B)**
  Pediatric: <18 years: not recommended; ≥18 years
    Humulin 70/30 *(human, recombinant)* **(OTC)** onset 30 minutes; peak 2-12 hours; duration up to 24 hours; SC only
      Vial: 100 U/ml (10 ml)
    Novolin 70/30 *(recombinant)* **(OTC)** onset 30 minutes; peak 2-12 hours; duration up to 24 hours; SC only
      Vial: 100 U/ml (10 ml)
▷ *NPH* 50%+*regular* 50% **(B)**
  Pediatric: <18 years: not recommended; ≥18 years: same as adult
    Humulin 50/50 *(human)* **(OTC)** onset 30 minutes; peak 3-5 hours; duration up to 24 hours; SC only
      Vial: 100 U/ml (10 ml)

Insulin Lispro Protamine+Insulin Lispro Combinations

▷ *insulin lispro protamine* 75%+*insulin lispro* 25% **(B)**
  Pediatric: <18 years: not recommended; ≥18 years: same as adult
    Humalog Mix 75/25 *(recombinant)* onset 15 minutes; peak 30-90 minutes; duration 24 hours; SC only
      Vial: 100 U/ml (10 ml); *Prefilled disposable KwikPen:* 100 U/ml (3 ml, 5/pck) (zinc, m-cresol); *HumaPen Memoir* and *HumaPen LUXURA* HD inj device for *Humalog cartridges* (100 U/ml, 3 ml 5/pck) (zinc, m-cresol)
▷ *insulin lispro protamine* 50%+*insulin lispro* 50% **(B)**
  Pediatric: <18 years: not recommended; ≥18 years: same as adult
    Humalog Mix 50/50 *(recombinant)* onset 15 minutes; peak 1 hour; duration up to 16 hours; SC only
      Vial: 100 U/ml (10 ml); *Prefilled disposable KwikPen:* 100 U/ml (3 ml, 5/pck) (zinc, m-cresol); *HumaPen Memoir* and *HumaPen LUXURA* HD inj device for *Humalog cartridges* (100 U/ml, 3 ml 5/pck) (zinc, m-cresol); U/ml (3 ml, 5/pck) (zinc, m-cresol); *HumaPen Memoir* and *HumaPen LUXURA* HD inj device for *Humalog cartridges* (100 U/ml, 3 ml 5/pck) (zinc, m-cresol); (100 U/ml, 3 ml 5/pck (zinc, m-cresol)

Basal Insulin+GLP-1 RA Combinations

▷ *insulin degludec (insulin analog)+liraglutide* **(C)** for treatment of type 2 diabetes only in adults inadequately controlled on <50 units of basal insulin daily <u>or</u> ≤1.8 mg of *liraglutide* daily; administer by SC injection once daily, with <u>or</u> without food, into the upper arm, abdomen, <u>or</u> thigh; titrate every 3-4 days
  Pediatric: <18 years: not recommended; ≥18 years: same as adult
    Xultophy *Prefilled pen:* 100/3.6 U/ml (3 ml, 5 pens/carton)
▷ *insulin glargine (insulin analog)+lixisenatide* **(C)** for treatment of type 2 diabetes only in adults inadequately controlled on <60 units of basal insulin daily <u>or</u> *lixisenatide*; administer by SC injection once daily, with <u>or</u> without food, into the upper arm, abdomen, <u>or</u> thigh; titrate every 3-4 days
  Pediatric: <18 years: not recommended; ≥18 years: same as adult
    Soliqua *Prefilled pen:* 100/33 U/ml (3 ml, 5 pens/carton) covering 15-60 mg *insulin glargine* 100 units/ml and 15-20 mcg of *lixisenatide (m-cresol)*

◯ TYPE 2 DIABETES MELLITUS (T2DM)

Comment: Normal fasting glucose is <100 mg/dL. Impaired glucose tolerance is a risk factor for type 2 diabetes and a marker for cardiovascular disease risk; it occurs early in the natural history of these two diseases. Impaired fasting glucose is >100 mg/dL and <125 mg/dL. Impaired glucose tolerance is OGTT, 2 hour post-load 75 gm glucose >140 mg/dL and <200 mg/dL. Target pre-prandial glucose is 80 mg/dL to 120 mg/dL. Target bedtime glucose is 100 mg/dL to 140 mg/dL. Target glycosylated hemoglobin (HbA1c) is <7.0%. Additional medications to be considered for initiation at onset of T2DM, particularly in the presence of hypertension, include an angiotensin-converting enzyme inhibitor (ACEI), angiotensin II receptor blocker (ARB), thiazide-like diuretic, or a calcium channel blocker (CCB). Consider diabetes screening at age 25 years for persons in high-risk groups (non-Caucasian, positive family history for DM, obesity). Hypertension and hyperlipidemia are common comorbid conditions. Macrovascular complications include cerebral vascular disease, coronary artery disease, and peripheral vascular disease. Microvascular complications include retinopathy, nephropathy, neuropathy, and cardiomyopathy. Oral hypoglycemics are contraindicated in pregnancy.

REFERENCE

American Diabetes Association. (2017). Standards of medical care in diabetes—2017. *Diabetes Care*, 40(Suppl. 1), S1–S135. Retrieved from http://care.diabetesjournals.org/content/diacare/suppl/2016/12/15/40. Supplement_1.DC1/DC_40_S1_final.pdf

Insulins *see Type 1 Diabetes Mellitus page* 497

TREATMENT FOR ACUTE HYPOGLYCEMIA

▷ *glucagon (recombinant)* (B) administer SC, IM, or IV; if patient does not respond in 15 minutes, may administer a single or 2 divided doses
Adults and Children: <20 kg: 0.5 mg or 20-30 mg/kg; ≥20 kg: 1 mg

SULFONYLUREAS

Comment: Sulfonylureas are secretagogues (i.e., stimulate pancreatic insulin secretion); therefore, the patient taking a sulfonylurea should be alerted to the risk for hypoglycemia. Action is dependent on functioning beta cells in the pancreatic islets.

First Generation Sulfonylureas

▷ *chlorpropamide* (C)(G) initially 250 mg/day with breakfast; max 750 mg
Pediatric: <12 years: not recommended; ≥12 years: same as adult
   Diabinese *Tab:* 100*, 250*mg
▷ *tolazamide* (C)(G) initially 100-250 mg/day with breakfast; increase by 100-250 mg/day at weekly intervals; maintenance 100 mg 1 gm/day; max 1 gm/day
Pediatric: <12 years: not recommended; ≥12 years: same as adult
   Tolinase *Tab:* 100, 250, 500 mg
▷ *tolbutamide* (C) initially 1-2 gm in divided doses; max 2 gm/day
Pediatric: <12 years: not recommended; ≥12 years: same as adult
   Tab: 500 mg

Second Generation Sulfonylureas

▷ *glimepiride* (C) initially 1-2 mg once daily with breakfast; after reaching dose of 2 mg, increase by 2 mg at 1-2 week intervals as needed; usual maintenance 1-4 mg once daily; max 8 mg/day
Pediatric: <12 years: not recommended; ≥12 years: same as adult
   Amaryl *Tab:* 1*, 2*, 4*mg
▷ *glipizide* (C)(G)
Pediatric: <12 years: not recommended; ≥12 years: same as adult
   Glucotrol initially 5 mg before breakfast; increase by 2.5-5 mg every few days if needed; max 15 mg/day; max 40 mg/day in divided doses
      Tab: 5*, 10*mg
   Glucotrol XL initially 5 mg with breakfast; usual range 5-10 mg/day; max 20 mg/day
      Tab: 2.5, 5, 10 mg ext-rel
▷ *glyburide* (C)(G) initially 2.5-5 mg/day with breakfast; increase by 2.5 mg at weekly intervals; maintenance 1.25-20 mg/day in a single or 2 divided doses; max 20 mg/day
Pediatric: <12 years: not recommended; ≥12 years: same as adult
   DiaBeta, Micronase *Tab:* 1.25*, 2.5*, 5*mg
▷ *glyburide, micronized* (B)
Pediatric: <12 years: not recommended; ≥12 years: same as adult
   Glynase PresTab initially 1.5-3 mg/day with breakfast; increase by 1.5 mg at weekly intervals if needed; usual maintenance 0.75-12 mg/day in single or divided doses; max 12 mg/day
      Tab: 1.5*, 3*, 6*mg

ALPHA-GLUCOSIDASE INHIBITORS

Comment: Alpha-glucosidase inhibitors block the enzyme that breaks down carbohydrates in the small intestine, delaying digestion and absorption of complex carbohydrates, and lowering peak post-prandial glycemic concentrations. Use as monotherapy or in combination with a sulfonylurea. Contraindicated in inflammatory bowel disease, colon ulceration, and intestinal obstruction. Side effects include flatulence, diarrhea, and abdominal pain.

▸ *acarbose* (B) initially 25 mg tid ac, increase at 4-8 week intervals; or initially 25 mg once daily, increase gradually to 25 mg tid; usual range 50-100 mg tid; max 100 mg tid
  Pediatric: <12 years: not recommended; ≥12 years: same as adult
    Precose *Tab:* 25, 50, 100 mg

▸ *miglitol* (B) initially 25 mg tid at the start of each main meal, titrated to 50 mg tid at the start of each main meal; max 100 mg tid
  Pediatric: <12 years: not recommended; ≥12 years: same as adult
    Glyset *Tab:* 25, 50, 100 mg

BIGUANIDE

Comment: The biguanides decrease gluconeogenesis by the liver in the presence of insulin. Action is dependent on the presence of circulating insulin. Lower hepatic glucose production leads to lower overnight, fasting, and pre-prandial plasma glucose levels. Common side effects include GI distress, nausea, vomiting, bloating, and flatulence which usually eventually resolve. May be used as monotherapy (in adults only) or with a sulfonylurea or insulin. The only biguanide is *metformin*.

▸ *metformin* (B)(G) take with meals
  Comment: *metformin* is contraindicated with renal impairment, metabolic acidosis, ketoacidosis. *Metformin* is contraindicated in patients with decreased tissue perfusion or hemodynamic instability, alcohol abuse, advanced liver disease, acute unstable acute congestive heart failure, or any condition that may lead to lactic acidosis. Suspend *metformin*, prior to, and for 48 hours after, surgery or receiving IV iodinated contrast agents. *Metformin* is associates with weight loss. Clinicians should consider adding either a sulfonylurea, a thiazolidindione (TZD), an SGLT-2 inhibitor, or a DPP-4 inhibitor to metformin to improve glycemic control when a second oral therapy is considered.
    Fortamet initially 500 mg by mouth every evening; may increase by 500 mg/day at 1 week intervals; max 2 gm/day
    Pediatric: <10 years: not recommended; ≥10-16 years: use immediate release form; >16 years: same as adult
      Tab: 500, 1000 mg ext-rel
    Glucophage initially 500 mg bid; may increase by 500 mg/day at 1 week intervals; max 1 gm bid or 2.5 gm in 3 divided doses; or initially 850 mg once daily in AM; may increase by 850 mg/day in divided doses at 2 week intervals; max 2000 mg/day; take with meals
    Pediatric: <10 years: not recommended; ≥10-16 years: use only as monotherapy; >16 years: same as adult dose same as adult
      Tab: 500, 850, 1000*mg
    Glucophage XR initially 500 mg by mouth every evening; may increase by 500 mg/day at 1 week intervals; max 2 gm/day
    Pediatric: <10 years: not recommended; ≥10-16 years: use immediate release form; >16 years: same as adult
      Tab: 500, 750 mg ext-rel
    Glumetza ER (G) initially 1000 mg once daily; may increase by 500 mg/day at week intervals; max 2 gm/day
    Pediatric: <18 years: not recommended; ≥18 years: same as adult
      Tab: 500, 1000 mg ext-rel
    Riomet XR initially 500 mg once daily; may increase by 500 mg/day at 1 week intervals; max 2 gm/day in divided doses; take with meals
    Pediatric: <10 years: not recommended; ≥10 years: monotherapy only
      Oral soln: 500 mg/ml (4 oz; cherry)

MEGLITINIDES

Comment: Meglitinides are secretagogues (i.e., stimulate pancreatic insulin secretion) in response to a meal. Action is dependent on functioning beta cells in the pancreatic islets. Use as monotherapy or in combination with *metformin*.

▷ *nateglinide* (C) 60-120 mg tid ac 1-30 minutes prior to start of the meal
    Pediatric: <12 years: not recommended; ≥12 years: same as adult
        Starlix *Tab:* 60, 120 mg
▷ *repaglinide* (C)(G) initially 0.5 mg with 2-4 meals/day; take 30 minutes ac; titrate by doubling dose at intervals of at least 1 week; range 0.5-4 mg with 2-4 meals/day; max 16 mg/day
    Pediatric: <12 years: not recommended; ≥12 years: same as adult
        Prandin *Tab:* 0.5, 1, 2 mg

THIAZOLIDINEDIONES (TZDs)

Comment: The TZDs decrease hepatic gluconeogenesis and reduce insulin resistance (i.e., increase glucose uptake and utilization by the muscles). Liver function tests are indicated before initiating these drugs. Do not start if ALT more than 3 times greater than normal. Recheck ALT monthly for the first six months of therapy; then every two months for the remainder of the first year and periodically thereafter. Liver function tests should be obtained at the first symptoms suggestive of hepatic dysfunction (nausea, vomiting, fatigue, dark urine, anorexia, abdominal pain).

▷ *pioglitazone* (C)(G) initially 15-30 mg once daily; max 45 mg/day as a monotherapy; usual max 30 mg/day in combination with *metformin*, insulin, or a sulfonylurea
    Pediatric: <18 years: not recommended; ≥18 years: same as adult
        Actos *Tab:* 15, 30, 45 mg
▷ *rosiglitazone* (C)(G) initially 4 mg/day in a single or 2 divided doses; may increase after 8-12 weeks; max 8 mg/day as a monotherapy or combination therapy with *metformin* or a sulfonylurea; not for use with *insulin*
    Pediatric: <18 years: not recommended; ≥18 years: same as adult
        Avandia *Tab:* 2, 4, 8 mg

DIPEPTIDYL PEPTIDASE-4 (DPP-4) INHIBITOR+THIAZOLIDINEDIONE COMBINATION

Comment: The FDA has reported that *alogliptin*-containing drugs may increase the risk of heart failure, especially in patients who already have cardiovascular or renal disease. The drug **Oseni** (*alogliptin+pioglitazone*) is in this risk group.
▷ *alogliptin+pioglitazone* (C) take 1 dose once daily with first meal of the day; max: *rosiglitazone* 8 mg and max *glimepiride* per day; same precautions as *alogliptin* and *pioglitazone*
    Pediatric: <18 years: not recommended; ≥18 years: same as adult
        Oseni
            Tab: **Oseni 12.5/15** alo 12.5 mg+pio 15 mg;
                Oseni 12.5/30 alo 12.5 mg+pio 30 mg
                Oseni 12.5/45 alo 12.5 mg+pio 45 mg
                Oseni 25/15 alo 25+pio 15 mg
                Oseni 25/30 alo 25+pio 30 mg
                Oseni 25/45 alo 25 mg+pio 45 mg

SECOND GENERATION SULFONYLUREA+BIGUANIDE COMBINATIONS

Comment: *Metaglip* and *Glucovance* are combination secretagogues (sulfonylureas) and insulin sensitizers (biguanides). *Sulfonylurea:* Action is dependent on functioning beta cells in the pancreatic islets; patient should be alerted to the risk for hypoglycemia. Common side effects of the biguanide include GI distress, nausea, vomiting, bloating, and flatulence which usually eventually resolve. Take with food. *metformin* is contraindicated with renal impairment, metabolic acidosis, ketoacidosis. Suspend *metformin*, prior to, and for 48 hours after, surgery or receiving IV iodinated contrast agents.

▷ *glipizide+metformin* (C) take with meals; *Primary therapy:* 2.5/250 once daily or if FBS is 280-320 mg/dL, may start at 2.5/250 bid; may increase by 1 tab/day every 2 weeks; max 10/2000 per day in 2 divided doses; *Second Line Therapy:* 2.5/500 or 5/500 bid; may increase by up to 5/500 every 2 weeks; max: 20/2000 per day; Same precautions as *glipizide* and *metformin*
    Pediatric: <12 years: not recommended; ≥12 years: same as adult
        Metaglip
            Tab: **Metaglip 2.5/250** glip 2.5 mg+met 250 mg
                Metaglip 2.5/500 glip 2.5 mg+met 500 mg
                Metaglip 5/500 glip 5 mg+met 500 mg

▶ *glyburide+metformin* (B) take with meals; *Primary therapy (initial therapy if HgbA1c <9.0%):* initially 1.25/250 once daily; max *glyburide* 20 mg and *metformin* 2000 mg per day; *Primary therapy (initial therapy if HbA1c >9.0% or FBS >200):* initially 1.25/250 bid; max *glyburide* 20 mg and *metformin* 2000 mg per day; *Second line therapy (initial therapy if HbA1c >7.0%):* initially 2.5/500 or 5/500 bid; max *glyburide* 20 mg and *metformin* 2000 mg per day; *Previously treated with a sulfonylurea and metformin:* dose to approximate total daily doses of *glyburide* and *metformin* already being taken; max: *glyburide* 20 mg and *metformin* 2000 mg per day; Same precautions as *glyburide* and *metformin*
Pediatric: <12 years: not recommended; ≥12 years: same as adult

    Glucovance
      Tab: Glucovance **1.25/250** glyb 1.25 mg+met 250 mg
           Glucovance **2.5/500** glyb 2.5 mg+met 500 mg
           Glucovance **5/500** glyb 5 mg+met 500 mg

Comment: *metformin* is contraindicated with renal impairment, metabolic acidosis, ketoacidosis. Suspend *metformin*, prior to, and for 48 hours after, surgery or receiving IV iodinated contrast agents.

THIAZOLIDINEDIONE (TZD)+BIGUANIDE COMBINATION

▶ *pioglitazone+metformin* (C) take in divided doses with meals; *Previously on metformin alone:* initially 15 mg/500 mg or 15 mg/850 mg once or twice daily; *Previously on pioglitazone alone:* initially 15 mg/500 mg bid; *Previously on pioglitazone and metformin:* switch on a mg/mg basis; may increase after 8-12 weeks; max: *pioglitazone* 45 mg and *metformin* 2000 mg per day; Same precautions as *pioglitazone* and *metformin*
Pediatric: <12 years: not recommended; ≥12 years: same as adult

    Actoplus Met, Actoplis Met R (G)
      Tab: Actoplus Met **15/500** pio 15 mg+met 500 mg
           Actoplus Met **15/850** pio 15 mg+met 850 mg
           Actoplus Met XR **15/1000** pio 15 mg+met 1000 mg
           Actoplus Met XR **30/1000** pio 30 mg+met 1000 mg

Comment: *metformin* is contraindicated with renal impairment, metabolic acidosis, ketoacidosis. Suspend *metformin*, prior to, and for 48 hours after, surgery or receiving IV iodinated contrast agents.

▶ *rosiglitazone+metformin* (C)(G) take in divided doses with meals; *Previously on metformin alone:* add *rosiglitazone* 4 mg/day; may increase after 8-12 weeks; *Previously on rosiglitazone alone:* add *metformin* 1000 mg/day; may increase after 1-2 weeks; *Previously on rosiglitazone and metformin:* switch on a mg/mg basis; may increase *rosiglitazone* by 4 mg and/or *metformin* by 500 mg per day; max: *rosiglitazone* 8 mg and *metformin* 2000 mg per day; Same precautions as *rosiglitazone* and *metformin*
Pediatric: <12 years: not recommended; ≥12 years: same as adult

    Avandamet
      Tab: Avandamet **2/500** rosi 2 mg+met 500 mg
           Avandamet **2/1000** rosi 2 mg+met 1000 mg
           Avandamet **4/500** rosi 4 mg+met 500 mg
           Avandamet **4/1000** rosi 4 mg+met 1000 mg

Comment: *rosiglitazone* has been withdrawn from retail pharmacies. In order to enroll and receive *rosiglitazone*, healthcare providers and patients must enroll in the *Avandia-Rosiglitazone Medicines Access Program*. The program limits the use of *rosiglitazone* to patients already being treated successfully, and those whose blood sugar cannot be controlled with other antidiabetic medicines. *metformin* is contraindicated with renal impairment, metabolic acidosis, ketoacidosis. Suspend *metformin*, prior to, and for 48 hours after, surgery or receiving IV iodinated contrast agents.

THIAZOLIDINEDIONE (TZD)+SULFONYLUREA COMBINATIONS

▶ *pioglitazone+glimepiride* (C)(G) take 1 dose daily with first meal of the day; *Previously on sulfonylurea alone:* initially 30 mg/2 mg; *Previously on pioglitazone and glimepiride:* switch on a mg/mg basis; max: *pioglitazone* 30 mg and *glimepiride* 4 mg per day; Same precautions as *pioglitazone* and *glimepiride*
Pediatric: <18 years: not recommended; ≥18 years: same as adult

    Duetact
      Tab: Duetact **30/2** pio 30 mg+glim 2 mg
           Duetact **304** pio 30 mg+glim 4 mg

▷ **rosiglitazone+glimepiride** (C) take 1 dose daily with first meal of the day; max: *rosiglitazone* 8 mg and *glimepiride* 4 mg per day; Same precautions as *rosiglitazone* and *glimepiride*
Pediatric: <18 years: not recommended; ≥18 years: same as adult
> Avandaryl
> > *Tab:* Avandaryl 4/1 rosi 4 mg+glim 1 mg
> > Avandaryl 4/2 rosi 4 mg+glim 2 mg
> > Avandaryl 4/4 rosi 4 mg+glim 4 mg
> > Avandaryl 8/2 rosi 8 mg+glim 2 mg
> > Avandaryl 8/4 rosi 8 mg+glim 4 mg

GLUCAGON-LIKE PEPTIDE-1 (GLP-1) RECEPTOR AGONISTS

Comment: GLP-1 receptor agonists act as an agonist at the GLP-1 receptors. They have a longer half-life than the native protein allowing them to be dosed once daily. They increase intracellular cAMP resulting in *insulin* release in the presence of increased serum concentration, decrease *glucagon* secretion, and delay gastric emptying, thus, reducing fasting, pre-meal, and post-prandial glucose throughout the day. GLP-1 receptor agonists are not a substitute for *insulin*, not for treatment of DKA, and not for post-prandial administration.

▷ **dulaglutide** (C) administer by SC injection into the upper arm, abdomen, or thigh once weekly on the same day and the same time of day, with or without food; initially 0.75 mg SC once weekly; may increase to 1.5 mg SC once weekly
Pediatric: <18 years: not established; ≥18 years: same as adult
> **Trulicity** *Prefilled pen/syringe:* 0.75, 1.5 mg/0.5 ml single-dose disposable autoinjector (4/pck)

▷ **exenatide** (C) administer by SC injection into the upper arm, abdomen, or thigh once weekly
Pediatric: <12 years: not recommended; ≥12 years: same as adult
> **Bydureon** inject immediately after mixing; administer 2 mg SC once weekly; administer on the same day, at any time of day; with or without meals; if switching from **Byetta**, discontinue **Byetta** and instead administer **Bydureon** and continue the same once weekly administration schedule with **Bydureon**
> > *Vial:* 2 mg w. 0.65 ml diluent, single-dose; *Prefilled pen:* 2 mg w. 0.65 ml diluent, single-dose
> **Bydureon BCise** administer 2 mg by SC injection once weekly; at any time of day; with or without meals; if switching from **Byetta** to **Bydureon**, discontinue **Byetta** and start **Bydureon BBCise** SC once weekly on the same day of the week
> > *Autoinjector:* 2 mg (0.85 ml) single-dose
> **Byetta** inject within 60 minutes before AM and PM meals, or before the 2 main meals of the day, approximately ≥6 hours apart; initially 5 mcg/dose; may increase to 10 mcg/dose after one month
> > *Prefilled pen:* 250 mcg/ml (5, 10 mcg/dose; 60 doses, needles not included) (m-cresol, mannitol)

Comment: *exenatide* is indicated as an adjunctive therapy to basal insulin among patients whose blood sugar remains uncontrolled on one or more antidiabetic medications, along with diet and exercise.

▷ **liraglutide** (C) administer by SC injection into the upper arm, abdomen, or thigh once daily; initially 0.6 mg/day for 1 week; then 1.2 mg/day; may increase to 1.8 mg/day
Pediatric: <18 years: not recommended; ≥18 years: same as adult
> **Victoza** *Prefilled pen:* 6 mg/ml (3 ml; needles not included)

▷ **lixisenatide** (C) administer SC in the upper arm, abdomen, or thigh once daily; initially 10 mcg SC x 14 days; maintenance: 20 mcg beginning on day 15; administer within one hour of the first meal of the day and the same meal of the day
Pediatric: <18 years: not established; ≥18 years: same as adult
> **Adlyxin** *Soln for SC inj; Starter Pen:* 50 mcg/ml (14 doses of 10 mcg; 3 ml); *Maintenance Pen:* 100 mcg/ml (14 doses of 20 mcg); *Starter Pack:* 1 prefilled starter pen and 1 prefilled maintenance pen; *Maintenance Pack:* 2 prefilled maintenance pens
> Comment: **Adlyxin** is indicated as an adjunct to diet and exercise for T2DM. Not indicated for treatment of T1DM. Do not use with **Victoza, Saxenda,** other GLP-1 receptor agonists, or insulin. Contraindicated with gastroparesis and GFR <15 mL/min. Poorly controlled diabetes in pregnancy increases the maternal risk for diabetic ketoacidosis, pre-eclampsia, spontaneous abortions, preterm delivery, stillbirth and delivery complications. Poorly controlled diabetes increases the fetal risk for major birth defects, still birth, and macrosomia related morbidity. **Adlyxin** should be used during pregnancy only if the potential benefit justifies the potential risk to the

fetus. Estimated background risk of major birth defects and miscarriage in clinically recognized pregnancies is 2-4% and 15-20%, respectively.

▶ *semaglutide* administer SC in the upper arm, abdomen, or thigh once weekly at any time of day, with or without meals; initially 0.25 mg once weekly; after 4 weeks, increase the dose to 0.5 mg once weekly; if after at least 4 weeks additional glycemic control is needed, increase to 1 mg once weekly (usual main-maintenance dose); if a dose is missed, administer within 5 days of the missed dose

Pediatric: <18 years: not recommended: ≥18 years: same as adult

　　Ozempic *Prefilled pen:* 2 mg/1.5 ml (1.34 mg/ml) single-patient-use; 0.25, 0.5, 1 mg/ injection

Comment: *semaglutide* is contraindicated with personal or family history of medullary thyroid carcinoma or with multiple endocrine neoplasia syndrome type 2. **Ozempic** has not been studied in patients with a history of pancreatitis. Consider another antidiabetic therapy. **Ozempic** is not recommended in females or males with reproductive potential. Discontinue in women at least 2 months before a planned pregnancy due to the long washout period for *semaglutide*. Not recommended as first-line therapy for patients inadequately controlled on diet and exercise. There are no data on the presence of *semaglutide* in human milk or the effects on the breastfed infant.

BASAL INSULIN+GLP-1 RA COMBINATIONS

▶ *insulin degludec (insulin analog)+liraglutide* (C) for treatment of type 2 diabetes only when inadequately controlled on <50 units of basal *insulin* daily or ≤1.8 mg of *liraglutide* daily; administer by SC injection once daily, with or without food, into the upper arm, abdomen, or thigh; titrate every 3-4 days

Pediatric: <18 years: not recommended: ≥18 years: same as adult

　　Xultophy *Prefilled pen:* 100/3.6 U/ml (3 ml, 5 pens/carton)

▶ *insulin glargine (insulin analog)+lixisenatide* (C) for treatment of type 2 diabetes only when inadequately controlled on <60 units of basal *insulin* daily or *lixisenatide*; administer by SC injection once daily, with or without food, into the upper arm, abdomen, or thigh; titrate every 3-4 days

Pediatric: <18 years: not recommended: ≥18 years: same as adult

　　Soliqua *Prefilled pen:* 100/33 U/ml (3 ml, 5 pens/carton) covering 15-60 mg *insulin glargine* 100 units/ml and 15-20 mcg of *lixisenatide (m-cresol)*

SODIUM-GLUCOSE CO-TRANSPORTER 2 (SGLT2) INHIBITORS

Comment: SGLT2 inhibitors block the SGLT2 protein involved in 90% of glucose reabsorption in the proximal renal tubule, resulting in increased renal glucose excretion (typically >2000 mg/dL), and lower blood glucose levels (low risk of hypoglycemia), modest weight loss, and mild reduction in blood pressure (probably due to sodium loss). These agents probably also increase insulin sensitivity, decrease gluconeogenesis, and improve *insulin* release from pancreatic beta cells. SGLT2 inhibitors are contraindicated in T1DM, and are decreased or contraindicated with decreased GFR, increased SCr, renal failure, ESRD, renal dialysis, metabolic acidosis, or diabetic ketoacidosis. The most common ASEs are increased urination, UTI, and female genital mycotic infection (due to the glycosuria). These effects may be managed with adequate oral hydration and post-voiding genital hygiene. OTC **Vagisil** wet wipes are recommended to completely remove any post-voiding glucose film, and, thus, reduce potential risk of UTI and vaginal candidiasis, and reverse initial signs/symptoms of candida vaginalis. The SGLT2 inhibitors are not recommended in nursing women. There is potential for a hypersensitivity reaction to include angioedema and anaphylaxis. Caution with SGLT2 use due to reports of increased risk of treatment-emergent bone fractures. Serious, life-threatening cases of necrotizing fasciitis (Fournier's gangrene) have been reported in both females and males taking an SGLT2 inhibitor. Assess patients presenting with pain or tenderness, erythema, or swelling in the genital or perineal area, along with fever or malaise. If suspected, initiate prompt diagnosis and treatment.

▶ *canagliflozin* (C) take one tab before the first meal of the day; initially 100 mg; may titrate up to max 300 mg once daily; *GFR <45 mL/min:* do not initiate

Pediatric: <18 years: not established; ≥18 years: same as adult

　　Invokana *Tab:* 100, 300 mg

　　Comment: Invokana is contraindicated with GFR <45 mL/min; If GFR 45-≤60 mL/ min, max 100 mg once daily or consider other antihyperglycemic

▶ *dapagliflozin* (C) take one tab before the first meal of the day; initially 5 mg; may increase to max 10 mg once daily

Pediatric: <18 years: not established; ≥18 years: same as adult

    Farxiga *Tab:* 5, 10 mg

    Comment: **Farxiga** is contraindicated with GFR <60 mL/min.

▶ *empagliflozin* (C) take one tab before the first meal of the day; initially 10 mg; may increase to max 25 mg once daily

Pediatric: <18 years: not established; ≥18 years: same as adult

    Jardiance *Tab:* 10, 25 mg

    Comment: **Jardiance** is contraindicated with GFR <45 mL/min.

▶ *ertugliflozen* (C) take one tab before the first meal of the day; initially 5 mg; may increase to max 15 mg once daily

Pediatric: <18 years: not established; ≥18 years: same as adult

    Steglatro *Tab:* 5, 15 mg

SODIUM-GLUCOSE CO-TRANSPORTER 2 (SGLT2) INHIBITOR+BIGUANIDE COMBINATIONS

Comment: Caution with **SGLT2** use due to reports of increased risk of treatment-emergent bone fractures. *metformin* is contraindicated with renal impairment, metabolic acidosis, ketoacidosis. Suspend *metformin*, prior to, and for 48 hours after, surgery or receiving IV iodinated contrast agents.

▶ *canagliflozin+metformin* (C) take 1 dose twice daily with meals; max daily dose 300/2000; *GFR 45-≤60 mL/min:* canagliflozin max 100 mg once daily or consider other antihyperglycemic; *GFR <45 mL/min:* do not initiate

Pediatric: <18 years: not established; ≥18 years: same as adult

    Invokamet

        Tab: **Invokamet 50/500** cana 50 mg+met 500 mg

                Invokamet 50/1000 cana 50 mg+met 1000 mg

                Invokamet 150/500 cana 150 mg+met 500 mg

                Invokamet 150/1000 cana 150 mg+met 1000 mg

▶ *dapagliflozin+metformin* (C) swallow whole; do not crush or chew; take once daily first meal of the day; max daily dose 10/2000

Pediatric: <18 years: not established; ≥18 years: same as adult

    Xigduo XR

        Tab: **Xigduo XR 5/500** dapa 5 mg+met 500 mg ext-rel

                Xigduo XR 5/1000 dapa 5 mg+met 1000 mg ext-rel

                Xigduo XR 10/500 dapa 10 mg+met 500 mg ext-rel

                Xigduo XR 10/1000 dapa 10 mg+met 1000 mg ext-rel

    Comment: **Xigduo** is contraindicated with GFR <60 mL/min, SCr >1.5 (men) or SCr >1.4 (women)

▶ *empagliflozin+metformin* (C) take 1 dose twice daily with meals; max daily dose 25/2000

Pediatric: <18 years: not established; ≥18 years: same as adult

    Synjardy

        Tab: **Synjardy 5/500** empa 5 mg+met 500 mg

                Synjardy 5/1000 empa 5 mg+met 1000 mg

                Synjardy 12.5/500 empa 12.5 mg+met 500 mg

                Synjardy 12.5/1000 empa 12.5 mg+met 1000 mg

    Synjardy XR

        Tab: **Synjardy XR 5/1000** empa 5 mg+met 1000 mg

                Synjardy XR 12.5/1000 empa 12.5 mg+met 1000 mg

                Synjardy XR 10/1000 empa 10 mg+met 1000 mg

                Synjardy XR 25/1000 empa 25 mg+met 1000 mg

    Comment: **Synjardy** is contraindicated with GFR <45 mL/min, SCr >1.5 (men), or SCr >1.4 (women).

▶ *ertugliflozin+metformin* (C) take 1 dose twice daily with meals; max daily dose 15/2000

Pediatric: <18 years: not established; ≥18 years: same as adult

    Segluormet

        Tab: **Segluormet 2.5/500** ertu 2.5 mg+met 500 mg

                Segluormet 2.5/1000 ertu 2.5 mg+met 1000 mg

                Segluormet 7.5/500 ertu 7.5 mg+met 500 mg

                Segluormet 7.5/1000 ertu 7.5 mg+met 1000 mg

    Comment: **Steglatro** is contraindicated with GFR <30 mL/min. Do not initiate or continue with eGFR <60 mL/min.

SODIUM-GLUCOSE CO-TRANSPORTER 2 (SGLT2) INHIBITOR+DIPEPTIDYL PEPTIDASE-4 (DPP-4) INHIBITOR COMBINATIONS

Comment: Caution with SGLT2 use due to reports of increased risk of treatment-emergent bone fractures and increased risk for UTI and Candida vaginalis secondary to drug-associated glycosuria.

▷ *dapagliflozin+saxagliptin* (C) initially 5/10 once daily, at any time of day, with or without food; if a dose is missed and it is ≥12 hours until the next dose, the dose should be taken; if a dose is missed and it is <12 hours until the next dose, the missed dose should be skipped and the next dose taken at the usual time.
 Pediatric: <18 years: not recommended: ≥18 years: same as adult
   Qtern *Tab:* dapa 10 mg+saxa 5 mg film-coat
   Comment: Qtern should not be used during pregnancy. If pregnancy is detected, treatment with Qtern should be discontinued. It is unknown whether Qtern and/or its metabolites are excreted in human milk. Do not use with CrCl <60 mL/min or eGFR <60 mL/min/1.73 m² or ESRD or severe hepatic impairment or history of pancreatitis.

▷ *empagliflozin+linagliptin* (C) initially 10/5 once daily with the first meal of the day; max daily dose 25/5
 Pediatric: <18 years: not established; ≥18 years: same as adult
   Glyxambi
     Tab: Glyxambi 10/5 empa 10 mg+lina 5 mg
              Glyxambi 25/5 empa 25 mg+lina 5 mgss
   Comment: Glyxambi is contraindicated with GFR <45 mL/min.

▷ *ertugliflozin+sitagliptin* (C) initially 5/100 once daily with the first meal of the day; max daily dose 15/100
 Pediatric: <18 years: not established; ≥18 years: same as adult
   Steglujan
     Tab: Steglujan 5/100 ertu 5 mg+sita 100 mg
              Steglujan 15/100 ertu 15 mg+sita 100 mg
   Comment: Steglujan is contraindicated with GFR <45 mL/min.

DIPEPTIDYL PEPTIDASE-4 (DPP-4) INHIBITOR

Comment: DPP-4 is an enzyme that degrades incretin hormones glucagon-like peptide-1 (GLP-1) and glucose-dependent insulinotropic polypeptide (GIP). Thus, DPP-4 inhibitors increase the concentration of active incretin hormones, stimulating the release of *insulin* in a glucose-dependent manner and decreasing the levels of circulating *glucagon*. The FDA has reported that *saxagliptin*- and *alogliptin*-containing drugs may increase the risk of heart failure, especially in patients who already have cardiovascular or renal disease. Drugs in this risk group include Nesina (*alogliptin*) and Onglyza (*saxagliptin*)

▷ *alogliptin* (B) take twice daily with meals; max 25 mg day
 Pediatric: <18 years: not recommended; ≥18 years: same as adult
   Nesina *Tab:* 6.25, 12.5, 25 mg
▷ *linagliptin* (B) 5 mg once daily
 Pediatric: <18 years: not recommended; ≥18 years: same as adult
   Tradjenta *Tab:* 5 mg
▷ *saxagliptin* (B) 2.5-5 mg once daily
 Pediatric: <18 years: not recommended; ≥18 years: same as adult
   Onglyza *Tab:* 2.5, 5 mg
▷ *sitagliptin* (B) as monotherapy or as combination therapy with metformin or a TZD
 Pediatric: <18 years: not recommended; ≥18 years: same as adult
   Januvia 25-100 mg once daily
     Tab: 25, 50, 100 mg

DIPEPTIDYL PEPTIDASE-4 (DPP-4) INHIBITOR+BIGUANIDE COMBINATIONS

Comment: DPP-4 inhibitor+*metformin* combinations are contraindicated with renal impairment (men: SCr ≥1.5 mg/dL; women: SCr ≥1.4 mg/dL) or abnormal CrCl, metabolic acidosis, ketoacidosis, or history of angioedema. Suspend *metformin*, prior to, and for 48 hours after, surgery or receiving IV iodinated contrast agents. Avoid in the elderly, malnourished, dehydrated, or with clinical or lab evidence of hepatic disease. For other DPP-4 and/or *metformin* precautions, see mfr pkg insert. The FDA has reported that *saxagliptin*- and *alogliptin*-containing drugs may increase the risk of heart failure, especially in patients who already have cardiovascular or renal disease. These drugs include: Onglyza (*saxagliptin*), Kombiglyze XR (*saxagliptin+metformin*), Nesina (*alogliptin*), Kazano (*alogliptin+metformin*), and Oseni (*alogliptin+pioglitazone*).

▶ *alogliptin+metformin* (B) take twice daily with meals; max *alogliptin* 25 mg/day, max *metformin* 2000 mg/day

Pediatric: <18 years: not recommended; ≥18 years: same as adult

    Kazano

        Tab: **Kazano 12.5/500** algo 12.5 mg+met 500 mg

            Kazano 2.5/1000 algo 12.5 mg+met 1000 mg

▶ *linagliptin+metformin* (B)

Pediatric: <18 years: not recommended; ≥18 years: same as adult

    Jentadueto take twice daily with meals; max *linagliptin* 5 mg/day, max *metformin* 2000 mg/day

        Tab: **Jentadueto 2.5/500** lina 2.5 mg+met 500 mg film-coat

            Jentadueto 2.5/850 lina 2.5 mg+met 850 mg film-coat

            Jentadueto 2.5/1000 lina 2.5 mg+met 1000 mg film-coat

    Jentadueto XR *Currently not treated with* *metformin*: initiate **Jentadueto XR 5/1000** once daily; *Already treated with* *metformin*: initiate **Jentadueto XR 5 mg** *linagliptin* total daily dose and a similar total daily dose of *metformin* once daily; *Already treated with* *linagliptin and* *metformin* or *Jentadueto*: switch to **Jentadueto XR** containing 5 mg of *linagliptin* total daily dose and a similar total daily dose of *metformin* once daily; max *linagliptin* 5 mg and *metformin* 2,000 mg; take as a single dose once daily; take with food; do not crush or chew *eGFR <30 mL/min*: contraindicated; *eGFR 30-45 mL/min*: not recommended

        Tab: **Jentadueto 2.5/1000** lina 2.5 mg+met 1,000 mg film-coat ext-rel

            Jentadueto 5/1000 lina 5 mg+met 1,000 mg film-coat ext-rel

▶ *saxagliptin+metformin* (B) take once daily with meals; max *saxagliptin* 5 mg/day, max *metformin* 2,000 mg/day; do not crush or chew

Pediatric: <18 years: not recommended; ≥18 years: same as adult

    Kombiglyze XR

        Tab: **Kombiglyze XR 5/500** saxa 5 mg+met 500 mg

            Kombiglyze XR 2.5/1000 saxa 2.5 mg+met 1,000 mg

            Kombiglyze XR 5/1000 saxa 5 mg+met 1,000 mg

Comment: The FDA has reported that *saxagliptin*-containing drugs may increase the risk of heart failure, especially in patients who already have cardiovascular or renal disease. The drug Kombiglyze XR (*saxagliptin+metformin*) is in this risk group. *metformin* is contraindicated with renal impairment, metabolic acidosis, ketoacidosis. Suspend *metformin*, prior to, and for 48 hours after, surgery or receiving IV iodinated contrast agents.

▶ *sitagliptin+metformin* (B) take twice daily with meals; max *sitagliptin* 100 mg/day, max *metformin* 2000 mg/day

Pediatric: <18 years: not recommended; ≥18 years: same as adult

    Janumet

        Tab: **Janumet 50/500** sita 50 mg+met 500 mg

            Janumet 50/1000 sita 50 mg+met 1,000 mg

    Janumet XR

        Tab: **Janumet XR 50/500** sita 50 mg+met 500 mg ext-rel

            Janumet XR 50/1000 sita 50 mg+met 1,000 mg ext-rel

            Janumet XR 100/1000 sita 100 mg+met 1,000 mg ext-rel

Comment: *metformin* is contraindicated with renal impairment, metabolic acidosis, ketoacidosis. Suspend *metformin*, prior to, and for 48 hours after, surgery or receiving IV iodinated contrast agents.

MEGLITINIDE+BIGUANIDE COMBINATION

▶ *repaglinide+metformin* (C)(G) take in 2-3 divided doses within 30 minutes before food; max 4/1000 per meal and 10/2000 per day

Pediatric: <18 years: not recommended; ≥18 years: same as adult

    Prandimet

        Tab: **Prandimet 1/500** repa 1 mg+met 500 mg

            Prandimet 2/500 repa 2 mg+met 500 mg

Comment: *metformin* is contraindicated with renal impairment, metabolic acidosis, ketoacidosis. Suspend *metformin*, prior to, and for 48 hours after, surgery or receiving IV iodinated contrast agents.

DIPEPTIDYL PEPTIDASE-4 (DPP-4) INHIBITOR+HMG-COA REDUCTASE INHIBITOR COMBINATION

▶ *sitagliptin+simvastatin* (B) take once daily in the PM; swallow whole; adjust dose if needed after 4 weeks; *Concomitant* **verapamil** *or* **diltiazem**: max 100/10 once daily; *Concomitant* **amiodarone, amlodipine,** *or* **ranolazine**: max 100/20 once daily; *Homogenous familial hyper-cholesterolemia*: max 100/40 once daily; *Chinese patients taking lipid-modifying doses (>1 gm/ day niacin) of niacin-containing products*: caution with 100/40 dose; increase risk of myopathy
Pediatric: <18 years: not recommended; ≥18 years: same as adult
> Juvisync
> > *Tab*: **Juvisync 100/10** sita 100 mg+simva 10 mg
> > **Juvisync 100/20** sita 100 mg+simva 20 mg
> > **Juvisync 100/40** sita 100 mg+simva 40 mg

DOPAMINE RECEPTOR AGONIST

▶ *bromocriptine mesylate* (B) take with food in the morning within 2 hours of waking; ini-tially 0.8 mg once daily; may increase by 0.8 mg/week; max 4.8 mg/week; *Severe psychotic disorders*: not recommended
Pediatric: <12 years: not recommended; ≥12 years: same as adult
> Cycloset *Tab*: 0.8 mg
> Comment: Cycloset is an adjunct to diet and exercise to improve glycemic control. Contraindicated with syncopal migraines, nursing mothers, and other ergot-related drugs.

Bile Acid Sequestrant

▶ *colesevelam* (B)(G)
> WelChol recommended dose is 6 tablets once daily *or* 3 tablets twice daily; take with a meal and liquid
> *Pediatric*: <10 years: not recommended; ≥10 years: same as adult
> > *Tab*: 625 mg
> WelChol for Oral Suspension recommended dose is one 3.75 gm packet once daily *or* one 1.875 gm packet twice daily; empty one packet into a glass or cup; add 1/2 to 1 cup (4 to 8 ounces) of water, fruit juice, *or* diet soft drink; stir well and drink immediately; do not swallow dry form; take with meals
> *Pediatric*: <12 years: not established; ≥12 years: same as adult
> > *Pwdr*: 3.75 gm/pkt (30 pkt/carton), 1.875 gm/pkt (60 pkt/carton) for oral suspension
> Comment: WelChol is indicated as adjunctive therapy to improve glycemic control in adults with type 2 diabetes. It can be added to **metformin**, sulfonylureas, *or* insulin alone *or* in combination with other antidiabetic agents

TYPHOID FEVER (*SALMONELLA TYPHI*)

PRE-EXPOSURE PROPHYLAXIS

▶ *typhoid* vaccine, oral, live, attenuated strain
> Vivotif Berna 1 cap every other day, 1 hour before a meal, with a lukewarm (not > body temperature) *or* cold drink for a total of 4 doses; do not crush *or* chew; complete therapy at least 1 week prior to expected exposure; re-immunization recommended every 5 years if repeated exposure
> > *Pediatric*: <6 years: not recommended; ≥6 years: same as adult
> > *Cap*: ent-coat
▶ *typhoid Vi polysaccharide* vaccine (C)
> *Pediatric*: <2 years: not recommended; ≥2 years: same as adult
> > Typhim Vi 0.5 ml IM in deltoid; re-immunization recommended every 2 years if repeated exposure
> > > *Vial*: 20, 50 dose; *Prefilled syringe*: 0.5 ml
> Comment: Febrile illness may require delaying administration of the vaccine; have *epinephrine* 1:1000 readily available.

TREATMENT

▶ *azithromycin* (B)(G) 8-10 mg/kg/day; *Mild Illness*: treat x 7 days; *Severe Illness*: treat x 14 days
Pediatric: 8-10 mg/kg/day; max 500 mg/day; *Mild Illness*: treat x 7 days; *Severe Illness*: treat x 14 days; *see page 619 for dose by weight*

Zithromax *Tab:* 250, 500, 600 mg; *Oral susp:* 100 mg/5 ml (15 ml); 200 mg/5 ml (15, 22.5, 30 ml) (cherry); *Pkt:* 1 gm for reconstitution (cherry-banana)

Zithromax Tri-pak *Tab:* 3 x 500 mg tabs/pck

Zithromax Z-pak *Tab:* 6 x 250 mg tabs/pck

Zmax *Oral susp:* 2 gm ext-rel for reconstitution (cherry-banana) (148 mg Na⁺)

▷ *cefixime* (B)(G) *Mild Illness:* 15-20 mg/kg/day x 7-14 days; *Severe Illness:* 20 mg/kg/day x 10-14 days

Pediatric: <6 months: not recommended; 6 months-12 years, <50 kg: *Mild Illness:* 15-20 mg/kg/day x 7-14 days; *Severe Illness:* 20 mg/kg/day x 10-14 >50 kg: same as adult; *see page 621 for dose by weight*

Suprax *Tab:* 400 mg; *Cap:* 400 mg; *Oral susp:* 100, 200, 500 mg/5 ml (50, 75, 100 ml) (strawberry)

▷ *ciprofloxacin* (C) 15 mg/kg/day; *Mild Illness:* treat x 5-7 days; *Severe Illness:* treat x 10-14 days

Pediatric: <18 years: not recommended; ≥18 years: same as adult

Cipro (G) *Tab:* 250, 500, 750 mg; *Oral susp:* 250, 500 mg/5 ml (100 ml) (strawberry)

Cipro XR *Tab:* 500, 1000 mg ext-rel

ProQuin XR *Tab:* 500 mg ext-rel

Comment: *ciprofloxacin* is contraindicated <18 years-of-age, and during pregnancy and lactation. Risk of tendonitis or tendon rupture.

▷ *ofloxacin* (C) 15 mg/kg/day; *Mild Illness:* treat x 5-7 days; *Severe Illness:* treat x 10-14 days

Pediatric: <18 years: not recommended; ≥18 years: same as adult

Floxin *Tab:* 200, 300, 400 mg

Comment: *ofloxacin* is contraindicated <18 years-of-age, and during pregnancy and lactation. Risk of tendonitis or tendon rupture.

▷ *cefotaxime* 80 mg/kg/day IM/IV x 10-14 days; max 2 gm/day

Pediatrics: 80 mg/kg/day IM/IV x 10-14 days; max 2 gm/day

Claforan *Vial:* 500 mg; 1, 2 gm

▷ *ceftriaxone* (B)(G) 75 mg/kg/day IM/IV x 10-14 days; max 2 gm/day

Pediatrics: 75 mg/kg/day IM/IV x 10-14 days; max 2 gm/day

Rocephin *Vial:* 250, 500 mg; 1, 2 gm

▷ *trimethoprim+sulfamethoxazole* (TMP-SMX) (D)(G) 8-40 mg/kg/day x 14 days

Pediatric: <2 months: not recommended; ≥2 months: 8-40 mg/kg/day of *sulfamethoxazole* in 2 divided doses bid x 10 days; *see page 630 for dose by weight*

Bactrim, Septra 2 tabs bid x 10 days

Tab: trim 80 mg+sulfa 400 mg*

Bactrim DS, Septra DS 1 tab bid x 10 days

Tab: trim 160 mg+sulfa 800 mg*

Bactrim Pediatric Suspension, Septra Pediatric Suspension 20 ml bid x 10 days

Oral susp: trim 40 mg+sulfa 200 mg per 5 ml (100 ml) (cherry) (alcohol 0.3%)

Comment: Sulfonamides are contraindicated in the first trimester of pregnancy, the final month of pregnancy, and infants <8 weeks-of-age. *CrCl 15-30 mL/min:* reduce dose by 1/2; *CrCl <15 mL/min:* not recommended. Contraindicated with G6PD deficiency. A high fluid intake is indicated during sulfonamide therapy to avoid crystallization in the kidneys.

ULCER: DIABETIC, NEUROPATHIC (LOWER EXTREMITY); VENOUS INSUFFICIENCY (LOWER EXTREMITY)

NUTRITIONAL SUPPLEMENT

▷ *L-methylfolate calcium (as metafolin)+pyridoxyl 5-phosphate+methylcobalamin* take 1 cap daily

Pediatric: <12 years: not recommended; ≥12 years: same as adult

Metanx *Cap:* metafo 3 mg+pyrid 35 mg+methyl 2 mg (gluten-free, yeast-free, lactose-free)

Comment: Metanx is indicated as adjunct treatment of endothelial dysfunction and/or hyperhomocysteinemia in patients who have lower extremity ulceration.

DEBRIDING+CAPILLARY STIMULANT AGENT

▷ *trypsin+balsam peru+castor oil* apply at least twice daily; may cover with a wet bandage

Granulex *Aerosol liq:* tryp 0.12 mg+bal peru 87 mg+cast 788 mg per 0.82 ml

GROWTH FACTOR

▶ **becaplermin** (C) apply once daily with a cotton swab or tongue depressor; then cover with saline moistened gauze dressing; rinse after 12 hours; then re-cover with a clean saline dressing

    Regranex *Gel:* 0.01% (2, 7.5, 15 gm) (parabens)

Comment: Store in refrigerator; do not freeze. Not for use in wounds that close by primary intention.

 ULCER: PRESSURE, DECUBITUS

DEBRIDING/CAPILLARY STIMULANT AGENT

    Granulex (*trypsin* 0.1 mg+*balsam peru* 72.5 mg+*castor oil* 650 mg per 0.82 ml) apply at least twice daily; may cover with a wet bandage

      Aerosol liq: (2, 4 oz)

GROWTH FACTOR

▶ **becaplermin** (C) apply once daily with a cotton swab or tongue depressor; then cover with saline moistened gauze dressing; rinse after 12 hours; then recover with a clean saline dressing

    Regranex *Gel:* 0.01% (2, 7.5, 15 gm) (parabens)

Comment: Store in refrigerator; do not freeze. Not for use in wounds that close by primary intention.

 ULCERATIVE COLITIS (UC)

Comment: Standard treatment regimen is anti-infective, anti-spasmodic, and bowel rest; progressing to clear liquids; then to high fiber.

Parenteral Corticosteroids *see page 577*

Oral Corticosteroids *see page 577*

▶ **budesonide micronized** (C)(G) 9 mg once daily in the AM for up to 8 weeks; may repeat an 8-week course; *Maintenance of remission:* 6 mg once daily for up to 3 months; taper other systemic steroids when transferring to **budesonide**

Pediatric: <12 years: not recommended; ≥12 years: same as adult

    Entocort EC *Cap:* 3 mg ent-coat granules

    Uceris *Tab:* 9 mg ext-rel

RECTAL CORTICOSTEROIDS

▶ **hydrocortisone** rectal (C)

Pediatric: <12 years: not recommended; ≥12 years: same as adult

    Anusol-HC Suppositories 1 supp rectally 3 x/day or 2 supp rectally 2 x/day for 2 weeks; max 8 weeks

      Rectal supp: 25 mg (12, 24/pck)

    Cortenema 1 enema q HS x 21 days or until symptoms controlled

      Enema: 100 mg/60 ml (1, 7/pck)

    Cortifoam 1 applicator full once daily-bid x 2-3 weeks and every 2nd day thereafter until symptoms are controlled

      Aerosol: 80 mg/applicator (14 application/container)

    Proctocort 1 supp rectally in AM and PM x 2 weeks; for more severe cases, may increase to 1 supp rectally 3 times daily or 2 supp rectally twice daily; max 4-8 weeks

      Rectal supp: 30 mg (12, 24/pck)

Comment: Use **hydrocortisone** foam as adjunctive therapy in the distal portion of the rectum when **hydrocortisone** enemas cannot be retained.

RECTAL CORTICOSTEROID+ANESTHETIC

Hydrocortisone+Pramoxine

    Proctofoam HC apply to anal/rectal area 3-4 times daily; max 4-8 weeks

      Rectal foam: hydrocort 1%+pram 1% (10 gm w. applicator)

SALICYLATES

Comment: symptoms of salicylate toxicity include hematemesis, tachypnea, hyperpnea, tinnitus, deafness, lethargy, seizures, confusion, or dyspnea. Severe intoxication may lead to electrolyte and blood pH imbalance and potentially to other organ (e.g., renal and liver) involvement. There is no specific antidote for mesalamine overdose; however, conventional therapy for salicylate toxicity may be beneficial in the event of acute overdosage. This includes prevention of further gastrointestinal tract absorption by emesis and, if necessary, by gastric lavage. Fluid and electrolyte imbalance should be corrected by the administration of appropriate intravenous therapy. Adequate renal function should be maintained.

▷ *balsalazide disodium* (B)

   Comment: *balsalazide* 6.75 gm provides 2.4 gm of *mesalazine* to the colon.

      Colazal 3 x 750 mg caps/day (6.75 gm/day), with or without food, x 8 weeks; may require treatment for up to 12 weeks; swallow whole or may be opened and sprinkled on applesauce, then chewed or swallowed immediately

      Pediatric: <5 years: not recommended; 5-17 years: 1 x 750 mg cap 3 x/day (2.25 gm/day), with or without food for up to 8 weeks or 3 x 750 mg caps/day (6.75 gm/day), with or without food, x 8 weeks; swallow whole or may be opened and sprinkled on applesauce, then chewed or swallowed immediately

        Cap: 750 mg

      Comment: Colazal is a locally-acting aminosalicylate indicated for the treatment of mildly to moderately active ulcerative colitis in patients ≥5 years. Safety and effectiveness of Colazal >8 weeks in children (5-17 years) and >12 weeks in patients ≥18 years has not been established.

      Giazo is a locally-acting aminosalicylate indicated for the treatment of mildly to moderately active ulcerative colitis only in male patients ≥18 years; take 3 x 1.1 gm tabs bid (6.6 gm/day) for up to 8 weeks

      Pediatric: <18 years: not recommended; >18 years: same as adult

        Tab: 1.1 gm (sodium 126 mg/tab) film-coat

      Comment: Effectiveness of Giazo in female patients has not been demonstrated in clinical trials. Safety and effectiveness of Giazo > 8 weeks has not been established.

▷ *mesalamine* (B)

   Apriso *Maintenance: of Remission* 4 x 0.375 gm caps (1.5 gm/day) once daily in the morning, for maintenance of remission with or without food; do not co-administer with antacids

   Pediatric: <18 years: not recommended; ≥18 years: same as adult

     Cap: 0.375 gm ext-rel (phenylalanine 0.56 mg/cap)

   Comment: Apriso is a locally-acting aminosalicylate indicated for the maintenance of remission of ulcerative colitis in adults.

   Asacol HD (G) Induction of Remission: 2 x 800 mg tab (1600 mg) tid x 6 weeks; *Maintenance of Remission:* 1.6 gm/day in divided doses; take on an empty stomach, at least 1 hour before or 2 hours after a meal; swallow whole; do not crush, break, or chew

   Pediatric: <18 years: not recommended; ≥18 years: same as adult

     Tab: 800 mg del-rel

   Comment: Asacol HD is an aminosalicylate indicated for the treatment of moderately active ulcerative colitis in adults. Do not substitute one Asacol HD 800 tablet for two mesalamine delayed-release 400 mg oral products

   Canasa 1 x 1,000 mg suppository administered rectally once daily at bedtime for 3 to 6 weeks.

   Pediatric: <18 years: not recommended; ≥18 years: same as adult

     Rectal supp: 1 gm del-rel (30, 42/pck)

   Comment: Canasa is an aminosalicylate indicated in adults for the treatment of mildly to moderately active ulcerative proctitis. Safety and effectiveness of Canasa beyond 6 weeks have not been established.

   Delzicol Treatment: 2 x 400 mg caps (800 mg/day) 3 x/day x 6 weeks; *Maintenance:* 4 x 400 mg caps (1.6 gm/day) in 2-4 divided doses once daily; swallow whole; take with or without food; do not crush or chew

   Pediatric: ≥5-17 years: twice daily dosing for 6 weeks; see mfr pkg **insert** for weight-based dosing table; ≥18 years: same as adult

     Cap: 400 mg del-rel

   Comment: 2 x 400 mg Dezlicol caps have not been shown to be interchangeable or substitutable with one *mesalamine* delayed-release 80 mg tablet. Evaluate renal function prior to initiation of Dezlicol.

   Lialda (G) Induction of Remission: 2-4 x 1.2 gm tabs (2.4-4.8 gm) once daily for up to 8 weeks; *Maintenance: of Remission:* 2 x 1.2 gm tabs (2.4 gm) once daily; swallow whole; do not crush or chew

Pediatric: <18 years: not recommended; ≥18 years: same as adult
    Tab: 1.2 gm del-rel

Comment: **Lialda** is a locally-acting 5-aminosalicylic acid (5-ASA) indicated for the induction of remission in adults with active, mild to moderate ulcerative colitis and for the maintenance of remission of ulcerative colitis. Safety and effectiveness of **Lialda** in pediatric patients have not been established.

Pentasa Induction of Remission: 1 gm qid for up to 8 weeks
Pediatric: <18 years: not recommended; ≥18 years: same as adult
    Cap: 250, 500 mg ext-rel

Comment: **Pentasa** is an aminosalicylate anti-inflammatory agent indicated for the induction of remission and for the treatment of patients with mildly to moderately active ulcerative colitis.

Rowasa Suppository 1 supp rectally bid x 3-6 weeks; retain for 1-3 hours <u>or</u> longer
Pediatric: <18 years: not recommended; ≥18 years: same as adult
    Rectal supp: 500 mg (12, 24/pck)

Rowasa Rectal Suspension 4 gm (60 ml) rectally by enema q HS; retain for 8 hours x 3-6 weeks (sulfite-free)
Pediatric: <18 years: not recommended; ≥18 years: same as adult
    Enema: 4 gm/60 ml (7, 14, 28/pck; kit, 7, 14, 28/pck w. wipes)

Comment: *RowasaRectal Suspension Enema* is indicated for the treatment of active mild to moderate distal ulcerative colitis, proctosigmoiditis, and proctitis.

▷ *olsalazine* (C) **Maintenance of Remission:** 1 gm/day in 2 divided doses; take with food
Pediatric: <18 years: not recommended; ≥18 years: same as adult
    Dipentum *Cap:* 250 mg

Comment: *osalazine* is the sodium salt of a salicylate, disodium 3,3'-azobis (6-hydroxybenzoate) a compound that is effectively bioconverted to 5-amino-salicylic acid (5-ASA), which has anti-inflammatory activity in ulcerative colitis. The conversion of *olsalazine* to *mesalamine* (5-ASA) in the colon is similar to that of *sulfasalazine*, which is converted into *sulfapyridine* and *mesalamine*. *olsalazine* is indicated for the maintenance of remission of ulcerative colitis in patients who are intolerant of *sulfasalazine*.

▷ *sulfasalazine* (B; D in 2nd, 3rd)(G) **Induction of Remission:** 3-4 gm/day in evenly divided doses with dosage intervals not exceeding eight hours; in some cases, it is advisable to initiate therapy with a smaller dosage, e.g., 1-2 gm/day, to reduce possible gastrointestinal intolerance. If daily doses exceeding 4 gm are required to achieve desired effects, the increased risk of toxicity should be kept in mind; **Maintenance of Remission: 4 gm/day in divided doses**
Pediatric: <2 years: not recommended; 2-16 years: initially 40-60 mg/kg/day in 3 to 6 divided doses; max 30 mg/kg/day in 4 divided doses; max 2 gm/day in divided doses; >16 years: same as adult
    Azulfidine *Tab:* 500*mg
    Azulfidine EN-Tabs *Tab:* 500 mg ent-coat

TUMOR NECROSIS FACTOR (TNF) BLOCKER

▷ *adalimumab* (B) initially 180 mg SC (as 4 injections in 1 day <u>or</u> divided over 2 days) on week 0; then 80 mg at week 2; start 40 mg every other week maintenance at week 4; only continue if evidence of clinical remission by 8 weeks; administer in abdomen <u>or</u> thigh; rotate sites
Pediatric: <18 years: not recommended; ≥18 years: same as adult
    Humira *Prefilled syringe:* 20 mg/0.4 ml; 40 mg/0.8 ml single-dose (2/pck; 2, 6/starter pck) (preservative-free)

▷ *adalimumab-adbm* (B) *First dose (Day 1):* 160 mg SC (4 x 40 mg injections in one day or 2 x 40 mg injections per day for two consecutive days); *Second dose two weeks later (Day 15):* 80 mg SC; *Two weeks later (Day 29):* begin a maintenance dose of 40 mg SC every other week (only continue in patients who have shown evidence of clinical remission by eight weeks (Day 57) of therapy.
Pediatric: <18 years: not recommended; ≥18 years: same as adult
    Cyltezo *Prefilled syringe:* 40 mg/0.8 ml single-dose (preservative-free)
    Comment: **Cyltezo** is biosimilar to **Humira** (*adalimumab*).

▷ *infliximab (tumor necrosis factor-alpha blocker)* must be refrigerated at 2°C to 8°C (36°F to 46°F); administer dose via IV infusion over a period of not less than 2 hours; do not use beyond the expiration date as this product contains no preservative; 5 mg/kg at 0, 2 and 6 weeks, then every 8 weeks.

Pediatric: <6 years: not studied; ≥6-17 years: mg/kg at 0, 2 and 6 weeks, then every 8 weeks; ≥18 years: same as adult

Remicade *Vial:* 100 mg for reconstitution to 10 ml administration volume, single-dose (preservative-free)

Comment: **Remicade** is indicated to reduce signs and symptoms, and induce and maintain clinical remission, in adults and children ≥6 years-of-age with moderately to severely active disease who have had an inadequate response to conventional therapy and reduce the number of draining enterocutaneous and rectovaginal fistulas, and maintain fistula closure, in adults with fistulizing disease. Common adverse effects associated with **Remicade** included abdominal pain, headache, pharyngitis, sinusitis, and upper respiratory infections. In addition, **Remicade** might increase the risk for serious infections, including tuberculosis, bacterial sepsis, and invasive fungal infections. Available data from published literature on the use of *infliximab* products during pregnancy have not reported a clear association with *infliximab* products and adverse pregnancy outcomes. *infliximab* products cross the placenta and infants exposed *in utero* should not be administered live vaccines for at least 6 months after birth. Otherwise, the infant may be at increased risk of infection, including disseminated infection which can become fatal. Available information is insufficient to inform the amount of *infliximab* products present in human milk or effects on the breast-fed infant. To report suspected adverse reactions, contact Merck Sharp & Dohme Corp., a subsidiary of Merck & Co. at 1-877-888-4231 or FDA at 1-800-FDA1088 or www.fda.gov/medwatch.

▷ *infliximab-abda (tumor necrosis factor-alpha blocker)* **(B)**

Renflexis: see *infliximab* (**Remicade**) above for full prescribing information

Comment: **Renflexis** is a biosimilar to **Remicade** for the treatment of immune-disorders including Crohn's disease, ulcerative colitis, rheumatoid arthritis, ankylosing spondylitis, psoriatic arthritis and plaque psoriasis. **Renflexis** was approved under the FDA category for biosimilars and demonstrated no clinically meaningful differences for use, dosing regimens, strengths, dosage forms, and routes of administration from the FDA-approved biological product **Remicade**.

▷ *infliximab-dyyb (tumor necrosis factor-alpha blocker)* **(B)**

Inflectra: see *infliximab* (**Remicade**) above for full prescribing information

Comment: **Inflectra** is a biosimilar to **Remicade** for the treatment of immune-disorders including Crohn's disease, ulcerative colitis, rheumatoid arthritis, ankylosing spondylitis, psoriatic arthritis and plaque psoriasis. **Inflectra** was approved under the FDA category for biosimilars and demonstrated no clinically meaningful differences for use, dosing regimens, strengths, dosage forms, and routes of administration from the FDA-approved biological product **Remicade**.

▷ *infliximab-qbtx (tumor necrosis factor-alpha blocker)* **(B)**

Ifixi: see *infliximab* (**Remicade**) above for full prescribing information

Comment: **Ifixi** is a biosimilar to **Remicade** for the treatment of immune disorders including Crohn's disease, ulcerative colitis, rheumatoid arthritis, ankylosing spondylitis, psoriatic arthritis and plaque psoriasis. **Ifixi** was approved under the FDA category for biosimilars and demonstrated no clinically meaningful differences for use, dosing regimens, strengths, dosage forms, and routes of administration from the FDA-approved biological product **Remicade**.

JANUS KINASE (JAK) INHIBITOR (JAKI)

▷ *tofacitinib* **(C)** 5 mg twice daily; reduce to 5 mg once daily for moderate-to-severe renal impairment or moderate hepatic impairment, concomitant potent CYP3A4 inhibitors, or drugs that result in both CYP3A4 and potent CYP2C19 inhibition and/or CYP3A4 inhibitors; in patients with moderate or severe renal impairment or moderate hepatic impairment, and patients with lymphopenia, neutropenia, or anemia; use of **Xeljanz/Xeljanz XR** in patients with severe hepatic impairment is not recommended in any patient population

Comment: FDA has issued a MedWatch Alert to the public that a recent safety clinical trial found an increased risk of blood clots in the lungs and death when a 10 mg twice daily dose of *tofacitinib* (**Xeljanz, Xeljanz XR**) was administered to patients with rheumatoid arthritis (RA). FDA has **not** approved the 10 mg twice daily dosing regimen for RA; this dosing regimen is only approved for patients with ulcerative colitis (UC).

Pediatric: <12 years: not established; ≥12 years: same as adult

Xeljanz *Tab:* 5, 10 mg

Xeljanz XR *Tab:* 11 mg ext-rel

Comment: Xeljanz is the first oral JAKI approved for chronic treatment of moderately-to-severely active UC. Other FDA-approved treatments for the treatment of moderately-to-severely active UC must be administered through an IV infusion or SC injection. Use with caution in patients that may be at increased risk for gastrointestinal perforation. The most common adverse events associated with Xeljanz treatment for UC are diarrhea, elevated cholesterol level, headache, herpes zoster (shingles), increased blood creatine phosphokinase, nasopharyngitis, rash, and upper respiratory tract infection (URI). Avoid use of Xeljanz/Xeljanz XR during an active serious infection, including localized infection. Patients treated with Xeljanz are at increased risk for developing serious infections that may lead to hospitalization or death. Xeljanz has a BBW for serious infections (e.g., opportunistic infections), and malignancy (e.g., lymphoma). Use of Xeljanz in combination with biological therapies for ulcerative colitis or with potent immunosuppressants, such as *azathioprine* and *cyclosporine*, is not recommended. Avoid live vaccines administration during treatment with Xeljanz. Prior to starting Xeljanz, perform a test for latent tuberculosis; if it is positive, start treatment for tuberculosis prior to starting Xeljanz. Monitor all patients for active tuberculosis during treatment, even if the initial latent tuberculosis test is negative. Recommend lab monitoring due to potential for changes in lymphocytes, neutrophils, hemoglobin, liver enzymes, and lipids. Do not initiate Xeljanz if absolute lymphocyte count <500 cells/mm^3, an absolute neutrophil count (ANC) <1000 cells/mm3 or Hgb <9 g/dL. The safety and effectiveness of Xeljanz/Xeljanz XR in pediatric patients have not been established. Available data with Xeljanz use in pregnancy are insufficient to establish a drug associated risk of major birth defects, miscarriage, or adverse maternal or fetal outcomes. In animal reproduction studies, fetocidal, and teratogenic effects were noted. There is a pregnancy exposure registry that monitors pregnancy outcomes in women exposed to Xeljanz/Xeljanz XR during pregnancy. Consider pregnancy planning and prevention for females of reproductive potential. Patients should be encouraged to enroll in the Xeljanz/Xeljanz XR pregnancy registry if they become pregnant. To enroll or obtain information from the registry, patients can call the toll free number 1-877-311-8972. There are no data on the presence of *tofacitinib* in human milk or the effects on a breastfed infant; however, patients should be advised not to breastfeed. To report suspected adverse reactions, contact Pfizer at 1-800-438-1985 or FDA at 1-800-FDA-1088 or visit www.fda.gov/medwatch.

INTEGRIN RECEPTOR ANTAGONIST

▷ *vedolizumab* (B) administer by IV infusion over 30 minutes; 300 mg at weeks 0, 2, 6; then once every 8 weeks
Pediatric: <12 years: not established; ≥12 years: same as adult
Entyvio *Vial:* 300 mg (20 ml) single-dose, pwdr for IV infusion after reconstitution (preservative-free)
Comment: To report suspected adverse reactions, contact Takeda Pharmaceuticals at 1-877-TAKEDA-7 (1-877-825-3327) or FDA at 1800-FDA-1088 or www.fda.gov/medwatch.

ANTI-DIARRHEAL AGENTS

▷ *difenoxin+atropine* (C) 2 tabs; then 1 tab after each loose stool or 1 tab q 3-4 hours; max 8 tabs/day x 2 days
Motofen *Tab:* dif 1 mg+atro 0.025 mg
▷ *diphenoxylate+atropine* (C)(G) 2 tabs or 10 ml qid
Lomotil *Tab:* diphen 2.5 mg+atro 0.025 mg; *Liq:* diphen 2.5 mg+atro 0.025 mg/5 ml (2 oz w. dropper)
▷ *loperamide* (B)(G)
Imodium (OTC) 4 mg initially; then 2 mg after each loose stool; max 16 mg/day
Cap: 2 mg
Imodium A-D (OTC) 4 mg initially; then 2 mg after each loose stool; usual max 8 mg/day x 2 days
Cplt: 2 mg; *Liq:* 1 mg/5 ml (2, 4 oz)
▷ loperamide+simethicone (B)(G)
Imodium Advanced (OTC) 2 tabs chewed after first loose stool; then 1 after the next loose stool; max 4 tabs/day
Chew tab: loper 2 mg+simeth 125 mg

URETHRITIS: NONGONOCOCCAL (NGU)

Comment: The following treatment regimens for NGU are published in the **2015 CDC Sexually Transmitted Diseases Treatment Guidelines**. Treatment regimens are for adults only; consult a specialist for treatment of patients less than 18 years-of-age. Treatment regimens are presented by generic drug name first, followed by information about brands and dose forms. All persons who have confirmed or suspected urethritis should be tested for gonorrhea and chlamydia. Men treated for NGU should be instructed to abstain from sexual intercourse for 7 days after a single dose regimen or until completion of a 7-day regimen.

RECOMMENDED REGIMEN: UNCOMPLICATED NGU

▷ *azithromycin* 1 gm in a single dose or 100 mg orally bid x 7 days
   plus
▷ *doxycycline* 100 mg bid x 7 days

PERSISTENT-RECURRENT NGU

Men Initially Treated With Azithromycin+Doxycycline

▷ *azithromycin* 1 gm PO in a single dose

Men Who Fail a Regimen of Azithromycin

▷ *moxifloxacin* 400 mg PO once daily x 7 days

Heterosexual Men Who Live in Areas Where *T. Vaginalis* is Highly Prevalent

▷ *metronidazole* 2 gm PO in a single dose
   or
▷ *tinidazole* 2 gm PO in a single dose

ALTERNATIVE REGIMENS

▷ *erythromycin base* 500 mg PO qid x 7 days

   or

▷ *erythromycin ethylsuccinate* 800 mg PO qid x 7 days

   or

▷ *levofloxacin* 500 mg once daily x 7 days

   or

▷ *ofloxacin* 300 mg PO bid x 7 days

DRUG BRANDS AND DOSE FORMS

▷ *azithromycin* (B)(G)
   Zithromax *Tab:* 250, 500, 600 mg; *Oral susp:* 100 mg/5 ml (15 ml); 200 mg/5 ml (15, 22.5, 30 ml) (cherry); *Pkt:* 1 gm for reconstitution (cherry-banana)
   Zithromax Tri-pak *Tab:* 3 x 500 mg tabs/pck
   Zithromax Z-pak *Tab:* 6 x 250 mg tabs/pck
   Zmax *Oral susp:* 2 gm ext-rel for reconstitution (cherry-banana) (148 mg Na⁺)

▷ *doxycycline* (D)(G)
   Acticlate *Tab:* 75, 150**mg
   Adoxa *Tab:* 50, 75, 100, 150 mg ent-coat
   Doryx *Tab:* 50, 75, 100, 150, 200 mg del-rel
   Doxteric *Tab:* 50 mg del-rel
   Monodox *Cap:* 50, 75, 100 mg
   Oracea *Cap:* 40 mg del-rel
   Vibramycin *Tab:* 100 mg; *Cap:* 50, 100 mg; *Syr:* 50 mg/5 ml (raspberry-apple) (sulfites); *Oral susp:* 25 mg/5 ml (raspberry)
   Vibra-Tab *Tab:* 100 mg film-coat

▷ *erythromycin base* (B)
   Ery-Tab *Tab:* 250, 333, 500 mg ent-coat
   PCE *Tab:* 333, 500 mg

Comment: *erythromycin* may increase INR with concomitant *warfarin*, as well as increase serum level of *digoxin*, benzodiazepines, and statins.

➤ *erythromycin ethylsuccinate* (B)(G)

> **EryPed** *Oral susp:* 200 mg/5 ml (100, 200 ml) (fruit); 400 mg/5 ml (60, 100, 200 ml) (banana); *Oral drops:* 200, 400 mg/5 ml (50 ml) (fruit); *Chew tab:* 200 mg wafer (fruit)
> **E.E.S.** *Oral susp:* 200, 400 mg/5 ml (100 ml) (fruit)
> **E.E.S. Granules** *Oral susp:* 200 mg/5 ml (100, 200 ml) (cherry)
> **E.E.S. 400 Tablets** *Tab:* 400 mg

Comment: *erythromycin* may increase INR with concomitant *warfarin,* as well as increase serum level of *digoxin,* benzodiazepines, and statins.

➤ *levofloxacin* (C)

> **Levaquin** *Tab:* 250, 500, 750 mg; *Oral soln:* 25 mg/ml (480 ml) (benzyl alcohol); *Inj conc:* 25 mg/ml for IV infusion after dilution (20, 30 ml single-use vial) (preservative-free); *Premix soln:* 5 mg/ml for IV infusion (50, 100, 150 ml) (preservative-free)

➤ *metronidazole* (not for use in 1st; B in 2nd, 3rd)(G)

> **Flagyl** *Tab:* 250*, 500*mg
> **Flagyl 375** *Cap:* 375 mg
> **Flagyl ER** *Tab:* 750 mg ext-rel

➤ *moxifloxacin* (C)(G)

> **Avelox** *Tab:* 400 mg

Comment: *moxifloxacin* is contraindicated <18 years-of-age, and during pregnancy and lactation. Risk of tendonitis or tendon rupture.

➤ *ofloxacin* (C)(G)

> **Floxin** *Tab:* 200, 300, 400 mg

Comment: *ofloxacin* is contraindicated <18 years-of-age, and during pregnancy and lactation. Risk of tendonitis or tendon rupture.

➤ *tinidazole* (not for use in 1st; B in 2nd, 3rd)

> **Tindamax** *Tab:* 250*, 500*mg

URINARY RETENTION: UNOBSTRUCTIVE

➤ *bethanechol* (C) 10-30 mg tid

> **Urecholine** *Tab:* 5, 10, 25, 50 mg

Comment: Contraindicated in presence of urinary obstruction. *atropine* 0.4 mg administered SC reverses *bethanechol* toxicity.

URINARY TRACT INFECTION, COMPLICATED (cUTI)

➤ *ceftazidime+avibactam* (B) infuse dose over 2 hours; recommended duration of treatment: 5 to 4 days; *CrCl 31-50 mL/min:* 1.25 gm every 8 hours; *CrCl 16-30 mL/min:* 0.94 gm every 12 hours; *CrCl 6-15 mL/min:* 0.94 gm every 24 hours; *CrCl ≤5 mL/min:* 0.94 gm every 48 hours; both *ceftazidime* and *avibactam* are hemodialyzable; thus, administer **Avycaz** after hemodialysis on hemodialysis days

Pediatric: <18 years: not recommended; ≥18 years: same as adult

> **Avycaz** *Vial:* 2.5 gm, single-dose, pwdr for reconstitution and IV infusion

Comment: **Avycaz** 2.5 gm contains *ceftazidime* (a cephalosporin) 2 grams (equivalent to 2.635 grams of *ceftazidime pentahydrate/sodium carbonate powder*) and *avibactam* (a beta lactam inhibitor) 0.5 grams (equivalent to 0.551 grams of *avibactam sodium*). As only limited clinical safety and efficacy data for **Avycaz** are currently available, reserve **Avycaz** for use in patients who have limited or no alternative treatment options. To reduce the development of drug-resistant bacteria and maintain the effectiveness of **Avycaz** and other antibacterial drugs, **Avycaz** should be used only to treat infections that are proven or strongly suspected to be caused by susceptible bacteria. Seizures and other neurologic events may occur, especially in patients with renal impairment. Adjust dose in patients with renal impairment. Decreased efficacy in patients with baseline CrCl 30--≤50 mL/min. Monitor CrCl at least daily in patients with changing renal function and adjust the dose of **Avycaz** accordingly. Monitor for hypersensitivity reactions, including anaphylaxis and serious skin reactions. Cross-hypersensitivity may occur in patients with a history of penicillin allergy. If an allergic reaction occurs, discontinue **Avycaz**. *Clostridium difficile*-associated diarrhea CDAD) has been reported with nearly all systemic antibacterial agents, including **Avycaz**. There are no adequate and well-controlled studies of **Avycaz**, *ceftazidime*, or *avibactam* in pregnant females.

ceftazidime is excreted in human milk in low concentrations. It is not known whether *avibactam* is excreted into human milk. There are no studies to inform effects on the breastfed infant.

 URINARY TRACT INFECTION (UTI, CYSTITIS: ACUTE)

URINARY TRACT ANALGESIA

Comment: Except when contraindicated, *ibuprofen* or other inflammatory agent of choice is a recommended adjunct or monotherapy in the treatment of UTI dysuria, frequency, and urgency which is due to inflammation and associated smooth muscle spasms/colic.
OTC AZO Standard
OTC AZO Standard Maximum Strength
OTC Prodium
OTC Uristat

ANTISPASMODIC AGENT

▷ *flavoxate* (B)(G) 100-200 mg tid-qid
 Pediatric: <12 years: not recommended; >12 years: same as adult
  Urispas *Tab:* 100 mg
 Comment: *flavoxate* hydrochloride tablets are indicated for symptomatic relief of dysuria, urgency, nocturia, suprapubic pain, frequency and incontinence as may occur in cystitis, prostatitis, urethritis, urethrocystitis/urethrotrigonitis. *flavoxate* is not indicated for definitive treatment, but is compatible with drugs used for the treatment of UTI. *flavoxate* is contraindicated in patients who have any of the following obstructive conditions: pyloric or duodenal obstruction, obstructive intestinal lesions, ileus, achalasia, GI hemorrhage, and obstructive uropathies of the lower urinary tract. Used with caution with glaucoma. It is not known whether *flavoxate* is excreted in human milk.

URINARY TRACT ANALGESIC-ANTISPASMODIC AGENTS

▷ *hyoscyamine* (C)(G)
  Anaspaz 1-2 tabs q 4 hours prn; max 12 tabs/day
   Tab: 0.125*mg
  Pediatric: <2 years: not recommended; 2-12 years: 0.0625-0.125 mg q 4 hours prn; max 0.75 mg/day; >12 years: same as adult
  Levbid 1-2 tabs q 12 hours prn; max 4 tabs/day
  Pediatric: <12 years: not recommended; ≥12 years: same as adult
   Tab: 0.375*mg ext-rel
  Levsin 1-2 tabs q 4 hours prn; max 12 tabs/day
  Pediatric: <6 years: not recommended; 6-12 years: 1 tab q 4 hours prn; ≥12 years: same as adult
   Tab: 0.125*mg
  Levsin Drops Use SL or PO forms
  Pediatric: 3.4 kg: 4 drops q 4 hours prn; max 24 drops/day; 5 kg: 5 drops q 4 hours prn; max 30 drops/day; 7 kg: 6 drops q 4 hours prn; max 36 drops/day; 10 kg: 8 drops q 4 hours prn; max 40 drops/day
   Oral drops: 0.125 mg/ml (15 ml) (orange) (alcohol 5%)
  Levsin Elixir 5 ml q 4 hours prn ←fix raised font left
  Pediatric: <10 kg: use drops; 10-19 kg: 1.25 ml q 4 hours prn; 20-39 kg: 2.5 ml q 4 hours prn; 40-49 kg: 3.75 ml q 4 hours prn; >50 kg:
   Elix: 0.125 mg/5 ml (16 oz) (orange) (alcohol 20%)
  Levsinex SL 1-2 tabs q 4 hours; max 12 tabs/day
  Pediatric: <2 years: not recommended; 2-12 years: 1 tab q 4 hours; max 6 tabs/day; >12 years: same as adult
   Tab: 0.125 mg sublingual
  Levsinex Timecaps 1-2 caps q 12 hours; may adjust to 1 cap q 8 hours
  Pediatric: <2 years: not recommended; 2-12 years: 1 cap q 12 hours; max 2 caps/day; >12 years: same as adult
   Cap: 0.375 mg time-rel
  NuLev dissolve 1-2 tabs on tongue, with or without water, q 4 hours prn; max 12 tabs/day

Pediatric: <2 years: not recommended; 2-12 years: dissolve 1 tab on tongue, with or without water, q 4 hours prn; max 6 tabs/day; >12 years:
    ODT: 0.125 mg (mint) (phenylalanine)

▷ *methenamine+phenyl salicylate+methylene blue+benzoic acid+atropine sulfate+hyoscyamine* (C)(G) 2 tabs qid prn
  Pediatric: <6 years: not recommended; ≥6 years: same as adult
    Urised *Tab:* meth 40.8 mg+phenyl salic 18.1 mg+meth blue 5.4 mg+benz acid 4.5 mg+atro sulf 0.03 mg+hyoscy 0.03 mg
  Comment: **Urised** imparts a blue-green color to urine which may stain fabrics.

▷ *methenamine+phenyl salicylate+methylene blue+sod phosphate monobasic+hyoscyamine* (C) 1 cap qid prn
  Pediatric: <6 years: not recommended; ≥6 years: same as adult
    Uribel *Cap:* meth 118 mg+phenyl salic 36 mg+meth blue 10 mg+sod phos mono 40.8 mg+hyoscy 0.12 mg

▷ *methenamine+phenyl salicylate+methylene blue+sod biphosphate+hyoscyamine* (C) 1 tab qid prn
  Pediatric: <6 years: not recommended; ≥6 years: same as adult
    Urelle *Cap:* meth 81 mg+phenyl salic 32.4 mg+meth blue 10.8 mg+sod biphos 40.8 mg+hyoscy 0.12 mg

▷ *phenazopyridine* (B)(G) 100-200 mg q 6 hours prn; max 2 days
  Pediatric: <12 years: not recommended; ≥12 years: same as adult
    AZO Standard, Prodium, Uristat (OTC) *Tab:* 95 mg
    AZO Standard Maximum Strength (OTC) *Tab:* 97.5 mg
    Pyridium, Urogesic *Tab:* 100, 200 mg
  Comment: *phenazopyridine* imparts an orange-red color to urine which may stain fabrics.

ANTI-INFECTIVES

▷ *acetyl sulfisoxazole* (C)(G)
    Gantrisin initially 2-4 gm in a single or divided doses; then, 4-8 gm/day in 4-6 divided doses x 3-10 days
    Pediatric: <12 years: not recommended; ≥12 years: same as adult
      Tab: 500 mg
    Gantrisin initially 2-4 gm in a single or divided doses; then, 4-8 gm/day in 4-6 divided doses x 3-10 days
    Pediatric: <2 months: not recommended; 2 months-12 years: initial dose 75 mg/kg/day; then 150 mg/kg/day in 4-6 divided doses x 3-10 days; max 6 gm/day; >12 years: same as adult
      Oral susp: 500 mg/5 ml (4, 16 oz); *Syr:* 500 mg/5 ml (16 oz)

▷ *amoxicillin* (B)(G) 500-875 mg bid or 250-500 mg tid x 3-10 days
  Pediatric: <40 kg (88 lb): 20-40 mg/kg/day in 3 divided doses x 10 days or 25-45 mg/kg/day in 2 divided doses 3-10 days; *see page* 617 *for dose by weight table;* ≥40 kg: same as adult
    Amoxil *Cap:* 250, 500 mg; *Tab:* 875*mg; *Chew tab:* 125, 200, 250, 400 mg (cherry-banana-peppermint) (phenylalanine); *Oral susp:* 125, 250 mg/5 ml (80, 100, 150 ml) (strawberry); 200, 400 mg/5 ml (50, 75, 100 ml) (bubble gum); *Oral drops:* 50 mg/ml (30 ml) (bubble gum)
    Moxatag *Tab:* 775 mg ext-rel
    Trimox *Tab:* 125, 250 mg; *Cap:* 250, 500 mg; *Oral susp:* 125, 250 mg/5 ml (80, 100, 150 ml) (raspberry-strawberry)

▷ *amoxicillin+clavulanate* (B)(G)
    Augmentin 500 mg tid or 875 mg bid x 3-10 days
    Pediatric: <40 kg: 40-45 mg/kg/day divided tid x 3-10 days or 90 mg/kg/day divided bid x 10 days; *see page* 618 *for dose by weight table;* ≥40 kg: same as adult
      Tab: 250, 500, 875 mg; *Chew tab:* 125, 250 mg (lemon-lime); 200, 400 mg (cherry-banana) (phenylalanine); *Oral susp:* 125 mg/5 ml (banana), 250 mg/5 ml (75, 100, 150 ml) (orange); 200, 400 mg/5 ml (50, 75, 100 ml) (orange) (phenylalanine)
    Augmentin ES-600 <3 months: not recommended; ≥3 months, <40 kg: 90 mg/kg/day divided q 12 hours x 3-10 days; *see page* 618 *for dose by weight table;* ≥40 kg: not recommended
      Oral susp: 600 mg/5 ml (50, 75, 100, 125, 150, 200 ml) (strawberry cream) (phenylalanine)
    Augmentin XR <16 years: use other forms; ≥16 years: 2 tabs q 12 hours x 3-10 days
      Tab: 1000*mg ext-rel

▷ *ampicillin* (B) 500 mg qid x 3-10 days
  Pediatric: <12 years: 50-100 mg/kg/day in 4 divided doses x 3-10 days; *see page 619 for dose by weight table;* ≥12 years: same as adult
    Omnipen, Principen *Cap:* 250, 500 mg; *Oral susp:* 125, 250 mg/5 ml (100, 150, 200 ml) (fruit)

▷ *carbenicillin* (B) 1-2 tabs qid x 3-10 days
  Pediatric: <12 years: not recommended; ≥12 years: same as adult
    Geocillin *Tab:* 382 mg
      Tab: 375, 500 mg ext-rel

▷ *cefaclor* (B)(G) 250-500 mg q 8 hours x 3-10 days; max 2 gm/day
  Pediatric: <1 month: not recommended; 1 month-12 years: 20-40 mg/kg divided bid x 10 days; *see page 620 for dose by weight table;* max 1 gm/day; >12 years: same as adult
    Tab: 500 mg; *Cap:* 250, 500 mg; *Susp:* 125 mg/5 ml (75, 150 ml) (strawberry); 187 mg/5 ml (50, 100 ml) (strawberry); 250 mg/5 ml (75, 150 ml) (strawberry); 375 mg/5 ml (50, 100 ml) (strawberry)
    Cefaclor Extended Release 500 mg bid x 3-10 days (clinically equivalent to 250 mg immed-rel caps tid); swallow whole; take with meals
    Pediatric: <16 years: not recommended; ≥16 years: same as adult
      Tab: 375, 500 mg ext-rel

▷ *cefadroxil* (B) 1-2 gm in a single or 2 divided doses x 3-10 days
  Pediatric: <12 years: 30 mg/kg/day in 2 divided doses x 3-10 days; *see page 620 for dose by weight table;* ≥12 years: same as adult
    Duricef *Cap:* 500 mg; *Tab:* 1 gm; *Oral susp:* 250 mg/5 ml (100 ml); 500 mg/5 ml (75, 100 ml) (orange-pineapple)

▷ *cefixime* (B)(G) 400 mg once daily x 5 days
  Pediatric: <6 months: not recommended; 6 months-12 years, <50 kg: 8 mg/kg/day in 1-2 divided doses x 5 days; *see page 621 for dose by weight table;* >12 years, >50 kg: same as adult
    Suprax *Tab:* 400 mg; *Cap:* 400 mg; *Oral susp:* 100, 200, 500 mg/5 ml (50, 75, 100 ml) (strawberry)

▷ *cefpodoxime proxetil* (B) 100 mg bid x 3-10 days
  Pediatric: <2 months: not recommended; 2 months-12 years: 10 mg/kg/day (max 400 mg/dose) or 5 mg/kg/day bid (max 200 mg/dose) x 3-10 days: *see page 622 for dose by weight table;* ≥12 years: same as adult
    Vantin *Tab:* 100, 200 mg; *Oral susp:* 50, 100 mg/5 ml (50, 75, 100 mg) (lemon creme)

▷ *cephalexin* (B)(G) 500 mg bid x 3-10 days
  Pediatric: <12 years: 25-50 mg/kg/day in 4 divided doses x 3-10 days; *see page 623 for dose by weight table;* ≥12 years:
    Keflex *Cap:* 250, 333, 500, 750 mg; *Oral susp:* 125, 250 mg/5 ml (100, 200 ml) (strawberry)

▷ *ciprofloxacin* (C) 500 mg bid or 1000 mg XR once daily x 3-7 days
  Pediatric: <18 years: not recommended; ≥18 years: same as adult
    Cipro (G) *Tab:* 250, 500, 750 mg; *Oral susp:* 250, 500 mg/5 ml (100 ml) (strawberry)
    Cipro XR *Tab:* 500, 1000 mg ext-rel
    ProQuin XR *Tab:* 500 mg ext-rel
  Comment: *ciprofloxacin* is contraindicated <18 years-of-age, and during pregnancy and lactation. Risk of tendonitis or tendon rupture.

▷ *doxycycline* (D)(G) 100 mg bid x 3-10 days
  Pediatric: <8 years: not recommended; ≥8 years, <100 lb: 2 mg/lb on first day in 2 divided doses, followed by 1 mg/lb/day in a single or 2 divided doses x 3-10 days; ≥8 years, ≥100 lb: same as adult
    Acticlate *Tab:* 75, 150**mg
    Adoxa *Tab:* 50, 75, 100, 150 mg ent-coat
    Doryx *Tab:* 50, 75, 100, 150, 200 mg del-rel
    Doxteric *Tab:* 50 mg del-rel
    Monodox *Cap:* 50, 75, 100 mg
    Oracea *Cap:* 40 mg del-rel
    Vibramycin *Tab:* 100 mg; *Cap:* 50, 100 mg; *Syr:* 50 mg/5 ml (raspberry-apple) (sulfites); *Oral susp:* 25 mg/5 ml (raspberry)
    Vibra-Tab *Tab:* 100 mg film-coat
  Comment: *doxycycline* is contraindicated <8 years-of-age, in pregnancy, and lactation (discolors developing tooth enamel). A side effect may be photosensitivity (photophobia).

Do not take with antacids, calcium supplements, milk or other dairy, or within 2 hours of taking another drug.

➤ *enoxacin* (C) 200 mg q 12 hours x 3-10 days
Pediatric: <18 years: not recommended; ≥18 years: same as adult
  Penetrex *Tab:* 200, 400 mg
Comment: *enoxacin* is contraindicated <18 years-of-age, and during pregnancy and lactation. Risk of tendonitis or tendon rupture.

➤ *fosfomycin* (B) take as a single dose on an empty stomach; dissolve 1 sachet pkt in 3-4 oz cold water and drink immediately
Pediatric: <12 years: not established; ≥12 years: same as adult
  Monurol *Single-dose sachet pkts:* 3 gm (mandarin orange) (saccharin, sucrose)
Comment: *fosfomycin tromethamine* is a single-dose synthetic, broad spectrum, bactericidal antibiotic for treatment of uncomplicated UTI. Repeat dosing does not improve clinical efficacy. Safety and effectiveness in children ≥12 years have not been established in adequate and well-controlled studies.

➤ *levofloxacin* (C) 250 mg once daily x 3-7 days
Pediatric: <18 years: not recommended; ≥18 years: same as adult
  Levaquin *Tab:* 250, 500, 750 mg; *Oral soln:* 25 mg/ml (480 ml) (benzyl alcohol); *Inj conc:* 25 mg/ml for IV infusion after dilution (20, 30 ml single-use vial) (preservative-free); *Premix soln:* 5 mg/ml for IV infusion (50, 100, 150 ml) (preservative-free)
Comment: *levofloxacin* is contraindicated <18 years-of-age, and during pregnancy and lactation. Risk of tendonitis or tendon rupture.

➤ *lomefloxacin* (C) 400 mg once daily x 3-7 days
Pediatric: <18 years: not recommended; ≥18 years: same as adult
  Maxaquin *Tab:* 400 mg
Comment: *lomefloxacin* is contraindicated <18 years-of-age, and during pregnancy and lactation. Risk of tendonitis or tendon rupture.

➤ *minocycline* (D)(G) 100 mg q 12 hours x 3-10 days
Pediatric: <8 years: not recommended; <8 years, <100 lb: 1-2 mg/lb in 2 divided doses x 3-10 days; ≥8 years, ≥100 lb: same as adult
  Dynacin *Cap:* 50, 100 mg
  Minocin *Cap:* 50, 75, 100 mg; *Oral susp:* 50 mg/5 ml (60 ml) (custard) (sulfites, alcohol 5%)
Comment: *minocycline* is contraindicated <8 years-of-age, in pregnancy, and lactation (discolors developing tooth enamel). A side effect may be photo-sensitivity (photophobia). Do not take with antacids, calcium supplements, milk or other dairy, or within two hours of taking another drug.

➤ *nalidixic acid* (B) 1 gm qid x 3-10 days
Pediatric: <3 months: not recommended; ≥3 months-<12 years: 25 mg/lb/day in 4 divided doses x 3-10 days; ≥12 years: same as adult
  NegGram *Tab:* 250, 500 mg; 1 gm; *Cap:* 250, 500 mg; *Oral susp:* 250 mg/5 ml

➤ *nitrofurantoin* (B)(G)
  Furadantin 50-100 mg qid x 3-10 days
  Pediatric: <1 month: not recommended; ≥1 month-12 years: 5-7 mg/kg/ day in 4 divided doses x 3-10 days; *see page 629 for dose by weight table;* >12 years: same as adult
    Oral susp: 25 mg/5 ml (60 ml)
  Macrobid 100 mg q 12 hours x 3-10 days
  Pediatric: <12 years: not recommended; ≥12 years: same as adult
    Cap: 100 mg
  Macrodantin 50-100 mg qid x 3-10 days
  Pediatric: <12 years: not recommended; ≥12 years: same as adult
    Cap: 25, 50, 100 mg

➤ *norfloxacin* (C) 400 mg once daily x 3-7 days
Pediatric: <18 years: not recommended; ≥18 years: same as adult
  Noroxin *Tab:* 400 mg
Comment: *norfloxacin* is contraindicated <18 years-of-age, and during pregnancy and lactation. Risk of tendonitis or tendon rupture.

➤ *ofloxacin* (C)(G) 200 mg q 12 hours x 3-7 days
Pediatric: <18 years: not recommended; ≥18 years: same as adult
  Floxin *Tab:* 200, 300, 400 mg
  Floxin UroPak *Tab:* 200 mg (6/pck)

Comment: *ofloxacin* is contraindicated <18 years-of-age, and during pregnancy and lactation. Risk of tendonitis or tendon rupture.

▷ *trimethoprim* (C)(G)

Primsol 100 mg q 12 hours or 200 mg once daily x 10 days
Pediatric: <6 months: not recommended; ≥6 months-12 years: 10 mg/kg/ day in 2 divided doses x 10 days; >12 years: same as adult
Oral soln: 50 mg/5 ml (bubble gum) (dye-free, alcohol-free)
Proloprim 100 mg q 12 hours or 200 mg once daily x 10 days
Pediatric: <12 years: not recommended; ≥12 years: same as adult
Tab: 100, 200 mg
Trimpex 100 mg q 12 hours or 200 mg once daily x 10 days
Pediatric: <12 years: not recommended; ≥12 years: same as adult
Tab: 100 mg

▷ *trimethoprim+sulfamethoxazole (TMP-SMX)* (D)(G)

Bactrim, Septra 2 tabs bid x 3-10 days
Pediatric: <12 years: not recommended; ≥12 years: same as adult
Tab: trim 80 mg+sulfa 400 mg*
Bactrim DS, Septra DS 1 tab bid x 3-10 days
Pediatric: <12 years: not recommended; ≥12 years: same as adult
Tab: trim 160 mg+sulfa 800 mg*
Bactrim Pediatric Suspension, Septra Pediatric Suspension use tabs
Pediatric: <2 months: not recommended; ≥2 months-12 years: 40 mg/kg/day of *sulfa-methoxazole* in 2 doses bid; >12 years: use tabs
Oral susp: trim 40 mg+sulfa 200 mg per 5 ml (100 ml) (cherry) (alcohol 0.3%)

Comment: Sulfonamides are contraindicated in the first trimester of pregnancy, the final month of pregnancy, and infants <8 weeks-of-age. *CrCl 15-30 mL/min:* reduce dose by 1/2; *CrCl <15 mL/min:* not recommended. Contraindicated with G6PD deficiency. A high fluid intake is indicated during sulfonamide therapy to avoid crystallization in the kidneys.

PARENTERAL THERAPY FOR COMPLICATED cUTI

▷ *ertapenem* (B) 1 gm once daily; *CrCl <30 mL/min:* 500 mg once daily; treat x 10-14 days; may switch to an oral antibiotic after 3 days if warranted; *IV infusion:* administer over 30 minutes; *IM injection:* reconstitute
Pediatric: <18 years: not recommended; ≥18 years same as adult
Invanz *Vial:* 1 gm pwdr for reconstitution

▷ *meropenem+vaborbactam* administer 4 gm (*meropenem* 2 gm and *vaborbactam* 2 gm) every 8 hours by IV infusion; administer over 3 hours; treat for up to 14 days; monitor urine cultures and eGFR; *eGFR 30-49 mL/min:* 2 gm (*meropenem* 1 gm and *vaborbactam* 1 gm) every 8 hours; *eGFR 15-29 mL/min:* 2 gm (*meropenem* 1 gm and *vaborbactam* 1 gm) every 12 hours; *eGFR <15 mL/min:* 1 gm (*meropenem* 0.5 gm and *vaborbactam* 0.5 gm) every 12 hours; *ESRD:* administer 1 gm (*meropenem* 0.5 gm and *vaborbactam* 0.5 gm) every 12 hours *after* dialysis
Pediatric: <18 years: not recommended; ≥18 years same as adult
Vabomere *Vial:* mero 1 gm+vabor 1 gm pwdr for reconstitution and dilution

Comment: Vabomere (formerly **Carbavance**) is a carbapenem (*meropenem)* and beta-lactamase inhibitor *(vaborbactam)* combination indicated for the treatment of complicated urinary tract infections (cTIs). Administer **abomere** with caution with history of hyper-sensitivity to penicillin, cephalosporin, other betalactams or other allergens. Discontinue immediately if allergic reaction occurs. Vabomere is not recommended with concomitant *valproic acid* or *divalproex sodium.* Discontinue Vabomere if *C. difficile*-associated diarrhea is suspected or confirmed. Monitor, and reevaluate risk/ benefit if signs of neuromotor impairment (e.g., seizures, focal tremors, myoclonus, delirium, paresthesias), renal impairment, thrombocytopenia, and/or superinfection.

LONG-TERM PROPHYLACTIC-SUPPRESSION THERAPY

▷ *methenamine hippurate* (C) 1 gm once daily
Pediatric: <6 years: 0.25 gm/30 lb once daily; 6-12 years: 25-50 mg/kg/day once daily or 0.5-1 gm once daily; >12 years:
Hiprex *Tab:* 1 gm; *Oral susp:* 500 mg/5 ml (480 ml)
Urex *Tab:* 1 gm; *Oral susp:* 500 mg/5 ml (480 ml)

▷ *nitrofurantoin* (B)(G)

> **Furadantin** 50-100 mg as a single dose at bedtime
> *Pediatric:* <1 month: not recommended; ≥1 month-12 years: 1 mg/kg as a single dose at bedtime; >12 years: same as adult
>> *Oral susp:* 25 mg/5 ml (60 ml)
> **Macrobid** 50-100 mg as a single dose at bedtime
> *Pediatric:* <12 years: not recommended; ≥12 years: same as adult
>> *Cap:* 100 mg
> **Macrodantin** 50-100 mg as a single dose at bedtime
> *Pediatric:* <12 years: not recommended; ≥12 years: same as adult
>> *Cap:* 25, 50, 100 mg
> **Furadantin** 50-100 mg as a single dose at bedtime
> *Pediatric:* <12 years: not recommended; ≥12 years: same as adult
>> *Oral susp:* 25 mg/5 ml (60 ml)
> **Macrobid** 100 mg as a single dose at bedtime
> *Pediatric:* <12 years: not recommended; ≥12 years: same as adult
>> *Cap:* 100 mg
> **Macrodantin** 50-100 mg as a single dose at bedtime
> *Pediatric:* <12 years: not recommended; ≥12 years: same as adult
>> *Cap:* 25, 50, 100 mg

UROLITHIASIS (RENAL CALCULI, KIDNEY STONES)

Acetaminophen for IV Infusion *see Pain page 352*
NSAIDs *see page 571*
Opioid Analgesics *see Pain page 354*

PREVENTION OF CALCIUM STONES

▷ *chlorothiazide* (B)(G) 50 mg bid
> *Pediatric:* <6 months: up to 15 mg/lb/day in 2 divided doses; ≥6 months-12 years: 10 mg/lb/day in 2 divided doses; max 375 mg/day; >12 years: Same as adult
>> **Diuril** *Tab:* 250*, 500*mg; *Oral susp:* 250 mg/5 ml (237 ml)
▷ *hydrochlorothiazide* (B)(G) 50 mg bid
> *Pediatric:* <12 years: not recommended; ≥12 years: same as adult
>> **Esidrix** *Tab:* 25, 50 mg
>> **Microzide** *Cap:* 12.5 mg

PREVENTION OF CYSTINE STONES

▷ *penicillamine* administer on an empty stomach, at least one hour before meals or two hours after meals, and at least one hour apart from any other drug, food, milk, antacid, zinc or iron-containing preparation; usual dose is 2,000-4,000 mg/day; maintenance dosage must be individualized, and may require adjustment during the course of treatment; initially, a single daily dose of 125-250 mg; then, increase at 1-3 month intervals by 125-250 mg/day, as patient response and tolerance indicate; if a satisfactory remission of symptoms is achieved, the dose associated with the remission should be continued as the patient's maintenance therapy; if there is no improvement, and there are no signs of potentially serious toxicity after 2-3 months of treatment with doses of 500-750 mg/day, increase by 250 mg/day at 2-3 month intervals until a satisfactory remission occurs or signs of toxicity develop; if there is no discernible improvement after 3-4 months of treatment, discontinue **Cuprimine**. Changes in maintenance dosage levels may not be reflected clinically or in the erythrocyte sedimentation rate (ESR) for 2-3 months after each dosage adjustment.

> **Cuprimine** *Cap:* 125, 250 mg
> **Depen:** 250 mg

Comment: The use of *penicillamine* has been associated with fatalities due to certain diseases such as aplastic anemia, agranulocytosis, thrombocytopenia, Goodpasture's syndrome, and myasthenia gravis. Because of the potential for serious hematological and renal adverse reactions to occur at any time, routine urinalysis, white and differential blood cell count, hemoglobin, and direct platelet count must be checked twice weekly, together with monitoring of the patient's skin, lymph nodes and body temperature, during the first month of therapy, every two weeks for the next five months, and monthly thereafter.

Patients should be instructed to report promptly the development of signs and symptoms of granulocytopenia and/or thrombocytopenia such as fever, sore throat, chills, bruising or bleeding; the above laboratory studies should then be promptly repeated.

▷ *potassium citrate* (C)(G) 30 mEq qid
  Pediatric: <12 years: not recommended; ≥12 years: same as adult
    Urocit-K *Tab:* 5, 10, 15 mEq ext-rel
    Comment: *potassium citrate* is contraindicated in hyperkalemia. Encourage patients to limit salt intake and maintain liberal hydration (urine volume should be at least 2 liters/day). Target urine pH is 6.0-7.0 and urine citrate at least 320 mg/day and close to the normal mean of 640 mg/day. Take with food.

PREVENTION OF URIC ACID STONES

▷ *allopurinol* (C)(G) 200-300 mg in 1-3 doses; max 800 mg/day; max single dose 300 mg
  Pediatric: <6 years: max 150 mg/day; 6-10 years: max 400 mg/day; max single dose 300 mg; >10 years: same as adult
    Zyloprim *Tab:* 100*, 300*mg
▷ *potassium citrate* (C)(G) 30 mEq qid
    Urocit-K *Tab:* 5, 10, 15 mEq ext-rel
    Comment: *potassium citrate* is contraindicated in hyperkalemia. Encourage patients to limit salt intake and maintain liberal hydration (urine volume should be at least 2 liters/day). Target urine pH is 6.0-7.0 and urine citrate at least 320 mg/day and close to the normal mean of 640 mg/day. Take with food.

ALPHA-1A BLOCKERS

Comment: Alpha-1A blockers facilitate stone passage.
▷ *alfuzosin* (B)(G) 10 mg once daily taken immediately after the same meal each day
    UroXatral *Tab:* 10 mg ext-rel
▷ *tamsulosin* (B)(G) initially 0.4 mg once daily; may increase to 0.8 mg once daily after 2-4 weeks if needed
  Pediatric: ≤18 years: with radiopaque lower ureteral stones of 10-12 mm or smaller have received the following doses: *tamsulosin* 0.2 mg PO at bedtime (≤4 years) and 0.4 mg PO at bedtime (>4 years); administer x 28 days or until definite stone passage (i.e., evidence of stone on urine straining); >18 years:
    Flomax *Cap:* 0.4 mg
    Comment: *tamsulosin* 0.4 mg may be taken with **Avodart** 0.5 mg once daily as combination therapy. *tamsulosin* is taken with standard analgesia (e.g., ibuprofen); mild somnolence is common. If pain is controlled with oral analgesia, clear liquids are tolerated, and there is no evidence of infection, monitor closely for spontaneous passage for 3 to 4 weeks prior to definitive therapy, since most data demonstrate safe lower uretal stone expulsion in the first 10 days of conservative medical management.

ANTISPASMODIC AGENT

▷ *flavoxate* (B)(G) 100-200 mg tid-qid
  Pediatric: <12 years: not recommended; >12 years: same as adult
    Urispas Tab: 100 mg
    Comment: *flavoxate* hydrochloride tablets are indicated for symptomatic relief of dysuria, urgency, nocturia, suprapubic pain, frequency and incontinence as may occur in cystitis, prostatitis, urethritis, urethrocystitis/urethrotrigonitis. *flavoxate* is not indicated for definitive treatment, but is compatible with drugs used for the treatment of UTI. flavoxate is contraindicated in patients who have any of the following obstructive conditions: pyloric or duodenal obstruction, obstructive intestinal lesions, ileus, achalasia, GI hemorrhage, and obstructive uropathies of the lower urinary tract. Used with caution with glaucoma. It is not known whether *flavoxate* is excreted in human milk.

ACETAMINOPHEN FOR IV INFUSION

▷ *acetaminophen* injectable (B) administer by IV infusion over 15 minutes; 1,000 mg q 6 hours prn or 650 mg q 4 hours prn; max 4,000 mg/day
  Pediatric: <2 years: not recommended; 2-13 years <50 kg: 15 mg/kg q 6 hours prn or 2.5 mg/kg q 4 hours prn; max 750 mg/single dose; max 75 mg/kg per day; >13 years: same as adult
    Ofirmev *Vial:* 10 mg/ml (100 ml) (preservative-free)

Comment: The **Ofirmev** vial is intended for single-use. If any portion is withdrawn from the vial, use within 6 hours. Discard the unused portion. For pediatric patients, withdraw the intended dose and administer via syringe pump. Do not admix **Ofirmev** with any other drugs. **Ofirmev** is physically incompatible with *diazepam* and *chlorpromazine hydrochloride*.

IBUPROFEN FOR IV INFUSION

▷ *ibuprofen* (B) dilute dose in 0.9% NS, D5W, or Lactated Ringers (LR) solution; administer by IV infusion over at least 10 minutes; do not administer via IV bolus or IM; 400-800 mg q 6 hours prn; maximum 3,200 mg/day
Pediatric: <6 months; not recommended; 6 months-<12 years: 10 mg/kg q 4-6 hours prn; max 400 mg/dose; max 40 mg/kg or 2,400 mg/24 hours, whichever is less; 12-17 years: 400 mg q 4-6 hours prn; max 2,400 mg/24 hours
  Caldolor *Vial:* 800 mg/8 ml single-dose

  Comment: Prepare **Caldolor** solution for IV administration as follows: 100 mg dose: dilute 1 ml of **Caldolor** in at least 100 ml of diluent (IVF); 200 mg dose: dilute 2 ml of **Caldolor** in at least 100 ml of diluent; 400 mg dose: dilute 4 ml of **Caldolor** in at least 100 ml of diluent; 800 mg dose: dilute 8 ml of **Caldolor** in at least 200 ml of diluent. **Caldolor** is also indicated for management of fever. For adults with fever, 400 mg via IV infusion, followed by 400 mg q 4-6 hours or 100-200 mg q 4 hours prn.

MU OPIOID ANALGESICS

▷ *tramadol* (C)(IV)(G)
  Comment: *tramadol* is known to be excreted in breast milk. The FDA and the European Medicines Agency (EMA) are investigating the safety of using *tramadol*-containing medications to treat pain in children 12-18 years because of the potential for serious side effects, including slowed or difficult breathing.
  Rybix ODT initially 100 mg once daily; may increase by 100 mg every 5 days; max 300 mg/day; *CrCl <30 mL/min or severe hepatic impairment:* not recommended; *Cirrhosis:* max 50 mg q 12 hours
  Pediatric: <12 years: contraindicated; 12-<18: use extreme caution; not recommended for children and adolescents with obesity, asthma, obstructive sleep apnea, or other chronic breathing problem, or for post-tonsillectomy/adenoidectomy pain; ≥18 years: same as adult
    ODT: 50 mg (mint) (phenylalanine)
  Ryzolt initially 100 mg once daily; may increase by 100 mg every 5 days; max 300 mg/day; CrCl <30 mL/min or severe hepatic impairment: not recommended
  Pediatric: <12 years: contraindicated; 12-<18: use extreme caution; not recommended for children and adolescents with obesity, asthma, obstructive sleep apnea, or other chronic breathing problem, or for post-tonsillectomy/adenoidectomy pain; ≥18 years: same as adult
    Tab: 100, 200, 300 mg ext-rel
  Ultram 50-100 mg q 4-6 hours prn; max 400 mg/day; *CrCl <30 mL/min,* max 100 mg q 12 hours; cirrhosis, max 50 mg q 12 hours
  Pediatric: <12 years: contraindicated; 12-<18: use extreme caution; not recommended for children and adolescents with obesity, asthma, obstructive sleep apnea, or other chronic breathing problem, or for post-tonsillectomy/ adenoidectomy pain; ≥18 years: same as adult
    Tab: 50*mg
  Ultram ER initially 100 mg once daily; may increase by 100 mg every 5 days; max 300 mg/day; *CrCl <30 mL/min or severe hepatic impairment*: not recommended
  Pediatric: <12 years: contraindicated; 12-<18: use extreme caution; not recommended for children and adolescents with obesity, asthma, obstructive sleep apnea, or other chronic breathing problem, or for post-tonsillectomy/adenoidectomy pain; ≥18 years: same as adult
    Tab: 100, 200, 300 mg ext-rel
▷ *tramadol+acetaminophen* (C)(IV)(G) 2 tabs q 4-6 hours; max 8 tabs/day x 5 days; *CrCl <30 mL/min:* max 2 tabs q 12 hours; max 4 tabs/day x 5 days
  Pediatric: <12 years: contraindicated; 12-<18: use extreme caution; not recommended for children and adolescents with obesity, asthma, obstructive sleep apnea, or other chronic breathing problem, or for post-tonsillectomy/adenoidectomy pain; same as adult
    Ultracet *Tab:* tram 37.5+acet 325 mg

Comment: *tramadol* is known to be excreted in breast milk. The FDA and the European Medicines Agency (EMA) are investigating the safety of using *tramadol*-containing medications to treat pain in children 12-18 years because of the potential for serious side effects, including slowed or difficult breathing.

INTRANASAL (TRANSMUCOSAL) OPIOID ANALGESICS

▷ *butorphanol tartrate* nasal spray (C)(IV) initially 1 spray (1 mg) in one nostril and may repeat after 60-90 minutes in opposite nostril if needed or 1 spray in each nostril and may repeat q 3-4 hours prn
Pediatric: <18 years: not recommended; ≥18 years: same as adult
    Butorphanol Nasal Spray *Nasal spray:* 1 mg/actuation (10 mg/ml, 2.5 ml)
    Stadol Nasal Spray *Nasal spray:* 1 mg/actuation (10 mg/ml, 2.5 ml)

▷ *fentanyl* nasal spray (C)(II) initially 1 spray (100 mcg) in one nostril and may repeat after 2 hours; when adequate analgesia is achieved, use that dose for subsequent breakthrough episodes; *Titration steps:* 100 mcg using 1 x 100 mcg spray; 200 mcg using 2 x 100 mcg spray (1 spray in each nostril); 400 mcg using 1 x 400 mcg spray; 800 mcg using 2 x 400 mcg (1 spray in each nostril); max 800 mcg; limit to ≤4 doses per day
Pediatric: <18 years: not recommended; ≥18 years: same as adult
    Lazanda Nasal Spray *Nasal spray:* 100, 400 mcg/100 mcl (8 sprays/bottle)
    Comment: **Lazanda Nasal Spray** is available by restricted distribution program. Call 855-841-4234 or visit https://www.fda.gov/downloads/drugs/drugsafety/ postmarketdrugsafetyinformationforpatientsandproviders/ucm261983.pdf to enroll. **Lazanda Nasal Spray** is indicated for the management of breakthrough pain in cancer patients who are already receiving and who are tolerant to opioid therapy for their underlying persistent cancer pain. Patients considered opioid tolerant are those who are taking at least 60 mg of oral morphine/day, 25 mcg of transdermal *fentanyl*/hour, 30 mg oral *oxycodone*/day, 8 mg oral *hydromorphone*/day, 25 mg oral *oxymorphone*/day, or an equianalgesic dose of another opioid for a week or longer. Patients must remain on around-the-clock opioids when using **Lazanda Nasal Spray**. As such, it is contraindicated in the management of acute or post-op pain, including headache/migraine, or dental pain.

Comment: The Transmucosal Immediate Release **Fentanyl** (TIRF) Risk Evaluation and Mitigation Strategy (REMS) program is an FDA-required program designed to ensure informed risk-benefit decisions before initiating treatment, and while patients are treated to ensure appropriate use of TIRF medicines. The purpose of the TIRF REMS Access program is to mitigate the risk of misuse, abuse, addiction, overdose and serious complications due to medication errors with the use of TIRF medicines. You must enroll in the TIRF REMS Access program to prescribe, dispense, or distribute TIRF medicines. To register, call the TIRF REMS Access program at 1-866-822-1483 or register online at https://www .tirfremsaccess.com/TirfUI/rems/home.action.

URTICARIA: MILD-TO-ACUTE HIVES AND CHRONIC SPONTANEOUS/ IDIOPATHIC URTICARIA (CSU/CIU)

Topical Corticosteroids *see page 574*
Oral Corticosteroids *see page 577*
Parenteral Corticosteroids *see page 577*

MILD-TO-MODERATE URTICARIA (HIVES, ANGIOEDEMA)
Second Generation Oral Antihistamines

Comment: The following drugs are second generation antihistamines. As such they minimally sedating, much less so than the first generation antihistamines. All antihistamines are excreted into breast milk.

▷ *cetirizine* (C)(OTC)(G) initially 5-10 mg once daily; 5 mg once daily; ≥65 years: use with caution
Pediatric: <6 years: not recommended; ≥6 years: same as adult
    cetirizine Cap: 10 mg
    Children's Zyrtec Chewable *Chew tab:* 5, 10 mg (grape)
    Children's Zyrtec Allergy Syrup *Syr:* 1 mg/ml (4 oz) (grape, bubble gum) (sugar-free, dye-free)
    Zyrtec *Tab:* 10 mg

Zyrtec Hives Relief *Tab:* 10 mg
Zyrtec Liquid Gels *Liq gel:* 10 mg
▷ *desloratadine* (C)
Clarinex 1/2-1 tab once daily
Pediatric: <6 years: not recommended; ≥6 years: same as adult
Tab: 5 mg
Clarinex RediTabs 5 mg once daily
Pediatric: <6 years: not recommended; 6-12 years: 2.5 once daily; ≥12 years: same
as adult
ODT: 2.5, 5 mg (tutti-frutti) (phenylalanine)
Clarinex Syrup 5 mg (10 ml) once daily
Pediatric: <6 months: not recommended; 6-11 months: 1 mg (2 ml) once daily; 1-5 years:
1.25 mg (2.5 ml) once daily; 6-11 years: 2.5 mg (5 ml) once daily; ≥12 years: same as adult
Syr: 0.5 mg per ml (4 oz) (tutti-frutti) (phenylalanine)
Desloratadine ODT 1 tab once daily
Pediatric: <6 years: not recommended; 6-11 years: 1/2 tab once daily; ≥12 years: same
as adult
ODT: 5 mg
▷ *fexofenadine* (C)(OTC)(G) 60 mg once daily-bid <u>or</u> 180 mg once daily; *CrCl <90 mL/min:*
60 mg once daily
Pediatric: <6 months: not recommended; 6 months-2 years: 15 mg bid; *CrCl ≤90 mL/min:*
15 mg once daily; 2-11 years: 30 mg bid; *CrCl ≤90 mL/min:* 30 mg once daily; ≥12 years:
same as adult
Allegra *Tab:* 30, 60, 180 mg film-coat
Allegra Allergy *Tab:* 60, 180 mg film-coat
Allegra ODT *ODT:* 30 mg (phenylalanine)
Allegra Oral Suspension *Oral susp:* 30 mg/5 ml (6 mg/ml) (4 oz)
▷ *levocetirizine* (B)(OTC)(G) administer dose in the PM; *Seasonal Allergic Rhinitis:* <2
years: not recommended; may start at ≥2 years; *Chronic Idiopathic Urticaria (CIU),
Perennial Allergic Rhinitis:* <6 months: not recommended; may start at ≥ 6 months;
Dosing by Age: 6 months-5 years: max 1.25 mg once daily; 6-11 years: max 2.5 mg once
daily; ≥12 years: 2.5-5 mg once daily; *Renal Dysfunction <12 years:* contraindicated;
Renal Dysfunction ≥12 years: CrCl 50-80 ml/min: 2.5 mg once daily; CrCl 30-50 mL/
min: 2.5 mg every other day; CrCl: 10-30 mL/min: 2.5 mg twice weekly (every 3-4 days);
CrCl <10 mL/min, ESRD <u>or</u> hemodialysis: contraindicated
Children's Xyzal Allergy 24HR *Oral Soln:* 0.5 mg/ml (150 ml)
Xyzal Allergy 24HR *Tab:* 5*mg
▷ *loratadine* (C)(OTC)(G) 5 mg bid <u>or</u> 10 mg once daily; *Hepatic <u>or</u> Renal Insufficiency:* see
mfr pkg insert
Pediatric: <2 years: not recommended; 2-5 years: 5 mg once daily; ≥6 years: same as adult
Children's Claritin Chewables *Chew tab:* 5 mg (grape) (phenylalanine)
Children's Claritin Syrup 1 mg/ml (4 oz) (fruit) (sugar-free, alcohol-free, dye-free;
sodium 6 mg/5 ml)
Claritin *Tab:* 10 mg
Claritin Hives Relief *Tab:* 10 mg
Claritin Liqui-Gels *Liq gel:* 10 mg
Claritin RediTabs 12 Hours *ODT:* 5 mg (mint)
Claritin RediTabs 24 Hours *ODT:* 10 mg (mint)

First Generation Oral Antihistamines

▷ *diphenhydramine* (B)(G) 25-50 mg q 6-8 hours; max 100 mg/day
Pediatric: <2 years: not recommended; 2-6 years: 6.25 mg q 4-6 hours; max 37.5 mg/day;
>6-12 years: 12.5-25 mg q 4-6 hours; max 150 mg/day; >12 years: same as adult
Benadryl (OTC) *Chew tab:* 12.5 mg (grape) (phenylalanine); *Liq:* 12.5 mg/ 5 ml (4, 8
oz); *Cap:* 25 mg; *Tab:* 25 mg; *Dye-free soft gel:* 25 mg; *Dye-free liq:* 12.5 mg/5 ml (4, 8 oz)
▷ *hydroxyzine* (C)(G) 50 mg/day divided qid prn; 50-100 mg/day divided qid prn
Pediatric: <6 years: 50 mg/day divided qid prn; ≥6 years: same as adult
Atarax *Tab:* 10, 25, 50, 100 mg; *Syr:* 10 mg/5 ml (alcohol 0.5%)
Vistaril *Cap:* 25, 50, 100 mg; *Oral susp:* 25 mg/5 ml (4 oz) (lemon)
Comment: *hydroxyzine* is contraindicated in early pregnancy and in patients with a
prolonged QT interval. It is not known whether this drug is excreted in human milk;
therefore, *hydroxyzine* should not be given to nursing mothers.

SEVERE URTICARIA

Parenteral Antihistamine

▷ *diphenhydramine* injectable (B)(G) 25-50 mg IM immediately; then q 6 hours prn
Pediatric: <12 years: *See mfr pkg insert:* 1.25 mg/kg up to 25 mg IM x 1 dose; then q 6 hours prn; ≥12 years: same as adult
Benadryl Injectable *Vial:* 50 mg/ml (1 ml single-use); 50 mg/ml (10 ml multi-dose); *Amp:* 10 mg/ml (1 ml); *Prefilled syringe:* 50 mg/ml (1 ml)

Parenteral Epinephrine

▷ *epinephrine* (C) 1:1000 0.01 ml/kg SC; max 0.3 ml
Pediatric: 0.01 mg/kg SC

CHRONIC SPONTANEOUS/IDIOPATHIC URTICARIA

IgE Blocker (IgG1k Monoclonal Antibody)

Comment: Xolair *(omalizumab)* is a humanized monoclonal antibody that specifically binds to free immunoglobulin E in the blood and on the surface of selected B lymphocytes, but not on the surface of mast cells, antigen-presenting dendritic cells, or basophils. In the US *omalizumab* is approved for adults at 150 mg or 300 mg subcutaneously administered every 4 weeks for the treatment of CSU not responsive to high-dose antihistamines. In three published, pivotal, phase 3 randomized trials, the clinical response rate to **omalizumab** at 300 mg every 4 weeks, as defined by a weekly 7-day Urticaria Activity Score (UAS7) ≤6 at 12 weeks, was 52% in ASTERIA I, 66% in ASTERIA II, and 52% in GLACIAL. Good control of disease activity was defined as a UAS7 score of ≤6 on the 0- to 42-point UAS7, which correlates well with minimal or no patient symptoms

REFERENCE
Finlay, A. Y., Kaplan, A. P., Beck, L. A., Antonova, E. N., Balp, M.-M., Zazzali, J., … Maurer, M. (2017). Omalizumab substantially improves dermatology-related quality of life in patients with chronic spontaneous urticaria. *Journal of the European Academy of Dermatology and Venereology*, 31(10), 1715–1721. doi:10.1111/jdv.14384

Comment: A multicenter open-label study of 286 patients with CSU, conducted by the Catalan and Balearic Chronic Urticaria Network (XUrCB) at 15 hospitals, found about two-thirds of patients with CSU treated with the approved dose of *omalizumab* achieved good disease control. Three-quarters of the non-responders achieved good disease control upon up-dosing to 450 or 600 mg (twice the approved dose) every 4 weeks, without increase in adverse events.

REFERENCE
Jancin, B. (2018, January 8). Updosing omalizumab for chronic urticaria pays off. *Dermatology News*. Retrieved from https://www.mdedge.com/dermatology/article/155732/urticaria/updosing-omalizumab-chronic-urticaria-pays

▷ *omalizumab* (B) 150-375 mg SC every 2-4 weeks based on body weight and pre-treatment serum total IgE level; max 150 mg/injection site; should be administered only by a qualified health care provider
Pediatric: <12 years: not recommended; ≥12 years: 30-90 kg + IgE >30-100 IU/ml 150 mg q 4 weeks; 90-150 kg + IgE >30-100 IU/ml or 30-90 kg + IgE >100-200 IU/ml or 30-60 kg + IgE >200-300 IU/ml 300 mg q 4 hours; >90-150 kg + IgE >100-200 IU/ml or >60-90 kg + IgE >200-300 IU/ml or 30-70 kg + IgE >300-400 IU/ml 225 mg q 2 weeks; >90-150 kg + IgE >200-300 IU/ml or >70-90 kg + IgE >300-400 IU/ml or 30-70 kg + IgE >400-500 IU/ml or 30-60 kg + IgE >500-600 IU/ml or 30-60 kg + IgE >600-700 IU/ml 375 mg q 2 weeks
Xolair *Vial:* 150 mg, single-dose, pwdr for SC injection after reconstitution; *Prefilled syringe:* 75 mg/0.5 ml, 150 mg/1 ml, single-dose (preservative-free)

 UTERINE FIBROIDS

See **Progesterone-only Contraceptives** *page 567*

▷ *medroxyprogesterone acetate* (X) 10 mg daily
Provera *Tab:* 2.5, 5, 10 mg
▷ *Oral contraceptives* (X) with 35 mcg estrogen equivalent

SELECTIVE PROGESTERONE RECEPTOR MODULATOR

▶ *ulipristal acetate (UPA)* (X)(G) 5-10 mg once daily

Comment: Ulipristal acetate is currently approved in the United States as an emergency contraceptive (a single 30 mg dose), but is marketed for treating symptomatic fibroids in Canada and Europe. It is not yet available in a dose form appropriate for treatment of uterine fibroids (i.e., 5, 10 mg). The drug reduced dysfunctional uterine bleeding in about 90% of patients in the European trials. Women with uterine fibroids taking UPA experienced significant improvement of quality of life, compared with those taking placebo according to researchers' reported outcomes of VENUS II, a phase 3, prospective, randomized, double-blind, double-dummy, placebo-controlled study. Its design incorporated both parallel and crossover elements: Some patients who were on placebo crossed over to one of two doses of UPA after a washout period, and some patients on each active arm crossed over to placebo. The women (n = 432) were between 18 and 50 years and premenopausal. At 13 weeks, uterine bleeding was controlled in 91% of the women receiving 5 mg of *ulipristal acetate*, 92% of those receiving 10 mg of *ulipristal* acetate, and 19% of those receiving placebo (P<0.001). Of women taking 5 mg of UPA, 91% achieved control (40.5%-42% became amenorrheic); of those taking 10 mg, 92% achieved control (54.8%-57.3% became amenorrheic) (controlled in 92%). These results compared to amenorrhea rates of 0%-8% (controlled in 19%) for women on placebo (*p*< .0001 for all values).

Ella *Tab:* 30 mg
Logilia *Tab:* 30 mg

REFERENCE

Donnez, J., Tatarchuk, T. F., Bouchard, P., Puscasiu, L., Zakharenko, N. F., Ivanova, T., . . . Loumaye, E. (2012). Ulipristal acetate versus placebo for fibroid treatment before surgery. *New England Journal of Medicine, 366*(5), 409–420. doi:10.1056/nejmoa1103182

 VAGINAL IRRITATION: EXTERNAL

OTC Replens Vaginal Moisturizer
OTC Vagisil Intimate Moisturizer

Comment: Vagisil has no effect on condom integrity.

VERTIGO

▶ *meclizine* (B)(G) 25-100 mg/day in divided doses
Pediatric: <12 years: not established; ≥12 years: same as adult
Antivert *Tab:* 12.5, 25, 50*mg
Bonine (OTC) *Cap:* 15, 25, 30 mg; *Tab:* 12.5, 25, 50 mg; *Chew tab/Film-coat tab:* 25 mg
Dramamine II (OTC) *Tab:* 25*mg
Zentrip *Strip:* 25 mg orally-disint

▶ *methscopolamine bromide* (B) 1 tab q 6 hours prn
Pediatric: <12 years: not recommended; ≥12 years: same as adult
Pamine *Tab:* 2.5 mg
Pamine Forte *Tab:* 5 mg

▶ *scopolamine* (C) 0.4-0.8 mg tab (may repeat in 8 hours) or 1 x 1.5 mg transdermal patch behind ear (effective x 3 days; may replace every 4th day)
Pediatric: <12 years: not recommended; ≥12 years: same as adult
Scopace *Tab:* 0.4 mg
Transderm Scop *Transdermal patch:* 1.5 mg (4/carton)

VITILIGO

RE-PIGMENTATION AGENTS

▶ *methoxsalen* (C) Apply to well-defined area of vitiligo; then expose area to source of UVA (ultraviolet A) or sunlight; initial exposure no more than 1/2 predicted minimal erythemal dose; repeat weekly
Pediatric: <12 years: not recommended; ≥12 years: same as adult
Oxsoralen *Lotn:* 1% (30 ml)

Comment: *methoxsalen* may only be applied by a health care provider. Do not dispense to patient.

▷ *trioxsalen* (C) 10 mg daily, taken 2-4 hours before ultraviolet light exposure; max 14 days and 28 tabs
   Pediatric: <12 years: not recommended; ≥12 years: same as adult
      Trisoralen *Tab:* 5 mg

DEPIGMENTING AGENTS

▷ *hydroquinone* (C)(G) apply sparingly to affected area and rub in bid
      Lustra *Crm:* 4% (1, 2 oz) (sulfites)
      Lustra AF *Crm:* 4% (1, 2 oz) (sunscreen, sulfites)
▷ *monobenzone* (C) apply sparingly to affected area and rub in bid-tid; depigmentation occurs in 1-4 months
   Pediatric: same as adult
      Benoquin *Crm:* 20% (1.25 oz)
▷ *tazarotene* (X)(G) apply daily at HS
   Pediatric: <12 years: not recommended; ≥12 years: same as adult
      Avage Cream *Crm:* 0.1% (30 gm)
      Tazorac Cream *Crm:* 0.05, 0.1% (15, 30, 60 gm)
      Tazorac Gel *Gel:* 0.05, 0.1% (30, 100 gm)
▷ *tretinoin* (C) apply daily at HS
   Pediatric: <12 years: not recommended; ≥12 years: same as adult
      Avita *Crm/Gel:* 0.025% (20, 45 gm)
      Renova *Crm:* 0.02% (40 gm); 0.05% (40, 60 gm)
      Retin-A Cream *Crm:* 0.025, 0.05, 0.1% (20, 45 gm)
      Retin-A Gel *Gel:* 0.01, 0.025% (15, 45 gm) (alcohol 90%)
      Retin-A Liquid *Liq:* 0.05% (28 ml) (alcohol 55%)
      Retin-A Micro *Microspheres:* 0.04, 0.1% (20, 45 gm)

COMBINATION AGENTS

▷ *hydroquinone+fluocinolone+tretinoin* (C) apply sparingly to affected area and rub in daily at HS
   Pediatric: <12 years: not recommended; ≥12 years: same as adult
      Tri-Luma *Crm:* hydroquin 4%+fluo 0.01%+tretin 0.05% (30 gm) (parabens, sulfites)
▷ *hydroquinone+padimate o+oxybenzone+octyl methoxycinnamate* (C) apply sparingly to affected area and rub in bid
   Pediatric: <12 years: not recommended; ≥16 years: same as adult
      Glyquin *Crm:* 4% (1 oz jar)
▷ *hydroquinone+ethyl dihydroxypropyl PABA+dioxybenzone+oxybenzone* (C) apply sparingly to affected area and rub in bid; max 2 months
   Pediatric: <12 years: not recommended; ≥12 years: same as adult
      Solaquin *Crm:* hydroquin 2%+PABA 5%+dioxy 3%+oxy 2% (1 oz) (sulfites)
▷ *hydroquinone+padimate+dioxybenzone+oxybenzone* (C) apply sparingly to affected area and rub in bid; max 2 months
   Pediatric: <12 years: not recommended; ≥12 years: same as adult
      Solaquin Forte *Crm:* hydroquin 4%+pad 0.5%+dioxy 3%+oxy 2% (1oz) (sunscreen, sulfites)
▷ *hydroquinone+padimate+dioxybenzone* (C) apply sparingly to affected area and rub in bid; max 2 months
   Pediatric: <12 years: not recommended; ≥12 years: same as adults
      Solaquin Forte Gel: hydroquin 4%+pad 0.5%+dioxy 3% (1 oz) (alcohol, sulfites)

WART: COMMON (*VERRUCA VULGARIS*)

▷ *salicylic acid* (G)
   Pediatric: same as adult
      Duo Film (OTC) apply daily-bid; max 12 weeks; *Liq:* 17% (1/2 oz w. applicator)
      Duo Film Patch for Kids (OTC) apply 1 patch q 48 hours; max 12 weeks
         Patch: 40% (18/pck)
      Occlusal HP (OTC) apply daily-bid; max 12 weeks
         Liq: 17% (10 ml w. applicator)
      Wart-Off (OTC) apply one drop at a time to sufficiently cover wart, let dry; repeat 1-2 times daily; max 12 weeks
         Liq: 17% (0.45 oz)

➤ *trichloroacetic acid* apply after wart is pared and repeat weekly
➤ Cryotherapy with liquid nitrogen or cryoprobe or cryospray; repeat applications every 1-2 weeks as needed to destroy lesion
   Histofreeze (see pkg insert for application freeze time

ORAL RETINOID

➤ *acitretin* (X)(G) 25-50 mg once daily with main meal
   Pediatric: <18 years: not recommended; ≥18 years: same as adult
      Soriatane *Cap:* 10, 25 mg

REFERENCES

Hoffman, K. (2017, October 31). Can oral retinoids have an impact for recalcitrant warts? *Podiatry Today*. Retrieved from https://www.podiatrytoday.com/blogged/can-oral-retinoids-have-impact-recalcitrant-warts
Joshipura, D., Goldminz, A., Greb, J., & Gottlieb A. (2017). Acitretin for the treatment of recalcitrant plantar warts. *Dermatology Online Journal, 23*(3). Retrieved from https://escholarship.org/uc/item/721426pm

WART: PLANTAR (*VERRUCA PLANTARIS*)

➤ *salicylic acid* (G)
   Duo Plant Gel (OTC) apply daily bid; max 12 weeks
      Gel: 17% (1/2 oz)
   Mediplast cut to size of wart and apply; remove q 1-2 days, peel keratin, and reapply; repeat as long as needed
   Occlusal-HP (OTC) apply once daily-bid; max 12 weeks
      Liq: 17% (10 ml w. applicator)
   Wart-Off (OTC) apply one drop at a time to sufficiently cover wart, let dry; repeat 1-2 times daily; max 12 weeks
      Liq: 17% (0.45 oz)
➤ *trichloroacetic acid* apply after wart is pared and repeat weekly

ORAL RETINOID

➤ *acitretin* (X)(G) 25-50 mg once daily with main meal
   Pediatric: <12 years: not recommended; ≥12 years: same as adult
      Soriatane *Cap:* 10, 25 mg

REFERENCES

Can Oral Retinoids Have An Impact For Recalcitrant Warts? https://www.podiatrytoday.com/blogged/can-oral -retinoids-have-impact-recalcitrant-warts
Joshipura, D., Goldminz, A., Greb, J., & Gottlieb A. (2017). Acitretin for the treatment of recalcitrant plantar warts. *Dermatology Online Journal, 23*(3).

WART: VENEREAL, HUMAN PAPILLOMAVIRUS (HPV), CONDYLOMA ACUMINATA

Comment: This section contains treatment regimens for genital warts published in the **2015 CDC Sexually Transmitted Diseases Treatment Guidelines** as well as other treatment options. Due to the increased risk of cervical cancer with HPV, Pap smears should be done q 3 months during active disease and then q 3-6 months for the next 2 years.

PATIENT-APPLIED AGENTS
Regimen 1

➤ *imiquimod* (C)
   Pediatric: <12 years: not recommended; ≥12 years: same as adult
      Aldara (G) rub into lesions before bedtime and remove with soap and water 6-10 hours later; treat 3 times per week; max 16 weeks
         Crm: 5% (12 single-use pkts/carton)
      Zyclara rub into lesions before bedtime and remove with soap and water 8 hours later; treat 3 times per week; max 1 packet per treatment; max 8 weeks
         Crm: 3.75% (28 single-use pkts/carton) (parabens)

Regimen 2

▷ *podofilox 0.5% cream* (C) apply bid (q 12 hours) x 3 days; then discontinue for
  4 days; may repeat if needed; max 4 treatment cycles
    Condylox *Soln:* 0.5% (3.5 ml); *Gel:* 0.5% (3.5 gm)

Regimen 3

▷ *sinecatechins 15% ointment* (C) apply to each lesion tid for up to 16 weeks
    Veregen *Oint:* 15% (15, 30 gm)

PROVIDER-ADMINISTERED AGENTS

Regimen 1

▷ Cryotherapy with liquid nitrogen or cryoprobe; repeat applications every 1-2 weeks as
  needed

Regimen 2

▷ *trichloroacetic acid (TCA) 80-90%* (C) apply to warts; repeat weekly if needed
Comment: TCA is the preferred treatment during pregnancy. Immediate application of
sodium bicarbonate paste following treatment decreases pain.

Regimen 3

▷ *podofilox 0.5% cream* (C) apply bid (q 12 hours) x 3 days; then discontinue for 4 days; may
  repeat if needed; max 4 treatment cycles
    Condylox *Soln:* 0.5% (3.5 ml); *Gel:* 0.5% (3.5 gm)

Regimen 4

▷ *interferon alfa-n3* (C) 0.05 ml injected into base of wart twice weekly for up to 8 weeks;
  max 0.5 ml/session (20 warts/session)
    Alferon N *Vial:* 5 million units/ml (1 ml)

Regimen 5

▷ *interferon alfa-2b* (C) 0.1 ml injected into base of wart three times weekly for up to 3 weeks;
  max 0.5 ml/session (5 warts/session)
    Intron A *Vial:* 1 million units/0.1 ml (0.5, 1 ml)

Regimen 6

▷ Surgical removal either by tangential scissor excision, tangential shave excision, curettage,
  or electrosurgery

WEST NILE VIRUS (WNV)

Comment: The principal route of human infection with West Nile virus is through the bite of
an infected mosquito. Additional routes of infection have become a parent during the 2002
West Nile epidemic. It is important to note that these other methods of transmission represent
a very small proportion of cases. Other methods of transmission include blood transfusion,
organ transplantation, mother-to-child (ingestion of breast milk and transplacental) and
occupational. Symptoms of mild disease will generally last a few days. Symptoms of severe
disease may last several weeks, although neurological effects may be permanent. There is no
specific treatment for West Nile virus infection; treatment is symptomatic and supportive.
About 8 in 10 infected with West Nile virus do not develop any symptoms. About 1 in 5
develop a fever with other symptoms such as headache, body aches, joint pains, vomiting,
diarrhea, or rash. Most people with this level of disease recover completely, but fatigue and
weakness can last for weeks to months. About 1 in 150 people who are infected develop
a severe illness affecting the central nervous system (encephalitis meningitis. Symptoms
of severe illness include high fever, headache, neck stiffness, stupor, disorientation, coma,
tremors, convulsions, muscle weakness, vision loss, numbness and paralysis. About 1 in
10 who develop severe illness affecting the central nervous system die. There is currently
no preventive vaccine. However, the National Institutes of Health have announced that
an experimental vaccine to protect against West Nile Virus has entered human trial. The
developers say because the vaccine uses inactivated virus it should be suitable for a wide
range of people. The trial tested the safety of the vaccine, called **HydroVax-001**, and its ability

to produce an immune response in human subjects. The randomized, placebo-controlled, double-blind clinical trial was conducted by researchers at Duke University School of Medicine, Durham, NC, and enrolled 50 healthy volunteers, men and women 18-50 years-of-age. Participants were randomly assigned to one of the three groups. One group volunteers (n = 20) received a low dose of the vaccine (1 mcg), another group (n = 20) received a higher dose (4 mcg), and a third group (n = 10) received a placebo. All participants received their doses via IM injection on day 1 and day 29 of the trial and are followed for 14 months. Results of the completed trial are pending.

REFERENCE

https://www.cdc.gov/westnile/symptoms/index.html

 WHIPWORM (TRICHURIASIS)

ANTHELMINTICS

▷ *albendazole* (C) 400 mg as a single dose; may repeat in 3 weeks; take with a meal
  Pediatric: <2 years: 200 mg daily x 3 days; may repeat in 3 weeks; 2-12 years: 400 mg daily x 3 days; may repeat in 3 weeks; >12 years: same as adult
    Albenza *Tab:* 200 mg
▷ *mebendazole* (C) chew, swallow, or mix with food; 100 mg bid x 3 days; may repeat in 3 weeks if needed; take with a meal
  Pediatric: <2 years: not recommended; ≥2 years: same as adult
    Emverm *Chew tab:* 100 mg
    Vermox (G) *Chew tab:* 100 mg
▷ *pyrantel pamoate* (C) 11 mg/kg x 1 dose; max 1 gm/dose; take with a meal
  Pediatric: 25-37 lb: 1/2 tsp x 1 dose; 38-62 lb: 1 tsp x 1 dose; 63-87 lb: 1 tsp x 1 dose; 88-112 lb: 2 tsp x 1 dose; 113-137 lb: 2 tsp x 1 dose; 138-162 lb: 3 tsp x 1 dose; 163-187 lb: 3 tsp x 1 dose; >187 lb: 4 tsp x 1 dose
    Antiminth (OTC) *Cap:* 180 mg; *Liq:* 50 mg/ml (30 ml); 144 mg/ml (30 ml); *Oral susp:* 50 mg/ml (60 ml)
    Pin-X (OTC) *Cap:* 180 mg; *Liq:* 50 mg/ml (30 ml); 144 mg/ml (30 ml); *Oral susp:* 50 mg/ml (30 ml)
▷ *thiabendazole* (C) 25 mg/kg bid x 7 days; max 1.5 gm/dose; take with a meal
  Pediatric: same as adult; <30 lb: consult mfr pkg insert; >30 lb: 2 doses/day with meals; 30-50 lb: 250 mg bid with meals; >50 lb: 10 mg/lb/dose bid with meals; max 3 gm/day
    Mintezol *Chew tab:* 500*mg (orange); *Oral susp:* 500 mg/5 ml (120 ml) (orange)
  Comment: *thiabendazole* is not for prophylaxis. May impair mental alertness. May not be available in the US.

WILSON'S DISEASE

Comment: Wilson's disease (hepatolenticular degeneration) occurs in individuals who have inherited an autosomal recessive defect that leads to an accumulation of copper far in excess of metabolic requirements. The excess copper is deposited in several organs and tissues, and eventually produces pathological effects primarily in the liver, where damage progresses to post-necrotic cirrhosis, and in the brain, where degeneration is widespread. Copper is also deposited as characteristic, asymptomatic, golden-brown Kayser-Fleischer rings in the corneas of all patients with cerebral symptomatology. Treatment has two objectives: (1) to minimize dietary intake of copper; (2) to promote excretion and complex formation (i.e., detoxification) of excess tissue copper.

COPPER CHELATING AGENTS

▷ *penicillamine* administer on an empty stomach, at least one hour before meals or two hours after meals, and at least one hour apart from any other drug, food, milk, antacid, zinc or iron-containing preparation; dosage must be individualized, and may require adjustment during the course of treatment; initially, a single daily dose of 125-250 mg; then, increase at 1-3 month intervals by 125-250 mg/day, as patient response and tolerance indicate; if a satisfactory remission of symptoms is achieved, the dose associated with the remission should be continued as the patient's maintenance therapy; if there is no improvement, and there are no signs of potentially serious toxicity after 2-3 months of treatment with doses of 500-750 mg/day, increase by 250 mg/day at 2-3 month intervals until a satisfactory remission occurs or signs of toxicity develop; if there is no discernible improvement after 3-4 months of treatment with 1000-1500 mg/day, discontinue **Cuprimine**; changes in maintenance dosage levels may not be reflected clinically or in the erythrocyte sedimentation rate (ESR) for 2-3 months after each dosage adjustment

    Cuprimine *Cap:* 125, 250 mg

    Depen: 250 mg

    Comment: Taking *penicillamine* on an empty stomach permits maximum absorption and reduces the likelihood of inactivation by metal binding in the GI tract. Optimal dosage can be determined by measurement of urinary copper excretion and the determination of free copper in the serum. The urine must be collected in copper-free glassware, and should be quantitatively analyzed for copper before and soon after initiation of therapy with **Cupramine**. Determination of 24-hour urinary copper excretion is of greatest value in the first week of therapy with *penicillamine*. In the absence of any drug reaction, a dose between 0.75 and 1.5 gm that results in an initial 24-hour cupriuresis of over 2 mg should be continued for about three months, by which time the most reliable method of monitoring maintenance treatment is the determination of free copper in the serum. This equals the difference between quantitatively determined total copper and ceruloplasmin-copper. Adequately treated patients will usually have less than 10 mcg free copper/dL of serum. It is seldom necessary to exceed a dosage of 2 gm/day. In patients who cannot tolerate as much as 1 g/day initially, initiating dosage with 250 mg/day, and increasing gradually to the requisite amount, gives closer control of the effects of the drug and may help to reduce the incidence of adverse reactions. If the patient is intolerant to therapy with **Cuprimine**, alternative treatment is *trientine* (**Syprine**).

The use of *penicillamine* has been associated with fatalities due to certain diseases such as aplastic anemia, agranulocytosis, thrombocytopenia, Goodpasture's syndrome, and myasthenia gravis. Because of the potential for serious hematological and renal adverse reactions to occur at any time, routine urinalysis, white and differential blood cell count, hemoglobin, and direct platelet count must be checked twice weekly, together with monitoring of the patient's skin, lymph nodes and body temperature, during the first month of therapy, every two weeks for the next five months, and monthly thereafter. Patients should be instructed to report promptly the development of signs and symptoms of granulocytopenia and/or thrombocytopenia such as fever, sore throat, chills, bruising or bleeding; the above laboratory studies should then be promptly repeated.

▷ *trientine* (C)(G) recommended initial dose is 500-750 mg/day for pediatric patients and 750-1250 mg/day for adults administered in divided doses 2, 3 or 4 x/day; may be increased to max 2000 mg/day for adults or 1500 mg/day for patients ≤12 years-of-age; the daily dose of **Syprine** should be increased only when the clinical response is not adequate or the concentration of free serum copper is persistently above 20 mcg/dL; optimal long-term maintenance dose should be determined at 6-12 month intervals; administer on an empty stomach, at least one hour before meals or two hours after meals and at least one hour apart from any other drug, food, or milk; swallow whole with water; do not open the cap or chew the contents

    Syprine *Cap:* 250 mg

    Comment: **Syprine** is a chelating agent indicated in the treatment of patients with Wilson's disease who are intolerant of *penicillamine*. Clinical experience with **Syprine** is limited and alternate dosing regimens have not been well-characterized; all endpoints in determining an individual patient's dose have not been well defined. **Syprine** and *penicillamine* cannot be considered interchangeable. **Syprine** should be used when continued treatment with *penicillamine* is no longer possible because of intolerable or life-endangering side effects. Unlike *penicillamine*, **Syprine** is not recommended in cystinuria or rheumatoid arthritis. The absence of a sulfhydryl moiety renders it incapable of binding cystine and, therefore, it is of no use in cystinuria. In 15 patients with rheumatoid arthritis, **Syprine** was reported not to be effective in improving any clinical or biochemical parameter after 12 weeks of treatment. The most reliable index for monitoring treatment is the determination of free copper in the serum, which equals the difference between quantitatively determined total copper and ceruloplasmin-copper. Adequately treated patients will usually have less than 10 mcg free copper/dL of serum. Therapy may be monitored with a 24-hour urinary copper analysis periodically (i.e., every 6-12 months). Urine must be collected in copper-free glassware. Since a low copper diet should keep copper absorption down to less than one milligram a day, the patient probably will be in the desired state of negative copper balance if 0.5 to 1.0 milligram of copper is present in a 24-hour collection of urine. In general, mineral supplements should <u>not</u> be used since they may block the absorption of **Syprine**. However, iron deficiency may develop, especially in children and menstruating or pregnant women, <u>or</u> as a result of the low copper diet recommended for Wilson's disease. If necessary, iron may be given in short courses, but since iron and **Syprine** each inhibit absorption of the other, two hours should elapse between administration of **Syprine** and iron. *trientine* was teratogenic in animals at doses similar to the human dose. The frequencies of both resorptions and fetal abnormalities, including hemorrhage and edema, increased while fetal copper levels decreased when *trientine* was given in the maternal diets. There are no adequate and well-controlled studies in pregnant women. **Syprine** should be used during pregnancy <u>only</u> if the potential benefit justifies the potential risk to the fetus. It is not known whether this drug is excreted in human milk. Caution should be exercised when **Syprine** is administered to a nursing mother. Clinical studies of **Syprine** did not include sufficient numbers of subjects ≥65 years-of-age to determine whether they respond differently from younger subjects. Other reported clinical experience is insufficient to determine differences in responses between the elderly and younger patients. In general, dose selection should be cautious, usually starting at the low end of the dosing range, reflecting the greater frequency of decreased hepatic, renal, <u>or</u> cardiac function, and of concomitant disease <u>or</u> other drug therapy. Clinical experience with **Syprine** has been limited.

The following adverse reactions have been reported in a clinical study in patients with Wilson's disease who were on therapy with *trientine*: iron deficiency, systemic lupus erythematosus. In addition, the following adverse reactions have been reported in marketed use: dystonia, muscular spasm, myasthenia gravis. To report suspected adverse reactions, contact Valeant Pharmaceuticals North America at 1-800-321-4576 <u>or</u> FDA at 1-800-FDA-1088 <u>or</u> www.fda.gov/medwatch.

WOUND: INFECTED, NONSURGICAL, MINOR

TETANUS PROPHYLAXIS VACCINE

Previously Immunized (within previous 5 years)

▷ *tetanus toxoid* vaccine (C) 0.5 ml IM x 1 dose
   Vial: 5 Lf units/0.5 ml (0.5, 5 ml); *Prefilled syringe:* 5 Lf units/0.5 ml (0.5 ml)

Not Previously Immunized

see Tetanus page 478

TOPICAL ANTI-INFECTIVES

▷ *mupirocin* (B)(G) apply to lesions bid
   Pediatric: same as adult
      Bactroban *Oint:* 2% (22 gm); *Crm:* 2% (15, 30 gm)
      Centany *Oint:* 2% (15, 30 gm)

ORAL ANTI-INFECTIVES

▷ *azithromycin* (B)(G) 500 mg x 1 dose on day 1, then 250 mg daily on days 2-5 <u>or</u> 500 mg daily x 3 days <u>or</u> Zmax 2 gm in a single dose
   Pediatric: 10 mg/kg x 1 dose on day 1, then 5 mg/kg/day on days 2-5; max 500 mg/day; *see page 619 for dose by weight*
      Zithromax *Tab:* 250, 500, 600 mg; *Oral susp:* 100 mg/5 ml (15 ml); 200 mg/5 ml (15, 22.5, 30 ml) (cherry); *Pkt:* 1 gm for reconstitution (cherry-banana)
      Zithromax Tri-pak *Tab:* 3 x 500 mg tabs/pck
      Zithromax Z-pak *Tab:* 6 x 250 mg tabs/pck
      Zmax *Oral susp:* 2 gm ext-rel for reconstitution (cherry-banana) (148 mg Na+)
▷ *amoxicillin+clavulanate* (B)(G)
      Augmentin 500 mg tid or 875 mg bid x 10 days
      Pediatric: 40-45 mg/kg/day divided tid x 10 days or 90 mg/kg/day divided bid x 10 days
      see pages 618 for dose by weight
      Tab: 250, 500, 875 mg; *Chew tab:* 125, 250 mg (lemon-lime); 200, 400 mg (cherry-banana) (phenylalanine); *Oral susp:* 125 mg/5 ml (banana), 250 mg/5 ml (75, 100, 150 ml) (orange); 200, 400 mg/5 ml (50, 75, 100 ml) (orange) (phenylalanine)

Augmentin ES-600 not recommended for adults
Pediatric: <3 months: not recommended; ≥3 months, <40 kg: 90 mg/kg/day in 2 divided doses x 10 days; ≥40 kg: not recommended
Oral susp: 42.9 mg/5 ml (50, 75, 100, 125, 150, 200 ml) (strawberry cream) (phenylalanine)
Augmentin XR 2 tabs q 12 hours x 10 days
Pediatric: <16 years: use other forms; ≥16 years: same as adult
Tab: 1000*mg ext-rel

► *cefaclor* (B)(G) 250-500 mg q 8 hours x 10 days; max 2 gm/day
Pediatric: <1 month: not recommended; 20-40 mg/kg bid or q 12 hours x 10 days; max 1 gm/day; *see page 620 for dose by weight*
Tab: 500 mg; *Cap:* 250, 500 mg; *Susp:* 125 mg/5 ml (75, 150 ml) (strawberry); 187 mg/5 ml (50, 100 ml) (strawberry); 250 mg/5 ml (75, 150 ml) (strawberry); 375 mg/5 ml (50, 100 ml) (strawberry)
Cefaclor Extended Release *Tab:* 375, 500 mg ext-rel
Pediatric: <16 years: ext-rel not recommended

► *cefadroxil* 1 gm/day in 1-2 divided doses x 10 days
Pediatric: 15-30 mg/kg/day in 2 divided doses x 10 days; *see page 620 for dose by weight*
Duricef *Cap:* 500 mg; *Tab:* 1 gm; *Oral susp:* 250 mg/5 ml (100 ml); 500 mg/5 ml (75, 100 ml) (orange-pineapple)

► *cefdinir* (B) 300 mg bid or 600 mg daily x 10 days
Pediatric: <6 months: not recommended; 6 months-12 years: 14 mg/kg/day in 1-2 divided doses x 10 days; *see page 621 for dose by weight*
Omnicef *Cap:* 300 mg; *Oral susp:* 125 mg/5 ml (60, 100 ml) (strawberry)

► *cefpodoxime proxetil* (B) 400 mg bid x 7-14 days
Pediatric: <2 months: not recommended; 2 months-12 years: 10 mg/kg/day (max 400 mg/dose) or 5 mg/kg/day bid (max 200 mg/dose) x 7-14 days; *see page 622 for dose by weight*
Vantin *Tab:* 100, 200 mg; *Oral susp:* 50, 100 mg/5 ml (50, 75, 100 mg; lemon creme)
Pediatric: see page 622 for dose by weight

► *cefprozil* (B) 250-500 mg q 12 hours or 500 mg daily x 10 days
Pediatric: <2 years: not recommended; 2-12 years: 7.5 mg/kg-15 mg/kg q 12 hours x 10 days; *see page 622 for dose by weight;* >12 years: same as adult
Cefzil *Tab:* 250, 500 mg; *Oral susp:* 125, 250 mg/5 ml (50, 75, 100 ml) (bubble gum, phenylalanine)

► *cephalexin* (B)(G) 2 gm 1 hour before procedure
Pediatric: 50 mg/kg/day in 4 divided doses x 10 days; *see page 623 for dose by weight*
Keflex *Cap:* 250, 333, 500, 750 mg; *Oral susp:* 125, 250 mg/5 ml (100, 200 ml) (strawberry)
Pediatric: see page 623 for dose by weight

► *clarithromycin* (C)(G) 500 mg bid or 500 mg ext-rel once daily x 7-10 days
Pediatric: see page 624 for dose by weight
Biaxin *Tab:* 250, 500 mg
Biaxin Oral Suspension *Oral susp:* 125, 250 mg/5 ml (50, 100 ml) (fruit-punch)
Biaxin XL *Tab:* 500 mg ext-rel
Comment: The FDA is advising caution before prescribing *clarithromycin* to patients with heart disease because of a potential increased risk of heart problems or death that can occur years later. This recommendation is based on a review of the results of a 10-year follow-up study of patients with coronary heart disease from a large clinical trial that first observed this safety issue. Consider risk benefit and the use of other antibiotics in such patients.

► *dirithromycin* (C)(G) 500 mg daily x 7 days
Pediatric: <12 years: not recommended
Dynabac *Tab:* 250 mg

► *erythromycin base* (B)(G) 500 mg qid x 14 days
Pediatric: 30-50 mg/kg/day in 2-4 divided doses x 10 days
Ery-Tab *Tab:* 250, 333, 500 mg ent-coat
PCE *Tab:* 333, 500 mg
Comment: *erythromycin* may increase INR with concomitant *warfarin*, as well as increase serum level of *digoxin*, benzodiazepines, and statins.

► *erythromycin ethylsuccinate* (B)(G) 400 mg qid x 7 days
Pediatric: 30-50 mg/kg/day in 4 divided doses x 7 days; may double dose with severe infection; max 100 mg/kg/day; *see page 626 for dose by weight*

EryPed *Oral susp:* 200 mg/5 ml (100, 200 ml) (fruit); 400 mg/5 ml (60, 100, 200 ml) (banana); *Oral drops:* 200, 400 mg/5 ml (50 ml) (fruit); *Chew tab:* 200 mg wafer (fruit)

E.E.S. *Oral susp:* 200, 400 mg/5 ml (100 ml) (fruit)

E.E.S. Granules *Oral susp:* 200 mg/5 ml (100, 200 ml) (cherry)

E.E.S. 400 Tablets *Tab:* 400 mg

Comment: *erythromycin* may increase INR with concomitant *warfarin*, as well as increase serum level of *digoxin,* benzodiazepines, and statins.

▷ *gemifloxacin* (C)(G) 320 mg daily x 5-7 days

Pediatric: <18 years: not recommended; ≥18 years: same as adult

Factive *Tab:* 320*mg

▷ *levofloxacin* (C) *Uncomplicated:* 500 mg daily x 7 days; *Complicated:* 750 mg daily x 7 days

Pediatric: <18 years: not recommended; ≥18 years: same as adult

Levaquin *Tab:* 250, 500, 750 mg

Comment: *levofloxacin* is contraindicated <18 years-of-age, and during pregnancy and lactation. Risk of tendonitis or tendon rupture.

▷ *loracarbef* (B) 200-400 mg bid x 7 days

Pediatric: 15 mg/kg/day in 2 divided doses x 7 days; *see page 628 for dose by weight*

Lorabid *Pulvule:* 200, 400 mg; *Oral susp:* 100 mg/5 ml (50, 100 ml); 200 mg/5 ml (50, 75, 100 ml) (strawberry bubble gum)

▷ *ofloxacin* (C)(G) 400 mg bid x 10 days

Pediatric: <18 years: not recommended; ≥18 years: same as adult

Floxin *Tab:* 200, 300, 400 mg

Comment: *levofloxacin* is contraindicated <18 years-of-age, and during pregnancy and lactation. Risk of tendonitis or tendon rupture.

◯ WRINKLES: FACIAL

TOPICAL RETINOIDS

Comment: Wash the affected area with a soap-free cleanser; pat dry and wait 20 to 30 minutes; then apply topical retinoid sparingly to affected area. Use only once daily in the PM. Avoid eyes, ears, nostrils, and mouth.

▷ *adapalene* (C)(G)

Pediatric: <12 years: not recommended; ≥12 years: same as adult

Differin *Crm:* 0.1% (15, 45 gm); *Gel:* 0.1% (15, 45 gm); *Pad:* 0.1% (30/pck) (alcohol 30%)

Differin Solution *Soln:* 0.1% (30 ml; alcohol 30%)

▷ *tazarotene* (X)(G) apply daily at HS

Pediatric: <12 years: not recommended; ≥12 years: same as adult

Avage Cream *Crm:* 0.1% (5, 30 gm)

Tazorac Cream *Crm:* 0.05, 0.1% (15, 30, 60 gm)

Tazorac Gel *Gel:* 0.05, 0.1% (30, 100 gm)

▷ *tretinoin* (C) apply daily at HS

Pediatric: <12 years: not recommended; ≥12 years: same as adult

Atralin Gel *Gel:* 0.05% (45 gm)

Avita *Crm:* 0.025% (20, 45 gm); *Gel:* 0.025% (20, 45 gm)

Renova *Crm:* 0.02% (40 gm); 0.05% (40, 60 gm)

Retin-A Cream *Crm:* 0.025, 0.05, 0.1% (20, 45 gm)

Retin-A Gel *Gel:* 0.01, 0.025% (15, 45 gm; alcohol 90%)

Retin-A Liquid *Soln:* 0.05% (alcohol 55%)

Retin-A Micro Gel *Gel:* 0.04, 0.08, 0.1% (20, 45 gm)

Tretin-X Cream *Crm:* 0.075% (35 gm) (parabens-free, alcohol-free, propylene glycol-free)

Retin-A Micro *Microspheres:* 0.04, 0.1% (20, 45 gm)

Comment: topical *treatinoin* is effective for mitigation of fine wrinkles, mottled hyperpigmentation, and tactile roughness of skin. No mitigating effect on deep wrinkles, skin yellowing, lentigines, telangiectasia, skin laxity, keratinocytic atypia, melanocytic atypia, or dermal elastosis. Avoid sun exposure. Cautious use of concomitant astringents, alcohol-based products, sulfur-containing products, salicylic acid-containing products, soap, and other topical agents.

BOTULISM TOXIN PRODUCT

▶ **prabotulinumtoxina-xvfs** *Glabellar Lines Administration:* using a 30-33 guage needle, 0.1 ml (4 Units) by IM injection into each of 5 sites, for a max total dose of 20 Units; consult pkg insert for exact injection sites; must be administered by a qualified healthcare provider with knowledge of the relevant neuromuscular and/or orbital anatomy of the area involved and any alterations to the anatomy due to prior surgical procedures; avoid injection near the levator palpebrae superioris, particularly in patients with larger brow depressor complexes; lateral corrugator injections should be placed at least 1 cm above the bony supraorbital ridge; ensure the injected volume/dose is accurate and where feasible kept to a minimum; avoid injecting toxin closer than 1 centimeter above the central eyebrow

Jeuveau *Vial:* 100 Units vacuum-dried pwdr, single-use, for reconstitution with 2.5 ml sterile, preservative-free 0.9% NaCl diluent, to obtain a solution concentration of 4 Units/0.1 ml (total 20 Units in 0.5 ml)

Comment: **Jeuveau** is an acetylcholine release inhibitor and a neuromuscular blocking agent indicated for the temporary improvement in the appearance of moderate to severe glabellar lines ("worry lines" between the brows) associated with corrugator and/or procerus muscle activity in adult patients. The effects of all botulinum toxin products may spread from the area of injection to produce symptoms consistent with botulinum toxin effects. These symptoms have been reported hours to weeks after injection. Swallowing and breathing difficulties can be life threatening. Adverse event reports have also involved the cardiovascular system, some with fatal outcomes. Use caution when administering to patients with pre-existing cardiovascular disease. **Jeuveau** is not approved for the treatment of spasticity or any conditions other than glabellar lines. Potency Units of **Jeuveau** are not interchangeable with other preparations of botulinum toxin products. Animal studies have not demonstrated treatment-related effects to the developing fetus when administered intramuscularly during organogenesis at doses up to 12 times the maximum recommended human dose (MRHD). There is no information regarding the presence of **prabotulinumtoxinA** in human or its effects on the breastfed infant.

 XEROSIS

MOISTURIZING AGENTS

Aquaphor Healing Ointment (OTC) *Oint:* 1.75, 3.5, 14 oz (alcohol)
Eucerin Daily Sun Defense (OTC) *Lotn:* 6 oz (fragrance-free)
Comment: **Eucerin Daily Sun Defense** is a moisturizer with SPF 15 sunscreen.
Eucerin Facial Lotion (OTC) *Lotn:* 4 oz
Eucerin Light Lotion (OTC) *Lotn:* 8 oz
Eucerin Lotion (OTC) *Lotn:* 8, 16 oz
Eucerin Original Creme (OTC) *Crm:* 2, 4, 16 oz (alcohol)
Eucerin Plus Creme (OTC) *Crm:* 4 oz
Eucerin Plus Lotion (OTC) *Lotn:* 6, 12 oz
Eucerin Protective Lotion (OTC) *Lotn:* 4 oz (alcohol)

Comment: **Eucerin Protective** is a moisturizer with SPF 25 sunscreen.
Lac-Hydrin Cream (OTC) *Crm:* 280, 385 gm
Lac-Hydrin Lotion (OTC) *Lotn:* 225, 400 gm
Lubriderm Dry Skin Scented (OTC) *Lotn:* 6, 10, 16, 32 oz
Lubriderm Dry Skin Unscented (OTC) *Lotn:* 3.3, 6, 10, 16 oz (fragrance-free)
Lubriderm Sensitive Skin Lotion (OTC) *Lotn:* 3.3, 6, 10, 16 oz (lanolin-free)
Lubriderm Dry Skin (OTC) *Lotn:* 2.5, 6, 10, 16 oz (scented); 1, 2.5, 6, 10, 16 oz (fragrance-free)
Lubriderm Bath & Shower Oil (OTC) 1-2 capfuls in bath or rub onto wet skin as needed, then rinse; *Oil:* 8 oz
Moisturel *Crm:* 4, 16 oz; *Lotn:* 8, 12 oz; *Clnsr:* 8.75 oz

Topical Oil

▶ **fluocinolone acetonide** 0.01% topical oil (C)
Pediatric: <6 years: not recommended; ≥6 years: apply sparingly bid for up to 4 weeks

Derma-Smoothe/FS Topical Oil apply sparingly tid
Topical oil: 0.01% (4 oz; peanut oil)

 YELLOW FEVER

Comment: The yellow fever vaccine is recommended for people ≥ 9 months-of-age who are traveling to or living in areas at risk for the yellow fever virus in https://www.cdc.gov/yellowfever/maps/africa.html Africa and South America (www.cdc.gov/yellowfever/maps/africa.html). The vaccine is a live, weakened form of the virus. A single dose provides lifelong protection for most people. Sanofi Pasteur, the manufacturer of the only yellow fever vaccine (**YF-Vax**) licensed in the United States, announced that **YF-Vax** for civilian use is expected to be available from the manufacturer again by mid-2019. However, **YF-VAX** might be available at some clinics, until remaining supplies at those sites are used up. Sanofi Pasteur applied and received approval from the US Food and Drug Administration (FDA) to make another yellow fever vaccine available in the United States under an investigational new drug (IND) program. Although the name of the FDA program is "investigational new drug," **Stamaril** is not investigational or experimental. **Stamaril** has been used in European and other countries for decades but is not licensed in the United States. IND is the mechanism through which FDA gives approval for **Stamaril** to be imported. Manufactured by Sanofi Pasteur in France, this vaccine, **Stamaril**, is registered and distributed in more than 70 countries. It is comparable in safety and efficacy to **YF-Vax**. In order to meet the requirements of the IND program, Sanofi Pasteur can provide **Stamaril** to only a limited number of clinics. Sanofi has identified sites throughout the United States to include in the program so patients can have continued access to yellow fever vaccine. Travelers and health care providers can find locations that can administer **Stamaril**, and those clinics with remaining doses of **YF-VAX**, by visiting the yellow fever vaccination clinic search page. For information about which countries require yellow fever vaccination for entry and which countries the CDC recommends yellow fever vaccination, visit the CDC Travelers' Health website (www.cdc.gov/travel). For more information, contact Sanofi Pasteur at 1-800-VACCINE (1-800-822-2463).

RESOURCE

https://wwwnc.cdc.gov/travel/news-announcements/yellow-fever-vaccine-access

 ZIKA VIRUS

Comment: The Zika virus is transmitted via the bite of an infected mosquito and is associated with severe teratogenicity: a unique and distinct pattern of birth defects, called congenital Zika syndrome, characterized by the following five features: (1) Severe microcephaly in which the skull has partially collapsed; (2) Decreased brain tissue with a specific pattern of brain damage, including subcortical calcifications; (3) Damage to the back of the eye, including macular scarring and focal pigmentary retinal mottling; (4) Congenital contractures, such as clubfoot and arthrogryposis; (5) Hypertonia restricting body movement. Congenital Zika virus infection has also been associated with other abnormalities, including but not limited to brain atrophy and asymmetry, abnormally formed or absent brain structures, hydrocephalus, and neuronal migration disorders. Other anomalies include excessive and redundant scalp skin. Reported neurologic findings include, hyperreflexia, irritability, tremors, seizures, brainstem dysfunction, and dysphagia. Reported eye abnormalities include, but are not limited to, focal pigmentary mottling and chorioretinal atrophy in the macula, optic nerve hypoplasia, cupping, and atrophy, other retinal lesions, iris colobomas, congenital glaucoma, microphthalmia, lens subluxation, cataracts, and intraocular calcifications. **A synthetic DNA-based preventive vaccine showed promising immune responses with no severe adverse reactions in humans,** an interim analysis of a phase I trial found. Following three doses of vaccine, 100% of patients produced binding antibodies, and 95% of patients produced binding antibodies following two doses of the vaccine, Examining immunogenicity, 41% of participants had detectable binding antibody responses 4 weeks after the first dose, the authors said, with a 74% antibody response at week 6 (2 weeks after the second dose). **The vaccine is not yet available to the public.** The FDA formally approved Roche's cobas Zika molecular test for use on whole donor blood and blood products and living organ donors; it's the first such approval granted.

REFERENCES

Paz-Bailey, GM, et al. Zika virus persistence in body fluids, final report in body fluids-Final report. ASTMH 2017. Paper presented at the 66th Annual Meeting of the American Society of Tropical Medicine and Hygiene, November 5-9, Baltimore, MD

Rosenberg, E, Doyle, K., Munoz-Jordan, J. L., Klein, L., Adams, L., Lozier, M., . . . Paz-Bailey, G. (2017, November). Prevalence and incidence of Zika virus infection among household contacts of Zika patients, Puerto Rico, 2016–2017. Paper presented at the 66th Annual Meeting of the American Society of Tropical Medicine and Hygiene, Baltimore, MD

Tebas, P., Roberts, C. C., Muthumani, K., Reuschel, E. L., Kudchodkar, S. B., Zaidi, F. I., . . . Maslow, J. N. (2017). Safety and immunogenicity of an anti–zika virus DNA vaccine—preliminary report. *New England Journal of Medicine*. doi:10.1056/nejmoa1708120

ZOLLINGER-ELLISON SYNDROME

Comment: Zollinger-Ellison Syndrome is a condition in which a gastrin-secreting tumor or hyperplasia of the islet cells in the pancreas causes overproduction of gastric acid, resulting in recurrent peptic ulcers.

PROTON PUMP INHIBITORS (PPIs)

Comment: If hepatic impairment, or if patient is Asian, consider reducing the PPI dose.

▶ *dexlansoprazole* (B)(G) 30-60 mg daily for up to 4 weeks
Pediatric: <18 years: not recommended; ≥18 years: same as adult
  Dexilant *Cap:* 30, 60 mg ent-rel del-rel granules; may open and sprinkle on apple-sauce; do not crush or chew granules
  Dexilant SoluTab *Tab:* 30 mg del-rel orally-disint

▶ *esomeprazole* (B)(OTC)(G) 20-40 mg daily; max 8 weeks; take 1 hour before food; swallow whole or mix granules with food or juice and take immediately; do not crush or chew granules
Pediatric: <1 year: not recommended; 1-11 years, <20 kg: 10 mg; ≥20 kg: 10-20 mg once daily; 12-17 years: 20-40 mg once daily; max 8 weeks
  Nexium *Cap:* 20, 40 mg ent-coat del-rel pellets
  Nexium for Oral Suspension *Oral susp:* 10, 20, 40 mg ent-coat del-rel granules/pkt; mix in 2 tbsp water and drink immediately; 30 pkt/carton

▶ *esomeprazole+aspirin* (D) take one dose daily; max 8 weeks; take 1 hour before food
  Yosprala
    Tab: **Yosprala 40/81** esom 40 mg+asp 81 mg del-rel
      Yosprala 40/325 esom 40 mg+asp 325 mg del-rel
Comment: *aspirin*-containing medications are contraindicated with history of allergic-type reaction to *aspirin*, children and adolescents with *Varicella* or other viral illness, and 3rd trimester of pregnancy.

▶ *lansoprazole* (B)(OTC)(G) 15-30 mg daily for up to 8 weeks; may repeat course; take before eating
Pediatric: <1 year: not recommended; 1-11 years, <30 kg: 15 mg once daily; >11 years: same as adult
  Prevacid *Cap:* 15, 30 mg ent-coat del-rel granules; swallow whole or mix granules with food or juice and take immediately; do not crush or chew granules; follow with water
  Prevacid for Oral Suspension *Oral susp:* 15, 30 mg ent-coat del-rel granules/pkt; mix in 2 tbsp water and drink immediately; 30 pkt/carton (strawberry)
  Prevacid SoluTab *ODT:* 15, 30 mg (strawberry) (phenylalanine)
  Prevacid 24HR *Oral granules:* 15 mg ent-coat del-rel granules; swallow whole or mix granules with food or juice and take immediately; do not crush or chew granules; follow with water

▶ *omeprazole* (C)(OTC)(G) 20-40 mg daily; take before eating; swallow whole or mix granules with applesauce and take immediately; do not crush or chew; follow with water
  Prilosec *Cap:* 10, 20, 40 mg ent-coat del-rel granules
  Pediatric: <18 years: not recommended; ≥18 years: same as adult
  Prilosec *Tab:* 20 mg del-rel (regular, wild berry)
  Pediatric: <1 year: not recommended; 5-<10 kg: 5 mg daily; 10-<20 kg: 10 mg daily; ≥20 kg: same as adult

▶ *pantoprazole* (B)(G) initially 40 mg bid
Pediatric: <12 years: not recommended; ≥12 years: same as adult
  Protonix *Tab:* 40 mg ent-coat del-rel

Protonix for Oral Suspension *Oral susp:* 40 mg ent-coat del-rel granules/pkt; mix in 1 tsp apple juice for 5 seconds <u>or</u> sprinkle on 1 tsp apple sauce, and swallow immediately; do not mix in water <u>or</u> any other liquid <u>or</u> food; take approximately 30 minutes prior to a meal; 30 pkt/carton any other liquid <u>or</u> food; take approximately 30 minutes prior to a meal; 30 pkt/carton

▷ *rabeprazole* (B)(OTC)(G) initially 20 mg daily; then titrate; may take 100 mg daily in divided doses <u>or</u> 60 mg bid

Pediatric: <12 years: not recommended; ≥12 years: 20 mg once daily; max 8 weeks

AcipHex *Tab:* 20 mg ent-coat del-rel

SECTION II

APPENDICES

APPENDIX A. U.S. FDA PREGNANCY CATEGORIES

Comment: For drugs FDA-approved *after June 30, 2015*, the 5-letter categories are no longer used and there is no replacement (categorical nomenclature) at this time. Rather, information regarding special populations, including pregnant and breastfeeding females, is addressed in a structured narrative format. Prescribers should refer to the drug's FDA labeling (https://www.fda.gov/Drugs/default.htm) or the manufacturer's package insert for this information. Prescription drugs submitted for FDA approval after June 30, 2015 use the new format immediately, while labeling for prescription drugs approved on or after June 30, 2015 are phased in gradually. Although drugs approved prior to June 29, 2015 are not subject to the FDA's **Pregnancy and Lactation Labeling Final Rule (PLLR)**, the *pregnancy letter category must be removed by June 29, 2018.* Labeling for over-the-counter (OTC) medicines will not change, as OTC drugs are not affected by the new FDA pregnancy labeling. For a more detailed explanation of the final rule **and** new narrative format, **visit** https://www.drugs.com/pregnancy-categories.html

Category	Description
A	Controlled studies in women have failed to demonstrate risk to the fetus in the first trimester of pregnancy and there is no evidence of risk in later trimesters.
B	Animal reproduction studies have not demonstrated risk to the fetus, but there are no controlled studies in pregnant women, or animal studies have demonstrated an adverse effect, but controlled studies in pregnant women have not documented risk to the fetus in the first trimester of pregnancy and there is no evidence of risk in later trimesters.
C	Risk to the fetus cannot be ruled out. Animal reproduction studies have demonstrated adverse effects on the fetus (i.e., teratogenic or embryocidal effects or other) but there are no controlled studies in pregnant women or controlled studies in women and animals are not available.
D	There is positive evidence of human fetal risk, but benefits from use by pregnant women may be acceptable despite the potential risk (e.g., if the drug is needed in a life-threatening situation or for a serious disease for which safer drugs cannot be used or are ineffective.
X	Studies in animals or humans have demonstrated fetal abnormalities or there is evidence of fetal risk based on human experience, or both, and the risk of using the drug in pregnant women clearly outweighs any possible benefit. The drug is contraindicated in women who are pregnant or who may become pregnant.

APPENDIX B. U.S. SCHEDULE OF CONTROLLED SUBSTANCES

Schedule	Description
I	High potential for abuse and of no currently accepted medical use. Not obtainable by prescription, but may be legally procured for research, study, or instructional use. (Examples: *heroin, LSD, marijuana, mescaline, peyote*)
II	High abuse potential and high liability for severe psychological or physical dependence potential. Prescription required and cannot be refilled. Prescription must be written in ink or typed and signed. A verbal prescription may be allowed in an emergency by the dispensing pharmacist, but must be followed by a written prescription within 72 hours. Includes opium derivatives, other opioids, and short-acting barbiturates.

(continued)

Appendix B (*continued*)

Schedule	Description
III	Potential for abuse is less than that for drugs in schedules I and II. Moderate to low physical dependence and high psychological dependence potential. Prescription required. May be refilled up to 5 times in 6 months. Prescription may be verbal (telephone) or written. Includes certain stimulants and depressants not included in the above schedules, and preparations containing limited quantities of certain opioids.
IV	Lower potential for abuse than Schedule III drugs. Prescription required. May be refilled up to 5 times in 6 months. Prescription may be verbal (telephone) or written.
V	Abuse potential less than that for Schedule IV drugs. Preparations contain limited quantities of certain narcotic drugs. Generally intended for antitussive and anti-diarrheal purposes and may be distributed without a prescription provided that • such distribution is made only by a pharmacist; • not more than 240 ml or not more than 48 solid dosage units of any substance containing opium, nor more than 120 ml or not more than 24 solid dosage units of any other controlled substance may be distributed at retail to the same purchaser in any given 48-hour period without a valid prescription order; • the purchaser is at least 18 years old; • the pharmacist knows the purchaser or requests suitable identification; • the pharmacist keeps an official written record of: name and address of purchaser, name, and quantity of controlled substance purchased, date of sale, initials of dispensing pharmacist. This record is to be made available for inspection and copying by the U.S. officers authorized by the Attorney General; • other federal, state, or local law does not reuire a prescription order. Under jurisdiction of the Federal Controlled Substances Act. Refillable up to 5 times within 6 months.

APPENDIX C. BLOOD PRESSURE GUIDELINES

APPENDIX C.1. BLOOD PRESSURE CLASSIFICATIONS (≥18 YEARS)

Classification	SBP mmHg		DBP mmHg
Normal	<120	and	<80
Elevated BP	120-129	and	<80
Stage I Hypertension	130-139	or	80-89
Stage 2 Hypertension	≥140	or	≥90
Hypertensive Crisis	>180	and/or	>120

Adapted from Vogt, C. (n.d.). New AHA/ACC guidelines lower high BP threshold. *Consultant360*. November 14, 2017. Retrieved from https://www.consultant360.com/exclusives/new-ahaacc-guidelines-lower-high-bp-threshold; Whelton, P. K., Carey, R. M., Aronow, W. S., Casey, D. E., Jr., Collins, K. J., Dennison Himmelfarb, C., . . . Wright, J. T., Jr. (2017). 2017 ACC/AHA/AAPA/ABC/ACPM/AGS/APhA/ASH/ASPC/NMA/PCNA Guideline for the prevention, detection, evaluation, and management of high blood pressure in adults: A report of the American College of Cardiology/American Heart Association Task Force on Clinical Practice Guidelines. *Hypertension*, 71(6), e13–e115. doi:10.1161/HYP.0000000000000065

APPENDIX C.2. BLOOD PRESSURE CLASSIFICATIONS (<18 YEARS)

Age Group	Significant		Severe	
	SBP	DBP	SBP	DBP
Newborn <7 days	>96		>106	
Newborn 8-30 days	>104		>110	
Infant 30 days-2 years	>112	>74	>118	>82
Children 3-5 years	>116	>76	>124	>84
Children 6-9 years	>122	>78	>130	>86
Children 10-12 years	>126	>82	>134	>90
Adolescents 13-15 years	>136	>86	>144	>92
Adolescents 16-18 years	>142	>92	>150	>98

Adapted from American Pharmacists Association. (2015). *Pediatric and neonatal dosage handbook: A universal resource for clinicians treating pediatric and neonatal patients* (22nd ed.). Hudson, OH: Lexicomp.

APPENDIX C.3. IDENTIFIABLE CAUSES OF HYPERTENSION (JNC-8)

• Obstructive sleep apnea • Chronic kidney disease • Primary aldosteronism • Renovascular disease	• *Prescription Drugs:* oral contraceptives, sympathomimetics, venlafaxine, bupropion, clozapine, buspirone, bromocriptine, carbamazepine, metoclopramide
• Excess sodium ingestion • Herbal supplements • Coarctation of the aorta • Pheochromocytoma • Thyroid disease • Parathyroid disease • Cushing's syndrome	• *Illicit, Over-the-Counter Drugs, and Herbal Products:* excess alcohol consumption, alcohol withdrawal, anabolic steroids, cocaine, cocaine withdrawal, phenylpropanolamine analogs, ephedra alkalois, ergot containing herbal products, St. John's wart, nicotine withdrawal

APPENDIX C.4. CVD RISK FACTORS (JNC-8)

• Hypertension • Obesity (BMI ≥30 kg/m^2) • Dyslipidemia • Diabetes mellitus • Cigarette smoking • Physical inactivity	• Microalbuminuria, GFR <60 mL/min • Age (men >55 yrs, women >65 yrs) • Family History of premature CVD (men <55 yrs, women <65 yrs)

APPENDIX C.5. DIAGNOSTIC WORKUP OF HYPERTENSION (JNC-8)

- Assess risk factors and comorbidities
- Reveal identifiable causes of hypertension
- Assess for presence of target organ damage
- History and physical examination
- Urinalysis, blood glucose, hematocrit, lipid panel, potassium, creatinine, calcium, (*optional* urine albumin/Cr ratio), EKG

APPENDIX C.6. RECOMMENDATIONS FOR MEASURING BLOOD PRESSURE (JNC-8)

- Blood pressure should be measured after the patient has emptied their bladder and has been seated for 5 minutes with back supported and legs resting on the ground (not crossed)

(*continued*)

Appendix C.6. (*continued*)

- Arm used for measurement should rest on a table, at heart level.
- Use a sphygmomanometer/stethoscope or automated electronic device (preferred) with the correct size arm cuff
- Take two readings one to two minutes apart, and average the readings (preferred)
- Measure blood pressure in both arms at initial valuation; use the higher reading for measurements thereafter
- Confirm the diagnosis of HTN at a subsequent visit one to four weeks after the first
- If blood pressure is very high (e.g., systolic 180 mmHg or higher), or timely follow-up unrealistic, treatment can be started after just one set of measurements

APPENDIX C.7. PATIENT-SPECIFIC FACTORS TO CONSIDER WHEN SELECTING DRUG TREATMENT FOR HYPERTENSION (JNC-8 AND ASH)

JNC-8:

- Nonblack, including those with diabetes: thiazide, CCB, ACEI, or ARB
- African American, including those with diabetes: thiazide or CCB
- CKD; regimen should include an ACEI or ARB (including African Americans)
- Can initiate with two agents, especially if systolic >20 mmHg above goal or diastolic >10 mmHg above goal
- If goal not reached: stress adherence to medication and lifestyle, increase dose or add a second or third agent from one of the recommended classes
- Choose a drug outside of the classes recommended above only if these options have been exhausted. Consider specialist referral

ASH:

- **Nonblack <60 years of age:** *First-line:* ACEI or ARB; *Second-line (add-on):* CCB or thiazide; *Third-line:* CCB plus ACEI or ARB plus thiazide
- **Nonblack 60 years of age and older:** *First-line:* CCB or thiazide preferred, ACEI, or ARB; *Second-line (add-on):* CCB, thiazide, ACEI, or ARB (don't use ACEI plus ARB); *Third-line:* CCB plus ACEI or ARB plus thiazide
- **African American:** *First-line:* CCB or thiazide; *Second-line (add-on):* ACEI or ARB. *Third-line:* CCB plus ACEI or ARB plus thiazide

Comorbidities (ASH):

- **Diabetes:** *First-line:* ACEI or ARB (can start with CCB or thiazide in African Americans); *Second-line:* add CCB or thiazide (can add ACEI or ARB in African Americans); *Third-line:* CCB plus ACEI or ARB plus thiazide
- **CKD:** *First-line:* ARB or ACEI (ACEI for African Americans) *Second-line (add-on):* CCB or thiazide; *Third-line:* CCB plus ACEI or ARB plus thiazide
- **CAD:** *First-line:* BB plus ARB or ACEI; *Second-line (add-on):* CCB or thiazide; *Third-line:* BB plus ARB or ACEI plus CCB plus thiazide
- **Stroke history:** *First-line:* ACEI or ARB; *Second-line:* add CCB or thiazide; *Third-line:* CCB plus ACEI or ARB plus thiazide
- **Heart failure:** ACEI or ARB plus BB plus diuretic plus aldosterone antagonist. Amlodipine can be added for additional BP control (Start with ACEI, BB, diuretic. Can add BB even before ACE-I optimized. Use diuretic to manage fluid.)
- In patients 60 years of age or older who do not have diabetes or chronic kidney disease, the goal blood pressure level is now <150/90 mmHg
- In patients 18 to 59 years of age without major comorbidities, and in patients 60 years of age or older who have diabetes, chronic kidney disease, or both conditions, the new goal blood pressure level is <140/90 mmHg

APPENDIX C.8. BLOOD PRESSURE TREATMENT RECOMMENDATIONS (JNC-8)¶

- First-line and later-line treatments should now be limited to 4 classes of medications: thiazide-type diuretics, calcium channel blockers (CCBs), ACEIs, and ARBs

(*continued*)

Appendix C.8. (*continued*)

- Second- and third-line alternatives included higher doses or combinations of ACEIs, ARBs, thiazide-type diuretics, and CCBs
- Several medications are now designated as later-line alternatives, including the following:
  - Beta-blockers
  - Alpha-blockers
  - Alpha₁/beta-blockers (e.g., *carvedilol*)
  - Vasodilating beta-blockers (e.g., *nebivolol*)
  - Central alpha₂-adrenergic agonists (e.g., *clonidine*)
  - Direct vasodilators (e.g., *hydralazine*)
  - Loop diuretics (e.g., *furosemide*)
  - Aldosterone antagonists (e.g., *spironolactone*)
  - Peripherally acting adrenergic antagonists (e.g., *reserpine*)
- When initiating therapy, patients of African descent without chronic kidney disease should use CCBs and thiazides instead of ACEIs.
- Use of ACEIs and ARBs is recommended in all patients with chronic kidney disease regardless of ethnic background, either as first-line therapy or in addition to first-line therapy.
- ACEIs and ARBs should not be used in the same patient simultaneously.
- CCBs and thiazide-type diuretics should be used instead of ACEIs and ARBs in patients over the age of 75 with impaired kidney function due to the risk of hyperkalemia, increased creatinine, and further renal impairment.

¶Adapted from: PL Detail-Document, Treatment of hypertension: JNC 8 and more [PL detail document #300201]. (2014). *Pharmacist's Letter/Prescriber's Letter*. http://pharma-smart.com/wp-content/uploads/2015/03/JNC-8-Guidelines.pdf

APPENDIX D. TARGET LIPID RECOMMENDATIONS (ATP-IV)

APPENDIX D.1. TARGET TC, TG, HDL-C, NON-HDL-C

Total cholesterol (TC)	<200 mg/dL
Triglyceride (TRG)	<150 mg/dL
High-density lipoprotein (HDL-C)	>40 mg/dL (male) >50 mg/dL (female)
Non-high-density lipoprotein (Non-HDL-C)	<130 mg/dL; 30 mg/dL above the LDL-C treatment target

Adapted from the National Cholesterol Education Program Expert Panel on Detection, Evaluation, and Treatment of High Blood Cholesterol in Adults (Adult Treatment Panel IV, 2012)

APPENDIX D.2. TARGET LDL-C (ATP-IV)†

Risk Assessment††	LDL Target	Initiate TLC†††	Initiate Drug Therapy
0-1	<160 mg/dL	≥160 mg/dL	≥190 mg/dL (optional at 160-189 mg/dL)
2 or more plus 10-year risk <10%	<130 mg/dL	≥130 mg/dL	≥160 mg/dL
2 or more plus 10-year risk <20%	<130 mg/dL <100 mg/dL optional	≥130 mg/dL	≥130 mg/dL
CHD or CHD risk equivalents 10-year risk >20%	<100 mg/dL <70 mg/dL optional	≥100 mg/dL	≥100 mg/dL

†Treatment decisions based on LDL-C

Calculation: LDL-C = TC - [(TRG ÷ 5) + HDL-C]

††Risk factors include age (men ≥45 years and women ≥55 years)

†††Therapeutic lifestyle changes (e.g., exercise, weight loss, low fat diet)

APPENDIX D.3. NON-HDL-C CLASSIFICATIONS (ATP-IV)

Desirable	<130 mg/dL	Non-HDL-C is calculated as total cholesterol minus HDL-C. The addition of non-HDL-C to the Lipid Panel reflects the recognition of this calculated value as a predictive factor in cardiovascular disease based on the National Cholesterol Education III studies. The reference ranges for non-HDL-C are based on National Cholesterol Education III guidelines: Non-HDL-C is thought to be a better predictor of CVD than LDL-C; treatment goal for non-HDL-C is usually 30 mg/dL above the LDL-C treatment target. For example, if the LDL-C treatment goal is <70 mg/dL, the non-HDL-C treatment target would be <100 mg/dL.
Borderline high	139-159 mg/dL	
High	160-189 mg/dL	
Very high	≥190 mg/dL	

Adapted from the National Cholesterol Education Program Expert Panel on Detection, Evaluation, and Treatment of High Blood Cholesterol in Adults (Adult Treatment Panel IV, 2012).

APPENDIX E. EFFECTS OF SELECTED DRUGS ON INSULIN ACTIVITY

Hyper- and Hypoglycemic Drug Effects	
Drugs That May Cause Hyperglycemia	Drugs That May Cause Hypoglycemia
Calcium channel blockers	Alcohol
Thiazide diuretics	Beta-blockers
Corticosteroids	MAO inhibitors
Nicotinic acid	Salicylates
Oral contraceptives	NSAIDs
Phenytoin	Warfarin
Sympathomimetics diazoxide	Phenylbutazone

APPENDIX F. GLYCOSYLATED HEMOGLOBIN (HBA1C) AND AVERAGE BLOOD GLUCOSE EQUIVALENT

HbA1c and Average Blood Glucose Equivalent			
HbA1c	GLU	HbA1c	GLU
4%	60 mg/dL	14%	360 mg/dL
5%	90 mg/dL	15%	390 mg/dL
6%	120 mg/dL	16%	420 mg/dL
7%	150 mg/dL	17%	450 mg/dL
8%	180 mg/dL	18%	480 mg/dL
9%	210 mg/dL	19%	510 mg/dL
10%	240 mg/dL	20%	540 mg/dL
11%	270 mg/dL	21%	570 mg/dL
12%	300 mg/dL	22%	600 mg/dL
13%	330 mg/dL	23%	630 mg/dL

APPENDIX G. ROUTINE IMMUNIZATION RECOMMENDATIONS

APPENDIX G.1. ADMINISTRATION OF VACCINES[1]

- Prior to 1 year-of-age, administer IM vaccinations in the vastus lateralis muscle
- After 1 year-of-age, administer vaccinations in the posterolateral upper arm
- Influenza vaccine should be administered annually for all ages ≥6 months
- Inactivated vaccines (e.g., pneumococcal, meningococcal, and inactivated influenza vaccines), are generally acceptable and live vaccines are generally avoided, in persons with immune deficiencies or immunocompromising conditions
- Additional information about routine vaccinations, unknown vaccination status, travel vaccinations, vaccinations in pregnancy, and other vaccines, is available at:
  www.cdc.gov/vaccines/hcp/acip-recs/index.html
  www.cdc.gov/mmwr/preview/mmwrhtml rr6002a1/htm
  wwwnc.cdc.gov/travel/destinations/list
  www.cdc.gov/vaccines/adult/rec-vac/pregnant.html
  www.cdc.gov/flu/protect/vaccine/vaccines/htm
- **DTaP** (*diphtheria-tetanus-toxoid, acellular pertussis*); minimum age 6 wks
- **DTaP** should not be administered at or after the 7th birthday
- The 4th dose of **DTaP** vaccine can be administered as early as age 12 months, provided that the interval between doses 3 and 4 is at least 6 months
- **DTaP** and **IPV** should be administered at or before school entry
- **HAV** (*hepatitis A vaccine*) is recommended for all children at 1 year (12-23 months) of age
- **HAV** 2-dose series should be administered at least 6 months apart
- **HBV** (*hepatitis B vaccine*) is a 3-dose series initiated at birth; administer 2nd dose at 1-2 months; administer the 3rd dose at age 6 months (not before ≥24 weeks)
- **HBV** should be offered to all children who have not received the full series
- Infants born to HVsAG-positive mothers should be tested for HBsAG and antibody to HBsAg after completion of the **HBV** series (at age 9-18 months)
- **Hib** (*hemophilus influenzae* type b conjugate vaccine) minimum age 6 months
- **Hib** is not recommended if age >5 years
- **HPV** (*human papillomavirus vaccine*) vaccine should be administered anytime between 11 and 12 years-of-age
- **HPV** is a 3-series vaccine administered months 0, 1, 6; females may receive HPV/4 or HPV/2; males should receive HPV/2
- **HPV** if not previously received at 11 or 12 years-of-age, may be initiated at any time between 13 and 26 years-of-age
- **IIV** (*inactivated influenza vaccine*) can be administered >6 months (use age-appropriate formulation), pregnant women, and persons with hives-only allergy to eggs
- **IHD** (*influenza high dose*) (**Fluzone High Dose**) may be recommended to persons ≥65 years of age
- **IPV** (*inactivated poliovirus vaccine*) minimum age 4 weeks
- An all-**IPV** schedule is recommended to eliminate the risk of vaccine-associated paralytic polio (VAPP) associated with **OPV** (*oral poliovirus vaccine*)
- **LAIV** (*live attenuated influenza vaccine*) may be administered intranasally (**FluMist**)
- **Men** (*meningococcal vaccine*) should be administered to all children at the 11-12 year old visit as well as to unvaccinated adolescents 15 years-of-age (usually at high school entry)
- **Men** should be administered to all college freshmen living in dormitories\
- Use MPSV4 for children aged 2-10 years and MCV4 for older children, although MPSV4 is an acceptable alternative for prophylaxis in men
- **MMR** (*mumps-measles-rubella*) should be administered at age 12 months in high-risk areas; if indicated, tuberculin testing can be done at the same visit
- **MMR** should be administered at age 11-12 years unless 2 doses were given after the first birthday; the interval between doses should be at least 4 weeks
- **MMR** adults born <1957 are generally considered immune to measles and mumps; all adults born ≥1957 should have documentation of at least I dose of MMR vaccine unless there is a medical contraindication or laboratory evidence of immunity to each of the 3 disease components; documentation of provider-diagnosed disease is not acceptable evidence of immunity to any of the 3 disease components

(continued)

Appendix G (*continued*)

- **PCV-13** (*pneumococcal vaccine*) does not replace 23-valent pneumococcal polysaccharide in children age ≥24 months
- **PCV-13** when PCV-13 and PCV-23 are indicated, administer PCV-13 first; do not administer PCV-13 and PCV-23 in the same visit
- **PCV-13** adults ≥65 years-of-age, who have not received PCV-13 or PCV-23, should receive PCV-13 followed by PCV-23 6-12 months later
- **PCV-23** (*pneumococcal vaccine 23 trivalent*) minimum age 6 weeks
- **PCV-23** adults ≥65 years of age, who have received **PCV-23**, but not received PCV-13, should receive. **PCV-13** at least I year later; adults ≥65 years of age, who have not received **PCV-23**, should receive
- **PCV-13** followed by **PCV-23** 6-12 months later
- **RIV** (*recombinant influenza vaccine*; **FluBlok**) may be administered to any adult >18 years-of-age, including pregnant women
- **RIV** does not contain any egg protein; can be administered to anyone with egg allergy at any severity
- Older infants and children previously vaccinated with **PCV** should receive 3 doses (if age 7-11 months), 2 doses (if age 12-23 months) or 1 dose (if age >24 months)
- **Rot** (*rotavirus vaccine*) is a live attenuated oral vaccine for infants age >6 weeks or <32 weeks *only*; administer the 1st dose at 6-12 weeks-of-age; administer 2nd and 3rd doses at 4-10-week intervals for a total of 3 doses
- **Rot** If an incomplete dose is administered, *do not* administer a replacement dose, but continue with the remaining doses in the recommended series
- **Td** (*tetanus-diphtheria vaccine*) should be repeated every 10 years throughout life (or if at-risk injury ≥5 years after previous dose)
- **Td** should *not* be administered until minimum age ≥7 years
- **TdaP** (*tetanus-diphtheria-acellular pertussis*) administer 1 dose to pregnant women during each pregnancy, preferably during 27-36 weeks gestation, regardless of interval since prior Td or TdaP
- **TdaP** persons ≥11 years of age who have not received **Tdap** vaccine or for whom vaccine status is unknown, should receive 1 dose of **TdaP** followed by a **Td** booster every 10 years
- **Var** should be administered to children at age 11-12 years who have not had chicken-pox or who report having had chickenpox but do not have laboratory documentation of immunity
- **Var** If not received between age 11 and 12 years, administer 2 doses at least 4 weeks apart anytime after 12 years-of-age or a 2nd dose if previously only received 1 dose
- **VarZ** (*herpes zoster vaccine*) should be administered in a single dose once at ≥60 years-of-age, whether or not the person reports a prior episode of active herpes zoster infection
- **VarZ** is contraindicated in pregnancy and immune deficiency
- DTaP and IPV can be initiated as early as 4 weeks in areas of high endemicity or outbreak.

¶Adapted from DHHS CDC 2015.

APPENDIX G.2. CONTRAINDICATIONS TO VACCINES

All vaccines	Previous anaphylactic reaction to the vaccine, moderate or severe illness with or without fever
Live or live attenuated (LAVs)	Immunocompromised, receiving immunosuppressive doses of corticosteroids
TDaP/DTaP, Td	Encephalopathy within 7 days of following previous dose
Hib	Previous anaphylactic reaction to the vaccine, moderate or severe illness with or without fever
HBV	Anaphylactic reaction to baker's yeast

(*continued*)

Appendix G.2. (*continued*)

HAV	Previous anaphylactic reaction to the vaccine Moderate or severe illness with or without fever
Influenza	Allergy to eggs (*except* **FluBlok** which does not contain any egg protein)
IPV	Anaphylactic reaction to neomycin or streptomycin
Pneumococcal	Hypersensitivity to diphtheria toxoid
MMR	Anaphylactic reaction to eggs or neomycin, pregnancy, immunocompromised (mumps, measles, rubella are LAVs)
Meningococcal	Encephalopathy within 7 days following previous dose
Rotavirus	<6 months or >32 months, (Rotavirus is an LAV)
HPV	Pregnancy (pregnancy testing is not required); however, if administered, defer the remaining dose(s) until completion or termination of pregnancy
Varicella	Pregnancy, immunocompromised (Varicella is an LAV)
Herpes zoster	Pregnancy (HZ is a live vaccine)

Adapted from DHHS CDC 2015.

APPENDIX G.3. ROUTE OF ADMINISTRATION AND DOSE OF VACCINES

Vaccine	Route	Dose
Single Vaccines		
Diphtheria-Tetanus-Pertussis (DTaP, Dtap, DT)	IM	0.5 ml
Haemophilus influenza type b (Hib)	IM	0.5 ml
Hepatitis A vaccine (HAV)	IM	0.5 ml: age <18 yrs 1.0 ml: age ≥19 yrs
Hepatitis B vaccine (HBV)	IM	0.5 ml: age <18 yrs 1.0 ml: age ≥19 yrs
Human Papillomavirus (HPV)	IM	0.5 ml
Influenza (**Fluzone Intradermal**)	ID	0.5 ml
Influenza, inactivated (IIV), recombinant (RIV)	IM	0.25 ml: age 6-35 months 0.5 ml: age ≥3 yrs
Influenza, live attenuated (LAIV)	NS	0.2 ml; 0.1 ml in each nostril
Meningococcal conjugate	IM	0.5 ml
Meningococcal polysaccharide (MPSV)	SC	0.5 ml
Meningococcal sero group B (Men B)	IM	0.5 ml
Mumps-Measles-Rubella (MMR)	SC	0.5 ml
Pneumococcal conjugate (PCV)	IM	0.5 ml
Pneumococcal polysaccharide (PPSV)	IM/SC	0.5 ml
Polio, Inactivated (IPV)	IM/SC	0.5 ml

(continued)

Appendix G.3. (*continued*)

Vaccine	Route	Dose
Rotavirus (**Rotarix**)	PO	1 ml
Rotavirus (**Rotateq**)	PO	2 ml
Tetanus (Td)	IM	0.5 ml
Varicella	SC	0.5 ml
Herpes Zoster	SC	0.65 ml: age ≥60 yrs
Combination Vaccines		
MMR-Var (**ProQuad**)	SC	0.5 ml: age ≤12 yrs
HBV-HAV (**Twinrix**)	IM	1 ml: >18 yrs
DTaP-HBV-IPV (**Pediarix**)	IM	0.5 ml
DTaP-IPV-Hib (**Pentacel**)	IM	0.5 ml
DTaP-IPV (**Kinrix, Quadracel**)	IM	0.5 ml
Hib-HBV (**Comvax**)	IM	0.5 ml
Hib-MenCY (**MenHibrix**)	IM	0.5 ml

Adapted from DHHS CDC 2015

APPENDIX G.4. ADVERSE REACTIONS TO VACCINES

Vaccine	Signs and Symptoms	Treatment
Inactivated antigens: DTP, Dtap, DTaP, Td, IPV, influenza inactivated (IIV) recombinant (RIV) Live attenuated viruses: MMR, Meningococcal, rotavirus, varicella, herpes zoster	Local tenderness Erythema Swelling Low-grade fever Drowsiness Fretfulness Decreased appetite Prolonged crying Unusual cry	*acetaminophen* or *ibuprofen* for age and/or weight; *aspirin* and *aspirin*-containing products are contraindicated

Adapted from DHHS CDC 2015.

APPENDIX G.5. MINIMUM INTERVALS BETWEEN VACCINE DOSES

Type	#1 to #2	#2 to #3	#3 to #4	#4 to #5
HBV	4 weeks	5 months		
HAV	6 months			
DTaP	4 weeks	4 weeks	6 months	6 months
IPV	4 weeks	4 weeks	4 weeks	
MMR	4 weeks			
Var	4 weeks			
Rotavirus	4 weeks	4 weeks; do not administer >32 weeks of age		

(*continued*)

Appendix G.5. *(continued)*

Type	#1 to #2	#2 to #3	#3 to #4	#4 to #5
PCV-13	4 weeks (if #1 at age <12 months and current age <24 months); 8 weeks (as last dose if #1 at age >12 months or current age 24-59 months); No more doses needed if healthy and #1 at age ≥24 months	4 weeks if age <12 months; 8 weeks (as last dose if age ≥12 months); No more doses needed if healthy and previous dose at age ≥24 months	8 weeks (as last dose; only necessary for age 12 months to 5 years who received 3 doses before age 12 months)	
Hib	4 weeks (if #1 at age <12 months); 8 weeks (as last dose if #1 at age 12-14 months); No more doses needed if healthy and #1 at age ≥15 months	4 weeks if age 12 months; 8 weeks (as last dose if age ≥12 months); No more doses needed if previous dose at age ≥15 months	8 weeks (as last dose; only necessary for age 12 months to 2 years who received 3 doses before age 12 months)	
HPV	4 weeks	20 weeks (24 weeks after #1		

Adapted from DHHS CDC 2015

APPENDIX G.6. RECOMMENDED CHILDHOOD (BIRTH-12 YEARS) IMMUNIZATION SCHEDULE

Type	Birth	1 month	2 months	4 months	6 months	6-18 months	12-15 months	15-18 months	4-6 years	11-12 years
HBV	✔	✔			✔					
DTaP			✔	✔	✔		✔		✔	
IPV			✔	✔		✔			✔	
Hib			✔	✔	✔		✔			
Rotavirus			✔	✔	✔					
MMR							✔		✔	
TDaP										✔
Varicella							✔		✔	
PVC-13			✔	✔	✔		✔			
HAV							✔	✔		
Meningitis										✔
HPV										✔✔✔

Adapted from DHHS CDC 2015.

✔ = immunization due.

✔✔✔ = HPV 3-dose series, months 0, 1, 6.

APPENDIX G.7. RECOMMENDED CHILDHOOD (BIRTH-12 YEARS) IMMUNIZATION CATCH-UP SCHEDULE

Vaccine	Minimum Interval Between Doses			
	#1 to #2	#2 to #3	#3 to #4	#4 to #5
HBV	4 weeks	8 weeks (16 weeks after #1)		
DTaP	4 weeks	4 weeks	6 months	6 months
IPV	4 weeks	4 weeks	4 weeks	
MMR	4 weeks			
Var	4 weeks			
Rotavirus	4 weeks	4 weeks; do not administer >32 weeks of age		
PCV	2 months	2 months	2 months	6-15 months
HPV	4 weeks	20 weeks (24 weeks after #1		

Adapted from DHHS CDC 2015

APPENDIX G.8. RECOMMENDED ADULT IMMUNIZATION SCHEDULE

Type	19-21 yrs	22-26 yrs	27-49 yrs	50-59 yrs	60-65 yrs	≥65 yrs
Influenza	1 dose annually					
HBV	3 dose series: months 0, 1, 6					
Td/TdaP	Substitute Tdap for Td one time; then continue Td once every 10 years					
MMR*	Born >1957: 2 doses, 4 weeks apart					
Varicella*	Without evidence of immunity: 2 doses, 4 weeks apart					
Herpes zoster*					1 time dose	
PVC-13/ PVC-23					1 time dose	
HAV	Single Antigen, 2 doses: months 0, 6-12 (**Havrix**); 0, 6-18 (**Vaqta**)					
Meningitis	1 or more doses					
HPV (female)*β	3 doses; months 0, 1, 6					
HPV (male)β	3 doses; months 0, 1, 6					

Adapted from DHHS CDC 2015
* Contraindicated in pregnancy
β Only if not previously vaccinated between 11-12 years-of-age

APPENDIX H. CONTRACEPTIVES

APPENDIX H.1. CONTRAINDICATIONS AND RECOMMENDATIONS

- All contraceptives are pregnancy category X
- No non-barrier contraceptives protect against STDs
- **Absolute Contraindication:**
  - HTN >35 years-of-age
  - DM >35 years-of-age
  - LDL-C >160 or TG >250
  - Known or suspected pregnancy
  - Known or suspected carcinoma of the breast
  - Known or suspected carcinoma of the endometrium
  - Known or suspected estrogen-dependent neoplasia
  - Undiagnosed abnormal genital bleeding
  - Cerebral vascular or coronary artery disease
  - Cholestatic jaundice of pregnancy or jaundice with prior use
  - Hepatic adenoma or carcinoma or benign liver tumor
  - Active or past history of thrombophlebitis or thromboembolic disorder
- **Relative Contraindications**
  - Lactation
  - Asthma
  - Ulcerative colitis
  - Migraine or vascular headache
  - Cardiac or renal dysfunction
  - Gestational diabetes, prediabetes, diabetes mellitus
  - Diastolic BP 90 mmHg or greater or hypertension by any other criteria
  - Psychic depression
  - Varicose veins
  - Smoker >35 years-of-age
  - Sickle-cell or sickle-hemoglobin C disease
  - Cholestatic jaundice during pregnancy, active gallbladder disease
  - Hepatitis or mononucleosis during the preceding year
  - First-order family history of fatal or nonfatal rheumatic CVD or diabetes prior to age 50 years
  - Drug(s) with known interaction(s)
  - Elective surgery or immobilization within 4 weeks
  - Age >50 years
- **Recommendations**
  - Start the first pill on the first Sunday after menses begins. Thereafter, each new pill pack will be started on a Sunday.
  - Take each daily pill in the same 3-hour window (e.g., 9A-12N, 12N-3P; a 4-hour window prior to bedtime is not recommended).
  - If 1 pill is missed, take it as soon as possible and the next pill at the regular time.
  - If 2 pills are missed, take both pills as soon as possible and then two pills the following day. A barrier method should be used for the remainder of the pill pack.
  - If 3 pills are missed before 10th cycle day, resume taking OCs on a regular schedule and take precautions.
  - If 3 pills are missed after the 10th cycle day, discard the current pill pack and begin a new one 7 days after the last pill was taken.
  - If very low-dose OCs are used or if combination OCs are begun after the 5th day of the menstrual cycle, an additional method of birth control should be used for the first 7 days of OC use.
  - If nausea occurs as a side effect, select an OC with *lower **estrogen*** content.

(continued)

Appendix H.1. (*continued*)

- If breakthrough bleeding occurs during the first half of the cycle, select an OC with *higher progesterone* content.
- Symptoms of a serious nature include loss of vision, diplopia, unilateral numbness, weakness, or tingling, severe chest pain, severe pain in left arm or neck, severe leg pain, slurring of speech, and abdominal tenderness or mass.

APPENDIX H.2. 28-DAY ORAL CONTRACEPTIVES WITH ESTROGEN AND PROGESTERONE CONTENT

Comment: Beyaz, Loryna, Rajani, Syeda, Safyral, Tydemy, Yasmin, and Yaz are contraindicated with renal insufficiency and adrenal insufficiency. Monitor k$^+$ level during the first cycle if the patient is at risk for hyperkalemia for any reason. If the patient is taking drugs that increase potassium (e.g., ACEIs, ARBS, NSAIDs, K$^+$ sparing diuretics), the patient is at risk for hyperkalemia.

Combined Oral Contraceptive	Estrogen (mcg)	Progesterone (mg)
Alesse-21, Alesse-28 (X)(G) *ethinyl estradiol+levonorgestrel*	20	0.1
Altavera (X) *ethinyl estradiol+levonorgestrel*	30	0.15
Apri (X)(G) *ethinyl estradiol+desogestrel*	30	0.15
Aranelle (X)(G) *ethinyl estradiol+norethindrone*	35	0.5 1 0.5
Aviane (X)(G) *ethinyl estradiol+levonorgestrel*	20	0.1
Balcoltra (X) *ethinyl estradiol+levonorgestrel* plus *ferrous bisglycinate* 36.5 mg	20	0.1
Balziva (X)(G) *ethinyl estradiol+norethindrone*	35	0.4
Beyaz (X)(G) *ethinyl estradiol+drospirenone* plus levomefolate calcium 0.451 mcg (28 tabs)	20	3
Blisovi 24Fe (X)(G) *ethinyl estradiol+norethindrone* plus *ferrous fumarate* 75 mg (4 tabs)	20	1
Brevicon-21, Brevicon-28 (X)(G) *ethinyl estradiol+norethindrone*	35	0.5
Camrese (X) *ethinyl estradiol+levonorgestrel*	30 10	0.15
Camrese Lo (X) *ethinyl estradiol+levonorgestrel*	20 10	0.1
Cesia (X)(G) *ethinyl estradiol+desogestrel*	25 25 25	0.1 0.125 0.15

(*continued*)

Appendix H.2. (continued)

Combined Oral Contraceptive	Estrogen (mcg)	Progesterone (mg)
Cryselle (X)(G) *ethinyl estradiol+norgestrel*	30	0.3
Cyclessa (X)(G) *ethinyl estradiol+desogestrel*	25 25 25	0.1 0.125 0.15
Demulen 1/35-21, Demulen 1/35-28 (X)(G) *ethinyl estradiol+ethynodiol diacetate*	35	1
Demulen 1/50-21, Demulen 1/50-28 (X)(G) *ethinyl estradiol+ethynodiol diacetate*	50	1
Desogen (X)(G) *ethinyl estradiol+desogestrel diacetate*	30	0.15
Enpresse (X)(G) *ethinyl estradiol+levonorgestrel*	30 40 30	0.05 0.075 0.125
Estrostep Fe (X) *ethinyl estradiol+norethindrone* plus *ferrous fumarate* 75 mg	20 30 35	1 1 1
Femcon Fe (X)(G) *ethinyl estradiol+norethindrone* <u>plus</u> *ferrous fumarate* 75 mg	35	0.4
Generess Fe Chew tab (X)(G) *ethinyl estradiol+norethindrone* <u>plus</u> *ferrous fumarate* 75 mg	25	0.8
Genora (X)(G) *ethinyl estradiol+norethindrone*	35 35 35	0.5 1 0.5
Gianvi (X)(G) *ethinyl estradiol+drospirenone*	20	3
Gildess 1.5/30 (X)(G) *ethinyl estradiol+norethindrone*	30	1.5
Introvale (X) *ethinyl estradiol+levonorgestrel*	30	0.15
Jenest-28 (X) *ethinyl estradiol+norethindrone*	35 35	0.5 1
Jolessa (X)(G) *ethinyl estradiol+levonorgestrel*	30	0.15
Junel 1/20 (X)(G) *ethinyl estradiol+norethindrone*	20	1
Junel 1.5/30 (X)(G) *ethinyl estradiol+norethindrone*	30	1.5
Junel Fe 1/20 (X)(G) *ethinyl estradiol+norethindrone* <u>plus</u> *ferrous fumarate* 75 mg	20	1

(continued)

Appendix H.2. *(continued)*

Combined Oral Contraceptive	Estrogen (mcg)	Progesterone (mg)
Junel Fe 1.5/30 (X)(G) *ethinyl estradiol+norethindrone* plus *ferrous fumarate* 75 mg	30	1.5
Kaitlib Fe Chew Tab (X)(G) *ethinyl estradiol+norethindrone* plus *ferrous fumarate* 75 mg	25	0.8
Kariva (X)(G) *ethinyl estradiol+desogestrel*	20 10	0.15 0.15
Kelnor 1/35 (X)(G) *ethinyl estradiol+ethynodiol diacetate*	35	1
Leena (X) *ethinyl estradiol+norethindrone*	35 35 35	0.5 1 0.5
Lessina 28 (X)(G) *ethinyl estradiol+levonorgestrel*	20	0.1
Levlen 21, Levlen 28 (X)(G) *ethinyl estradiol+levonorgestrel*	30	0.15
Levlite 28 (X)(G) *ethinyl estradiol+levonorgestrel*	20	0.1
Levora-21, Levora-28 (X)(G) *ethinyl estradiol+levonorgestrel*	30	0.15
Loestrin 21 1/20 (X)(G) *ethinyl estradiol+norethindrone*	20	1
Loestrin 21 1.5/30 (X)(G) *ethinyl estradiol+norethindrone*	30	1.5
Loestrin Fe 1/20 (X)(G) *ethinyl estradiol+norethindrone* plus *ferrous fumarate* 75 mg	20	1
Loestrin Fe 1.5/30 (X)(G) *ethinyl estradiol+norethindrone* plus *ferrous fumarate* 75 mg (4 tabs)	30	1.5
Loestrin 24 Fe (X)(G) *ethinyl estradiol+norethindrone* plus *ferrous fumarate* 75 mg (4 tabs)	20	1
Lo Loestrin Fe (X) *ethinyl estradiol+norethindrone* plus *ferrous fumarate* 75 mg (2 tabs)	10	1
Lomedia 24 Fe (X)(G) *ethinyl estradiol+norethindrone* plus *ferrous fumarate* 75 mg	20	1
Lo/Ovral-21, Lo/Ovral-28 (X)(G) *ethinyl estradiol+norgestrel*	30	0.3
Loryna (X) *ethinyl estradiol+drospirenone*	20	3

(continued)

Appendix H.2. (*continued*)

Combined Oral Contraceptive	Estrogen (mcg)	Progesterone (mg)
Low-Ogestrel-21, Low-Ogestrel-28 (X)(G) *ethinyl estradiol/norgestrel*	30	0.3
Lutera (X)(G) *ethinyl estradiol+levonorgestrel*	20	0.1
Lybrel (X) *ethinyl estradiol+levonorgestrel*	20	0.09
Mibelas 24 FE (X)(G) *ethinyl estradiol+norethindrone* plus *ferrous fumarate 75 mg*	20	1
Microgestin 1/20 (X)(G) *ethinyl estradiol+norethindrone*	20	1
Microgestin Fe 1/20 (X)(G) *ethinyl estradiol+norethindrone* plus *ferrous fumarate 75 mg*	20	1
Microgestin 1.5/30 (X)(G) *ethinyl estradiol+norethindrone*	30	1.5
Microgestin Fe 1.5/30 (X)(G) *ethinyl estradiol+norethindrone* plus *ferrous fumarate 75 mg*	30	1.5
Mircette (X)(G) *ethinyl estradiol+desogestrel diacetate*	20 10	0.15
Minastrin 24 FE (X)(G) *ethinyl estradiol+norethindrone* plus *ferrous fumarate 75 mg*	20	1
Modicon 0.5/35-28 (X)(G) *ethinyl estradiol+norethindrone*	35	0.5
MonoNessa (X)(G) *ethinyl estradiol+norgestimate*	35	0.25
Natazia (X)(G) *estradiol valerate+dienogest*	30 20 20 10	— 2 3 —
Necon 0.5/35-21, Necon 0.5/35-28 (X)(G) *ethinyl estradiol+norethindrone*	35	0.5
Necon 1/35-21, Necon 1/35-28 (X)(G) *ethinyl estradiol+norethindrone*	35	0.5
Necon 10/11-21, Necon 10/11-28 (X)(G) *ethinyl estradiol+norethindrone*	35 35	0.5 1
Necon 1/50-21, Necon 1/50-28 (X)(G) *mestranol+norethindrone*	50	1
Nelova 0.5/35-21, Nelova 0.5/35-28 (X)(G) *ethinyl estradiol+norethindrone*	35	0.5

(*continued*)

Appendix H.2. (*continued*)

Combined Oral Contraceptive	Estrogen (mcg)	Progesterone (mg)
Nelova 1/35-21, Nelova 1/35-28 (X)(G) *ethinyl estradiol+norethindrone*	35	1
Nelova 10/11-21, Nelova 10/11-28 (X)(G) *ethinyl estradiol/norethindrone*	35 35	0.5 1
Nelova 1/50-21, Nelova 1/50-28 (X)(G) *mestranol+norethindrone*	50	1
Neocon 7/7/7 (X)(G) *ethinyl estradiol+norethindrone*	35 35 35	0.5 0.75 1
Nordette-21, Nordette-28 (X)(G) *ethinyl estradiol+levonorgestrel*	30	0.15
Norinyl 1/35-21, Norinyl 1/35-28 (X)(G) *ethinyl estradiol+norethindrone*	35	1
Norinyl 1/50-21, Norinyl 1/50-28 (X)(G) *mestranol+norethindrone*	50	1
Nortrel 0.5/35 (X)(G) *ethinyl estradiol/norethindrone*	35	0.5
Nortrel 1/35-21, Nortrel 1/35-28 (X)(G) *ethinyl estradiol+norethindrone*	35	1
Nortrel 7/7/7-28 (X)(G) *ethinyl estradiol+norethindrone*	35 35 35	0.5 0.75 1
Ocella (X)(G) *ethinyl estradiol+drospirenone*	30	3
Ortho-Cept 28 (X)(G) *ethinyl estradiol+desogestrel*	30	0.15
Ortho-Cyclen 28 (X)(G) *ethinyl estradiol+norgestimate*	35	0.25
Ortho-Novum 1/35-21, Ortho-Novum 1/35-28 (X)(G) *ethinyl estradiol+norethindrone*	35	1
Ortho-Novum 1/50-21, Ortho-Novum 1/50-28 (X)(G) *mestranol+norethindrone*	50	1
Ortho-Novum 7/7/7-28 (X)(G) *ethinyl estradiol+norethindrone*	35 35 35	0.5 0.75 1
Ortho-Novum 10/11-28 (X) *ethinyl estradiol+norethindrone*	35 35	0.5 1
Ortho Tri-Cyclen 21, Ortho Tri-Cyclen 28 (X)(G) *ethinyl estradiol+norgestimate*	35 35 35	0.18 0.215 0.25

(*continued*)

Appendix H.2. (*continued*)

Combined Oral Contraceptive	Estrogen (mcg)	Progesterone (mg)
Ortho Tri-Cyclen Lo (X)(G) *ethinyl estradiol+norgestimate*	25 25 25	0.18 0.215 0.25
Ovcon 35 Fe (X)(G) *ethinyl estradiol+norethindrone* <u>plus</u> *ferrous fumarate* 75 mg (4 tabs)	35	0.4
Ovcon 50-28, Ovcon 50-28 (X)(G) *ethinyl estradiol+norethindrone*	50	1
Ovral-21, Ovral-28 (X)(G) *ethinyl estradiol+norgestrel*	50	0.5
Portia (X)(G) *ethinyl estradiol+levonorgestrel*	30	0.15
Previfem (X) *ethinyl estradiol+norgestimate*	35	0.25
Quasense (X) *ethinyl estradiol+levonorgestrel*	30	0.15
Rajani *ethinyl estradiol + drospirenone* <u>plus</u> *levomefolate calcium* 0.451 mg	20	3
Reclipsen (X)(G) *ethinyl estradiol+desogestrel* <u>plus</u> *ferrous fumarate* 75 mg (4 tabs)	30	0.15
Safyral (X)(G) *ethinyl estradiol+drospirenone* <u>plus</u> *levomefolate calcium* 0.451 mg	30	3
Sprintec 28 (X)(G) *ethinyl estradiol+norgestimate*	35	0.25
Syeda (X) *ethinyl estradiol+drospirenone*	30	3
Tarina Fe 1/20 (X)(G) *ethinyl estradiol+norethindrone* <u>plus</u> *ferrous fumarate* 75 mg (7 tabs)	20	1
Taytulla Fe 1/20 (X)(G) (Softgel caps) *ethinyl estradiol+norethindrone* <u>plus</u> *ferrous fumarate* 75 mg (4 Softgel caps)	20	1
Tilia Fe (X)(G) *ethinyl estradiol+norethindrone* <u>plus</u> *ferrous fumarate* 75 mg (7 tabs)	20 30 35	1 1 1
Tri-Legest 21 (X)(G) *ethinyl estradiol+norethindrone*	20 30 35	1 1 1

(*continued*)

Appendix H.2. (*continued*)

Combined Oral Contraceptive	Estrogen (mcg)	Progesterone (mg)
Tri-Legest Fe (X)(G) *ethinyl estradiol+norethindrone* plus *ferrous fumarate* 75 mg (7 tabs)	20 30 35	1 1 1
Tri-Levlen 21, Tri-Levlen 28 (X)(G) *ethinyl estradiol+levonorgestrel*	30 40 30	0.05 0.075 0.125
Tri-Lo-Estarylla (X)(G) *ethinyl estradiol+norgestimate*	25 25 25	0.18 0.215 0.25
Tri-Lo-Sprintec (X)(G) *ethinyl estradiol+norgestimate*	25 25 25	0.18 0.215 0.25
TriNessa (X)(G) *ethinyl estradiol+norgestimate*	35 35 35	0.18 0.215 0.25
Tri-Norinyl 21, Tri-Norinyl 28 (X)(G) *ethinyl estradiol+norethindrone*	35 35 35	0.5 1 0.5
Triphasil-21, Triphasil-28 (X)(G) *ethinyl estradiol+levonorgestrel*	30 40 30	0.050 0.075 0.125
Tri-Previfem (X)(G) *ethinyl estradiol+norgestimate*	35 35 35	0.18 0.215 0.25
Tri-Sprintec (X)(G) *ethinyl estradiol+norgestimate*	35 35 35	0.18 0.215 0.25
Trivora (X)(G) *ethinyl estradiol+levonorgestrel*	30 40 30	0.05 0.075 0.125
Tydemy *ethinyl estradiol+drospirenone* plus *levomefolate calcium* 0.451 mg	30	3
Velivet (X)(G) *ethinyl estradiol+desogestrel*	25 25 25	0.1 0.125 0.15
Yasmin (X)(G) *ethinyl estradiol+drospirenone*	30	3
Yaz (X)(G) *ethinyl estradiol+drospirenone*	20	3
Zovia 1/35E-28 (X)(G) *ethinyl estradiol+ethynodiol diacetate*	35	1
Zovia 1/50E-28 (X)(G) *ethinyl estradiol+ethynodiol diacetate*	50	1

APPENDIX H.3. EXTENDED-CYCLE ORAL CONTRACEPTIVES

91 Day

▶ *ethinyl estradiol+levonorgestrel* (X) 1 tab daily x 91 days; repeat (no tablet-free days)

Ashlyna (G) *Tab:* levonor 15 mcg+eth est 30 mcg (84)+eth est 10 mcg (7) (91 tabs/pck)

Jolessa (G) *Tab:* levonor 15 mcg+eth est 30 mcg (84)+inert tabs (7m91 tabs/pck)

LoSeasonique *Tab:* levonor 0.1 mcg+eth est 20 mcg (84)+eth est 10 mcg (7) (91 tabs/pck)

Quartette (G) *Tab:* levonor 15 mcg+eth est 30 mcg (84)+eth est 10 mcg (7) (91 tabs/pck)

Quasense (G) *Tab:* levonor 15 mcg+eth est 30 mcg (84)+eth est 10 mcg (7) (91 tabs/pck)

Seasonale (G) *Tab:* levonor 15 mcg+eth est 30 mcg (84)+inert tabs (7) (91 tabs/pck)

Seasonique (G) *Tab:* levonor 15 mcg+eth est 30 mcg (84)+eth est 10 mcg (7) (91 tabs/pck)

365 Day

▶ *ethinyl estradiol+levonorgestrel* (X) 1 tab daily x 28 days; repeat (no tablet-free days)

Lybrel *Tab:* levonor 0.09 mcg+eth est 20 mcg (28 tabs/pck)

APPENDIX H.4. PROGESTERONE-ONLY ORAL CONTRACEPTIVES ("MINI-PILL")

Brand	Progesterone	mcg
Comment: Take progestin-only pills at the same time each day (within a 3-hour time window). If a pill is missed, another method of contraception should be used for the remainder of the pill pack.		
Camila (X)(G)	*norethindrone*	35
Errin (X)(G)	*norethindrone*	35
Jolivette (X)(G)	*norethindrone*	35
Micronor (X)(G)	*norethindrone*	35
Nora-BE (X)(G)	*norethindrone*	35
Nor-QD (X)(G)	*norethindrone*	35
Ortho Micronor (X)(G)	*norethindrone*	35
Ovrette (X)(G)	*norgestrel*	7.5

APPENDIX H.5. INJECTABLE CONTRACEPTIVES

Injectable Progesterone

90 Days

Comment: Administer first dose within 5 days of onset of normal menses, within 5 days postpartum if not breastfeeding, or at 6 weeks postpartum if breastfeeding exclusively. Do not use for >2 years unless other methods are inadequate.

▶ *medroxyprogesterone* (X)(G)

Depo-Provera 150 mg deep IM q 3 months
Vial: 150 mg/ml (1 ml); *Prefilled syringe:* 150 mg/ml

Depo-SubQ 104 mg SC q 3 months
Prefilled syringe: 104 mg/ml (0.65 ml) (parabens)

APPENDIX H.6. TRANSDERMAL CONTRACEPTIVE

Ethinyl Estradiol+Norelgestromin

Comment: Apply the transdermal patch to the abdomen, buttock, upper-outer arm, or upper torso. *Do* not apply the transdermal patch to the breast. Rotate the site (however, may use the same anatomical area).

▶ *ethinyl estradiol+norelgestromin* (X)(G) apply one patch once weekly x 3 weeks; then 1 patch-free week; then repeat sequence

Ortho Evra
Transdermal patch: eth est 20 mcg+norel 150 mcg per day (1, 3/pck)

APPENDIX H.7. CONTRACEPTIVE VAGINAL RINGS

Ethinyl Estradiol+Etonogestrel

Comment: The vaginal ring should be inserted prior to, or on 5th day, of the menstrual cycle. Use of a backup method is recommended during the first week. When switching from oral contraceptives, the vaginal ring should be inserted anytime within 7 days after the last active tablet and no later than the day a new pill pack would have been started (no back up method is needed). If the ring is accidently expelled for less than 3 hours, it should be rinsed with cool to lukewarm water and reinserted promptly. If ring removal lasts for more than 3 hours, an additional contraceptive method should be used. If the ring is lost, a new ring should be inserted and the regimen continued without alteration.

▷ *etonogestrel+ethinyl estradiol* (X) insert 1 ring vaginally and leave in place for 3 weeks; then remove for 1 ring-free week; then repeat
    NuvaRing *Vag ring:* eth est 2.7 mg (0.015 mg/day)+*etonnorgestrel* 11.7mg (0.12 mg/ day) (1, 3/pck) (polymeric)

▷ *segesterone acetate+ethinyl estradiol* (X) insert 1 ring vaginally and leave in place for 3 weeks (21 on-days); then, remove, clean, and store in the compact storage case suppled; after 7 off-days, clean and re-insert for the next 21 on-day/7 off-day cycle; discard the ring after 13 cycles
    Annovera *Vag ring:* eth est 17.4 mg (0.013 mg/day)+segest 103 mg (0.15 mg/day) (1/ pck w. compact case)(silicone elastomer)

Comment: Contraindications to **Annovera/NuvaRing** include co-administration with hepatitis C drug combinations containing *ombitasvir+paritaprevir+ritonavir,* with or without *dasabuvir,* age >35 years, smoking, risk of arterial or venous thrombotic diseases, breast cancer or other estrogen or progestin-sensitive cancer, liver tumors or liver disease, acute hepatitis or cirrhosis, undiagnosed abnormal uterine bleeding, pregnancy. Stop **Annovera/NuvaRing** at least 4 weeks before and through 2 weeks after major surgery. **Annovera/NuvaRing** are not recommended with breastfeeding. Start no earlier than 4 weeks after delivery in females who are not breastfeeding. Drugs or herbal products that induce certain enzymes, including CYP3A4, may decrease the effectiveness of **Annovera/NuvaRing** or increase breakthrough bleeding. Counsel patients to use a back-up or alternative method of contraception when enzyme inducers are used.

Comment: **NuvaRing** is a polymeric vaginal ring containing 11.7 mg *etonogestrel* and 2.7 mg *ethinyl estradiol,* which releases on average 0.12 mg/day of *etonogestrel* and 0.015 mg/ day of *ethinyl estradiol.* Do not re-use **NuvaRing** (discard after 3 weeks in-use and after 7 days, start the next cycle with a new **NuvaRing.**

Comment: The **Annovera** vaginal system (ring) is a silicone elastomer vaginal system containing 103 mg *segesterone acetate* and 17.4 mg *ethinyl estradiol,* which releases on average 0.15 mg/day of *segesterone acetate* and 0.013 mg/day of *ethinyl estradiol.* **Annovera** is the first and only vaginal system/ring that provides contraception for 13 cycles. The removed vaginal system should be cleaned with mild soap and warm water, patted dry with a clean cloth towel or paper towel, and stored in the case provided during the one-week dose-free interval. At the end of the dose-free interval, the vaginal system should be cleaned prior to being placed back in the vagina for the next cycle.

APPENDIX H.8. SUBDERMAL CONTRACEPTIVES

Comment: Implants must be inserted within 7 days of the onset of menses. A complete physical examination is required annually. Remove if pregnancy, thromboembolic disorder including thrombophlebitis, jaundice, visual disturbances. Not for use by patients with hypertension, diabetes, hyperlipidemia, impaired liver function, epilepsy, asthma, migraine, depression, cardiac or renal insufficiency, thromboembolic disorder including thrombophlebitis, pro-longed immobilization, or who are smokers.

▷ *etonogestrel* (X) implant rod subdermally in the upper inner non-dominant arm; remove and replace at the end of 3 years
    Implanon, Nexplanon
    Implantable rod: 68 mg implant for subdermal insertion (w. insertion device; latex-free)

(continued)

Appendix H.8. (*continued*)

➤ *levonorgestrel* (X) implant rods subdermally in the upper inner non-dominant arm; remove and replace at the end of 5 years

    Norplant

        Implantable rods: 6-36 mg implants (total 216 mg) for subdermal insertion (1 kit w. sterile supplies)

APPENDIX H.9. INTRAUTERINE CONTRACEPTIVES

Comment: Indicated in women who have had at least one child and who are in a stable, mutually monogamous relationship. Reexamine after menses within 3 months (recommend 4-6 weeks) to check placement.

➤ *levonorgestrel* (X)

    Kyleena *IUD:* 19.5 mg (replace at least every 5 years)

    Liletta *IUD:* 52 mg (replace at least every 3 years)

    Mirena *IUD:* 52 mg (replace at least every 5 years)

    Skyla *IUD:* 13.5 mg (replace at least every 3 years)

APPENDIX H.10. EMERGENCY CONTRACEPTION

Comment: Emergency contraception must be started within 72 hours after unprotected intercourse following a negative urine hCG pregnancy test. If vomiting occurs within 1 hour of taking a dose, repeat the dose.

➤ *ethinyl estradiol+levonorgestrel* (X) 2 tabs as soon as possible after unprotected intercourse or contraceptive failure, then 2 more 12 hours after first dose

    Premenarchal: not applicable

    Preven *Tab:* eth est 50 mcg+levonor 250 mcg (4/pck) *plus Pregnancy test:* 1 hCG home pregnancy test

    Yuzpe Regimen *Tab:* eth est 50 mcg+levonor 250 mcg (4/pck)

➤ *levonorgestrel* (X)(OTC)(G) 1 tab as soon as possible, within 72 hours, after unprotected sex or suspected contraceptive failure

    Premenarchal: not applicable; <17 years (prescription required); ≥17 years (OTC)

    EContra EZ *Tab:* 1.5 mg single-dose

    My Way *Tab:* 1.5 mg single-dose

    Plan B One Step *Tab:* 1.5 mg single-dose

    EContra EZ *Tab:* 1.5 mg single-dose

    Preventeza *Tab:* 1.5 mg single-dose

➤ *ulipristal* (X)(G) take 1 tab as soon as possible within 120 hours (5 days) after unprotected intercourse or contraceptive failure; may repeat dose if vomiting occurs within 3 hours

    Pediatric: premenarchal: not applicable

    ella *Tab:* 30 mg (1/pck)

    Logilia *Tab:* 30 mg (1/pck)

APPENDIX I. ANESTHETIC AGENTS FOR LOCAL INFILTRATION AND DERMAL/MUCOSAL MEMBRANE APPLICATION

Agents and Indications	
Brand/*generic*	**Indication(s)**
AnaMantle HC *lidocaine 3%+hydrocortisone 0.5%*	Local anesthetic+steroid; for hemorrhoids, pruritus ani, anal fissure
Decadron Phosphate with Xylocaine *dexamethasone 4 mg+lidocaine 10 mg/ml (5 ml)*	Local anesthetic+steroid; infiltration by injection
Dyclone *dyclonine 0.5%, 0.1%*	Local anesthetic; infiltration by injection

(continued)

Appendix I (*continued*)

Agents and Indications	
Brand/*generic*	**Indication(s)**
Duranest (B) *etidocaine 1% (30 ml)* **Duranest (B) w. Epinephrine** *Inj:* etido 1.5%+epi *1:200,000* (30 ml) *Dental Cartridge:* etido 1.5%+epi *1:200,000* (1.8 ml)	Nerve block and local anesthetic; mouth, pharynx, larynx, trachea, esophagus, anogenital area, urethra Local anesthetic: dental procedures
Ela-Max 4% Cream (B) *lidocaine 4%* **Ela-Max 5% Cream (B)** *lidocaine 5%*	Local dermal anesthetic and for anorectal irritation and pain
Emla Cream (B) (5, 30 gm) **Emla Anesthetic Disc (B)** (2 discs/box) *lidocaine 2.5%+prilocaine 2.5%*	Local dermal anesthetic; preparation for phlebotomy, PIV starts, injections
Flector Patch (C/D) (30/box) *diclofenac epolamine 180 mg*	Local dermal NSAID analgesic
Exparel (B) *Vial:* 13.3 mg/ml (20 ml) *bupivacaine liposome 1.3% susp for inj*	Surgical site injection for postop pain management
LidaMantle (B) cream (1, 2 oz) **LidaMantle (B)** lotion (177 ml) **Lidoderm cream (B)** (85 gm) *lidocaine 3%* **Lidoderm (B)(G)** adhesive patch (10 cm x14 cm; 30/box) *lidocaine 5%*	Local dermal anesthetic lotion, cream, and adhesive patch
Ophthaine (B) (15 ml) *proparacaine 0.5% ophthalmic solution*	Ophthalmic anesthetic for examination and removal of foreign body (eye)
Pliaglis Cream (B) (30 g) *lidocaine 7%+tetracaine 7%*	Local dermal anesthetic for superficial dermatological procedures
Qutenza (B) (1, 2 patches, each *with 50 g tube of cleansing gel*) *capsaicin 8% patch*	Local dermal NSAID analgesic for postherpetic neuralgia
Septocaine, Ultican (G) *articaine hcl+epinephrine 4%/1:200,000*	Local, infiltrate, or conductive anesthesia in both simple and complex dental procedures
Synera Topical Patch (B) (2, 10/pck) *lidocaine 70 mg+tetracaine 70 mg*	Local dermal anesthetic for venous access or skin lesion removal
Tetracaine Ophthalmic Solution (B) (15 ml) *proparacaine 0.5% ophthalmic solution*	Ophthalmic anesthetic for examination/removal of foreign body (eye)
Xylocaine Jelly (B) (5, 10, 20, 30 ml) *lidocaine 2% aqueous*	For procedures of the urethra, painful urethritis, and endotracheal intubation
Xylocaine Ointment (B) (3.5, 35 gm) *lidocaine 5% water miscible*	For procedures of the urethra, painful urethritis, and endotracheal intubation

(*continued*)

Appendix I (*continued*)

Agents and Indications	
Brand/*generic*	**Indication(s)**
Xylocaine Topical Solution (B) (100 ml) *lidocaine 2% solution* **Xylocaine Viscous (B)** (50 ml) *lidocaine 2% viscous solution*	Anesthetic for the nasal and oropharyngeal mucosa and the proximal portions of the GI tract
Zingo *lidocaine monohydrate 0.5 mg*	Hand-held, needle-free device, helium-powered delivery system that numbs site in 1-3 minutes delivers 0.5 mg sterile lidocaine HCL monohydrate sterile lidocaine HCL pwdr for intradermal injection for the management of venous access pain
Zostrix (B) (0.7, 1.5, 3 oz) *capsaicin 0.025% cream* **Zostrix HP (B)** (1, 2 oz) *capsaicin 0.075% emollient cream*	Local dermal NSAID analgesic

APPENDIX J. NSAIDs

Comment: NSAIDs should be taken with food to decrease gastric upset. Dosing of NSAIDs should be scheduled rather than PRN for maximal benefit. NSAIDs are contraindicated with sulfonamide or *aspirin* allergy, 3rd trimester pregnancy (causes premature closure of the ductus arteriosus), and coronary artery bypass graft (CABG) surgery. Concomitant use of *misoprostol* (**Cytotec**) with NSAIDs reduces gastric upset and potential for ulceration; however, *misoprostol* is pregnancy category X. Administration of *misoprostol* in pregnancy can cause spontaneous abortion, premature birth, birth defects, and uterine rupture (beyond the 8th week of pregnancy). NSAIDs and *warfarin* (**Coumadin**) are synergistic. With all patients, use the lowest effective dose for the shortest time necessary. NSAIDs should be taken with food to reduce the risk of gastrointestinal adverse side effects (GIASE).

Legend: GI Adverse Side Effects:
(+) mild; (++) frequent; (+++) more frequent/severe

▷ *celecoxib* (C/D)(G)(+) 100 mg twice daily or 200 mg once daily or 200 mg twice daily or 400 mg once daily; <50 kg, start at lowest dose
Pediatric: <2 years: not recommended; ≥2 years, >10<25 kg: 50 mg twice daily; ≥25 kg: 100 mg once daily
Celebrex *Cap:* 50, 100, 200, 400 mg

▷ *diclofenac potassium* (C/D)(G)(+++) 50 mg tid or qid or 25 mg tid or qid and may add 25 mg at HS
Pediatric: <12 years: not recommended; ≥12 years: same as adult
Cataflam *Tab:* 50 mg
Zipsor *Gel cap:* 25 mg

▷ *diclofenac sodium* (D)(+++)
Pediatric: <12 years: not recommended; ≥12 years: same as adult
Dyloject administer 37.5 mg IV bolus over 15 seconds q 6 hours; max 150 mg/day
Vial: 37.5 mg/ml (25/box)
Pennsaid 1% in 10 drop increments, dispense and rub into front, side, and back of knee: usually 40 drops (40 mg) qid
Topical soln: 1.5% (150 ml)
Pennsaid 2% apply 2 pump actuations (40 mg) and rub into front, side, and back of knee bid
Topical soln: 2% (20 mg/pump actuation; 112 g)

(*continued*)

Appendix J (continued)

       Solaraze Gel apply to affected areas bid
         Gel: 3% (30 mg (100 g)
       Voltaren 50 mg bid <u>or</u> qid <u>or</u> 75 mg bid <u>or</u> 25 mg qid with an additional 25 mg at HS if necessary
         Tab: 25, 50, 75 mg ent-coat
       Voltaren XR 100 mg once daily; rarely, 100 mg bid may be used
         Tab: 100 mg ext-rel
       Zorvolex 35 mg tid
         Gelcap: 18, 35 mg ext-rel

▷ *diclofenac sodium+misoprostol* (X)(++)
   Pediatric: <12 years: not recommended; ≥12 years: same as adult
      Arthrotec *Tab:* 50, 75 mg

▷ *diflunisal* (C/D)(G)(+++) initially 1 gm as a single dose followed by 500 mg q 8-12 hours <u>or</u> 500 mg as a single dose followed by 250 mg q 8-12 hours
   Pediatric: <12 years: not recommended; ≥12 years: same as adult
      Dolobid *Tab:* 500*mg

▷ *etodolac* (C/D)(G)(+)
   Pediatric: <12 years: not recommended; ≥12 years: same as adult
      Lodine initially 600 mg to 1 gm/day in 2-3 divided doses; usual max 1 gm/day in divided doses; may increase to 1.2 g/day when needed
         Tab: 400, 500 mg; *Cap:* 200, 300 mg
      Lodine XL 400 mg to 1 gm once daily; max 1.2 g/day
         Tab: 400, 500, 600 mg ext-rel

▷ *fenoprofen* (B/D)(++) 300-600 mg tid-qid; max 3.2 g/day
   Pediatric: <12 years: not recommended; ≥12 years: same as adult
      Nalfon *Tab:* 200 mg

▷ *flurbiprofen* (B/D)(G)(++) 200-300 mg/day in 2-4 divided doses; max single dose 100 mg; reduce dosage for renal impairment
   Pediatric: <12 years: not recommended; ≥12 years: same as adult
      Ansaid *Tab:* 50, 100 mg

▷ *ibuprofen+famotidine* (B/D)(++) 1 tab 3 times daily; swallow whole; use lowest effective dose for the shortest duration
   Pediatric: <12 years: not recommended; ≥12 years: same as adult
      Duexis *Tab:* ibu 800 mg/fam 26.6 mg

▷ *indomethacin* (B/D)(G)(+++) 75-100 mg daily in 3-4 divided doses; max 200 mg/day
   Pediatric: <14 years: not recommended; ≥14 years: same as adult
      Indocin *Cap:* 25, 50 mg; *Rectal supp:* 50 mg; *Oral susp:* 25 mg/5 ml; *Vial:* 1 mg pwdr for reconstitution and IV infusion
      Indocin SR *Cap:* 75 mg ext-rel
      Tivorbex *Cap:* 20, 40 mg

▷ *ketoprofen* (C/D)(G)(++) 75 mg tid <u>or</u> 50 mg qid; max 300 mg/day
   Pediatric: <18 years: not recommended; ≥18 years: same as adult
      Orudis *Cap:* 50, 75 mg
      Oruvail *Cap:* 100, 150, 200 mg ext-rel

▷ *ketorolac tromethamine* (C/D)(G)(+++)
   Pediatric: <17 years: not recommended; ≥17 years: same as adult
      Sprix *17-64 years:* 1 spray each nostril (total dose 31,5 mg) every 6-8 hours prn; max 4 doses/24 hours (total daily dose 126 mg); *≥65 years, renal impairment or <50 kg:* 1 spray in one nostril (total dose 15.75 mg) every 6-8 hours; max 4 doses/24 hours (63 mg); discard used bottle after 24 hours
       Nasal spray: 15.75 mg/100 mcl nasal spray (8 sprays, 1.7 g)
      Toradol 60 mg as a single IM dose; max 30 mg as a single IV dose; may administer 30 mg IV and 30 mg IM as a single dose; oral dosing is indicated <u>*only*</u> as continuation therapy to IM <u>or</u> IV dosing; oral formulation should <u>*never*</u> be administered as an initial

(continued)

Appendix J (*continued*)

dose; initiate oral dosing at 20 mg followed by 10 mg q 4-6 hours prn; max oral dosing 40 mg/day; >65 years, initiate oral dosing at 10 mg followed by 10 mg q 4-6 hours prn; max 40 mg/day; the combined duration of IV/IM/PO dosing is not to exceed 5 days
> Tab: 10 mg; *Inj* 15, 30, 60 mg/ml

▷ *magnesium choline trisalicylate* (C/D)(G)(+)
Pediatric: <12 years: not recommended; ≥12 years: same as adult
> **Trilisate** *Tab:* 500*, 750*mg; 1*gm; *Oral susp:* 5 mg/5 ml (cherry cordial)

▷ *meclofenamate sodium* (B/D)(G)(++) 50-100 mg q 4-6 hours *or* 300-400 mg/day in 3-4 equal doses; max 400 mg/day
Pediatric: <14 years: not recommended; ≥14 years: same as adult
> **Meclofen** *Cap:* 50, 100 mg

▷ *mefenamic acid* (C)(G)(++) 500 mg once; then, 250 mg q 6 hours
Pediatric: <14 years: not recommended; ≥14 years: same as adult
> **Ponstel** *Cap:* 250 mg

▷ *meloxicam* (C/D)(G)(+) 7.5 mg once daily; max 15 mg/day; hemodialysis max 7.5 mg/day
Pediatric: <2 years: not recommended; ≥2 years: 0.125 mg/kg; max 7.5 mg once daily
> **Mobic** *Tab:* 7.5, 15 mg; *Oral susp:* 7.5 mg/5 ml (100 ml) (raspberry)

▷ *nabumetone* (C/D)(G)(+) 1-2 gm/day in a single dose *or* 2 divided doses; max 2 gm/day; <50 kg, max 1 gm/day
Pediatric: <12 years: not recommended; ≥12 years: same as adult
> *Tab:* 500, 750 mg

▷ *naproxen* (B)(G)(++) 275-550 mg twice daily *or* 275 mg every 6-8 hours; max 1.375 gm first day; then, max 1.1 gm/day; acute gout: 825 mg once, then 275 mg every 8 hours
Pediatric: <2 years: not recommended; ≥2 years: 5 mg/kg bid; max 15 mg/kg/day has been used; use suspension
> **Naprosyn** *Tab:* 250, 375, 500 mg
> **Naprosyn Suspension** *Oral susp:* 125 mg/5 ml

▷ *naproxen+esomeprazole (as magnesium trihydrate)* (C/D)(++)(G) one 375/20 *or* one 500/20 tab twice daily; take at least 30 minutes before meals; take lowest effective dose
Pediatric: <18 years: not recommended; ≥18 years: same as adult
> **Vimovo 375/20** *Tab:* nap 375 mg+eso 20 mg
> **Vimovo 500/20** *Tab:* nap 500 mg+eso 20 mg

▷ *oxaprozin* (C/D)(++) 1.2 gm once daily; max 1.8 gm *or* 26 mg/kg daily, whichever is less, in divided doses; low body weight, milder disease, *or* on dialysis: initially 600 mg once daily; max 1.2 gm daily
Pediatric: <6 years: not recommended; 6-16 years, 21-31 kg: 600 mg once daily; 32-54 kg: 900 mg once daily; ≥55 kg: 1.2 gm once daily
> **Daypro** *Tab:* 600*

▷ *piroxicam* (C/D)(G)(+++) 20 mg once daily
Pediatric: <12 years: not recommended; ≥12 years: same as adult
> **Feldene** *Cap:* 10, 20 mg

Comment: Because of the long half-life, steady state blood levels of *piroxicam* are not reached for 7-12 days. Therefore, expect a progressive response over several weeks.

▷ *salsalate* (C/D)(G)(+) 1.5 gm bid *or* 1 gm tid
Pediatric: <12 years: not recommended; ≥12 years: same as adult: 500*, 750*mg
> *Cap:* 500 mg

▷ *sulindac* (B/D)(G)(+++) 150-200 mg bid; max 400 mg/day; usually x 7-14 days
Pediatric: <14 years: not recommended; ≥14 years: same as adult
> **Clinoril** *Tab:* 150*, 200*mg

▷ *tolmetin* (C/D)(G)(+++) initially 400 mg tid; usual range 600 mg to 1.8 gm/day in divided doses; max 1,800 mg/day
Pediatric: <2 years: not recommended; ≥2 years: 20 mg/kg divided tid to qid; usual range 15-30 mg/kg/day divided tid to qid: max 30 mg/kg/day
> *Tab:* 200*mg

(*continued*)

Appendix J (*continued*)

▷ *piroxicam* (C/D)(G)(+++) 20 mg once daily
  Pediatric: not recommended
    Feldene *Cap:* 10, 20 mg

 APPENDIX K. TOPICAL CORTICOSTEROIDS BY POTENCY

Comment: All topical, oral, and parenteral corticosteroids are pregnancy category C. Use with caution in infants and children. Steroids should be applied sparingly and for the shortest time necessary. Do not use in the diaper area. Do not use an occlusive dressing. Systemic absorption of topical corticosteroids can induce reversible hypothalamic-pituitary-adrenal (HPA) axis suppression with the potential for clinical glucocorticoid insufficiency.

Potency guide: Face: Low potency
                  Ears/Scalp margin: Intermediate potency
                  Eyelids: Hydrocortisone in ophthalmic ointment base 1%
                  Chest/Back: Intermediate potency
                  Skin folds: Low potency

Generic Name and Pregnancy Category	Brands, Formulation, and Dosing Frequency	Strength and Volume
Low Potency		
alclometasone dipropionate (C)	**Aclovate** Crm bid-tid **Aclovate** Oint bid-tid	0.05% (15,45, 60 gm) 0.05% (15,45, 60 gm)
fluocinolone acetonide (C)	**Synalar** Crm bid-qid	0.025% (15, 60 gm)
hydrocortisone base or acetate (C)(G)	**Anusol-HC** Crm bid-qid **Hytone** Crm bid-qid **Hytone** Oint bid-qid **Hytone** Lotn bid-qid	2.5% (30 gm) 1% (1, 2 oz) 1% (1 oz) 1% (2 oz)
	Hytone Crm bid-qid **Hytone** Oint bid-qid **Hytone** Lotn bid-qid **U-cort** Crm bid-qid	2.5% (1, 2 oz) 2.5% (1 oz) 2.5% (1 oz) 1% (7, 28, 35 gm)
triamcinolone acetonide (C)(G)	**Kenalog** Crm bid-qid **Kenalog** Lotn bid-qid **Kenalog** Oint bid-qid	0.025% (15, 80 gm) 0.025% (60 ml) 0.025% (15, 60, 80 gm)
Intermediate Potency		
betamethasone valerate (C)(G)	**Luxiq** Foam bid	0.12% (100 gm)
clocortolone pivalate (C)	**Cloderm** Crm bid	0.1% (30, 45, 75, 90 gm)
desonide (C)(G)	**Desonate** Gel/Formulation bid-tid **DesOwen** Crm bid-tid **DesOwen** Lotn bid-tid **DesOwen** Oint bid-tid **Tridesilon** Crm bid-qid **Tridesilon** Oint bid-qid **Verdeso** Foam	0.05% (15, 60 gm) 0.05% (15, 60 gm) 0.05% (2, 4 fl oz) 0.05% (15, 60 gm) 0.05% (15, 60 gm) 0.05% (15, 60 gm)
desoximetasone (C)(G)	**Topicort-LP** Emol Crm bid	0.05% (15, 60 gm; 4 oz)

(*continued*)

Appendix K (*continued*)

Generic Name and Pregnancy Category	Brands, Formulation, and Dosing Frequency	Strength and Volume
fluocinolone acetonide (C) (G)	**Capex** Shampoo **Derma-Smoothe/FS** Oil tid **Derma-Smoothe/FS** Shampoo **Synalar** Crm bid-qid **Synalar** Oint bid-qid	0.01% (4 oz) 0.01% (4 oz) 0.01% (4 oz) 0.025% (15, 30, 60 gm) 0.025% (15, 60 gm)
flurandrenolide (C)(G)	**Cordran-SP** Crm bid to tid **Cordran** Oint bid-tid **Cordran-SP** Crm bid-tid **Cordran** Lotn bid-tid **Cordran** Oint bid-tid	0.025% (30, 60 gm) 0.025% (30, 60 gm) 0.05% (15, 30, 60 gm) 0.05% (15, 60 ml) 0.05% (15, 30, 60 gm)
fluticasone propionate (C) (G)	**Cutivate** Oint bid **Cutivate** Crm qd-bid **Cutivate** Lotn qd-bid	0.005% (15, 30, 60 gm) 0.05% (15, 30, 60 gm) 0.05%
hydrocortisone probutate (C)	**Pandel** Crm qd-bid	0.1% (15, 45 gm)
hydrocortisone butyrate (C)(G)	**Locoid** Crm bid-tid **Locoid** Oint bid-tid **Locoid** Soln bid-tid	0.1% (15, 45 gm) 0.1% (15, 45 gm) 0.1% (30, 60 ml)
hydrocortisone valerate (C) (G)	**Westcort** Crm bid-tid **Westcort** Oint bid-tid	0.2% (15, 45, 60, 120 gm) 0.2% (15, 45, 60 gm)
mometasone furoate (C)	**Elocon** Crm qd **Elocon** Lotn qd **Elocon** Oint qd	0.1% (15, 45 gm) 0.1% (30, 60 ml) 0.1% (15, 45 gm)
prednicarbate	**Dermatop** Emol Crm bid **Dermatop** Oint bid	0.1% (15, 60 gm)
triamcinolone acetonide (C)(G)	**Kenalog** Crm bid-tid **Kenalog** Lotn bid-tid **Kenalog** Emul Spray bid-tid	0.1% (15, 60, 80 gm) 0.1% (60 ml) 0.2% (63, 100 gm)
High Potency		
amcinonide (C)(G)	Crm bid-tid Lotn bid Oint bid	0.1% (15, 30, 60 gm) 0.1% (20, 60 ml) 0.1% (15, 30, 60 gm)
Betamethasone dipropionate (C)	**Sernivo Spray** Emul Spray bid	0.05% (60, 120 ml)
betamethasone dipropionate, augmented (C)	**Diprolene AF** Emol Crm qd-bid **Diprolene** Lotn qd-bid	0.05% (15, 50 gm) 0.05% (30, 60 ml)
clobetasol propionate (C)(G)	**Bryhali** Lotn bid **Impoyz** Crm bid	0.01% (60, 112 gm) 0.025% (60, 112 gm)

(*continued*)

Appendix K (*continued*)

Generic Name and Pregnancy Category	Brands, Formulation, and Dosing Frequency	Strength and Volume
desoximetasone (C)(G)	**Topicort** Gel bid **Topicort** Emol Crm bid **Topicort** Oint bid	0.05% (15, 60 gm) 0.25% (15, 60 gm) 0.25% (15, 60 gm)
diflorasone diacetate (C)	**Psorcon e** Emol Crm bid **Psorcon e** Emol Oint qd-tid	0.05% (15, 30, 60 gm) 0.05% (15, 30, 60 gm)
fluocinonide (C)	**Lidex** Crm bid-qid **Lidex** Gel bid-qid **Lidex** Oint bid-qid **Lidex** Soln bid-qid **Lidex-E** Emol Crm bid-qid	0.05% (15, 30, 60, 120 gm) 0.05% (15, 30, 60 gm) 0.05% (15, 30, 60, 120 gm) 0.05% (20, 60 ml) 0.05% (15, 30, 60 gm)
flurandrenolide (C)	**Cordan** Oint bid-tid **Cordan** Crm bid-tid	0.05% (15, 30, 60 gm) 0.025% (30, 60, 120 gm) 0.05% (15, 30, 60, 120 gm)
halcinonide (C)	**Halog** Crm bid-tid **Halog** Oint bid-tid **Halog** Soln bid-tid **Halog-E** Emol Crm qd-tid	0.1% (15, 30, 60, 240 gm) 0.1% (15, 30, 60, 120 gm) 0.1% (20, 60 ml) 0.1% (15, 30, 60 gm)
triamcinolone acetonide (C)(G)	**Kenalog** Crm bid-tid	0.5% (20 gm)
Super High Potency		
betamethasone dipropionate, augmented (C)(G)	**Diprolene** Oint qd-bid **Diprolene** Gel qd-bid	0.05% (15, 50 gm) 0.05% (15, 50 gm)
clobetasol propionate (C)(G)	**Bryhali** Lotn bid **Clobex** Shampoo daily **Clobex** Spray bid **Cormax** Oint bid **Cormax** Scalp App **Olux** Foam **Olux E** Foam **Temovate** Crm bid **Temovate** Gel bid **Temovate** Oint bid	0.01% (60, 112 gm) 0.05% (4 oz) 0.05% (2, 4.5 oz) 0.05% (15, 45 gm) 0.05% (15, 45 gm) 0.05% (50, 100 gm) 0.05% (50, 100 gm) 0.05% (15, 30, 45, 60 gm) 0.05% (15, 30, 60 gm) 0.05% (15, 30, 45, 60 gm)
	Temovate Scalp App bid **Temovate-E** Emol Crm bid	0.05% (25, 50 ml) 0.05% (15, 30, 60 gm)
fluocinonide (C)(G)	**Vanos** Oint qd-tid	0.1% (30, 60, 120 gm)
flurandrenolide (C)	**Cordran** Tape q 12 hours	4 mcg/sq cm (roll of 3″x 80″)
halobetasol propionate (C)	**Ultravate** Crm qd-bid **Ultravate** Oint qd to bid	0.05% (15, 45 gm) 0.05% (15, 45 gm)

APPENDIX L. ORAL CORTICOSTEROIDS

Comment: Systemic corticosteroids increase glucose intolerance, reduce the action of insulin and oral hypoglycemic agents, reduce adrenal cortex activity, decrease immunity, mask signs of infection, impair wound healing, suppress growth in children, and promote osteoporosis, fluid retention, and weight gain. Use systemic steroids with caution, using the lowest possible dose to affect clinical response, and withdraw (wean) gradually in tapering doses to avoid adrenal insufficiency. The American Academy of Rheumatology (AAR) recommends the following daily doses for anyone on a chronic systemic corticosteroid regimen: Calcium 1,200-1,500 mg/day and vitamin D 800-1,000 IU/day.

ORAL CORTICOSTEROIDS

▷ *betamethasone* (C)(G) initially 0.6-7.2 mg daily
   Pediatric: <12 years: not recommended; ≥12 years: same as adult
      Celestone *Tab:* 0.6 mg; *Syr:* 0.6 mg/5 ml (120 ml)

▷ *cortisone* (D)(G) initially 25-300 mg daily or every other day
   Pediatric: <12 years: not recommended; ≥12 years: same as adult
      Cortone Acetate *Tab:* 25 mg

▷ *dexamethasone* (C)(G) initially 0.75-9 mg/day
   Pediatric: <12 years: not recommended; ≥12 years: same as adult
      Decadron *Tab:* 0.5*, 0.75*, 4*mg; *Syr:* 0.5 mg/5 ml (100 ml)
      Decadron 5-12 Pak *Tabs:* 0.75*mg (12/pck)

▷ *hydrocortisone* (C)(G) 20-240 mg daily
   Pediatric: <12 years: 2-8 mg/day; ≥12 years: same as adult
      Cortef *Tab:* 5, 10, 20 mg; *Oral susp:* 10 mg/5 ml
      Hydrocortone *Tab:* 10 mg

▷ *methylprednisolone* (C)(G) 4-48 mg/day
   Pediatric: <12 years: not recommended; ≥12 years: same as adult
      Medrol *Tab:* 2*, 4*, 8*, 16*, 24*, 32*mg
      Medrol Dosepak *Dosepak:* 4*mg tabs (21/pck)

▷ *prednisolone* (C)(G) initially 5-60 mg/day in 1-2 doses x 3-5 days
   Pediatric: 0.14-2 mg/kg/day in 3-4 doses x 3-5 days
      Flo-Pred *Susp:* 5, 15 mg/5 ml
      Orapred *Soln:* 15 mg/5 ml (grape) (dye-free, alcohol 2%)
      Orapred ODT *Tab:* 10, 15, 30 mg orally disintegrating (grape)
      Pediapred *Soln:* 5 mg/5 ml (raspberry) (sugar-, alcohol-, dye-free)
      Prelone *Syr:* 15 mg/5 ml
      Comment: Flo-Pred does not require refrigeration or shaking prior to use.

▷ *prednisone* (C)(G) initially 5-60 mg/day in 1-2 doses x 3-5 days
   Pediatric: 0.14-2 mg/kg/day in 3-4 doses x 3-5 days
      Deltasone *Tab:* 2.5*, 5*, 10*, 20*, 50*mg

▷ *prednisone* (*delayed release*) (C)(G) initially 5-60 mg/day in 1-2 doses x 3-5 days
   Pediatric: 0.14-**2 mg**/kg/day in 3-4 doses x 3-5 days
      Rayos *Tab:* 1, 2, 5 mg del-rel

▷ *triamcinolone* (C)(G) initially 4-48 mg/day in 1-2 doses x 3-5 days
   Pediatric: 0.14-2 mg/kg/day in 3-4 doses x 3-5 days
      Aristocort *Tab:* 4*mg
      Aristocort Forte *Susp:* 40 mg/ml (benzoyl alcohol)
      Aristocort Aristopak *Tab:* 4*mg (16/pck)

APPENDIX M. PARENTERAL CORTICOSTEROIDS

Comment: Systemic glucocorticosteroids increase glucose intolerance, reduce the action of insulin and oral hypoglycemic agents, reduce adrenal cortex activity, decrease immunity, mask signs of infection, impair wound healing, suppress growth in children, and promote

(*continued*)

Appendix M (*continued*)

osteoporosis, fluid retention, and weight gain. Use systemic steroids with caution, using the lowest possible dose to affect clinical response, and withdraw (wean) gradually in tapering doses to avoid adrenal insufficiency. The American Academy of Rheumatology (AAR) recommends the following daily doses for anyone on a chronic systemic corticosteroid regimen: Calcium 1,200-1,500 mg/day and vitamin D 800-1,000 IU/day.

▷ *betamethasone* (C)(G)
   Celestone 0.5-9 mg IM/IV x 1 dose
      Vial: 3 mg/ml (10 ml)
   Celestone Soluspan 0.5-9 mg IM/IV x 1 dose; usual IM dose 6 mg
      Vial: 6 mg/ml (10 ml)

▷ *cortisone* (D)(G) 20-300 mg IM
   Pediatric: <12 years: not recommended; ≥12 years: same as adult
      Cortone Acetate *Vial:* 50 mg/ml (10 ml)

▷ *dexamethasone* (C)(G) initially 0.5-9 mg IM/IV daily
   Pediatric: <12 years: not recommended; ≥12 years: same as adult
      Decadron *Vial:* 4, 24 mg/ml for IM use (5 ml, sulfites)
      Dalalone D.P. *Vial:* 16 mg/ml (1, 5 ml)
      Decadron-LA *Vial:* 8 mg/ml (1, 5 ml)

▷ *hydrocortisone* (C)(G) initially 100-500 mg IM/IV daily
   Pediatric: 2-8 mg/kg loading dose (max 250 mg); then 8 mg/kg/day
      Hydrocortone *Vial:* 50 mg/ml (5 ml)
      Solu-Cortef *Vial:* 100 mg (2 ml); 250 mg (2 ml); 500 mg (4 ml); 1 gm (8 ml)

▷ *hydrocortisone phosphate* (C)(G) for IM, IV, and SC injection
   Pediatric: <12 years: not recommended; ≥12 years: same as adult
      Hydrocortone *Vial:* 50 mg/ml (2 ml)

▷ *methylprednisolone* (C)(G) 40-120 mg IM/week for 1-4 weeks
   Pediatric: <12 years: not recommended; ≥12 years: same as adult
      Depo-Medrol *Vial:* 20 mg/ml (5 ml); 40 mg/ml (5, 10 ml); 80 mg/ml (5 ml)

▷ *methylprednisolone sodium succinate* (C)(G) 10-40 mg IV initially; then, IM or IV
   Pediatric: 1-2 mg/kg loading dose; then 1.6 mg/kg/day in divided doses at least
   6 hours apart
      Solu-Medrol *Vial:* 40 mg (1 ml), 125 mg (2 ml), 500 mg (4 ml); 1 g (8 ml); 2 g (8 ml)

▷ *triamcinolone* (C)(G) 40 mg IM/week
   Pediatric: <12 years: not recommended; ≥12 years: same as adult
      Aristocort *Vial:* 25 mg/ml (5 ml)
      Aristocort Forte *Vial:* 40 mg/ml (1, 5 ml)(*do* not *administer IV*)
      Aristospan *Vial:* 5 mg/ml (5 ml); 20 mg/ml (1, 5 ml)
      TAC-3 *Vial:* 3 mg/ml (5 ml) for intralesional and intradermal use

Injectable Corticosteroid/Anesthetic

▷ *dexamethasone/lidocaine* (C) 0.1-0.75 ml into painful area
      Decadron Phosphate with Xylocaine *Vial:* dexa 4 mg/lido 10 mg per ml (5 ml)

◯ APPENDIX N. INHALATIONAL CORTICOSTEROIDS

Comment: Inhaled corticosteroids are indicated for the long-term control of asthma. Inhaled corticosteroids are not indicated for exercise induced asthma or for relief of acute symptoms (i.e., "rescue"). Low doses are indicated for mild persistent asthma, medium doses are indicated for moderate persistent asthma, and high doses are reserved for severe cases. Titrate to lowest effective dose. To reduce the potential for adverse effects with inhalers, the patient should use a spacer or holding chamber and rinse the mouth and spit after every inhalation treatment. Linear growth should be monitored in children. When inhaled doses exceed 1,000 mcg/day, consider supplements of calcium (1-1.5 gm/day), vitamin D (400 IU/day).

(*continued*)

Appendix M (*continued*)

▷ *beclomethasone* (C)

Beclovent 2 inhalations tid-qid <u>or</u> 4 inhalations bid; max 20 inhalations/day
Pediatric: <6 years: not recommended; 6-12 years: 1-2 inhalations tid-qid <u>or</u> 4 inhalations bid; max 10 inhalations/day

  Inhaler: 42 mcg/actuation (6.7 g, 80 inh); 16.8 g (200 inh)

Qvar *Previously using only bronchodilators:* initiate 40-80 mcg bid; max 320 mcg/day;
Previously using an inhaled corticosteroid: initiate 40-160 mcg bid; max 320 mcg/day;
Previously taking a systemic corticosteroid: attempt to wean off the systemic drug after approximately 1 week after initiating Qvar
Pediatric: <12 years: not recommended; ≥12 years: same as adult

  Inhaler: 40, 80 mcg/actuation metered-dose aerosol w. dose counter (8.7 g, 120 inh) (CFC-free)

Vanceril 2 inhalations tid to qid <u>or</u> 4 inhalations bid
Pediatric: <6 years: not recommended; 6-12 years: 1-2 inhalations tid to qid

  Inhaler: 42 mcg/actuation (16.8 g, 200 inh)

Vanceril Double Strength 2 inhalations bid
Pediatric: <6 years: not recommended; 6-12 years: 1-2 inhalations bid; >12 years: same as adult

  Inhaler: 84 mcg/actuation (12.2 g, 120 inh)

▷ *budesonide* (B)(G)

Pulmicort Respules use turbuhaler
Pediatric: <12 months: not recommended; ≥12 months to 8 years: *Previously using only bronchodilators:* initiate 0.5 mg/day once daily <u>or</u> in 2 divided doses; may start at 0.25 mg/day; *Previously using inhaled orticosteroids:* initiate 0.5 mg/day daily <u>or</u> in 2 divided doses; max 1 mg/day; *Previously using oral orticosteroids:* initiate 1 mg/day daily <u>or</u> in 2 divided doses

  Inhal susp: 0.25 mg/2 ml (30/box)

Pulmicort Turbuhaler 1-2 inhalations bid; *Previously on oral corticosteroids:* 2-4 inhalations bid
Pediatric: <6 years: not recommended; 6-12 years: 1-2 inhalations bid; >12 years: same as adult

  Turbuhaler: 200 mcg/actuation (200 inh)

▷ *flunisolide* (C)(G)

AeroBid, AeroBid M initially 2 inhalations bid; max 8 inhalations/day
Pediatric: <6 years: not recommended; 6-15 years: 2 inhalations bid; ≥16 years: same as adult

  Inhaler: 250 mcg/actuation (7 gm, 100 inh)

▷ *fluticasone* (C)(G)

Flovent HFA initially 88 mcg bid; if previously using an inhaled corticosteroid, initially 88-220 mcg bid; if previously taking an oral corticosteroid, initially 880 mcg/day
Pediatric: use **Rotadisk:** initially 50-88 mcg inh bid; <4 years: not recommended; 4-11 years: initially 50-88 mcg bid; >11 years: initially 100 mcg bid; if previously using an inhaled corticosteroid, initially 100-200 mcg bid; *Previously taking an oral corticosteroid;* initially 1000 mcg bid

  Inhaler: 44 mcg/actuation (7.9 g, 60 inh; 13 g, 120 inh); 110 mcg/actuation (13 g, 120 inh); 220 mcg/actuation (13 g, 120 inh)

Rotadisk 50 mcg/actuation (60 blisters/disk); 100 mcg/actuation (60 blisters/disk); 250 mcg/actuation (60 blisters/disk)
Pediatric: <12 years: not recommended; ≥12 years: same as adult

▷ *mometasone furoate* (C) *Previously using a bronchodilator <u>or</u> inhaled corticosteroid:* 220 mcg q PM <u>or</u> bid; max 440 mcg q PM <u>or</u> 220 mcg bid; *Previously using an oral corticosteroid:* 440 mcg bid; max 880 mcg/day
Pediatric: <12 years: not recommended; ≥12 years: same as adult
  Asmanex Twisthaler *Inhaler:* 220 mcg/actuation (6.7 gm, 80 inh); 16.8 gm (200 inh)

APPENDIX O. ANTIARRHYTHMIA DRUGS

Antiarrhythmics by Classification With Dose Forms		
Brand/Generic and Pregnancy Category	**Class and Indication(s)**	**Dose Form(s)**
Betapace *sotalol* (B)	*Class:* Class II and III Antiarrhythmic *Indications:* Documented life-threatening ventricular arrhythmias	Tab: 80*, 120*, 160*, 240*mg
Betapace AF *sotalol* (B)	*Class:* Class II and III Antiarrhythmic *Indications:* Maintenance of normal sinus rhythm in patients with highly symptomatic atrial fibrillation or atrial flutter who are currently in sinus rhythm	Tab: 80*, 120*, 160*mg
Calan *verapamil* (C)(G)	*Class:* Calcium Channel Blocker *Indications:* Control (with *digitalis*) of ventricular rate in patients with chronic atrial fibrillation or atrial flutter; prophylaxis of repetitive paroxysmal supraventricular tachycardia	Tab: 40, 80*, 120*mg
Cordarone *amiodarone* (D)(G)	*Class:* Class III Antiarrhythmic *Indications:* Documented life-threatening recurrent refractory ventricular fibrillation or hemodynamically unstable ventricular tachycardia	Tab: 200*mg
Quinidex *quinidine sulfate* (C) (G)	*Class:* Class I Antiarrhythmic *Indications:* Atrial and ventricular arrhythmias	Tab: 300 mg ext-rel
Inderal *propranolol* (C)(G) **Inderal XL** *propranolol ext-rel* (C)(G) **InnoPran XL** *Propranolol ext-rel* (C)	*Class:* Beta-Blocker *Indications:* Atrial and ventricular arrhythmias; tachyarrhythmias due to *digitalis* intoxication; reduce mortality and risk of reinfarction in stabilized patients after myocardial infarction	Tab: 10*, 20*, 40*, 60*, 80* mg; Cap: 60, 80, 120, 160 mg sust-rel Cap: 80, 120 mg ext-rel
Mexitil *mexiletine* (C)	*Class:* Class IB Antiarrhythmic *Indications:* Documented life-threatening ventricular arrhythmias	Cap: 150, 200, 250 mg
Multaq *dronedarone* (C)	*Class:* IB Antiarrhythmic *Indications:* Paroxysmal or persistent atrial fibrillation or atrial flutter	Tab: 400 mg
Norpace *disopyramide* (C)	*Class:* Class I Antiarrhythmic *Indications:* Documented life-threatening ventricular arrhythmias	Cap: 100, 150 mg
Procanbid *procainamide* (C)(G)	*Class:* Class IA Antiarrhythmic *Indications:* Life-threatening ventricular arrhythmias	Tab: 500, 1000 mg ext-rel

(continued)

Appendix O (*continued*)

Antiarrhythmics by Classification With Dose Forms		
Brand/Generic and Pregnancy Category	Class and Indication(s)	Dose Form(s)
Quinaglute *quinidine gluconate* (C)(G)	*Class:* Class I Antiarrhythmic *Indications:* Atrial and ventricular arrhythmias	*Tab:* 324 mg ext-rel
Rythmol *propafenone* (C)(G)	*Class:* Class IC Antiarrhythmic *Indications:* Documented life-threatening ventricular arrhythmias; prolonged recurrence of paroxysmal atrial fibrillation and/or atrial flutter or paroxysmal supraventricular tachycardia associated with disabling symptoms in patients without structural heart disease	*Tab:* 150*, 225*, 300*mg *Cap:* 225, 325, 425 mg ext-rel
Sectral *acebutolol* (B)(G)	*Class:* Beta-Blocker *Indications:* Ventricular arrhythmias	*Cap:* 200, 400 mg
Sotylize *sotalol* (B)	*Class:* Class II and III Antiarrhythmic *Indications:* Documented life-threatening ventricular arrhythmias, and highly symptomatic A-flutter/A-fib	*Oral soln:* 5 mg/ml
Tambocor *flecainide acetate* (C)(G)	*Class:* Class IC Antiarrhythmic *Indications:* Documented life-threatening ventricular arrhythmias; paroxysmal atrial fibrillation and/or atrial flutter or paroxysmal supraventricular tachycardia in patients without structural heart disease	*Tab:* 50, 100*, 150* mg
Tenormin *atenolol* (C)(G)	*Class:* Beta-Blocker *Indications:* Reduce mortality and in stabilized patients after myocardial infarction	*Tab:* 25, 50, 100 mg *Inj:* 5 mg/ml (10 ml) for IV administration
timolol maleate (C) (G)	*Class:* Beta-Blocker *Indications:* Reduce mortality and in stabilized patients after myocardial infarction	*Tab:* 5, 10*, 20*mg
dofetilide (C)(G)	*Class:* Class III Antiarrhythmic *Indications:* Maintenance of normal sinus rhythm in patients with atrial fibrillation or atrial flutter of >1 week duration who were converted to normal sinus rhythm (only for highly symptomatic patients); conversion to normal sinus rhythm	*Cap:* 125, 250, 500 mcg
Tonocard *tocainide* (C)(G)	*Class:* Class I Antiarrhythmic *Indications:* Documented life-threatening ventricular arrhythmias	*Tab:* 400*, 600*mg
Toprol XL *metoprolol* (C)(G)	*Class:* Beta-Blocker *Indications:* Ischemic, hypertensive, or cardiomyopathic heart failure	*Tab:* 25*, 50*, 100*, 200*mg

APPENDIX P. ANTINEOPLASIA DRUGS

Comment: A new lab test offers potential for early detection of multiple cancer types with a single blood sample. Researchers studied 1,005 persons with non-metastatic, clinically-detected, stage 2 and 3 cancers of the ovary, liver, stomach, pancreas, esophagus, colorectum, lung, or breast. The blood test, CancerSEEK, accurately identified cancer cases 33-98% (M = 70%) of the time in the study cohort, with accuracy reportedly 69-98% for the five cancers that currently have no widely used screening test: ovarian, pancreatic, stomach, liver and esophageal cancers. CancerSEEK combines tests that look for 16 genes and 10 proteins (mutations in cell-free DNA), linked to cancer. The researchers also tested blood samples from 812 healthy people, to see how often the test gave false-positive results, and were reported to be less than 1%. These findings represent a promising future for screening and early detection of cancer in asymtomatic persons. Optimally, cancers would be detected early enough that they could be cured by surgery alone, but even cancers that are not curable by surgery alone will respond better to systemic therapies when there is less advanced disease.

Anne Marie Lennon, MD, PhD, Johns Hopkins Kimmel Cancer Center, Baltimore and Len Lichtenfeld, MD, Deputy Chief Medical Officer, American Cancer Society, Atlanta. Online and print announcements, January 2018: PR Newswire, Science, U.S. News & World Report, Los Angeles Times, Forbes, The Guardian, Chicago Tribune

REFERENCE

Cohen, J. D., Li, L., Wang, Y., Thoburn, C., Afsari, B., Danilova, L., . . . Papadopoulos, N. (2018). Detection and localization of surgically resectable cancers with a multi-analyte blood test. *Science, 359*(6378), 926–930. doi:10.1126/science.aar3247

Antineoplastics With Classification and Dose Forms		
Brand, Generic and Pregnancy Category	**Class and Indications**	**Dose Form(s)**
Adcetris *brentuximab vedotin*	CD30-directed Antibody-Drug Conjugate	*Vial:* 50 mg single-use, pwdr for reconstitution
Afinitor *everolimus (D)*	Kinase Inhibitor	*Tab:* 2.5, 5, 7.5, 10 mg
Afinitor Disperz *everolimus (D)*	Kinase Inhibitor	*Tab:* 2, 3, 5 mg for oral suspension
Alecensa *alectinib*	Kinase Inhibitor	*Cap:* 150 mg
Aliqopa *copanlisib*	Kinase Inhibitor	*Vial:* 60 mg pwdr for injection, single dose
Alkeran *melphalan (D)(G)*	Alkylating Agent	*Tab:* 2*mg
Alunbrig *brigatinib*	Kinase Inhibitor	*Tab:* 30, 90 mg
Arimidex *anastrozole (D)*	Aromatase Inhibitor	*Tab:* 1 mg
Aromasin *exemestane (D)*	Aromatase Inactivator	*Tab:* 25 mg
Arranon *nelarabine (D)*	Nucleoside Analog	*Vial:* 250 mg for IV infusion

(continued)

Appendix P (continued)

Antineoplastics With Classification and Dose Forms		
Brand, Generic and Pregnancy Category	Class and Indications	Dose Form(s)
Asparlas *calaspargase pegol-mknl*	Asparagine-Specific Enzyme	*Vial:* 3,750 units/5 ml (750 units/ml, 5 ml) single-dose for IV infusion
Azedra *iobenguane I*[131]	Radioactive Therapeutic Agent	*Vial:* 555 MBq/ml (15 mCi/ml) single-dose for IV infusion
Bavencio *avelumab* (D)	Programmed Death Ligand-1 (PD-L1) Blocking Antibody	*Vial:* 200 mg/10 ml (20 mg/ml), single-dose
Besponsa *inotuzumab ozogamicin*	CD22-Directed Antibody-Drug Drug Conjugate Mixture of	*Vial:* 0.9 mg single-dose
Bevyxxa *betrixiban*	Factor Xa (FXa) Inhibitor	*Cap:* 40, 80 mg
bleomycin sulfate (G)	Cytotoxic Glycopeptide Antibiotics Isolated from a Strain of *Streptomyces verticillus*	*Vial:* 15, 30 units; pwdr for reconstitution and IV, IM, SC, intrapleural administration
Blincyto *blinatumomab*	Bispecific CD19-directed CD3 T-cell Engager	*Vial:* 35 mcg pwdr for reconstitution, single-dose
bortizomib	Kinase Inhibitor	*Vial:* 3.5 mg pwdr for reconstitution, single-dose
Bosulif *bosutinib*	Kinase Inhibitor	*Tab:* 100, 400, 500 mg
Braftovi *encorafenib*	Kinase Inhibitor	*Cap:* 50, 75 mg
Cabometyx *cabozantinib*	Kinase Inhibitor	*Tab:* 20, 40, 60 mg
Calquence *acalabrutinib*	Kinase Inhibitor	*Cap:* 100 mg
Casodex *bicalutamide*	Antiandrogen	*Tab:* 50 mg
Clolar *clofarabine* (X)	Purine Nucleoside Metabolic Inhibitor	*Vial:* 20 mg/20 ml single-dose
Copiktra *duvelisib*	Dual phosphoinositide-3-kinase (PI3K)-delta/PI3K-gamma Inhibitor	*Cap:* 15, 25 mg
Cytoxan *Cyclophosphamide* (D)	Alkylating Agent	*Tab:* 25, 50 mg
Daralex *daratumumab*	Human CD38-directed Monoclonal Antibody	*Vial:* 100 mg/5 ml, 400 mg/20 ml, single-dose

(continued)

Appendix P (*continued*)

Antineoplastics With Classification and Dose Forms		
Brand, Generic and Pregnancy Category	**Class and Indications**	**Dose Form(s)**
Daurismo *glasdegib*	Hedgehog Pathway Inhibitor	*Tab*: 25, 100 mg
Doxil (D) *doxorubicin HCl*	Anthracycline Topoisomerase Inhibitor	Vial: 10 mg/10 ml, 50 mg/30 ml (10 mg/ml) single-use
Eligard *leuprolide acetate* **(X)**	GnRH Analog	*Inj*: 7.5 mg ext-rel per monthly SC injection
Elzonris *tagraxofusp-erzs*	CD123-directed Cytotoxin	*Vial*: 1,000 mcg/ml (1 ml) single-dose for IV infusion
Endari *l-glutamine*	Amino Acid	*Oral Pwdr*: 5 grams of L-glutamine pwdr per paper-foil-plastic laminate pkt
Eulexin *flutamide* **(D)**	Antiandrogen	*Cap*: 125 mg
Fareston *toremifene* **(D)(G)**	Selective Estrogen Receptor Modulator (SERM)	*Tab*: 60 mg
Faslodex *fulvestrant* **(D)(G)**	Estrogen Receptor Antagonist	*Prefilled syringe for IM inj*: 50 mg/ml (2.5, 5 ml/syringe)
Femara *letrozole* **(D)**	Aromatase Inhibitor	*Tab*: 2.5 mg
Gleevec *imatinib mesylate* **(D)**	Signal Transduction Inhibitor	*Cap*: 100 mg
Herceptin *trastuzumab*	HER2/neu Receptor Antagonist	*Vial*: 420 mg multi-dose pwdr for reconstitution and IV infusion
Herzuma *trastuzumab-pkrb*	HER2/neu Receptor Antagonist	*Vial*: 420 mg multi-dose for reconstitution, dilution, and IV infusion
Hydrea *hydroxyurea* **(D)(G)**	Substituted Urea	*Cap*: 500 mg
Ibrance *palbociclib*	Kinase Inhibitor	*Cap*: 75, 100, 150 mg
Imbruvica *imbrutinib*	Kinase Inhibitor	*Tab*: 140 mg
Imfinzi *durvalumab*	Programmed Death Ligand-1 (PD-L1) Blocking Antibody	*Vial*: 120 mg/2.4 ml, 500 mg/10 ml (50 mg/ml) single-dose
Inhifa *enasidenib*	Isocitrate Dehydrogenase-2 Inhibitor	*Tab*: 50, 100 mg

(*continued*)

Appendix P (*continued*)

Antineoplastics With Classification and Dose Forms		
Brand, Generic and Pregnancy Category	**Class and Indications**	**Dose Form(s)**
Iressa *gefitinib* (D)	Epidermal Growth Factor Receptor Tyrosine Kinase Inhibitor	*Tab:* 250 mg
Jakafi *ruxolitinib*	Kinase Inhibitor	*Tab:* 5, 10, 15, 20, 25 mg
Keytruda *pembrolizumab*	Programmed Death Receptor-1 (PD-1)-Blocking Antibody	*Vial:* 50 mg, single-dose for reconstitution; 100 mg/4 ml (25 mg/ml) single dose
Kisquali Femara Co-Pack *ribociclib+letrozole*	Cyclin-dependent Kinase Inhibitor+Aromatase Inhibitor	*Tab:* 600/2.5, 400/2.5, 200/2.5 mg
Kymriah *tisagenlecleucel*	CD19-directed Genetically Modified Autologous T cell Immunotherapy	*IV bag:* frozen suspension for IV infusion after thawing
Kyprolis, *carfilzomib*	Protease Inhibitor	*Vial:* 30, 60 mg, single-dose, pwdr for reconstitution
Lartruvo *olaratumab*	Platelet-derived Growth Factor Receptor Alpha (PDGFR-α) Blocking Antibody	*Vial:* 500 mg/50 ml (10 mg/ml, single-dose)
Lemvina *lenvatinib*	Kinase Inhibitor	*Cap:* 4, 10 mg
Leukeran *chlorambucil* (D)(G)	Alkylating Agent	*Tab:* 2 mg
Leupron *leuprolide* (X)	GnRH Analog	*Susp for IM inj:* 1 mg (daily); 7.5 mg depot (monthly); 22.5 mg depot (every 3 months); 30 mg depot (every 4 months)
Libtayo *cemiplimab-rwle*	Programmed Death Receptor-1 (PD-1) Blocking Antibody	*Vial:* 350 mg/7 ml (50 mg/ml single-dose for IV infusion
Lobrena *lorlatinib*	Kinase Inhibitor	*Tab:* 25, 100 mg
Lumoxiti *moxetumomab pasudotox-tdfk*	Anti-CD22 Recombinant Immunotoxin	*Vial:* 1 mg single-dose for reconstitution and IV infusion
Lynparza *olaparib*	Poly (ADP-ribose) Polymerase (PARP)-Inhibitor	*Tab:* 100, 150 mg

(*continued*)

Appendix P (*continued*)

Antineoplastics With Classification and Dose Forms		
Brand, Generic and Pregnancy Category	**Class and Indications**	**Dose Form(s)**
Megace, Megace Oral Suspension, Megace ES, *megestrol acetate* (D) (G)	Progestin	*Tab:* 20*, 40*mg; *Susp:* 40 mg/ml; ES concentrate: 125 mg/ml, 625 mg/5 ml
Mekinist *trametinib*	Kinase Inhibitor	*Tab:* 0.5, 2 mg
Mektovi *binimetinib*	Kinase Inhibitor	*Tab:* 15 mg
Nerlynx *neratinib*	Kinase Inhibitor	*Tab:* 40 mg
Nexavar *sorafenib* (D)	Multikinase Inhibitor	*Tab:* 200 mg
Nilandron *nilutamide*	Nonsteroidal Orally Active Antiandrogen	*Tab:* 150 mg
Ogivri *trastuzumab-dkst*	HER2/neu Receptor Antagonist	*Vial:* 420 mg multi-dose pwdr for reconstitution and IV infusion
Opdivo *nivolumab*	Anti-PD1 Monoclonal Antibody	*Vial:* 40 mg/4 ml, 100 mg/10 ml, 240 mg/24 ml (10 mg/ml) single-use
Perjeta *pertuzumab*	HER2/neu Receptor Antagonist	*Vial:* 420 mg/14 ml single-dose
Poteligeo *mogamulizumab*	CC Chemokine Receptor Type 4 (CCR4)-Directed Monoclonal Antibody	*Vial:* 420 mg multi-dose pwdr for reconstitution and IV infusion
Revlimid *lenalidomide*	Thalidomide Analogue	*Cap:* 2.5, 5, 10, 15, 20, 25 mg
Responsa *inotuzumab ozogamicin*	CD22-directed Antibody-Drug Conjugade (ADC)	*Vial:* 0.9 mg, single-dose, for reconstitution
Rituxan Hyclea *rituximab+ hyaluronidase*	Combination of ***rituximab***, a CD20-directed Cytolytic Antibody and ***hyaluronidase human***, an Endoglycosidase	*Vial:* 1,400 mg ***rituximab*** and 23,400 Units ***hyaluronidase human*** per 11.7 ml (120 mg/2,000 Units per ml) single-dose; 1,600 mg ***rituximab*** and 26,800 Units ***hyaluronidase human*** per 13.4 ml (120 mg/2,000 Units per ml) single-dose
Rubraca *rucaparib*	Poly ADP-ribose Polymerase (PARP)-Inhibitor	*Tab:* 200, 300 mg

(*continued*)

Appendix P (*continued*)

Antineoplastics With Classification and Dose Forms		
Brand, Generic and Pregnancy Category	**Class and Indications**	**Dose Form(s)**
Rydapt *midostaurin*	Kinase Inhibitor	*Tab:* 40 mg
Stivarga *regorafenib*	Kinase Inhibitor	*Tab:* 40 mg
Sutent *sunitinib malate*	Kinase Inhibitor	*Cap:* 12.5, 25, 37.5, 50 mg
Tagrisso *osimertinib*	Kinase Inhibitor	*Tab:* 40, 80 mg
Talzenna *talazoparib*	Poly (ADP-ribose) (PARP) Inhibitor	*Tab:* 0.5, 1 mg
tamoxifen citrate (G)	Antiestrogen	*Tab:* 10, 20 mg
Tarceva *erlotinib* (D)	Kinase Inhibitor	*Tab:* 25, 100, 150 mg
Tasigna *nilotinib*	Kinase Inhibitor	*Cap:* 50, 150, 200 mg
Taxotere *docetaxel* (G)	Microtubule Inhibitor	*Vial:* 20 mg/2 ml (10 mg/ml) single-dose, 80 mg/8 ml (10 mg/ml), 160 mg/16 ml (10 mg/ml) multi-dose
Tecentriq *atezolizumab*	Programmed Death Ligand-1 (PD-L1) Blocking Antibody	*Vial:* 1,200 mg/20 ml (60 mg/ml, single-dose)
Tibsovo *ivosidenib*	Isocitrate Dehydrogenase-1 (IDH1) Inhibitor	*Tab:* 250 mg
Treanda *bendamustine*	Alkylating Agent	*Vial:* 45 mg/0.5 ml, 180 mg/2 ml solution, single-dose; 25, 100 mg pwdr for reconstitution, single-dose
Trisenox *arsenic trioxide*	Arsenical	*Vial:* 12 mg/6 ml single-dose
Truxima *rituximab-abbs*	CD20-directed Cytolytic Antibody (biosimilar to **Rituxan**)	*Vial:* 100 mg/10 ml, 500 mg/50 ml (10 mg/ml) single-use for dilution and IV infusion
Vectibix *panitumumab*	Epidermal Growth Factor Receptor (EGFR) Antagonist	*Vial:* 100 mg/5 ml, 200 mg/10 ml, 400 mg/20 ml (20 mg/ml, single-use)
Velcade *bortezomib* (D)	Proteasome Inhibitor	*Vial:* 3.5 mg (pwdr for IV infusion after reconstitution)
Venclexta *venetoclax*	BCL-2 Inhibitor	*Tab:* 10, 50, 100 mg

(*continued*)

Appendix P (*continued*)

Antineoplastics With Classification and Dose Forms		
Brand, Generic and Pregnancy Category	**Class and Indications**	**Dose Form(s)**
Viadur (X) *leuprolide acetate*	GnRH Analog	*SC implant:* 65 mg depot (replace every 12 months)
Vitrakvi *larotrectinib*	Selective Tropomyosin Receptor Kinase (TRK) Inhibitor	*Caps:* 25, 100 mg; *Oral soln:* 20 mg/ml (100 ml)
Vizimpro *dacomitib*	Irreversible Pan-human Epidermal Growth Factor Receptor Tyrosine Kinase Inhibitor (TKI)	*Tab:* 15, 30, 45 mg
Vyxeos *daunorubicin+ cytarabine*	*daunorubicin:* Anthracycline Topoisomerase Inhibitor; *cytarabine:* Nucleoside Metabolic Inhibitor	*Vial:* daun 44 mg/cytar 100 mg (pwdr for IV injection after reconstitution)
Xalkori *crizotinib*	Kinase Inhibitor	*Cap:* 25, 100 mg
Xeloda (D) *capecitabine*	*Fluoropyrimidine* (prodrug of *5-fluorouracil*)	*Tab:* 150, 500 mg
Xospata *gilteritinib*	Kinase Inhibitor	*Tab:* 40 mg
Yervoy *ipilimumab*	CD19-Directed Genetically Human Cytotoxic T-lymphocyte Antigen 4 (CTLA-4)-Blocking Antibody	*Vial:* 50 mg/10 ml, 200 mg/40 ml (5 mg/ml) single-dose
Yescarta *axicabtagene*	CD19-Directed Genetically Modified Autologous T cell	*Infusion bag:* 68 ml single autologous use Immunotherapy
Zejula *niraparib*	Poly ADP-ribose Polymerase (PARP)-Inhibitor	*Cap:* 100 mg
Zelboraf *vemurafenib*	Kinase Inhibitor	*Tab:* 240 mg
Zoladex *goserelin acetate*	GnRH Analog	*SC implant:* 3.6 mg depot (28 days), 10.8 mg depot (3-month)
Zometa *zoledronic acid* (D)	Bisphosphonate	*Vial:* 4 mg pwdr for reconstitution for IV infusion, single-dose
Zykadia *ceritinib*	Kinase Inhibitor	*Cap:* 150 mg

APPENDIX Q. ANTIPSYCHOSIS DRUGS

ANTIPSYCHOTICS WITH DOSE FORMS

Comment: Patients receiving an antipsychotic agent should be monitored closely for the following adverse side effects: neuroleptic malignant syndrome, extrapyramidal reactions, tardive dyskinesia, blood dyscrasias, anticholinergic effects, drowsiness, hypotension, photo-sensitivity, retinopathy, and lowered seizure threshold. Use lower doses for elderly or debilitated patients. Prescriptions should be written for the smallest practical amount. Foods and beverages containing alcohol are contraindicated for patients receiving any psychotropic drug. *Neuroleptic Malignant Syndrome* (NMS) and *Tardive Dyskinesia* (TD) are adverse side effects (ASEs) most often associated with the older antipsychotic drugs. Risk is decreased with the newer "atypical" antipsychotic drugs. However, these syndromes can develop, although much less commonly, after relatively brief treatment periods at low doses. Given these considerations, antipsychotic drugs should be prescribed in a manner that is most likely to minimize the occurrence. NMS, a potentially fatal symptom complex, is characterized by hyperpyrexia, muscle rigidity, altered mental status and evidence of autonomic instability (irregular pulse or blood pressure, tachycardia, diaphoresis, and cardiac dysrhythmia). Additional signs may include elevated creatine phosphor-kinase (CPK), myoglobinuria (rhabdomyolysis), and acute renal failure (ARF). TD is a syndrome consisting of potentially irreversible, involuntary, dyskinetic movements that can develop in patients with antipsychotic drugs. Characteristics include repetitive involuntary movements, usually of the jaw, lips and tongue, such as grimacing, sticking out the tongue and smacking the lips. Some affected people also experience involuntary movement of the extremities or difficulty breathing. The syndrome may remit, partially or completely, if antipsychotic treatment is withdrawn. If signs and symptoms of NMS and/or TD appear in a patient, management should include immediate discontinuation of antipsychotic drugs and other drugs not essential to concurrent therapy, intensive symptomatic treatment, medical monitoring, and treatment of any concomitant serious medical problems. The risk of developing NMS and/or TD, and the likelihood that either syndrome will become irreversible, is believed to increase as the duration of treatment and the total cumulative dose of antipsychotic drugs administered to the patient increase. The first and only FDA-approved treatment for TD is *valbenazine* (**Ingrezza**) (*see page 473*)

ANTIPSYCHOTICS WITH DOSE FORMS

▷ *aripiprazole* (C)(G)

> **Abilify** *Tab:* 2, 5, 10, 15, 20, 30 mg; *Oral soln:* 1 mg/ml (150 ml) (orange crèam; parabens)
> **Abilify Discmelt** *Tab:* 15 mg orally disintegrating (vanilla) (phenylalanine)
> **Abilify Maintena** *Vial:* 300, 400 mg ext-rel pwdr for IM injection after reconstitution; 300, 400 mg single-dose prefilled dual chamber syringes w. supplies
> **Aristada** *Prefilled syringe:* 441, 662, 882, 1064 mg, ext-rel susp for IM injection, single-dose w. safety needle

▷ *aripiprazole lauroxil* (C)

> **Aristada** Prefilled *syringe:* single-use, ext-rel injectable suspension: 441mg (1.6 ml), 662 mg (2.4 ml), 882 mg (3.2 ml), 1064 mg (3.9 ml)

▷ *asenapine* (C)

> **Saphris** *SL tab:* 2.5, 5, 10 mg

▷ *brexpizole* (C)

> **Rexulti** *Tab:* 0.25, 0.5, 1, 2, 3, 4 mg

▷ *bupropion* (C)

> **Forfivo XL** *Tab:* 450 mg ext-rel

▷ *cariprazine* (NE)

> **Vraylar** *Cap:* 1.5, 3, 4.5, 6 mg

▷ *chlorpromazine* (C)(G)

> **Thorazine** *Tab:* 10, 25, 50, 100, 200 mg; *Cap:* 30, 75, 150 mg sust-rel; *Syr:* 10 mg/5 ml (4 oz) (orange-custard); *Vial/Amp:* 25 mg/ml (1, 2 ml) (sulfites)

(continued)

Appendix Q (*continued*)

▷ *clozapine* (B)(G)
　　Clozapine ODT (G) *ODT:* 150, 200 mg
　　Clozaril (G) *Tab:* 25*, 100*mg; *ODT:* 150, 200 mg
　　FazaClo ODT (G) *ODT:* 12.5, 25, 100, 150, 200 mg (phenylalanine)
　　Versacloz *Oral susp:* 50 mg/ml (100 ml)

▷ *fluphenazine* (C)(G)
　　Prolixin *Tab:* 1, 2.5, 5*, 10 mg (tartrazine); *Conc:* 5 mg/ml (4 oz w. calib dropper) (alcohol 14%); *Elix:* 5 mg/ml (2 oz w. calib dropper) (alcohol 14%); *Vial:* 25 mg/ml (10 ml)

▷ *fluphenazine decanoate* (C)(G)
　　Prolixin Decanoate *Vial:* 25 mg/ml (5 ml) (benzyl alcohol)

▷ *fluphenazine* (C)(G)
　　Prolixin Ethanate *Vial:* 25 mg (5 ml) (benzyl alcohol)

▷ *fluphenazine decanoate* (C)(G)
　　Prolixin Decanoate *Vial:* 25 mg/ml (5 ml) (benzyl alcohol)

▷ *haloperidol* (B)(G)
　　Haldol *Tab:* 0.5*, 1*, 2*, 5*, 10*, 20*mg
　　Haldol Lactate *Vial:* 5 mg for IM injection, single-dose
　　Haldol Decanoate *Vial:* 50, 100 mg for IM injection, single-dose

▷ *iloperidone* (C)
　　Fanapt *Tab:* 1, 2, 4, 6, 8, 10, 12 mg

▷ *loxapine* (C)
　　Adasuve *Oral inhal pwdr:* 10 mg single-use disposable inhaler (5/box)

▷ *lurasidone* (B)(G)
　　Latuda *Tab:* 20, 40, 80 mg

▷ *olanzapine fumarate* (C)(G)
　　Zyprexa *Tab:* 2.5, 5, 7.5, 10, 15, 20 mg
　　Zyprexa Zydis *ODT:* 5, 10, 15, 20 mg (phenylalanine)

▷ *paliperidone palmitate* (C)(G)
　　Invega *Tab:* 3, 6, 9 mg ext-rel
　　Invega Sustenna *Prefilled syringe:* 39, 78, 117, 156, 234 mg ext-rel suspension w. needle
　　Invega Trinza *Prefilled syringe:* 273, 410, 546, 819 mg ext-rel suspension

▷ *pimozide* (C)(G)
　　Orap *Tab:* 1, 2 mg

▷ *prochlorperazine* (C)(G)
　　Compazine *Tab:* 5, 10 mg; *Cap:* 10, 15 mg sus-rel; *Syr:* 5 mg/5 ml (4 oz) (fruit); *Supp:* 2.5, 5, 25 mg

▷ *quetiapine* (C)(G)
　　Seroquel *Tab:* 25, 100, 200, 300 mg
　　Seroquel XR *Tab:* 50, 150, 200, 300, 400 mg ext-rel

▷ *risperidone* (C)(G)
　　Risperdal *Tab:* 0.25, 0.5, 1, 2, 3, 4 mg; *Soln:* 1 mg/ml (30 ml w. pipette); *Consta Inj:* 25, 37.5, 50 mg
　　Risperdal M-Tabs *M-tab:* 0.5, 1, 2, 3, 4 mg orally-disint (phenylalanine)

▷ *thioridazine* (C)(G) *Tab:* 10, 25, 50, 100 mg

▷ *trifluoperazine* (C)(G)
　　Stelazine *Tab:* 1, 2, 5, 10 mg; *Conc:* 10 mg/ml; (2 oz w. calib dropper (banana-vanilla) (sulfites); *Vial:* 2 mg/ml (10 ml)

▷ *ziprasidone* (C)(G)
　　Geodon *Cap:* 20, 40, 60, 80 mg

APPENDIX R. ANTICONVULSANT DRUGS

ANTICONVULSANTS WITH DOSE FORMS

▷ *brivaracetam* (C)
　　Briviact *Tab:* 10, 25, 50, 75, 100 mg; *Oral soln:* 10 mg/ml (300 ml); *Vial:* 50 mg/
　　　5 ml single-dose for IV inj

▷ *carbamazepine* (D)(G)
　　Carbatrol *Cap:* 200, 300 mg ext-rel
　　Carnexiv *Vial:* 200 mg/20 ml (10 mg/ml) single-dose for IV infusion
　　Equetro *Cap:* 100, 200, 300 mg ext-rel
　　Tegretol *Tab:* 100*, 200*mg; *Chew tab:* 100*mg
　　Tegretol Suspension *Oral susp:* 100 mg/5 ml (450 ml) (citrus vanilla) (sorbitol)
　　Tegretol-XR *Tab:* 100, 200, 400 mg ext-rel

▷ *clobazam* (C)(IV)
　　Onfi *Tab:* 10*, 20*mg
　　Onfi Oral Suspension *Oral susp:* 2.5 mg/ml (120 ml w. 2 dosing syringes) (berry)

▷ *clonazepam* (D)(IV)(G)
　　Clonazepam ODT *ODT:* 0.125, 0.25, 0.5, 1, 2, oral-disint
　　Klonopin *Tab:* 0.5*, 1, 2 mg

▷ *diazepam* (D)(IV)(G)
　　Diastat *Rectal gel delivery system:* 2.5 mg
　　Diastat AcuDial *Rectal gel delivery system:* 10, 20 mg
　　Valium *Tab:* 2*, 5*, 10*mg
　　Valium Injectable *Vial:* 5 mg/ml (10 ml); *Amp:* 5 mg/ml (2 ml); *Prefilled syringe:* 5 mg/
　　　ml (5 ml)
　　Valium Intensol *Conc oral soln:* 5 mg/ml (30 ml w. dropper) (alcohol 19%)
　　Valium Oral Solution *Oral soln:* 5 mg/5 ml (500 ml) (winter green-spice)

▷ *divalproex sodium* (D)(G)
　　Depakene *Cap:* 250 mg; *Syr:* 250 mg/5 ml (16 oz)
　　Depakote *Tab:* 125, 250, 500 mg
　　Depakote ER *Tab:* 250, 500 mg ext-rel
　　Depakote Sprinkle *Cap:* 125 mg

▷ *eslicarbazepine* (C)
　　Aptiom *Tab:* 200*, 400, 600*, 800*mg

▷ *felbamate* (C)(G)
　　Felbatol *Tab:* 400*, 600*mg
　　Felbatol Oral Suspension *Oral susp:* 600 mg/5 ml (4, 8, 32 oz)
　　Peganone *Tab:* 250, 500 mg

▷ *bapentin* (C)
　　Horizant *Tab:* 300, 600 ext-rel
　　Neurontin (G) *Cap:* 100, 300, 400 mg; *Tab:* 600*, 800*mg
　　Neurontin Oral Solution *Oral soln:* 250 mg/5 ml (480 ml) (strawberry-anise)

▷ *lacosamide* (C)(V)(G)
　　Vimpat *Tab:* 50, 100, 150, 200 mg; *Oral soln:* 10 mg/ml (200, 465 ml); *Vial:* 10 mg/ml
　　soln for IV infusion, single-use (20 ml)

▷ *lamotrigine* (C)(G)
　　Lamictal *Tab:* 25*, 100*, 150*, 200*mg
　　Lamictal Chewable Dispersible Tab *Chew tab:* 2, 5, 25, 50 mg (black current)
　　Lamictal ODT *ODT:* 25, 50, 100, 200 mg oral-disint
　　Lamictal XR *Tab:* 25, 50, 100, 200, 250, 300 mg ext-rel

▷ *levetiracetam* (C)(G)
　　Elepsia *Tab:* 1000, 1500 mg ext-rel
　　Keppra *Tab:* 250*, 500*, 750*, 1000*mg

(continued)

Appendix R (*continued*)

       Keppra Oral Solution *Oral soln:* 100 mg/ml (16 oz) (grape) (dye-free)
       Keppra XR *Tab:* 500, 750 mg ext-rel
       Levitiracetam IV *Premixed:* 500, 1,000, 1,500 mg for IV infusion (100 ml)
       Roweepra *Tab:* 250, 500, 750 mg; 1 gm

▷ *mephobarbital* (D)(II)
       Mebaral *Tab:* 32, 50, 100 mg

▷ *methsuximide* (C)
       Celontin Kapseals *Cap:* 150, 300 mg

▷ *oxcarbazepine* (C)(G)
       Trileptal *Tab:* 150, 300, 600 mg; *Oral susp:* 300 mg/5 ml (lemon) (alcohol)
       Oxtellar XR *Tab:* 150, 300, 600 mg ext-rel

▷ *perampanel* (C)(III)
       Fycompa *Tab:* 2, 4, 6, 8, 10, 12 mg
       Fycompa Oral Suspension *Oral susp:* 0.5 mg/ml (340 ml w. dosing syringe)

▷ *phenytoin* (D)(G), *primidone* (D)(G)
       Dilantin *Cap:* 30, 100 mg ext-rel
       Dilantin Infatabs *Chew tab:* 50 mg
       Dilantin Oral Suspension *Oral susp:* 125 mg/5 ml (237 ml) (alcohol 6%)
       Phenytek *Cap:* 200, 300 mg ext-rel

▷ *pregabalin* (C)(V)
       Lyrica *Cap:* 25, 50, 75, 100, 200, 225, 300 mg
       Lyrica CR *Tab:* 82.5, 165, 330 mg ext-rel
       Lyrica Oral Solution *Oral soln:* 20 mg/ml

▷ *primidone* (C)
       Mysoline *Tab:* 50*, 250*mg
       Mysoline Oral Solution *Oral susp:* 250 mg/5 ml (8 oz)

▷ *rufinamide* (C)(G)
       Banzel *Tab:* 200*, 400*mg
       Banzel Oral Solution *Susp:* 40 mg/ml (orange) (lactose-free, gluten-free, dye-free)

▷ *stiripentol*
       Diacomit *Cap:* 250, 500 mg; *Pwdr for oral susp:* 250, 500 mg/pkt (60/carton) (fruit)

▷ *tiagabine* (C)(G)
       Gabitril *Tab:* 2, 4, 12, 16 mg

▷ *topiramate* (D)(G)
       Topamax *Tab:* 25, 50, 100, 200 mg
       Topamax Sprinkle Caps *Cap:* 15, 25, 50 mg
       Trokendi XR *Cap:* 25, 50, 100, 200 mg ext-rel
       Qudexy *Tab:* 25, 50, 100, 150, 200 mg ext-rel
       Qudexy XR *Cap:* 25, 50, 100, 150, 200 mg ext-rel

▷ *vigabatrin* (C)(G)
       Sabril *Tab:* 500 mg
       Sabril for Oral Solution 500 mg/pkt pwdr for reconstitution

▷ *zonisamide* (C)
       Zonegran *Cap:* 25, 50, 100 mg

◯ APPENDIX S. ANTI-HIV DRUGS

ANTI-HIV DRUGS WITH DOSE FORMS

▷ **Aptivus** (C) *tipranavir*
    Gel cap: 250 mg (alcohol); *Oral soln:* 100 mg/ml (95 ml w. dosing syringe) (Vit E 116 IU/ml) (buttermint-butter, toffee)

(*continued*)

Appendix S (*continued*)

➤ **Atripla (D)** *efavirenz+emtricitabine+tenofovir disoproxil*
  Tab: efa 600 mg+emtri 200 mg+teno diso 300 mg

➤ **Biktarvy** *bictegravir+emtricitabine+tenofovir alafenamide*
  Tab: bict 50 mg+emtri 200 mg+teno alaf 25 mg

➤ **Cimduo** *lamivudine+tenofovir disoproxil fumarate*
  Tab: lami 300 mg+teno teno diso 300 mg

➤ **Combivir (C)(G)** *lamivudine+zidovudine*
  Tab: aba+lami 150+zido 300 mg

➤ **Complera (B)** *emtricitabine+tenofovir disoproxil*
  Tab: emtri 200 mg+teno diso 300 mg+rilpiv 25 mg

➤ **Crixivan (C)** *indinavir sulfate*
  Cap: 100, 200, 333, 400 mg

➤ **Cytovene (C)(G)** *ganciclovir*
  Cap: 250, 500 mg; *Vial:* 50 mg/ml single-dose (500 mg, 10 ml)

➤ **Delstrigo** *doravirine+lamivudine+tenofovir disoproxil fumarate*
  Tab: dora 100 mg+lami ala 300 mg+teno dis 300 mg

➤ **Descovy (D)** *emtricitabine+tenofovir alafenamide+rilpivirine*
  Tab: emtri 200 mg+teno ala 25 mg

➤ **Edurant (B)** *rilpivirine*
  Tab: 25 mg

➤ **Emtriva (B)(G)** *emtricitabine*
  Cap: 200 mg; *Oral soln:* 10 mg/ml (170 ml) (cotton candy)

➤ **Epivir (C)(G)** *lamivudine*
  Tab: 150*, 300*mg; *Oral soln:* 10 mg/ml (240 ml) (strawberry-banana) (sucrose
  3 gm/15 ml)

➤ **Epzicom (B)** *abacavir sulfate+lamivudine*
  Tab: aba 600 mg+lami 300 mg

➤ **Evotaz (B)** *atazanavir+cobicistat*
  Tab: ataz 300+cobi 150 mg

➤ **Fortovase (B)** *aquinavir*
  Soft gel cap: 200 mg

➤ **Fuzeon (B)** *enfuvirtide*
  Vial: 90 mg/ml pwdr for SC inj after reconstitution (1 ml, 60 vials/kit) (preservative-free)

➤ **Genvoya (B)** *elvitegravir+cobicistat+emtricitabine+tenofovir alafenamide (TAF)*
  Tab: elv 150 mg+cob 150 mg+emtri 200 mg+teno alafen 10 mg

➤ **Intelence (C)** *etravirine*
  Tab: 25*, 100, 200 mg

➤ **Invirase (B)** *saquinavir mesylate*
  Hard gel cap: 200 mg

➤ **Isentress (C)** *raltegravir (potassium)*
  Tab: 400 mg film-coat; *Chew tab:* 25, 100*mg (orange-banana) (phenylalanine); *Oral susp:*
  100 mg/pkt pwdr for oral susp (banana)

➤ **Juluca** *dolutegravir+rilpivirine*
  Tab: dolu 50 mg+rilp 25 mg

(*continued*)

Appendix S (*continued*)

▷ **Kaletra (C)** *lopinavir plus ritonavir*
Cap: lopin 100 mg+riton 25 mg, lopin 200 mg+riton 50 mg; *Oral soln:* lopin 80 mg+riton
20 mg per ml (160 ml w. dose cup) (cotton candy) (alcohol 42%)
Hard gel cap: 200 mg

▷ **Lexiva (C)(G)** *fosamprenavir*
Tab: 700 mg; *Oral soln:* 50 mg/ml (grape, bubble gum) (peppermint)

▷ **Norvir (B)** *ritonavir*
Soft gel cap: 100 mg (alcohol); *Oral soln:* 80 mg/ml (8 oz) (peppermint-caramel) (alcohol)

▷ **Odefsey (D)** *emtricitabine+rilpivirine+tenofovir alafenamide*
Tab: emtri 200 mg+rilpiv 25 mg+tenof alafen 25 mg

▷ **Pifeltro** *doravirine*
Tab: 100 mg

▷ **Prezcobix (B)** *darunavir+cobicistat*
Tab: daru 800+cobi 150 mg

▷ **Prezista (C)(G)** *darunavir*
Tab: 75, 150, 600, 800 mg; *Oral susp:* 100 mg/ml (200 ml) (strawberry cream)

▷ **Rescriptor (C)** *delavirdine mesylate*
Tab: 100, 200 mg

▷ **Retrovir (C)(G)** *zidovudine*
Tab: 300 mg; *Cap:* 100 mg; *Syr:* 50 mg/5 ml (240 ml) (strawberry); *Vial:* 10 mg/ml (20 ml
vial for IV infusion) (preservative-free)

▷ **Reyataz (B)** *atazanavir*
Cap: 100, 150, 200, 300 mg

▷ **Selzentry (B)** *maraviroc*
Tab: 150, 300 mg

▷ **Stribild (B)** *elvitegravir+cobicistat+emtricitabine+tenofovir disoproxil fumarate*
Tab: elv 150 mg+cob 150 mg+emtri 200 mg+teno diso fumar 300 mg

▷ **Sustiva (C)** *efavirenz*
Tab: 75, 150, 600, 800 mg; *Cap:* 50, 200 mg

▷ **Symfi** *efavirenz+lamivudine+tenofovir disoproxil fumarate*
Tab: efav 600 mg+lami 300 mg+teno diso fum 300 mg

▷ **Symfi Lo** *efavirenz+lamivudine+tenofovir disoproxil fumarate*
Tab: efav 400 mg+lami 300 mg+teno diso fum 300 mg

▷ **Temixys** *lamivudine+tenofovir disoproxil fumarate*
Tab: lami 300 mg+teno diso fum 300mg

▷ **Tivicay (B)** *dolutegavir*
Tab: 50 mg

▷ **Temixys** *lamivudine+tenofovir disoproxil fumarate*
Tab: lami 300 mg+teno diso fum 300mg

▷ **Triumeq (C)** *abacavir sulfate+dilutegravir+lamivudine*
Tab: aba 600 mg+dilu 50 mg+lami 300 mg

▷ **Trizivir (C)(G)** *abacavir sulfate+lamivudine+zidovudine*
Tab: aba 300 mg+lami 150 mg+zido 300 mg

(*continued*)

Appendix S (*continued*)

▷ **Trogarzo** *ibalizumab-uiyk* **administer as an IV injection once every 14 days**
Vial: 200 mg/1.33 ml (1.33 ml), single-dose

▷ **Truvada (B)(G)** *emtricitabine+tenofovir disoproxil fumarate*
Tab: emt 100 mg+teno 150 mg, 133 mg+teno 200 mg, emt 167 mg+teno 250 mg, emt 200 mg+teno 300 mg

▷ **Valcyte (C)(G)** *valganciclovir*
Tab: 450 mg
Comment: *valganciclovir* is indicated for the treatment of AIDS-related cytomegalovirus (CMV) retinitis.

▷ **Videx EC (C)(G)** *didanosine*
Cap: 125, 200, 250, 400 mg ent-coat del-rel; *Chew tab:* 25, 50, 100, 150, 200 mg (mandarin orange; buffered with calcium carbonate and magnesium hydroxide) (phenylalanine); *Pwdr for oral soln:* 2, 4 gm (120, 240 ml)

▷ **Videx Pediatric Pwdr for Oral Solution (C)** *didanosine*
Pwdr for oral soln: 2, 4 gm (120, 240 ml)

▷ **Viracept (B)** *nelfinavir mesylate*
Tab: 250, 625 mg; *Pwdr for oral soln:* 50 mg/gm (144 gm) (phenylalanine)

▷ **Viramune (C)(G)** *nevirapine*
Tab: 200*mg; *Oral susp:* 50 mg/5 ml (240 ml)

▷ **Viramune XR (C)** *nevirapine*
Tab: 100, 400 mg ext-rel

▷ **Viread (C)(G)** *tenofovir disoproxil fumarate*
Tab: 150, 200, 250, 300 mg; *Oral pwdr:* 40 mg/1 gm pwdr (60 gm w. dosing scoop)

▷ **Vistide (C)** *cidofovir*
Inj: 75 mg/ml (5 ml vials for IV infusion) (preservative free)
Comment: *cidofovir* is indicated for the treatment of AIDS-related *Cytomegalo-virus* (CMV) retinitis.

▷ **Vitekta (C)** *elvitegravir*
Inj: 75 mg/ml (5 ml vials for IV infusion) (preservative free)

▷ **Zerit (C)(G)** *stavudine*
Cap: 15, 20, 30, 40 mg; *Oral soln:* 1 mg/ml pwdr for reconstitution (200 ml) (fruit) (dye-free)

▷ **Ziagen (C)(G)** *abacavir sulfate*
Tab: 300*mg; *Oral soln:* 20 mg/ml (240 ml) (strawberry-banana) (parabens, propylene glycol)

APPENDIX T. COUMADIN (WARFARIN)

T.1. COUMADIN TITRATION AND DOSE FORMS

▷ *warfarin* **(X)(G)** dosage initially 2-5 mg/day; usual maintenance 2-10 mg/day; adjust dosage to maintain INR in therapeutic range:
Venous thrombosis: 2.0-3.0
Atrial fibrillation: 2.0-3.0
Post MI: 2.5-3.5
Mechanical and bioprosthetic heart valves: 2.0-3.0 for 12 weeks after valve insertion, then 2.5-3.5 long-term
Pediatric: not recommended <18 years
Coumadin *Tab:* 1*, 2*, 2.5*, 3*, 4*, 5*, 6*, 7.5*, 10*mg
Coumadin for Injection *Vial:* 2 mg/ml (2.5 ml)
Comment: **Coumadin for Injection** is for peripheral IV administration only.

T.2. COUMADIN OVER-ANTICOAGULATION REVERSAL

▷ *phytonadione (vitamin K)*(G) 2.5-10 mg PO or IM; max 25 mg
　　AquaMEPHYTON *Vial:* 1 mg/0.5 ml (0.5 ml); 10 mg/ml (1, 2.5, 5 ml)
　　Mephyton *Tab:* 5 mg

T.3. AGENTS THAT INHIBIT COUMADIN'S ANTICOAGULATION EFFECTS

Increase Metabolism	Decrease Absorption	Other Mechanism(s)
azathioprine	azathioprine	coenzyme Q10
carbamazepine	cholestyramine	estrogen
dicloxacillin	colestipol	griseofulvin
ethanol	sucralfate	oral contraceptives
griseofulvin		ritonavir
nafcillin		spironolactone
pentobarbital		trazodone
phenobarbital		vitamin C (high dose)
phenytoin		vitamin K
primidone		
rifabutin		
rifampin		

APPENDIX U. LOW MOLECULAR WEIGHT HEPARINS

Comment: Administer by subcutaneous injection *only*, in the abdomen, and rotate sites. Avoid concomitant drugs that affect hemostasis (e.g., oral anti-coagulants and platelet aggregation inhibitors, including **aspirin**, NSAIDs, **dipyridamole**, **sulfinpyrazone**, **ticlopidine**). Not recommended <18 years-of-age.

LOW MOLECULAR WEIGHT HEPARINS WITH DOSE FORMS

▷ *ardeparin* (C)
　　Normiflo *Soln for inj:* 5,000 anti-Factor Xa U/0.5 ml; 10,000 anti-Factor Xa U/0.5 ml (sulfites, parabens)

▷ *dalteparin* (B)
　　Fragmin *Prefilled syringe:* 2500 IU/0.2 ml, 5000 IU/0.2 ml (10/box) (preservative-free); *Multi-dose vial:* 1,000 IU/ml (95,000 IU, 9.5 ml) (benzyl alcohol)

▷ *danaparoid* (B)
　　Organ *Amp:* 750 anti-Xa units/0.6 ml (0.6 ml, 10/box); *Prefilled syringe:* 750 anti-Xa units/0.6 ml (0.6 ml, 10/box) (sulfites)

▷ *enoxaparin* (B)(G)
　　Lovenox *Prefilled syringe:* 30 mg/0.3 ml, 40 mg/0.4 ml, 60 mg/0.6 ml, 80 mg/0.8 ml (100 mg/ml) (preservative-free); *Vial:* 100 mg/ml (3 ml)

▷ *tinzaparin* (B)
　　Innohep *Vial:* 20,000 *anti-Factor Xa* IU/ml (2 ml) (sulfites, benzyl alcohol)

APPENDIX V. FACTOR XA INHIBITORS

FACTOR Xa INHIBITOR DOSE FORMS AND THERAPY

▷ *apixaban* (C) 5 mg bid; reduce to 2.5 mg bid if any two of the following: ≥80 years, ≤60 kg, serum Cr ≥1.5
Pediatric: not recommended
　　Eliquis *Tab:* 2.5, 5 mg

(continued)

Appendix V (*continued*)

Comment: Eliquis is indicated to reduce the risk of stroke and systemic embolism in patients with nonvalvular atrial fibrillation (NVAF).

▸ ***betrixaban*** *Recommended dose:* is an initial single dose of 160 mg, followed by 80 mg once daily, taken at the same time each day with food;
Recommended duration of treatment: 35 to 42 days; reduce dose with severe renal impairment or with P-glycoprotein (P-gp) inhibitors
Pediatrics: not established
    Bevyxxa *Cap:* 40, 80 mg

Comment: Bevyxxa is indicated for the prophylaxis of venous thromboembolism (VTE) in adults who are hospitalized for acute mental illness and at risk for thromboembolic complications due to moderate or severe restricted mobility and other VTE risk factors. There are no data with the use of ***betrixaban*** in pregnancy, but treatment is likely to increase the risk of hemorrhage during pregnancy and delivery. No data are available regarding the presence of ***betrixaban*** or its metabolites in human milk or the effects of the drug on the breastfed infant.

▸ ***edoxaban*** (C) transition to and from **Savaysa**; assess CrCl prior to initiation:
NVAF CrCl >50 mL/min: 60 mg once daily; *CrCl 15-50 mL/min:* 30 mg once daily
DVT/PE CrCl >50 mL/min: 60 mg once daily following initial parental anticoagulant; *CrCl 15-50 mL/min, <60 kg,* or *concomitant Pgp inhibitors:* 30 mg once daily
Pediatric: not established
    Savaysa *Tab:* 15, 30, 60 mg

Comment: Savaysa is indicated to reduce the risk of stroke and systemic embolism in patients with nonvalvular atrial fibrillation (NVAF), treatment of DVT and pulmonary embolism (PE) following 5-10 days of initial therapy with parenteral anticoagulant. Not for use in persons with NVAF with CrCl >95 mL/min.

▸ ***fondaparinux*** (B) Administer SC; administer first dose no earlier than 6-8 hours after hemostasis is achieved, start warfarin usually within 72 hours of last dose of *fondaparinux*
Post-op: 2.5 mg once daily x 5-9 days
Hip/Knee Replacement: once daily x 11 days
Hip Fracture: once daily x 32 days
Abdominal Surgery: once daily x 10 days
Prophylaxis: do not use <50 kg
Treatment: once daily for at least 5 days until INR = 2-3 (usually 5-9 days); max 26 days; <50 kg: 5 mg; 50-100 kg: 7.5 mg; >100 kg: 10 mg
Pediatric: not established
    Arixtra *Soln for SC inj:* 2.5 mg/0.5 ml, 5 mg/0.4 ml, 7.5 mg/0.6 ml, 10 mg/0.8 ml *prefilled syringe* (10/box) (preservative-free)

▸ ***prasugrel*** (B)(G) *Loading dose:* 60 mg once in a single-dose; *Maintenance:* 10 mg once daily; *<60 kg:* consider 5 mg once daily; take with aspirin 75-325 mg once daily
Pediatric: not recommended
    Effient *Tab:* 5, 10 mg

Comment: Effient is indicated to reduce the risk of thrombotic cardiovascular events in persons with acute coronary syndrome (ACS) who are to be managed with percutaneous coronary intervention (PCI) including unstable angina, non-ST elevation myocardial infarction (NSTEMI) and STEMI. Do not start if active pathological bleeding (e.g., peptic ulcer, intracranial hemorrhage), prior TIA or stroke, or if patient likely to undergo urgent CABG. Discontinue 7 days before surgery and if TIA or stroke occurs.

▸ ***rivaroxaban*** (C) take with food
Treatment of DVT or *PE:* 15 mg twice daily for the first 21 days; then 20 mg once daily
Reduction in risk of DVT or *PE recurrence:* 20 mg once daily with the evening meal; *CrCl <30 mL/min:* avoid
Prophylaxis of DVT: take 6-10 hours after surgery when hemostasis established, then 10-20 mg once daily with the evening meal; *CrCl 30-50 mL/min:* 10 mg; *CrCl <30 mL/min:* avoid; discontinue if acute renal failure develops; monitor closely for blood loss
Hip: treat for 35 days; *Knee:* treat for 12 days

(*continued*)

Appendix V (*continued*)

Nonvalvular AF: take once daily with the evening meal; *CrCl >50 mL/min:* 20 mg; *CrCl 15-50 mL/min:* 15 mg; *CrCl >15 mL/min:* avoid
Pediatric: not recommended
    Xarelto *Cap:* 10, 15, 20 mg

Comment: **Xarelto** is indicated to reduce the risk of stroke and systemic embolism in nonvalvular atrial fibrillation (AF), to treat deep vein thrombosis (DVT) and pulmonary embolism (PE), to reduce the risk of recurrence of DVT and/or PE following 6 months treatment for DVT and/or PE, and prophylaxis of DVT which may lead to PE in patients undergoing knee or hip replacement surgery. **Xarelto** eliminates the need for bridging with heparin or low molecular heparin; no need for routine monitoring of INR or other coagulation parameters; no need for dose adjustments for age, weight, or gender; no known dietary restrictions. Switching from *warfarin* or other anticoagulant, see mfr pkg insert.

FACTOR Xa INHIBITOR REVERSAL AGENT

Comment: Andexxa *(coagulation factor Xa [recombinant] inactivated-zhzo)* is indicated to reverse the anticoagulation effects of factor Xa inhibitors (i.e., reversal agent specific to *rivaroxaban* [Xarelto] and *apixaban* [Eliquis]) when needed due to life-threatening or uncontrolled bleeding or emergency surgery. **Andexxa** was approved under the FDA's accelerated approval pathway based on effects in healthy volunteers, and continued approval may be contingent on post-marketing studies to demonstrate an improvement in hemostasis in patients. A clinical trial comparing this agent or usual care is scheduled to start in 2019 and to be reported in 2023.

▷ *coagulation factor Xa [recombinant] inactivated-zhzo* administer as an IV bolus, with a target rate of 30 mg/min, followed by continuous infusion for up to 120 minutes; select a high dose or low dose regimen based on the specific FXa inhibitor, dose of FXa inhibitor, and time since the patient's last dose of FXa inhibitor (see pkg insert); resume anticoagulant therapy as soon as medically appropriate following treatment with **Andexxa**.
High Dose Regimen: Initial IV Bolus: 800 mg at a target rate of 30 mg/min; *Follow-on IV infusion:* 8 mg/min for up to 120 min
Low Dose Regimen: Initial IV Bolus: 400 mg at a target rate of 30 mg/min; *Follow-on IV infusion:* 4 mg/min for up to 120 min
Pediatric: >18 years: not studied; ≥18 years: same as adult
    Andexxa *Vial:* 100 mg single dose pwdr for reconstitution and IV infusion

Comment: There are no adequate and well-controlled studies of **Andexxa** in pregnant women to inform patients of associated risks. The safety and effectiveness of **Andexxa** during labor and delivery have not been evaluated. There is no information regarding the presence of **Andexxa** in human milk or effects on the breastfed infant. Safety and efficacy of **Andexxa** in the pediatric population have not been studied. BBW: Treatment with **Andexxa** has been associated with serious and life-threatening adverse events, including arterial and venous thromboembolic events, ischemic events, including myocardial infarction and ischemic stroke, cardiac arrest, and sudden deaths.

APPENDIX W. DIRECT THROMBIN INHIBITORS

DIRECT THROMBIN INHIBITOR DOSING AND DOSE FORMS

▷ *aspirin* (D) single dose once daily
Pediatric: not established
    Durlaza *Cap:* 162.5 mg 24-hr ext-rel (30, 90/bottle)
▷ *dabigatran etexilate mesylate* (C) swallow whole; *CrCl >30 mL/min:* 150 mg bid; *CrCl 15-30 mL/min:* 75 mg twice daily; *CrCl <15 mL/min:* not recommended
Pediatric: not recommended
    Pradaxa *Cap:* 75, 150 mg
    Comment: **Pradaxa** is indicated to reduce the risk of stroke and systemic embolism in nonvalvular AF, DVT prophylaxis, PE prophylaxis in patients who have undergone hip

(*continued*)

Appendix W (*continued*)

replacement surgery, treatment of DVT and PE in patients who have been treated with a parenteral anticoagulant for 5-10 days, and to reduce the risk of recurrent DVT and PE in patients who have been previously treated. **Pradaxa** is contraindicated in patients with a mechanical prosthetic heart valve and not recommended with a bioprosthetic heart valve. Presently there is only one reversal agent for this drug class. *idarucizumab* (**Praxbind**) is a specific reversal agent for *dabigatran* (**Pradaxa**). It is a humanized monoclonal antibody fragment (Fab) that binds to dabigatran and its acylglucuronide metabolites with higher affinity than the binding affinity of dabigatran to thrombin, neutralizing its anticoagulant effects. [See **Pradaxa** reversal agent, *idarucizumab* (**Praxbind**) at the end of this appendix].

▷ *desirudin (recombinant hirudin)* (C) 15 mg SC every 12 hours, preferably in the abdomen <u>or</u> thigh, starting up to 5-15 minutes before surgery (after induction of regional block anesthesia, if used); may continue for 9-12 days post-op; *CrCl <60 mL/min:* reduce dose (see mfr pkg insert)
    Pediatric: not recommended
        Iprivask *Pwdr for SC inj after reconstitution:* 15 mg/single-use vial (10/box) (preservative-free, diluent contains mannitol)
Comment: **Iprivask** is indicated for DVT prophylaxis in patients undergoing hip replacement surgery. It is not interchangeable with other hirudins.

IDARUCIZUMAB REVERSAL AGENT: HUMANIZED MONOCLONAL–ANTIBODY FRAGMENT (FAB)

▷ *idarucizumab* (NE) administer 5 gm (2 vials) IV drip <u>or</u> push; administer within 1 hour of removal from vial
    Pediatric: not established
        Praxbind *Vial:* 2.5 g/50 ml, single-use (preservative-free)
Comment: Presently, there is inadequate human and animal data to assess risk of *idarucizumab* (**Praxbind**) use in pregnancy. Risk/benefit should be considered prior to use.

APPENDIX X. PLATELET AGGREGATION INHIBITORS

PLATELET AGGREGATION INHIBITOR DOSING AND DOSE FORMS

▷ *cilostazol* (B) 100 mg bid
    Pediatric: not recommended
        Pletal *Tab:* 50, 100 mg
Comment: **Pletal** is an antiplatelet/vasodilator (PDE III inhibitor)

▷ *clopidogrel* (B) 75 mg once daily
    Pediatric: not recommended
        Plavix *Tab:* 75, 300 mg
Comment: **Plavix** is indicated for the reduction of atherosclerotic events in recent MI <u>or</u> stroke, established PAD, non-ST-segment elevation acute coronary syndrome (unstable angina/non-STEMI), <u>or</u> STEMI.

▷ *dipyridamole* (B)(G) 75-100 mg qid
    Pediatric: not recommended
        Persantine *Tab:* 25, 50, 75 mg
Comment: *dipyridamole* is indicated as an adjunct to oral anticoagulants after cardiac valve replacement surgery to prevent thromboembolism.

▷ *dipyridamole+aspirin* (B)(G) swallow whole; one cap bid
    Pediatric: not recommended
        Aggrenox *Cap:* dipyr 200 mg+asa 25 mg

▷ *pentoxifylline* (C) [hemorrheologic (xanthine)]
    Pediatric: not recommended
        Trental *Tab:* 400 mg sust-rel

(*continued*)

Appendix X (*continued*)

▷ *prasugrel* (C)(G)
   Pediatric: not recommended
      Efficient *Tab:* 5, 10 mg
Comment: **Efficient** is indicated to reduce the risk of cardiovascular events in patients with acute coronary syndrome (ACS) who are to be managed with percutaneous coronary intervention (unstable angina or non-STEMI), and STEMI when managed with either primary or delayed PCI.

▷ *ticagrelor* (C) initiate 180 mg loading dose once in a single dose with *aspirin* 325 mg loading dose in a single dose; maintenance 90 mg twice daily with *aspirin* 75-100 mg once daily; ACS patients may start *ticagrelor* after a loading dose of *clopidogrel*
      Brilinta *Tab:* 90 mg
Comment: **Brilinta** is indicated to reduce the risk of cardiovascular events in patients with acute coronary syndrome (ACS) (unstable angina, Non-ST elevation (NSTEMI), myocardial infarction, or STEMI).

▷ *ticlopidine* (B) 250 mg bid
   Pediatric: not recommended
      Ticlid *Tab:* 250 mg
Comment: **Ticlid** is indicated to reduce the risk of thrombotic stroke in selected patients intolerant of *aspirin*.

APPENDIX Y. PROTEASE-ACTIVATED RECEPTOR-1 (PAR-1) INHIBITOR

PROTEASE-ACTIVATED RECEPTOR-1 (PAR-1) INHIBITOR DOSING AND DOSE FORM

▷ *vorapaxar* (B) administer 2.08 mg once daily; use with *aspirin* or *clopidogrel*
   Pediatric: <12 years: not established; ≥12 years: same as adult
      Zontivity *Tab:* 2.08 mg (equivalent to 2.5 mg vorapaxar sulfate)
Comment: **Zontivity** is indicated to reduce thrombotic cardiovascular events in patients with a history of myocardial infarction or with peripheral arterial disease (PAD). Contraindicated with active pathological bleeding (e.g., peptic ulcer, intra-cranial hemorrhage), prior TIA or stroke. Not recommended with severe hepatic impairment.

APPENDIX Z. PRESCRIPTION PRENATAL VITAMINS

Comment: It is recommended that prenatal vitamins be started at least 3 months prior to conception to improve preconception nutritional status, and continued throughout pregnancy and the postnatal period, in lactating and nonlactating women, and throughout the childbearing years.

▷ **CitraNatal 90 DHA** take 1 tab* and 1 DHA cap daily
   Tab: thiamine 3 mg, riboflavin 3.4 mg, niacinamide 20 mg, pyridoxine HCL 20 mg, folic acid 1 mg, Vit C 120 mg, Vit D3 400 IU, Vit E 30 IU, calcium (as citrate) 160 mg, copper (as oxide) 2 mg, iodine (as potassium iodide) 150 mcg, iron (as carbonyl) 90 mg, zinc (as oxide) 25 mg, docusate sodium 50 mg
   Cap: docosahexaenoic acid (DHA) 300 mg

▷ **CitraNatal Assure** take 1 tab and 1 DHA cap daily
   Tab: thiamine 3 mg, riboflavin 3.4 mg, niacinamide 20 mg, pyridoxine HCL 25 mg, folic acid 1 mg, Vit C 120 mg, Vit D3 400 IU, Vit E 30 IU, calcium (as citrate) 125 mg, copper (as oxide) 2 mg, iodine (as potassium oxide) 150 mcg, iron (as carbonyl and ferrous gluconate) 35 mg, zinc (as oxide) 25 mg, docusate sodium 50 mg
   Cap: docosahexaenoic acid (DHA) 300 mg

▷ **CitraNatal B-Calm** take 1 tab every 8 hours; begin with tab #1.
   Tab: pyridoxine HCL 25 mg, folic acid 1 mg, Vit C 120 mg, Vit D3 400 IU, calcium (as citrate) 120 mg, iron (as carbonyl) 20 mg
   Tab: pyridoxine 25 mg
Comment: **Citranatal B-Calm** may be used as an adjunct treatment to help minimize pregnancy-related nausea and vomiting.

(*continued*)

Appendix Z (*continued*)

▷ **CitraNatal DHA** take 1 tab and 1 DHA cap daily
Tab: thiamine 3 mg, riboflavin 3.4 mg, niacinamide 20 mg, pyridoxine HCL 20 mg, folic acid 1 mg, Vit C 120 mg, Vit D3 400 IU, Vit E 30 IU, calcium (as citrate) 125 mg, copper (as oxide) 2 mg, iodine (as potassium oxide) 150 mcg, iron (as carbonyl and gluconate) 27 mg, zinc (as oxide) 25 mg, docusate sodium 50 mg
Cap: docosahexaenoic acid (DHA) 250 mg

▷ **CitraNatal Harmony** take 1 gelcap daily
Gelcap: pyridoxine HCL 25 mg, folic acid 1 mg, Vit D3 400 IU, Vit E 30 IU, calcium (as citrate) 104 mg, iron (as carbonyl and ferrous fumarate) 27 mg, docusate sodium 50 mg, docosahexaenoic acid (DHA) 260 mg

▷ **CitraNatal Rx** take 1 tab* and 1 DHA cap daily
Tab: thiamine 3 mg, riboflavin 3.4 mg, niacinamide 20 mg, pyridoxine HCL 20 mg, folic acid 1 mg, Vit C 120 mg, Vit D3 400 IU, Vit E 30 IU, calcium (as citrate) 125 mg, copper (as oxide) 2 mg, iodine (as potassium iodide) 150 mcg, iron (as carbonyl and gluconate) 27 mg, zinc (as oxide) 25 mg, docusate sodium 50 mg

▷ **Duet DHA Balanced** take 1 tab and 1 gelcap daily
Tab: Vit A (as beta carotene) 2800 IU, thiamine 1.5 mg, riboflavin 2 mg, niacinamide 20 mg, pyridoxine HCL 50 mg, Vit B12 12 mcg, folic acid 1 mg, Vit C 120 mg, Vit D3 640 IU, Vit E 15 IU, calcium (as carbonate) 215 mg, iron (as polysaccharide iron complex and sodium iron EDTA, Ferrazone) 25 mg, copper (as oxide) 1.8 mg, magnesium (as oxide) 25 mg, zinc (as oxide) 25 mg, iodine (as potassium iodide) 210 mcg, selenium 65 mcg, choline (as bartrate) 55 mg
Gelcap: omega 3 fatty acids 267 mg (includes docosahexaenoic acid [DHA], eicosapentaenoic acid [EPA], alpha-linolenic acid [ALA], docasapentaeoic acid [DPA]) (gelatin, gluten-free)

▷ **Duet DHA Complete** take 1 tab and 1 gelcap daily
Tab: Vit A (as beta carotene) 3000 IU, thiamine 1.8 mg, riboflavin 4 mg, niacinamide 20 mg, pyridoxine HCL 50 mg, Vit B12 12 mcg, folic acid 1 mg, Vit C 120 mg, Vit D3 800 IU, Vit E 3 mg, calcium (as carbonate) 230 mg, iron (as polysaccharide iron complex and sodium iron EDTA, ferrazone) 27 mg, copper (as oxide) 2 mg, magnesium (as oxide) 25 mg, zinc (as oxide) 25 mg, iodine 220 mcg
Gelcap: omega 3 fatty acids ≥430 mg (as docosahexaenoic acid (DHA) ≥295 mg, as other omega-3 fatty acids ≥135 mg (eicosapentaenoic acid (EPA), docasapentaenoic acid (DHA) (gluten-free)

▷ **Natachew** take 1 chew tab daily
Chew tab: Vit A 1000 IU (as beta carotene), thiamine 2 mg, riboflavin 3 mg, niacinamide 20 mg, pyridoxine HCL 10 mg, B12 12 mcg, folic acid 1 mg, Vit C 120 mg, Vit D3 400 IU, Vit E 11 IU, iron (as ferrous fumarate) 29 mg (wildberry)

▷ **Natafort** take 1 tab daily
Tab: Vit A 1000 IU (as acetate and beta carotene), thiamine 2 mg, riboflavin 3 mg, niacinamide 20 mg, pyridoxine HCL 10 mg, B12 12 mcg, folic acid 1 mg, Vit C 120 mg, Vit D3 400 IU, Vit E 11 IU, iron (as carbonyl and sulfate) 60 mg

▷ **Neevo DHA** take 1 cap daily
Cap: l-methylfolate (as Metafolin) 1.3 mg, thiamin 1.4 mg, riboflavin 1.4 mg, niacinamide 18 mg, pyridoxine HCL 25 mg, B12 1 mg, Vit C 85 mg, Vit D3, 5 mcg, Vit E 15 IU, calcium (as carbonate) 110 mg, iron (ferrous fumarate) 27 mg, iodine (as potassium iodide) 220 mcg, magnesium (as oxide) 60 mg, docosahexaenoic acid (DHA, vegetarian source (algal oil) 581.92 mg (soy, gelatin, sorbitol, glycerin)

Comment: Neevo DHA is indicated as a nutritional supplement during pregnancy, and the prenatal and postnatal periods, in women with dietary needs for the biologically active form of folate, who are at risk for hyperhomocysteinemia, impaired folic acid absorption, <u>and/or</u> impaired folic acid metabolism due to 667C >T mutations in the MTHFR gene.

▷ **Nexa Plus** take 1 cap daily
Cap: pyridoxine HCL 25 mg, folic acid 1.25 mg, Vit C 28 mg, Vit D3 800 IU, Vit E 30 IU, biotin 250 mcg, calcium (as carbonate [158 mg]+docusate calcium [2 mg] 160 mg, iron (as

(*continued*)

Appendix Z (*continued*)

ferrous fumarate) 29 mg, docosahexaenoic acid (DHA, plant-based source [algal oil]) 350 mg (soy)

▷ **Nexa Select** take 1 softgel cap daily
Softgel cap: pyridoxine HCL 25 mg, folic acid 1.25 mg, Vit C 28 mg, Vit D3 800 IU, Vit E 30 IU, calcium (as phosphate) 160 mg, iron (as ferrous fumarate) 29 mg, docosahexaenoic acid (DHA) plant-based source (algal oil) 325 mg, docusate sodium 55 mg (soy)

▷ **Prenate AM** take 1 tab daily
Tab: pyridoxine HCL 75 mg, folate (as folic acid 400 mcg+Quatrefolic 1.1 mg [equivalent to 600 mcg folic acid]) 1 mg, Vit B12 12 mcg, calcium (as carbonate) 200 mg, ginger extract 500 mg, lingon-berry 25 mg

▷ **Prenate Chewable** take 1 chew tab daily
Chew tab: pyridoxine HCL 10 mg, Vit B12 125 mcg, calcium (as carbonate) 500 mg, Vit D3 300 IU, biotin 280 mcg, boron amino acid chelate 250 mcg, folate (as Quatrefolic) 1 mg, magnesium (as oxide) 50 mg, blueberry extract 25 mg (Dutch chocolate)

▷ **Prenate DHA** take 1 gel cap daily
Gelcap: pyridoxine HCL 26 mg, folate (as folic acid) 400 mcg+Quatrefolic 1.1 mg [equivalent to 600 mcg folic acid]) 1 mg, Vit B12 13 mcg, Vit C 90 mg, Vit D3 220 IU, Vit E 10 IU, calcium (as carbonate) 145 mg, iron (as ferrous fumarate) 28 mg, magnesium (as oxide) 50 mg, docosahexaenoic acid (DHA) 300 mg (fish oil, soy, gelatin)

▷ **Prenate Elite** take 1 gel cap daily
Gelcap: Vit A (as beta-carotene) 2600 IU, thiamine 3 mg, riboflavin 3.5 mg, pyridoxine HCl 21 mg, niacinamide 21 mg, pantothenic acid 6 mg, folate (as folic acid 400 mcg+Quatrefolic 1.1 mg [equivalent to 600 mcg folic acid]) 1 mg, Vit B12 13 mcg, Vit C 75 mg, Vit D3 450 IU, Vit E 10 IU, biotin 330 mcg, calcium (as carbonate) 100 mg, iron (as ferrous fumarate) 27 mg, magnesium (as oxide) 25 mg, copper (as oxide) 1.5 mg, iodine 150 mcg, iron (as ferrous fumarate) 26 mg, zinc (as oxide) 15 mg

▷ **Prenate Enhance** take 1 gel cap daily
Gelcap: pyridoxine HCL 25 mg, folate (as folic acid 400 mcg+Quatrefolic 1.1 mg [equivalent to 600 mcg folic acid]) 1 mg, Vit B12 12 mcg, Vit C 85 mg, Vit D3 1000 IU, Vit E 10 IU, biotin 500 mcg, calcium (as carbonate+Formical) 155 mg, iodine (as potassium) 150 mcg, iron (as ferrous fumarate) 28 mg, magnesium (as oxide) 50 mg, docosahexaenoicacid (DHA) 400 mg (soy, gelatin)

▷ **Prenate Essential** take 1 gel cap daily
Gelcap: pyridoxine HCL 26 mg, folate (as folic acid 400 mcg+Quatrefolic 1.1 mg [equivalent to 600 mcg folic acid]) 1 mg, Vit B12 13 mcg, Vit C 90 mg, Vit D3 220 IU, Vit E 10 IU, biotin 280 mcg, calcium (as carbonate) 145 mg, iodine (as potassium iodide) 150 mcg, iron (as ferrous fumarate) 29 mg, magnesium (as oxide) 50 mg, docosahexaenoic acid (DHA) 300 mg, eicosapentaenoic acid (EPA) 40 mg (fish oil, soy, gelatin)

▷ **Prenate Mini** take 1 gel cap daily
Gelcap: pyridoxine HCL 26 mg, folate (as folic acid 400 mcg+Quatrefolic 1.1 mg [equivalent to 600 mcg folic acid]) 1 mg, Vit B12 13 mcg, Vit C 60 mg, Vit D3 220 IU, Vit E 10 IU, calcium (as carbonate) 100 mg, iron (as carbonyl iron) 29 mg, iodine (as potassium iodide) 150 mcg, biotin 280 mcg, magnesium (as oxide) 25 mg, docosahexaenoic acid (DHA) 300 mg, blueberry extract 25 mg (fish oil, soy, gelatin)

▷ **Prenate Restore** take 1 gel cap daily
Gelcap: pyridoxine HCL 25 mg, folate (as folic acid 400 mcg+Quatrefolic 1.1 mg [equivalent to 600 mcg folic acid]) 1 mg, Vit B12 12 mcg, Vit C 85 mg, Vit D3 1000 IU, Vit E 10 IU, biotin 500 mcg, calcium (as carbonate+Formical) 155 mg, iron (as ferrous fumarate) 27 mg, magnesium (as oxide) 45 mg, docosahexaenoic acid (DHA) 400 mg, *Bacillus coagulans* 150 million CFU (as lactospore) 10 mg (soy, gelatin)

▷ **Prenexa** take 1 gel cap daily
Gelcap: pyridoxine HCL 25 mg, folic acid 1.25 mg, Vit C 28 mg, Vit D3 400 IU, Vit E 30 IU, calcium (as phosphate) 160 mg, iron (as ferrous fumarate) 27 mg, docosahexaenoic acid (DHA) plant-based source (algal oil) 300 mg, docusate sodium 55 mg (soy)

APPENDIX AA. DRUGS FOR THE MANAGEMENT OF ALLERGY, COUGH, AND COLD SYMPTOMS

Comment: Oral prescription drugs for the management of allergy symptoms, cough, and symptoms of the common cold are listed in alphabetical order by brand name.

LEGEND

acriv	*acrivastine*
benzo	*benzonatate*
brom	*brompheniramine*
carb	*carbinoxamine*
carbeta	*carbetapentane*
chlor	*chlorpheniramine*
cod	*codeine*
cypro	*cyproheptadine*
deslorat	*desloratadine*
dexchlo	*dexchlorpheniramine*
dextro	*dextromethorphan*
diphen	*diphenhydramine*
hydrox	*hydroxyzine*
guaiac	*potassium guaiacolsulfonate*
guaif	*guaifenesin*
homat	*homatropine*
hydro	*hydrocodone*
hydrox	*hydroxyzine*
levocetir	*levocetirizine*
meth	*methscopolamine*
phenyle	*phenylephrine*
prometh	*promethazine*
pseud	*pseudoephedrine*
pyril	*pyrilamine tannate*

➤ **Allerex (C)** 1 AM tab in the morning and 1 PM tab in the evening prn
  Pediatric: <12 years: not recommended; ≥12 years: same as adult
  AM tab: meth 2.5 mg+pseud 120 mg ext-rel; *PM tab:* meth 2.5 mg+chlor 8 mg+phenyle 10 mg* ext-rel (*Dose Pack 20:* 10 AM tabs+10 PM tabs; *Dose Pack 60:* 30 AM tabs+30 PM tabs)
➤ **Allures-D (C)** 1 tab q 12 hours prn
  Pediatric: <12 years: not recommended; ≥12 years: same as adult
  Tab: meth 2.5 mg+pseud 120 mg ext-rel
➤ **Allerex DF (C)** 1 AM tab in the morning and 1 PM tab in the evening prn
  Pediatric: <12 years: not recommended; ≥12 years: same as adult
  AM tab: meth 2.5 mg+chlor 4 mg; *PM tab:* meth 2.5 mg+chlor 8 mg* (*Dose Pack 20:* 10 AM tabs+10 PM tabs; *Dose Pack 60:* 30 AM tabs+30 PM tabs)
➤ **Allerex PE (C)** 1 AM tab in the morning and 1 PM tab in the evening prn
  Pediatric: <12 years: not recommended; ≥12 years: same as adult
  AM tab: meth 2.5 mg+phenyle 40 mg/*PM tab:* meth 8 mg+phenyle 10 mg* (*Dose Pack 20:* 10 AM tabs+10 PM tabs; *Dose Pack 60:* 30 AM tabs+30 PM tabs)
➤ **Allerex Suspension (C)** 15 ml q 12 hours prn
  Pediatric: <6 years: not recommended; 6-12 years: 2.5-5 ml q 12 hours prn; >12 years: same as adult
  Susp: chlor 3 mg+phenyle 7.5 mg ext-rel (raspberry)
➤ **Atarax (B)(G)** 25 mg tid or qid prn
  Pediatric: <2 years: not recommended; 2-6 years: 6.25 mg q 4-6 hours prn; 6-12 years: 12.5-25 mg q 4-6 hours prn; >12 years: same as adult
  Tab: hydrox 10, 25, 50, 100 mg; *Syr:* hydrox 10 mg/5 ml (alcohol 0.5%)

(continued)

Appendix AA (*continued*)

▶ **Bromfed DM (C)(G)** 2 tsp q 4 hours prn: max 6 doses/day
Pediatric: <2 years: not recommended; 2-6 years: 2 tsp q 4 hours prn; 6-12 years: 1 tsp q 4 hours prn; max 6 doses/day; >12 years: same as adult
Susp: brom 2 mg+pseudo 30 mg+dextro 10 mg per 5 ml (butterscotch; alcohol 0.95%)

▶ **Bromfed DM Sugar-Free (C)(G)** 2 tsp q 4 hours prn: max 6 doses/day
Pediatric: <2 years: not recommended; 2-6 years: 1/2 tsp q 4 hours prn; 6-12 years: 1 tsp q 4 hours prn; >12 years: same as adult
max 6 doses/day
Susp: brom 2 mg+pseudo 30 mg+dextro 10 mg per 5 ml (butterscotch) (alcohol 0.95%)

▶ **Clarinex (C)** 1 tab daily prn
Pediatric: <6 years: not recommended; ≥6 years: 1/2-1 tab once daily
Tab: deslorat 5 mg

▶ **Clarinex RediTabs (C)** 5 mg daily prn
Pediatric: <6 years: not recommended; 6-12 years: 2.5 mg once daily; >12 years: same as adult
ODT: deslorat 2.5, 5 mg (tutti-frutti) (phenylalanine)

▶ **Clarinex Syrup (C)** 1 tab daily prn
Pediatric: <6 months: not recommended; 6-11 months: 1 mg (2 ml) daily prn; 1-5 years: 1.25 mg (2.5 ml) daily prn; 6-11 years: 2.5 mg (5 ml) daily prn; ≥11 years: 5 mg (10 ml) daily prn
Tab: deslorat 0.5 mg per ml (4 oz) (tutti-frutti) (phenylalanine)

▶ **Duratuss AC 12 (C)** 1-2 tsp q 12 hours prn
Pediatric: <2 years: not recommended; 2-6 years: 1/2 tsp q 12 hrs prn; 6-12 years: 1 tsp q 12 hours prn; >12 years: same as adult
Susp: diphen 12.5 mg+dextro 15 mg+phenyle 15 mg per 5 ml (strawberry banana) (sugar-free, alcohol-free, phenylalanine)

▶ **Duratuss DM (C)** 1 tsp q 4 hours prn
Pediatric: <2 years: not recommended; 2-6 years: 1/4 tsp q 4 hrs prn; >6 years: 1/2 tsp q 4 hours prn
Susp: dextro 25 mg+guaif 225 mg per 5 ml (grape) (sugar-free, alcohol-free)

▶ **Duratuss DM 12 (C)** 1-2 tsp q 12 hours prn; max 6 tabs/day
Pediatric: <2 years: not recommended; 2-6 years: 1/2 tsp q 12 hrs prn; >6 years: 1/2-1 tsp q 12 hours prn; >6 years: same as adult
Susp: dextro 15 mg+guaif 225 mg per 5 ml (grape) (sugar-free, alcohol-free)

▶ **Flowtuss Oral Solution (C)(II)(G)** 1-2 tsp q 4-6 hours prn; max 6 tsp/24 hours
Pediatric: <6 years: not recommended; 6-12 years: 1/2 tsp q 4-6 hours prn; max 15 ml/day; >12 years: same as adult
Oral soln: hydro 2.5 mg+guaif 200 mg per 5 ml (black raspberry)
Comment: *hydrocodone* is known to be excreted in human milk.

▶ **Hycodan (C)(III)** 1 tab q 4-6 hours prn; max 6 tabs/day
Pediatric: <6 years: not recommended; 6-12 years: 1/2 tab q 4-6 hours prn; max 3 tabs/day; >12 years: same as adult
Tab: hydro 5 mg+homat 1.5 mg
Comment: *hydrocodone* is known to be excreted in human milk.

▶ **Hycodan Syrup (C)(II)(G)** 1 tsp q 4-6 hours prn
Pediatric: <6 years: not recommended; 6-12 years: 1/2 tsp q 4-6 hours prn; max 15 ml/day; >12 years: same as adult
Syr: hydro 5 mg+homat 1.5 mg per 5 ml
Comment: *hydrocodone* is known to be excreted in human milk.

▶ **Hycofenix Oral Solution (C)(II)** 1 tsp q 4-6 hours prn
Pediatric: <6 years: not recommended; 6-12 years: 1/2 tsp q 4-6 hours prn; max 15 ml/day; >12 years: same as adult
Oral soln: hydro 2.5 mg+pseudo 30 mg+quaf 200 mg per 5 ml (black raspberry)
Comment: *hydrocodone* is known to be excreted in human milk.

▶ **Obredon Oral Solution (C)(II)** 10 ml q 4-6 hours prn cough; max 60 ml/day
Pediatric: <18 years: not recommended; >18 years: same as adult
Oral soln: hydro 2.5 mg+guaif 200 mg per 5 ml

(continued)

Appendix AA (*continued*)

Comment: **Obredon** is indicated only for short term treatment of cough due to the common cold. **Obredon** is not indicated for persistent or chronic cough such as occurs with smoking, asthma, chronic bronchitis, or emphysema, or where cough is accompanied by excessive phlegm. Use with caution in patients with diabetes, thyroid disease, Addison's disease, BPH or urethral stricture, and asthma. **Obredon** is contraindicated with paralytic ileus, anticholinergics, TCAs, and within 14 days of an MAOI. *hydrocodone* is known to be excreted in human milk. There is no FDA-approved generic form of *hydrocodone+guaifenesin*.

➤ **Palgic (C)** 4 mg daily prn; max 24 mg/day in divided doses 6-8 hours apart
  Pediatric: <2 year: not recommended; 2-3 years: 2 mg tid or qid prn or 0.2-0.4 mg/kg/day divided tid or qid; 3-6 years: 2-4 mg daily prn or 0.2-0.4 mg/kg/day divided tid or qid; >6 years: same as adult
  Tab: carb 4*mg; *Syr:* carb 4 mg per 5 ml (bubble gum)

➤ **Periactin (B)(G)** initially 4 mg tid prn, then adjust as needed; usual range 12-16 mg/day; max 32 mg/day
  Pediatric: <2 years: not recommended; 2-6 years: 2 mg 2-3 times/day: max 12 mg daily; 7-14 years: 4 mg 2-3 times/day: max 16 mg daily; >14 years: same as adult
  Tab: cypro 4*mg; *Syr:* cypro 2 mg per 5 ml

➤ **Prolex-DH (C)(III)** 1-1½ tsp qid prn
  Pediatric: <3 years: not recommended; 3-6 years: 1/4-1/2 tsp qid prn; 6-12 years: 1/2-1 tsp qid prn; >12 years: same as adult
  Liq: hydro 4.5 mg+pot guaiac 300 mg per 5 ml (tropical fruit punch) (alcohol-free, sugar-free)

➤ **Phenergan (C)(G)** 25 mg po or rectally tid ac and HS prn
  Pediatric: <2 years: not recommended; 2-12 years: 0.5 mg/lb or 6.25-25 mg po or rectally tid; ≥12 years: same as adult
  Tab: prometh 12.5*, 25*, 50 mg; *Syr:* prometh 6.25 mg per 5 ml; *Syr fortis:* prometh 25 mg per 5 ml; *Rectal supp:* prometh 12.5, 25, 50 mg

➤ **Promethazine DM (C)(V)(G)** 1 tsp q 4-6 hours prn
  Pediatric: <6 years: not recommended; 6-12 years: 1/2-1 tsp q 4-6 hours prn; >12 years: same as adult
  Syr: prometh 6.25 mg+dextro 15 mg per 5 ml (alcohol 7%)
  Comment: *promethazine* is contraindicated in children with uncomplicated nausea, dehydration, Reye's syndrome, history of sleep apnea, asthma, and lower respiratory disorders in children. *promethazine* lowers the seizure threshold in children, may cause cholestatic jaundice, anticholinergic effects, extrapyramidal effects, and potentially fatal respiratory depression.

➤ **Promethazine VC (C)(V)(G)** 1 tsp q 4-6 hours prn; max 30 ml/day
  Pediatric: 2-6 years: 1.25 ml q 4-6 hours prn; max 7.5 ml/day; 6-12 years: 2.5 ml q 4-6 hours prn; max 15 ml/day; >12 years: same as adult
  Syr: prometh 6.25 mg+phenyle 5 mg per 5 ml (alcohol 7%)
  Comment: *promethazine* is contraindicated in children with uncomplicated nausea, dehydration, Reye's syndrome, history of sleep apnea, asthma, and lower respiratory disorders in children. *promethazine* lowers the seizure threshold in children, may cause cholestatic jaundice, anticholinergic effects, extrapyramidal effects, and potentially fatal respiratory depression.

➤ **Promethazine VC w. Codeine (C)(V)(G)** 1 tsp q 4-6 hours prn; max 30 ml/day
  Pediatric: <6 years: not recommended; 6-12 years: 1/2-1 tsp q 4-6 hours prn; max 30 ml/day; >12 years: same as adult
  Syr: prometh 6.25 mg+phenyle 5 mg+cod 10 mg per 5 ml (alcohol 7%)
  Comment: *codeine* is known to be excreted in breast milk. <12 years: not recommended; 12-<18: use extreme caution; not recommended for children and adolescents with asthma or other chronic breathing problem. The FDA and the European Medicines Agency (EMA) are investigating the safety of using *codeine*-containing medications to treat pain, cough and colds, in children 12-<18 years because of the potential for serious side effects, including slowed or difficult breathing. *promethazine* is contraindicated in children with uncomplicated nausea, dehydration, Reye's syndrome, history of sleep apnea, asthma, and lower respiratory disorders in children. *promethazine* lowers the seizure threshold in children, may cause cholestatic jaundice, anticholinergic effects, extrapyramidal effects, and potentially fatal respiratory depression.

(*continued*)

Appendix AA (*continued*)

➤ **Promethazine w. Codeine (C)(V)(G)** 1 tsp q 4-6 hours prn
  Pediatric: <6 years: not recommended; 6-12 years: 1/2-1 tsp q 4-6 hours prn; >12 years: same as adult
    Liq: prometh 6.25 mg+cod 10 mg per 5 ml (alcohol 7%)
  Comment: *codeine* is known to be excreted in breast milk. <12 years: not recommended; 12-<18: use extreme caution; not recommended for children and adolescents with asthma or other chronic breathing problem. The FDA and the European Medicines Agency (EMA) are investigating the safety of using *codeine*-containing medications to treat pain, cough and colds, in children 12-<18 years because of the potential for serious side effects, including slowed or difficult breathing. *promethazine* is contraindicated in children with uncomplicated nausea, dehydration, Reye's syndrome, history of sleep apnea, asthma, and lower respiratory disorders in children. *promethazine* lowers the seizure threshold in children, may cause cholestatic jaundice, anticholinergic effects, extrapyramidal effects, and potentially fatal respiratory depression.

➤ **Rynatan (C)** 1-2 tabs q 12 hours prn
  Pediatric: not recommended
    Tab: chlor 9 mg+phenyle 25 mg

➤ **Rynatan Pediatric Suspension (C)**
  Pediatric: <2 years: not recommended; 2-6 years: 1/2-1 tsp q 12 hours prn; 6-12 years: 1-2 tsp q 12 hours prn; >12 years: same as adult
    Susp: chlor 4.5 mg+phenyle 5 mg

➤ **Ryneze (C)** 1 tab q 12 hours prn
  Pediatric: <6 years: not recommended; 6-12 years: 1/2 tab q 12 hours prn; >12 years: same as adult
  Tab: chlor 8 mg+meth 2.5 mg

➤ **Robitussin AC (C)(III)(G)** 2 tsp q 4 hours prn; max 60 ml/day
  Pediatric: <2 years: not recommended; 2-6 years: 1/4-1/2 tsp q 4 hours prn; 6-12 years: 1 tsp q 4 hours prn; >12 years: same as adult
    Liq: cod 10 mg+guaif 100 mg per 5 ml

➤ **Rondec Syrup (C)(G)** 1 tsp qid prn; max 30 ml/day
  Pediatric: <2 years: not recommended; 2-6 years: 1/4 tsp q 4-6 hours prn; max 7.5 ml/day; 6-12 years: 1/2 tsp q 4-6 hours prn; max 15 ml/day; ≥12 years: same as adult
    Syr: phenyle 12.5 mg+chlor 4 mg per 5 ml (bubblegum) (sugar-free, alcohol-free)

➤ **Semprex-D (B)** 1 cap q 4-6 hours prn; max 4 doses/day
  Pediatric: <12 years: not recommended; ≥12 years: same as adult
    Cap: acriv 8 mg+pseud 60 mg

➤ **Tanafed DMX (C)(G)** 2-4 tsp q 12 hours prn
  Pediatric: <2 years: not recommended; 2-6 years: 1/2-1 tsp q 12 hours prn; 6-12 years: 1-2 tsp q 12 hours prn; >12 years: same as adult
    Susp: dexchlor 2.5 mg+pseud 75 mg+dextro 25 mg per 5 ml (cotton candy) (alcohol-free)

➤ **Tessalon Caps (C)** 100-200 mg tid prn; max 600 mg/day
  Pediatric: <10 years: not recommended; ≥10 years: same as adult
    Cap: benzo 200 mg
  Comment: Swallow whole. Do not suck or chew.

➤ **Tessalon Perles (C)** 100-200 mg tid prn; max 600 mg/day
  Pediatric: <10 years: not recommended; ≥10 years: same as adult
    Perles: benzo 100 mg
  Comment: Swallow whole. Do not suck or chew.

➤ **Tussi-12 D Tablets (C)** 1-2 tabs q 12 hours prn
  Pediatric: <6 years: use susp; 6-11 years: 1/2-1 tab q 12 hours prn; >11 years: same as adult
    Tab: carbeta 60 mg+pyril 40 mg+phenyle 10*mg

➤ **Tussi-12 DS (C)** 1-2 tsp q 12 hours prn
  Pediatric: <2 years: individualize; 2-6 years: 1/2-1 tsp q 12 hours prn; 6-12 years: 1-2 tsp q 12 hours prn; >12 years: same as adult
    Liq: carbeta 30 mg+pyril 30 mg+phenyle 5 mg per 5 ml (strawberry-currant) (tartrazine)

(*continued*)

Appendix AA (*continued*)

➤ **TussiCaps 5 mg/4 mg (C)(III)** 2 caps q 12 hours prn; max 4 caps/day
Pediatric: <6 years: not recommended; 6-12 years: 1 cap q 12 hours prn; max 2 caps/day;
>12 years: same as adult
  Cap: hydro 5 mg+chlor 4 mg ext-rel (alcohol)

➤ **TussiCaps 10 mg/8 mg (C)(III)** 1 cap q 12 hours prn; max 2 caps/day
Pediatric: <12 years: not recommended; >12 years: same as adult
  Cap: hydro 10 mg+chlor 8 mg ext-rel (alcohol)

➤ **Tussionex (C)(III)** 1 tsp q 12 hours prn
Pediatric: <6 years: not recommended; 6-12 years: 1/2 tsp q 12 hours prn; >12 years: same
as adult
  Susp: hydro 10 mg+chlor 8 mg per 5 ml ext-rel

➤ **Tussi-Organidin DM NR Liquid (C)(III)** 5 ml q 4 hours prn; max 40 ml/day
Pediatric: <6 months: not recommended; 6-23 months: 0.6 ml q 4 hours prn; max 3.7 ml/
day; 2-5 years: 1.25 ml q 4 hours prn; max 7.5 ml/day; 6-12 years: 2.5 ml q 4 hours prn; max
15 ml/day; ≥12 years: same as adult
  Liq: dextro 10 mg+guaif 300 mg per 5 ml (grape) (sugar-free, alcohol-free)

➤ **Tussi-Organidin NR (C)(V)** 1 tsp q 4 hours prn; max 40 ml/day
Pediatric: <2 years: not recommended; 2 years: 1.5 ml q 4-6 hours prn; max 6 ml/day; 3
years: 1.75 ml q 4-6 hours prn; max 7 ml/day; 4 years: 2 ml q 4-6 hours prn; max 8 ml/day;
5 years: 2.25 ml q 4-6 hours prn; max 9 ml/day; 6-11 years: 2.5 ml q 4 hours prn; max 20
ml/day; ≥12 years: same as adult
  Liq: cod 10 mg+guaif 300 mg per 5 ml (grape) (sugar-free, alcohol-free)

➤ **Tuzistra XR (C)(III)** 1-2 tsp q 12 hours prn; max 20 ml/day
Pediatric: <18 years: not recommended; ≥18 years: same as adult
  Liq: cod 14.7 mg+chlor 2.8 mg per 5 ml (cherry)

➤ **Vistaril (C)(G)** 25 mg tid or qid prn
Pediatric: <6 years: 50 mg/day prn; 6-12 years: 50-100 mg daily prn; >12 years: same as
adult
  Cap: hydrox 25, 50, 100 mg; *Susp:* hydrox 25 mg/5 ml (lemon)

➤ **Xyzal, Xyzal Oral Solution (B)** 2.5-5 mg in the evening prn
CrCl 30-50 mL/min: 2.5 mg every other day
CrCl 10-30 mL/min: 2.5 mg twice weekly
CrCl <10 mL/min or hemodialysis: contraindicated
Pediatric: <6 months: not recommended; 6 months-6 years: max 1.25 mg once daily in the
PM prn; 6-12 years: max 2.5 mg once daily in the PM prn; >12 years: same as adult
  Tab: levocetir 5*mg film-coat; *Oral soln:* levocetir 0.5 mg/ml (150 ml)

APPENDIX BB. SYSTEMIC ANTI-INFECTIVES

Comment:
- Adverse effects of aminoglycosides include nephrotoxicity and ototoxicity.
- Use cephalosporins with caution in persons with penicillin allergy due to potential cross
  allergy.
- Sulfonamides are contraindicated with sulfa allergy and G6PD deficiency. A high fluid
  intake is indicated during sulfonamide therapy.
- Tetracyclines should be taken on an empty stomach to facilitate absorption. Tetracyclines
  should not be taken with milk.
- Tetracyclines are contraindicated during pregnancy and breastfeeding, and in children <8
  years of age, due to the risk of developing tooth enamel discoloration.
- Systemic quinolones and fluoroquinolones are contraindicated in pregnancy and children
  <18 years of age due to the risk of joint dysplasia.

(*continued*)

Appendix BB (*continued*)

Anti-infectives by Class With Dose Forms		
Generic Name	**Brand Name**	**Dose Form/Volume**
Amebicides		
chloroquine phosphate (C)(G)	**Aralen**	*Tab:* 500 mg
chloroquine phosphate+ primaquine phosphate (C)(G)	Aralen Phosphate+ Primaquine Phosphate	*Tab:* chlor 300 mg+prim 45 mg
iodoquinol (C)	**Yodoxin**	*Tab:* 210, 650 mg
metronidazole (**not for use in 1st; B in 2nd, 3rd**)(G)	**Flagyl**	*Tab:* 250*, 500*mg
	Flagyl 375	*Cap:* 375 mg
	Flagyl ER	*Tab:* 750 mg ext-rel
tinidazole (C)	**Tindamax**	*Tab:* 250*, 500*mg
Aminoglycosides		
amikacin (C)(G)	**Amikin**	*Vial:* 500 mg, 1 gm (2 ml)
gentamicin (C)(G)	**Garamycin**	*Vial:* 20, 80 mg/2 ml
streptomycin (D)(G)	**Streptomycin**	*Amp:* 1 gm/2.5 ml or 400 mg/ml (2.5 ml)
Antifungals		
atovaquone (C)	**Mepron**	*Susp:* 750 mg/5ml (210 ml)
clotrimazole (B)(G)	**Mycelex Troche**	10 mg (70, 40/bottle)
fluconazole (C)(G)	**Diflucan**	*Tab:* 50, 100, 150, 200 mg; *Oral susp:* 10, 40 mg/ml (35 ml) (orange)
griseofulvin, microsize (C)(G)	**Grifulvin V**	*Tab:* 250, 500 mg; *Oral susp:* 125 mg/ 5 ml (120 ml) (alcohol 0.02%)
griseofulvin, ultramicrosize (C)(G)	**Gris-PEG**	*Tab:* 125, 250 mg
itraconazole (C)	**Sporanox**	*Cap:* 100 mg; *Soln:* 10 mg/ml (150 ml); *Pulse Pack:* 100 mg caps (7/pck)
ketoconazole (C)(G)	**Nizoral**	*Tab:* 200 mg
nystatin (C)(G)	**Mycostatin**	*Pastille:* 200,000 units/pastille (30 pastilles/pck); *Oral susp:* 100,000 units/ml (60 ml w. dropper)
posaconazole	**Noxafil**	*Tab:* 100 mg ext-rel; *Oral susp:* 40 mg/ml (105 ml); *Vial:* 300 mg/16.7 ml (18 mg/ ml) soln for IV infusion
terbinafine (B)(G)	**Lamisil**	*Tab:* 250 mg
voriconazole (D)(G)	**Vfend**	*Tab:* 50, 200 mg
Antihelmintics		
albendazole (C)(G)	**Albenza**	*Tab:* 200 mg
ivermectin (C)(G)	**Stromectol**	*Tab:* 3 mg
mebendazole (C)(G)	**Emverm, Vermox**	*Chew tab:* 100 mg

(*continued*)

Appendix BB (*continued*)

Anti-infectives by Class With Dose Forms		
Generic Name	**Brand Name**	**Dose Form/Volume**
pyrantel pamoate (C)(G)	**Antiminth** Pin-X	*Cap:* 180 mg; *Liq:* 50 mg/ml (30 ml); 144 mg/ml (30 ml); *Oral susp:* 50 mg/ml (30 ml) (caramel) (sodium benzoate, tartrazine-free)
thiabendazole (C)(G)	**Mintezol** (currently not available in the United States)	*Chew tab:* 500*mg (orange); *Oral susp:* 500 mg/5 ml (120 ml) (orange)
Antimalarials		
atovaquone (C)	**Mepron**	*Susp:* 750 mg/5 ml
atovaquone+proguanil (C)	**Malarone**	*Tab:* atov 250 mg+proq 100 mg
	Malarone Pediatric	*Tab:* atov 62.5 mg+proq 25 mg
chloroquine (C)(G)	**Aralen**	*Tab:* 500 mg; *Amp:* 50 mg/ml (5 ml)
doxycycline (D)(G)	**Acticlate**	*Tab:* 75, 150**mg
	Adoxa	*Tab:* 50, 75, 100, 150 mg ent-coat
	Doryx	*Cap:* 100 mg; *Tab:* 50, 75, 100, 150, 200 mg
	Doxsteric	*Tab:* 50 mg del-rel
	Monodox	*Cap:* 50, 75, 100 mg
	Oracea	*Cap:* 40 mg del-rel
	Vibramycin	*Cap:* 50, 100 mg; *Syr:* 50 mg/5 ml (raspberry-apple) (sulfites); *Oral susp:* 25 mg/5 ml (raspberry)
	Vibra-Tab	*Tab:* 100 mg film-coat
	Xerava	*Vial:* 50 mg pwdr for IV infusion
hydroxychloroquine (C)(G)	**Plaquenil**	*Tab:* 200 mg
mefloquine (C)	**Lariam**	*Tab:* 250 mg
minocycline (D)(G)	**Dynacin**	*Cap:* 50, 100 mg
	Minocin	*Cap:* 50, 75, 100 mg; *Oral susp:* 50 mg/5 ml (60 ml) (custard) (sulfites, alcohol 5%)
	Minolira	*Tab:* 105, 135 mg ext-rel
	Solodyn	*Tab:* 55, 65, 80, 105, 115 mg ext-rel
Antiprotozoal/Antibacterials		
quinine sulfate (C)(G)	**Qualaquin**	*Cap:* 324 mg
metronidazole (not for use in 1st; B in 2nd, 3rd)(G)	**Flagyl, Protostat**	*Tab:* 250*, 500*mg
	Flagyl 375	*Cap:* 375 mg
	Flagyl ER	*Tab:* 750 mg ext-rel

(*continued*)

Appendix BB (*continued*)

Anti-infectives by Class With Dose Forms		
Generic Name	**Brand Name**	**Dose Form/Volume**
nitazoxanide (C)(G)	**Alinia**	*Tab:* 500 mg; *Oral susp:* 100 mg/5 ml (60 ml) (strawberry)
tinidazole (C)	**Tindamax**	*Tab:* 250*, 500*mg
Antituberculars		
ethambutol (EMB) (B)(G)	**Myambutol**	*Tab:* 100, 400*mg
isoniazid (INH) (C) (G)	*generic only*	*Tab:* 100, 300*mg; *Syr:* 50 mg/5 ml; *Inj:* 100 mg/ml
pyrazinamide (PZA) (C)	*generic only*	*Tab:* 500*mg
rifampin (C)(G)	**Priftin**	*Tab:* 150 mg
	Rifadin	*Cap:* 150, 300 mg
Rifampin+isoniazid (C)	**Rifamate**	*Cap:* rif 300 mg+iso 150 mg
rifampin+isoniazid+ pyrazinamide (C)	**Rifater**	*Tab:* rif 120 mg+iso 50 mg+pyr 300 mg
Antivirals (*for HIV-specific antiviral drugs see page 592*)		
acyclovir (C)(G)	**Zovirax**	*Cap:* 200 mg; *Tab:* 400, 800 mg; *Oral susp:* 200 mg/5 ml (banana)
amantadine (C)(G)	**Symmetrel**	*Tab:* 100 mg; *Syr:* 50 mg/5ml (16 oz) (raspberry)
famciclovir (B)	**Famvir**	*Tab:* 125, 250, 500 mg
lamivudine (C)	**Epivir-HBV**	*Tab:* 100 mg; *Oral soln:* 5 mg/ml (240 ml) (strawberry-banana)
oseltamivir (C)	**Tamiflu**	*Cap:* 75 mg
rimantadine (C)	**Flumadine**	*Tab:* 100 mg
valacyclovir (B)	**Valtrex**	*Tab:* 500 mg; 1 gm
zanamivir	**Relenza**	*Tab:* lami 150+zido 300 mg
Cephalosporins		
• **1st Generation Cephalosporins**		
cefadroxil (B)	**Duricef**	*Cap:* 500 mg; *Tab:* 1 gm; *Oral susp:*250 mg/5 ml (100 ml); 500 mg/5 ml (75, 100 ml) (orange-pineapple)
cefazolin (B)	**Ancef, Zolicef**	*Vial:* 500 mg; 1, 10 gm
cephalexin (B)	**Keflex**	*Cap:* 250, 333, 500, 750 mg; *Oral susp:*125, 250 mg/5 ml (100, 200 ml)

(*continued*)

Appendix BB (*continued*)

Anti-infectives by Class With Dose Forms		
Generic Name	Brand Name	Dose Form/Volume
• *2nd Generation Cephalosporins*		
cefaclor (B)(G)	*generic only*	*Tab:* 500 mg; *Cap:* 250, 500 mg; *Susp:* 125 mg/5 ml (75, 150 ml) (strawberry); 187 mg/5 ml (50, 100 ml) (strawberry); 250 mg/5 ml (75, 150 ml) (strawberry); 375 mg/5 ml (50, 100 ml) (strawberry)
cefaclor ext-rel (B)(G)	Cefaclor Extended Release	*Tab:* 375, 500 mg ext-rel
cefamandole (B)	Mandol	*Vial:* 1, 2 gm
cefotetan (B)	Cefotan	*Vial:* 1, 2 gm
cefoxitin (B)	Mefoxin	*Vial:* 1, 2 gm
cefprozil (B)	Cefzil	*Tab:* 250, 500 mg; *Oral susp:* 125, 250 mg/5 ml (50, 75, 100 ml) (bubble gum) (phenylalanine)
ceftaroline (B)	Teflaro	*Vial:* 400, 600 mg
cefuroxime sodium (B)(G)	Zinacef	*Vial:* 750 mg; 1.5 gm
loracarbef (B)	Lorabid	*Pulvule:* 200, 400 mg; *Oral susp:* 100 mg/5 ml (50, 100 ml); 200 mg/5 ml (50, 75, 100 ml) (strawberry bubble gum)
• *3rd Generation Cephalosporins*		
cefoperazone (B)	Cefobid	*Vial:* 1, 2 gm pwdr for reconstitution
cefotaxime (B)	Claforan	*Vial:* 500 mg; 1, 2 gm pwdr for reconstitution
cefpodoxime (B)	Vantin	*Tab:* 100, 200 mg; *Oral susp:* 50, 100 mg/5 ml (50, 75, 100 ml) (lemon creme)
ceftazidime (B)	Ceptaz	*Vial:* 1, 2 gm pwdr for reconstitution
	Fortaz	*Vial:* 500 mg; 1, 2 gm pwdr for reconstitution
	Tazicef	*Vial:* 1, 2 gm pwdr for reconstitution
	Tazidime	*Vial:* 1, 2 gm pwdr for reconstitution
Ceftazidime/ avibactam (B)	Avycaz	*Vial:* 2.5 gm pwdr for reconstitution
ceftibuten (B)	Cedax	*Cap:* 400 mg; *Oral susp:* 90 mg/5 ml (30, 60, 90, 120 ml); 180 mg/5 ml (30, 60, 120 ml) (cherry)
• *3rd/4th Generation Cephalosporins*		
cefdinir (B)	Omnicef	*Cap:* 300 mg; *Oral susp:* 125 mg/5 ml (60, 100 ml) (strawberry)
cefditoren pivoxil (C)	Spectracef	*Tab:* 200 mg

(*continued*)

Appendix BB (*continued*)

Anti-infectives by Class With Dose Forms		
Generic Name	**Brand Name**	**Dose Form/Volume**
cefepime (B)	**Maxipime**	*Vial:* 1 gm pwdr for reconstitution
cefixime (B)(G)	**Suprax**	*Tab/Cap:* 400 mg; *Oral Susp:* 100 mg/5 ml (50, 75, 100 ml) (strawberry)
ceftaroline (B)	**Teflaro**	*Vial:* 400, 600 mg
ceftriaxone (B)(G)	**Rocephin**	*Vial:* 250, 500 mg; 1, 2 gm
cytolozane+ tazobactam (B)	**Zerbaxa**	*Vial:* 1.5 gm pwdr for reconstitution
Penicillins		
amoxicillin (B)(G)	**Amoxil**	*Cap:* 250, 500 mg; *Tab:* 500, 875* mg; *Chew tab:* 125, 200, 250, 400 mg (cherry-banana-peppermint) (phenylalanine); *Oral susp:*125, 250 mg/ml (80, 100, 150 ml) (bubble gum); 200, 400 mg/5 ml (50, 75, 100 ml) (bubble gum); *Oral drops:* 50 mg/ml (30 ml) (bubble gum)
	Moxatag	*Tab:* 775 mg ext-rel
	Trimox	*Cap:* 250, 500 mg; *Oral susp:* 125, 250 mg/5ml (80, 100, 150 ml) (raspberry-strawberry)
amoxicillin+ clavulanate (B)(G)	**Augmentin**	*Tab:* 250, 500, 875 mg; *Chew tab:* 125, 250 mg (lemon lime); 200, 400 mg (cherry-banana; phenylalanine); *Oral susp:* 125 mg/5 ml (banana), 250 mg/5 ml (orange) (75, 100, 150 ml); 200, 400 mg/5 ml (50, 75, 100 ml) (orange)
	Augmentin ES-600	*Oral susp:* 600 mg/5 ml (50, 75, 100, 125, 150, 200 ml) (strawberry cream) (phenylalanine)
	Augmentin XR	*Tab:* 1000*mg ext-rel
ampicillin (B)(G)	**Omnipen**	*Cap:* 250, 500 mg; *Oral susp:* 125, 250 mg/ml (100, 150, 200 ml)
	Principen	*Cap:* 250, 500 mg; *Syr:* 125, 250 mg/5 ml
ampicillin+ sulbactam (B)(G)	**Unasyn**	*Vial:* 1.5, 3 gm
carbenicillin (B)	**Geocillin**	*Tab:* 382 mg film-coat
dicloxacillin (B)(G)	**Dynapen**	*Cap:* 125, 250, 500 mg; *Oral susp:* 62.5 mg/5 ml (80, 100, 200 ml)
ertapenem (B)	**Invanz**	*Vial:* 1 gm pwdr for reconstitution
meropenem (B)(G)	**Merrem**	*Vial:* 500 mg; 1 gm pwdr for reconstitution (sodium 3.92 mEq/gm)

(*continued*)

Appendix BB (*continued*)

Anti-infectives by Class With Dose Forms		
Generic Name	Brand Name	Dose Form/Volume
penicillin g benzathine (B)(G)	**Bicillin LA, Bicillin C-R**	*Cartridge-needle unit:* 600,000 million units (1 ml); 1.2 million units (2 ml); 2.4 million units (4 ml)
	Permapen	*Prefilled syringe:* 1.2 million units
penicillin g potassium (B)(G)	*generic only*	*Vial:* 5, 20 MU pwdr for reconstitution; *Premixed bag:* 1, 2, 3 MU (50 ml)
penicillin g procaine (B)(G)	*generic only*	*Prefilled syringe:* 1.2 million units
penicillin v potassium (B)(G)	**Pen-Vee K**	*Tab:* 250, 500 mg; *Oral soln:* 125 mg/5 ml (100, 200 ml); 250 mg/5 ml (100, 150, 200 ml)
piperacillin+ tazobactam (B)(G)	**Zosyn**	*Vial:* 2, 3, 4 gm pwdr for reconstitution
Quinolone and Fluoroquinolones		
• 1st Generation Quinolone		
enoxacin (C)	**Penetrex**	*Tab:* 200, 400 mg
• 1st Generation Fluoroquinolones		
ciprofloxacin (C)(G)	**Cipro**	*Tab:* 250, 500, 750 mg; *Oral susp:* 250, 500 mg/5 ml (100 ml) (strawberry); *IV conc:* 10 mg/ml after dilution (20, 40 ml); *Premixed bag:* 2 mg/ml (100, 200 ml)
	Cipro XR	*Tab:* 500, 1000 mg ext-rel
	ProQuin XR	*Tab:* 500 mg ext-rel
lomefloxacin (C)	**Maxaquin**	*Tab:* 400 mg
norfloxacin (C)(G)	**Noroxin**	*Tab:* 400 mg
ofloxacin (C)(G)	**Floxin**	*Tab:* 200, 300, 400 mg
lomefloxacin (C)	**Floxin**	*Tab:* 200, 300, 400 mg
• 3rd Generation Fluoroquinolone		
levofloxacin (C)(G)	**Levaquin**	*Tab:* 250, 500, 750 mg
• 4th Generation Fluoroquinolone		
delafloxacin (C)	**Baxdela**	*Tab:* 400 mg; *Vial:* 300 mg pwdr for reconstitution
gemifloxacin (C)(G)	**Factive**	*Tab:* 320*mg
moxifloxacin (C)(G)	**Avelox**	*Tab:* 400 mg
Ketolide		
telithromycin (C)	**Ketek**	*Tab:* 300, 400 mg

(*continued*)

Appendix BB (continued)

Anti-infectives by Class With Dose Forms		
Generic Name	Brand Name	Dose Form/Volume
Macrolides		
azithromycin (B)	Zithromax	*Tab:* 250, 500, 600 mg; *Granules:* 1 gm/pck for reconstitution (cherry-banana)
	ZithPed Syr	*Oral susp:* 100 mg/5 ml, (15 ml); 200 mg/5 ml (15, 22.5, 30 ml) (cherry)
	Zithromax Tri-Pak	*Tab:* 3 x 500 mg tabs/pck
	Zithromax Z-Pak	*Tab:* 6 x 250 mg tabs/pck
	Zmax	*Granules:* 2 gm/pkt for reconstitution (cherry-banana)
clarithromycin (C)(G)	Biaxin	*Tab:* 250, 500 mg; *Oral susp:* 125, 250 mg/5 ml (50, 100 ml) (fruit punch)
	Biaxin XL	*Tab:* 500 mg ext-rel
dirithromycin (C)(G)	*generic only*	*Tab:* 250 mg
erythromycin base (B)(G)	Ery-Tab	*Tab:* 250, 333, 500 mg ent-coat
	PCE	*Tab:* 333, 500 mg
erythromycin estolate (B)(G)	Ilosone	*Pulvule:* 250 mg; *Tab:* 500 mg; *Liq:* 125, 250 mg/5 ml (100 ml)
erythromycin ethylsuccinate (B)(G)	E.E.S.	*Tab:* 400 mg; *Oral susp:* 200 mg/5 ml (100, 200 ml) (cherry); 200, 400 mg/5 ml (100 ml) (fruit)
erythromycin ethylsuccinate (B)(G)	EryPed	*Oral susp:* 200 mg/5 ml (100, 200 ml) (fruit); 400 mg/5 ml (60, 100, 200 ml) (banana); *Oral drops:* 200, 400 mg/5 ml (50 ml) (fruit); *Chew tab:* 200 mg (fruit)
erythromycin stearate (B)(G)	Erythrocin	*Film tab:* 250, 500 mg
Macrolide+Sulfonamide		
erythromycin ethylsuccinate+ sulfisoxazole (C)(G)	Pediazole	*Oral susp:* eryth 200 mg+sulf 600 mg per 5 ml (100, 150, 200 ml) (strawberry-banana)
Sulfonamides		
sulfamethoxazole (B/D)(G)	Gantrisin Pediatric	*Oral susp:* 500 mg/5 ml; *Syr:* 500 mg/5 ml
trimethoprim (C)(G)	Primsol	*Oral soln:* 50 mg/5 ml (bubble gum) (dye-free, alcohol-free)
	Trimpex	*Tab:* 100 mg
	Proloprim	*Tab:* 100, 200 mg

(continued)

Appendix BB (*continued*)

Anti-infectives by Class With Dose Forms		
Generic Name	**Brand Name**	**Dose Form/Volume**
trimethoprim+ sulfamethoxazole (C)(G)	**Bactrim, Septra**	*Tab:* trim 80 mg+sulfa 400 mg*
	Bactrim DS, Septra DS	*Tab:* trim 160 mg+sulfa 800 mg*; *Oral susp:* trim 40 mg+sulfa 200 mg per 5 ml (100 ml) (cherry) (alcohol 0.3%)
Tetracyclines		
demeclocycline (D)	**Declomycin**	*Tab:* 300 mg
doxycycline (D)(G)	**Adoxa**	*Tab:* 50, 100 mg ent-coat
	Doryx	*Cap:* 100 mg
	Monodox	*Cap:* 50, 100 mg
doxycycline (D)(G)	**Vibramycin**	*Cap:* 50, 100 mg; *Syr:* 50 mg/5 ml; (raspberry) (sulfites); *Oral susp:* 25 mg/5 ml (raspberry-apple); *IV conc:* doxy 100 mg+asc acid 480 mg after dilution; doxy 200 mg+asc acid 960 mg after dilution
	Vibra-Tab	*Tab:* 100 mg film-coat
	Xerava	*Vial:* 50 mg pwdr for IV infusion
minocycline (D)(G)	**Dynacin**	*Cap:* 50, 100 mg
	Minocin	*Cap:* 50, 100 mg; *Oral susp:* 50 mg/5 ml (60 ml) (custard) (sulfites, alcohol 5%); *Vial:* 100 mg soln for inj
	Minolira	*Tab:* 105, 135 mg ext-rel
tetracycline (D)(G)	**Achromycin V**	*Cap:* 250, 500 mg
	Sumycin	*Tab:* 250, 500 mg; *Oral susp:* 125 mg/5 ml (fruit) (sulfites)
Unclassified/Miscellaneous		
aztreonam (B)	**Cayston**	*Vial:* 75 mg pwdr for reconstitution (preservative-free)
chloramphenicol (C) (G)	**Chloromycetin**	*Vial:* 1 gm
clindamycin (B)(G)	**Cleocin**	*Cap:* 75 (tartrazine), 150 (tartrazine), 300 mg; *Oral susp:* 75 mg/5 ml (100 ml) (cherry); *Vial:* 150 mg/ml (2, 4 ml) (benzyl alcohol)
dalbavancin (C)	**Dalvance**	*Vial:* 500 mg pwdr for reconstitution (preservative-free)
daptomycin (B)(G)	**Cubicin**	*Vial:* 500 mg pwdr for reconstitution
doripenem (B)	**Doribax**	*Vial:* 500 mg pwdr for reconstitution
fosfomycin (B)	**Monurol**	*Sachet:* 3 gm single-dose (mandarin orange; sucrose)

(*continued*)

Appendix BB (*continued*)

Anti-infectives by Class With Dose Forms		
Generic Name	Brand Name	Dose Form/Volume
imipenem+ cilastatin (C)(G)	Primaxin	*Vial:* imip 500 mg+cila 500 mg; imip 750 mg+cila 750 mg pwdr for reconstitution
lincomycin (B)(G)	Lincocin	*Vial:* 300 mg/ml (10 ml)
linezolid (C)(G)	Zyvox	*Tab:* 400, 600 mg; *Oral susp:* 100 mg/5 ml (orange) (phenylalanine); *IV:* 2 mg ml (100, 200, 300 ml)
meropenem (B)	Merrem	*Vial:* 500 mg; 1 gm (sodium 3.92 mEq/gm)
meropenem+ vaborbactam	Vabomere	*Vial:* mero 1 gm+vabor 1 gm pwdr for reconstitution, single-dose
nitrofurantoin (B)(G)	Furadantin	*Oral susp:* 25 mg/5 ml (60 ml)
	Macrobid	*Cap:* 100 mg
	Macrodantin	*Cap:* 25, 50, 100 mg
quinupristin+ dalfopristin (B)	Synercid	*Vial:* quin 150 mg+dalfo 350 mg, quin 180 mg+dalfo 420 mg single-dose
tygecycline (D)(G)	Tygacil	*Vial:* 50 mg pwdr for reconstitution
rifaximin (C)	Xifaxan	*Tab:* 200, 550 mg
telavancin (C)	Vibativ	*Vial:* 250, 750 mg pwdr for reconstitution (preservative-free)
vancomycin (C)(G)	Vancocin	*Cap:* 125, 250 mg; *Vial:* 500 mg, 1 gm pwdr for reconstitution

APPENDIX CC.1. *ACYCLOVIR* (ZOVIRAX SUSPENSION)

Weight												
Pounds	15	20	25	30	35	40	45	50	55	60	65	70
Kilograms	6.8	9	11.4	13.6	15.9	18.2	20.5	22.7	25	27.3	29.5	31.8
Single Dose (ml)/Frequency/Strength/5-Day Volume (ml)												
20 mg/kg/d ml/dose qid	3.5	4.5	5.5	6.5	8	9	10	11.5	12.5	13.5	14.5	16
mg/5 ml	200	200	200	200	200	200	200	200	200	200	200	200
Volume (ml)	70	90	110	130	160	180	200	230	250	270	290	320

Zovirax Oral Suspension <2 years: not recommended; >2 years, <40 kg: 20 mg/kg dosed qid x 5 days; ≥2 years, >40 kg: 800 mg dosed qid x 5 days; *Oral susp:* 200 mg/5 ml (banana).

APPENDIX CC.2. *AMANTADINE* (SYMMETREL SYRUP)

Weight												
Pounds	15	20	25	30	35	40	45	50	55	60	65	70
Kilograms	6.8	9	11.4	13.6	15.9	18.2	20.5	22.7	25	27.3	29.5	31.8
Single Dose (ml)/Frequency/Strength/10-Day Volume (ml)												
4 mg/kg/d ml/dose bid	3	4	5	6	7	8	9	10	11	12	13	14
mg/5 ml	50	50	50	50	50	50	50	50	50	50	50	50
Volume (ml)	30	40	50	60	70	80	90	100	110	120	130	140
8 mg/lb/d ml/dose bid	6	8	10	12								
mg/5 ml	50	50	50	50								
Volume (ml)	60	80	100	60								

Symmetrel Suspension (C)(G) Symmetrel <1 year: not recommended; 1-8 years: max 150 mg/day; 9-12 years: 2 tsp bid; >12 years: 100 mg bid <u>or</u> 200 mg once daily; *Syr:* 50 mg/5 ml (raspberry).

 APPENDIX CC.3. *AMOXICILLIN* (AMOXIL SUSPENSION, TRIMOX SUSPENSION)

Weight												
Pounds	15	20	25	30	35	40	45	50	55	60	65	70
Kilograms	6.8	9	11.4	13.6	15.9	18.2	20.5	22.7	25	27.3	29.5	31.8
Single Dose (ml)/Frequency/Strength/10-Day Volume (ml)												
20 mg/kg/d ml/dose tid	2	2.5	3	3.5	4	5	5.5	6	7	7.5	8	9
mg/5 ml	125	125	125	125	125	125	125	125	125	125	125	125
Volume (ml)	60	75	90	105	120	150	165	180	210	225	240	270
30 mg/kg/d ml/dose tid	3	3.5	2.5	3	3	3.5	4	4.5	5	5.5	6	6.5
mg/5 ml	125	125	250	250	250	250	250	250	250	250	250	250
Volume (ml)	90	105	75	90	90	105	120	135	150	165	180	195
40 mg/kg/d ml/dose bid	5	7	4.5	5	6	7	8	9	10	11	12	13
mg/5 ml	125	125	250	250	250	250	250	250	250	250	250	250
Volume (ml)	100	140	90	100	120	140	160	180	200	220	240	250
45 mg/kg/d ml/dose bid	4	2.5	3	4	4.5	5	6	6.5	7	7.5	8.5	9
mg/5 ml	200	400	400	400	400	400	400	400	400	400	400	400
Volume (ml)	80	50	60	80	90	100	120	130	140	150	170	180
90 mg/kg/d ml/dose bid	8	5	6	7	9	10	12	13	14	15	17	18

(continued)

Appendix CC.3. (*continued*)

mg/5 ml	200	400	400	400	400	400	400	400	400	400	400	400
Volume (ml)	160	100	120	140	180	200	240	260	280	300	340	360

<40 kg (88 lb): 20-30 mg/kg/day in 3 divided doses or 40-90 mg/kg/day in 2 divided doses; >40 kg: same as adult.

Amoxil Suspension (B)(G) 125, 250 mg/5 ml (80, 100, 150 ml) (strawberry); 200, 400 mg/5 ml (50, 75, 100 ml) (bubble gum).

Trimox Suspension (B)(G) 125, 250 mg/5 ml (80, 100, 150 ml) (raspberry-strawberry).

APPENDIX CC.4. *AMOXICILLIN+CLAVULANATE* (AUGMENTIN SUSPENSION)

Weight												
Pounds	15	20	25	30	35	40	45	50	55	60	65	70
Kilograms	6.8	9	11.4	13.6	15.9	18.2	20.5	22.7	25	27.3	29.5	31.8
Single Dose (ml)/Frequency/Strength/10-Day Volume (ml)												
40 mg/kg/d ml/dose bid	5.5	7	4.5	5.5	6.5	7	8	9	10	11	12	13
mg/5 ml	125	125	250	250	250	250	250	250	250	250	250	250
Volume (ml)	110	140	90	110	130	140	160	180	200	220	240	260
45 mg/kg/d ml/dose bid	3	4	5	6	7	8	9	10	11.5	12.5	13.5	14.5
mg/5 ml	250	250	250	250	250	250	250	250	250	250	250	250
Volume (ml)	60	80	100	120	140	160	180	200	230	250	270	290
45 mg/kg/d ml/dose bid	4	2.5	3	4	4.5	5	6	6.5	7	7.5	8.5	9
mg/5 ml	200	400	400	400	400	400	400	400	400	400	400	400
Volume (ml)	80	50	60	80	90	100	120	130	140	150	170	180
90 mg/kg/d ml/dose bid	4	5	6.5	8	9	10	11.5	13	14	15.5	16.5	18
mg/5 ml	400	400	400	400	400	400	400	400	400	400	400	400
Volume (ml)	80	100	130	160	180	200	240	260	280	300	340	360

Augmentin Suspension (B)(G) 40-45 mg/kg/day divided tid or 90 mg/kg/day divided bid; 125 mg/5 ml (75, 100, 150 ml) (banana), 250 mg/5 ml (75, 100, 150 ml) (orange); 200, 400 mg/5 ml (50, 75, 100 ml) (orange-raspberry) (phenylalanine).

APPENDIX CC.5. *AMOXICILLIN+CLAVULANATE* (AUGMENTIN ES 600 SUSPENSION)

Weight												
Pounds	15	20	25	30	35	40	45	50	55	60	65	70
Kilograms	6.8	9	11.4	13.6	15.9	18.2	20.5	22.7	25	27.3	29.5	31.8
Single Dose (ml)/Frequency/Strength/10-Day Volume (ml)												
40 mg/kg/d ml/dose bid	1	1.5	2	2	2.5	3	3.5	4	4	4.5	5	5

(*continued*)

Appendix CC.5. (*continued*)

mg/5 ml	600	600	600	600	600	600	600	600	600	600	600	600
Volume (ml)	30	40	40	40	50	60	70	80	80	90	100	100
45 mg/kg/d ml/dose bid	1.25	1.5	2	2.5	3	3.5	4	4.5	5	5	5.5	6
mg/5 ml	600	600	600	600	600	600	600	600	600	600	600	600
Volume (ml)	25	30	40	50	60	70	80	90	100	100	110	120
90 mg/kg/d ml/dose bid	2.5	3.5	4	5	6	7	8	8.5	9.5	10	11	12
mg/5 ml	600	600	600	600	600	600	600	600	600	600	600	600
Volume (ml)	50	70	80	100	120	140	160	170	190	200	220	240

Augmentin ES 600 Suspension (B) <3 months: not recommended; ≥3 months, <40 kg: 90 mg/kg/day in 2 divided doses; ≥40 kg: not recommended; 600 mg/5 ml (50, 75, 100, 125, 150, 200 ml) (strawberry cream) (phenylalanine).

APPENDIX CC.6. *AMPICILLIN* (OMNIPEN SUSPENSION, PRINCIPEN SUSPENSION)

Weight												
Pounds	15	20	25	30	35	40	45	50	55	60	65	70
Kilograms	6.8	9	11.4	13.6	15.9	18.2	20.5	22.7	25	27.3	29.5	31.8
Single Dose (ml)/Frequency/Strength/10-Day Volume (ml)												
50 mg/kg/d ml/dose q6h	3.5	4.5	3	3.5	4	4.5						
mg/5 ml	125	125	250	250	250	250						
Volume (ml)	140	180	120	140	160	180						
100 mg/kg/d ml/dose q6h	3.5	4.5	6	7	8	9						
mg/5 ml	250	250	250	250	250	250						
Volume (ml)	140	180	240	280	320	360						

Omnipen Suspension, Principen Suspension (B)(G) >20 kg: 250-500 mg q 6 h 125, 250 mg/5 ml (100, 150, 200 ml) (fruit).

APPENDIX CC.7. *AZITHROMYCIN* (ZITHROMAX SUSPENSION, ZMAX SUSPENSION)

Weight								
Pounds	11	22	33	44	55	66	77	88
Kilograms	5	10	15	20	25	30	35	40
Single Dose (ml)/Frequency/Strength/Volume (ml)								
3 Day Regimen								
10 mg/kg qd	2.5	5	7.5	5	6	7.5	9	10

(continued)

Appendix CC.7. (*continued*)

mg/5 ml	100	100	100	200	200	200	200	200
Volume (ml)	7.5	15	22.5	15	18	22.5	27	30
5 Day Regimen								
10 mg/kg qd								
Day 1	2.5	5	7.5	5	6	7.5	7.5	10
Days 2–5	1.25	2.5	4	2.5	3	4	4	5
Volume (ml)	10	15	23.5	15	18	23.5	23.5	30

Zithromax ES 600 Suspension (B)(G) 100 mg/5 ml (15 ml), 200 mg/5 ml (15, 22.5, 30 ml) (cherry-vanilla-banana).

APPENDIX CC.8. *CEFACLOR* (CECLOR SUSPENSION)

Weight												
Pounds	15	20	25	30	35	40	45	50	55	60	65	70
Kilograms	6.8	9	11.4	13.6	15.9	18.2	20.5	22.7	25	27.3	29.5	31.8
Single Dose (ml)/Frequency/Strength/10-Day Volume (ml)												
20 mg/kg/d ml/dose tid	2	2.5	3	3.5	4	5	5.5	6	7	7.5	8	8.5
mg/5 ml	125	125	125	125	125	125	125	125	125	125	125	125
Volume (ml)	60	75	90	105	120	150	165	180	210	225	240	255
20 mg/kg/d ml/dose tid	1.5	1.5	2	2.5	3	3	4	4	4.5	5	5.5	6
mg/5 ml	187	187	187	187	187	187	187	187	187	187	187	187
Volume (ml)	45	45	60	75	90	90	105	120	135	150	165	180
40 mg/kg/d ml/dose tid	2	2.5	3	3.5	4	5	5.5	6	6.5	7	8	8.5
mg/5 ml	250	250	250	250	250	250	250	250	250	250	250	250
Volume (ml)	60	75	90	105	120	150	165	180	195	210	240	255
40 mg/kg/d ml/dose tid	1.5	1.5	2	2.5	3	3	3.5	4	4.5	5	5	5.5
mg/5 ml	375	375	375	375	375	375	375	375	375	375	375	375
Volume (ml)	45	45	60	75	90	90	105	120	135	150	150	165

Ceclor Suspension (B) <6 months: not recommended; 125, 250 mg/5 ml (75, 150 ml) (strawberry); 187, 375 mg/5 ml (50, 100 ml) (strawberry).

APPENDIX CC.9. *CEFADROXIL* (DURICEF SUSPENSION)

Weight												
Pounds	15	20	25	30	35	40	45	50	55	60	65	70
Kilograms	6.8	9	11.4	13.6	15.9	18.2	20.5	22.7	25	27.3	29.5	31.8
Single Dose (ml)/Frequency/Strength/10-Day Volume (ml)												
30 mg/kg/d ml/dose bid	2	3	3.5	4	5	5.5	6	7	7.5	8	9	9.5

(*continued*)

Appendix CC.9. (*continued*)

mg/5 ml	250	250	250	250	250	250	250	250	250	250	250	250
Volume (ml)	40	60	75	80	100	110	120	140	150	160	180	190
30 mg/kg/d ml/dose qd	2	3	3.5	4	5	5.5	6	7	7.5	8	9	9.5
mg/5 ml	500	500	500	500	500	500	500	500	500	500	500	500
Volume (ml)	20	30	35	40	50	55	60	70	75	80	90	95

Duricef Suspension (B) 250 mg/5 ml (100 ml) (orange-pineapple); 500 mg/5 ml (75, 100 ml) (orange-pineapple).

APPENDIX CC.10. *CEFDINIR* (OMNICEF SUSPENSION)

Weight												
Pounds	15	20	25	30	35	40	45	50	55	60	65	70
Kilograms	6.8	9	11.4	13.6	15.9	18.2	20.5	22.7	25	27.3	29.5	31.8
Single Dose (ml)/Frequency/Strength/10-Day Volume (ml)												
7 mg/kg/d ml/dose bid	2	2.5	3	4	4.5	5	6	6.5	7	7.5	8	9
mg/5 ml	125	125	125	125	125	125	125	125	125	125	125	125
Volume (ml)	40	50	60	80	90	100	120	130	140	150	160	180
14 mg/kg ml/dose bid	4	5	6	8	9	10	12	13	14	15	16	18
mg/5 ml	125	125	125	125	125	125	125	125	125	125	125	125
Volume (ml)	40	50	60	80	90	100	120	130	140	150	160	180

Omnicef Suspension (B) <6 months: not recommended; 125 mg/5 ml (60, 100 ml) (strawberry).

APPENDIX CC.11. *CEFIXIME* (SUPRAX ORAL SUSPENSION)

Weight												
Pounds	15	20	25	30	35	40	45	50	55	60	65	70
Kilograms	6.8	9	11.4	13.6	15.9	18.2	20.5	22.7	25	27.3	29.5	31.8
Single Dose (ml)/Frequency/Strength/10-Day Volume (ml)												
8 mg/kg/d ml/dose bid	1.3	1.8	2.2	2.5	3.1	3.5	4	4.5	5	5.5	6	6.5
mg/5 ml	100	100	100	100	100	100	100	100	100	100	100	100
8 mg/kg/d ml/dose qd	2.7	3.6	4.5	5.5	6.3	7.2	8.2	9	10	11	12	13
mg/5 ml	100	100	100	100	100	100	100	100	100	100	100	100
Volume (ml)	27	36	45	55	65	70	80	90	100	110	120	130

Supra Oral Suspension (B)(G) <6 months: not recommended; 100 mg/5 ml (50, 75, 100 ml) (strawberry).

APPENDIX CC.12. *CEFPODOXIME PROXETIL* (VANTIN SUSPENSION)

Weight												
Pounds	15	20	25	30	35	40	45	50	55	60	65	70
Kilograms	6.8	9	11.4	13.6	15.9	18.2	20.5	22.7	25	27.3	29.5	31.8
Single Dose (ml)/Frequency/Strength/10-Day Volume (ml)												
5 mg/kg/d ml/dose bid	3.5	4.5	5.5	7	8	9	10	11	12.5	13.5	15	16
mg/5 ml	50	50	50	50	50	50	50	50	50	50	50	50
Volume (ml)	70	90	110	140	160	180	200	220	250	270	300	320
5 mg/kg/d ml/dose bid	2	2	3	3.5	4	4.5	5	5.5	6	7	7.5	8
mg/5 ml	100	100	100	100	100	100	100	100	100	100	100	100
Volume (ml)	40	40	60	70	80	90	100	110	120	140	150	160

Vantin Suspension (B) <2 months: not recommended; 50, 100 mg/5 ml (50, 75, 100 ml) (lemon-crème).

 APPENDIX CC.13. *CEFPROZIL* (CEFZIL SUSPENSION)

Weight												
Pounds	15	20	25	30	35	40	45	50	55	60	65	70
Kilograms	6.8	9	11.4	13.6	15.9	18.2	20.5	22.7	25	27.3	29.5	31.8
Single Dose (ml)/Frequency/Strength/10-Day Volume (ml)												
7.5 mg/kg/d ml/dose bid	2	3	3.5	4	5	5.5	6	7	7.5	4	4.5	5
mg/5 ml	125	125	125	125	125	125	125	125	125	250	250	250
Volume (ml)	40	60	70	80	100	110	120	140	150	80	90	100
15 mg/kg/d ml/dose bid	2	3	3.5	4	5	5	6	7	7.5	8	9	9.5
mg/5 ml	250	250	250	250	250	250	250	250	250	250	250	250
Volume (ml)	40	60	70	80	100	100	120	140	150	160	180	190
20 mg/kg/d ml/dose qd	3	3.5	4.5	5.5	6.5	7	8	9	10	11	12	13
mg/5 ml	250	250	250	250	250	250	250	250	250	250	250	250
Volume (ml)	60	70	90	110	130	140	160	180	200	220	240	260

Cefzil Suspension (B) ≤6 months: not recommended; 2-12 years: 7.5-20 mg/kg bid >12 years: same as adult, 250-500 mg bid or 500 mg once daily; 125, 250 mg/5 ml (50, 75, 100 ml) (bubble gum) (phenylalanine).

APPENDIX CC.14. *CEFTIBUTEN* (CEDAX SUSPENSION)

Weight												
Pounds	15	20	25	30	35	40	45	50	55	60	65	70
Kilograms	6.8	9	11.4	13.6	15.9	18.2	20.5	22.7	25	27.3	29.5	31.8
Single Dose (ml)/Frequency/Strength/10-Day Volume (ml)												
9 mg/kg/d ml/dose qd	3.5	4.5	6	7	8	9	10	11.5	12.5	13.5	15	16
mg/5 ml	90	90	90	90	90	90	90	90	90	90	90	90
Volume (ml)	35	45	60	70	80	90	100	115	125	135	150	160
9 mg/kg/d ml/dose qd	1.75	2.3	3	3.5	4	4.5	5	5.4	6.2	6.6	7.5	8
mg/5 ml	180	180	180	180	180	180	180	180	180	180	180	180
Volume (ml)	20	25	30	35	40	45	50	55	60	65	70	80

Cefzil Suspension (B) 90 mg/5 ml (30, 60, 90, 120 ml) (cherry); 180 mg/5 ml (30, 60, 120 ml) (cherry).

APPENDIX CC.15. *CEPHALEXIN* (KEFLEX SUSPENSION)

Weight												
Pounds	15	20	25	30	35	40	45	50	55	60	65	70
Kilograms	6.8	9	11.4	13.6	15.9	18.2	20.5	22.7	25	27.3	29.5	31.8
Single Dose (ml)/Frequency/Strength/10-Day Volume (ml)												
25 mg/kg/d ml/dose tid	1	1.5	2	2	3	3	3.5	4	4	4.5	5	5
mg/5 ml	125	125	125	125	125	125	125	125	125	125	125	125
Volume (ml)	30	45	60	60	90	90	105	120	120	135	150	150
25 mg/kg/d ml/dose qid	1	1	1.5	2	2	2.5	2.5	3	3	3.5	4	4
mg/5 ml	250	250	250	250	250	250	250	250	250	250	250	250
Volume (ml)	40	40	60	80	80	100	100	120	120	140	160	160
50 mg/kg/d ml/dose tid	2	3	4	4.5	5	6	7	7.5	8	9	10	10.5
mg/5 ml	250	250	250	250	250	250	250	250	250	250	250	250
Volume (ml)	60	90	120	135	150	180	210	225	240	270	300	315
50 mg/kg/d ml/dose qid	2	2	3	3.5	4	4.5	5	6	6	7	7.5	8
mg/5 ml	250	250	250	250	250	250	250	250	250	250	250	250
Volume (ml)	80	80	120	140	160	180	200	240	240	280	300	320

Keflex Suspension (B)(G) <2 months: not recommended; 125, 250 mg/5 ml (100, 200 ml) (strawberry).

APPENDIX CC.16. *CLARITHROMYCIN* (BIAXIN SUSPENSION)

Weight												
Pounds	15	20	25	30	35	40	45	50	55	60	65	70
Kilograms	6.8	9	11.4	13.6	15.9	18.2	20.5	22.7	25	27.3	29.5	31.8
Single Dose (ml)/Frequency/Strength/10-Day Volume (ml)												
7.5 mg/kg/d ml/dose bid	2	3	3.5	4	5	5.5	6	7	7.5	8	9	10
mg/5 ml	125	125	125	125	125	125	125	125	125	125	125	125
Volume (ml)	40	60	70	80	100	110	120	140	150	160	180	200
7.5 mg/kg/d ml/dose bid	1	1.5	2	2	2.5	3	3	3.5	4	4	4.5	5
mg/5 ml	250	250	250	250	250	250	250	250	250	250	250	250
Volume (ml)	20	30	40	40	50	60	60	70	80	80	90	100

Biaxin Suspension (B) <6 months: not recommended; 125, 250 mg/5 ml (50, 100 ml) (fruit-punch).

APPENDIX CC.17. *CLINDAMYCIN* (CLEOCIN PEDIATRIC GRANULES)

Weight												
Pounds	15	20	25	30	35	40	45	50	55	60	65	70
Kilograms	6.8	9	11.4	13.6	15.9	18.2	20.5	22.7	25	27.3	29.5	31.8
Single Dose (ml)/Frequency/Strength/10-Day Volume (ml)												
8 mg/kg/d ml/dose tid	1	1.5	2	2.5	3	3	3.5	4	4.5	5	5	5.5
mg/5 ml	75	75	75	75	75	75	75	75	75	75	75	75
Volume (ml)	30	45	60	75	90	90	105	120	135	150	150	165
16 mg/kg/d ml/dose tid	2.5	3	4	5	5.5	6.5	7	8	9	9.5	10.5	11
mg/5 ml	75	75	75	75	75	75	75	75	75	75	75	75
Volume (ml)	75	90	120	150	165	105	210	240	270	285	315	330

Cleocin Pediatric Granules (B)(G) 75 mg/5 ml (100 ml) (cherry).

APPENDIX CC.18. *DICLOXACILLIN* (DYNAPEN SUSPENSION)

Weight												
Pounds	15	20	25	30	35	40	45	50	55	60	65	70
Kilograms	6.8	9	11.4	13.6	15.9	18.2	20.5	22.7	25	27.3	29.5	31.8
Single Dose (ml)/Frequency/Strength/10-Day Volume (ml)												
12.5 mg/kg/d ml/dose qid	2	2.5	3	3.5	4	4.5	5	6	6	7	7.5	8

(continued)

Appendix CC.18. (*continued*)

mg/5 ml	62.5	62.5	62.5	62.5	62.5	62.5	62.5	62.5	62.5	62.5	62.5	62.5
Volume (ml)	80	100	120	140	160	180	200	240	240	280	300	320
25 mg/kg/d ml/dose qid	3.5	4.5	6	7	8	9	10	11.5	12.5	13.5	15	16
mg/5 ml	62.5	62.5	62.5	62.5	62.5	62.5	62.5	62.5	62.5	62.5	62.5	62.5
Volume (ml)	140	180	240	280	320	360	400	460	500	540	600	640

Dynapen Suspension (B)(G) 6.25 mg/5 ml (80, 100 ml) (raspberry-strawberry).

APPENDIX CC.19. *DOXYCYCLINE* (VIBRAMYCIN SYRUP/SUSPENSION)

Weight												
Pounds	15	20	25	30	35	40	45	50	55	60	65	70
Kilograms	6.8	9	11.4	13.6	15.9	18.2	20.5	22.7	25	27.3	29.5	31.8
Single Dose (ml)/Frequency/Strength/10-Day Volume (ml)												
1 mg/lb/d ml/dose qd	1.5	2	2.5	3	3.5	4	4.5	5	5.5	6	6.5	7
50 mg/5 ml	50	50	50	50	50	50	50	50	50	50	50	50
Volume (ml)	15	20	25	30	35	40	45	50	55	60	65	70
1 mg/lb/d ml/dose qd	3	4	5	6	7	8	9	10	11	12	13	14
25 mg/5 ml	25	25	25	25	25	25	25	25	25	25	25	25
Volume (ml)	30	40	50	60	70	80	90	100	110	120	130	140

Vibramycin Syrup (B)(G) <8 years: not recommended; double dose first day; 50 mg/5 ml (80, 100, ml) (raspberry-apple) (sulfites).

Vibramycin Suspension (B)(G) <8 years: not recommended; double dose first day; 25 mg/5 ml (80, 100, ml) (raspberry).

APPENDIX CC.20. *ERYTHROMYCIN ESTOLATE* (ILOSONE SUSPENSION)

Weight												
Pounds	15	20	25	30	35	40	45	50	55	60	65	70
Kilograms	6.8	9	11.4	13.6	15.9	18.2	20.5	22.7	25	27.3	29.5	31.8
Dose/Volume (10 days) in ml												
10 mg/kg/d ml/dose bid	3	3.5	4.5	5.5	6	7	8	9	10	5.5	6	6.5
mg/5 ml	125	125	125	125	125	125	125	125	125	250	250	250
Volume (ml)	60	70	90	110	120	140	160	180	200	110	120	130
15 mg/kg/d ml/dose bid	4	5.5	7	8	9.5	5.5	6	7	7.5	8	9	9.5
mg/5 ml	125	125	125	125	125	250	250	250	250	250	250	250

(*continued*)

Appendix CC.20. (*continued*)

Volume (ml)	80	110	140	160	190	110	120	140	150	160	180	190
20 mg/kg/d ml/dose bid	3	3.5	4.5	5.5	6.5	7	8	9	10	11	12	13
mg/5 ml	250	250	250	250	250	250	250	250	250	250	250	250
Volume (ml)	60	70	90	110	120	140	160	180	200	220	240	260
25 mg/kg/d ml/dose bid	3.5	4.5	5.5	7	8	9	10	11.5	12.5	13.5	15	16
mg/5 ml	250	250	250	250	250	250	250	250	250	250	250	250
Volume (ml)	70	90	110	140	160	180	200	230	250	280	300	320

Ilosone Suspension (B)(G) 125, 250 mg/5 ml (100 ml).

APPENDIX CC.21. *ERYTHROMYCIN ETHYLSUCCINATE* (E.E.S. SUSPENSION, ERY-PED DROPS/SUSPENSION)

Weight												
Pounds	15	20	25	30	35	40	45	50	55	60	65	70
Kilograms	6.8	9	11.4	13.6	15.9	18.2	20.5	22.7	25	27.3	29.5	31.8
Single Dose (ml)/Frequency/Strength/10-Day Volume (ml)												
30 mg/kg/d ml/dose qid	1.5	2	2	2.5	3	3.5	4	4	4.5	5	5.5	6
mg/5 ml	200	200	200	200	200	200	200	200	200	200	200	200
Volume (ml)	60	80	80	100	120	140	160	160	180	200	220	240
30 mg/kg/d ml/dose qid			1	1.5	1.5	2	2	2	2.5	2.5	3	3
mg/5 ml			400	400	400	400	400	400	400	400	400	
Volume (ml)			60	60	80	80	80	100	100	120	120	
50 mg/kg/d ml/dose qid	2	3	3.5	4.5	5	5.5	6.5	7	8	8.5	9	10
mg/5 ml	200	200	200	200	200	200	200	200	200	200	200	200
Volume (ml)	80	120	140	180	200	220	260	280	320	340	360	400
50 mg/kg/d ml/dose qid	1	1.5	2	2	2.5	3	3	3.5	4	4.5	4.5	5
mg/5 ml	400	400	400	400	400	400	400	400	400	400	400	400
Volume (ml)	40	60	80	80	100	120	140	140	160	180	180	200

Ery-Ped Drops/Suspension (B)(G) 200 mg/5 ml (100, 200 ml) (fruit); 400 mg/5 ml (60, 100, 200 ml) (banana); Oral drops: 200, 400 mg/5 ml (50 ml) (fruit).

E.E.S. Suspension (B)(G) 200 mg/5 ml, 400 mg/5 ml (100 ml) (fruit).

E.E.S. Granules (B)(G) 200 mg/5 ml (100, 200 ml) (cherry).

APPENDIX CC.22. *ERYTHROMYCIN+SULFAMETHOXAZOLE* (ERYZOLE, PEDIAZOLE)

Weight												
Pounds	15	20	25	30	35	40	45	50	55	60	65	70
Kilograms	6.8	9	11.4	13.6	15.9	18.2	20.5	22.7	25	27.3	29.5	31.8
Single Dose (ml)/Frequency/Strength/10-Day Volume (ml)												
10 mg/kg/d ml/dose bid	3	4	5	6	6.5	7.5	8.5	9.5	10	11	12	13.5
mg/5 ml	200	200	200	200	200	200	200	200	200	200	200	200
Volume (ml)	90	120	150	180	200	225	255	285	300	330	360	400

Eryzole (C)(G) <2 months: not recommended; *eryth* 200 mg/*sulf* 600 mg/5 ml (100, 150, 200, 250 ml).

Pediazole (C)(G) <2 months: not recommended; *eryth* 200 mg/*sulf* 600 mg/5 ml (100, 150, 200 ml) (strawberry-banana).

APPENDIX CC.23. *FLUCONAZOLE* (DIFLUCAN SUSPENSION)

Weight												
Pounds	15	20	25	30	35	40	45	50	55	60	65	70
Kilograms	6.8	9	11.4	13.6	15.9	18.2	20.5	22.7	25	27.3	29.5	31.8
Single Dose (ml)/Frequency/Strength/21-Day Volume (ml)												
3 mg/kg/d ml/dose qd	2	3	3.5	4	5	5.5	6	7	7.5	8	9	9.5
mg/ml	10	10	10	10	10	10	10	10	10	10	10	10
Volume (ml)	44	66	77	88	110	121	132	154	165	176	198	209
6 mg/kg/d ml/dose qd	4	5.5	2	2	2.5	3	3	3.5	4	4	4.5	5
mg/ml	10	10	40	40	40	40	40	40	40	40	40	40
Volume (ml)	88	121	44	44	55	66	66	77	88	88	99	110

Diflucan Suspension (B)(G) double-dose first day; 10, 40 mg/5 ml (35 ml) (orange).

APPENDIX CC.24. *FURAZOLIDONE* (FUROXONE LIQUID)

Weight												
Pounds	15	20	25	30	35	40	45	50	55	60	65	70
Kilograms	6.8	9	11.4	13.6	15.9	18.2	20.5	22.7	25	27.3	29.5	31.8
Single Dose (ml)/Frequency/Strength/7-Day Volume (ml)												
5 mg/kg/d ml/dose qid	2.5	3.5	4	5	6	7	8	8.5	9.5	10	11	12
mg/15 ml	50	50	50	50	50	50	50	50	50	50	50	50
Vol	100	140	160	200	240	280	320	340	380	400	440	480

Furoxone Liquid (C)(G) double-dose first day; 50 mg/15 ml (35 ml).

APPENDIX CC.25. *GRISEOFULVIN, MICROSIZE* (GRIFULVIN V SUSPENSION)

Weight												
Pounds	15	20	25	30	35	40	45	50	55	60	65	70
Kilograms	6.8	9	11.4	13.6	15.9	18.2	20.5	22.7	25	27.3	29.5	31.8
Single Dose (ml)/Frequency/Strength/30-Day Volume (ml)												
5 mg/lb/d ml/dose day	3	4	5	6	7	8	9	10	11	12	13	14
mg/5 ml	125	125	125	125	125	125	125	125	125	125	125	125
Volume (ml)	90	120	150	180	210	240	270	300	330	360	390	420

Grifulvin V Suspension (C)(G) double-dose first day; 125 mg/5 ml (120 ml) (orange) (alcohol 0.02%).

APPENDIX CC.26. *ITRACONAZOLE* (SPORANOX SOLUTION)

Weight												
Pounds	15	20	25	30	35	40	45	50	55	60	65	70
Kilograms	6.8	9	11.4	13.6	15.9	18.2	20.5	22.7	25	27.3	29.5	31.8
Single Dose (ml)/Frequency/Strength/7-Day Volume (ml)												
5 mg/kg/d ml/dose qd	3.5	4.5	6	7	8	9	10	11.5	12.5	14	15	16
mg/ml	10	10	10	10	10	10	10	10	10	10	10	10
Volume (ml)	25	32	42	49	56	63	70	71	88	98	105	112

Sporanox V Solution (C)(G) double-dose first day; 10 mg/ml (150 ml) (cherry-caramel).

APPENDIX CC.27. *LORACARBEF* (LORABID SUSPENSION)

Weight												
Pounds	15	20	25	30	35	40	45	50	55	60	65	70
Kilograms	6.8	9	11.4	13.6	15.9	18.2	20.5	22.7	25	27.3	29.5	31.8
Single Dose (ml)/Frequency/Strength/10-Day Volume (ml)												
15 mg/kg/d ml/dose bid	2.5	3.5	4	5	3	3.5	4	4	5	5	5.5	6
mg/5 ml	100	100	100	100	200	200	200	200	200	200	200	200
Volume (ml)	50	70	80	100	60	70	80	80	100	100	110	120
30 mg/kg/d ml/dose bid	2.5	3.5	4	5	6	7	8	8.5	9.5	10	11	12
mg/5 ml	200	200	200	200	200	200	200	200	200	200	200	200
Volume (ml)	50	70	80	100	120	140	160	170	190	200	220	240

Lorabid Suspension (B) 100 mg/5 ml (50, 100 ml) (strawberry bubble gum); 200 mg/5 ml (50, 75, 100 ml) (strawberry bubble gum).

APPENDIX CC.28. *NITROFURANTOIN* (FURADANTIN SUSPENSION)

Weight												
Pounds	15	20	25	30	35	40	45	50	55	60	65	70
Kilograms	6.8	9	11.4	13.6	15.9	18.2	20.5	22.7	25	27.3	29.5	31.8
Single Dose (ml)/Frequency/Strength/10-Day Volume (ml)												
5 mg/kg ml/dose qid	1.5	2.5	3	3.5	4	4.5	5	5.5	6	7	7.5	8
mg/5 ml	25	25	25	25	25	25	25	25	25	25	25	25
Volume (ml)	60	100	120	140	160	190	200	220	240	280	300	320

Furadantin Suspension (B)(G) 25 mg/5 ml (60 ml).

APPENDIX CC.29. *PENICILLIN V POTASSIUM* (PEN-VEE K SOLUTION, VEETIDS SOLUTION)

Weight												
Pounds	15	20	25	30	35	40	45	50	55	60	65	70
Kilograms	6.8	9	11.4	13.6	15.9	18.2	20.5	22.7	25	27.3	29.5	31.8
Single Dose (ml)/Frequency/Strength/10-Day Volume (ml)												
25 mg/kg/d ml/dose qid	2	2.5	3	3.5	4	4.5	5	5.5	6	7	7.5	8
mg/5 ml	125	125	125	125	125	125	125	125	125	125	125	125
Volume (ml)	80	90	120	140	160	180	200	220	240	280	300	320
25 mg/kg/d ml/dose qid	1	1	1.5	2	2	2.5	2.5	3	3	3.5	4	4
mg/5 ml	250	250	250	250	250	250	250	250	250	250	250	250
Volume (ml)	40	40	60	80	80	100	100	120	120	140	160	160
50 mg/kg/d ml/dose qid	2	2.5	3	3.5	4	4.5	5	6	6.5	7	7.5	8
mg/5 ml	250	250	250	250	250	250	250	250	250	250	250	250
Volume (ml)	80	100	120	140	160	180	200	240	260	280	300	320

Pen-Vee K Solution (B)(G) 125 mg/5 ml (100, 200 ml), 250 mg/5 ml (100, 150, 200 ml).

Veetids Solution (B)(G) 125, 250 mg/5 ml (100, 200 ml).

APPENDIX CC.30. *RIMANTADINE* (FLUMADINE SYRUP)

Weight												
Pounds	15	20	25	30	35	40	45	50	55	60	65	70
Kilograms	6.8	9	11.4	13.6	15.9	18.2	20.5	22.7	25	27.3	29.5	31.8
Single Dose (ml)/Frequency/Strength/10-Day Volume (ml)												
5 mg/kg/d ml/dose qd	3.5	4.5	6	7	8	9	10	11.5	12.5	13.5	15	16

(continued)

Appendix CC.30. (*continued*)

mg/5 ml	50	50	50	50	50	50	50	50	50	50	50	50
Volume (ml)	35	45	60	70	80	90	100	115	125	135	150	160

Flumadine Syrup (B) >10 years: same as adult; 50 mg/5 ml (2, 8, 16 oz) (raspberry).

APPENDIX CC.31. *TETRACYCLINE* (SUMYCIN SUSPENSION)

Weight												
Pounds	15	20	25	30	35	40	45	50	55	60	65	70
Kilograms	6.8	9	11.4	13.6	15.9	18.2	20.5	22.7	25	27.3	29.5	31.8
Single Dose (ml)/Frequency/Strength/10-Day Volume (ml)												
25 mg/kg/d ml/dose qid	1.5	2.5	3	3.5	4	4.5	5	6	6.5	7	7.5	8
mg/5 ml	125	125	125	125	125	125	125	125	125	125	125	125
Volume (ml)	60	100	120	140	160	180	200	240	260	280	300	320
50 mg/kg/d ml/dose qid	3.5	4.5	6	7	8	9	10	11.5	12.5	13.5	15	16
mg/5 ml	125	125	125	125	125	125	125	125	125	125	125	125
Volume (ml)	140	180	240	280	320	360	400	460	500	540	600	640

Sumycin Suspension (D)(G) <8 years: not recommended; 125 mg/5 ml (100, 200 ml) (fruit) (sulfites).

APPENDIX CC.32. *TRIMETHOPRIM* (PRIMSOL SUSPENSION)

Weight												
Pounds	15	20	25	30	35	40	45	50	55	60	65	70
Kilograms	6.8	9	11.4	13.6	15.9	18.2	20.5	22.7	25	27.3	29.5	31.8
Single Dose (ml)/Frequency/Strength/10-Day Volume (ml)												
5 mg/kg/d ml/dose bid	3.5	4.5	6	7	8	9	10	11.5	12.5	13.5	15	16
mg/5 ml	50	50	50	50	50	50	50	50	50	50	50	50
Volume (ml)	70	90	120	140	160	180	200	230	250	270	300	320

Primsol Suspension (C)(G) 50 mg/5 ml (50 mg/5 ml) (bubble gum) (dye-free, alcohol-free).

APPENDIX CC.33. *TRIMETHOPRIM+SULFAMETHOXAZOLE* (BACTRIM SUSPENSION, SEPTRA SUSPENSION)

Weight												
Pounds	15	20	25	30	35	40	45	50	55	60	65	70
Kilograms	6.8	9	11.4	13.6	15.9	18.2	20.5	22.7	25	27.3	29.5	31.8
Single Dose (ml)/Frequency/Strength/10-Day Volume (ml)												
10 mg/kg/d ml/dose bid	2	2	3	3.5	4	4.5	5	5.5	6	7	7.5	8

(*continued*)

Appendix CC.33. (*continued*)

mg/5 ml	200	200	200	200	200	200	200	200	200	200	200	200
Volume (ml)	40	40	60	70	80	90	100	110	120	140	150	160
20 mg/kg/d ml/dose bid	4	4	6	7	8	9	10	11	12	14	15	16
mg/5 ml	200	200	200	200	200	200	200	200	200	200	200	200
Volume (ml)	80	80	120	140	160	180	200	220	240	280	300	320

Bactrim Pediatric Suspension, Septra Pediatric Suspension (C)(G) trim 40 mg/sulfa 200 mg/5 ml (100 ml) (cherry) (alcohol 0.3%).

APPENDIX CC.34. *VANCOMYCIN* (VANCOCIN SUSPENSION)

Weight												
Pounds	15	20	25	30	35	40	45	50	55	60	65	70
Kilograms	6.8	9	11.4	13.6	15.9	18.2	20.5	22.7	25	27.3	29.5	31.8
Single Dose (ml)/Frequency/Strength/10-Day Volume (ml)												
40 mg/kg/d ml/dose tid	2	2.5	3	3.5	4.5	5	5.5	6	7	7.5	8	8.5
mg/5 ml	250	250	250	250	250	250	250	250	250	250	250	250
Volume (ml)	60	75	90	105	135	150	165	180	210	225	240	255
40 mg/kg/d ml/dose qid	1.5	2	2.5	3	3	3.5	4	4.5	5	5.5	6	6.5
mg/5 ml	250	250	250	250	250	250	250	250	250	250	250	250
Volume (ml)	60	80	100	120	120	140	160	180	200	220	240	260
40 mg/kg/d ml/dose tid	1	1	1.5	2	2	2.5	3	3	3.5	3.5	4	4
mg/6 ml	500	500	500	500	500	500	500	500	500	500	500	500
Volume (ml)	30	30	45	60	60	75	90	90	105	105	120	120
40 mg/kg/d ml/dose qid	1	1	1.5	1.5	1.5	2	2	2.5	2.5	3	3	3.5
mg/6 ml	500	500	500	500	500	500	500	500	500	500	500	500
Volume (ml)	40	40	60	60	60	80	80	100	100	120	120	140

Vancomycin Suspension (C)(G).

2017 ACC/AHA/AAPA/ABC/ACPM/AGS/APhA/ASH/ASPC/NMA/PCNA Guideline for the Prevention, Detection, Evaluation, and Management of High Blood Pressure in Adults: A report of the American College of Cardiology/American Heart Association Task Force on Clinical Practice Guidelines
http://hyper.ahajournals.org/content/hypertensionaha/early/2017/11/10/HYP.0000000000000065.full.pdf

ACR Guidelines on Prevention & Treatment of Glucocorticoid-induced Osteoporosis [press release, June 7, 2017]. Atlanta, GA: American College of Rheumatology
https://www.rheumatology.org/About-Us/Newsroom/Press-Releases/ID/812/ACR-Releases-Guideline-on-Prevention-Treatment-of-Glucocorticoid-Induced-Osteoporosis

Advance for Nurse Practitioners
http://nurse-practitioners.advanceweb.com

Advanced Practice Education Associates
www.apea.com

Ake, J. A., Schuetz, A., Pegu, P., Wieczorek, L., Eller, M. A., Kibuuka, H., . . . Robb, M. L. (2017). Safety and immunogenicity of PENNVAX-G DNA prime administered by biojector 2000 or CELLECTRA electroporation device with modified vaccinia Ankara-CMDR boost. *The Journal of Infectious Diseases*, 216(9), 1080–1090. doi:10.1093/infdis/jix456

American Academy of Dermatology
https://www.aad.org/home

American Academy of Pediatrics (AAP)
http://aapexperience.org

American Association of Nurse Practitioners
www.aanp.org

American College of Cardiology. Then and now: ATP III vs. IV: Comparison of ATP III and ACC/AHA guidelines.
http://www.acc.org/latest-in-cardiology/articles/2014/07/18/16/03/then-and-now-atp-iii-vs-iv

American Diabetes Association (ADA), Professional Diabetes Resources Online.
http://professional.diabetes.org/content/clinical-practice-recommendations/?loc=rp-slabnav

American Diabetes Association. (2018). Children and adolescents: Standards of medical care in diabetes—2018. *Diabetes Care*, 41(Suppl 1), S126–S136. doi.org/10.2337/dc18-S012

American Diabetes Association. (2018). Management of diabetes in pregnancy: Standards of medical care in diabetes—2018. *Diabetes Care*, 41(Suppl 1), S137–S143. doi.org/10.2337/dc18-S013

American Diabetes Association. (2018). Microvascular complications and foot care: Standards of medical care in diabetes—2018. *Diabetes Care*, 41(Suppl 1), S105-S118. doi.org/10.2337/dc18-S010

American Diabetes Association. (2018). Older adults: Standards of medical care in diabetes—2018. *Diabetes Care*, 41(Suppl 1), S119–S125. doi.org/10.2337/dc18-S011

American Diabetes Association. (2018). Pharmacologic approaches to glycemic treatment: Standards of medical care in diabetes—2018. *Diabetes Care*, 41(Suppl 1), S73–S85. doi.org/10.2337/dc18-S008

American Diabetes Association. (2018). Summary of revisions: Standards of medical care in diabetes—2018. *Diabetes Care*, 41(Suppl 1), S4–S6. doi.org/10.2337/dc18-Srev01

American Family Physician
http://www.aafp.org/online/en/home.html

American Geriatrics Society 2015 updated Beers criteria for potentially inappropriate medication use in older adults. *Journal of the American Geriatrics Society, 63*(11), 2227–2246

American Headache Society
www.americanheadachesociety.org

American Pain Society
http://americanpainsociety.org

American Pharmacists Association. (2018). *Pediatric and neonatal dosage handbook: A universal resource for clinicians treating pediatric and neonatal patients* (25th ed.). Hudson, OH: Lexicomp.

American Trypanosomiasis Centers for Disease Control and Prevention. *Parasites—American Trypanosomiasis (also known as Chagas disease). Resources for health professionals.*

Anderson, E., Fantus, R. J., & Haddadin, R. I. (2017). Diagnosis and management of herpes zoster ophthalmicus. *Disease-a-Month, 63*(2), 38–44.

Andorf, S., Purington, N., Block, W. M., Long, A. J., Tupa, D., Brittain, E., . . . Chinthrajah, R. S. Anti-IgE treatment with oral immunotherapy in multi-food allergic participants: A double-blind, randomised, controlled trial [published online December 12, 2017]. *Lancet Gastroenterology Hepatology, 3*(2), 85–94 doi:10.1016/S2468-1253(17)30392-8

Antiretroviral Pregnancy Registry at http://www.apregistry.com/index.htm; Research Park, 1011 Ashes Drive, Wilmington, NC 28405; telephone: 800-258-4263; fax: 800-800-1052; e-mail: registies@kendle.com

Aronow, W. S. *Initiation of antihypertensive therapy.* Presented at: American Heart Association (AHA) Scientific Sessions 2017; November 11-15, 2017; Anaheim, CA. http://www.abstractsonline.com/pp8/ - !/4412/presentation/55060

ATP III and ACC/AHA Guidelines
http://www.acc.org/latest-in-cardiology/articles/2014/07/18/16/03/then-and-now-atp-iii-vs-iv

Auron, M., & Raissouni, N. (2015). Adrenal insufficiency. *Pediatric Review, 36*(3), 92–102.

Belknap, R., Holland, D., Feng P., *et al.* Self-administered versus directly observed once-weekly isoniazid and rifapentine treatment of latent tuberculosis infection: A randomized trial. [Published online ahead of print November 7, 2017]. *Annals of Internal Medicine.* doi:10.7326/M17-1150

Bosworth, T. (2017) *Testosterone deficiency treatment recommendation.*
https://www.medpagetoday.com/resource-center/hypogonadism/treatment-recommendations/a/64511

Bradley, J. S., & Nelson, J. D. (2018). *Nelson's pediatric antimicrobial therapy (24th ed.).* Itasca, IL: American Academy of Pediatrics.

Brody, A. A., Gibson, B., Tresner-Kirsch, D., Kramer, H., Thraen, I., Coarr, M. E., & Rupper, R. (2016). High prevalence of medication discrepancies between home health referrals and Centers for Medicare and Medicaid Services home health certification and plan of care and their potential to affect safety of vulnerable elderly adults. *Journal of the American Geriatrics Society, 64*(11), e166–e170.

Brunk, D. Learn 'four Ds' approach to heart failure in diabetes. Clinician Reviews [Posted online January 28, 2018]. https://www.mdedge.com/clinicalendocrinologynews/article/157198/diabetes/learn-four-ds-approach-heart-failure-diabetes

Canestaro, W. J., Forrester, S. H., Raghu, G., Ho, L., & Devine, B. E. (2016). Drug treatment of idiopathic pulmonary fibrosis: Systematic review and network meta-analysis. *Chest, 149*, 756–766.

CDC 2015 Sexually Transmitted Diseases Treatment Guidelines
http://www.cdc.gov/std/tg2015/default.htm

CDC Cases of Public Health Importance (COPHI) Coordinator (for reporting HIV infections in HCP and failures of PEP); telephone 404-639-2050

CDC Guidelines for Conception in HIV Positive Women Stress the Use of PrEP in Sexual Partners
https://www.medpagetoday.com/resource-centers/contemporary-hiv-prevention/cdc-guide-lines-conception-hiv-positive-women-stress-use-prep-sexual- partners/775?xid=NL_MPT_MPT_HIV_2017-09-26&eun=g766320d0r

CDC Guideline for Prescribing Opioids for Chronic Pain—United States. (2016).
https://jamanetwork.com/learning/article-quiz/10.1001/jama.2016.1464#qundefined

CDC: Morbidity and Mortality Weekly Report (MMWR)
http://www.cdc.gov/mmwr/mmwr_wk.html

CDC Provider Information Sheet–PrEP During Conception, Pregnancy, and Breast-feeding Information for Clinicians Counseling Patients About PrEP Use During Conception, Pregnancy, and Breastfeeding.
https://www.cdc.gov/hiv/pdf/prep_gl_clinician_factsheet_pregnancy_english.pdf

CDC Travelers' Health
https://wwwnc.cdc.gov/travel/destinations/list

CDC. (2017). *Recommended Immunization Schedule for Children and Adolescents Aged 18 Years or Younger, United States.*
https://www.cdc.gov/vaccines/schedules/downloads/child/0-18yrs-child-combined-schedule.pdf

Centers for Disease Control and Prevention. (2017). *Adult Immunization Schedule by Medical and other Indications.*
http://www.cdc.gov/vaccines/schedules/hcp/imz/adult-conditions.html

Centers for Disease Control and Prevention. (2016). *Diphtheria, Tetanus, and Pertussis Vaccine Recommendations.*
http://www.cdc.gov/vaccines/vpd/dtap-tdap-td/hcp/recommendations.htm

Centers for Disease Control and Prevention. (2016). *Facts About ADHD.*
www.cdc.gov/ncbddd/adhd/facts.html

Centers for Disease Control and Prevention. (2016). *Pneumococcal vaccination: summary of who and when to vaccinate.*
http://www.cdc.gov/vaccines/vpd/pneumo/hcp/who-when-to-vaccinate.html

Chang, A., Martins, K. A. O., Encinales, L., Reid, S. P., Acuña, M., & Encinales, C., . . . Firestein, G. S. (2017). A cross-sectional analysis of chikungunya arthritis patients 22 months post-infection demonstrates no detectable viral persistence in synovial fluid. *Arthritis Rheumatology.* doi:10.1002/art.40383

Chang, A., Encinales, L., Porras, A., Pachecho, N., Reid, S. P., Martins, K. A. O., . . . Simon, G. L. (2017). Frequency of chronic joint pain following chikungunya infection: A Colombian cohort study. *Arthritis Rheumatology,* doi:10.1002/art.40384

Chow, A. W., Benninger, M. S., Brook, I., Brozek, J. L., Goldstein, E. J., Hicks, L. A., . . . Infectious Disease Society of America. (2012). IDSA clinical practice guideline for acute and bacterial rhinosinusitis in children and adults. *Clinical Infectious Diseases, 54*(8), e72–e112.

Chutka, D. S., Takahashi, P. Y., & Hoel, R. W. (2004). Inappropriate medications for elderly patients. Mayo Clinic Proceedings. 79(1), 122–139.

Clinician Reviews
http://www.clinicianreviews.com

Cohen, J. D., Li, L., Wang, Y., Thoburn, C., Afsari, B., Danilova, L., . . . Papadopoulos, N. (2018). Detection and localization of surgically resectable cancers with a multi-analyte blood test. *Science*, eaar3247. doi:10.1126/science.aar3247

Coker, T. J., & Dierfeldt, D. M. (2016). Acute bacterial prostatitis: Diagnosis and management. *American Family Physician, 93*(2), 114–120.

Consultant 360
http://www.consultant360.com/home

Daily Med: NIH. US Library of Medicine
https://dailymed.nlm.nih.gov/dailymed/index.cfm

Davis, M. C., Miller, B. J., Kalsi, J. K., Birkner, T., & Mathis, M. V. (2017). Efficient trial design—FDA approval of valbenazine for tardive dyskinesia. *New England Journal of Medicine, 376*, 2503–2506.

Dhadwal, G., & Kirchhof, M. G. The risks and benefits of cannabis in the dermatology clinic. [Published online ahead of print October 23, 2017]. *Journal of Cutaneous Medicine and Surgery*. doi:10.1177/1203475417738971

Dietrich, E. A., & Davis, K. (2017). Antibiotics for acute bacterial prostatitis: Which agent, and for how long? *Consultant, 57*(9), 564–565.

Domino, F. J., Baldor, R. A., Golding, J., & Stephens, M. B. (2016). *The 5-minute clinical consult standard 2016*. Philadelphia, PA: Wolters Kluwer.

Dowell, D., Haegerich, T. M., & Chou, R. (2016). CDC guidelines for prescribing opi-oids for chronic pain. *Journal of the American Medical Association, 315*(15), 1624–1645. doi:10.1001/jama.2016.1464

DRUGS.COM
www.drugs.com

DRUGS.COM: Drugs Interaction Checker
https://www.drugs.com/drug_interactions.php

DRUGS at FDA: FDA Approved Drug Products
http://www.accessdata.fda.gov/scripts/cder/drugsatfda/index.cfm

Durkin, M. J., Jafarzadeh, S. R., Hsueh, K., Sallah, Y. H., Munshi, K. D., Henderson, R. R., & Fraser, V. J. (2018). Outpatient Antibiotic Prescription Trends in the United States: A National Cohort Study. *Infection Control & Hospital Epidemiology, 39*(05), 584–589. doi:10.1017/ice.2018.26

Emer, J. J., Bernardo, S. G., Kovalerchik, O., & Ahmad, M. (2013). Urticaria multiforme. *The Journal of Clinical and Aesthetic Dermatology, 6*(31), 34–39.

eMPR: Monthly Prescribing Reference (new FDA approved products, new generics, new drug withdrawals, safety alerts)
http://www.empr.com

Endocrinology on the comprehensive type 2 diabetes management algorithm —2017 executive summary. (2017). *Endocrine Practice, 23*(2), 207–238. doi:10.4158/ep161682.cs

Engorn, B., & Flerlage, J. (Eds.). (2015). *The Harriet Lane handbook: A handbook for pediatric house officers* (20th ed.). Philadelphia, PA: Elsevier.
https://online.epocrates.com/drugs

epocrates
https://online.epocrates.com/drugs

FDA Drug Safety Communication. *FDA review finds additional data supports the potential for increased long-term risks with antibiotic clarithromycin (Biaxin) in patients with heart disease.* (02/22/18)
https://www.fda.gov/downloads/Drugs/DrugSafety/ucm597723.pdf

FDA: News Release: FDA Approves Drug to Treat Duchenne Muscular Dystrophy. (2017) https://www.fda.gov/NewsEvents/Newsroom/PressAnnouncements/ucm540945.htm

FDA: Recalls, Market Withdrawals, and Safety Alerts http://www.fda.gov/Safety/Recalls/default.htm

FDA, Reporting Unusual or Severe Toxicity to Antiretroviral Agents); http://www.fda.gov/ medwatch/; telephone: 800-332-1088; address: MedWatch, The FDA Safety Information and Adverse Event Reporting Program, Food and Drug Administration, 5600 Fishers Lane, Rockville, MD 20852

Fleming, J. E., & Lockwood, S. (2017). Cannabinoid hyperemesis syndrome. *Federal Practitioner, 34*(10), 33–36.

Flynn, J. T., Kaelber, D. C., Baker-Smith, C. M., Blowey, D., Carroll, A. E., Daniels, S. R., . . . Subcommittee On Screening And Management Of High Blood Pressure In Children. (2017). Clinical practice guideline for screening and management of high blood pressure in children and adolescents. [Published online ahead of print August 22, 2017]. *Pediatrics, 140*(3), e20171904.

Freedberg, D. E., Kim, L. S., & Yang, Y.-X. (2017). The risks and benefits of long-term use of proton pump inhibitors: Expert review and best practice advice from the American Gastroenterological Association. *Gastroenterology, 152*(4), 706–715. doi:10.1053/j.gastro.2017.01.031

Garber, A. J., Abrahamson, M. J., Barzilay, J. I., Blonde, L., Bloomgarden, Z. T., Bush, M. A., . . . Umpierrez, G. E. (2017). Consensus statement by the American Association of Clinical Endocrinologists and American College of Endocrinology on the comprehensive type 2 diabetes management algorithm – 2017 executive summary. *Endocrine Practice, 23*(2), 207–238. doi:10.4158/ep161682.cs

Gilbert, D. N., Chambers, H. F., Eliopoulos, G. M., Gilbert, D. N., Chambers, H. F., Eliopoulos, S. M., & Pavia, A. (2016). *The Sanford guide to antimicrobial therapy, 2016* (48th ed.). Sperryville, VA: Antimicrobial Therapy.

Gordon, C., Amissah-Arthur, M. B., Gayed, M., Brown, S., Bruce, I. N., D'Cruz D., . . . British Society for Rheumatology Standards, Audit and Guidelines Working Group. (2017). The British Society for Rheumatology guideline for the management of systemic lupus erythematosus in adults: Executive Summary. *Rheumatology (Oxford).* doi:10.1093/rheumatology/kex291. [Epub ahead of print]

Gordon, C., Amissah-Arthur, M. B., Gayed, M., Brown, S., Bruce, I. N., D'Cruz D., . . . British Society for Rheumatology Standards, Audit and Guidelines Working Group. The British Society for Rheumatology guideline for the management of systemic lupus erythematosus in adults. *Rheumatology (Oxford).* 2017 Oct 6. doi:10.1093/rheumatology/kex286

Greenhawt, M., Turner, P. J., & Kelso, J. M. (2018). Allergy experts set the record straight on flu shots for patients with egg sensitivity. *Annals of Allergy, Asthma & Immunology, 120*(1), 49–52. doi:10.1016/j.anai.2017.10.020

Groot, N., de Graaff, N., Avcin, T., Bader-Meunier, B., Brogan, P., Dolezalova, P., . . . Beresford, M. W. (2017). European evidence-based recommendations for diagnosis and treatment of childhood-onset systemic lupus erythematosus [cSLE]: The [Single Hub and Access point for paediatric Rheumatology in Europe] SHARE initiative. *Annals of the Rheumatic Diseases, 76*(11), 1788–1796. doi:10.1136/annrheumdis-2016-210960

Groot, N., de Graeff, N., Marks, S. D., Brogan, P., Avcin, T., Bader-Meunier, B., . . . Kamphuis, S. (2017). European evidence-based recommendations for the diagnosis and treatment of childhood-onset lupus nephritis [cLN]: The SHARE initiative. *Recommendation.* doi. org/10.1136/annrheumdis-2017-211898

Guidelines updated for thyroid disease in pregnancy and postpartum. (2017). *American Journal of Nursing, 4*(117), 16.

Handbook of Antimicrobial Therapy (20th ed.). (2015). New Rochelle, NY: The Medical Letter

Harrison's Infectious Diseases (3rd ed.). (2016). New York, NY: McGraw Hill Education

Huang, A. R., Mallet, L., Rochefort, C. M. (2012). Medication-related falls in the elderly: Causative factors and preventive strategies. *Drugs & Aging. 29*(5), 359–376.

Hughes, H. K., & Kahl, K. (Eds.). (2018). *The Johns Hopkins Hospital: The Harriet Lane handbook for pediatric house officers (21st ed.).* Philadelphia, PA: Elsevier.

International Diabetes Federation (IDF) Clinical Practice Guidelines
http://www.idf.org/guidelines

Inzucchi, S. E., Iliev, H., Pfarr, E., & Zinman, B. Empagliflozin and assessment of lower-limb amputations in the EMPA-REG OUTCOME Trial [published online November 13, 2017]. *Diabetes Cares, 41*(1), e4–e5. doi:10.2337/dc17-1551

James, P. A., Oparil, S, Carter, B. L, Cushman, W. C., Dennison-Himmelfarb, C., Handler, J., . . . Ortiz, E. (2014). Evidence-based guidelines for the management of high blood pressure in adults: Report from the panel members appointed to the eighth joint national committee (JNC 8). *Journal of the American Medical Association, 311*(5), 507–520.

Jarrett, J. B., & Moss, D. Oral agent offers relief from generalized hyperhidrosis–An inexpensive and well-tolerated anticholinergic reduces sweating in patients with localized—and generalized— hyperhidrosis. *Clinician Reviews.* July 2017 [posted online]
https://www.mdedge.com/sites/default/files/Document/June-2017/CR02707024.PDF

JNC 8 Guideline Summary. *Pharmacist's Letter/Prescriber's Letter.*
https://www.scribd.com/doc/290772273/JNC-8-guideline-summary

Journal of the American Academy of Nurse Practitioners
https://www.aanp.org/publications/jaanp

Journal of the American Medical Association (JAMA) Internal Medicine
http://archinte.jamanetwork.com/journal.aspx

Journal of the American Geriatrics Society
http://onlinelibrary.wiley.com/journal/10.1111/(ISSN)1532–5415

Justesen, K., & Prasad, S. (2016). On-demand pill protocol protects against HIV. *Clinician Reviews, 26*(9), 18–19, 22.
https://www.mdedge.com/authors/kathryn-justesen-md
https://www.mdedge.com/authors/shaliendra-prasad-mbbs-mph

Kasper, D. L., & Fauci, A. S. (2017). Listeria monocytogenes infections. In: *Harrison's Infectious Diseases (3rd ed.).* New York, NY: McGraw Hill Education

Khera, M., Adaikan, G., Buvat, J, Carrier, S., El-Meliegy, A., Hatzimouratidis, K., . . (2016). Diagnosis and treatment of testosterone deficiency: Recommendations from the Fourth International Consultation for Sexual Medicine (ICSM 2015). *The Journal of Sexual Medicine, 13*, 1787–1804.

Kim, D. K., Riley, L. E., Harriman, K. H., Hunter, P., & Bridges, C. B. (2017). Advisory Committee on Immunization Practices recommended immunization schedule for adults aged 19 years or older—United States, 2017. *Morbidity and Mortality Weekly Report, 66*, 136–138. doi:10.15585/mmwr.mm6605e2

Kuhar, D. T., Henderson, D. K., Struble, K. A., Heneine, W., Thomas, V., . . . Cheever, L. W. (2013). Updated US Public Health Service Guidelines for the Management of Occupational Exposures to Human Immunodeficiency Virus and Recommendations for Postexposure Prophylaxis. *Infection Control & Hospital Epidemiology, 34*(09), 875–892. doi:10.1086/672271

Kumar, S., Yegneswaran, B., & Pitchumoni, C. S. (2017). Preventing the adverse effects of glucocorticoids: A reminder. *Consultant, 57*(12), 726–728.

Langer, R., Simon, J. A., Pines, A., Lobo, R. A., Hodis, H. N., Pickar, J. H., . . . Utian, W. H. (2017). Menopausal hormone therapy for primary prevention: Why the USPSTF is wrong. *The North American Menopause Society*, *24*(10), 1101–1112. doi:10.1097/GME.0000000000000983

Leach, M. Z. (November 7, 2017). First UK guidelines for adults with lupus. *Rheumatology Network* http://www.rheumatologynetwork.com/article/first-uk-guidelines-adults-lupus

Lieberthal, A. S., Carroll, A. E., Chonmaitree, T., Ganiats, T. G., Hoberman, A., Jackson, M. A., & Tunkel, D. E. (2013). The diagnosis and management of acute otitis media. *Pediatrics*, *131*(3), e964–e999.

Lortscher, D, Admani, S, Satur, N, & Eichenfield, LF. (2016). Hormonal contraceptives and acne: a retrospective analysis of 2147 patients. *J Drugs Dermatol*, *15*(6), 670–674. http://jddonline.com/articles/dermatology/S1545961616P0670X

Mallick, J., Devi, L., & Malik, P. K., & Mallick J. (2016). Update on normal tension glaucoma. *Journal of Ophthalmic and Vision Research*, *11*(2), 204–208. doi:10.4103/2008-322X. 183914

Manchikanti, L., Kaye, A. M., Knezevic, N. N., McAnally, H., Slavin, K., Trescot, A. M., . . . Hirsch, J. A. (2017). Responsible, safe, and effective prescription of opioids for chronic non-cancer pain: American Society of Interventional Pain Physicians (ASIPP) guidelines. *Pain Physician*, *20*(2S), S3–S92.

Mandell, L. A., Wunderink, R. G., Anzueto, A., Bartlett, J. G., Campbell, G. D., Dean, N. C., . . . American Thoracic Society. (2007). Infectious diseases society of America/American Thoracic Society consensus guidelines on the management of community-acquired pneumonia in adults. *Clinical Infectious Diseases*, *44*(Suppl 2), S27–S72. https://enp-network.s3.amazonaws.com/NPA_Long_Island/pdf/Pneumonia.pdf

McDonald, J., & Mattingly, J (2016). Chagas disease: Creeping into family practice in the United States. *Clinician Reviews*, *26*(11), 38–45.

McLean, A. J., & Le Couteur, D. G. (2004). Aging biology and geriatric clinical pharmacology. *Pharmacological Reviews*, *56*(2), 63–84.

McMillan, J. A., Lee, C. K. K., Siberry, G. K., & Carroll, K. (2013). *The Harriet Lane handbook of pediatric antimicrobial therapy*. Philadelphia, PA: Elsevier Saunders.

McNeill, C., Sisson, W., & Jarrett, A. (2017). Listerosis: A resurfacing menace. *International Journal of Nursing Practice*, *13*(10), 647–654.

MDedge: Family Practice News https://www.mdedge.com/familypracticenews/

MedlinePlus https://www.nlm.nih.gov/medlineplus/ency/article/000165.htm

MedPage Today http://www.medpagetoday.com

Medscape http://www.medscape.com

Medscape: Drug Interaction Checker http://reference.medscape.com/drug-interactionchecker?src=wnl_drugguide _170410_mscpref &uac=123859AY&impID=1324737&faf=1

Merel, S. E., & Paauw, D. S. (2017). Common drug side effects and drug-drug interactions in elderly adults in primary care. *Journal of the American Geriatrics Society*, *65*(7), 1578–1585.

Miller, G. E., Sarpong, E. M., Davidoff, A. J., Yang, E. Y., Brandt, N. J., Fick, D. M. (2016). Determinants of potentially inappropriate medication use among community-dwelling older adults. *Health Services Research*, *52*(4), 1534–1549.

Molina, J. M., Capitant, C., Spire, B., Pialoux, G., Cotte, L., Charreau, I., . . . ANRS IPERGAY Study Group. (2015). On-demand preexposure prophylaxis in men at high risk for HIV-1 infection. *The New England Journal of Medicine, 373,* 2237–2246.

Monaco, K. *HRT benefits outweigh risks for certain menopausal women—Menopause Society statement aims to clear up confusion.* https://www.medpagetoday.com/Endocrinology/Menopause/66158?xid=NL_MPT_IRXHealthWomen_2017-12-27&eun=g766320d0r

Morales, A., Bebb, R. A., Manoo, P., Assimakopoulos, P., Axler, J., Collier, C., . . . Lee, J. (2015). Appendix 1 (as supplied by the authors): Full-text guidelines Multidisciplinary Canadian Clinical Practice Guideline on the diagnosis and management of testosterone deficiency syndrome in adult males. http://www.cmaj.ca/content/suppl/2015/10/26/cmaj.150033.DC1/15-0033-1-at.pdf

National Academy of Medicine http://nam.edu

National Center for Emerging and Zoonotic Infectious Diseases (NCEZID) https://www.cdc.gov/ncezid/index.html

National Cholesterol Education Program Expert Panel on Detection, Evaluation, and Treatment of High Blood Cholesterol in Adults (Adult Treatment Panel IV, 2012) http://circ.ahajournals.org/content/circulationaha/106/25/3143.full.pdf

National Heart Lung and Blood Institute (NHLBI) http://www.nhlbi.nih.gov

National Institute of Diabetes and Digestive and Kidney Diseases. *Adrenal Insufficiency and Addison's Disease.* http://www.nidk.nih.gov/health-infromation/health-topics/endocrine/adren [Accessed May 31, 2016]

New England Journal of Medicine (NEJM) Journal Watch General Medicine http://www.jwatch.org/general-medicine

Ní Chróinín, D., Neto, H. M., Xiao, D., Sandhu, A., Brazel, C., Farnham, N., . . . Beveridge, A. (2016). Potentially inappropriate medications (PIMs) in older hospital in-patients: Prevalence, contribution to hospital admission and documentation of rationale for continuation. *Australasian Journal on Ageing, 35*(4), 262–265.

NIH, HIV/AIDS Treatment Information Service http://aidsinfo.nih.gov/

Ostergaard, L., Vesikari, T., Absalon, J., Beeslaar, J., Ward, B. J., . . . B1971009 and B1971016 Trial Investigators. A bivalent meningococcal b vaccine in adolescents and young adults [published online December 14, 2017]. *The New England Journal of Medicine, 35*(4), 262–265. doi:10.1111/ajag.12312

Paz-Bailey, G, et al. Zika virus persistence in body fluids, final report in body fluids: Final report. ASTMH 2017. Paper presented at the 66th Annual Meeting of the American Society of Tropical Medicine and Hygiene, November 5–9, Baltimore, MD.

PEPline; http://www.nccc.ucsf.edu/about_nccc/pepline/; telephone: 888-448-4911

Pharmacist's Letter www.pharmacistsletter.com

Physician's Desk Reference (PDR) http://www.pdr.net

Pregnancy and Lactation Labeling Final Rule (PLLR)
https://www.drugs.com/pregnancy-categories.html

Prescriber's Letter
http://prescribersletter.therapeuticresearch.com/pl/sample.
aspx?cs=&s=PRL&AspxAutoDetectCookieSupport=1

Psychopharmacology
http://link.springer.com/journal/213

Reference for Interpretation of Hepatitis C Virus (HCV) Test Results
www.cdc.gov/hepatitis

Robinson, C. L., Romero, J. R., Kempe, A., & Pellegrini, C. (2017). Advisory committee on immunization practices recommended immunization schedule for children and adolescents aged 18 years or younger—United States, 2017. *MMWR. Morbidity and Mortality Weekly Report, 66*(5), 134–135. doi:10.15585/mmwr. mm6605e1

Rosenberg, E., et al. (2017, November 5–9). *Prevalence and incidence of Zika virus infection among household contacts of Zika patients, Puerto Rico, 2016-2017. ASTMH 2017* . Paper presented at the 66th Annual Meeting of the American Society of Tropical Medicine and Hygiene, Baltimore, MD

RxLIST
http://www.rxlist.com/script/main/hp.asp

RxLIST: Drugs A-Z
http://www.rxlist.com/drugs/alpha_a.htm

Sáez-Llorens, X., Tricou, V., Yu, D., Rivera, L., Jimeno, J., Villarreal, A. C., … Wallace, D. (2018). Immunogenicity and safety of one versus two doses of tetravalent dengue vaccine in healthy children aged 2–17 years in Asia and Latin America: 18-month interim data from a phase 2, randomised, placebo-controlled study. *The Lancet Infectious Diseases, 18*(2), 162–170. doi:10.1016/s1473-3099(17)30632-1

Sanford Guide Web Edition
https://webedition.sanfordguide.com

Saunders, K. H., Shukla, A. P., Igel, L. I., & Aronne, L. J. (2017). Obesity: When to consider medication. *The Journal of Family Practice, 66*(10), 608–616.
http://www.mdedge.com/sites/default/files/Document/September-2017/JFP06610608.PDF

Schaeffer, A. J., & Nicolle, L. E. (2016). Urinary tract infections in older men. *The New England Journal of Medicine. 374*(6), 562–571.

Schwartz, S. R., Magit, A. E., Rosenfeld, R. M., Ballachanda, B. B., Hackell, J. M., Krouse, H. J., … Cunningham, E. R. (2017). Clinical practice guideline (update): Earwax (cerumen impaction). *Otolaryngology Head Neck Surgery, 156*(1S), S1–S29.

Solutions for safer ER/LA opioid prescribing in a new Era of Health Care. *American Nurses Credentialing Center, Post Graduate Institute of Medicine.*
www.cmeuniversity.com

Sterling, T. R., Villarino, M. E., Borisov, A. S., Shang, N., Gordin, F., Bliven-Sizemore, E., … TB trials consortium PREVENT TB study team. (2011). Three months of rifapentine and isoniazid for latent tuberculosis infection. *The New England Journal of Medicine, 365*, 2155–2166. doi:10.1056/NEJMoa1104875

Stone, N. J., Robinson, J. G., Lichtenstein, A. H., Bairey Merz, C. N., Blum, C. B., Eckel, R. H., … American College of Cardiology/American Heart Association Task Force on Practice Guidelines. (2014). 2013 ACC/AHA guideline on the treatment of blood cholesterol to reduce atherosclerotic cardiovascular risk in adults: A report of the American College of Cardiology/American Heart Association Task Force on Practice Guidelines. *Circulation, 129*(25 suppl 2), S1–S45.

Taipale, H., Mittendorfer-Rutz, E., Alexanderson, K., Majak, M., Mehtälä, J., Hoti, F., ... Tiihonen, J. Antipsychotics and mortality in a nationwide cohort of 29,823 patients with schizophrenia [published online December 20, 2017]. *Schizophrenia Research, pii: S0920–9964*(17), 30762–30764. doi:10.1016/j.schres.2017.12.010

Taketomo, C. K., Hodding, J. H., & Kraus, D. M. (2015). *Pediatric and neonatal dosage handbook: A universal resource for clinicians treating pediatric and neonatal patients (22nd ed.).* Wolters Kluwer.

Tebas, P., Roberts, C. C., Muthumani, K., Reuschel, E. L., Kudchodkar, S. B., Zaidi, F. I., ... Maslow, J. N. (2017). Safety and immunogenicity of an anti–zika virus DNA vaccine—Preliminary Report. *New England Journal of Medicine.* doi:10.1056/nejmoa1708120

The 2017 hormone therapy position statement of The North American Menopause Society. (2017). *Menopause: The North American Menopause Society.* doi:10.1097/GME.0000000000000921

The American Congress of Obstetrics and Gynecology (ACOG)
http://www.acog.org

The American Geriatrics Society
http://www.americangeriatrics.org

The JAMA Network.com
www.jamanetwork.com

The Journal for Nurse Practitioners
www.elsevier.com/locate/tjnp

The Medical Letter on Drugs and Therapeutics
http://secure.medicalletter.org

The Nurse Practitioner Journal
www.tnpj.com

Third Report of the National Cholesterol Education Program (NCEP) expert panel on detection, evaluation, and treatment of high blood cholesterol in adults (Adult Treatment Panel III) final report.
http://www.ncbi.nlm.nih.gov/pubmed/12485966

Tomaselli, G. F., Mahaffey, K. W., Cuker, A., Dobesh, P. P., Doherty, J. U., Eikelboom, J. W., ... Wiggins, B. S. (2017). 2017 ACC expert consensus decision pathway on management of bleeding in patients on oral anticoagulants. *Journal of the American College of Cardiology, 70*(24), 3042–3067. doi:10.1016/j.jacc.2017.09.1085

Tricou, V, et al. *Progress in development of Takeda's tetravalent dengue vaccine. ASTMH 2017.* Paper presented at the 2017 American Society of Tropical Medicine & Hygiene

Turner, P. J., Southern, J., Andrews, N. J., Miller, E., Erlewyn-Lajeunesse, M., & Doyle, C. (2015). Safety of live attenuated influenza vaccine in atopic children with egg allergy. *Journal of Allergy and Clinical Immunology, 136*(2), 376–381. doi:10.1016/j.jaci.2014.12.1925

Updated CDC guidance: Superbugs threaten hospital patients. *Medscape Education Clinical Briefs.* (2016, March 31)
http://www.medscape.org/viewarticle/859361?nlid=105320_2713&src=wnl_cmemp_160523_mscpedu_nurs&impID=1106718&faf=1

UpToDate.com
http://www.uptodate.com

U.S. Pharmacist Weekly Newsletter
http://www.uspharmacist.com

Vogt, C. (2017, November 14). New AHA/ACC guidelines lower high BP threshold. Consultant360
https://www.consultant360.com/exclusives/new-ahaacc-guidelines-lower- high-bp-threshold

Vrcek, I., Choudhury, E., & Durairaj, V. (2017). Herpes zoster ophthalmicus: A review for the internist. *The American Journal of Medicine, 130*(1), 21–26.

Wald, E. R., Applegate, K. E., Bordley, C., Darrow, D. H., Glode, M. P., Marcy, S. M., . . . American Academy of Pediatrics. (2013). Clinical practice guidelines for the diagnosis and management of acute bacterial sinusitis in children 1 to 18 years. *Pediatrics, 132*(1), e262–280.

Wallace, D. V., Dykewicz, M. S., Oppenheimer, J., Portnoy, J. M., & Lang, D. M. (2017). Pharmacologic treatment of seasonal allergic rhinitis: Synopsis of guidance from the 2017 joint task force on practice parameters. *Annals of Internal Medicine, 167*(12), 876. doi:10.7326/m17-2203

Watkins, S. L., Glantz, S. A., & Chaffee, B. W. (2018). Association of Noncigarette Tobacco Product Use With Future Cigarette Smoking Among Youth in the Population Assessment of Tobacco and Health (PATH) Study, 2013-2015. *JAMA Pediatrics, 172*(2), 181. doi:10.1001/jamapediatrics.2017.4173

Watson, T., Hickok, J., Fraker, S., Korwek, K., Poland, R. E., & Septimus, E. (2017). Evaluating the risk factors for hospital-onset Clostridium difficile infections in a large healthcare system. *Clinical Infectious Diseases.* doi:10.1093/cid/cix1112

WebMD: Drugs and Medications A to Z. Latest Drug News
http://www.webmd.com/drugs

Wimmer, B. C., Cross, A. J., Jokanovic, N., Wiese, M. D., George, J., Johnell, K., . . . Bell, J. S. (2016). Clinical Outcomes Associated with Medication Regimen Complexity in Older People: A Systematic Review. *Journal of the American Geriatrics Society, 65*(4), 747–753. doi:10.1111/jgs.14682

Winkel, P., Hilden, J., Hansen, J. F., Kastrup, J., Kolmos, H. J., Kjøller, E., . . . Gluud, C. (2015). Clarithromycin for stable coronary heart disease increases all-cause and cardiovascular mortality and cerebrovascular morbidity over 10years in the CLARICOR randomised, blinded clinical trial. *International Journal of Cardiology, 182*, 459–465. doi:10.1016/j.ijcard.2015.01.020

Wong, J., Marr, P., Kwan, D., Meiyappan, S., & Adcock, L. (2014). Identification of inappropriate medication use in elderly patients with frequent emergency department visits. *Canadian Pharmacists Journal/Revue Des Pharmaciens Du Canada, 147*(4), 248–256. doi:10.1177/1715163514536522

World Health Organization. *Growing Antibiotic Resistance Forces Updates to Recommended Treatments for Sexually Transmitted Infections. August 30 2016.*
http://www.who.int/mediacentre/news/releases/2016/antibiotics-sexual-infections/en

World Health Organization. (2016). *WHO Guidelines for the Treatment of Chlamydia trachomatis.*
http://www.who.int/reproductivehealth/publications/rtis/chlamydia-treatment-guidelines/en

World Health Organization. (2016). *WHO Guidelines for the Treatment of Neisseria gonorrhoeae.*
http://www.who.int/reproductivehealth/publications/rtis/gonorrhoea-treatment-guidelines/en

World Health Organization. *WHO Guidelines for the Treatment of Treponema pallidum (Syphilis)—2016.*
http://www.who.int/reproductivehealth/publications/rtis/syphilis-treatment-guidelines/en

World Health Organization. (2017, March). *WHO Model List of Essential Medicines (20th list).* Geneva, Switzerland: Author
http://www.who.int/medicines/publications/essentialmedicines/20th_EML2017.pdf?ua=1

World Health Organization. (2017, March). *WHO Model List of Essential Medicines for Children (6th list).* Geneva, Switzerland: Author
http://www.who.int/medicines/publications/essentialmedicines/6th_EMLc2017.pdf?ua=1

World Health Organization. (2017, June 6). *WHO Updates Essential Medicines List with New Advice on Use of Antibiotics, and Adds Medicines for Hepatitis C, HIV, Tuberculosis and Cancer.* Geneva, Switzerland: Author
http://www.who.int/mediacentre/news/releases/2017/essential-medicines-list/en

Xie, Y., Bowe, B., Li, T., Xian, H., Yan, Y., & Al-Aly, Z. Long-term kidney outcomes among users of proton pump inhibitors without intervening acute kidney injury [published online february 22, 2017]. *Kidney International, 91*(6), 1482–1494. Dx.doi.org/10.1016/j.kint.2016.12.021

Yılmaz, D, Heper, Y, & Gözler, L. (2017). Effect of the use of buzzy during phlebotomy on pain and individual satisfaction in blood donors. *Pain Management Nursing, 18*(4), 260–267.

Yoon, I.-K., & Thomas, S. J. (2017). Encouraging results but questions remain for dengue vaccine. *The Lancet Infectious Diseases, 18*(2), 125–126doi:10.1016/S1473-3099(17)30634-5

Zarrabi, H., Khalkhali, M., Hamidi, A., Ahmadi, R., & Zavarmousavi, P. (2016). Clinical features, course and treatment of methamphetamine-induced psychosis in psychiatric inpatients. *BMC Psychiatry, 16*, 44. doi:10.1186/s12888-016-0745-5

NOTE: Generic names are in italics; FDA pregnancy categories and controlled drug categories appear in parentheses after the entry. * indicates no assigned pregnancy category.

narcolepsy, 318
Cyltezo, *adalimumab-adbm* (B)
  Crohn's disease, 110
  juvenile idiopathic arthritis, 284
  osteoarthritis, 339
  psoriatic arthritis, 424
  rheumatoid arthritis, 437
  ulcerative colitis, 515
Cymbalta, *duloxetine* (C)
  anxiety disorder, 26
  fibromyalgia, 166
  major depressive disorder, 119
  peripheral neuritis, 379–380
  post-traumatic stress disorder, 407
cyproheptadine, Periactin (B)
  anorexia/cachexia, 19
cystic fibrosis (CF)
  acetylcysteine, Mucomyst (B), 112
  ciprofloxacin, Cipro, Cipro XR, ProQuin XR
    (C), 113
  ivacaftor, Kalydeco (B), 112
  lumacaftor+ivacaftor, Orkambi (B), 113
  tezacaftor+ivacaftor plus ivacaftor, Symdeko
    (B), 113
  ursodeoxycholic acid (UDCA), Ursofalk (G), 113
cytomegalovirus (CMV) retinitis
  cidofovir, Vistide V (C), 432
  letermovir, Prevymis (*), 433
  valganciclovir, Valcyte (C)(G), 432, 433
Cytomel, *liothyronine* (A)
  hypothyroidism, 261–262
Cytotec, *misoprostol* (X)
  peptic ulcer disease (PUD), 379
Cytoxan, *Cyclophosphamide* (D), 584

daclatasvir, Daklinza (X)
  hepatitis C (HCV), 210
Daklinza, *daclatasvir* (X)
  hepatitis C (HCV), 210
dalbavancin, Dalvance (C)
  cellulitis, 77
dalfampridine, Ampyra (C)
  multiple sclerosis (MS), 309
Daliresp, *roflumilast* (C)
  chronic obstructive pulmonary disease, 67
Dalmane, *flurazepam* (X)(IV)
  fibromyalgia, 167
  insomnia, 274
Dalvance, *dalbavancin* (C)
  cellulitis, 77
danazol, Danocrine (X)
  endometriosis, 156
  fibrocystic breast disease, 165
  hereditary angioedema, 213
Danocrine, *danazol* (X)
  endometriosis, 156
  fibrocystic breast disease, 165
  hereditary angioedema, 213
dantrolene, Dantrium (C)
  muscle strain, 312
  temporomandibular joint disorder, 474
  temporomandibular joint (TMJ) disorder, 474
dapagliflozin, Farxiga (C)
  type 2 diabetes mellitus, 507–508
dapsone, Aczone (C)
  acne vulgaris, 5

folliculitis barbae, 169
Hansen's disease, 191
pemphigus vulgaris, 376
Daralex, *daratumumab*, 584
darbepoetin alpha, Aranesp (C)
  anemia of chronic kidney disease, 15
darifenacin, Enablex (C)
  urinary overactive bladder, 267
darunavir, Prezista (C)
  human immunodeficiency virus infection, 228
Daurismo, *glasdegib*, 585
Daytrana, *methylphenidate* (transdermal patch)
    (C)(II)
  attention deficit hyperactivity disorder (ADHD),
    44
  narcolepsy, 318
DDAVP, DDAVP Rhinal Tube, *desmopressin*
    acetate (DDAVP) (B)
  nocturnal enuresis, 156
  urinary overactive bladder, 267
Debrox, *carbamide peroxide* (G)
  cerumen impaction, 79
Decadron, *dexamethasone phosphate* (C)
  allergic (vernal) conjunctivitis, 101
Decadron Phosphate with Xylocaine,
    lidocaine+dexamethasone (B), 579
  atopic dermatitis, 125
  burn: minor, 69
  diabetic peripheral neuropathy (DPN), 132
  gouty arthritis, 187
  herpangina, 216
  indications, 569
  insect bite/sting, 272
  juvenile idiopathic arthritis, 282
  muscle strain, 314
  pain, 354
  peripheral neuritis, 381
  post-herpetic neuralgia, 404
Declomycin, *demeclocycline* (X)
  gonorrhea, 183
deep vein thrombosis (DVT) prophylaxis, 114
deferasirox (tridentate ligand), Exjade, Jadenu (C)
  iron overload, 278
deferoxamine mesylate, Desferal (C)
  lead poisoning, 289
deflazacort, Emflaza (B)
  duchenne muscular dystrophy (DMD), 142
dehydration
  oral electrolyte replacement (OTC),
    KaoLectrolyte, Pedialyte, Pedialyte Freezer
    Pops (G), 114
delafloxacin, Baxdela (*)
  cellulitis, 77–78
delavirdine mesylate, Rescriptor (C)
  human immunodeficiency virus infection,
    226–227
delirium
  haloperidol, Haldol, Haldol Lactate (C), 114
  lorazepam, Ativan, Lorazepam Intensol (D)
    (IV), 114
  mesoridazine, Serentil (C), 115
  olanzapine, Zyprexa, Zyprexa Zydis (C), 115
  quetiapine fumarate, SeroQUEL, SeroQUEL XR
    (C), 115
  risperidone, Risperdal, Risperdal M-Tab (C), 115
  thioridazine, Mellaril (C), 115